Diagnosis of Diseases of the Chest

THIRD EDITION

Robert G. Fraser, M.D.
Professor of Radiology
University of Alabama at Birmingham
Birmingham, Alabama

J.A. Peter Paré, M.D.C.M., F.A.C.P., F.R.C.P.(C)
Professor Emeritus
Department of Medicine
McGill University
Montreal, Canada

P.D. Paré, M.D.
Professor of Medicine
University of British Columbia
Head, Respiratory Division
University of British Columbia and
    St. Paul's Hospital
Vancouver, British Columbia, Canada

Richard S. Fraser, M.D.
Associate Professor of Pathology
McGill University
Pathologist, Montreal General Hospital
Head, Department of Pathology
Montreal Chest Hospital Institute
Montreal, Canada

George P. Genereux, M.D.
Professor of Radiology
University of Saskatchewan, Saskatoon
Radiologist, University of Saskatchewan Hospital
Saskatoon, Saskatchewan, Canada

1988
W.B. SAUNDERS COMPANY
Harcourt Brace Jovanovich, Inc.
Philadelphia   London   Toronto   Montreal   Sydney   Tokyo

W. B. SAUNDERS COMPANY
Harcourt Brace Jovanovich, Inc.

West Washington Square
Philadelphia, PA 19105

Library of Congress Cataloging-in-Publication Data

Diagnosis of diseases of the chest.

Rev. ed. of: Diagnosis of diseases of the chest/
Robert G. Fraser, J. A. Peter Paré. 2nd ed. 1977–

Includes bibliographies and index.

1. Chest—Diseases—Diagnosis. I. Fraser, Robert G.,
   1921–   . [DNLM: 1. Thoracic Diseases—diagnosis.
   2. Thoracic Radiography. WF 975 D536]

RC941.D52 1988   617'.54'07572   87–4678

ISBN 0–7216–3874–8 (set)
ISBN 0–7216–3870–8 (v. I)

Listed here are the latest translated editions of this book
together with the language of the translation and the
publisher.

Italian (2nd Edition)–Editrice Ambrosiana, Milan, Italy
Spanish (2nd Edition)–Salvat Editores S.A., Barcelona, Spain
Portuguese (2nd Edition)—Editora Manole Ltda., Sao Paulo, Brazil
German (2nd Edition, Vol. IV)—F. K. Schattauer Verlag, Stuttgart, West Germany

Editor: Dean Manke
Developmental Editor: David Kilmer
Designer: Terri Siegel
Production Manager: Bob Butler
Manuscript Editor: Wynette Kommer
Illustration Coordinator: Walt Verbitski
Indexer: Angela Holt/Dorothy Hoffman

Diagnosis of Diseases of the Chest

Volume I   ISBN   0–7216–3870–8
Set   ISBN   0–7216–3874–8

Last digit is the print number: 9   8   7   6   5   4   3   2

DEDICATION

This book is dedicated to the many scholars and scientists who over these many decades have applied themselves with diligence and devotion to the enrichment of our knowledge of the normal and diseased chest.

PREFACE TO
THE THIRD EDITION

—vanity of vanities; all is vanity.
What profit hath a man of all his labour which
he taketh under the sun?
One generation passeth away, and another
generation cometh.

—ECCLESIASTES 1:2

It has been 20 years since the two senior authors began writing the first edition of this book, and during the preliminary stages of planning for the third edition, we grudgingly acknowledged a mild but inescapable attrition in the motivation and initiative we possessed formerly. More importantly, we recognized the need to prepare to hand over the reins for the writing of future editions to dependable and tested hands. As a result, we felt obliged to augment the authorship of this edition with young, fertile minds, and we didn't have far to look: our two sons, RSF and PP, were devoting much of their professional lives to the pathologic and physiologic manifestations of chest disease respectively, and it was logical that they should take up the cudgel to prevent their fathers from wallowing in their own misconceptions. We also felt the need for the addition of a third creative mind, this time a radiologist, to bring about renewed vigor and enthusiasm to the description and illustration of roentgenologic pathology; again we had to look no further than our own back yard to find GG, an internationally renowned radiologist with a vast clinical experience in chest disease. As the first volume of this third edition has evolved, it has become abundantly clear that we possessed much wisdom in seeking the collaboration of these three. The new authors have reorganized many chapters and have greatly improved the text by preparing a much more accurate description and illustration of the pathologic manifestations of thoracic disease, a more thorough discussion of normal and pathologic physiology, and fresh new material on the roentgenologic manifestations of many conditions.

It was stated in the Preface to the First Edition that the book was written with the aim of emphasizing the value of the roentgenogram as the *first* rather than the *major* step in the diagnosis of chest disease. In the subsequent 15 year interval, we have not seen cause to alter this opinion. However, despite the usefulness of this approach from a practical day-to-day viewpoint, we have come to realize more fully that the ultimate foundation upon which diagnosis must be based is a knowledge of chest disease itself. In addition to a thorough familiarity with normal structure and function, this includes a detailed knowledge of physiologic and pathologic alterations as well as the etiologies and pathogenetic mechanisms behind them. Although intimated in the first two editions, this belief has reached full fruition in the present text in which all aspects of the normal and diseased chest have been given roughly equal coverage. Whatever emphasis was formerly placed on roentgenology is now of necessity less evident. This should not be interpreted as a diminution in our belief of the importance of the roentgenogram in diagnosis but rather as an extension of the previously unstated but implied importance of the broader view. This approach has necessarily involved the inclusion of a vast amount of new information and has resulted unavoidably in a comprehensive reference work rather than a textbook. The scope of the text is such that it will find its greatest use in the hands of specialists such as respirologists, thoracic surgeons, and radiologists and pathologists whose particular interest lies in diseases of the chest. However, those with a more general outlook, such as internists and house officers, will also find the book useful as an occasional reference source.

What will the reader find new? In addition to the more extensive coverage of pathology and physiology and the addition of new knowledge that has appeared in the literature over the seven or eight year span, fresh material has appeared on the control of breathing, the respiratory muscles in health and disease, breathing during sleep, the development of the lung, host defense mechanisms, opportunistic infections, pulmonary vasculitides, the acquired immunodeficiency syndrome, the lung in transplantation, and drug-induced pulmonary disease. In addition, there is a complete reorganization of the chapter on neoplasms based on the 1982 WHO classification, and there are extensive additions to the discussion of the obstructive airway diseases, particularly with regard to pathophysiology and bronchial reactivity. A number of illustrations have been replaced and many new ones added, with emphasis on computed tomography and, to a lesser extent, magnetic resonance imaging. Virtually all illustrations of gross and microscopic pathology are new, and it is hoped that they will provide new insights into pathologic/radiologic correlation.

Since the publication of the Second Edition, a spectacular expansion of knowledge has occurred concerning the structure and function of the lung in health and disease; as a result, it has proved impossible to carry out a simple revision, and in most areas the book has been almost completely rewritten. However, all attempts have been made not to increase its length: the addition of new material, particularly in sections dealing with pathology and pathophysiology, has been balanced by the removal of out-of-date text. To achieve a roughly equal size of the new volumes, it has been necessary to alter the order of chapters somewhat from that in the first two editions. The tables of differential diagnosis and decision trees have been incorporated into Volume IV rather than occupying a separate volume as in the second edition. The rapidity with which new knowledge is appearing has also made it necessary to publish the four volumes sequentially rather than simultaneously. We regret the necessity for this, but were we to await completion of the later volumes, the first volume would be long out of date, requiring thorough revision; the inevitable result would be a vicious cycle whereby none of the volumes would ever be published!

As anticipated, the writing style of each of the five authors has varied considerably, requiring considerable subediting in an attempt to unify syntax and nomenclature. In this regard, we and others have been concerned with the variable terminology employed by physicians in the description of the normal and diseased thorax. In an attempt to obviate this variability, in 1975 a joint committee of the American College of Chest Physicians and the American Thoracic Society published a glossary of pulmonary terms and symbols pertinent to the medical and physiologic aspects of the normal and diseased chest (Chest 67:583, 1975). At about the same time, the Fleischner Society formed a committee on nomenclature that designed and subsequently published a glossary of words and terms that they recommended for roentgenologic terminology (AJR 143:509, 1984). Since several of the terms recommended by the ACCP/ATS Committee for use in the classification of diseases, in physical examination, and in respiratory therapy are at variance with those used in this book, we have chosen to include only the terms and symbols used in respiratory physiology and pathophysiology. Both the modified ACCP/ATS and the Fleischner glossaries are printed before Chapter 1, and the reader is urged to review them and use them regularly.

The burgeoning of knowledge in the field of chest disease continues unabated. The 20-odd journals that the two senior authors reviewed in the preparation of the first and second editions have been expanded not only by the profligation of new biomedical publications and the inclusion of a number of recognized journals in other specialized clinical disciplines, but also by the many physiology and pathology journals that were not included in the original review. As a consequence, the near-10,000 references cited in the second edition will certainly be exceeded in the third. Bibliographies have been placed at the end of each chapter and their position indicated by a black slash on page edges, thus facilitating their identification.

Once again, we invite our readers to inform us of differences of opinion they may have with the contents of this book or to offer their advice as to how future editions may be improved. It is only through such interchange of information and opinion that we can hope to establish on a firm basis the knowledge necessary for a full understanding of respiratory disease.

RGF
JAPP
PDP
RSF
GPG

ACKNOWLEDGMENTS

Coordination of the contributions of two authors in the preparation of the first two editions of this book proved to be a formidable undertaking, but in fact was comparatively simple compared with the enormous problems created by attempts to assimilate material from five separate sources. The writing of the manuscript and the choice and preparation of new illustrations were the most formidable part of the undertaking, but the many steps necessary to the final product required the unselfish and enthusiastic contributions of many hands and minds, and the support and encouragement we received from many of our friends are greatly appreciated and duly acknowledged.

It is not possible to overstate our gratitude to our secretaries who handled magnificently the tedious and necessarily exacting task of listing and filing references, transcribing manuscript from tape, typing the several drafts up to and including the final, and cheerfully coping with the innumerable problems encountered. Anne Paré of Val Morin, Quebec; Peggy Stewart and Diane Ford of St. Paul's Hospital, Vancouver; Donna O'Conner and Wendy Segall of the Montreal General Hospital; Joan Matlock of the University of Saskatchewan Hospital; and Marianne Constantine of the Montreal Chest Hospital exhibited exemplary patience and devotion in accomplishing these thorny chores. Although these individuals have earned our heartfelt thanks, the efforts by RGF's secretaries, Shelley McCain, Marcia Segers, and Lynn Hogan of the Hospital of the University of Alabama at Birmingham deserve special praise since it was their lot to type not only the contributions from their boss but also the edited manuscript from the other four authors; they also carried out the tedious job of recording, filing, and checking the innumerable references, an extremely frustrating chore that they performed with meticulous accuracy. The devotion and diligence with which all these people carried out their tasks are deeply appreciated.

The majority of the case histories and roentgenograms reproduced here are of patients of staff members of the Royal Victoria Hospital, the Montreal General Hospital, the Montreal Chest Hospital Institute, the Hospital of the University of Alabama at Birmingham, and the Medical Center of the University of Saskatchewan, Saskatoon. All illustrations of pathology derived from patients in the Montreal General Hospital and the Montreal Chest Hospital Institute. Our indebtedness to our colleagues who were caring for these patients cannot be overemphasized, not only for their generosity in permitting us to publish these case reports but also for the benefit of their experience and guidance over the years.

The superb photographic work throughout these volumes was the accomplishment of the Department of Visual Aids of the Royal Victoria Hospital, Susie Gray of the Department of Radiology, UAB, David Mandeville of the University of Saskatchewan Hospital, and Joseph Donohue and Anthony Graham of Montreal. Their craftsmanship and rich experience in photography are readily apparent in these pages. We would also like to thank Sally Osborne of St. Paul's Hospital, Vancouver, for many of the physiologic illustrations, and Elizabeth Baile, also of St. Paul's, for her help in preparation of the section on the bronchial circulation.

Throughout our labors, we received much support and cooperation from the publishers, notably Suzanne Boyd, who effectively and sympathetically minimized the many obstacles we encountered. Jack Hanley, the former president of the company, gave us much encouragement during the formative stages, and we shall miss his enthusiasm and guidance. Since taking over as medical editor in 1986, Dean Manke has assisted us in many ways in our endeavors.

Finally, and with immense gratitude, we recall the patience and understanding displayed by our wives and children throughout our labors. Without their continuous encouragement, this book surely would not have been completed, and we acknowledge their many virtues with much love.

RGF
JAPP
PDP
RSF
GPG

PREFACE TO
THE FIRST EDITION

This book was written with the aim of defining an approach to the diagnosis of diseases of the chest based on the abnormal roentgenogram. Experience over the years has led the authors to the conclusion that the chest roentgenogram represents the focal point or sheet anchor in the diagnosis of the majority of pulmonary diseases, many patients presenting with either no symptoms and signs or entirely nonspecific ones. This emphasis on the roentgenogram as the first step in reaching a diagnosis does not represent an attempt to relegate history and physical examination to a position of no importance, but merely an effort to place them in proper perspective. In no other medical field is diagnosis so dependent upon the intelligent integration of information from roentgenologic, clinical, laboratory, and pathologic sources as in diseases of the chest. We submit that the roentgenogram is the starting point in this investigation; the knowledge of structural change thus obtained, when integrated with pertinent clinical findings and results of pulmonary function tests and other ancillary diagnostic procedures, enables one to arrive at a confident diagnosis. Some patients manifest symptoms and signs that themselves are virtually diagnostic of some chest disorders, but even in such cases the confirmation of diagnosis requires the presence of an appropriate roentgenographic pattern.

A glance through the pages will reveal an abundance of roentgenographic illustrations that might create the illusion that this book is written primarily for the roentgenologist, but this is not our intention. In fact, the clinical, morphologic, and laboratory aspects of many diseases are described at greater length than the roentgenologic, a fact pointing up the broad interest we hope the book will engender among internists, surgeons, and family practitioners interested in chest disease. The numerous illustrations reflect the aim of the book—to emphasize the value of the roentgenogram as the *first* rather than the *major* step in diagnosis.

During the writing of the book, our original plan was considerably modified as the format unfolded and we became even more aware of the complexities of design and organization. Originally, our approach to differential diagnosis suggested a division of chapters on the basis of specific roentgenographic patterns. It soon became apparent, however, that since many diseases give rise to various different roentgenographic patterns, this method of presentation would require tedious repetition of clinical and laboratory details in several chapters. To obviate this, we planned tables of differential diagnosis, listing etiologic classifications of diseases that produce specific roentgenographic patterns and describing briefly the clinical and laboratory characteristics of each disease, thus facilitating recognition of disease states. The tables are designed to be used with the text in the following manner. When a specific pattern of disease is recognized, the appropriate table should be scanned and those conditions selected that correspond most closely with the clinical picture presented by the patient. Additional information about the likeliest diagnostic possibilities can be obtained by referring to the detailed discussions in the relevant sections of the text (page numbers are cited after each diagnosis). The tables relate to 17 basic patterns of bronchopulmonary, pleural, and mediastinal disease; they are grouped together in Chapter 5 in Volume I and may be located with ease from the black marks found on the upper corners of their pages. Each table is preceded by a detailed description and representative illustrations of the specific roentgenographic pattern. An attempt has been made to indicate the relative incidence of the diseases.

Although our original plan called for a one volume presentation, it soon became apparent that the length of the text and the number and size of illustrations necessary for full coverage of the subject required two volumes. Volume I includes descriptions of the normal chest, methods and techniques of investigation, clinical features, and roentgenologic signs of chest diseases, the tables of differential diagnosis, and chapters devoted to diseases of developmental origin and the infectious diseases; in Volume II appear detailed discussions of the morphologic, roentgenologic, and clinical aspects of all other diseases of the thorax arranged in chapters according to etiology.

The roentgenograms have been reproduced by two different techniques, the majority in Volume I by the logEtronic method and those in Volume II by direct photography. The publishers have been generous in allotting sufficient space for the reproduction of the roentgenograms in a size adequate for good detail recognition.

Much of the material in the book has been based on our personal experience gained in the past almost two decades, during which we have had a predominant interest in pulmonary disease. Obviously, this experience has been greatly enhanced by the extensive literature that has accumulated during these years, and we are mindful of the tremendous help we have received from the contributions of others. Our free use of the literature is reflected in the extensive bibliography.

Certain differences from the contents of other books on respiratory disease will be noted. First, this text contains no reference to treatment. Since drug therapies and surgical techniques are constantly changing, any attempt to include them would make the book out of date almost before it was published. Second, we have intentionally made only passing reference to pulmonary disease peculiar to children, a full description of which would require a complete separate text.

The relative incidence of respiratory diseases has changed considerably over the last quarter century. In some diseases, such as tuberculosis and bronchiectasis, a decreased frequency reflects improved public health measures and therapeutic innovations; in others, man's therapeutic triumphs have proved a mixed blessing, enabling patients with disabling chronic respiratory disease to live longer despite formerly fatal pneumonias. Perhaps even more important, man himself is responsible for varying the spectrum of respiratory disease as a result of his irresponsible insistence upon increasing the amount and variety of atmospheric pollutants. Inhaled contaminated air not only is regarded as the major etiologic factor in chronic obstructive pulmonary disease and the inorganic dust pneumoconioses, but also has been incriminated in the etiology of several hypersensitivity diseases of the lungs. This last group comprises the "extrinsic" form of allergic alveolitis. The number of conditions involved, when added to the better known "intrinsic" counterpart—the collagen diseases—is largely responsible for the length of the chapter devoted to immunologic diseases. Other changes that have contributed to the "new face" of pulmonary disease include increasing knowledge of the hormonal effects of neoplasms; the discovery that various immunologic defects may reduce host resistance to infection; and finally the appearance in the western world of parasitic infestations and bacterial infections formerly considered so rare in those areas as to warrant little consideration in differential diagnosis, but now of some importance because of the modern day ease of intercontinental travel. Although the novelty of these recent changes may have led the authors to consider them in greater detail and length than is their due, the emphasis may serve to bring them into proper perspective.

Finally, we recognize our fallibility. It is inevitable that some observations in a text of this magnitude will prove erroneous in time or will find disagreement among our knowledgeable readers. This we expect and accept. We sincerely hope that such differences of opinion will be made known to us, so that they may be weighed and, where appropriate, introduced into subsequent editions or revisions. It is only through such interchange of information and opinion that we can hope to establish on a firm basis the knowledge necessary to a full understanding of respiratory disease.

R.G.F.
J.A.P.P.

CONTENTS

VOLUME I

Glossary of Words, Terms and Symbols in Chest Medicine and Roentgenology

"Then you should say what you mean," the March Hare went on.
"I do," Alice hastily replied; "at least—at least, I mean what I say—that's the same thing, you know."
"Not the same thing a bit!" said the Hatter. "Why, you might just as well say that 'I see what I eat' is the same thing as 'I eat what I see!'"

This well-known excerpt from Lewis Carroll's *Alice's Adventures in Wonderland* points out a problem that confronts many physicians in today's constantly expanding scientific literature—the use of words and terms that mean different things to different people. The frequency with which imprecise or frankly erroneous words are employed to describe roentgenographic images (for example) is astonishing; common usage has created a jargon that has led to confusion if not to actual communication breakdown. In 1975, a joint committee of the American College of Chest Physicians and the American Thoracic Society published a glossary of pulmonary

terms and symbols* pertinent to the medical and physiologic aspects of chest disease, but it omitted words that specifically related to chest roentgenology. As a consequence, the Fleischner Society formed a Committee on Nomenclature several years ago to draw up a glossary of roentgenologic words and terms and this task now has been completed and the glossary published.† We list herewith a number of words, terms, and symbols selected from the two publications that we hope our readers will refer to and use. The precise definition of some words has been altered slightly to coincide with usage in this book.

---

*Pulmonary Terms and Symbols; A report of the ACCP/ATS Joints Committee on Pulmonary Nomenclature. Chest 67:583, 1975.
†Glossary of Terms for Thoracic Radiology: Recommendations of the Nomenclature Committee of the Fleischner Society. Am J Roentgenol *143*:509, 1984.

WORDS OR TERMS USED IN ROENTGENOLOGY

Word or Term

Comments

abscess *n., pl.* -es. 1. (pathol.) An inflammatory mass, the central part of which has undergone purulent liquefaction necrosis. It may communicate with the bronchial tree. 2. (radiol.) Within the lung, a mass presumed to be caused by infection. The presence of gas within the mass, with or without a fluid level, represents a cavity (q.v.) and implies a communication with the bronchial tree. Otherwise, a pulmonary mass can be considered to represent an abscess in the morpholgic sense only by inference. *Qualifiers:* Expressing clinical course: acute, chronic. Expressing etiology: bacterial, fungal, etc. Expressing site of involvement: lung, mediastinum, etc.

Should be used only with reference to masses of presumed infectious etiology. The word is not synonymous with cavity (*q.v.*).

WORDS OR TERMS USED IN ROENTGENOLOGY *Continued*

Word or Term	Comments
acinar pattern *n.* (radiol.) A collection of round or elliptic, ill-defined, discrete or partly confluent opacities in the lung, each measuring 4 to 8 mm in diameter and together producing an extended, inhomogeneous shadow. *Synonyms:* Rosette pattern; acinonodose pattern (used specifically with reference to endobronchial spread of tuberculosis); alveolar pattern.	An inferred conclusion usually used as a descriptor. An acceptable term, preferred to cited synonyms (especially "alveolar pattern," which is an inaccurate descriptor).
acinar shadow *n.* (radiol.) A round or slightly elliptic pulmonary opacity 4 to 8 mm in diameter presumed to represent an anatomic acinus rendered opaque by consolidation. Usually employed in the presence of many such opacities (*see* acinar pattern).	An inferred conclusion sometimes applicable as a roentgenologic descriptor.
acinus *n.* (anat.) The portion of lung parenchyma distal to the terminal bronchiole and consisting of respiratory bronchioles, alveolar ducts, alveolar sacs, and alveoli (*see* acinar shadow, acinar pattern).	A specific feature of pulmonary anatomy.
aeration *n.* (physiol./radiol.) 1. The state of containing air. 2. The state or process of being filled or inflated with air. *Qualifiers:* overaeration (preferred) or hyperaeration; underaeration (preferred) or hypoaeration. *Synonym:* Inflation.	An acceptable term with reference to the inspiratory phase of respiration. Inflation is preferred in sense 2.
air, *n.* (radiol.) Inspired atmospheric gas. The word is sometimes used to describe gas within the body regardless of its composition or site.	With reference to pneumothorax, subcutaneous emphysema, or the content of the stomach, colon, etc., gas is the more accurate term and is preferred.
air bronchiologram *n.* (radiol.) The equivalent of air bronchogram but in airways assumed to be bronchioles because of their peripheral location and diameter.	An acceptable term.
air bronchogram *n.* (radiol.) The roentgenographic shadow of an air-containing bronchus peripheral to the hilum and surrounded by airless lung (whether by virtue of absorption of air, replacement of air, or both), a finding generally regarded as evidence of the patency of the more proximal airway. Hence, any bandlike tapering and/or branching lucency within opacified lung corresponding in size and distribution to a bronchus or bronchi and presumed to represent an air-containing segment of the bronchial tree.	A specific feature of roentgenologic anatomy whose identify is often inferred. A useful and recommended term.
air-fluid level *n.* (radiol.) A local collection of gas and liquid that, when traversed by a horizontal x-ray beam, creates a shadow characterized by a sharp horizontal interface between gas density above and liquid density below.	A useful roentgenologic descriptor. Since with rare exception (*e.g.,* fat-fluid level) the upper of the two absorbant media is "air" (gas), it is sufficient to describe such an appearance as a "fluid level."
air space *n.* (*adj.* air-space) (anat./radiol.) The gas-containing portion of lung parenchyma, including the acini and excluding the interstitium and purely conductive portions of the lung. *Synonyms:* Acinar consolidation, alveolar consolidation (when used as an adjective in relation to air-space consolidation).	An inferred conclusion usually used as a roentgenologic descriptor. An acceptable term whose use as an adjective is also appropriate.

WORDS OR TERMS USED IN ROENTGENOLOGY *Continued*

Word or Term

Comments

air-trapping *n*. (pathophysiol./radiol.) The retention of excess gas in all or part of the lung at any stage of expiration.

A specific roentgenologic sign to be employed only if excess air retention is demonstrated by a dynamic study, *e.g.*, inspiration-expiration roentgenography or fluoroscopy. *Not* to be used with reference to overinflation of the lung at full inspiration (total lung capacity).

airway *n., adj.* (anat./radiol.) A collective term for the air-conducting passages from the larynx to and including the respiratory bronchioles.

Synonyms: Conducting airway; tracheobronchial tree.

A useful anatomic term. May be used as an adjective in relation to disease or abnormality. Note that the respiratory bronchioles are both conducting and gas-exchanging airways and thus constitute the transitory zone.

alveolarization *n*. (radiol.) The opacification of groups of alveoli by a contrast medium.

A misnomer whose use is to be deplored. Excessive filling of peripheral lung structure by contrast media usually employed for bronchography may opacify respiratory bronchioles but not alveoli. Thus, the correct term is "bronchiolar filling or opacification."

anterior junction line *n*. (radiol.) A vertically oriented linear or curvilinear opacity approximately 1 to 2 mm wide, commonly projected on the tracheal air shadow. It is produced by the shadows of the right and left pleurae in intimate contact between the aerated lungs anterior to the great vessels (and sometimes the heart); hence, it never extends above the suprasternal notch (*cf.* posterior junction line).

Synonyms: Anterior mediastinal septum, line, or stripe.

A specific feature of roentgenologic anatomy; to be preferred to cited synonyms.

aortopulmonary window *n*. 1. (anat.) A mediastinal space bounded anteriorly by the posterior surface of the ascending aorta; posteriorly by the anterior surface of the descending aorta; superiorly by the inferior surface of the aortic arch; inferiorly by the superior surface of the left pulmonary artery; medially by the left side of the trachea, left main bronchus, and esophagus; and laterally by the left lung. Within it are situated fat, the ductus ligament, the left recurrent laryngeal nerve, and lymph nodes. 2. (radiol.) A zone of relative lucency in the mediastinal shadow that is seen to best advantage in the left anterior oblique or lateral projection and that corresponds to the anatomic space defined above. On a posteroanterior roentgenogram of the chest, the lateral margin of the space constitutes the aortopulmonary window interface.

Synonym: Aortic-pulmonic window.

A specific feature of roentgenologic anatomy.

atelectasis *n*. (pathophysiol./radiol.) Less than normal inflation of all or a portion of the lung with corresponding diminution in volume. *Qualifiers* may be employed to indicate severity (mild, moderate, severe), mechanism (resorption, relaxation, cicatrization, adhesive), or distribution (*e.g.*, lobar, platelike [*q.v.*], discoid).

Synonyms: Collapse, loss of volume, anectasis.

Generally this term is preferable to "collapse" in describing loss of volume. The word "collapse" connotes total atelectasis in which lung tissue has been reduced to its smallest volume. Anectasis is usually used in reference to failure of lung expansion in the neonate.

WORDS OR TERMS USED IN ROENTGENOLOGY *Continued*

Word or Term	Comments
azygoesophageal recess *n.* 1. (anat.) A space or recess in the right side of the mediastinum into which the medial edge of the right lower lobe (crista pulmonis) extends. It is limited superiorly by the arch of the azygos vein, inferiorly by the diaphragm, posteriorly by the azygos vein in front of the vertebral column, and medially by the esophagus and its adjacent structures. (The exact relationship between the medial edge of the lung and the mediastinal structures is variable.) 2. (radiol.) In a frontal chest roentgenogram, a vertically oriented interface between air in the right lower lobe and the adjacent mediastinum that represents the medial limit of the anatomic azygoesophageal recess.	A specific feature of roentgenologic anatomy. The use of the term "recess" to identify an interface is inappropriate; thus, azygoesophageal recess interface is preferred.
Synonyms: Infraazygos recess; right pleuroesophageal line or stripe; right paraesophageal line or stripe.	
bat's-wing distribution *n.* (radiol.) A spatial arrangement of roentgenographic opacities in a frontal roentgenogram that bears a vague resemblance to the shape of a bat in flight; said of coalescent, ill-defined opacities that are approximately bilaterally symmetric and that are confined to the medulla of the lungs (*q.v.*).	A roentgenologic descriptor of limited usefulness.
Synonym: Butterfly distribution.	
bleb *n.* 1. (pathol.) A gas-containing space within or contiguous to the visceral pleura of the lung. 2. (radiol.) A local, thin-walled lucency contiguous with the pleura, usually at the lung apex.	An inferred conclusion seldom justifiable by roentgenogram alone. Bulla or air cyst is preferred.
Synonyms: Type I bulla (pathol.); bulla; a form of pulmonary air cyst (radiol.)	
bronchiole *n.* (anat./radiol.) An airway that contains no cartilage in its wall. A bronchiole may be purely conducting (up to and including the terminal bronchiole) or transitory (the respiratory bronchioles that carry out both conduction and gas exchange).	A specific feature of pulmonary anatomy.
bronchocele *n. See* mucoid impaction.	
bronchus *n.* (anat./radiol.) A conducting airway distal to the tracheal bifurcation that contains cartilage in its wall.	A specific feature of pulmonary anatomy.
bulla *n., pl.* -lae. 1. (pathol.) A sharply demarcated region of emphysema; a gas-containing space that may contain nothing but gas or may contain overdistended and ruptured alveolar septa and blood vessels. 2. (radiol.) Sharply demarcated hyperlucent area of avascularity within the lung, measuring 1 cm or more in diameter and possessing a wall less than 1 mm in thickness. *Qualifiers:* small, medium, large.	The preferred term to describe all thin-walled air-containing spaces in the lung with the exception of pneumatocele (*q.v.*).
butterfly distribution *n.* (radiol.) *See* bat's-wing distribution.	To be distinguished from the use of this term in general medicine to describe the distribution of certain cutaneous lesions.

WORDS OR TERMS USED IN ROENTGENOLOGY *Continued*

Word or Term	Comments
calcification *n.* 1. (pathophysiol.) (a) The process by which one or more deposits of calcium salts are formed within lung tissue or within a pulmonary lesion. (b) Such a deposit of calcium salts. 2. (radiol.) A calcific opacity within the lung that may be organized (*e.g.*, concentric lamination), but which does not display the trabecular organization of true bone. *Qualifiers:* "eggshell," "popcorn," target, laminated, flocculent, nodular, etc.	An explicit conclusion; may be used as a descriptor. To be distinguished from ossification (*q.v.*).
carina *n.* (anat./radiol.) The keel-shaped ridge that separates the right and left main bronchi at the tracheal bifurcation.	A specific feature of pulmonary anatomy.
carinal angle *n.* (anat./radiol.) The angle formed by the right and left main bronchi at the tracheal bifurcation. *Synonyms:* Bifurcation angle; angle of tracheal bifurcation.	A definitive anatomic and roentgenologic measurement.
cavity *n.* 1. (pathol.) A mass within lung parenchyma, the central portion of which has undergone liquefaction necrosis and has been expelled via the bronchial tree, leaving a gas-containing space, with or without associated fluid. 2. (radiol.) A gas-containing space within the lung surrounded by a wall whose thickness is greater than 1 mm and usually irregular in contour.	A useful descriptor without etiologic connotation. The word must not be used interchangeably with abscess (*q.v.*), which may exist without bronchial communication and therefore without cavitation.
circumscribed *adj.* (radiol.) Possessing a complete or nearly complete visible border.	An acceptable descriptor.
clot *n.* (pathol.) A semisolidified mass of blood elements.	*Cf.* thrombus.
coalescence *n.* (radiol.) The joining together of a number of opacities into a single opacity; confluence (*q.v.*).	An acceptable descriptor.
coin lesion *n.* (radiol.) A sharply defined, circular opacity within the lung suggestive of the appearance of a coin and usually representing a spherical or nodular lesion. *Synonyms:* Pulmonary nodule, pulmonary mass.	A roentgenologic descriptor, the use of which is to be condemned. The term "coin" may be descriptive of the shadow, but certainly not of the lesion producing it.
collapse *n.* (radiol.) A state in which lung tissue has undergone complete atelectasis.	The term is acceptable when employed strictly as defined, but "atelectasis" is preferred, since the degree of loss of lung volume can be qualified by mild, moderate, or severe.
collateral ventilation *n.* (physiol./radiol.) The process by which gas passes from one lung unit (acinus, lobule, segment, or lobe) to a contiguous unit via alveolar pores (pores of Kohn), canals of Lambert, or direct airway anastomoses. *Synonym:* Collateral air drift.	An inferred conclusion usually based on fairly reliable signs. A useful term. The channels of peripheral airway communication also function as a mechanism for transmission of liquid from one unit to another (*e.g.*, in acute airspace pneumonia).
confluence *n.* (radiol.) The nature of opacities that are contiguous with or adjacent to one another. *Antonym:* Discrete (*q.v.*).	A useful descriptor; confluence is to be distinguished from coalescence (*q.v.*), which is the act of becoming confluent.

WORDS OR TERMS USED IN ROENTGENOLOGY *Continued*

Word or Term	Comments

consolidation *n.* 1. (pathophysiol.) The process by which air in the lung is replaced by the products of disease, rendering the lung solid (as in pneumonia). 2. (radiol.) An essentially homogeneous opacity in the lung characterized by little or no loss of volume, by effacement of pulmonary blood vessels, and sometimes by the presence of an air bronchogram (*q.v.*).

An inferred conclusion, applicable only in an appropriate clinical setting when the opacity can with reasonable certainty be attributed to replacement of alveolar air by exudate, transudate, or tissue. Not to be used with reference to all homogeneous opacities.

corona radiata *n.* (radiol.) A circumferential pattern of fine linear spicules, approximately 5 mm long, extending outward from the margin of a solitary pulmonary nodule through a zone of relative lucency.

A sign of limited usefulness in the differentiation of benign and malignant nodules.

cor pulmonale *n.* 1. (pathol./clin.) Right ventricular hypertrophy and/or dilatation occurring as a result of an abnormality of lung structure or function. 2. (radiol.) The combination of pulmonary arterial hypertension and chronic lung disease, with or without evidence of enlargement of right heart chambers. *Qualifiers:* acute, chronic.

An inferred roentgenologic conclusion based on usually reliable signs. An acceptable descriptor. Despite the pathologic definition, roentgenologic evidence of cardiomegaly need not be present.

cortex *n.* (radiol.) The peripheral 2 to 3 cm of lung parenchyma adjacent to the visceral pleura, either over the convexity of the thorax or in the interlobar fissures. (*See* medulla and hilum.)

The peripheral part of an arbitrary subdivision of the lung into three zones from the hilum to the visceral pleura. Of limited usefulness.

CT number *n.* (radiol./physics) In computed tomography, a quantitative numerical statement of the relative attenuation of the x-ray beam at a specified point; loosely, the relative attenuation of a specified tissue absorber, usually expressed in Hounsfield units (HU).

cyst *n.* 1. (pathol.) A circumscribed space whose contents may be liquid or gaseous and whose wall is generally thin and well defined and lined by epithelium. 2. (radiol.) A gas-containing space of any size possessing a thin wall. *Qualifiers:* foregut (bronchogenic, esophageal duplication); postinfectious.

This term is entirely nonspecific and should not possess inferred conclusion as to etiology. It is the preferred term to describe any thin-walled gas-containing space in the lung possessing a wall thickness greater than 1 mm.

defined *adj.* (radiol.) The character of the border of a shadow. *Qualifiers:* well, sharply, poorly, distinctly.

An acceptable descriptor.

demarcated *adj.* (radiol.) Distinct from adjacent structures. *Qualifiers:* well, sharply, poorly.

An acceptable descriptor. (*Cf.* defined.)

dense *adj.* (radiol.) Possessing density (*q.v.*). Usually used in describing or comparing roentgenographic shadows with respect to their light transmission.

A recommended term in the context defined. Should not be used in referring to the opacity of an absorber of x-radiation. (*See* opaque, opacity.)

density *n.* 1. (physics) The mass of a substance per unit volume. 2. (photometry/radiol.) The opacity of a roentgenographic shadow to visible light; film blackening. 3. (radiol.) The shadow of an absorber more opaque to x-rays than its surround; an opacity or radiopacity. 4. The degree of opacity of an absorber to x-rays, usually expressed in terms of the nature of the absorber (*e.g.*, bone, water, or fat density).

In sense 2, the term refers to a fundamental characteristic of the roentgenogram, and its use is recommended. In senses 3 and 4, it refers to the character of the absorber and has an exactly opposite connotation with respect to film blackening. Because of this potential confusion, the term should *never* be used to mean an "opacity" or "radiopacity."

WORDS OR TERMS USED IN ROENTGENOLOGY *Continued*

Word or Term

Comments

diffuse *adj.* 1. (pathophysiol.) Widely distributed through an organ or type of tissue. 2. (radiol.) Widespread and continuous (said of shadows and by inference of the states or processes producing them).

Synonyms: Disseminated, generalized, systemic, widespread.

A useful and acceptable term. In the context of chest radiology, "diffuse" connotes widespread, anatomically continuous but not necessarily complete involvement of the lung or other thoracic structure or tissue; "disseminated" connotes widespread but anatomically discontinuous involvement; and "generalized" connotes complete or nearly complete involvement whereas "systemic" connotes involvement of a thoracic structure or tissue as part of a process involving the entire body.

discrete *adj.* (radiol.) Separate, individually distinct; hence, with respect to opacities, usually circumscribed.

Antonyms: Confluent, coalescent.

An acceptable descriptor.

disseminated *adj.* 1. (pathophysiol.) Widely but discontinuously distributed through an organ or type of tissue. 2. (radiol.) Widespread but anatomically discontinuous (said of shadows and by inference of the states or processes producing them).

Synonyms: Diffuse (*q.v.*), generalized, systemic.

A useful and acceptable term.

doubling time *n.* (radiol.) The time span over which a pulmonary nodule or mass doubles in volume (increases its diameter by a factor of 1.25).

An acceptable term. The concept should be used with caution as a criterion for distinguishing benign from malignant nodules.

embolus *n.* 1. (pathol.) A clot or mass of foreign material that has been carried by the bloodstream to occlude partly or completely the lumen of a blood vessel. 2. (radiol.) (a) A lucent defect or obstruction within an opacified blood vessel presumed to represent an embolus in the pathologic sense. (b) An acutely dilated pulmonary artery persumed to represent the presence of blood clot or other embolic material. *Qualifiers:* acute, chronic; air, fat, amniotic fluid, parasitic, neoplastic, tissue, foreign material (*e.g.*, iodized oil, mercury, talc); septic, therapeutic, paradoxic.

In sense 2(a), an inferred conclusion based on reliable evidence (arteriography); in sense 2(b), based on highly suggestive evidence (conventional roentgenography) in the appropriate clinical setting. A useful descriptor, particularly in arteriography.

emphysema *n.* 1. (pathol.) (a) A morbid condition of the lung characterized by abnormally expanded air spaces distal to the terminal bronchiole, with or without destruction of the air-space walls (per Ciba Conference, 1959). (b) As above, but "with destruction of the walls of involved air spaces" specified (per World Health Organization, 1961, and American Thoracic Society, 1962). 2. (radiol.) Overinflation of all or a portion of one or both lungs, with or without associated oligemia (*q.v.*), presumed to represent morphologic emphysema.

In radiology, an inferred conclusion based on usually reliable signs (if the disease is moderate or advanced). Applicable only in an appropriate clinical setting and, in the sense of the ATS definition, not applicable to spasmodic asthma or compensatory overinflation.

fibrocalcific *adj.* (radiol.) Of or pertaining to sharply defined, linear, and/or nodular opacities containing calcification(s) (*q.v.*), usually occurring in the upper lobes and presumed to represent old granulomatous lesions.

A widely used and acceptable roentgenologic descriptor.

WORDS OR TERMS USED IN ROENTGENOLOGY *Continued*

Word or Term	Comments
fibronodular *adj.* (radiol.) Of or pertaining to sharply defined, approximately circular opacities occurring singly or in clusters, usually in the upper lobes, and associated with linear opacities and distortion (retraction) of adjacent structures. A finding usually presumed to represent old granulomatous disease.	An inferred conclusion usually employed as a roentgenologic descriptor. Its use is not recommended.
fibrosis *n.* 1. (pathol.) (a) Cellular fibrous tissue or dense acellular collagenous tissue. (b) The process of proliferation of fibroblasts leading to the formation of fibrous or collagenous tissue. 2. (radiol.) Any opacity presumed to represent fibrous or collagenous tissue; applicable to linear, nodular, or stellate opacities that are sharply defined, that are associated with evidence of loss of volume in the affected portion of the lung and/or with deformity of adjacent structures, and that show no change over a period of months or years. Also applicable with caution to a diffuse pattern of opacity if there is evidence of progressive loss of lung volume or if the pattern of opacity is unchanged over time.	In radiology, an inferred conclusion often used as a descriptor. An acceptable term if used in strict accordance with the criteria cited.
fissure *n.* 1. (anat.) The infolding of visceral pleura that separates one lobe or a portion of a lobe from another. 2. (radiol.) A linear opacity normally 1 mm or less in width that corresponds in position and extent to the anatomic separation of pulmonary lobes or portions of lobes. *Qualifiers:* minor, major, horizontal, oblique, accessory, anomalous, azygos, inferior accessory. *Synonym:* Interlobar septum.	A specific feature of anatomy.
Fleischner's line(s) *n.* (radiol.) A straight, curved, or irregular linear opacity that is visible in multiple projections; is usually situated in the lower half of the lung; is usually approximately horizontal but may be oriented in any direction; and may or may not appear to extend to the pleural surface. Such lines vary markedly in length and width; their exact pathologic significance is unknown.	An acceptable term. However, the term "linear opacity," properly qualified with respect to location, dimensions, and orientation, is preferred. There are no synonyms ("platelike," "discoid," and "platter" atelectasis should *not* be employed as synonyms; in the absence of clear histologic evidence of the significance of Fleischner's lines, the inferred identification of such lines with a form of atelectasis is unwarranted).
fluffy *adj.* (radiol.) In describing opacities: ill-defined, lacking clear-cut margins; resembling down. *Synonyms:* Shaggy, poorly defined.	An imprecise descriptor of limited usefulness.
ground-glass pattern *n.* (radiol.) Any extended, finely granular pattern of pulmonary opacity within which normal anatomic details are partly obscured. Term derived from a fancied resemblance to etched or abraded glass. *Synonym:* Granular pattern.	A nonspecific roentgenologic descriptor of limited usefulness; the synonym is preferred.
hernia *n.* (clin./morphol./radiol.) The protrusion of all or part of an organ or tissue through an abnormal opening.	An inferred conclusion to be used only within the precise terms of the definition. Thus, in the thorax the word is appropriate in relation to the diaphragm but should not be used with reference to pulmonary overinflation and mediastinal displacement.

WORDS OR TERMS USED IN ROENTGENOLOGY *Continued*

Word or Term	Comments
hilum, *n., pl.* -la. 1. (anat.) A depression or pit in that part of an organ where the vessels and nerves enter. 2. (radiol.) The composite shadow at the root of each lung composed of bronchi, pulmonary arteries and veins, lymph nodes, nerves, bronchial vessels, and associated areolar tissue. *Synonyms:* Lung root; hilus (hili).	A specific element of pulmonary anatomy. Hilum (hila) is preferred to hilus (hili).
homogeneous *adj.* (radiol.) Of uniform opacity or texture throughout. *Antonyms:* Inhomogeneous, nonhomogeneous, heterogeneous.	A useful roentgenologic descriptor. Inhomogeneous is the preferred antonym.
honeycomb pattern *n.* 1. (pathol.) A multitude of irregular cystic spaces in pulmonary tissue that are generally lined with bronchiolar epithelium and have markedly thickened walls composed of dense fibrous tissue, with or without associated chronic inflammation. 2. (radiol.) A number of closely approximated ring shadows representing air spaces 5 to 10 mm in diameter with walls 2 to 3 mm thick that resemble a true honeycomb; a finding whose occurrence implies "end-stage" lung.	It is recommended that the term be used strictly in accordance with the dimensional limits cited, in which case it possesses specific connotation.
hyperemia *n.* 1. (pathol./physiol.) An excess of blood in a part of the body; engorgement. 2. (radiol.) Increased blood flow. *Synonym:* Pleonemia (*q.v.*).	While semantically correct, this word has come through common usage to mean the increased blood flow that is part of the inflammatory response. We recommend that it be used as a descriptor only in arteriography. The synonym is preferred when indicating increased blood flow to the lungs.
hypertension *n.* (clin./radiol.) Elevation above normal levels of systolic and/or diastolic pressure within the systemic or pulmonary vascular bed. Generally accepted empiric levels of pressure for systemic arterial hypertension are 140 systolic, 90 diastolic; systemic venous hypertension, 12 mm Hg; pulmonary arterial hypertension, 30 mm Hg systolic; 15 diastolic; pulmonary venous hypertension, 12 mm Hg. *Synonym:* High blood pressure.	With the exception of systemic arterial hypertension, roentgenologic assessment of hypertension in each of the four vascular compartments constitutes an inferred conclusion, although based on usually reliable signs.
infarct *n.* (Literally, a portion of tissue stuffed with extravasated blood or serum.) 1. (pathol.) A zone of ischemic necrosis surrounded by hyperemic lung resulting from occlusion of the region's feeding vessel, usually by an embolus. 2. (radiol.) A pulmonary opacity that, by virtue of its temporal development and in the appropriate clinical setting, is considered to result from thromboembolic occlusion of a feeding vessel. The opacity is commonly but not exclusively hump-shaped and pleura-based when viewed in profile and poorly defined and round when viewed *en face*.	An inferred roentgenologic conclusion acceptable in the proper clinical setting and with appropriate signs. Subsequent events may establish that the opacity was the result of either hemorrhage or tissue necrosis. The word should not be used in the absence of an opacity (*e.g.,* with oligemia).

WORDS OR TERMS USED IN ROENTGENOLOGY *Continued*

Word or Term	Comments

infiltrate *n.* 1. (pathophysiol.) Any substance or type of cell that occurs within or spreads through the interstices (interstitium and/or alveoli) of the lung, which is foreign to the lung or which accumulates in greater than normal quantity within it. 2. (radiol.) (a) An ill-defined opacity in the lung that neither destroys nor displaces the gross morphology of the lung and is presumed to represent an infiltrate in the pathophysiologic sense. (b) Any ill-defined opacity in the lung.

An inferred and often unwarranted conclusion used as a descriptor. The term is almost invariably used in sense 2(b), in which it serves no useful purpose, and, lacking a specific connotation, is so variably used as to cause great confusion. The term's use as a descriptor is to be condemned. The preferred word is "opacity," properly qualified with respect to location, dimensions, and definition.

inflation *n.* (physiol./radiol.) The state or process of being expanded or filled with gas; used specifically with reference to the expansion of the lungs with air. *Qualifiers:* overinflation (preferred) or hyperinflation; underinflation (preferred) or hypoinflation.

Synonyms: Aeration, inhalation, inspiration.

"Inflation" connotes expansion with gas or air. "Aeration" connotes the admission of air, exposure to air. "Inhalation" refers specifically to the act of drawing air into the lungs in the process of breathing (as opposed to exhalation); "inspiration," with reference to breathing, is similar in connotation. The word "inflation" is the preferred term, since it avoids the confusion that surrounds the meaning of aeration as a result of common misusage.

interface *n.* (radiol.) The common boundary between the shadows of two juxtaposed structures or tissues of different texture or opacity (*e.g.*, lung and heart).

Synonyms: Edge, border.

A useful roentgenologic descriptor.

interstitium *n.* (anat./radiol.) A continuum of loose connective tissue throughout the lung consisting of three subdivisions: (a) bronchoarterial (axial), surrounding the bronchoarterial bundles from the hila to the point at which bronchiolar walls become intimately related to lung parenchyma; (b) parenchymal (acinar), situated between alveolar and capillary basement membranes; and (c) subpleural, situated between the pleura and lung parenchyma and continuous with the interlobular septa and perivenous interstitial space that extends from the lung periphery to the hila.

Synonym: Interstitial space.

A useful anatomic term. The interstitium of the lung is not normally visible roentgenographically and only becomes visible when disease (*e.g.*, edema) increases its volume and attenuation.

Kerley line *n.* (radiol.) A linear opacity, which, depending on its location, extent, and orientation, may be further classified as follows: Kerley A line—an essentially straight linear opacity 2 to 6 cm in length and 1 to 3 mm in width, usually situated in an upper lung zone, that points toward the hilum centrally and is directed toward but does not extend to the pleural surface peripherally. Kerley B line—a straight linear opacity 1.5 to 2 cm in length and 1 to 2 mm in width, usually situated at the lung base, and oriented at right angles to the pleural surface with which it is usually in contact. Kerley C lines—a group of branching, linear opacities producing the appearance of a fine net, situated at the lung base and representing Kerley B lines seen *en face*.

Synonym: Septal line(s).

A specific feature of pathologic/roentgenologic anatomy. Except when it is essential to distinguish A, B, and C lines, the term "septal line" is preferred. "Lymphatic line" is anatomically inaccurate and should never be used.

WORDS OR TERMS USED IN ROENTGENOLOGY *Continued*

Word or Term	Comments
line *n.* (radiol.) A longitudinal opacity no greater than 2 mm in width (*cf.* stripe).	A useful word appropriately employed in the description of roentgenographic shadows within the mediastinum (*e.g.,* anterior junction line) or lung (interlobar fissures).
linear opacity *n.* (radiol.) A shadow resembling a line; hence, any elongated opacity of approximately uniform width. *Synonyms:* Line, line shadow, linear shadow, band shadow.	A generic roentgenologic descriptor of great usefulness. "Band shadow" and "line shadow" have been employed by some to identify elongated shadows more than 2 mm wide and less than 2 mm wide, respectively; "linear opacity," qualified by a statement of specific dimensions, is the preferred term. The length, width, anatomic location, and orientation of such a shadow should be specified.
lobe *n.* (anat./radiol.) One of the principal divisions of the lungs (usually three on the right, two on the left), each of which is enveloped by the visceral pleura except at the hilum and in areas of developmental deficiency where fissures are incomplete. The lobes are separated in whole or in part by pleural fissures.	A specific feature of pulmonary anatomy.
lobule *n.* (anat./radiol.) A unit of lung structure. A subdivision of lung parenchyma that is of two types: (a) primary, arising from the last respiratory bronchiole and consisting of a series of alveolar ducts, atria, alveolar sacs, and alveoli, together with their accompanying blood vessels and nerves; (b) secondary, composed of a variable number of acini (usually 3 to 5) and bounded in most cases by connective tissue septa.	Acinus is the preferred anatomic/physiologic unit of lung structure. Since a primary lobule is not visible roentgenographically, the use of the term has been largely abandoned. When unmodified, the word "lobule" refers to a secondary lobule. A secondary pulmonary lobule occasionally becomes visible when it is either selectively consolidated or its surrounding connective tissue septa become visible from a process such as edema.
lucency *n.* (radiol.) The shadow of an absorber that attenuates the primary x-ray beam less effectively than do surrounding absorbers. Hence, in a roentgenogram, any circumscribed area that appears more nearly black (of greater photometric density) than its surround. Usually applied to local shadows of air density whose attenuation is less than that of surrounding lung (*e.g.,* a bulla) or of fat density when surrounded by a more effective absorber such as muscle. *Synonyms:* Radiolucency, translucency, transradiancy.	This term employed by analogy with "opacity," is acceptable in American usage, although it is etymologically indefensible. In British usage, "transradiancy" is preferred.
lymphadenopathy *n.* (clin./pathol./radiol.) Any abnormality of lymph nodes; by common usage usually restricted to enlargement of lymph nodes. *Synonym:* Lymph node enlargement.	Since "adeno-" specifically relates to a glandular structure and since lymph nodes are not glands, the term is a misnomer and its use is to be condemned in favor of its synonym.
marking(s) *n.* (radiol.) A descriptor variously used with reference to the shadows produced by a combination of normal pulmonary structures (blood vessels, bronchi, etc.). Usually used in the plural and following "lung" or "bronchovascular." *Synonym:* Linear opacity.	When used alone, a vague descriptor of little value and not recommended. With proper qualification, the term is acceptable.

WORDS OR TERMS USED IN ROENTGENOLOGY *Continued*

Word or Term	Comments

mass *n.* (radiol.) Any pulmonary or pleural lesion represented in a roentgenogram by a discrete opacity greater than 30 mm in diameter (without regard to contour, border characteristics, or homogeneity), but explicitly shown or presumed to be extended in all three dimensions.

Synonym: Tumor (*q.v.*).

A useful and recommended descriptor. Should always be qualified with respect to size, location, contour, definition, homogeneity, opacity, and number. Its use as a qualifier of "lesion" is to be deplored.

medulla *n.* (radiol.) That portion of the lung situated between the hilum and cortex (*q.v.*).

A term and concept of limited usefulness.

miliary pattern *n.* (radiol.) A collection of tiny discrete opacities in the lungs, each measuring 2 mm or less in diameter, and generally uniform in size and widespread in distribution.

Synonym: Micronodular pattern.

An acceptable descriptor without etiologic connotation.

mucoid impaction *n.* (radiol.) A broad I-, Y-, or V-shaped roentgenographic opacity caused by the presence within a proximal airway (lobar, segmental, or subsegmental bronchus) of thick, tenaceous mucus, usually associated with airway dilatation. The shape of the opacity depends upon the branching pattern of airway involved.

Synonym: Bronchocele (*q.v.*).

An inferred conclusion based on usually reliable signs. A useful descriptor preferred to its synonym.

Mueller maneuver *n.* (physiol.) Inspiration against a closed glottis, usually but not necessarily from a position of residual volume.

A useful technique for producing transient decrease in intrathoracic pressure.

nodular pattern *n.* (radiol.) A collection of innumerable, small discrete opacities ranging in diameter from 2 to 10 mm, generally uniform in size and widespread in distribution, and without marginal spiculation (*cf.* reticulonodular pattern).

An acceptable roentgenologic discriptor without specific pathologic or etiologic implications. The size of the nodules should be specified, either as a range or as an average.

nodule *n.* (radiol.) Any pulmonary or pleural lesion represented in a roentgenogram by a sharply defined, discrete, approximately circular opacity 2 to 30 mm in diameter (*cf.* mass).

Synonym: Coin lesion (*q.v.*).

A useful and recommended descriptor to be used in preference to its synonym, which is a colloquial abomination. Should always be qualified with respect to size, location, border characteristics, number, and opacity.

oligemia *n.* 1. (pathol./physiol.) Reduced blood flow to the lungs or a portion thereof. 2. (radiol.) General or local decrease in the apparent width of visible pulmonary vessels, suggesting less than normal blood flow. *Qualifiers:* acute, chronic; local, general.

Synonym: Reduced blood flow.

An inferred conclusion usually used as descriptor and appropriately based on reliable signs. An acceptable term.

opacity *n.* (radiol.) The shadow of an absorber that attenuates the x-ray beam more effectively than do surrounding absorbers. Hence, in a roentgenogram, any circumscribed area that appears more nearly white (of lesser photometric density) than its surround. Usually applied to the shadows of nonspecific pulmonary collections of fluid, tissue, etc., whose attenuation exceeds that of the surrounding aerated lung.

Synonym: Radiopacity (*cf.* density).

An essential and recommended roentgenologic descriptor. In the context of roentgenologic reporting, "radiopaque" is acceptable but seems redundant; however, it is preferred in British usage. "Density" (*q.v.*) should *never* be used in this context.

WORDS OR TERMS USED IN ROENTGENOLOGY *Continued*

Word or Term	Comments
opaque *adj.* (radiol.) Impervious to x-rays. *Synonym:* Radiopaque.	Opaque and radiopaque are both acceptable terms, although the former is preferred (*see* opacity).
ossification *n.* (radiol.) Calcific opacities within the lung that represent trabecular bone; applicable to calcific opacities that either display morphologic characteristics of trabecular bone (trabeculation and a defined cortex) or occur in association with a lesion known histologically to produce trabecular bone within lung (*e.g.,* mitral stenosis). *Synonyms:* Ossific nodulation, ossific nodule(s).	A useful roentgenologic term, although usually an inferred conclusion. To be distinguished from "calcification" (*q.v.*).
paraspinal line *n.* (radiol.) A vertically oriented interface usually seen in a frontal chest roentgenogram to the left (rarely to the right) of the thoracic vertebral column. It extends from the aortic arch to the diaphragm and represents contact between aerated lower lobe and adjacent mediastinal tissues. The anatomic interface is situated posterior to the descending aorta and is seen between the left lateral margin of the aorta and the spine. *Synonyms:* Left paraspinal pleural reflection; left paraspinal interface.	A specific feature of roentgenologic anatomy. Either of the synonyms cited is preferred inasmuch as the shadow represents an interface, not a line.
parenchyma *n.* 1. (anat.) The gas-exchanging portion of the lung consisting of the alveoli and their capillaries, estimated to comprise approximately 90 per cent of total lung volume. 2. (radiol.) All lung tissue exclusive of visible pulmonary vessels and airways.	A useful anatomic concept and an acceptable roentgenologic descriptor.
perfusion *n.* (physiol./radiol.) The passage of blood into and out of the lung. *Synonym:* Pulmonary blood flow.	A useful and recommended term.
phantom tumor *n.* (radiol.) A shadow produced by a local collection of fluid in one of the interlobar fissures (most often the minor fissure), usually possessing an elliptic configuration in one roentgenographic projection and a rounded configuration in the other, thus resembling a tumor. It is commonly caused by cardiac decompensation and usually disappears with appropriate therapy. *Synonyms:* Vanishing tumor, pseudotumor.	An explicit diagnostic conclusion from serial roentgenograms but only an inferred conclusion from a single examination. An acceptable descriptor.
platelike atelectasis *n.* (radiol.) A linear or planar opacity presumed to represent diminished volume in a portion of the lung; usually situated in lower lung zones. *Synonyms:* Platter, linear, or discoid atelectasis.	An inferred conclusion usually not subject to proof and often unwarranted. Its use as a descriptor is not recommended. "Linear opacity" is preferred.
pleonemia *n.* (pathol./physiol./radiol.) Increased blood flow to the lungs or a portion thereof, manifested roentgenologically by a general or local increase in the width of visible pulmonary vessels. *Synonyms:* Increased blood flow, hyperemia.	An inferred conclusion often used as a descriptor and based on usually reliable signs. An acceptable term preferrable to hyperemia (*q.v.*).
pneumatocele *n.* (pathol./radiol.) A thin-walled, gas-filled space within the lung usually occurring in association with acute pneumonia (most commonly of staphylococcal etiology) and almost invariably transient.	An inferred conclusion. An acceptable descriptor if used in accordance with the precise definition.

WORDS OR TERMS USED IN ROENTGENOLOGY *Continued*

Word or Term	**Comments**

pneumomediastinum *n.* (pathol./radiol.) A state characterized by the presence of gas in mediastinal tissues outside the esophagus, tracheobronchial tree, or pericardium. *Qualifiers:* spontaneous, traumatic, diagnostic.

Synonym: Mediastinal emphysema.

An appropriate descriptor based on roentgenologic signs alone; preferred to its synonym.

pneumonia *n.* (pathol./radiol.) Infection (or noninfectious inflammation) of the air spaces and/or interstitium of the lung. *Qualifiers* may be employed to indicate temporal course (acute, chronic), predominant anatomic involvement (air-space or lobar, interstitial, bronchial), or etiology (bacterial, viral, fungal).

Synonym: Pneumonitis.

An inferred conclusion, based on usually reliable signs. Generally preferred to its synonym, although the latter is sometimes used to designate infection caused by viruses or *Mycoplasma pneumoniae.*

pneumothorax *n.* (pathol./radiol.) A state characterized by the presence of gas within the pleural space. *Qualifiers:* spontaneous, traumatic, diagnostic, tension (*q.v.*).

A diagnostic conclusion appropriately based on roentgenologic evidence alone.

popcorn calcification *n.* (radiol.) A cluster of sharply defined, irregularly lobulated, calcific opacities, usually within a pulmonary nodule, suggesting the appearance of popcorn.

An acceptable descriptor.

posterior junction line *n.* (radiol.) A vertically oriented, linear or curvilinear opacity approximately 2 mm wide, commonly projected on the tracheal air shadow, and usually slightly concave to the right. It is produced by the shadows of the right and left pleurae in intimate contact between the aerated lungs. It represents the plane of contact between the lungs posterior to the trachea and esophagus and anterior to the spine; hence, in contrast to the anterior junction line, it may project both above and below the suprasternal notch.

Synonyms: Posterior mediastinal septum; posterior mediastinal line; supraaortic posterior junction line or stripe; mesentery of the esophagus.

A specific feature of roentgenologic anatomy; to be preferred to cited synonyms.

posterior tracheal stripe *n.* (radiol.) A vertically oriented linear opacity ranging in width from 2 to 5 mm, extending from the thoracic inlet to the bifurcation of the trachea, and visible only on lateral roentgenograms of the chest. It is situated between the air shadow of the trachea and the right lung and is formed by the posterior tracheal wall and contiguous mediastinal interstitial tissue.

Synonym: Posterior tracheal band.

A specific feature of radiologic anatomy; to be preferred to its synonym.

primary complex *n.* 1. (pathol.) The combination of a focus of pneumonia due to a primary infection (*e.g.,* tuberculosis or histoplasmosis) with granulomas in the draining hilar or mediastinal lymph nodes. 2. (radiol.) (a) One or more irregular opacities of variable extent and location assumed to represent consolidation of lung parenchyma, associated with enlargement of hilar or mediastinal lymph nodes, an appearance presumed to represent active infection. (b) One or more small, sharply defined parenchymal opacities (often calcified) associated with calcification of hilar or mediastinal lymph nodes, an appearance usually regarded as evidence of an inactive process.

A useful inferred conclusion. "Primary complex" is to be preferred to "Ranke complex," which is acceptable but rarely used. "Ghon complex" represents an inappropriate use of the eponym and is unacceptable (Ghon described the pulmonary abnormality alone, which thus becomes a Ghon focus or Ghon lesion).

WORDS OR TERMS USED IN ROENTGENOLOGY *Continued*

Word or Term	Comments
profusion *n.* (radiol.) The number of small opacities per unit area or zone of lung. In the ILO classification of radiographs of the pneumoconioses, the qualifiers 0 through 3 subdivide the profusion into 4 categories. The profusion categories may be further subdivided by employing a 12-point scale.	A useful word to describe the number of opacities in any diffuse disease, including the pneumoconioses.
pseudocavity *n.* (radiol.) A state in which a pulmonary nodule or mass possesses a central portion that is more lucent than its periphery (thus suggesting cavitation) but in which subsequent computed tomography or pathologic examination reveals only the presence of necrotic tissue high in lipid content, with no true cavity. *Synonym:* Simulated cavity.	An inferred conclusion sometimes used as a descriptor. The term is without etiologic connotation.
pulmonary edema *n.* 1. (pathophysiol.) The accumulation of liquid in the interstitial compartment of the lung with or without associated alveolar filling. Specifically, the accumulation of water, protein, and solutes (transudate), usually due to one or a combination of the following: (a) increased pressure in the microvascular bed, (b) increased microvascular permeability, or (c) impaired lymphatic drainage. Also, the accumulation of water, protein, solutes, and inflammatory cells (exudate) in response to inflammation of any type (*e.g.,* infection, allergy, trauma, or circulating toxins). 2. (radiol.) A pattern of opacity (usually bilaterally symmetrical) believed to represent interstitial thickening or alveolar filling when associated findings and/or history suggest one of the processes enumerated above. *Qualifiers:* interstitial, air-space, alveolar. *Synonyms:* Wet, boggy, or moist lung.	An inferred conclusion often employed as a descriptor, based on usually reliable signs. A useful and acceptable term when used in an appropriate clinical setting. The synonyms are colloquialisms to be avoided.
respiratory failure *n.* (physiol.) A state characterized by an arterial P_{O_2} below 60 mm Hg or an arterial P_{CO_2} above 49 mm Hg, at rest at sea level, resulting from impaired respiratory function. *Synonym:* Pulmonary insufficiency.	A useful term that should be restricted to clinical and physiologic usage. It is preferred to its synonym.
reticular pattern *n.* (radiol.) A collection of innumerable small linear opacities that together produce an appearance resembling a net. *Qualifiers:* fine, medium, coarse. *Synonym:* Small irregular opacities (in the ILO classification of radiographs of the pneumoconioses).	A recommended descriptor that usually indicates predominant abnormality of the pulmonary interstitium. The synonym should be restricted to the roentgenographic characterization of pneumoconiosis.
reticulonodular pattern *n.* (radiol.) A collection of innumerable small, linear, and nodular opacities that together produce a composite appearance resembling a net with small superimposed nodules. In common usage, the reticular and nodular elements are dimensionally of similar magnitude. *Qualifiers:* fine, medium, coarse.	An acceptable roentgenologic descriptor that usually indicates predominant abnormality of the pulmonary interstitium.
right tracheal stripe *n.* (radiol.) A vertically oriented linear opacity approximately 2 to 3 mm wide extending from the thoracic inlet to the right tracheobronchial angle. It is situated between the air shadow of the trachea and the right lung and is formed by the right tracheal wall and contiguous mediastinal interstitial tissue and pleura. *Synonym:* Right paratracheal stripe or band.	A specific feature of radiologic anatomy; to be preferred to the cited synonym since the opacity is caused chiefly by the tracheal wall itself.

WORDS OR TERMS USED IN ROENTGENOLOGY *Continued*

Word or Term	Comments

segment *n.* (anat./radiol.) One of the principal anatomic subdivisions of the pulmonary lobes served by a major branch of a lobar bronchus. *Qualifier:* bronchopulmonary.

> A useful anatomic and roentgenologic descriptor.

septal line(s) *n.* (radiol.) Usually used in the plural, a generic term for linear opacities of varied distribution produced when the interstitium between pulmonary lobules is thickened (*e.g.,* by fluid, dust deposition, cellular material).

Synonym: Kerley line (*q.v.*).

> A specific feature of roentgenologic pathology, sometimes inferred. A recommended term. "Kerley line" is acceptable, particularly when seeking to identify a particular type of septal line (*e.g.,* Kerley B line).

shadow *n.* (radiol.) In clinical roentgenography, any perceptible discontinuity in film blackening (or fluoroscopic image or CRT display) attributed to the attenuation of the x-ray beam by a specific anatomic absorber or lesion on or within the body of the patient; an opacity or lucency. The word should always be qualified as precisely as possible with respect to size, contour, location, opacity, lucency, and so on.

> A useful and recommended descriptor to be employed only when more specific identification is not possible.

silhouette sign *n.* (radiol.) 1. The effacement of an anatomic soft tissue border by either a normal anatomic structure (*e.g.,* the inferior border of the heart and left hemidiaphragm) or a pathologic state such as airlessness of adjacent lung or accumulation of fluid in the contiguous pleural space. 2. A sign of conformity, and hence, of the probable adjacency of a pathologic opacity to a known structure.

> Useful in detecting and localizing an opacity along the axis of the x-ray beam. Although the physical basis underlying the production of this sign is contentious, the term is a widely accepted and useful descriptor. Despite the fact that the definition implies *loss* of silhouette, the term has acquired such common popularity that its continued use is recommended.

small irregular opacities *n.* (radiol.) A collection of innumerable small linear opacities that together produce an appearance resembling a net. In the ILO/1980 classification of radiographs of the pneumoconioses, the qualifiers s, t, and u subdivide the dimensions of the opacities into three diameter ranges—up to 1.5 mm, 1.5 to 3 mm, and 3 to 10 mm, respectively.

Synonym: Reticular pattern (*q.v.*).

> A term to be employed specifically to describe roentgenographic manifestations of the pneumoconioses; the synonym is preferred for nonpneumoconiotic disease.

small rounded opacities *n.* (radiol.) A collection of innumerable pulmonary nodules ranging in diameter from bare visibility up to 10 mm, usually widespread in distribution. In the ILO/1980 classification of radiographs of the pneumoconioses, the qualifiers p, q, and r subdivide the dimensions of the opacities into three diameter ranges—up to 1.5 mm, 1.5 to 3 mm, and 3 to 10 mm, respectively.

Synonym: Nodular pattern (*q.v.*).

> A term to be employed specifically to describe roentgenographic manifestations of the pneumoconioses; the synonym is preferred for nonpneumoconiotic disease.

WORDS OR TERMS USED IN ROENTGENOLOGY *Continued*

Word or Term	Comments
stripe *n.* (radiol.) A longitudinal composite opacity measuring 2 to 5 mm in width (*cf.* line).	An acceptable descriptor when limited to anatomic structures within the mediastinum (*e.g.,* right tracheal stripe).
subsegment *n.* (anat./radiol.) A unit of pulmonary tissue supplied by a bronchus of lesser order than a segmental bronchus.	A useful anatomic and roentgenologic descriptor.
tension *adj.* 1. (physiol./clin.) When used with reference to pneumo- or hydrothorax, a state characterized by cardiorespiratory functional impairment. 2. (radiol.) The accumulation of gas or fluid in a pleural space in an amount sufficient to cause airlessness of the ipsilateral lung, marked depression of the ipsilateral hemidiaphragm, and displacement of the mediastinum to the opposite side.	An inferred conclusion to be used only in the presence of clinical cardiorespiratory embarrassment. In fact, "tension" in relation to pneumothorax exists only during the expiratory phase of the respiratory cycle, since pleural pressure on inspiration is usually subatmospheric. The word should not be employed as in the term "tension cyst," which does not satisfy the criteria cited.
thromboembolism *n.* (pathol./clin./radiol.) Partial or complete occlusion of the lumen of a blood vessel by a thrombus (*q.v.*).	An inferred conclusion sometimes based on reliable signs (in conventional roentgenography) or a diagnostic conclusion based on roentgenologic evidence alone (in angiography).
thrombosis *n.* (pathol./radiol.) The state or process of thrombus formation within a blood vessel or heart chamber.	*Cf.* clot.
thrombus *n.* (pathol./radiol.) A mass of semisolidified blood, composed chiefly of platelets and fibrin with entrapped cellular elements, at the site of its formation in a blood vessel or heart chamber.	A useful descriptor to be employed only in the precise sense of the definition. (*Cf.* embolus.)
tramline shadow *n.* (radiol.) Parallel or slightly convergent linear opacities that suggest the planar projection of tubular structures and that correspond in location and orientation to elements of the bronchial tree. They are generally assumed to represent thickened bronchial walls. *Synonyms:* Thickened bronchial wall, tubular shadow (*q.v.*).	A roentgenologic descriptor which is not recommended in deference to either of the synonyms. Such shadows are of possible pathologic significance only when they occur outside the limits of the hilar shadows where bronchial walls may be seen normally.
tubular shadow *n.* (radiol.) 1. Paired, parallel, or slightly convergent linear opacities presumed to represent the walls of a tubular structure seen *en face* (*e.g.,* a bronchus). 2. An approximately circular opacity presumed to represent the wall of a tubular structure seen end-on. *Synonyms:* Tramline shadow (*q.v.*), thickened bronchial wall.	Acceptable if the anatomic nature of a shadow is obscure; otherwise the more precise "thickened bronchial wall" is to be preferred.
tumor *n.* 1. (general) A swelling or morbid enlargement. 2. (pathol./radiol.) Literally, a mass (*q.v.*), not differentiated as to its neoplastic or non-neoplastic nature. *Synonym:* Mass.	A useful descriptor, although "mass" is preferred. The use of the word as a synonym for neoplasm is to be condemned.

WORDS OR TERMS USED IN ROENTGENOLOGY *Continued*

Word or Term	Comments
Valsalva maneuver *n.* (physiol.) Forced expiration against a closed glottis, usually but not necessarily from a position of total lung capacity.	A useful technique to produce transient increase in intrathoracic pressure.
vasoconstriction *n.* 1. (physiol.) Narrowing of muscular blood vessels by contraction of their muscle layer. 2. (radiol.) Local or general reduction in the caliber of visible pulmonary vessels (oligemia [*q.v.*]), presumed to result from decreased flow occasioned by contraction of muscular pulmonary arteries. *Qualifiers:* hypoxic, reflex.	An inferred conclusion based on usually reliable signs. The word is not synonymous with oligemia; although the latter is a *sign* of vasoconstriction, it may also occur when vessel narrowing is organic (as in emphysema) rather than functional and potentially reversible.
vasodilation *n.* (radiol.) The local or general increase in the width of visible pulmonary vessels resulting from increased pulmonary blood flow. *Synonym:* Vasodilatation.	An inferred conclusion based on usually reliable signs.
ventilation *n.* (physiol./radiol.) The movement of air into and out of the lungs; inspiration and expiration. *Qualifiers:* hyperventilation (preferred), or overventilation; hypoventilation (preferred), or underventilation.	The term always implies a biphasic dynamic process of admission and expulsion; hence, it cannot be assessed from a single static image (*see* inflation).

TERMS AND SYMBOLS USED IN RESPIRATORY PHYSIOLOGY AND PATHOPHYSIOLOGY

GENERAL SYMBOLS

P	Pressure, blood, or gas
$\dot{X}$	A time derivative indicated by a dot above the symbol (rate). This symbol is used for both instantaneous flow and volume per unit time
%X	Per cent sign *preceding* a symbol indicates percentage of the predicted normal value
X/Y%	Per cent sign *following* a symbol indicates a ratio function with the ratio expressed as a percentage. Both components of the ratio must be designated; e.g., $FEV_1/FVC\% = 100 \times FEV_1/FVC$
X_A or Xa	A small capital letter or lower case letter on the same line following a primary symbol is a qualifier to further define the primary symbol. When small capital letters are not available on typewriters or to printers, large capital letters may be used as subscripts; e.g., $X_A = XA$

GAS PHASE SYMBOLS

PRIMARY SYMBOLS (LARGE CAPITAL LETTERS)

V	Gas volume. The particular gas as well as its pressure, water vapor conditions, and other special conditions must be specified in text or indicated by appropriate qualifying symbols
F	Fractional concentration of gas

COMMON QUALIFYING SYMBOLS

I	Inspired
E	Expired
A	Alveolar
T	Tidal
D	Dead space or wasted ventilation
B	Barometric
L	Lung
STPD	Standard conditions: Temperature 0 degrees Centigrade, pressure 760 mm Hg, and dry (0 water vapor)
BTPS	Body conditions: Body temperature, ambient pressure, and saturated with water vapor at these conditions
ATPD	Ambient temperature and pressure, dry
ATPS	Ambient temperature and pressure, saturated with water vapor at these conditions
an	Anatomic
p	Physiologic
rb	Rebreathing
f	Respiratory frequency per minute
max	Maximal
t	Time

BLOOD PHASE SYMBOLS

PRIMARY SYMBOLS (LARGE CAPITAL LETTERS)

Q	Blood volume
$\dot{Q}$	Blood flow, volume units and time must be specified
C	Concentration in the blood phase
S	Saturation in the blood phase

QUALIFYING SYMBOLS (LOWER CASE LETTERS)

b	Blood in general
a	Arterial
c	Capillary
ć	Pulmonary end-capillary
v	Venous
v̄	Mixed venous

VENTILATION AND LUNG MECHANICS TESTS AND SYMBOLS

LUNG VOLUME COMPARTMENTS*

RV	Residual volume; that volume of air remaining in the lungs after maximal exhalation. The method of measurement should be indicated in the text or, when necessary, by appropriate qualifying symbols
ERV	Expiratory reserve volume; the maximal volume of air exhaled from the end-expiratory level

---

*Primary components are designated as volumes. When volumes are combined they are designated as capacities. All are considered to be at BTPS unless otherwise specified.

V_T	Tidal volume; that volume of air inhaled or exhaled with each breath during quiet breathing, used only to indicate a subdivision of lung volume
IRV	Inspiratory reserve volume; the maximal volume of air inhaled from the end-inspiratory level
IC	Inspiratory capacity; the sum of IRV and V_T
IVC	Inspiratory vital capacity; the maximal volume of air inhaled from the point of maximal expiration
VC	Vital capacity; the maximal volume of air exhaled from the point of maximal inspiration
FRC	Functional residual capacity; the sum of RV and ERV (the volume of air remaining in the lungs at the end-expiratory position). The method of measurement should be indicated, as with RV
TLC	Total lung capacity; the sum of all volume compartments or the volume of air in the lungs after maximal inspiration. The method of measurement should be indicated, as with RV
RV / TLC%	Residual volume to total lung capacity ratio, expressed as a per cent
CV	Closing volume; the volume exhaled after the expired gas concentration is inflected from an alveolar plateau during a controlled breathing maneuver. Since the value obtained is dependent on the specific test technique, the method used must be designated in the text and, when necessary, specified by a qualifying symbol. Closing volume is often expressed as a ratio of the VC, i.e., (CV/VC%)
CC	Closing capacity; closing volume plus residual volume, often expressed as a ratio of TLC, i.e., (CC/TLC%)
VL	Actual volume of the lung, including the volume of the conducting airways
V_A	Alveolar gas volume

Forced Spirometry Measurements*

FVC	Forced vital capacity; vital capacity performed with a maximally forced expiratory effort
FIVC	Forced inspiratory vital capacity; the maximal volume of air inspired with a maximally forced effort from a position of maximal expiration

---

*All values are BTPS unless otherwise specified.

FEVt	Forced expiratory volume (timed). The volume of air exhaled in the specified time during the performance of the forced vital capacity; e.g., FEV_1 for the volume of air exhaled during the first second of the FVC
FEVt / FVC%	Forced expiratory volume (timed) to forced vital capacity ratio, expressed as a percentage
FEF25–75%	Mean forced expiratory flow during the middle of the FVC (formerly called the maximal mid-expiratory flow rate)
PEF	The highest forced expiratory flow measured with a peak flow meter
$\dot{V}maxX$	Forced expiratory flow, related to the total lung capacity or the vital capacity of the lung at which the measurement is made. *Modifiers refer to the amount of lung volume remaining when the measurement is made.* For example: $\dot{V}max75\%$ = Instantaneous forced expiratory flow when the lung is at 75% of its TLC
$\dot{V}max50$	Instantaneous forced expiratory flow when 50% of the vital capacity remains to be exhaled
$\dot{V}maxXp$	Forced expiratory flow at "X" percentage of vital capacity on a partial flow volume curve, initiated from a volume below TLC
MVVx	Maximal voluntary ventilation. The volume of air expired in a specified period during repetitive maximal respiratory effort

Measurements of Ventilation

$\dot{V}_E$	Expired volume per minute (BTPS)
$\dot{V}_I$	Inspired volume per minute (BTPS)
$\dot{V}_{CO_2}$	Carbon dioxide production per minute (STPD)
$\dot{V}_{O_2}$	Oxygen consumption per minute (STPD)
$\dot{V}_A$	Alveolar ventilation per minute (BTPS)
V_D	The physiologic dead space volume defined as V_D/f
$\dot{V}_D$	Ventilation per minute of the physiologic dead space (wasted ventilation), BTPS, defined by the following equation: $$\dot{V}D = \dot{V}E(PaCO_2 - PECO_2)/PaCO_2$$
V_{DAN}	Volume of the anatomic dead space (BTPS)
$\dot{V}_{DAN}$	Ventilation per minute of the anatomic dead space, that portion of conducting airway in which no significant gas exchange occurs (BTPS)

V_DA The alveolar dead space volume defined as V_DA/f

$\dot{V}_DA$ Ventilation of the alveolar dead space (BTPS), defined by the following equation: $V_DA = V_D - V_{DAN}$

MEASUREMENTS OF MECHANICS OF BREATHING*

PRESSURE TERMS

Paw   Pressure in the airway, level to be specified

Pao   Pressure at the airway opening

Ppl   Intrapleural pressure

P_A Alveolar pressure

P_L Transpulmonary pressure

Pbs   Pressure at the body surface

P(A-ao)   Pressure gradient from alveolus to airway opening

Pw   Transthoracic pressure

Ptm   Transmural pressure pertaining to an airway or blood vessel

Pes   Esophageal pressure used to estimate Ppl

Pga   Gastric pressure; used to estimate abdominal pressure

Pdi   Transdiaphragmatic pressure; used to estimate the tension across the diaphragm

Pdi Max   Maximal transdiaphragmatic pressure; used to measure the strength of diaphragmatic muscle contraction

PI Max (also MIP)   Maximal inspiratory pressure; measured at the mouth, used to assess the strength of inspiratory muscles

PE Max (also MEP)   Maximal expiratory pressure; measured at the mouth, used to assess the strength of the expiratory muscles

FLOW-PRESSURE RELATIONSHIPS†

R   A general symbol for resistance, pressure per unit flow

Raw   Airway resistance

Rti   Tissue resistance

R_L Total pulmonary resistance, measured by relating flow-dependent transpulmonary pressure to airflow at the mouth

Rus   Resistance of the airways on the alveolar side (upstream) of the point in the airways where intraluminal pressure equals Ppl, measured under conditions of maximal expiratory flow

Rds   Resistance of the airways on the oral side (downstream) of the point in the airways where intraluminal pressure equals Ppl, measured under conditions of maximal expiratory flow

Gaw   Airway conductance, the reciprocal of Raw

Gaw/V_L Specific conductance, expressed per liter of lung volume at which G is measured (also SGaw)

VOLUME-PRESSURE RELATIONSHIPS

C   A general symbol for compliance, volume change per unit of applied pressure

Cdyn   Dynamic compliance, compliance measured at points of zero gas flow at the mouth during active breathing. The respiratory frequency should be designated; e.g., Cdyn40

Cst   Static compliance, compliance determined from measurements made during conditions of interruption of air flow

C/V_L Specific compliance

E   Elastance, pressure per unit of volume change, the reciprocal of compliance

Pst   Static transpulmonary pressure at a specified lung volume; e.g., PstTLC is static recoil pressure measured at TLC (maximal recoil pressure)

PstTLC/TLC   Coefficient of lung reaction expressed per liter of TLC

W   A general symbol for mechanical work of breathing, which requires use of appropriate qualifying symbols and description of specific conditions

BREATHING PATTERN

T_I Inspiratory time

T_E Expiratory time

T_{Tot} Total respiratory cycle time

T_I/T_{Tot} Ratio of inspiratory to total respiratory cycle time—Duty cycle

V_T Tidal volume

---

*All pressures are expressed relative to ambient pressure and gases are at BTPS unless otherwise specified.
†Unless otherwise specified, the lung volume at which all resistance measurements are made is assumed to be FRC.

V_T/T_I	Mean inspiratory flow
V_T/T_E	Mean expiratory flow
V_E	$\dfrac{V_t \times T_i}{T_i \times T_{Tot}}$

DIFFUSING CAPACITY TESTS AND SYMBOLS

D_x — Diffusing capacity of the lung expressed as volume (STPD) of gas (x) uptake per unit alveolar-capillary pressure difference for the gas used. Unless otherwise stated, carbon monoxide is assumed to be the test gas: i.e., D is D_{CO}. A modifier can be used to designate the technique: e.g., Dsb is single breath carbon monoxide diffusing capacity and Dss is steady state CO diffusing capacity

D_M — Diffusing capacity of the alveolar capillary membrane (STPD)

θx — Reaction rate coefficient for red cells; the volume STPD of gas (x) which will combine per minute with 1 unit volume of blood per unit gas tension. If the specific gas is not stated, θ is assumed to refer to CO and is a function of existing O_2 tension

Q_c — Capillary blood volume (usually expressed as Vc in the literature, a symbol inconsistent with those recommended for blood volumes). When determined from the following equation, Qc represents the effective pulmonary capillary blood volume, i.e., capillary blood volume in intimate association with alveolar gas:

$$\frac{1}{D} = \frac{1}{D_M} + \frac{1}{\theta \cdot Q_c}$$

D/V_A — Diffusion per unit of alveolar volume with D expressed STPD and V_A expressed as liters BTPS. This method is preferred to the occasional practice of expressing both values STPD

BLOOD GAS MEASUREMENTS*

Pa_{CO_2} — Arterial carbon dioxide tension

Sa_{O_2} — Arterial oxygen saturation

$C\acute{c}_{O_2}$ — Oxygen content of pulmonary end-capillary blood

---

*Symbols for these measurements are readily composed by combining the general symbols recommended earlier.

$P(A-a)O_2$ — Alveolar-arterial oxygen pressure difference. The previously used symbol, A-aDO$_2$ is not recommended.

$C(a-\bar{v})O_2$ — Arteriovenous oxygen content difference

PULMONARY SHUNTS

$\dot{Q}sp$ — Physiologic shunt flow (total venous admixture) defined by the following equation when gas and blood gas data are collected during ambient air breathing:

$$\dot{Q}sp = \frac{C\acute{c}_{O_2} - Ca_{O_2}}{C\acute{c}_{O_2} - C\bar{v}_{O_2}} \cdot \dot{Q}$$

$\dot{Q}san$ — A special case of $\dot{Q}sp$ (often called anatomic shunt flow) defined by the above equation when blood and gas data are collected after sufficiently prolonged breathing of 100% O_2 to assure an alveolar N_2 less than 1%

$\dot{Q}s/\dot{Q}t$ — The ratio $\dot{Q}sp$ or $\dot{Q}_{SAN}$ to total cardiac output

BRONCHIAL REACTIVITY

PC_{20} — Provocative concentration of an inhaled agonist producing a 20% decrease in FEV_1

PD_{20} — Provocative dose of an inhaled agonist producing a 20% decrease in FEV_1

$PD_{40}SGaw$ — Provocative dose of an inhaled agonist producing a 40% decrease in SGaw

Isocapnic hyperventilation (eucapnic hyperventilation) = "hyperventilation" with addition of CO_2 to the inspired air to keep end tidal P_{CO_2} constant (Iso) and/or normal (Eu-). Used to assess bronchoconstrictive response to cold and/or dry air

SLEEP STUDIES

Polysomnography — The evaluation during sleep of vital functions and a quantitative evaluation of sleep parameters overnight

NREM — Nonrapid eye movement sleep

REM — Rapid eye movement sleep

Apnea — Cessation of air flow for greater than 10 seconds

Sleep apnea — The presence of 30 or greater apneas in an overnight, 7 hour sleep study. (Apnea frequency >4/hr)

Obstructive apnea — Apnea with respiratory effort

Central apnea — Apnea without respiratory effort

Mixed apnea — Apnea initially without, but later with, respiratory effort

Hypopnea — Reduced respiratory effort with associated decrease in arterial saturation

Apnea index — Number of apneas divided by the total sleep time in hours

Arousal — Short neurologic awakening

PULMONARY DYSFUNCTION

Terms Related to Altered Breathing

Many terms are in use, such as tachypnea, hyperpnea, hypopnea, and so on. Simple descriptive terms, such as rapid, deep, or shallow breathing, should be used instead.

Dyspnea — A subjective sensation of difficult or labored breathing

Overventilation — A general term indicating excessive ventilation. When unqualified, it refers to *alveolar overventilation*, excessive ventilation of the gas-exchanging areas of the lung manifested by a fall in arterial CO_2 tension. The term *total overventilation* may be used when the minute volume is increased regardless of the alveolar ventilation. (When there is increased wasted ventilation, total overventilation may occur when alveolar ventilation is normal or decreased)

Underventilation — A general term indicating reduced ventilation. When otherwise unqualified, it refers to alveolar underventilation, decreased effective alveolar ventilation manifested by an increase in arterial CO_2 tension. (Over- and underventilation are recommended in place of hyper- and hypoventilation to avoid confusion when the words are spoken)

Terms Describing Blood Gas Findings

Hypoxia — A term for reduced oxygenation

Hypoxemia — A reduced blood oxygen content or tension

Hypocarbia — (hypocapnia) A reduced arterial carbon dioxide tension

Hypercarbia — (hypercapnia) An increased arterial carbon dioxide tension

Terms Describing Acid-base Findings

Acidemia — A pH less than normal; the value should always be given

Alkalemia — A pH greater than normal; the value should always be given

Hypobasemia — Blood bicarbonate level below normal

Hyperbasemia — Blood bicarbonate level above normal

Acidosis — A clinical term indicating a disturbance that can lead to acidemia. It usually is indicated by hypobasemia when metabolic (nonrespiratory) in origin and by hypercarbia when respiratory in origin. There may or may not be accompanying acidemia. The term should always be qualified as metabolic (nonrespiratory) or respiratory

Alkalosis — A clinical term indicating a disturbance that can lead to alkalemia. It usually is indicated by hyperbasemia when metabolic (nonrespiratory) in origin and by hypocarbia when respiratory in origin. There may or may not be accompanying alkalemia. The term should always be qualified as metabolic (nonrespiratory) or respiratory

Other Terms

Pulmonary insufficiency — Altered function of the lungs that produces clinical symptoms, usually including dyspnea

Acute respiratory failure — Rapidly occurring hypoxemia or hypercarbia due to a disorder of the respiratory system. The duration of the illness and the values of arterial oxygen tension and arterial carbon dioxide tension used as criteria for this term should be given. The term *acute ventilatory failure* should be used only when the arterial carbon dioxide tension is increased. The term *pulmonary failure* has been used to indicate respiratory failure due specifically to disorders of the lungs

Chronic respiratory failure — Chronic hypoxemia or hypercarbia due to a disorder of the respiratory system. The duration of the condition and the values of arterial oxygen tension and arterial carbon dioxide tension used as criteria for this term should be given

Obstructive pattern — (Obstructive ventilatory defect) Slowing of air flow during forced ventilatory maneuvers

Restrictive pattern — (Restrictive ventilatory defect) Reduction of vital capacity not explainable by airways obstruction

Impairment — A measurable degree of anatomic or functional abnormality which may or may not have clinical significance. *Permanent impairment* is that which persists after maximal medical rehabilitation has been achieved

Disability — A legally determined state in which a patient's ability to engage in a specific activity under a particular circumstance is reduced or absent because of physical or mental impairment. *Permanent disability* exists when no substantial improvement of the patient's ability to engage in the specific activity can be expected

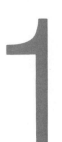

CHAPTER

The Normal Chest

1

THE AIRWAYS AND PULMONARY VENTILATION

ANATOMY OF THE AIRWAYS

The primary function of the bronchial tree is to conduct air to the alveolar surface, where gas transfer takes place between respired air and gas dissolved in the blood of the alveolar capillaries. The greater part of the length and the smaller part of the volume of the respiratory tract are concerned with this function. The trachea and bronchi (the walls of which contain cartilage) and nonalveolated bronchioles (with no cartilage) carry out this function. The remainder of the respiratory tract, comprising the large bulk of the lungs, is concerned with both conduction and gas exchange, the terminal unit (the alveolus) being the only structure whose unique function is gas exchange. Thus, the airway system can be subdivided into three zones, each with somewhat different but overlapping structural and functional characteristics.

The *conductive zone* includes the trachea, bronchi, and nonalveolated bronchioles in which air cannot diffuse through the well-developed wall. These structures, along with the pulmonary arteries and veins, lymphatic channels, nerves, connective tissues of the peribronchial and perivascular spaces, the interlobular septa, and the pleura constitute the nonparenchymatous portion of the lung.

The *transitory zone,* as its name implies, carries out both conductive and respiratory functions. It consists of the respiratory bronchioles, alveolar ducts, and alveolar sacs, all of which conduct air to the most peripheral alveoli. In addition, alveoli that arise from their walls are the sites of gas exchange. This zone and the respiratory zone constitute the parenchyma, the spongy respiratory portion of the lung.

The *respiratory zone* consists of the alveoli, whose primary function is the exchange of gases between air and blood.

Several excellent monographs on gross and microscopic morphology of the lungs are available for detailed study.[1-4]

THE CONDUCTIVE ZONE

Geometry and Dimensions

The basic branching pattern of the conductive zone is dichotomous (i.e., the parent branch divides into two parts). In any such system, the branching may be symmetric (two branches equal in all respects) or asymmetric (variation in the diameter or length of branches in a given generation, or in the number of divisions to the end branches, or a combination of these). In the conductive zone, there is variation in both branch diameter and the number of divisions; thus, the system is one of asymmetric dichotomy.

Branching systems can be analyzed geometrically by several methods. In the earliest investigations of the conductive zone, the trachea was designated the first branch, and subsequent bronchial and bronchiolar divisions were numbered sequentially. However, if one counts distally from the largest to the smallest branch along two pathways of different lengths in an asymmetric dichotomous branching system, at some point one reaches a generation whose number is the same in both airways but whose functional and morphologic characteristics are different: for example, compare a pathway in a lower lobe basal segment supplying parenchyma in the base of the lung with a "lateral pathway" arising from a large segmental branch supplying contiguous parenchyma in the inner third of the lung. For this reason, Horsfield and Cumming[6] suggested that the traditional method of numbering generations of bronchial branches is unsuitable. Instead, they proposed counting generations proximally from branches of an arbitrary but uniform diameter (0.7 mm in their study), a method that reveals a close relationship between the diameter of a branch, the number of distal respiratory bronchioles supplied, and its order number (Fig. 1–1).

Two methods, described by Strahler[7] and by Horsfield and Cumming,[6] employ this method of counting proximally from the smallest branch. In an analysis of the conductive zone, the terminal bronchiole is considered to be of order 1. When two of these join, they form a single branch (order 2); when two of order 2 join, they form an order 3, and so on. (For the sake of clarity, "generation" is applied to divisions counting distally from the trachea and "order" to divisions counting proximally.) Difficulties arise, however, when branches of two orders join, and it is at this point that the systems differ. In the Strahler system (Fig. 1–2), when different orders join the larger number continues unchanged, thereby providing little information about the total number of branching points; by contrast, in the Horsfield-Cumming system (Fig. 1–2) the larger order number increases by 1. Thus,

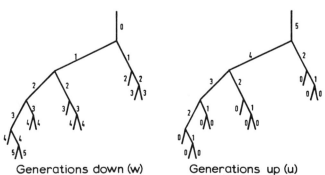

Generations down (w)   Generations up (u)

Figure 1–1. Generations in an Asymmetric Dichotomously Branching System. Two methods of numbering are shown: the branches may be numbered downward starting with the mainstem as 0 (*on the left*), or, alternatively, may be numbered upward starting with the end branches as 0 (*on the right*). (From Horsfield K, Cumming G: J Appl Physiol 24:373, 1968.)

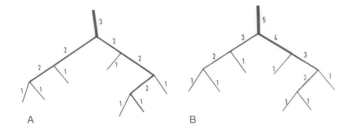

Figure 1–2. Orders Defined by the Methods of Strahler (A) and of Horsfield and Cumming (B). *A,* The most distal branches are order 1; two of these join to form an order 2 branch; subsequently the order increases only if branches of like order meet; e.g., two 4 orders produce an order 5 branch. If two different orders meet, the order of the higher one is continued. *B,* In the Horsfield/Cumming method, the most distal branches are of order 1; two of these meet to form an order 2 branch. When any two branches meet, they form a branch one order more than the higher of the two meeting branches. (From Cumming G, Horsfield K, Harding LK, et al: Bull Physiopathol Resp 7:31, 1971.)

the segment proximal to the junction of the second order and sixth order branch would be the sixth order according to the Strahler system and the seventh order according to the Horsfield-Cumming system.

Several investigators have analyzed the geometry and dimensions of the conductive system by inflating the lungs with plastic, polyester resin, or silicone rubber and taking detailed measurements of the resulting casts.[6–12]. Although the results of these studies have been extensively used in lung modeling, it is important to note that they come from a very small number of lungs fixed at a single lung volume; for example, the data of Horsfield and Cumming[6] and of Weibel[10] were derived from the lungs of only one and five subjects, respectively.

There is almost certainly considerable variability between individuals as well as change in dimensions at different lung volumes.

In their study of resin casts of human lungs inflated and fixed at a volume of 5 liters, Horsfield and Cumming[6] measured the length of each branch between two points of bifurcation and the diameter at midpoint of every structure from an arbitrary diameter of 0.7 mm (Table 1–1). One of the interesting findings was a roughly linear relationship between the order number and the logarithm of the number, diameter, and length of airway branches (Fig. 1–3). Thus, by measuring the slope of the line relating the two, the diameter and length of any order can be predicted by dividing the diameter and length of its parent by 1.4 and 1.49 respectively. Similarly, the number of branches is linearly related to order number (Fig. 1–3), the branching ratio of the conductive zone (average number of daughter branches per parent branch) being 2.8.

Although these "number laws" do not apply precisely at all airway levels (for example, the trachea clearly does not branch 2.8 times), their predictive accuracy over most of the system is quite good. Thus, the branching ratio of 2.8 is followed precisely from orders 6 through 15. Similarly, the diameter law is not applicable throughout the whole airway system. At order number 7 (approximately), diminution in airway diameter ceases and the more distal branches (to order 1) retain the parent's diameter. Cumming and his colleagues postulated functional significance for this change in branching pattern, which occurs at about the point at which conductive flow becomes the lesser and diffusive mixing the major property.

Counting distally from the trachea, Horsfield and Cumming[6] found the number of generations to a 0.7-mm airway to range from 8 to 25—i.e., the lobular branch with the shortest path length was reached after 8 dichotomous branchings and the longest path length after 25. It is likely that local spatial constraints are most important in determining the path length.

Analysis of the frequency distribution of divisions distal to the lobular branches (Fig. 1–4) showed a stepwise increase in division 8 to a peak at 14 and a decrease from 15 to 25. Path lengths distal to branches 0.7 mm in diameter ranged from 7.5 to 21.5 cm; beyond this point, they were very short, ranging from 0.2 to 0.9 cm, thus giving an

Table 1–1. Asymmetric Model of the Airways Derived from Measurements of a Cast

STRUCTURE	GENERATION UP	NO.	DIAMETER (mm)	LENGTH (mm)
Trachea	25	1	16.0	100
	24	1	12.0	40
	23	2	10.3	2
	22	2	8.9	18
	21	2	7.7	14
	20	3	6.6	11
	19	6	5.7	10
	18	8	4.9	10
	17	12	4.2	10
	16	14	3.5	10
	15	20	3.3	9.6
	14	30	3.1	9.1
	13	37	2.9	8.6
	12	46	2.8	8.2
	11	64	2.6	7.8
	10	85	2.4	7.4
	9	114	2.3	7.0
	8	158	2.2	6.7
	7	221	2.0	6.3
	6	341	1.78	5.7
	5	499	1.51	5.0
	4	760	1.29	4.4
	3	1104	1.10	3.9
	2	1675	0.93	3.5
	1	2843	0.79	3.1
Terminal bronchiole	(−2)*	27,992	0.60	
Distal respiratory bronchiole	(−5)*	223,941	0.40	

*Minus values for the terminal bronchiole and distal respiratory bronchiole are included to give an approximate indication of the number of divisions between the structures in a lobule. (Reprinted slightly modified from Horsfield K, Cumming G: J Appl Physiol *24*:373, 1968.)

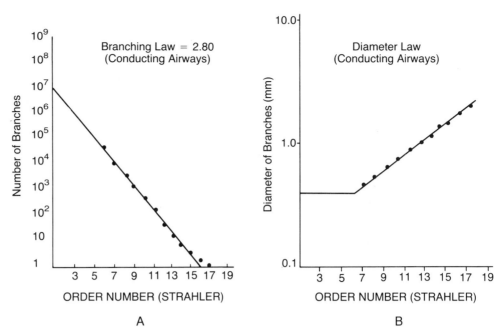

Figure 1–3. Number of Branches (A) and Their Diameter (B) Plotted Against Their Order Number. *B,* Note that orders 1 through 7 undergo no diameter change—diminution in caliber ceases at order 7, chiefly respiratory bronchioles. (From Cumming G, Horsfield K, Harding LK, et al: Bull Physiopathol Resp 7:31, 1971.)

overall range from carina to distal respiratory bronchioles of 7.7 to 22.4 cm. The volume of airways from the carina to 0.7-mm branches was computed to be 71 ml. This volume, added to that of the upper airways from the mouth to the carina (80 ml), gives a total volume of airways almost identical to the volume of anatomic dead space as determined by physiologic techniques.

As a general rule, the angles made by daughter branches with their parent vary with their diameter:[1] when they are of equal size, the angle itself tends to be equal, but when different, the smaller branch usually makes a larger angle with the parent. The branching angle has been found by some observers to be greater in the lower orders.[11]

Morphology

The basic morphology of the trachea, bronchi, and non-alveolated airways is the same and consists of a surface epithelium, composed largely of ciliated and secretory cells, and subepithelial tissue containing supporting connective tissues, inflammatory mediator cells, and glands. The proportion and type of these elements vary at different levels.

EPITHELIUM

The tracheal and proximal bronchial epithelium is composed of high columnar and smaller, somewhat triangular, basal cells. All are attached at their bases to a basement membrane, but since not all reach the luminal surface and since their nuclei are situated at varying levels, the epithelium possesses a pseudostratified appearance (Fig. 1–5). This is gradually lost in the distal bronchi and bronchioles as the epithelium becomes simple and low columnar in appearance. Ciliated and secretory cells, either goblet or Clara in type, constitute the bulk of the epithelium, with basal, intermediate, lymphoreticular, and specialized neuroendocrine cells interspersed in lesser numbers. The morphology and function of these various cell types have been reviewed in detail by Breeze and Wheeldon[13] and by Gail and Lenfant.[5]

The *ciliated cell* is the most prominent cell type in normal epithelium, comprising three to five times the number of goblet cells in the central airways (Fig. 1–6).[14, 15] It is columnar in shape and extends from the luminal surface to the basement membrane to which it is attached by a thin, tapering base. The cells are also attached firmly to one

Figure 1–4. Frequency Distribution of the Number of Divisions Down to the Lobular Branches. (From Horsfield K, Cumming G: J Appl Physiol 24:373, 1968.)

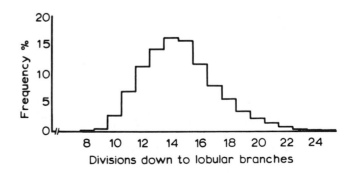

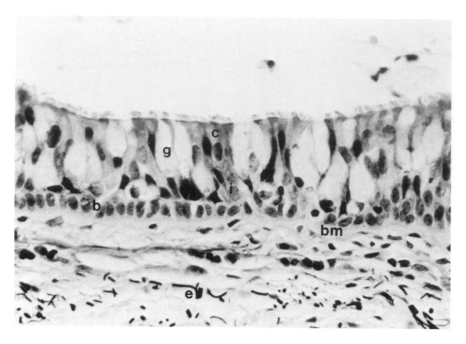

Figure 1–5. Normal Bronchial Epithelium. Ciliated (*c*), goblet (*g*), intermediate (*i*), and basal (*b*) cells are seen. Note also the thin basement membrane (*bm*), scattered elastic fibers (*e*), and inflammatory cells in the lamina propria. (Verhoeff–van Gieson, × 425.)

another at their apical surface by tight junctions, thus forming a physically impermeable barrier to most substances. Despite this, there is evidence in experimental animals that transport of particulates can occur across the epithelium by means of cyto-

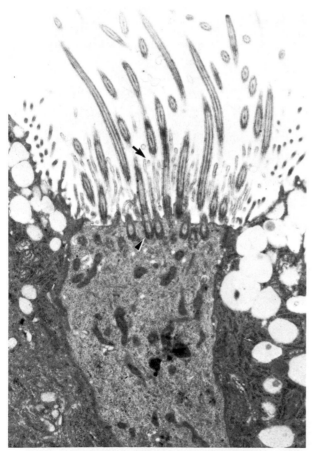

Figure 1–6. Ciliated Cell. Luminal portion showing cilia, surface microvilli (*arrow*) and apical mitochondria, and basal bodies (*arrowhead*). (Human bronchial epithelium, × 12,500.)

plasmic vesicles.[1143, 1144] Although also joined laterally to one another and to other epithelial cells by desmosomes, prominent intercellular spaces containing numerous microvillous projections can also be seen in this location, especially toward the basal aspect of the epithelium.[15, 16] There is evidence that these spaces and microvilli may be important in the transepithelial movement of fluid and electrolytes.[16, 335] Ultrastructurally, a prominent Golgi apparatus is situated above the centrally placed nucleus, a moderate amount of endoplasmic reticulum, and various other cell organelles.[15, 19] Although mitochondria are scattered throughout the cytoplasm, many are concentrated in a layer just under the apical basal bodies, presumably to provide an energy source for ciliary function. Emanating from the surface are approximately 200 to 250 cilia (Fig. 1–7).[5, 13] In the proximal airways, they measure 6 μm in length and 0.25 to 0.3 μm in diameter;[5, 13] distally, they decrease progressively in height so that at the level of the seventh generation bronchi they measure only 3.6 μm in length.[18] In addition to the cilia, numerous, shorter surface microvilli are present; they have been hypothesized to function either in the absorption of secretions emanating from more peripheral airways[19] or in the secretion of a portion of the periciliary mucous layer (*see* page 68).[20]

Each cilium is covered by a prolongation of the cell surface membrane and contains a complex structure called the *axoneme* (Fig. 1–8).[21, 22] This consists of two central microtubules surrounded by nine peripheral doublets, composed in turn of two intimately related microtubules termed A and B subfibers. Two small arms, composed of the protein dynein, project from the A subfiber of one doublet to the B subfiber of the next. Dynein has been shown to be the major source of ATPase activity in the axoneme,[23] and it is believed that the major

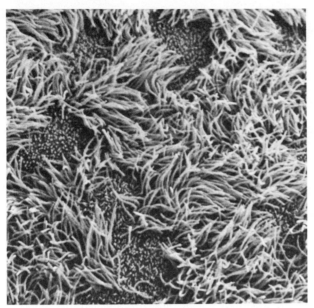

Figure 1–7. Normal Human Bronchial Epithelium. Scanning electron micrograph showing numerous cilia. (Courtesy of Dr. Nai-San Wang, McGill University, Montreal.)

focus of energy conversion into ciliary movement occurs in relation to it. Also attached to each A subfiber is an axillary-arranged radial spoke that joins it to a central sheath that surrounds the inner microtubules. Adjacent peripheral doublets are also joined by shorter nexin links. The apex of the cilium tapers to a fine tip from which small, hooklike structures have been observed to arise.[21, 24] It is thought that these function as anchoring sites within the surface mucous layer to aid in propulsion of

mucus. At the base of the cilium, the A and B subfibers continue into the apical cell cytoplasm and are joined by a third, or C, subfiber to form the *basal body*. Along with the numerous adjacent microtubules and actin filaments, this body serves to anchor the cilium firmly to the cell surface.[21] Occasional rudimentary cilia can be found in hyperplastic and metaplastic bronchial epithelial cells that are normally non-ciliated.[1145]

According to the sliding microtubule hypothesis,[21, 22] ciliary movement occurs by means of the coordinated movement of dynein arms of one doublet along an adjacent doublet, much like going up or down the rungs of a ladder. Since not all doublets move at the same time, this coordinated movement leads to a shortening of some peripheral microtubules relative to those that are either contiguous to or on the opposite side of the cilium. With the internal rigidity that is provided by the radial spokes and the basal anchoring system, the cilium will bend in the direction of shortening. The exact means by which the sliding microtubules are coordinated, both within a single cilium and with those of its neighbors, is not well understood.

Acquired abnormalities of ciliary structure are not uncommon and have been described in a high proportion of smokers[25, 26, 1146] and those with chronic bronchitis,[27] as well as in some apparently normal individuals who manifest neither acute nor chronic respiratory disease.[27-29, 1146] Derangements include compound cilia (showing partial or multiple complete axonemes within a single cell membrane), internalized cilia (projecting into cytoplasmic cavities in the cell apex rather than into the airway), cilia with disorganized axonemes, changes in the

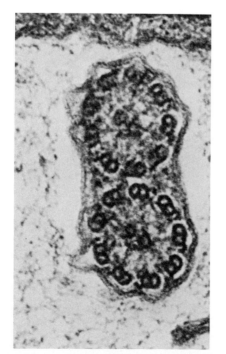

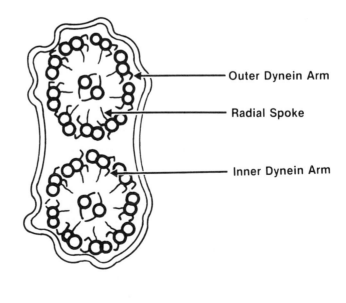

— Outer Dynein Arm

— Radial Spoke

— Inner Dynein Arm

Figure 1–8. Doublet Cilium from Chronic Smoker. Although paired within the same plasma membrane, the individual components of this cilium are normal, showing nine peripheral and two central doublets and the typical arrangement of dynein arms and radial spokes.

ciliary membrane or amount of cytoplasm, transposition of microtubules,[1146] radial spoke defects,[1146] and a variety of minor microtubular abnormalities.[27, 29]

Goblet cells (surface mucous cells) (see Fig. 1–5) comprise a considerable proportion of the epithelial population in the normal individual, representing about 20 to 30 per cent of cells in the more proximal airways[14, 15] and decreasing in number distally so that only occasional cells are present in normal bronchioles.[30, 31] They have been estimated to number 6900 per mm[2] in the normal adult trachea,[32] but in conditions of both acute and chronic airway irritation they may increase substantially in number in the proximal airways and may also appear in bronchioles.[32, 34] Ultrastructurally, the apical portion of the cytoplasm contains numerous membrane-bound, electron-lucent secretory granules; in one detailed study,[35] these were located in discrete clusters, each associated with a single Golgi apparatus. Although there may be considerable variation in cell shape,[34] the basal portion tends to become more attenuated as it approaches the basement membrane; the combination of tapered base and expanded apex provides the typical goblet shape from which the name of the cell is derived.

Histochemical studies have shown strong PAS positivity[36, 37] and somewhat weaker staining with toluidine blue,[36] alcian blue, and aldehyde fuchsin,[37] indicating predominantly neutral and sulfomucin content. However, a variation in both ultrastructural and histochemical features has been demonstrated at different locations in the tracheobronchial tree, and cells with a large proportion of nonsulfated sialomucins have also been identified.[38]

McDowell and colleagues have described a "small mucous granule" cell that is similar to the more typical goblet cell except that it does not show a distended apical cytoplasm and contains only a few small mucous granules.[14] They feel that this may represent a goblet cell at the beginning or end of a secretory cycle.

Basal cells (see Fig. 1–5) are relatively small, flattened, or triangular cells the bases of which are adjacent to the basement membrane and the apices of which normally do not reach the airway lumen. They are more abundant in the proximal airways, where they form a more or less continuous layer at the light microscopic level; they gradually diminish in number distally so as to become very difficult to identify in bronchioles.[24, 39] Most of the cytoplasm is occupied by nuclei whose basal location is largely responsible for the pseudostratified appearance of the proximal bronchial epithelium. Cytoplasmic contents show little evidence of cellular specialization, and it is widely believed that this is a reserve cell from which the epithelium is normally repopulated.[40, 41] Ultrastructural and enzymatic differences between basal cells of the bronchi and bronchioles have been described.[39]

The nuclei of *intermediate cells (see* Fig. 1–5) are located somewhat above the basal cell layer; these cells possess more cytoplasm than do basal cells and show evidence of either ciliogenesis or mucous granule accumulation. As their name implies, they are generally believed to represent an intermediate stage of differentiation between the basal cell and either the goblet or ciliated cell. However, this rather simplistic view of bronchial epithelial differentiation has been questioned: McDowell and her colleagues have postulated that the intermediate cell seen normally by light microscopy in fact represents a small mucous granule cell that is derived from basal cells and is capable of differentiation into mature goblet cells.[14] It has been suggested that a separate cell population, described as "indifferent cells" and also believed to be derived from basal cells, may be capable of developing directly into ciliated cells. There is also evidence that at least some ciliated cells may be derived directly from secretory cells.[42] The factors that determine the direction and rate of cellular differentiation are poorly defined, although inhaled agents such as cigarette smoke and nitrous oxide are known to increase numbers of goblet cells.

The response to epithelial injury is rapid. In one study in which the suprabasal epithelium of rat trachea was mechanically damaged, the basal cellular mitotic activity reached a peak between 26 and 30 hours post-injury, and the epithelium was virtually reconstituted with ultrastructurally mature cells by 90 hours.[40] A similar scanning electron microscopic investigation of acid-damaged mouse trachea showed complete epithelial recovery by 7 days.[43] The normal epithelial turnover rate has been variously estimated to be between 7 and 131 days.[13]

The *Clara* or *nonciliated bronchiolar secretory cell* is found primarily in bronchioles, in which it comprises the majority of the epithelium, along with ciliated cells. Originally described by Kölliker[44] and later by Clara,[44a] the cells showed pronounced interspecies differences in morphology, distribution, and possibly function.[45, 46] In humans, the cell is columnar and bulges into the airway lumen, projecting slightly above the surrounding ciliated cells (Fig. 1–9). Ultrastructurally, it has a deeply indented, centrally placed nucleus, prominent Golgi apparatus, and abundant granular endoplasmic reticulum and mitochondria.[47, 48] In addition, the apical portion contains membrane-bound, electron-dense, round granules, the chemical nature of which has been the subject of much debate. Early investigators[47, 49, 50] found that the granules stained positively with Luxol fast blue and Baker's acid hematin, implying phospholipid and lipoprotein composition, but since lipid solvents do not reduce staining activity, the significance of these findings has been questioned.[13] Despite this, a number of biochemical studies indicate that the normal Clara cell probably does synthesize lipids, although the precise nature and storage site of the lipids is not known.[46] The granules do not stain with alcian blue or mucicarmine,[47, 49] indicating lack of acid mucosubstance, and PAS staining is variable. More recent

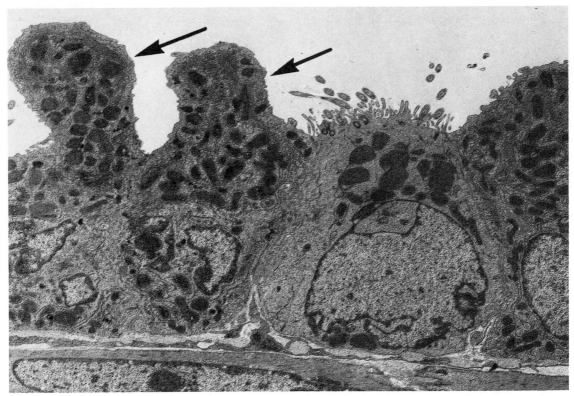

Figure 1–9. Clara Cells. These cells are low columnar in type and possess tongue- or flame-shaped cytoplasmic processes (*arrows*). Nuclei are basal in position and usually notched. Mitochondria are concentrated supranuclearly. A ciliated cell is also present. (Control × 4500.) (From Wang N-S, Huang SN, Sheldon H, et al: Am J Pathol 62:237, 1971.)

studies, summarized by Ebert and his colleagues[51] and by Widdicombe and Pack,[46] favor a prominent protein component. Although the structure of this is also unknown, one immunohistochemical investigation has shown the presence of surfactant-related glycoprotein within Clara cell cytoplasm.[1147]

Whatever the nature of the intragranular material, the morphologic features of Clara cells, their high level of oxidative enzymes,[49] and their response to pilocarpine[52] and catecholamine[46] stimulation are very suggestive of a secretory function, presumably involving the material in the apical granules. The potential mechanisms and factors affecting Clara cell secretion are not well understood and have been summarized by Widdicombe and Pack.[46] The precise function of the secretion is also uncertain. Both scanning[30] and transmission[17, 53] electron microscopic studies have shown a surface film covering the bronchiolar epithelium, and at least part of this may be derived from Clara cell secretion.[19, 53, 54] It has also been suggested that this secretion may enter the alveoli and either form the hypophase of alveolar surfactant[47] or serve as a source of lipase-phospholipase for its catabolism.[55]

Clara cells themselves have other important functions; for example, there is evidence that they act as progenitor cells in the regeneration of damaged bronchiolar[56] and alveolar[57] epithelium. In addition, they have been shown to contain a low-molecular-weight protease inhibitor[58] that may be important in maintaining the integrity of the bron-

chiolar epithelium. Finally, the presence in a number of species of abundant smooth endoplasmic reticulum as well as the cytochrome P-450 monooxygenase system has suggested that the cells might have a detoxification function, although possibly not of significance in human lungs.[45, 46]

Small, intraepithelial clear cells, originally described by Fröhlich[59] and by Feyrter,[60] are widely known as *K cells* because of their similarity to cells described by Kultschitzsky in the gastrointestinal tract (Fig. 1–10). Also known as *neuroendocrine (NE)*, *amine-containing*, or *small granules cells*, they have been the subject of much recent investigation as well as several reviews.[61-63] They are found infrequently in normal lung; although they have been estimated to constitute 1 to 2 per cent of bronchial epithelial cells in neonatal animals,[63] quantitative studies in adult human lungs suggest that their incidence is much smaller.[1148] They have been demonstrated at all levels of the conducting and transitory zone airways and within bronchial glands and their ducts, although they are more frequent in peripheral than in central airways and in younger than in older individuals.[13] They are especially prominent in fetuses and neonates.[13] Morphologically, these cells possess a roughly triangular shape, their base resting on the basement membrane, and their long, tapering apex pointing toward but infrequently reaching the luminal surface. By means of argyrophilic stains and electron microscopy, cytoplasmic processes can be seen emanating from the

10 THE NORMAL CHEST

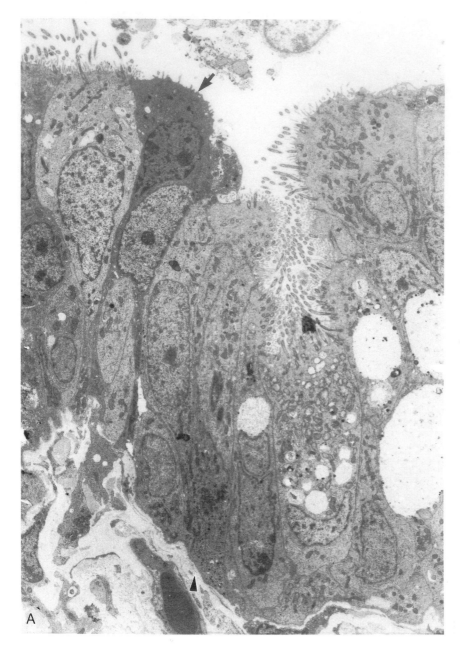

Figure 1–10. Neuroendocrine Cell. *A,* Bronchiolar epithelium showing ciliated, Clara (*arrow*), and basal neuroendocrine (*arrowhead*) cells. (Human bronchiole, × 4000.)
Illustration continued on opposite page

basal aspect and extending laterally between adjacent epithelial cells.[64, 65] The relationship of nerve fibers to cell bodies is controversial; some investigators find extensive innervation and others, little[66] or none.[13] Ultrastructurally,[13, 61, 63] the cytoplasm is electron-lucent and contains a prominent Golgi apparatus, abundant smooth endoplasmic reticulum and free ribosomes, prominent numbers of microtubules and microfilaments (at least some of which have been shown immunochemically to be neurofilaments[1149]), and most characteristically variable numbers of neurosecretory granules. The last-named are membrane-bound, and the majority range in diameter from 60 to 150 nm; they possess a central, electron-dense core surrounded by a thin, lucent halo. Different subtypes of neuroendocrine cells have been proposed, based on ultrastructurally different granules.[67]

Neuroendocrine cells are difficult to recognize at the light microscopic level with routine stains, and a variety of special techniques have been used to identify them.[68] One of the most common is based on their ability to retain silver ions and, with the addition of an appropriate reducing agent, to form metallic silver precipitates that can be seen as small, black, intracellular granules. This property, appropriately termed argyrophilia, is characteristic of pulmonary neuroendocrine or K cells and is the basis of the Grimelius and other silver stains used in their identification. The cells can also be identified by formaldehyde-induced fluorescence[61] and by immunohistochemical staining for a variety of peptides, including bombesin, calcitonin, serotonin, gastrin-releasing peptide, and leu-enkephalin.[63, 69]

Pearse and Takor have proposed that pulmonary neuroendocrine cells form a part of the pe-

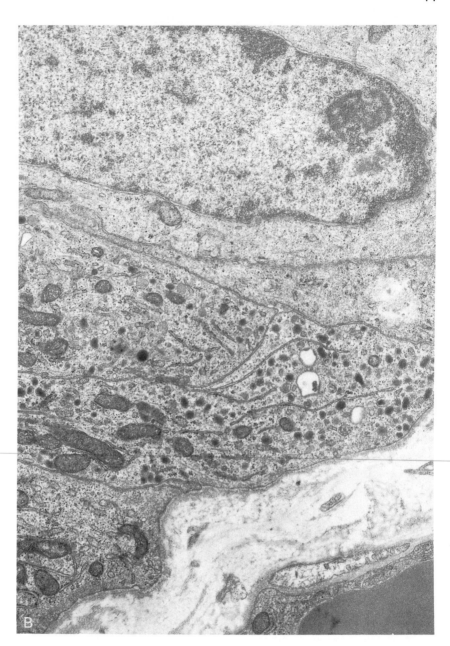

Figure 1–10 *Continued B,* Magnification of base of NE cell showing neurosecretory granules. (× 31,000.)

ripheral component of a diffuse neuroendocrine system also known as the Amine Precursor Uptake and Decarboxylase (APUD) system.[70] This system includes a variety of pancreatic, urogenital, gastrointestinal, and parenchymal endocrine cells, all of which (1) contain, or have the ability to take up from the blood, fluorogenic amines such as catecholamine or 5-hydroxytryptamine; (2) have the ability to extract from the blood amine precursors such as 5-hydroxytryptamine or DOPA; and (3) contain an acid decarboxylase for metabolic alteration of amine precursors. Pulmonary neuroendocrine cells have been shown to fulfill these criteria,[71] as well as others proposed by Pearse,[72] and are now widely believed to be part of the APUD system. It was initially hypothesized that all APUD cells were derived embryologically from a common neural crest ancestor that migrated to its appropriate end organ during fetal life.[72] However, this concept has

not been accepted by all,[63] and there is diverse experimental evidence[73, 74] suggesting that gastrointestinal and probably pulmonary neuroendocrine cells are derived from endoderm itself.

In addition to these biochemical attributes, all APUD cells are morphologically similar and functionally are believed to control other cellular functions by means of a variety of amine-related polypeptide hormones, either locally or at a distance. Although the precise function of pulmonary neuroendocrine cells is unknown, it has been suggested that they function either as neuroreceptors or as endocrine cells that are responsible at least in part for local control of airway or vascular function.[61] Their greater number in fetal lungs and their fairly rapid decrease in number after birth[75, 76] have suggested a role in regulation of the fetal or neonatal circulation. In hypoxic conditions, there is evidence that they may increase in number[75, 78] and may undergo ultrastructural changes similar to those found in carotid body chief cells;[76] as a consequence, it has also been suggested that they may be mediators of the pulmonary vascular hypoxic response.[61] A role in influencing the migration and growth of intraepithelial nerve fibers in both the developing and regenerating epithelium has also been proposed.[66] Apart from their possible functional importance in the normal individual, much attention has been focused on these cells because of a possible association with neuroendocrine-related pulmonary neoplasms such as carcinoid tumor and small cell carcinoma.[69]

A structure perhaps related to the solitary pulmonary neuroendocrine cell and known as the *neuroepithelial body* has been identified in the airways of human infants[79] and adults[82] and of several animal species (Fig. 1–11).[13] These are found throughout the tracheobronchial and bronchiolar epithelium, especially near branch points,[63] and consist of fairly well-demarcated, ovoid or triangular clusters of 4 to 10 large, columnar, non-ciliated cells with clear, strongly argyrophilic cytoplasm. Their apices reach the luminal surface and their bases rest on basement membrane in intimate contact with small nerve fibers[63, 81] and occasionally with fenestrated capillaries.[82] Ultrastructurally, they contain prominent dense-core neurosecretory granules that tend to be concentrated at their bases[81] and that have been shown by several techniques to contain serotonin and other peptides.[83, 84] Although individual cells of the neuroepithelial body resemble solitary neuroendocrine cells, their clustered arrangement and fairly consistent relationship to nerve fibers and possibly capillaries have suggested that the two may have different functions.[13] As with solitary neuroendocrine cells, the precise function of the neuroepithelial body is unknown. Lauweryns and Cokelaere have shown in hypoxic rabbits that the neurosecre-

tory granules are discharged,[84] and these investigators as well as others[61, 63] have suggested that the neuroepithelial body functions as a mediator of pulmonary hypoxic vasoconstriction.[83]

The number of neuroendocrine cells, whether solitary or clustered in neuroepithelial bodies, has been shown experimentally to be increased following fetal and neonatal nicotine exposure,[85] the administration of nitrosamine carcinogens,[86] and bronchial challenge after sensitization with a known antigen.[68] The relevance of these observations to human disease awaits further study.

Lymphoreticular cells may also be found within the epithelium, especially within extrapulmonary airways.[13] Although most of these have the morphologic appearance of mature lymphocytes, Langerhans' cells also occur uncommonly within the bronchiolar epithelium of otherwise normal lung.[87] Mast cells have also been identified within human bronchiolar epithelium,[88] and there is evidence that their number may increase with cigarette smoking.[88]

Submucosa and Lamina Propria

The subepithelial tissue can be subdivided into a lamina propria, situated between the basement membrane and muscularis mucosa, and a submucosa, comprising all the remaining airway tissue. The *lamina propria* is more prominent in the trachea and proximal bronchi than in distal airways; it consists principally of a delicate capillary network, a meshwork of fine reticulin fibers continuous with the basement membrane, and fairly prominent elastic tissue that is oriented primarily in a longitudinal direction. The elastic tissue is especially well developed in the noncartilaginous portions of the trachea and major bronchi where it forms thick, well-defined bundles that are easily visible to the naked eye as longitudinal ridges. These continue into the

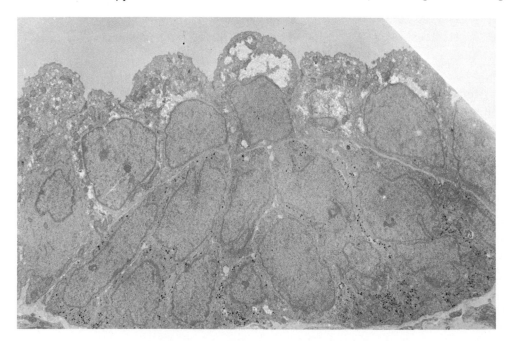

Figure 1–11. Neuroepithelial Body. Bronchiolar epithelium of neonatal rabbit showing well-defined aggregate of cells, each containing numerous neurosecretory granules. (Courtesy of Dr. Nai-San Wang, McGill University, Montreal.)

intrapulmonary airways as far as the distal branches where they can be seen over the whole circumference of the wall.[89] Prominent elastic thickening is also seen at bronchial branch points.

The *submucosa* contains cartilage, muscle, and other supportive connective tissue elements, the major portion of the tracheobronchial glands, and various cells related to airway function and defense mechanisms. The morphology of tracheobronchial cartilage has been reviewed in detail by Vanpeperstraete.[90] The tracheal cartilages consist of a series of 16 to 20 horseshoe-shaped rings oriented in a horizontal plane with their open ends directed posteriorly. Longitudinal sections show the spaces between the rings to contain numerous tracheal glands as well as dense collagenous and elastic tissue continuous with the perichondrium and binding the rings together. These U-shaped structures continue into the extrapulmonary main stem bronchi, but in lobar and segmental bronchi become quite irregular and platelike in shape (Fig. 1–12). At bronchial division points, the plates frequently take the shape of a saddle conforming to the branching angle, thus providing extra support at sites of increased turbulence. As the airway proceeds distally, the cartilages become smaller and less complete until they finally disappear altogether in airways 1 to 2 mm in diameter (bronchioles). The cartilage is hyaline in type and may become calcified; with advancing age,

it often contains foci of bone and bone marrow that may be visible roentgenographically.

The bronchial cartilages are tethered together by dense fibroelastic tissue arranged predominantly in a longitudinal direction. At numerous points, particularly in smaller airways, elastic fibers pass obliquely from these longitudinally arranged bundles to intermingle with the elastic tissue of the lamina propria.[1, 4] These obliquely arranged fibers are believed to help transmit to the more rigid and stronger cartilaginous-fibrous tissue the longitudinal tensions that arise in the surface epithelium and in the parenchyma as a whole during respiration.[1, 4] The development, structure, and function of the entire pulmonary elastic framework have been reviewed by Starcher.[1150]

Tracheal muscle is found predominantly in the membranous portion where it is arranged in transverse bundles that are attached to the inner perichondrium about 1 mm from the tip of the cartilaginous rings, joining each ring posteriorly. Although somewhat less prominent, transverse fibers can also be found between the cartilage rings in the anterior portion.[91] In addition, fairly prominent longitudinally oriented muscle fibers are present in most tracheas dorsal to the membranous transverse muscle layer, predominantly in the lower half.[92] In the intrapulmonary bronchi, the muscle coat lies close to the epithelium just deep to the

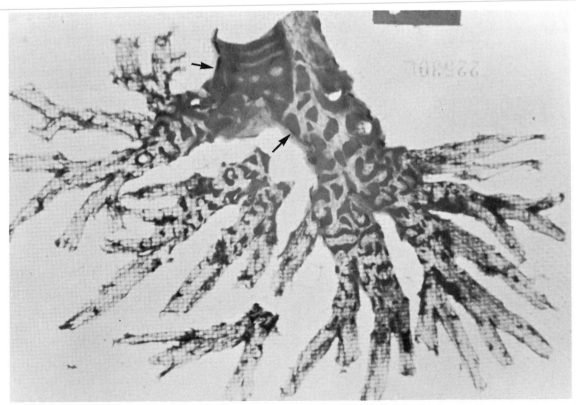

Figure 1–12. Cartilage Distribution in the Bronchial Tree. The bronchial tree of a normal left lung removed at necropsy has been dissected free, laid out on a wire mesh, and stained for cartilage. Note that the cartilages are horseshoe-shaped for a short distance in the main stem bronchus (*upper arrow*), but that in the lower lobe bronchus (*lower arrow*) and peripheral bronchi they form irregularly shaped, interconnecting, and discrete islands.

lamina propria. In the larger airways, the orientation is mainly transverse as in the trachea, but it soon becomes obliquely oriented and arranged in branching and anastomosing bundles that form irregular spirals down the airway. Because of this architecture, airway cross sections do not always show a complete muscle coat, especially in smaller bronchi. The proportion of muscle relative to airway diameter increases as the smaller airways are approached.[93] The ultrastructural, biophysical, and biochemical characteristics of airway smooth muscle have recently been reviewed.[94]

In addition to these more or less well-defined cartilaginous, fibroelastic, and muscular networks, loose connective tissue that is largely collagenous in type occupies the bulk of the remainder of the submucosa. This is continuous with adjacent periarterial connective tissue and with perivenous connective tissue near the hilum and thus, by extension, with interlobular and subpleural interstitial connective tissue. This interdependence of peribronchovascular connective tissue is important in maintaining the overall structure of the lung and in providing a scaffold for the more delicate connective tissue of the parenchyma. At all levels of the bronchial tree, adipose tissue, usually small in amount, can be found adjacent to cartilage plates and occasionally in association with mucous glands.[95]

Tracheobronchial glands (Fig. 1–13) are specialized extensions of the surface epithelium into the lamina propria and submucosa and are seen exclusively in the trachea and bronchi, roughly paralleling the distribution of cartilage. Both the number and size of the glands are greater in the more proximal airways; according to one study of three normal individuals, total gland volume per unit of airway surface area was greatest between the mid-trachea and main stem bronchi and decreased rapidly thereafter to relatively low levels in the subsegmental bronchi.[96] It has been calculated that the number of glands in the trachea ranges from 3500 to 6000[97, 98] (about 0.7 to 1.0 gland per mm^2).[1, 98] In the cartilaginous portion, they are located mainly in horizontal layers in the submucosa between cartilaginous rings, whereas in the membranous portion they lie both superficial and deep to transverse muscle layers and in a more craniocaudal orientation.[98] In the bronchi, the glands are more irregularly distributed and can be situated either between surface epithelium and cartilage or extending between cartilaginous plates into peribronchial interstitial tissue.

The secretory portion of the gland is connected with the surface by a duct of variable length whose lining contains both ciliated cells and goblet cells similar to surface airway epithelium. Meyrick and colleagues have proposed that, in addition to the main duct, a specialized "collecting duct" is interposed between the ciliated epithelium and the secretory portions of the gland.[99] They found this to be composed of tall, columnar, eosinophilic cells that ultrastructurally contain numerous mitochondria and a well-developed Golgi apparatus.[100] They interpreted these cells as being similar to the large mitochondria-laden, eosinophilic cells called "oncocytes" that are found frequently in other secretory organs and suggested that these cells may regulate water and ion concentration of the final gland secretion.[99] However, in our experience as well as that of others,[101] typical oncocytes can be found in other obviously secretory portions of the gland (Fig. 1–14) and in many cases are not interposed between ciliated and secretory portions. The number of oncocytes has been found to increase with age,[101] which suggests that they may simply represent a degenerative phenomenon similar to that seen in other secretory organs.

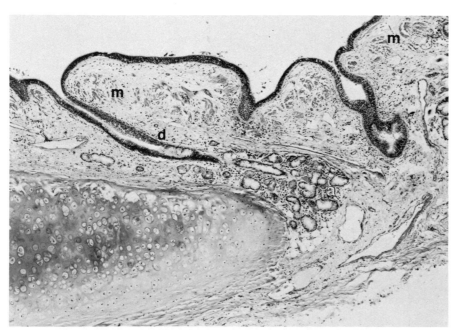

Figure 1–13. Normal Bronchial Wall. Section of lobar bronchus showing portion of cartilage plate, muscularis mucosa (*m*), bronchial gland ducts (*d*), and acini (*a*). (× 40.)

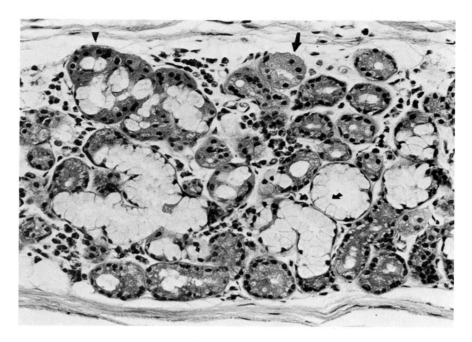

Figure 1–14. Bronchial gland. Note mucous (*small arrow*), serous (*arrowhead*), and oncocytic (*large arrow*) cells. Note also interstitial plasma cells. (× 240.)

Multiple, usually branched, secretory tubules arise from the ciliated duct and are lined at first by plump mucous cells and eventually near their termination by basophilic, frequently somewhat flattened, serous cells (Fig. 1–14). The ratio of serous to mucous cells is about 0.5 and is roughly the same from the trachea to medium-sized bronchi.[102] Fairly numerous myoepithelial cells are present between the basement membrane and epithelial cells, extending from the serous portions of the secretory tubules to the collecting duct;[100] these are presumably responsible in part for expulsion of glandular secretion. Solitary, unmyelinated axons are frequently seen beneath the basement membrane, interdigitating between glandular cells;[100] occasional neuroendocrine cells may also be found.

Histochemical and autoradiographic studies have shown two types of both sulfated mucin and sialomucin within the mucus-secreting portions.[103] All four varieties are present in older children and adults, but only sulfomucin can be identified in the fetus and in children up to the age of 4 years.[104] There is a tendency for the proportion of acid mucosubstance to total glandular tissue to increase from trachea to more distal airways and to be relatively greater in non-smokers at all airway levels.[102] Electron microscopic studies show morphologically different secretory granules, consistent with the variety of mucosubstances demonstrated histochemically.[1151]

The precise nature of the secretion of serous cells is not known. Histochemically, the secretion contains mucosubstances that are predominantly neutral rather than acidic.[38] However, the electron and light microscopic appearance of serous cells as well as their content of carbonic anhydrase[38] suggests that their principal secretion is a low-viscosity substance, possibly meant to flush out the secretion of the more distal mucous cells.[38] As in mucous

cells, cytoplasmic granules of serous cells show a variable morphology, implying that different types of cell may exist. Serous cells have also been shown to be a source of lysozyme,[106] lactoferrin,[107] and a low-molecular-weight protease inhibitor,[106]—substances that may be of importance in local antibacterial defense. There is also evidence that they may function both in the manufacture of secretory component and in its coupling with and ultimate secretion of dimeric IgA.[105]

Mucous glands can increase in size in conditions such as chronic bronchitis and asthma.[108, 109] Although the pathogenesis of this increase is unknown, it appears to be a true hyperplasia rather than simple hypertrophy of glandular cells.[110] It is not known why mucous secretion is divided between mucous glands and goblet cells, but since the volume of glands is estimated to be roughly 40 times that of total goblet cell mass,[108] mucous gland secretion is regarded as the more significant. The control of the tracheobronchial glands and the composition and function of their secretion are discussed in the section on mucous rheology (*see* page 65).

Many cells concerned with airway defense and other functions are found scattered in the airway lamina propria and submucosa. *Lymphocytes* are present in both subepithelial tissue and in the epithelium itself, either singly or in clusters, the latter being variously termed lymphoid nodules, lymphoid aggregates,[111] or bronchus-associated lymphoid tissue.[112] These clusters are not present at birth but appear during the neonatal period and progressively increase in number so as to be found in almost all lungs by the age of 5 years.[113] *Lymphoid nodules* (Fig. 1–15) are found most prominently at branch points of proximal bronchi and may extend from the lamina propria to the peribronchial connective tissue. Histologically, they are composed of well-defined but unencapsulated clusters of lympho-

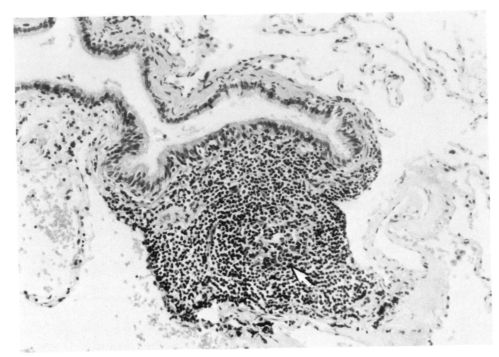

Figure 1–15. Peribronchiolar Lymphoid Tissue. A poorly defined nodule containing a mixture of mature and apparently stimulated lymphoid cells as well as scattered macrophages is present adjacent to and partly within bronchiolar epithelium.

cytes of small-to-medium size and of occasional larger histiocyte-like cells. Ultrastructural studies by Chamberlain and associates have shown them to have features similar to those of normal lymph node tissue.[114] Germinal centers are not present and cells with plasmacytoid differentiation are infrequent.[112] The overlying epithelium is often flattened and lacking in mucous or ciliary differentiation, and the basement membrane is frequently discontinuous.[112] Similar but somewhat less well-defined lymphocyte clusters in the peripheral bronchioles have been termed *lymphoid aggregates.*[111] Identical aggregates are found in relation to pulmonary arteries and in perivenous and subpleural interstitial tissue. It is not known whether these simply represent less organized lymphoid tissue that is functionally the same as lymphoid nodules. The precise function of peribronchial lymphoid tissue is not known. It has been hypothesized that it acts as a filter and repository for dust particles deposited in the periphery of the lung;[115] in one study, however, failure to find carbon particles in the lymphoid aggregates suggested that this is unlikely to be an important function.[113] Bienenstock and his associatess have recommended the descriptive term *bronchus-associated lymphoid tissue* (BALT) and have suggested that this is a component of a common epithelial mucosal IgA system that includes the gut, cervix, breast, and lung and is possibly involved in antigen processing and local IgA production.[116]

Plasma cells, primarily IgA in type, are commonly found in the tracheobronchial tree, particularly in relation to mucous glands, and in the lamina propria close to the basement membrane.[117] They are found in greatest density in major bronchi, being variably present in small bronchi and bronchioles.[117] *Macrophages* are found scattered singly throughout the lamina propria and submucosa and are especially prominent in heavy smokers and in individuals with occupational dust exposure. In the latter situation, they can be so numerous and can contain so much anthracotic pigment as to impart a gray or black appearance to the epithelium that can be seen by the naked eye. *Mast cells* are present throughout the lamina propria and submucosa,[118] and in both dog[119] and monkey[120] lung have been found to increase in number in distal airways.

THE TRANSITORY ZONE

Geometry and Dimensions

Detailed three-dimensional studies of peripheral pulmonary tissue have shown that the geometry of the airways at this level is much more complex than is usually appreciated by examining two-dimensional histologic sections.[6, 121-125] Although branching can occur in a more or less symmetric dichotomous fashion, trichotomous and even quadrivial (sometimes asymmetric) divisions of the respiratory bronchioles are frequently noted. Number, overall configuration, length, and diameter of airway generations from terminal bronchiole to alveolar sac are quite variable, both within the same acinus and between acini described by different investigators. The variability may be caused in part by different techniques of examination (discussed by Schreider and Raabe[123]) and by the rather limited number of acini investigated. However, some of the irregularity appears to be real and may be related to spatial constraints imposed by pleura, intralobular septa, and larger airways and vessels.

The number of airway generations from the

terminal bronchiole to the alveolar sac may be as many as 12, although 6 to 8 is probably representative of most pathways. The length and diameter of respiratory bronchioles and alveolar ducts have been found by some investigators to decrease progressively with generation number;[123] however, others have found the diameter to remain relatively constant despite a diminution in length.[6, 121, 124] Cumming and his associates[8] have suggested that, if true, this feature may relate to the physiologic function in this area: "Since the lungs have gas exchange as their function, the distribution of gas by the branching system consumes space without subserving gas exchange. Therefore the volume of the airways must be minimized, compatible with their requirement not to dissipate too much viscous work. These criteria are best satisfied by a branching system of the type described. When convective flow becomes less important and diffusive mixing more important, it is necessary to maximize the surface area of cross section in the airways, and this is done by preserving the same diameter while branching goes on as before."

The number of alveoli per respiratory bronchiole, alveolar duct, and alveolar sac also exhibits much variation. For example, the number of alveoli per alveolar sac has been calculated to be from 3.5[124] to 29,[1] with most studies documenting about 10.[6, 123, 125] The number of alveoli per alveolar duct has been estimated to be from 11[123] to 40;[126] the figures most closely representing the norm probably are 15 to 20. As in the other features of the transitional airways, this variation in number is likely caused by a combination of different techniques of examination and real differences due to local spatial constraints.

Morphology

As previously stated, the respiratory bronchioles, alveolar ducts, and alveolar sacs constitute the transitory zone and carry out the dual function of conduction and gas exchange. Respiratory bronchioles have a low columnar-to-cuboidal epithelium (comprised mostly of ciliated and Clara cells) that gradually decreases in extent as the number of alveoli increases. In the first- and second-order bronchioles, the epithelium is usually complete on one side, overlying a lamina propria and submucosa continuous with that of the terminal bronchiole and containing a prominent pulmonary artery branch. As the number of alveoli increases, the submucosa disappears, but the muscle and elastic tissue continue in fairly prominent bundles in a spiral fashion surrounding alveolar mouths. As the alveolar duct is reached, bronchiolar epithelium is lost altogether and only scanty alveolar interstitial tissue is present in the wall. Alveolar ducts terminate in a series of rounded enclosures called alveolar sacs, from each of which arise multiple alveoli. The contribution of transitory zone airways to gas exchange is substantial; Pump found from 36.5 to 41.6 per cent of all alveoli in three acini to be located along respiratory bronchioles and alveolar ducts.[121]

THE RESPIRATORY ZONE

Geometry

Weibel has greatly increased our knowledge of the geometry of the alveoli and their relationship to alveolar ducts,[10] and much of the following information is from his monograph on morphometry of the lung and reports of his earlier work with Gomez.[127]

Alveoli are small lateral outpouchings of respiratory bronchioles, alveolar ducts, and alveolar sacs (Fig. 16). Malpighi, in 1697, likened the shape of the alveolus to the cell of a honeycomb (Fig. 1–17), a similarity that has been emphasized more recently.[128] Weibel asserts that the honeycomb can serve as an acceptable alveolar model if one imagines it molded around the cylindric surface of the alveolar duct, thereby transforming the hexagonal prism of the cell into a pyramidal wedge of the air sleeve surrounding the duct (Fig. 1–18). The dome of a honeycomb cell consists of three equilateral rhombi, meeting at the characteristic Maraldi angle of 109° 27',[129] formed by two layers of cells in which the vertices of the cells of one side coincide with the junction of three lateral facets of the other side. The dome of an alveolus has a more complex structure, usually consisting of more than three facets, formed by close packing of several alveoli belonging to adjacent alveolar ducts; therefore, each alveolus may have more than one vertex. The size and shape of the facets vary considerably, the arrangement more nearly resembling that of closely packed bubbles of soap foam (irregular polyhedral configuration). In general, three facets have a common line of junction at an average angle of 120°, and it can be assumed that these facets are more or less flat if there is no pressure difference between contiguous alveoli. Although this idealized model is useful conceptually, it is important to note that some studies have shown considerable variation in both alveolar size and shape.[1153]

Dimensions

Until very recently it was generally accepted that the number of alveoli in the human lung remained fairly constant at about 300×10^6.[9, 10, 130, 131] In their study of the lungs of five patients ranging in age from 8 to 74 years, using a direct counting method, Weibel and Gomez[127] computed totals ranging from 286×10^6 to 310×10^6; the group mean was 296×10^6, with a 95 per cent confidence interval of about $\pm 13 \times 10^6$. More recently, however, in a study of 42 lungs free from chronic disease from 32 subjects aged 19 to 85 years, Angus and Thurlbeck[132] recorded much greater variation in the number of alveoli; their computed totals

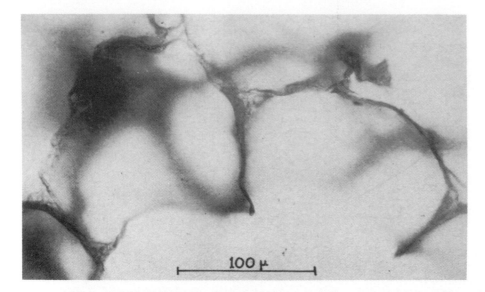

Figure 1–16. Thick Section of Human Lung Showing Two Alveoli That Open on an Alveolar Duct. Note the cuplike shape of the alveoli (× 330). (From Weibel ER, Gomez DM: Science 137:577, 1962. Copyright 1962 by the American Association for the Advancement of Science.)

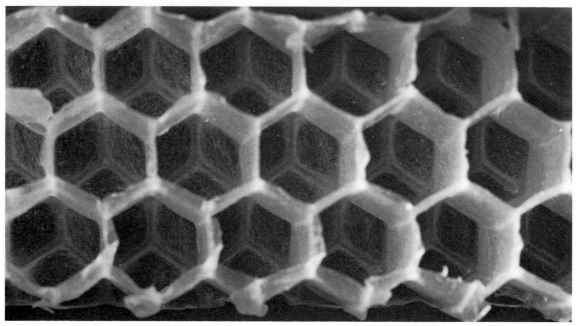

Figure 1–17. Photograph of the Cells of a Honeycomb. Cells have a hexagonal cross section. The three crests of the domes correspond to the lateral walls of the cells of the opposite layer. (From Weibel ER: Morphometry of the Human Lung. New York, Academic Press, 1963.)

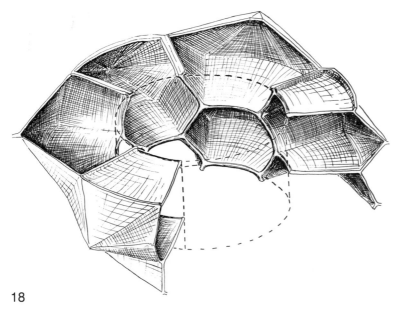

Figure 1–18. Schematic Model of the Arrangement of Alveoli Around an Alveolar Duct. Compare with photomicrograph in Figure 1–16 and with the honeycomb illustrated in Figure 1–17. (From Weibel ER: Morphometry of the Human Lung. New York, Academic Press, 1963.)

ranged from 212×10^6 to 605×10^6 (mean, 375×10^6). Further, they found a highly significant relationship ($P < 0.001$) between alveolar number and body length. Since it is generally believed that new alveoli are added after birth but that this multiplication ceases before somatic growth stops[130] (*i.e.*, alveolar number is determined before body length), it must be inferred that alveolar number is not governed solely by body length and lung volume. Angus and Thurlbeck[132] speculated that this might be genetically controlled and at least partly predetermined by future body height.

Alveolar *dimensions* were obtained by Weibel[10] by direct measurement with an eyepiece micrometer from thin histologic sections. In adults, both maximal diameter and total depth (measured from the opening onto the alveolar duct or sac) averaged 250 to 300 μ.

Total alveolar *surface area* was determined by Weibel[10] by three methods: the geometric method (honeycomb model), and by determining the mean cord length and the linear dimensions. These three independent methods provided estimates in close agreement in the five adult lungs studied: the area measured approximately 70 to 80 m², which Weibel considered consistent with an alveolar number of 300×10^6. In a study of nonemphysematous lungs, Thurlbeck estimated the total alveolar surface area to range from 40 to 100 m², depending upon body size.[133] In a more recent electron microscopic investigation, the total area was found to be 143 m²; however, when corrected for the smoothing effect of alveolar surface lining, the "true" surface area was estimated to be between 70 and 100 m².[123]

Morphology

Alveoli are demarcated by septa, or walls, that are lined by a markedly flattened, continuous layer of epithelial cells covering a thin interstitium. In humans, the epithelium consists primarily of two morphologically distinct cells, type I and type II, with occasional interspersed neuroendocrine cells.[13] A fourth cell, the brush cell, has been found in some animal species,[134, 135] but its presence in humans and its significance are uncertain and it will not be discussed further. The interstitium itself contains a variety of cell types as well as the connective tissue scaffold responsible in part for determining alveolar shape and patency. Finally, although not usually considered a part of the alveolar wall, the alveolar macrophage is in fact normally present on the alveolar epithelial surface and may be partly derived from septal interstitial cells;[134, 184, 1154] it is thus convenient to describe its morphology and function here.

TYPE I ALVEOLAR EPITHELIAL CELL

The type I alveolar cell (*synonyms:* small alveolar cell, squamous lining cell, membranous pneumo-

cyte, type A epithelial cell) (Figs. 1–19 and 1–20), although comprising only 8 per cent of all parenchymal lung cells and inconspicuous by light microscopy, covers approximately 95 per cent of the alveolar surface area and has a total volume twice that of the histologically more obvious type II cell.[137] Its nucleus is small, somewhat flattened, and covered by a thin rim of cytoplasm containing few organelles. The rest of the cytoplasm forms several broad sheets or plates that measure only 0.3 to 0.4 μm in thickness and that extend in all directions for 50 μm or more over the alveolar surface, covering approximately 5000 μm².[137] Sheets of adjacent type I cells interdigitate, and individual plates may reach into neighboring alveoli, either by winding around the septal tip or by extending through alveolar pores.[138] The plates are joined firmly to one another and to type II cells by occluding or tight junctions composed of 3 to 7 continuous, intermembranous fibrillar strands (Fig. 1–21; *see also* Fig. 1–67, page 76).[139] It is thought that these represent a more or less complete barrier to the diffusion of water-soluble substances into the alveolar lumen.[139, 140] Localized gap junctions have also been identified between adjacent type I cells and between type I and type II cells, usually in association with an occluding junction,[137, 139, 141] and it has been suggested that these may act as sites for intercellular communication, as in other epithelia.

The cytoplasm of the type I cell contains few organelles but fairly numerous pinocytotic vesicles. These have been hypothesized to transport fluid or proteins in either direction across the air-blood barrier and have been thought to be a means of resorbing neonatal or pathologic alveolar fluid;[142] they may also contribute to the intra-alveolar exudate in some cases of interstitial pneumonitis[143] and may form a part of the hypophase of alveolar surfactant.[140] Type I cells have also been shown to have the ability to take up intra-alveolar particulate material,[144, 145] possibly in association with actin-containing microfilaments.[146] Although the quantitative significance of these mechanisms in relation to total lung particle clearance or fluid flow is not known, it is probably small in comparison with alveolar macrophages and the mucociliary apparatus. It is possible, however, that the transport of materials into the alveolar interstitium by this route may be the mechanism by which particles are deposited in regional lymph nodes[1155] and may be important in the pathogenesis of some interstitial lung diseases.[146]

TYPE II ALVEOLAR EPITHELIAL CELL

The type II epithelial cell (*synonyms:* granular pneumocyte, great or large alveolar cell, type B alveolar epithelial cell) (Fig. 1–22) is roughly cuboidal in shape and frequently protrudes somewhat into the alveolar lumen, making it identifiable by light microscopy. It is usually isolated between type

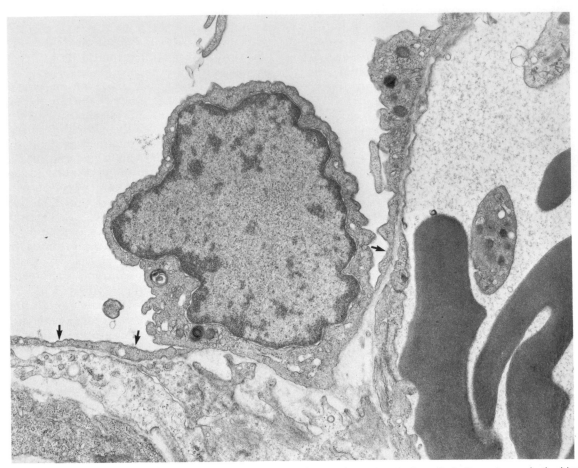

Figure 1–19. Type I Alveolar Epithelial Cell. Note the large nucleus and scanty cytoplasm that attenuates on both sides over the alveolar surface (*arrows*). (Courtesy of Dr. Nai-San Wang, McGill University, Montreal.)

I cells but may occur in groups of two or three, especially when the alveolus is adjacent to larger bronchovascular bundles or pleural connective tissue.[147] It is often located near corners where adjacent alveoli meet.[147] Ultrastructurally,[148] it maintains the roughly cuboidal shape seen on light microscopy, lacking the lateral extensions of the type I cell. The cytoplasm is rich in organelles, including a well-developed endoplasmic reticulum with many ribosomes, prominent Golgi complex, mitochondria, and numerous membrane-bound, osmiophilic granules.[135, 147] The last-named range in size from 0.2 to 1.0 μm and contain characteristic stacked, lamellar inclusions that are somewhat irregular in shape when seen on transmission electron microscopy but are highly uniform when viewed on freeze-etched specimens, with a spacing of about 5 nm.[135] There is some evidence that the number and density volume of such granules may decrease with age.[1156]

There is abundant evidence from ultrastructural, biochemical, autoradiographic, tissue culture, and immunologic studies that type II cells and specifically their osmiophilic granules are the source of alveolar surfactant.[148] The granules appear to function primarily as a storage depot, although it has been suggested that synthesis of some surfactant components may also occur within them.[149] Release of granule contents into the alveolar lumen has been shown to be by exocytosis (Fig. 1–23),[147, 150] but the possibility of an additional holocrine type of secretion involving disintegration of the cell similar to that seen in epidermal sebaceous glands has also been proposed.[151] The factors involved in the synthesis of surfactant and the control of its release are discussed further on (*see* page 58).

A second major function of the type II cell is its ability to repopulate both normal and damaged alveolar epithelium. The type I cell is thought to be incapable of replication, but, by contrast, in normal conditions about 1 per cent of the type II cell population is mitotically active and repopulates the surface.[152] In addition, the relative cytoplasmic simplicity and large surface area of type I cells makes them susceptible to damage from a wide variety of stimuli. In such circumstances, type II cells proliferate and temporarily repopulate the alveolar walls, providing epithelial integrity. With time, they transform into type I cells[153] and completely restore normal alveolar structure provided significant interstitial fibrosis has not occurred. This sequence has been demonstrated in tissue that has been damaged by a wide variety of noxious agents, including oxygen,[154] bleomycin,[155] nitrous oxide,[153] and various chemicals.[156, 157]

The surface of the type II cell is covered by numerous short microvilli. Experimental studies of type II cell tissue cultures,[158] the presence of surface anionic binding sites,[159] and the presence of microvilli all suggest that these cells may also function in the resorption of fluid or other substances from the alveolar airspace.

INTERALVEOLAR INTERSTITIUM

A more or less continuous basement membrane, antigenically similar to renal glomerular basement membrane,[160] underlies both type I and type II cells. Over about 50 per cent of its area, it is intimately apposed to the underlying endothelial basement membrane; interstitial connective tissue and cells and endothelial and epithelial cell nuclei tend to be absent from this region of apposition, so that the thickness of the air-blood barrier in this area is determined only by the thin type I cell sheet, endothelial cell wall, and fused basement membranes, the whole measuring only about 0.5 μm in thickness (Fig. 1–24). Elsewhere, endothelial and epithelial basement membranes are separated by an interstitial space of variable but much greater width. The interstitium is thus separated into two distinct anatomic compartments,[161, 162] one relatively thin, across which the major portion of gas transfer is presumed to take place, and the other thicker, functioning as both mechanical support for the alveolus and as a compartment for water transfer and a lodging place for various cells that regulate alveolar function (see below). Thus, any one alveolus consists of a multitude of alternating thin and thick sides, creating an undulating contour to the alveolar surface. This concept of alveolar wall structure is of considerable importance in pulmonary edema and is discussed in greater detail in that chapter.

In addition to the separated basement membranes, the thick portion of the interstitium contains connective tissue and several cell types. The former consists of a proteoglycan matrix in which are embedded tiny elastic fibers and small bundles of collagen that are intimately intertwined with and provide support for the capillary network. These fibers are also continuous with the fibroelastic tissue

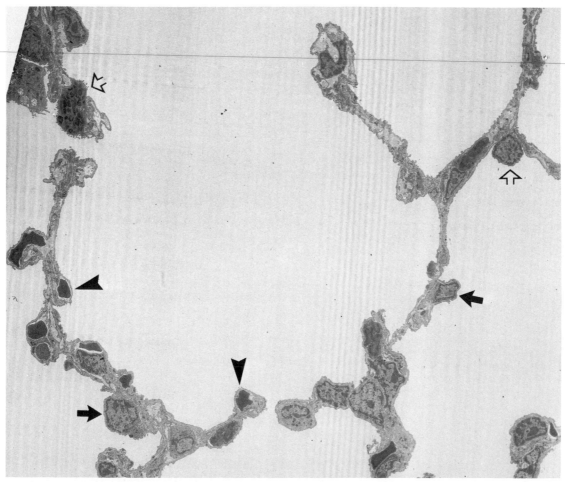

Figure 1–20. Single Pulmonary Alveolus. Visualized are type I (*solid arrows*) and type II (*open arrows*) cells, as well as alveolar capillaries (*arrowheads*). A pore of Kohn can be seen near the bottom of the figure. (Mouse lung, × 2300.) (From Wang N-S, Huang SN, Sheldon H, et al: Am J Pathol 62:237, 1971.)

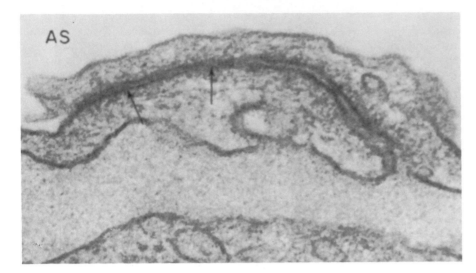

Figure 1–21. Epithelial Intercellular Cleft. The cleft extends roughly horizontally inward from the alveolar space (AS). In several areas (*arrows*) the outer leaflets of the bounding unit membranes appear fused. This fusion usually occurs toward the alveolar end of the cleft. (Uninjected mouse lung, TEM, × 140,000.) (From Schneeberger-Keeley EE, Karnovsky MJ: J Cell Biol 37:781, 1968.)

Figure 1–22. Type II Pneumocyte. Note the short surface microvilli, junctions with type I cells (*arrows*) and lamellated inclusion bodies. (Mouse lung, × 20,000.) (Courtesy of Dr. Nai-San Wang, McGill University, Montreal.)

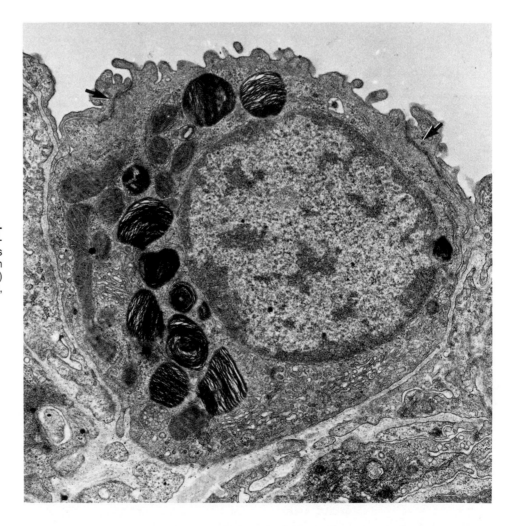

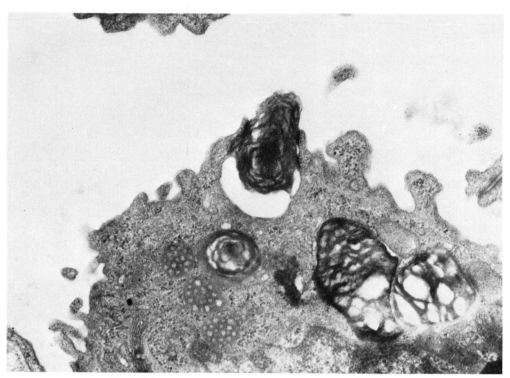

Figure 1–23. Type II Alveolar Epithelial Cell Releasing Osmiophilic Material into an Alveolar Space. (TEM, × 2800.) (Courtesy of Dr. Nai-San Wang, McGill University, Montreal.)

of the pleura, airways, and interlobular vessels, thus forming a complex, three-dimensional connective tissue framework traversing and interconnecting the whole of the pulmonary parenchyma.[161] Immunofluorescent analyses of collagen within the alveolar interstitium have shown the presence of both types I and III in an irregular pattern, the latter being somewhat more prominent.[163, 164] Types IV and V are also seen but in a linear distribution corresponding to their presence in alveolar and endothelial basement membranes.[163, 164] Fibronectin is also present in relation to both alveolar and capillary basement membranes and to interstitial collagen fibers themselves.[165] Although continuous over most of the alveolar wall, interstitial connective tissue is focally absent (Fig. 1–25; *see* also Figure 1–20, page 21). Many of these areas correspond to alveolar pores or fenestrae; some, however, show only a loss of connective tissue, the potential space being covered by normal-appearing type I cell processes.[166] The origin and significance of these discontinuities are unclear and are discussed in greater detail further on.

In addition to collagen-producing fibroblasts, the alveolar interstitium contains a variety of other cell types. One, termed the *contractile interstitial cell* by Kapanci and his colleagues,[167] can be seen ultrastructurally to contain a well-developed Golgi complex and abundant endoplasmic reticulum and free ribosomes suggestive of fibroblastic differentiation; in addition, there are prominent bundles of microfilaments resembling those found in smooth muscle.

Immunofluorescent studies have revealed the presence of actin within the cytoplasm, and pharmacologic investigations have shown hypoxia- and epinephrine-mediated contraction of strips of lung parenchyma, providing evidence for a contractile function.[167] These cells are present around pre- and post-capillary vessels and within the thick portion of the alveolar wall where they appear to cross the interstitial space and attach to the basement membrane of epithelial and endothelial cells by hemidesmosome-like structures.[161, 167] It has been suggested that their contraction may result in a reduction in capillary blood flow and that this may be the mechanism by which hypoxia causes decreased alveolar perfusion—thus, a possible means for local alveolar $\dot{V}A/\dot{Q}$ autoregulation.[167] It has also been proposed that these cells may function as compliance regulators of the interstitial space and that they may act to increase resistance to interstitial expansion by edema fluid,[161] thus propelling such fluid from the alveolar interstitium toward peribronchovascular lymphatics where it may be effectively removed.

Mast cells have been noted within both the interstitium and occasionally the alveolar epithelial lining and lumen.[168, 169] Although in some investigations they have been seen only sparsely in normal human lung,[169] one electron microscopic study[168] documented an average of 350 cells per mm^2 of alveolar wall, suggesting to the investigators that these cells may function in the local control of the pulmonary vasculature.[168] A reversible increase in

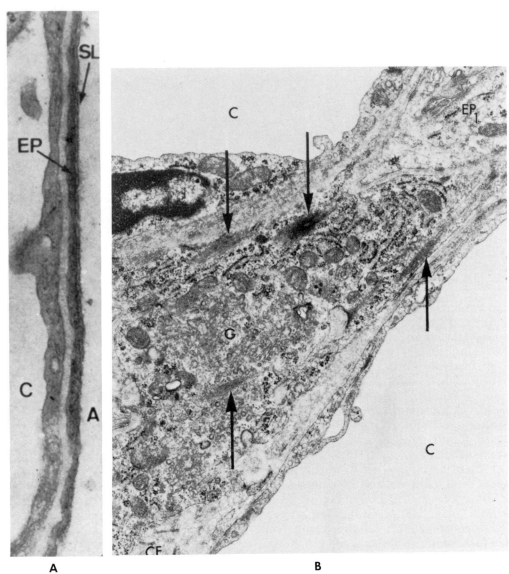

Figure 1–24. The Air-Blood Barrier. *A,* Thin portion. A capillary (*C*) is present on the left and the alveolar space (*A*) on the right. A type I alveolar epithelial cell (*EP*) is covered by a clearly extracellular osmiophilic layer (*SL*). (TEM, × 48,420.) (From Gil J, Weibel ER: Resp Physiol *8*:13, 1969.) *B,* Thick portion. Capillaries (*C*) and epithelial cells (*EP*₁) are separated by collagen fibers (*CF*) and a prominent interstitial cell containing a Golgi apparatus (*G*) and numerous fibrillar bundles (*arrows*). (Rat lung; TEM, × 24,000.) (From Kapanci Y, Assimacopoulos A, Irle C, et al: J Cell Biol *60*:375, 1974. Copyright The Rockefeller University Press.)

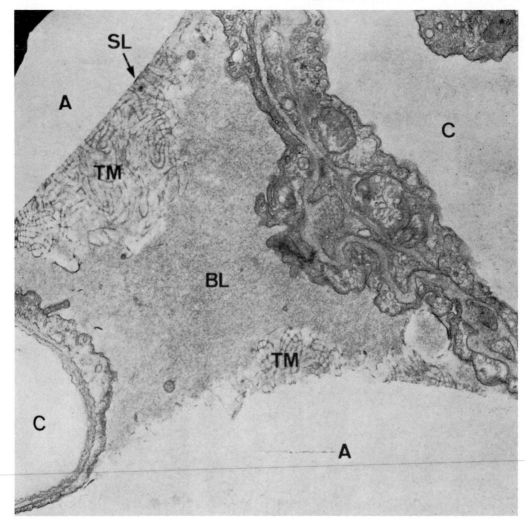

Figure 1–25. A Pore of Kohn. The pore is closed by lining material containing tubular myelin figures (*TM*) near the air-liquid interface. On the upper side, an osmiophilic outline (*SL*) is identified. *BL*, base layer of lining film; *A*, alveolus; *C*, capillary. (TEM, × 21,060.) (From Gil J, Weibel ER: Resp Physiol *8*:13, 1969.)

the number of alveolar septal and perivascular mast cells has been shown in chronically hypoxic rats,[17] an increase that has been correlated with a rise in right ventricular weight, lending further support to the hypothesis that mast cells may mediate the vascular hypoxic response.[171] Williams and colleagues have also speculated that an increase in mast cells may in fact be secondary to hypoxic pulmonary hypertension and that the increase may represent a protective response.[170] Finally, a marked increase in interstitial mast cell number, as well as a change in the ultrastructure of their granules, has been documented in chronic passive congestion secondary to mitral stenosis[172] and in fibrotic lung disorders of various etiologies.[169] The pathogenetic significance of these findings is uncertain, but it has been suggested that in these conditions a chronic partial release of mast cell contents may play a role in continuing alveolar injury and $\dot{V}/\dot{Q}$ irregularities.[169]

THE ALVEOLAR MACROPHAGE

Pulmonary macrophages have been divided into three groups on the basis of differing anatomic location: (1) the airway macrophage, situated within the lumen or beneath the epithelial lining of conducting airways; (2) the interstitial macrophage, found either isolated or in relation to lymphoid tissue within interstitial connective tissue throughout the lung; and (3) the alveolar macrophage, situated on the alveolar surface.[173] Although these cells are morphologically similar, it has been proposed that they may represent subpopulations with differing functional capabilities. However, because of its easy accessibility by bronchoalveolar lavage, the alveolar macrophage has been the most extensively studied and the following discussion deals principally with that cell.

As seen by light microscopy, the alveolar macrophage ranges from 15 to 50 μm in diameter, is

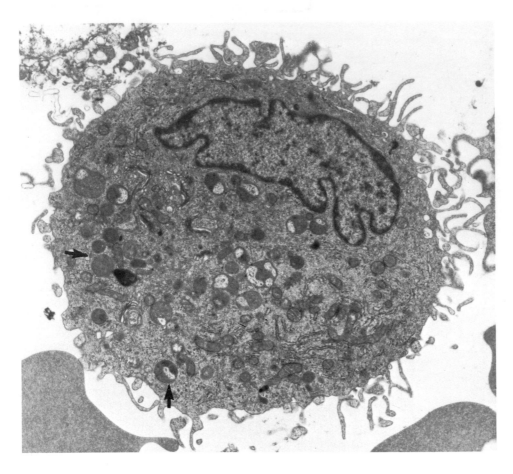

Figure 1–26. Alveolar Macrophage. Note numerous microvilli and lysosomes (*arrows*). (Human alveolar air space, × 8500.)

more or less round in shape, and has a foamy or finely granular cytoplasm. Nuclei are usually eccentric and may be multiple within one cell. Ultrastructurally (Fig. 1–26), macrophages show prominent surface cytoplasmic projections that appear as microvillus-like structures on transmission electron microscopy and as numerous ruffled folds on scanning electron microscopy.[174] The cytoplasm contains a well-developed Golgi apparatus, scattered mitochondria, endoplasmic reticulum, ribosomes, microtubules and microfilaments, and an abundance of characteristic membrane-bound granules of variable appearance, representing primary and secondary lysosomes.[175] Primary lysosomes are round or oval in shape, range in diameter from 0.1 to 0.5 μm, and contain an amorphous, electron-dense matrix.[175] Histochemical studies have revealed acid phosphatase[175] and numerous other lysosomal-associated enzymes within the granules.[176] Other granules that are more variable in size and shape contain portions of cytoplasmic material as well as poorly defined organic and possibly foreign substances; these represent the coalition of a primary lysosome with a phagosome, yielding a secondary lysosome. Such granules are especially prominent in the macrophages of cigarette smokers, where they may contain either "fibrillar" or "platelike" foreign material[175, 177] or lamellated lipid material ("sea-blue granules").[175, 178] The former has been shown to consist of kaolinite (an aluminum silicate found in

cigarette smoke)[177, 179] and the latter has been hypothesized to represent increased amounts of ingested alveolar surfactant. In addition to the increase in granule number in association with cigarette smoking, macrophages themselves typically increase in both size and number.[179]

Pulmonary alveolar macrophages differ somewhat from other body macrophages by having predominantly aerobic energy production, an increased number of mitochondria and mitochondrial enzymes, and more numerous and larger lysosomes.[180] These features are believed to be adaptations to its location within the alveolar airspaces where it is more or less continuously exposed to environmental toxins and a high oxygen concentration.

Multiple studies in humans and animals in which enzymatic, antigenic, karyotypic,[176] and ultrastructural[181] markers have been employed have shown that alveolar macrophages are ultimately derived from bone marrow precursors, presumably by way of the peripheral blood monocyte.[176] In addition, there is evidence for a population of alveolar interstitial macrophages that is capable of division and of replenishment or augmentation of the alveolar macrophage population, either in the absence of a functioning bone marrow[182, 183] or in times of increased need.[184] The average life span of the macrophage within the air space has been estimated to be about 80 days.[1157]

Various inhaled foreign materials have a deleterious effect on macrophage activity. For example, particulates such as silicon dioxide can rupture the lysosomal membrane, releasing enzymes into the cytoplasm and causing severe damage or death. A variety of insoluble compounds such as nitrogen dioxide, ozone, and a number of substances present in cigarette smoke are also toxic. They are not absorbed by the mucous blanket of the tracheobronchial tree and penetrate directly to the alveoli where they damage the macrophage through lipid peroxidation or by chemical combination on the cell membrane of the oxidant gas with susceptible enzymes such as sulfhydryl enzymes.[185] Cigarette smoke has also been reported to affect the alveolar macrophage by inhibiting metabolic activity and phagocytosis;[186-189] it has been suggested that its toxic effects are due to the inhibition of both glyceraldehyde dehydrogenase and anaerobic glycolysis.[185]

The functions of the alveolar macrophage are numerous and complex, and only a brief overview will be given here. They can be considered under three headings: (1) phagocytosis and clearance of unwanted intra-alveolar material; (2) immunologic interactions; and (3) production of inflammatory and other chemical mediators. There is evidence that different subpopulations of macrophages may have different capacities for one or more of these functions.[1158] This subject has been discussed in greater detail in several monographs.[176, 176a, 180, 190, 1157]

(1) Phagocytosis and clearance: Alveolar macrophages are motile and, in response to appropriate chemical stimuli, actively accumulate at the site of foreign material. Their surface possesses receptors for the Fc portion of IgG and IgE as well as C3.[180] In association with these and perhaps other opsonins such as fibronectin,[191] active phagocytosis of foreign material occurs. The latter may be particulate, such as silicates or anthracotic dust, and may remain largely unaltered within secondary lysosomes. On the other hand, ingested microorganisms are subjected to the full battery of lysosomal enzymes and in most cases are completely destroyed. The precise means of microbial killing are not understood but are believed to be predominantly oxygen-dependent and to be considerably more effective in activated macrophages (see following).[180] Possible mechanisms include a hydrogen peroxidase-peroxidase (catalase) system, superoxide anion, and lysosomal cationic proteins and other enzymes.[176]

In addition to inhaled foreign substances, alveolar macrophages ingest and eliminate endogenous pulmonary material, including the small number of dying type I and type II epithelial cells, alveolar surfactant,[192] and inflammatory exudate that may be produced during pneumonitis.

Although some macrophages containing foreign material enter the alveolar interstitium and either remain there or are transported via lymphatics to regional lymph nodes, there is evidence that few follow this route.[1155] Instead, the majority either die within the alveoli or make their way to the terminal bronchioles where they enter the mucociliary escalator and, along with their ingested material, are carried to the larynx and swallowed. Migration from the alveolar airspaces to the bronchioles may be partly due to inherent macrophage motility; the continual production of surfactant and its tendency to remain as a monolayer, possibly aided by respiratory excursion[193] and wave-like peristaltic movements,[194] may also be important.

(2) Immunologic interactions: Alveolar macrophages have important functions in both afferent and efferent immunologic mechanisms. Inhaled immunogens are phagocytosed and presented to T lymphocytes, which then develop specific immunity. Subsequent antigen presentation, again by macrophages, stimulates the T cells, which in time leads to both T and B cell and T cell and macrophage interaction. The latter, mediated via lymphokines, results in macrophage activation, which is manifested among other features by an increased number of surface receptors, increased amounts of lysosomal enzymes, and increased microbicidal activity. The great importance of these interactions is illustrated by the frequency and severity of pulmonary infections in immunocompromised individuals.

In addition to their obvious significance in pulmonary infections, macrophages either alone or in concert with T cells appear to have an important role in the destruction of neoplasms. The precise mechanisms and importance in relation to pulmonary cancer are not known.

(3) Production of mediators: Alveolar macrophages synthesize and probably secrete a variety of substances in both resting and activated conditions. Many of these may have important effects on local pulmonary defense and structural integrity. Fibronectin is present in fluid derived from bronchoalveolar lavage and has been shown immunochemically to be present in alveolar macrophages.[191] It has been hypothesized that it may act as a nonimmune opsonin to bind collagen fragments, fibrin, and some microorganisms.[191] Alpha-1-antitrypsin similarly has been identified within alveolar macrophages and may serve as a local intraluminal antiproteolytic agent.[195] Finally, alveolar macrophages are capable of producing highly active inflammatory mediators, such as prostaglandins[196] and leukotriene;[197] they also synthesize lysozyme and interferon,[180, 1159] substances that contribute to bacterial and viral defense.

THE LUNG UNIT

Of the subdivisions of lung parenchyma that have been proposed as the fundamental "unit" of lung structure, the primary and secondary lobules

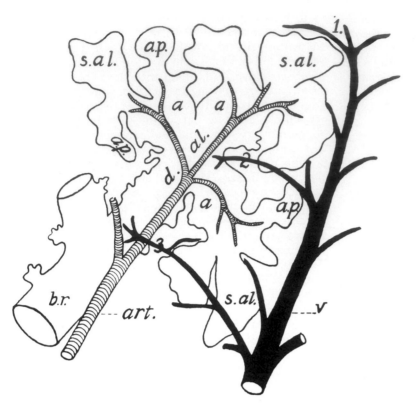

Figure 1–27. Schematic Longitudinal Section of a Primary Lobule of the Lung. Note the relation of the blood vessels to the air spaces. *b.r.*, respiratory bronchiole; *d.al.*, alveolar duct; *a*, atrium; *s.al.*, alveolar sac; *a.p.*, alveolus; *art.*, arteriole with branches to the atria and alveolar sacs; *v*, pulmonary venule with branches from the pleura (*1*), the alveolar ducts (*2*), and the respiratory bronchiole (*3*). (From Miller WS: The Lung. Springfield, IL, Charles C Thomas, 1937.)

of Miller[3] and the pulmonary acinus have gained the widest acceptance. The question of which most accurately represents the anatomic basis of normal and pathologic processes is controversial, since each possesses characteristics that suit one set of circumstances better than another. As we shall attempt to show, however, the one most uniformly acceptable for descriptive purposes, at least from the point of view of the roentgenologist and the physiologist, is the pulmonary acinus.

THE PRIMARY PULMONARY LOBULE OF MILLER

The primary lobule (Fig. 1–27) consists of all alveolar ducts, alveolar sacs, and alveoli, together with their accompanying blood vessels, nerves, and connective tissues, distal to the last respiratory bronchiole. Since there are approximately 23 million primary lobules in the human lung,[6] it is clear that this unit is too small to be seen roentgenographically when consolidated and thus is of no practical roentgenologic significance.

THE SECONDARY PULMONARY LOBULE OF MILLER

The secondary lobule is defined as the smallest discrete portion of the lung that is surrounded by connective tissue septa (Fig. 1–28).[3] It is composed of three to five terminal bronchioles, with their accompanying transitory airways and parenchyma, and has been estimated to contain between 30 and 50 primary lobules.[198] It is irregularly polyhedral in shape and generally ranges from 1 to 2.5 cm in diameter. Although Heitzman and his colleagues[199, 200] regard the secondary lobule as the basic unit of lung structure and function (a view held by others as well[201] and hold that most pulmonary diseases are best considered in terms of this unit's pathology), we take exception to this view for three reasons:

(1) The distribution of lobules is not uniform within the lung. Septa are most numerous in the lateral and anterior surfaces of the lower lobes, virtually nonexistent along the interlobar fissures and the posterior and mediastinal aspects of the lungs, and poorly developed in the central portion of the lungs. Thus, in disease affecting the latter regions a lobular distribution is usually impossible to detect.

(2) Even where visible, the size and extent of the septa are not uniform; the size of the lobules varies accordingly (Fig. 1–28), both within the same lung and between the lungs of different individuals.

(3) The secondary lobule seldom is recognizable roentgenographically as a structural unit (a fact, incidentally, with which Heitzman and his associates concur). Except for such uncommon events as the consolidation of a single secondary lobule—for example, by a pulmonary infarct—it is only when a pathologic process such as edema or infiltrating neoplasm distends the interlobular septa and renders them visible as septal lines that the volume of lung between two lines can be recognized as a secondary lobule.

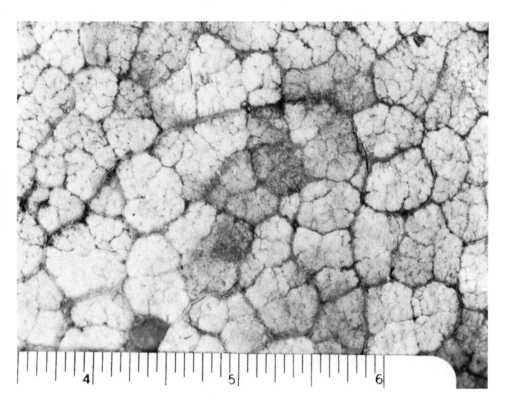

Figure 1–28. Secondary Lobule. Closeup view of the lower lobe visceral pleura showing the bases of numerous, irregularly shaped secondary lobules measuring from 0.5 to 1.5 cm in greatest dimension.

We feel that these limitations negate the usefulness of the secondary lobule for purposes of roentgenologic interpretation, and for most pathologic-roentgenologic correlation, and thus prefer to consider the acinus as the unit of lung structure.

THE PULMONARY ACINUS

The Acinus as an Anatomic Unit

Of the various definitions used for the same structures in the acinus (see the excellent review by Pump[202] and the more recent historical review by Raskin[203]), that suggested by Loeshcke[204] in 1921 is the most widely accepted. According to him the lung can be divided functionally into proximal conducting airways and distal gas-exchanging airways and air spaces; the acinus is meant to reflect the latter and is defined as *that portion of lung distal to the terminal bronchiole, comprising the respiratory bronchioles, alveolar ducts, alveolar sacs, and alveoli* (Figs. 1–29, 1–30).

According to Pump, the acinus measures approximately 7.5 × 8.5 mm on casts of lung inflated at a pressure equivalent to expiration;[121] these figures are somewhat higher than the 7.4-mm mean diameter reported by Gamsu and associates[205] in their roentgenographic study of the pulmonary acinus of lungs inflated and air-dried at a constant pressure of 30 cm of water, roughly equivalent to total lung capacity (*see* further on). In a morpho-

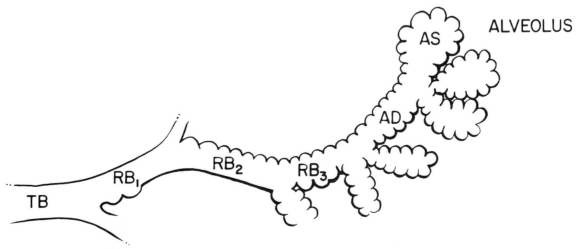

Figure 1–29. Component Parts of the Acinus. *TB*, terminal bronchiole; *RB*, respiratory bronchiole; *AD*, alveolar duct; *AS*, alveolar sac. (From Thurlbeck WM: *In* Sommers SC (ed): Pathology Annual: 1968. New York, Appleton-Century-Crofts, 1968, p 377.)

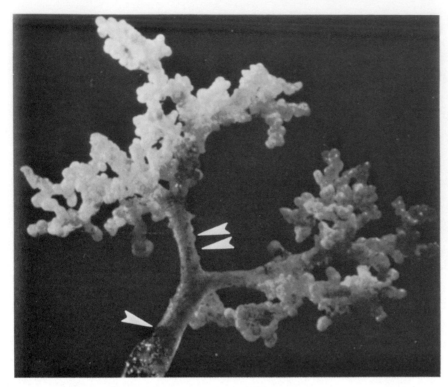

Figure 1–30. Cast of an Acinus Incompletely Filled with Resin. The smooth terminal bronchiole (*single arrowhead*) divides into two respiratory bronchioles, the upper one of which (*double arrowheads*) shows alveolar markings. After two or three generations the respiratory bronchioles divide to give rise to alveolar ducts, which are completely surrounded by alveoli. The rounded protuberances that are produced by partial filling of the alveoli with the resin are seen on the peripheral parts of the cast. (From Horsfield K, Cumming G: J Appl Physiol 24:373, 1968.)

metric study of a single acinus, Hansen and Ampaya[1153] estimated its volume to be 182.8 mm³ at three quarters TLC. To establish the postnatal growth pattern and size of the pulmonary acinus in humans, Osborne and his colleagues studied normal lungs from 4 adults and 11 children under 14 years of age who had died without evidence of pulmonary disease; the lungs were radiographed following inflation with intrabronchial neutral formalin at 25 cm of water pressure, air-drying at a similar pressure, and injection of contrast medium.[206] The following growth patterns were observed: the mean diameter of the pulmonary acinus at 1 month was 1 mm; at 1 year, 2.5 mm; at 2 years, 3 mm; at 12 years, 6 mm; and by late adolescence a normal adult range of 6 to 10 mm was seen.

In a study of two acini of a 32-year-old woman, Pump[121] found 3229 and 4041 alveoli; based on those findings, Boyden[122] estimated that the lungs of that particular individual contained a total of approximately 80,000 acini. Other estimates of alveolar number per acinus have been higher (7100 by Schreider and Raabe[123] and 15,000 to 20,000 by Hansen and his colleagues[124]), suggesting that the actual number of acini may be considerably less.

The Acinus as a Roentgenologic Unit

Since an acinus is visible macroscopically, it is reasonable to assume its visibility roentgenologically when completely or partially filled with contrast material or inflammatory exudate. In 1924 Aschoff[207] suggested that consolidation of a single acinus by tuberculous inflammatory exudate or granulation tissue results in a rosette-like appearance, which he termed the "acino-nodose" lesion (Fig. 31). Identical shadows were created by Twining[208] in 1931 by overfilling with Lipiodol the bronchial tree of lungs removed at necropsy (Fig. 1–32). Neither Aschoff nor Twining proved conclusively that the "acino-nodose" shadow represented a single acinus morphologically, and it was not until recently that the precise roentgenologic nature of the acinus was established. In an extension of their previously mentioned study of peripheral bronchographic morphology, Gamsu and his colleagues investigated the feasibility of roentgenographic identification of individual acini in human lung.[205] Using a special tantalum suspension, they progressively opacified two or more segments of normal excised lungs distal to a wedged catheter, obtaining sequential roentgenograms on fine-grain film until almost total opacification was achieved. By correlating roentgenographic, microradiographic, and histologic appearances, they identified and differentiated terminal and respiratory bronchioles and thus visualized individual acini (Fig. 1–33). Progressive filling of a single acinus initially produced a rosette appearance and eventually a spherical lesion (Fig. 1–34). Measurements of 25 acini revealed a mean diameter of 7.4 mm, in the range 6 to 10 mm. (These figures represent acinar caliber at a volume roughly equivalent to total lung capacity, since the lungs were fixed in inflation at a transpulmonary pressure of 30 cm of water.)

More recently, Lui and colleagues,[209] employing a different technique and injecting a mixture of barium sulfate and gelatin, opacified individual acini of normal human lung. They described the overall configuration as elliptic rather than spherical; however, their illustration of a single opacified acinus roentgenographed at 90° planes depicts a roughly spherical structure. Their measurements of acinar shadows ranged from 6 to 8 mm in diameter, similar to those of Gamsu and his associates.[205]

In the light of these observations and of previous discussions of the morphology and function of the lung parenchyma, we propose three reasons for accepting the acinus as a roentgenologic unit.

1. It is roentgenologically visible.

2. It is recognizable throughout the entire lung (in contrast to the secondary lobule, which is present in only the peripheral 2 to 3 cm or "cortex" of the lung).

3. It provides a useful correlation with function, since it constitutes the gas exchange (respiratory as well as transitory) portion of the lung.

A deserved interest in the pulmonary acinus as a roentgenologic unit was revived by Ziskind and his associates in the sixties.[210, 211] These investigators brought into proper perspective the importance of recognizing "alveolar filling" diseases that produce the roentgenographically visible rosette shadows or acinar pattern. In conditions such as pulmonary edema, acute alveolar pneumonia, and idiopathic pulmonary hemorrhage, recognition of this distinctive pattern enables the roentgenologist to narrow the differential diagnosis to the relatively few diseases capable of consolidating parenchymal air spaces.

The Acinus as a Functional Unit

The definition of the acinus as the fundamental lung unit is acceptable to both anatomists and roentgenologists, but is there evidence that this portion of the lung is also a functional unit? Most physiologists describe the alveolus as the unit of the lung. In so doing, however, they equate this not with the anatomic alveolus but with a hypothetic unit that, because of our lack of knowledge of correlation between physiology and anatomy, cannot be defined morphologically. In fact, it would be unrealistic to consider the structural alveolus as a physiologic unit. Each alveolus is one of a family of many that arise from a common alveolar sac, alveolar duct, or respiratory bronchiole and which receive from a common arteriole capillaries that interconnect the alveoli.[212] It is unlikely that, in normal circumstances, the behavior of any one alveolus differs from that of its "siblings." Thus it seems likely that Miller's primary lobule,[3] comprising the alveolar duct and its ramifications that arise from a last-order respiratory bronchiole, is the smallest portion that can be considered in the concept of a physiologic unit of lung function. Farther up the bronchial tree, at the level of the terminal bronchiole, a greater portion of the lung is included as a unit of function, since there are some 400 alveolar duct units distal to this point. Do all the alveoli that make up this acinus behave similarly? This question cannot be answered yet, although accumulating evidence in the areas of both structure and physiology suggests

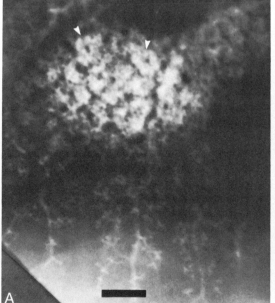 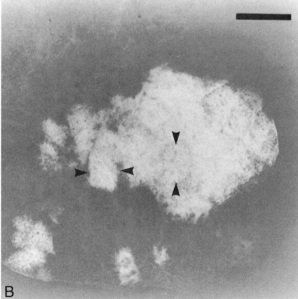

Figure 1–31. The "Acino-nodose" Shadow. *A,* An overfilled clinical bronchogram in anteroposterior projection demonstrates typical acinar shadows measuring up to 8 mm in diameter. Other views showed that the degree of filling did not extend beyond the millimeter pattern, indicating that contrast medium had not penetrated farther than respiratory bronchioles. Some nodules (two marked with *arrowheads*) possess a relatively large central radiolucency from which linear radiolucencies emanate (spoke-wheel appearance); this conceivably relates to axial imaging of air-containing distal bronchioles. *B,* A radiograph of a postmortem lung specimen injected with a barium/gelatin mixture shows contrast medium to have penetrated beyond the millimeter pattern to opacify intra-acinar components. Multiple nodular shadows (*arrowheads*) containing intra-acinar opacities are seen. This appearance was called the "acino-nodose" opacity by Aschoff (*see* text). Bars in *A* and *B* represent 1 cm. (From Genereux GP: Med Radiogr Photogr *61*:2, 1985. Courtesy of Eastman Kodak Company.)

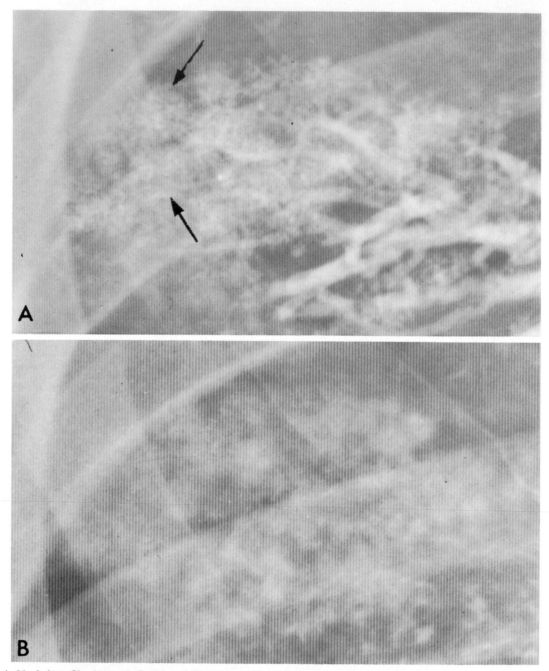

Figure 1–32. Acinar Shadows. *A*, Peripheral filling of respiratory bronchioles during bronchography (*arrows*). *B*, 24 hours later the contrast agent has absorbed but has incited an acute air space edema resulting in the "rosette" shadows of acinar consolidation.

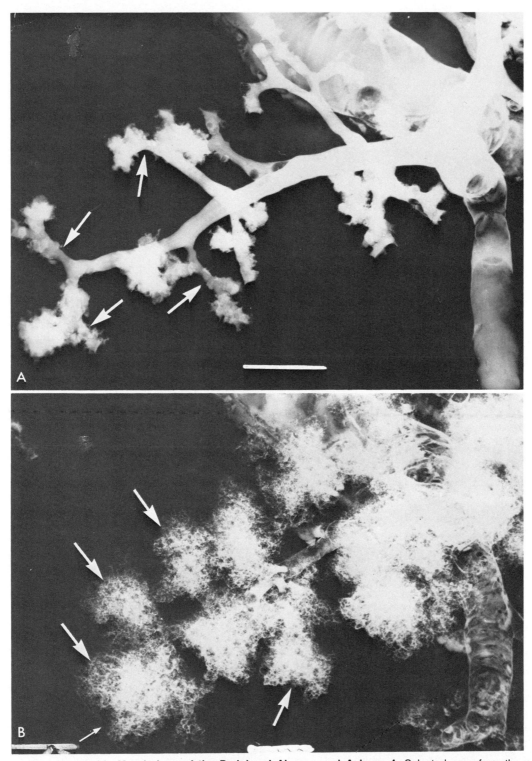

Figure 1–33. Bronchographic Morphology of the Peripheral Airways and Acinus. *A*, Selected area from the periphery of a bronchogram on a normal human lung removed at necropsy and opacified with a tantalum suspension. *Arrows* indicate terminal bronchioles, the majority of which are smooth walled. *B*, Roentgenograms after air drying of the lung. There has now been further opacification of the intra-acinar airways. *Arrows* indicate partially opacified acini that can be related to the terminal bronchioles in *A*. The bar in *A* represents 5 mm. (From Gamsu G, Thurlbeck WM, Macklem PT, et al: Invest Radiol 6:171, 1971.)

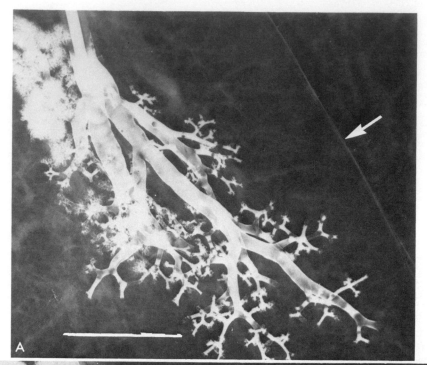

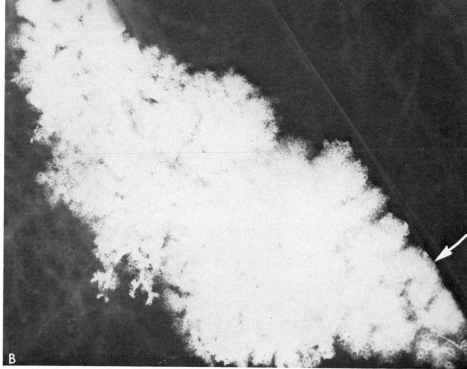

Figure 1–34. Bronchographic Morphology of the Peripheral Airways and Acinus. Roentgenograms showing progressive opacification of a segment of the bronchial tree distal to a wedged catheter (normal human lung removed at necropsy). *A*, Initially, mainly nonrespiratory bronchioles are visible with some early filling of acini producing stippling and rosettes; *B*, after further opacification, a mosaic of spherical, superimposed but distinct acini is visible. *Arrows* indicate the pleural surface. Bar in *A* represents 2.2 cm in both figures. (From Gamsu G, Thurlbeck WM, Macklem PT, et al: Invest Radiol *6*:171, 1971.)

that they do. For this reason, and in order to envisage a physiologic counterpart of the morphologic and roentgenologic unit, the basic functioning unit of the lung is taken to be the acinus—*i.e.,* all lung parenchyma distal to the terminal bronchiole.

Although peripheral lung parenchyma can be divided into anatomic, roentgenologic, and functional units as just discussed, a variety of communications exist at different levels.

Channels of Peripheral Airway and Acinar Communication

The first and probably the most studied of these structures are the *alveolar pores* (Fig. 1–35; *see also* Figure 1–25, page 25). Although first described by Adriani in 1847, these small discontinuities have come to be known as *pores of Kohn* after the latter's observation of fibrin strands traversing alveolar walls in cases of acute pneumonia. They are present in the lungs of most mammals,[214] in numbers varying with the species and with the technique of fixation and examination.[215] They tend to be more numerous in older animals and in the apex and subpleural regions of the lung.[216, 1156] In most cases, the size of the aperture ranges from 2 to 10 μm, although both the size of the pore and the number of pores per alveolus tend to be greater in lungs fixed via the airways than via the vasculature.[215, 217] Since the width of the alveolar wall is dependent on lung volume and the degree of capillary engorgement, the width of the pores can also vary with these factors.

Although the pores can be identified by light microscopy in 1- to 2-μm-thick sections, they are best studied by electron microscopy. Scanning electron microscopy of human lungs shows an average of nine pores per alveolus in airway-fixed tissue but only two per alveolus in lungs fixed by vascular channels.[217] The pores are round or oval, situated in intercapillary spaces, and lined by alveolar epithelium. Epithelial junctions are commonly present on both sides of the pores,[218] presumably representing a meeting of type I cells from adjacent alveoli. By transmission electron microscopy, the aperture is usually free of cellular or other material in airway-fixed material, but in vascular-perfused tissue the pore frequently is occluded by a thin film of material identical to and continuous with alveolar surfactant (*see* Fig. 1–25, page 25).[215, 217, 219] Since it is probable that vascular-perfused tissue more closely represents the normal state within the alveolar lumen, the presence of surfactant occlusion casts some doubt on the significance of alveolar pores as a mechanism for collateral ventilation. It is possible, however, that they represent an interacinar pathway for the spread of fluid, with or without pathogenic microorganisms.

The origin of the pores is unknown, but because of their rarity in children[216] most authorities believe that they are acquired. It has been suggested that they result from the desquamation of alveolar epithelial cells[220] or from the action of ventilatory stresses on alveolar walls.[216] It has also been hypothesized that the initial event might be loss of interstitial connective tissue,[166] possibly in association with the release of proteases from adjacent macrophages or neutrophils.[166, 221]

The relationship of so-called *fenestrae* (alveolar discontinuities measuring from 20 to 100 μm in diameter) to alveolar pores is unclear.[222] They are thought by most investigators[166, 215, 222] to represent a pathologic state of the alveolar wall, some believing them to be the earliest stage of pulmonary emphysema. It has also been speculated that alveolar pores may themselves be the precursors of

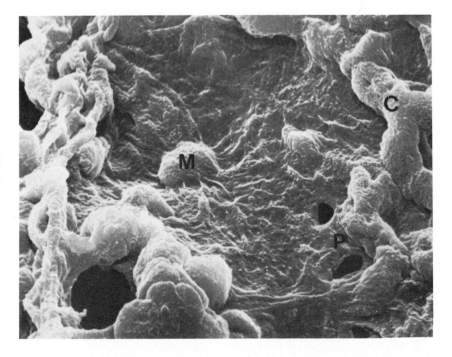

Figure 1–35. Surface of an Alveolus. Note surrounding capillaries (*C*), a macrophage (*M*), and alveolar pores (*P*). (SEM, × 3650.) (Courtesy of Dr. Nai-San Wang, McGill University, Montreal.)

fenestrae.[215, 222] Whatever their relationship, it is possible that these larger discontinuities are of greater significance than alveolar pores in providing a pathway for interacinar communication.

Direct communications between alveoli and respiratory, terminal, and preterminal bronchioles were first described by Lambert[223, 224] and their presence has been confirmed by others.[123, 225, 226] These *canals of Lambert* consist of epithelial-lined tubular structures that, in lungs fixed in deflation, range in diameter from "practically closed" to 30 μm; in one lung fixed in full inflation, a single communication measuring 150 μm in diameter was identified.[123] It is not known whether these "airways" provide solely intra-acinar accessory communications or whether interacinar connections capable of subserving collateral ventilation occur as well.

In both animals and humans, particles considerably larger than either alveolar pores or most canals of Lambert are able to pass through collateral channels in lung parenchyma. For example, polystyrene spheres 120 μm in diameter have been passed through collateral channels in dogs' lungs,[227] and spheres up to 64 μm have been passed in excised human lungs.[228] Several studies have attempted to localize and characterize these channels anatomically. Martin observed the passage of insufflated India ink aerosols from one segment of a dog's lobe into an adjacent segment, and reported that the particles were deposited on collateral channels that resembled respiratory bronchioles.[227] In a micropuncture injection study of cleared human lung, Raskin and Herman found interacinar and, occasionally, interlobular flow of silicon rubber through short, tubular channels approximately 200 μm in diameter (which were not further characterized).[201] In another study in which bronchial corrosion casts were utilized, intersegmental connections were identified in the form of small airways with a diameter of 80 to 150 μm that resembled first order respiratory bronchioles.[229] More distally, Boyden has shown histologic evidence of direct communication between two adjacent acini at the level of their alveolar sacs.[122]

In summary, it is apparent that collateral ventilation between adjacent acini, lobules, or segments can occur by several anatomic pathways. In addition to being poorly characterized, however, the frequency of these channels within an individual lung and their variation between different regions of the same lung are virtually unknown. The importance and mechanisms of collateral ventilation are thus more easily understood from a knowledge of physiologic data, discussed on page 64.

ROENTGENOLOGY OF THE AIRWAYS

Knowledge of segmental bronchial terminology and the mode of bronchial branching is important for two main reasons. (1) Surgical resection for localized disease, notably bronchiectasis, often can be limited to segments, and it is clearly desirable to remove no more pulmonary tissue than is necessary for cure. (2) The bronchoscopist may need assistance to determine which segment is affected; intrabronchial conditions such as a small peripheral pulmonary carcinoma or a small foreign body may be situated sufficiently far in the periphery of the lung as to remain undetected during standard bronchoscopic examination.

In this section, therefore, we will present a standard nomenclature of bronchopulmonary anatomy and describe the prevailing pattern of segmental bronchial branching. Minor variations in the pattern that occur fairly frequently will be indicated. The anatomy of the bronchi in the hila as seen on computed tomography is described in a later section (*see* page 86) along with hilar pulmonary vessels.

In 1943 Jackson and Huber[230] published a nomenclature of the bronchial segments that was widely adopted and remains the generally accepted terminology in North America (Table 1–2). The terminologies recommended by the Thoracic Society of Great Britain in 1949 introduced minor variations of the Jackson and Huber nomenclature.[231] In 1955 Boyden[232] proposed a numerical system for identification of bronchial segments which also is widely used. Although these three variations are included in the table, the Jackson-Huber nomenclature is used exclusively throughout this book.

No official nomenclature exists for the major bronchi interposed between the trachea and the segmental bronchi of the five pulmonary lobes. Through common usage, the designation "main bronchi" is applied to the bronchi arising from the bifurcation of the trachea down to the origin of the upper lobe bronchus on each side, and "intermediate bronchus" to the segment between the right upper lobe bronchus and the origins of the right middle and lower lobe bronchi.

The Trachea and Main Bronchi

The trachea is, to all intents and purposes, a midline structure; a slight deviation to the right after entering the thorax is a normal finding and should not be misinterpreted as evidence of displacement (*see* Figure 1–37A). Its walls are parallel except on the left side just above the bifurcation, where the aorta commonly impresses a smooth indentation. The air columns of the trachea, main bronchi, and intermediate bronchus have a smoothly serrated contour, created by the indentations of the horseshoe-shaped cartilage rings at regular intervals along these structures. In two computed tomographic studies,[233, 234] considerable variation was observed in the cross-sectional shape of the trachea. In their CT study of 50 subjects without tracheal or mediastinal abnormalities, Gamsu and Webb found the length of the intrathoracic trachea to range from 6 to 9 cm (mean, 7.5 ± 0.8 cm).[234] The most common shape was round or oval; a horseshoe shape with a flat posterior tracheal membrane was seen in only 12 subjects, an inverted pear shape in 6, and an almost square configuration in 2. Twenty-two of the 50 subjects had more than one distinct shape at different levels. The most inferior 1 to 2 cm of the intrathoracic trachea assumed an oval shape, the azygos arch usually being visible to the right of the trachea at this level. Kittridge emphasized the variation in the location of the trachea in an anteroposterior axis: while commonly more or less midway between the sternum and spine, it may rest against the vertebral bodies posteriorly or may be positioned more anteriorly than expected, mimicking forward displacement.[233] The relationship of the esophagus to the trachea is discussed in a subsequent section.

To determine the caliber of the normal trachea, Breatnach and his colleagues measured the coronal and sagittal diameters of the tracheal air column on posteroanterior and lateral chest roentgenograms of 808 patients with no clinical or roentgenographic evidence of respiratory disease.[235] The 430 male and 378 female subjects ranged in age from 10 to 79 years. Assuming a normative range that encompasses three standard deviations from the mean (99.7 per cent of the normal population), in men aged 20 to 79 years the upper limits of normal for coronal and sagittal diameters were 25 mm and 27 mm respectively; in women of the same age, they were 21 mm and 23 mm respectively. These investigators concluded that deviation from these figures reflects pathologic widening of the tracheal air column. The lower limit of normal for both dimensions was 13 mm in men and 10 mm in women. Of interest was the observation that no statistically significant correlation was found between tracheal caliber and body weight or body height. In the latter study, there were only negligible differences in coronal or sagittal dimensions on roentgenograms exposed at full inspiration and maximal expiration; the diameters were identical in most cases and rarely exceeded 1 mm. This rather surprising observation was confirmed more recently by a study carried out by Griscom and Wohl[236] in which computed tomography was used to examine the tracheas of two healthy adults at functional residual capacity, first at an intratracheal pressure of +20 cm H_2O and then at −20 cm H_2O: the intrathoracic portions of the tracheas showed little change in cross-sectional area between the two pressures, but by contrast the cross-sectional area of the cervical tracheas decreased by about one third from the higher pressure to the lower, the membranous posterior wall tending to bulge backward strikingly at the higher pressure and to draw well into the tracheal lumen at the lower pressure. The two tracheas were 6 per cent and 12 per cent shorter at the lower pressure. Pressure/area behavior of the extrathoracic trachea can be measured by performing CT scans during graded Valsalva and Mueller maneuvers (Fig. 1–36).[818]

Griscom and Wohl have also studied the dimensions of the growing trachea in relation to age and gender; they performed CT scans on 130 subjects in the first two decades of life and measured the lengths, AP and transverse diameters, cross-sectional areas, and contained volumes of the tracheas.[1132] They found no differences between boys and girls under the age of 14 years, at which time girls' tracheas stopped growing; by contrast, the

Table 1–2. Nomenclature of Bronchopulmonary Anatomy

JACKSON-HUBER	BOYDEN	BROCK	THORACIC SOCIETY OF GREAT BRITAIN
Upper Lobe			
Apical	B[1]	Apical	Apical
Anterior	B[2]	Pectoral	Anterior
Posterior	B[3]	Subapical	Posterior
Right Middle Lobe			
Lateral	B[4]	Lateral	Lateral
Medial	B[5]	Medial	Medial
Right Lower Lobe			
Superior	B[6]	Apical	Apical
Medial basal	B[7]	Cardiac	Medial basal
Anterior basal	B[8]	Anterior basal	Anterior basal
Lateral basal	B[9]	Middle basal	Lateral basal
Posterior basal	B[10]	Posterior basal	Posterior basal
Left Upper Lobe			
Upper division			Upper division
Apical-posterior	B[1&3]	Apical and subapical	Apicoposterior or apical and posterior
Anterior	B[2]	Pectoral	Anterior
Lower (lingular) division			Lingular (lower) division
Superior lingular	B[4]	Superior lingular	Superior lingular
Inferior lingular	B[5]	Inferior lingular	Inferior lingular
Left Lower Lobe			
Superior	B[6]	Apical	Apical
Anteromedial	B[7&8]	Anterior	Anterior basal
Lateral basal	B[9]	Middle basal	Lateral basal
Posterior basal	B[10]	Posterior basal	Posterior basal

(Modified slightly from Hinshaw HC: Diseases of the Chest. 3rd ed. Philadelphia, WB Saunders, 1969.)

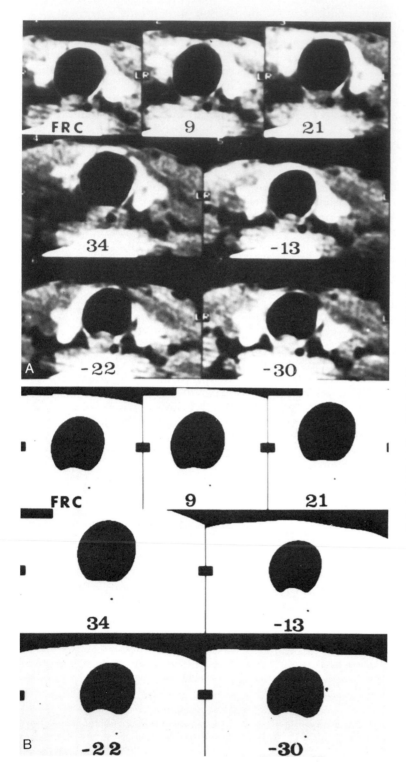

Figure 1–36. Pressure/Area Behavior of the Extrathoracic Trachea. These 5-mm CT cuts (*A* and *B* at different window settings) were made in a plane perpendicular to the long axis of the trachea 3 cm below the larynx. A normal subject performed graded Valsalva maneuvers resulting in the positive intratracheal (and therefore transmural) pressures of 9, 21, and 34 cm H_2O, as well as graded Mueller maneuvers that resulted in negative intratracheal (and therefore transmural) pressures of −13, −22, and −30 cm H_2O. It is apparent that with posterior transmural pressure the tracheal area increases and the posterior membranous portion flattens. With negative transmural pressure, there is an initial decrease in cross-sectional area and inward displacement of the posterior membranous portion of the trachea.

However, with progressively negative pressures further decrease in cross-sectional area does not occur. The extrathoracic esophageal pressure, presumably representing extratracheal pressure, becomes negative during the Mueller maneuvers, preventing further collapse. Such a procedure could conceivably be useful in delineating whether altered mechanical properties of large airways exist in disease. (From Muller N, Moreno R, Taylor R, et al: Clin Invest Med *8*:A202, 1986.)

tracheas of boys continued to enlarge (but not lengthen) for a time after growth in height ceased. Mean transverse diameters tended to be greater than mean AP diameters to the age of 6 years; thereafter, the diameters were nearly identical until age 18 years when AP diameters usually became slightly larger. The tracheas were nearly round in cross section, especially at high lung volumes.

The trachea divides into the two major bronchi at the carina. Two methods of measuring the angle of bifurcation are available: the interbronchial angle (the angle between the central axis of the right and left main stem bronchi) and the subcarinal angle (the angle of divergence of the right and left main stem bronchi measured along their inferior borders); the latter seems to us to be the most practical and is the one described here. Two roentgenologic studies have been performed to assess the subcarinal angle in adults. In the 58 adults aged 16 to 83 years studied by Alavi and associates, the carinal angle ranged from 41 to 71 degrees in men (mean, 56.4) and from 41 to 74 degrees in women (mean, 57.7).[237] In a more recent study by Haskin and Goodman of 100 normal adult subjects, the range of values was considerably wider—35 to 90.5 degrees, with a mean of 60.8 degrees (standard deviation, 11.8 degrees).[238] In the latter study, age and gender had no effect on the bifurcation angle, although there was a weak inverse correlation between the shape of the thorax and the angle of tracheal bifurcation: as the chest gets longer and narrower (i.e., the patient becomes more asthenic), the angle becomes more acute; however, this correlation was weak and of questionable predictive value. These researchers emphasized that there is such a wide range of normal values for the bifurcation angle that even gross deviation from the 60-degree average should not be interpreted as abnormal.

It has traditionally been accepted that the course of the right main bronchus distally is more direct than that of the left, an observation that is certainly true in adults and is attributable at least in part to the pressure on the left wall of the trachea by the aorta. However, noting that it is not unusual for the left lung to be affected by aspirated foreign bodies in young children, Cleveland measured the bronchial angles of 50 children and adolescents, ranging in age from birth to 18 years, and found symmetry of right and left bronchial angles in virtually all subjects to age 15 years.[239] Thus, the relatively equal incidence of right- and left-sided aspiration of foreign bodies in smaller children is readily explained.

The transverse diameter of the right main bronchus at total lung capacity is greater than that of the left (15.3 mm, compared with 13.0 mm[240]), although its length before the origin of the upper lobe bronchus as measured at necropsy is shorter (average 2.2 cm, compared with 5 cm on the left[241, 242]).

The air column of the trachea, both major bronchi, and the intermediate bronchus should be plainly visible on well-exposed standard roentgenograms of the chest in frontal projection. The right lateral and posterior walls of the trachea are usually identifiable on posteroanterior and lateral roentgenograms respectively as vertically oriented linear opacities or stripes—the right tracheal and posterior tracheal stripes; these are described in the mediastinal section (see page 230).

The Lobar Bronchi and Bronchopulmonary Segments

The pattern of bronchial branching shows considerable variation.[232, 243-250] In the great majority of instances, these are of no clinical significance and are discovered only during bronchoscopy or post mortem. In addition, despite the anatomic variation of segmental bronchi, the location of the bronchopulmonary segments is more or less constant; and since the recognition of these zones is more important roentgenographically than the identification of specific bronchi, anatomic differences in the latter are relatively unimportant. The exception is when surgery is being contemplated, in which case knowledge of any deviation may be important in determining the approach to pulmonary resection. For example, a tracheal bronchus or "mirror image" bronchial tree (bronchial isomerism) may be associated with cardiovascular anomalies or situs inversus, and their presence should be brought to the attention of the surgeon.

On this and the following pages, the anatomic distribution of the bronchial segments is described and illustrated. Each segmental bronchus is considered separately, preceded by reproductions of a right bronchogram and corresponding drawings in anteroposterior (Fig. 1–37) and lateral (Fig. 1–38) projections, and of a left bronchogram similarly depicted (Figs. 1–39 and 1–40).

RIGHT UPPER LOBE

The bronchus to the right upper lobe arises from the lateral aspect of the main stem bronchus approximately 2.5 cm from the carina. It divides at slightly more than 1 cm from its origin, most commonly into three branches designated anterior, posterior, and apical. The branching pattern is particularly variable in relation to the axillary portion of the lobe (Figs. 1–41 to 1–43). Of some interest, although of no definite significance, is the relatively infrequent origin of the upper lobe bronchus or of one of its branches (usually the apical bronchus) from the lateral wall of the trachea (the "tracheal bronchus").

RIGHT MIDDLE LOBE

The intermediate bronchus continues distally for 3 to 4 cm from the takeoff of the right upper

Text continued on page 49

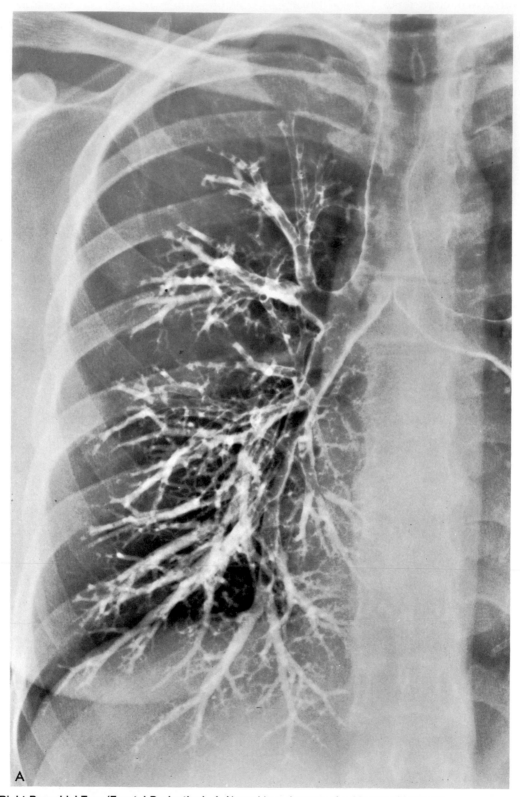

Figure 1–37. Right Bronchial Tree (Frontal Projection). *A*, Normal bronchogram of a 39-year-old woman.

Illustration continued on opposite page

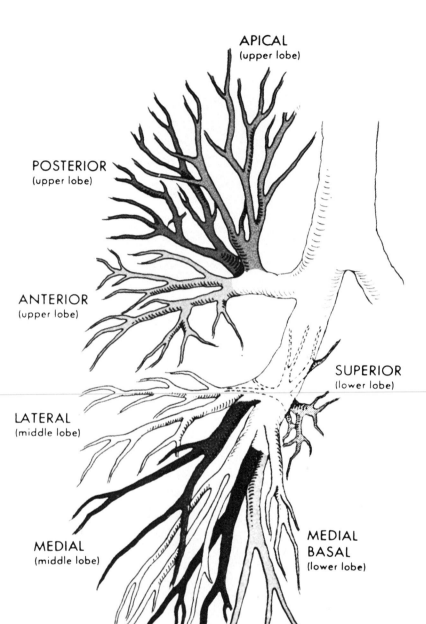

APICAL
(upper lobe)

POSTERIOR
(upper lobe)

ANTERIOR
(upper lobe)

SUPERIOR
(lower lobe)

LATERAL
(middle lobe)

MEDIAL
BASAL
(lower lobe)

MEDIAL
(middle lobe)

ANTERIOR
BASAL
(lower lobe)

LATERAL
BASAL
(lower lobe)

POSTERIOR
BASAL
(lower lobe)

B

Figure 1–37. *Continued. B,* The normal segments of the right bronchial tree in frontal projection. (*B* from Lehman JS, Crellin JA: Med Radiogr Photog *31*:81, 1955. Courtesy of Eastman Kodak Company.)

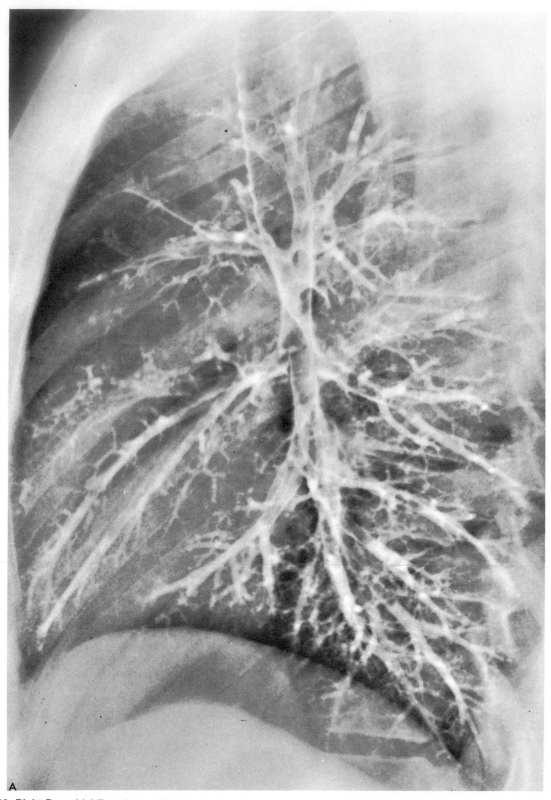

Figure 1–38. Right Bronchial Tree (Lateral Projection). *A,* Normal bronchogram of a 39-year-old woman.

Illustration continued on opposite page

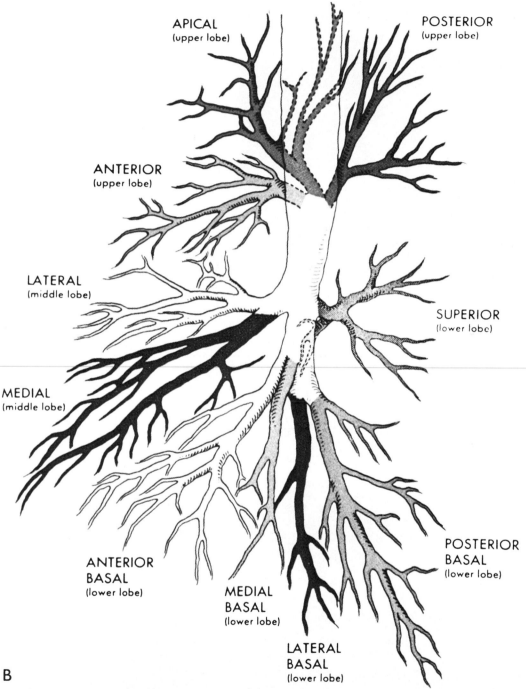

APICAL
(upper lobe)

POSTERIOR
(upper lobe)

ANTERIOR
(upper lobe)

LATERAL
(middle lobe)

SUPERIOR
(lower lobe)

MEDIAL
(middle lobe)

ANTERIOR
BASAL
(lower lobe)

MEDIAL
BASAL
(lower lobe)

POSTERIOR
BASAL
(lower lobe)

LATERAL
BASAL
(lower lobe)

B

Figure 1–38. *Continued. B*, The normal segments of the right bronchial tree in lateral projection. (*B* from Lehman JS, Crellin JA: Med Radiogr Photog *31*:81, 1955. Courtesy of Eastman Kodak Company.)

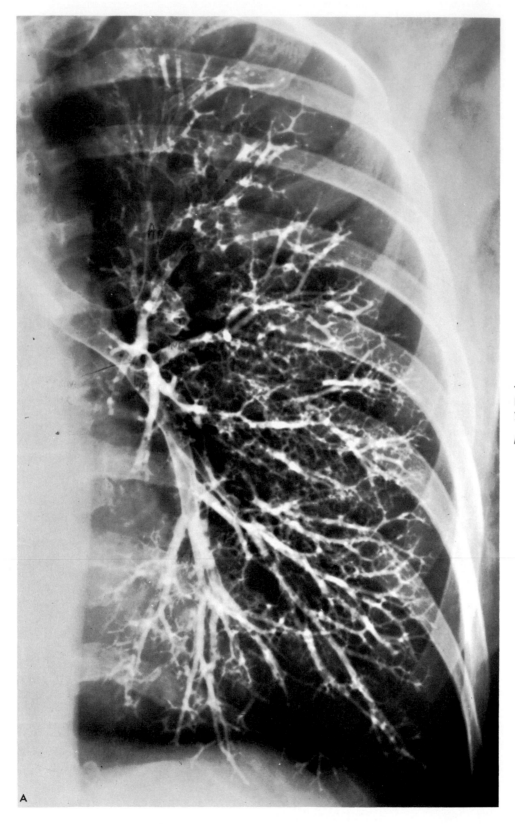

Figure 1–39. Left Bronchial Tree (Frontal Projection). *A,* Normal bronchogram of a 39-year-old woman.
Illustration continued on opposite page

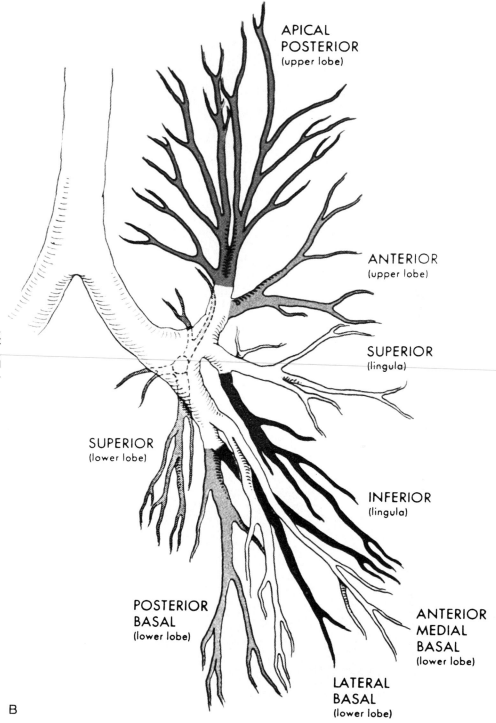

Figure 1–39. *Continued. B,* The normal segments of the left bronchial tree in frontal projection. (*B* from Lehman JS, Crellin JA: Med Radiogr Photog *31*:81, 1955. Courtesy of Eastman Kodak Company.)

APICAL
POSTERIOR
(upper lobe)

ANTERIOR
(upper lobe)

SUPERIOR
(lingula)

INFERIOR
(lingula)

SUPERIOR
(lower lobe)

POSTERIOR
BASAL
(lower lobe)

ANTERIOR
MEDIAL
BASAL
(lower lobe)

LATERAL
BASAL
(lower lobe)

B

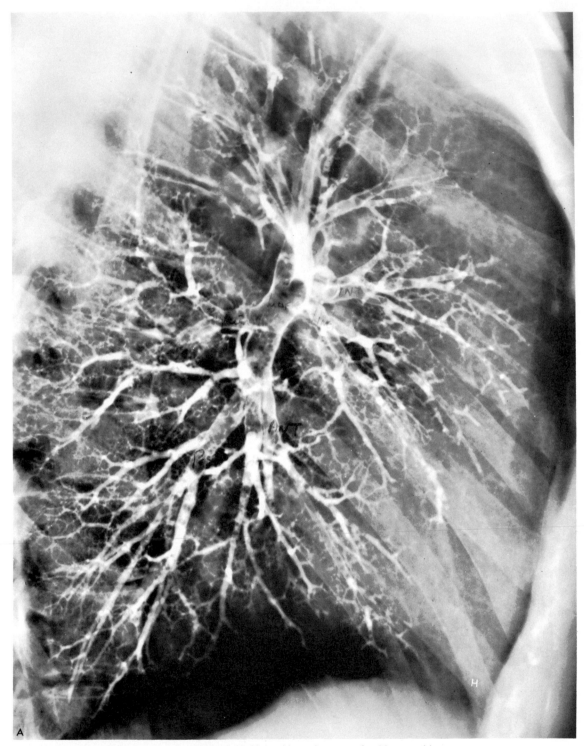

Figure 1–40. Left Bronchial Tree (Lateral Projection). *A*, Normal bronchogram of a 39-year-old woman.

Illustration continued on opposite page

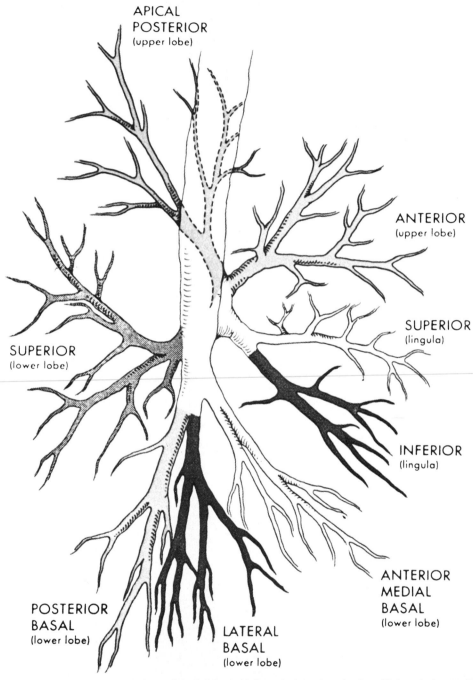

APICAL
POSTERIOR
(upper lobe)

ANTERIOR
(upper lobe)

SUPERIOR
(lingula)

SUPERIOR
(lower lobe)

INFERIOR
(lingula)

ANTERIOR
MEDIAL
BASAL
(lower lobe)

POSTERIOR
BASAL
(lower lobe)

LATERAL
BASAL
(lower lobe)

B

Figure 1–40. *Continued*. *B*, The normal segments of the left bronchial tree in lateral projection. (*B* from Lehman JS, Crellin JA: Med Radiogr Photog *31*:81, 1955. Courtesy of Eastman Kodak Company.)

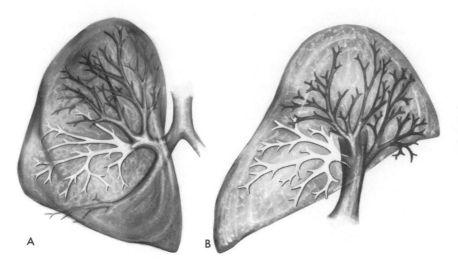

Figure 1–41. Anterior Segmental Bronchus, Right Upper Lobe. *A*, Frontal projection; *B*, lateral projection. This segment is directed anteriorly and laterally to supply that portion of the upper lobe contiguous to the minor fissure.

Figure 1–42. Posterior Segmental Bronchus, Right Upper Lobe. *A*, Frontal projection; *B*, lateral projection. This bronchus extends posteriorly, laterally, and somewhat superiorly to supply the posterolateral projection of the lobe.

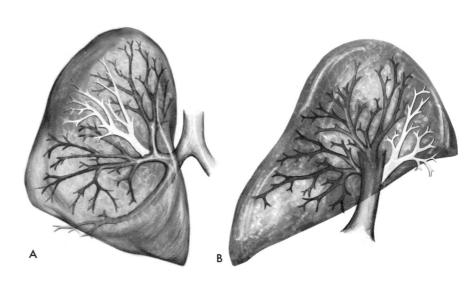

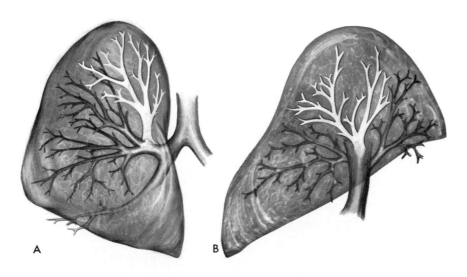

Figure 1–43. Apical Segmental Bronchus, Right Upper Lobe. *A*, Frontal projection; *B*, lateral projection. This bronchus supplies the superior paramediastinal zone, including the lung apex.

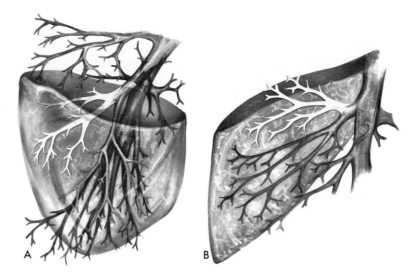

Figure 1–44. Lateral Segmental Bronchus, Right Middle Lobe. *A*, Frontal projection; *B*, lateral projection. This segment extends anterolaterally to supply that portion of the middle lobe that lies contiguous to the minor fissure and the anterior segment of the right upper lobe; its extreme lateral portion abuts against the chief fissure.

lobe bronchus and then bifurcates to become the bronchi to the middle and lower lobes. The middle lobe bronchus arises from the anterolateral wall of the intermediate bronchus, almost opposite the origin of the superior segmental bronchus of the lower lobe; 1 to 2 cm beyond its origin it bifurcates into lateral and medial segments (Figs. 1–44 and 1–45).

RIGHT LOWER LOBE

The first segment originating in the lower lobe, the superior segmental bronchus (Fig. 1–46), arises from the posterior aspect of the lower lobe bronchus immediately beyond its origin; thus, it is almost opposite the takeoff of the middle lobe bronchus. The four basal segments of the lower lobe can be readily identified roentgenologically by applying a few basic principles of anatomy. Reference to Figures 1–47 to 1–50 shows that in the frontal projection of a well-filled bronchogram, the order of the basal bronchi from the lateral to the medial aspect of the hemithorax is *anterior-lateral-posterior-medial*. As the patient is rotated into 45° oblique and lateral

projections, the relationship anterior-lateral-posterior is maintained; hence the mnemonic "ALP," which has been employed advantageously by Nelson.[251] As he pointed out, the relationship of one basal bronchus to another is easily recognized by use of the ALP designation, the medial basal segment being projected between the lateral and posterior segments in the 45° oblique projection and between the anterior and lateral segments in the lateral projection.

LEFT UPPER LOBE

About 1 cm beyond its origin from the anterolateral aspect of the main bronchus, the bronchus to the left upper lobe either bifurcates or trifurcates, usually the former. In the bifurcation pattern, the upper division almost immediately divides again into two segmental branches, the apical posterior and anterior (Figs. 1–51 and 1–52). The lower division is the lingular bronchus, which is roughly analogous to the middle lobe bronchus of the right lung. When trifurcation of the left upper lobe

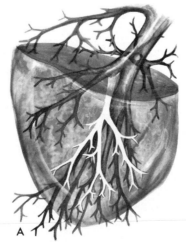
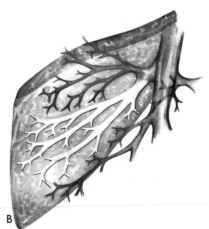

Figure 1–45. Medial Segmental Bronchus, Right Middle Lobe. *A*, Frontal projection; *B*, lateral projection. This bronchus extends anteromedially to supply the portion of the middle lobe that is contiguous to the heart and to the lower portion of the chief fissure.

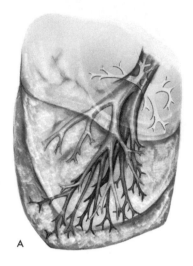
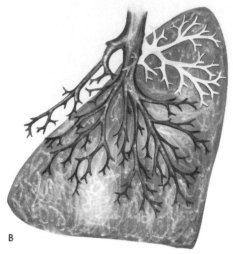

Figure 1–46. Superior Segmental Bronchus, Right Lower Lobe. *A*, Frontal projection; *B*, lateral projection. Usually this bronchus has three subsegments that extend superiorly, laterally, and inferiorly to supply the apical region of the lower lobe.

Figure 1–47. Medial Basal Bronchus, Right Lower Lobe. *A*, Frontal projection; *B*, lateral projection. This is the first branch of the lower lobe bronchus beyond the superior segmental bronchus; it is the smallest of the basal segments and the most medial in frontal projection. It arises from the medial aspect of the lower lobe bronchus to supply the anteromedial portion of the lower lobe contiguous to the posterior portion of the heart and the lower end of the chief fissure.

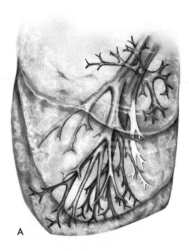
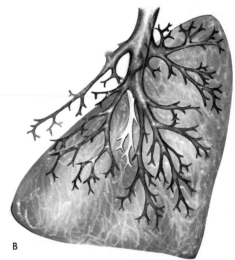

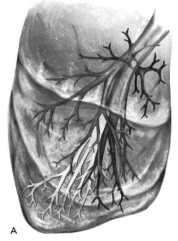
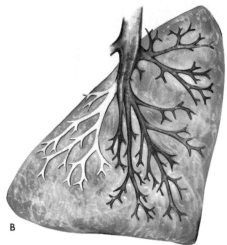

Figure 1–48. Anterior Basal Bronchus, Right Lower Lobe. *A,* Frontal projection; *B,* lateral projection. This bronchus is the most lateral of the basal bronchi, extending anterolaterally into the costophrenic sulcus.

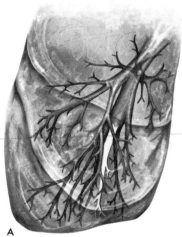
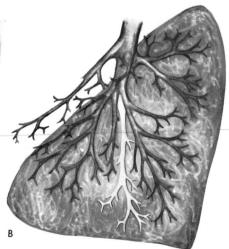

Figure 1–49. Lateral Basal Bronchus, Right Lower Lobe. *A,* Frontal projection; *B,* lateral projection. In frontal projection, this bronchus is projected just medial to the anterior basal bronchus; it extends laterally and slightly posteriorly to supply the portion of the lower lobe that lies behind the anterior basal bronchopulmonary segment. Neither the anterior nor the lateral bronchopulmonary segments relate to the major fissure, being separated from it by the medial segment.

Figure 1–50. Posterior Basal Bronchus, Right Lower Lobe. *A,* Frontal projection; *B,* lateral projection. In frontal projection this bronchus appears between the lateral and medial basal bronchi; it supplies the posteroinferior portion of the lower lobe and extends into the posterior costophrenic gutter.

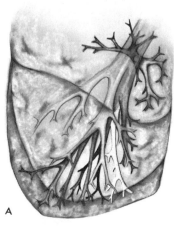
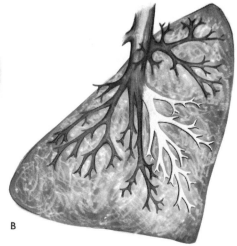

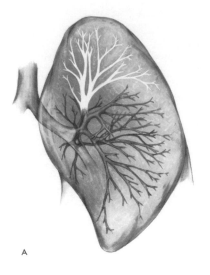

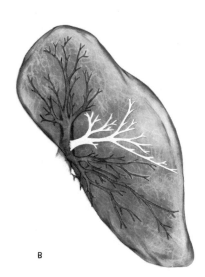

Figure 1–51. Apical Posterior Bronchus, Left Upper Lobe. *A,* Frontal projection; *B,* lateral projection. This bronchus bifurcates into apical and posterior segments that supply areas of the left upper lobe in a pattern similar to that of corresponding bronchi in the right upper lobe.

A   B

Figure 1–52. Anterior Segmental Bronchus, Left Upper Lobe. *A,* Frontal projection; *B,* lateral projection. The distribution is the same as in the right upper lobe.

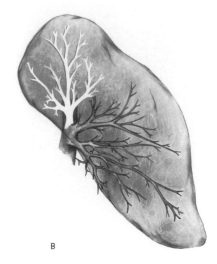

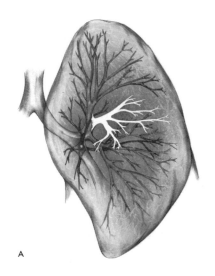

A   B

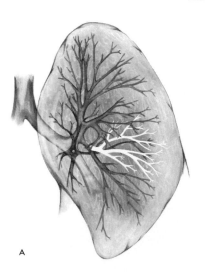

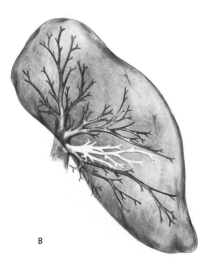

Figure 1–53. Superior Segmental Bronchus, Lingula. *A,* Frontal projection; *B,* lateral projection. This bronchus supplies the anterolateral portion of the lingula.

A   B

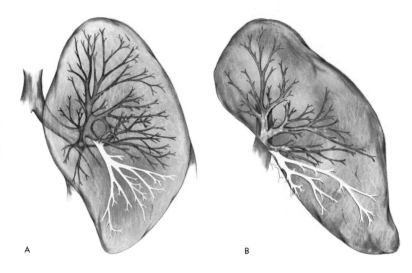

Figure 1–54. Inferior Segmental Bronchus, Lingula. *A*, Frontal projection; *B*, lateral projection. This segment supplies the inferomedial portion of the lingula contiguous to the left border of the heart. The lingula is somewhat larger in volume than the middle lobe of the right lung.

bronchus occurs, the apical posterior, anterior, and lingular bronchi originate simultaneously.

The lingular bronchus extends anteroinferiorly for 2 to 3 cm before bifurcating into superior and inferior divisions (Figs. 1–53 and 1–54).

LEFT LOWER LOBE

With one exception, the divisions of the left lower lobe bronchus are identical in name and anatomic distribution to those of the right lower lobe (Figs. 1–55 to 1–58). The exception lies in the absence of a separate medial basal bronchus, the anterior and medial portions of the lobe being supplied by a single anteromedial bronchus, although Boyden[232] prefers to designate two separate basal bronchi, the anterior and medial, as on the right side. The mnemonic ALP applies as well to the left lower lobe as to the right for identification of the order of basilar bronchi and their relationship to one another in frontal, oblique, and lateral projections.

The anatomy of the proximal airways as depicted on computed tomography is described in detail in the section on the pulmonary hila (*see* page 118).

FUNCTION OF THE AIRWAYS

PULMONARY VENTILATION

The purpose of respiration is to supply oxygen for the metabolic needs of cells and to remove carbon dioxide, one of the waste products of cellular metabolism. In the unicellular organism this is achieved simply by diffusion of these gases across the cell membrane; in humans, although the basic purpose is the same, a much more complex mechanism is necessary. To bring oxygen from the atmosphere into contact with the cell membrane requires not only passage of the air down a long system of branching tubes but also an additional means of transport to convey oxygen to even the most distant cells. This process utilizes two areas of diffusion, one in which oxygen is taken up by blood in pulmonary capillaries, and the other in which oxygen arrives at the tissue membrane. The elimi-

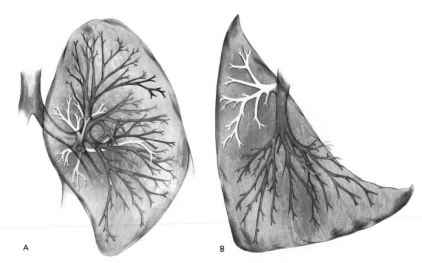

Figure 1–55. Superior Segmental Bronchus, Left Lower Lobe. *A*, Frontal projection; *B*, lateral projection. The distribution of this segment is similar to that of the corresponding segment of the right lower lobe.

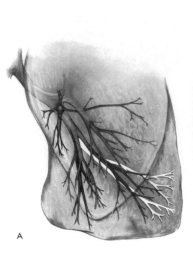

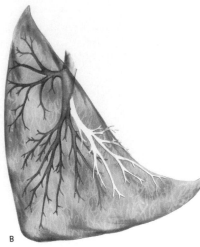

Figure 1–56. Anterior Basal Bronchus, Left Lower Lobe. *A*, Frontal projection; *B*, lateral projection. Distribution is similar to that of the corresponding segment of the right lower lobe. *See* text regarding medial basal bronchus.

Figure 1–57. Lateral Basal Bronchus, Left Lower Lobe. *A*, Frontal projection; *B*, lateral projection. Distribution is similar to that of the corresponding segment of the right lower lobe.

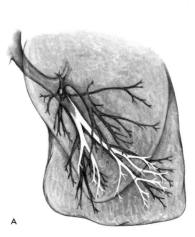

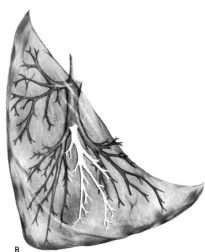

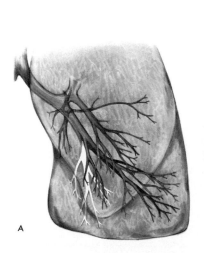

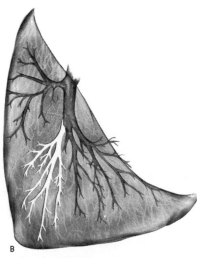

Figure 1–58. Posterior Basal Bronchus, Left Lower Lobe. *A*, Frontal projection; *B*, lateral projection. Distribution is similar to that of the corresponding segment of the right lower lobe.

nation of carbon dioxide is accomplished by the same procedure in reverse: diffusion from tissues into blood, and then conveyance to lung capillaries, where the gas diffuses from liquid to gas phase and moves up the tubular conducting system and is exhaled.

Normal lung function requires the provision at the alveoli of sufficient oxygen to satisfy the demands of the tissues and sufficient movement of gas in the tracheobronchial tree to eliminate carbon dioxide brought to the alveoli. The needs of the tissues for oxygen—and consequently, the quantity of carbon dioxide eliminated—vary considerably, owing mainly to muscle activity. At rest, the oxygen requirement may be 200 to 250 ml per min, whereas during maximal exercise it may increase to 20 times this amount. To satisfy this variation in oxygen need under normal circumstances, a similar increase in volume of ventilation is necessary. This is accomplished by stimuli from various sources, the origin depending upon the circumstances of the need: oxygen lack, carbon dioxide excess in the blood, nervous reflexes from the lungs themselves, chemoreceptors in blood vessels, and other reflexes from somatic and visceral tissues, including the cerebral cortex, act directly or indirectly on the respiratory center to induce movement of the diaphragm and intercostal muscles and, thus, an appropriate increase in ventilation. It follows that this increase in ventilation to satisfy the need for oxygen will be to no avail if there is not a parallel increase in circulating blood through the lungs to carry oxygen to the tissues. Accordingly, rate and stroke volume increase and, for example, during exercise, raise the cardiac output from, say, 5 liters per min to 25 to 30 liters per min.

Keeping in mind the chemical, nervous, and mechanical stimuli that act directly or indirectly on the respiratory center, cardiac muscle, airways, and pulmonary vessels and that vary the quantity of ventilation and perfusion of blood to the acinar unit, let us focus our attention on this unit, since it is here that the lung fulfills its role in respiration. To do this we shall consider (1) alveolar gas and its composition, (2) the mechanism by which this gas is moved in and out of the acinus, (3) perfusion of the acinus, (4) the process of diffusion of gas in the acinar unit and across the alveolocapillary membrane to red blood cells, (5) the matching of blood flow with ventilation in the acinar unit, and the end result of these processes, (6) blood gases and H ion concentration.

The Composition of Gas in Alveoli

The composition of this gas depends upon the rate and amount of oxygen removed and carbon dioxide added by capillary blood (which, in turn, depends upon aerobic metabolism of tissues) and the quantity and quality of the gas that reaches the acinus through the tracheobronchial tree.

VENTILATION OF THE ACINUS

Air contains approximately 21 per cent oxygen and 79 per cent nitrogen and at sea level has an atmospheric pressure of 760 mm Hg; the amount of carbon dioxide and other gases is negligible and can be disregarded. The partial pressures of these gases are approximately 159 mm Hg for oxygen ($PO_2 = 21/100 \times 760$) and 601 mm Hg for nitrogen ($PN_2 = 79/100 \times 760$). As air is inhaled into the tracheobronchial tree, it becomes fully saturated with water vapor at body temperature and a partial pressure of 47 mm Hg, so that the partial pressure of oxygen drops to 149 mm Hg ($[760 - 47] \times 21/100$). At sea level, therefore, the ventilation of alveoli depends upon the quantity of gas containing oxygen, at a PO_2 of 149 mm Hg, that the thoracic "bellows" moves per minute into the acinus.

The quantity of gas reaching the alveoli (alveolar ventilation—$\dot{V}A$) depends upon the depth of inspiration (tidal volume—VT), the volume of the conducting airways (the anatomic dead space—VD), and the number of breaths per minute (f).

$$\dot{V}A \ 1/min = (VT - VD) \times f$$

If a subject inhales 450 ml with each breath, has a respiratory dead space of 150 ml, and an f of 15 per min, total minute ventilation ($\dot{V}E$) will be $15 \times 450 = 6750$ ml per min, and alveolar ventilation will be $(450 - 150) \times 15 = 4500$ ml per min. VD ventilation is not considered alveolar ventilation because at the end of the previous expiration the dead space was filled not with atmospheric air but with expired air having a composition equivalent to that in the acinus.

The VA portion of each breath (ΔV) is added to the residual alveolar gas (VO), and rapid diffusive mixing occurs so that gas tensions approach a uniform alveolar concentration. Failure of complete diffusive mixing within the air spaces may occur with acinar enlargement (emphysema) and with a decreased time for mixing; this is termed series inhomogeneity.[252]

The ratios of VD/VT and $\Delta V/VO$ vary in different lung regions (interregional) and between closely adjacent acini (intraregional), even in normal lungs, and the resultant variation in alveolar gas composition is termed parallel inhomogeneity.[252] An additional mechanism that can result in parallel inhomogeneity of alveolar gas concentrations has recently been proposed:[253, 254] diffusive "Pendelluft" at branch points subtending different-sized parallel units within the acinus can be shown by model analysis to result in inhomogeneity despite proportionate and synchronous emptying and filling of units.[253, 254]

ALVEOLAR-CAPILLARY GAS EXCHANGE

In addition to the contribution of ventilation to the composition of gas in the acinus, blood flow in

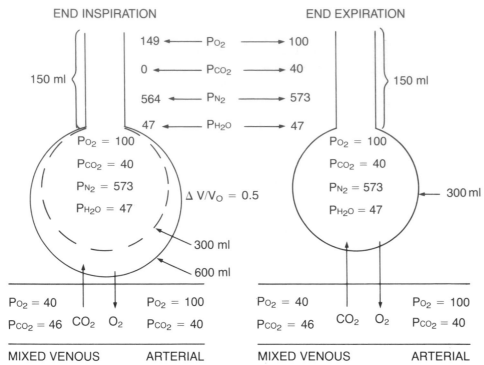

END INSPIRATION

END EXPIRATION

P_{O_2} 149 ← → 100
P_{CO_2} 0 ← → 40
P_{N_2} 564 ← → 573
P_{H_2O} 47 ← → 47

150 ml

$P_{O_2} = 100$
$P_{CO_2} = 40$
$P_{N_2} = 573$
$P_{H_2O} = 47$

$\Delta V/V_O = 0.5$

300 ml
600 ml

$P_{O_2} = 40$ $P_{O_2} = 100$
$P_{CO_2} = 46$ CO₂ O₂ $P_{CO_2} = 40$

MIXED VENOUS   ARTERIAL

150 ml

$P_{O_2} = 100$
$P_{CO_2} = 40$
$P_{N_2} = 573$
$P_{H_2O} = 47$

← 300 ml

$P_{O_2} = 40$ $P_{O_2} = 100$
$P_{CO_2} = 46$ CO₂ O₂ $P_{CO_2} = 40$

MIXED VENOUS   ARTERIAL

Figure 1–59. A Diagram Portraying the Conducting System and Alveolar Space. At the end of an inspiration of 450 ml of air, 150 ml of fresh air (saturated with water vapor) are situated within the conducting system, and the remaining 300 ml have entered and mixed with alveolar gas (*left panel*). At end expiration, the conducting system (dead space) is filled with alveolar air. The ventilation of the lung in this example is given by the $\Delta V/V_O$ ratio of 0.5.

the pulmonary capillaries varies the composition by continuous removal of oxygen and addition of carbon dioxide. The ratio of perfusion to alveolar ventilation ($\dot{V}A/\dot{Q}$) varies within the lung, and the interaction of these two dynamic processes results in fluctuation in alveolar gas tensions not only throughout the respiratory cycle but also from breath to breath, lobe to lobe, and even acinus to acinus (*see* $\dot{V}A/\dot{Q}$ mismatch, page 136). In our hypothetic example, if perfusion is matched evenly with ventilation ($\dot{V}A = 300$ ml per breath and $\dot{Q} = 300$ ml over the same time period), alveolar and mixed venous and arterial gas tensions will reach steady state values (Fig. 1–59). With normal resting mixed venous gas tensions, every 100 ml of blood delivers to the alveolar gas approximately 5.6 ml of CO_2 and at the same time carries away from it 7 ml of O_2. Thus, added to and removed from the 300 ml of fresh gas delivered to the unit by alveolar ventilation is 16.8 ml of CO_2 (5.6 × 3) and 21 ml of O_2 (7 × 3). Therefore, the partial pressure of carbon dioxide in the acinus is 40 mm Hg (16.5/300 × 713). The removal of O_2 decreases the fractional concentration from 21 to 14 per cent, giving a P_{O_2} of 100 mm Hg (42/300 × 713).

MECHANICS OF ACINAR VENTILATION

The movement of atmospheric air down the conducting system to the acinar unit requires force, measured as pressure (P), to overcome the elastic recoil of the lung parenchyma and chest wall (Pel), the frictional resistance of pulmonary tissues and chest wall, the frictional resistance to airflow through the tracheobronchial tree (P_{Fr}), and the

inertia of the gas. Since air has very little mass, the inertial component of the equation is negligible with normal breathing frequencies; the elastic recoil of the lung and chest wall and the frictional resistance to air flow in the tracheobronchial tree represent the major portion of the work of breathing and are chiefly affected in lung disease.[255]

The force necessary to inflate the lung is provided by contraction of the inspiratory muscles, mainly the diaphragm, to a lesser extent the external intercostal muscles, and in circumstances requiring greatly increased ventilation, the accessory respiratory muscles (*see* page 268). Normally, expiration is a passive phenomenon associated with relaxation of the inspiratory muscles; in fact, inspiratory muscle electrical activity may extend well into expiration to "brake" expiratory flow, especially during hyperinflation.[256]

In patients with obstructive airway disease and in normal subjects during periods of increased ventilation produced by exercise or CO_2 rebreathing, expiratory muscles, especially the abdominals, may be recruited.

ELASTIC RECOIL OF LUNG PARENCHYMA AND THORACIC CAGE

The static pressure-volume relationships of the lung and thoracic cage are depicted pictorially and graphically in Figure 1–60. At FRC (functional residual capacity), the chest wall recoils outward, exerting a force that is equal and opposite to the force exerted by the lung recoiling inward. These balanced forces result in a negative pleural pressure of approximately 4 to 5 cm H_2O. FRC is therefore

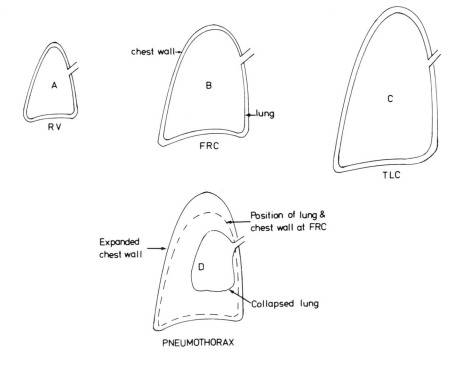

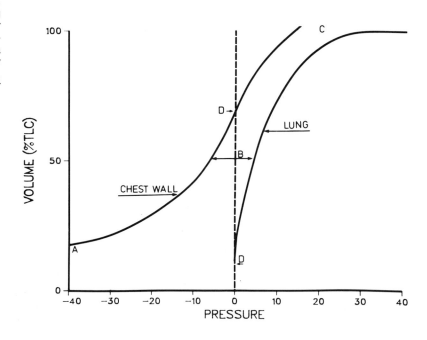

Figure 1–60. The Static Pressure/ Volume Relationships of the Lung and Chest Wall (illustrated schematically and graphically). In the lower panel, lung and chest wall volumes are plotted against pressure. Transpulmonary pressure (pleural pressure–alveolar pressure) is the appropriate pressure for the lung whereas transthoracic pressure (pleural pressure–atmospheric pressure) is the appropriate pressure for the chest wall. In the upper panel, drawing *B* shows the relationship of lung and chest wall at FRC; point *B* below shows that, at FRC, the transpulmonary and transthoracic pressures are equal and opposite in sign. At RV (*A* above and below), transpulmonary pressure is near zero as the lung deflates toward its resting position while the transthoracic pressure is very negative since the chest wall becomes stiffer at low lung volumes. At TLC (*C* above and below), both the lung and chest wall are expanded beyond their resting position and both exert recoil favoring deflation. With development of a complete pneumothorax, transpulmonary and transthoracic pressure become zero, and the lung and chest wall assume their unstressed and relaxed positions (*D*).

determined by the balance of static recoil forces exerted by the lung and chest wall. On inspiration the respiratory muscles act initially to overcome the elastic recoil of the lungs only; the chest wall and thoracic cage actually aid inflation by their outward recoil until a volume of about 70 per cent TLC (total lung capacity) is reached, at which point the chest wall is inflated beyond its resting position and the force of muscle contraction is then exerted against the recoil of both lung and chest wall. TLC is reached when the inspiratory forces achieved by the muscles is equaled by the combined recoil force of lung and chest wall. It is apparent from Figure 1–60 that as lung volume increases, the elastic recoil of the lung parenchyma increases in a nonlinear fashion.

During deflation of the lung from FRC toward RV (residual volume), the expiratory muscles are aided by the elastic recoil of the lung until its resting volume is reached. The chest wall curve becomes progressively nonlinear near RV as the chest wall becomes more difficult to distort; RV is finally set at the point at which outward recoil of the chest wall equals the force exerted by the expiratory muscles. In older subjects this point may not be reached, however, since the airways may narrow and limit expiration at higher lung volumes.[257, 817] In diseased lungs, RV may be determined by airway closure.

When air is introduced into the pleural space, the visceral and parietal pleura separate, and the lung and chest wall move along their respective pressure/volume curves, each assuming its resting volume (points D and D_1 in Figure 1–60).

The relationship between volume and pressure (V/P) is compliance, which can be calculated for lung and chest wall either separately or together (respiratory system compliance). In normal subjects, the compliance of the respiratory system is the major determinant of the work of breathing; in disease states, work of breathing can be altered by increases or decreases in the compliance of the lung or chest wall (Fig. 1–61).

During periods of no inspiratory or expiratory flow, the relationship between pressure and volume represents the static elastic properties of the lung and chest wall, but during flow extra pressure must be exerted to overcome flow resistance. This pressure is measurable, since it is reflected in the degree of change in intrapleural pressure. Measurement is made directly or, more conveniently, by use of an intraesophageal balloon that reflects changes in intrapleural pressure. As the normal lung becomes more inflated it becomes less compliant; for this reason it is more informative to express compliance as the change in intrapleural pressure required to produce a volume change at a specific degree of lung inflation, usually functional residual capacity (FRC). Interstitial edema, fibrosis, or cellular infiltration render the lungs stiffer and less compliant, so that more pressure is required to move a given

volume of gas; or, to put it differently, a given pressure moves a smaller volume. When the elastic architecture of the lung is faulty, as in emphysema, a given pressure may actually produce a greater volume change than in the normal lung; in such a case compliance is increased.

"Elastic" recoil of the lung has been attributed in part to the peculiar arrangement of collagenous and elastic fibers.[258, 259] The helical structure of this fibrous network gives the lungs an elastic behavior similar to that of a coil spring. However, tissue elasticity is not the only component of the elastic recoil of the lungs. This was first indicated by the work of von Neergaard[260] in 1929, who measured the pressure-volume relationships of a fluid-distended lung and an air-distended lung and found less elastic recoil in the former. Less pressure change was required to fully distend the fluid-filled lung than the air-filled lung. Von Neergaard deduced that a surface tension, a force that tended to contract alveolar spaces and to resist expansion, existed in each alveolus between its lining and its gas content. He suggested that this surface tension accounted for most of the lung's elastic recoil and that it was eliminated when gas was replaced by liquid.

SURFACE TENSION AND SURFACTANT

Macklin[261] also recognized the need for a substance to regulate "surface tension" in the alveoli and surmised that it was secreted by a large alveolar epithelial cell, which he called a "granular pneumocyte." Various anatomic methods have been employed to demonstrate this lining layer, but it is probable that at least some of these attempts have resulted in artifacts caused by staining of a mucopolysaccharide-containing cell coat, or to protein leakage into the alveoli during tissue preparation.[262, 263] More recent work employing rapid tissue freezing, perfusion-fixation through the vascular system, and immersion-fixation of subpleural alveoli, along with technical improvement in electron microscopy, has permitted definite identification of an osmiophilic 4.2-nm lining in all mammalian species studied, including humans (Fig. 1–62).[186, 219, 264-268] In contrast to their polyhedral or pentagonal shape after conventional methods of tissue preparation, the alveoli appear spherical after rapid freezing, when fixed by vascular perfusion, or when viewed through the pleura of living animals. The common denominator of the three methods of inspection is the presence of air in the alveoli, which molds macrophages, epithelium, capillaries, and alveolar lining fluid into a continuous curved surface that probably represents the configuration consistent with the lowest surface energy.[269] When the alveolar spaces are filled with fluid fixative, surface forces are eliminated and alveolar topography becomes dependent upon tissue and hemodynamic factors.

According to Gil and Weibel,[219] the acellular

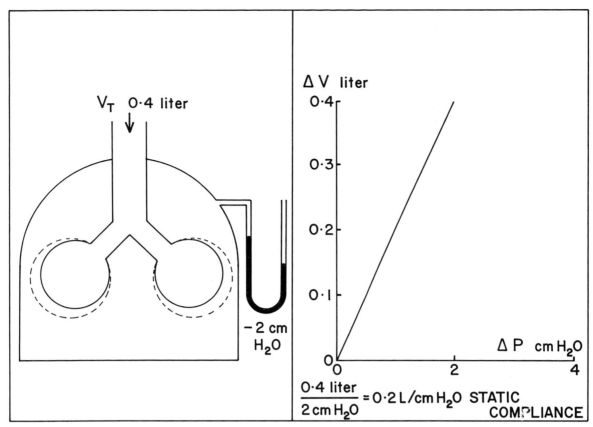

Figure 1–61. Pressure-Volume Relationships. A change of 2 cm H_2O in pleural pressure (ΔP) results in a volume change (ΔV) of 0.4 liter of tidal air (V_T) in two hypothetic acini. The diagram on the right depicts the change in volume of 0.4 liter and the change in pressure of 2 cm H_2O. The static compliance in this example is 0.2 liter/cm H_2O.

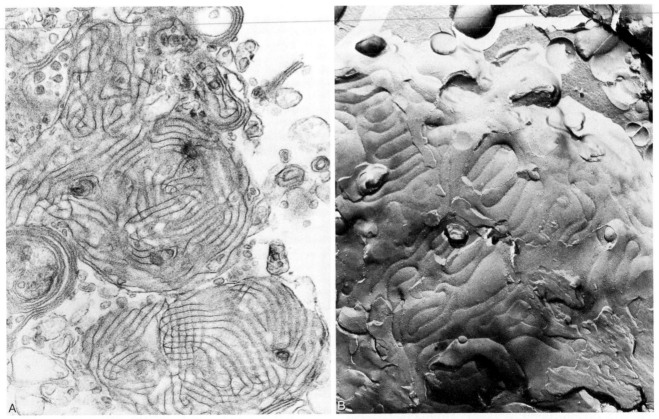

Figure 1–62. Surfactant. A, Transmission electron micrograph of free alveolar surfactant showing tubular myelin figures. B, Free surfactant within the alveolar space using the freeze etching method. (Courtesy of Dr. David Walker, University of British Columbia, Vancouver.)

layer covering the alveolar surface consists of two functionally different components: (1) a film facing the alveolar air space, which is composed of densely spaced, highly surface-active phospholipids, and (2) deep to this film, a layer containing surface-active phospholipids in a different physicochemical configuration, linked to proteins. This deep layer, known as the "base layer" of the surface lining material, represents the hypophase described by the physiologist[270] (see Fig. 1–25, page 25). Components of the superficial layer are thought to be recruited from the deeper hypophase during expansion of the lung and may re-enter the base layer at low lung volumes. The hypophase contains aggregates of lipid in the form of vesicles, lamellae, and lattice-like arrangements that are termed *tubular myelin figures*. The lipids in the hypophase include (a) newly secreted lamellar bodies *en route* to the surface film, (b) lipid molecules that have temporarily entered the hypophase from the surface film as the surface area of the alveoli reduces, and (c) aggregates of lipid and protein that are going to be removed by alveolar macrophages.[271] Most pores of Kohn are filled with extracellular material that appears to be supplied from the base layer (see Fig. 1–33).[272] The tubular myelin figures are particularly evident in the thickest portions of the hypophase and on section exhibit a characteristic fingerprint-like pattern (see Fig. 1–25, page 25); this material is believed to be a degeneration or breakdown product of lung surfactant.

The composition of the pulmonary surface-active material was first identified in 1961 by Klaus and associates,[273] who concluded that the main component of the alveolar phospholipid was dipalmitoyl phosphatidylcholine (DPPC), also known as dipalmitoyl lecithin (DPL). Phospholipids make up 90 per cent of the surfactant material, 45 per cent being saturated and 25 per cent unsaturated phosphatidylcholine; phosphatidylglycerol contributes 5 per cent, phosphatidylethanolamine 3 per cent, and neutral lipids 10 per cent. In some species, phosphatidylglycerol is not present at birth but appears within the first hour or day of life and is a marker of maturity; however, this substance is probably not absolutely necessary for surface-active properties. Surfactant is secreted with protein as a large-molecular-weight complex. Two specific surfactant proteins have been identified, apoprotein A with a molecular weight of 10,000 daltons and apoprotein B with a molecular weight of 34,000 to 35,000 daltons. Apoprotein B is secreted by type II cells with the same time course as dipalmotyl phosphatidylcholine (DPPC), but apoprotein A appears later and possibly is not secreted by type II cells. The lamellar bodies themselves do not contain apoprotein so that inhibition of protein synthesis by type II cells does not result in inhibition of DPPC secretion.[271, 274] Apoprotein B forms complexes whose molecular weight is greater than 400,000 daltons; immunoperoxidase staining has shown that this protein is specific to type II alveolar cells.[275] Although pure phospholipid and the complex of apoprotein and phospholipids have similar capabilities for lowering surface tension, the lipoprotein complex absorbs and spreads much more readily over the air-liquid interface and is probably necessary for efficient function; this quality possibly explains the greater efficacy of naturally occurring surfactants that has been observed in recent studies of exogenous replacement therapy (see subsequent discussion).[274, 276]

Electron microscopic and radioautographic studies have provided much evidence linking osmiophilic inclusion bodies of the granular pneumocyte with surfactant.[275] There is now overwhelming evidence that the type II granular pneumocyte is the site of synthesis and storage of pulmonary surfactant.[271] Type II cells are dispersed singly throughout the alveolar lining, and although they make up 14 per cent of peripheral lung cells in normal lung, they cover only about 3 per cent of the alveolar surface. The phospholipids are synthesized within the endoplasmic reticulum of type II cells and are formed into the storage or lamellar bodies in the Golgi–endoplasmic reticulum complex. They are discharged into the extracellular medium by the classic secretory exocytosis process that involves the microtubules; this process can be blocked by anticytochalasin B, a drug that disrupts filamentous actin.[271, 277] The kinetics of apoprotein secretion and the mechanism by which protein and phospholipid interact are as yet incompletely understood.[271]

The synthesis of DPPC in type II cells can be accomplished by two independent pathways: a "*de novo*" synthesis pathway that involves direct synthesis from dipalmitoyl diglyceride and cytidine-diphosphate-choline, and a "de- and reacetylation" or "remodeling" pathway that represents conversion of unsaturated phosphatidylcholine molecules to DPPC through acetylation of 1-palmitoyl, 2-lysophosphatidylcholine by palmitoyl-coenzyme A. It is likely that the contribution of each pathway can vary depending on substrate availability.[271]

Studies on 11 vertebrate species have shown that the amounts of surfactant and of saturated phosphatidylcholine in the lung are related to alveolar surface area.[278]

The ultimate metabolic fate of secreted surfactant is poorly understood. Very little passes up the airways. Some surface lipids are taken up by alveolar macrophages and enter into the pinocytotic vesicles of type I cells, and some find their way back into type II cells where they are presumably reutilized.[192, 271, 274] Surfactant secretion is under complex neural, humeral, and chemical control. Changes in phospholipid secretion during the perinatal period are of specific interest with respect to the development of the respiratory distress syndrome.

Surfactant has a very rapid rate of turnover: in studies with dipalmitoyl lecithin labeled with radioactive palmitic acid, its half-life in normal adults has been reported as ranging from 14 hours[186] to somewhat less than 2 days.[279] It has been known for some time through chemical analysis of lipids that the concentration of surfactant is higher in the neonate than in the adult;[280, 281] the rate of phospholipid synthesis reaches a peak at term and right after birth, declining rapidly to normal adult levels shortly thereafter.[282, 283] As pointed out by Avery,[284] pulmonary surfactant must be present at the moment of birth; otherwise every breath necessarily would resemble the first breath. Pulmonary surfactant allows for creation of a functional residual capacity.

The burst of phospholipid synthesis shortly before birth is associated with the rapid appearance of phosphatidylglycerol in the amniotic fluid and an increase above 2.0 in the ratio of lethicin to sphingomyelin. Both these measurements have proved invaluable in the assessment of fetal lung maturation and the likelihood of the development of the neonatal respiratory distress syndrome.[285, 286] Acceleration of lung maturation with stimulation of type II cells and the production of a mature pattern of phospholipid secretion can be produced by the administration of corticosteroids to the fetus or mother; such corticosteroid therapy may act by stimulating a fibroblast-derived peptide factor rather than by direct stimulation of the alveolar epithelium. There is evidence that thyroxine, estrogens, beta-adrenergic agonists, and other pharmacologic agents, including heroin, can stimulate maturation of the surfactant system; by contrast, insulin, phenobarbital, and metyrapone may retard fetal lung maturation.[271, 287] Beta-adrenergic and cholinergic agonists increase surfactant secretion. In adult animals,[271, 277, 288, 289] both beta-adrenergic and cholinergic stimulation can be demonstrated *in vivo* although the latter is not demonstrable with isolated type II cells; the *in vivo* cholinergic stimulation is attenuated by beta-blockers or indomethacin, suggesting that the cholinergic effect acts through the beta-adrenergic or prostaglandin system.[289]

Surfactant production in the lung is stimulated by an increase in ventilation and by an increase in tidal volume, an effect that has been demonstrated in animals by measurement of phospholipids[288] and by morphologic evidence of a decrease in lamellar body density and identifiable type II cells.[290] Breathing at low lung volumes results not only in decreased surfactant secretion but also in altered function as a result of diminished alveolar stability and the accumulation of large phospholipid aggregates; the formation of these aggregates is diminished by a deep breath.[291] The ventilation and sigh-induced secretion of phospholipids appears to be mediated through the beta-adrenergic system since this mechanical stimulatory effect can be blocked by propranolol.[288, 292] Vagotomy has been reported to alter surface-active properties in rat lungs.[293]

The function of surfactant includes prevention of alveolar collapse, decrease in the work of breathing, an anti-sticking action that prevents adherence of alveolar walls, and an anti-wetting action that may aid in keeping the alveolar lining layer dry.[274, 294] The forces that tend to decrease alveolar size are surface tension and tissue elasticity. The force generated by tissue elasticity is roughly proportional to lung volume but constitutes only one third of the total lung elastic recoil at total lung capacity. The pressure due to surface factors can be calculated from the Young-Laplace relationship: $P - \gamma = 2\gamma/r$, where γ is the surface tension of the alveolar air-liquid interface and r is the alveolar radius. Opposed to the lung elastic recoil and surface tension forces that tend to collapse alveoli is the transpulmonary pressure. Mechanical balance is achieved when the transpulmonary pressure equals the pressures generated by elastic recoil and surface tension. With lung deflation, transpulmonary pressure decreases at the same time that alveolar radius is decreasing, a situation that favors alveolar collapse. This is why a substance with the surface tension-lowering ability of surfactant is necessary to achieve alveolar stability.[274]

The second major role of surfactant is to decrease the work of breathing. The compliance of a lung with deficient or denatured surfactant is considerably reduced and the pressures necessary to achieve tidal ventilation are increased.[274] Surfactant's potential role in reducing adhesion between alveolar walls where they come in contact has not been experimentally evaluated.[274]

The reduction in surface tension imparted by surfactant may have an important role in fluid balance in the lung, distinct from its role in the mechanics of breathing. The reduced surface tension counteracts the tendency for fluid to be sucked into alveolar spaces from the capillary lumen.[295] The mechanism by which surfactant acts to decrease the driving force for the development of pulmonary edema is related to its ability to lower surface tension: since the pressure drop across a curved interface is proportional to the surface tension and inversely proportional to the radius of curvature, by decreasing surface tension lung surfactant decreases the pressure drop across the alveolar-interstitial compartment and leads to less-negative tissue pressures.[296] An additional anti-wetting function has been proposed by Hills, who has suggested that the strong hydrophobic nature of cationic surfactants induces a nonwettable alveolar surface that further aids in decreasing transepithelial fluid movement.[297, 298] Surface-active phospholipids have also been found in the pleural space where they presumably act as lubricants to facilitate pleural surface movement; the site of origin of the pleural surfactants has not been identified.[299]

In addition to the well-known mechanical functions of surfactant there is some evidence that the alveolar lining layer has other roles to play. For example, it has been reported to contain a protective factor that inhibits the lysis of alveolar macrophages; *in vitro* studies on rabbits have suggested that dipalmitoyl lecithin has a similar protective action.[300] Many environmental stresses, such as ozone, may exert their effects by inhibiting the protective factor; the resulting lysis of alveolar macrophages would destroy this defense mechanism against inhaled microorganisms and particulate matter.[300] This same mechanism may explain a property in alveolar lining material that aids the bactericidal activity of alveolar macrophages against *Staphylococcus aureus*.[301, 302] Lung lining material also aids alveolar macrophage migration and has been shown to be chemotactic for alveolar macrophages, a factor that could aid in their clearance from the air spaces up the mucociliary escalator.[303]

Disorders of surfactant metabolism are important in a number of disease states, including the respiratory distress syndrome (RDS) of the neonate (formerly termed hyaline membrane disease), pulmonary thromboembolism, adult respiratory distress syndrome (ARDS), alveolar proteinosis, oxygen toxicity, and atelectasis.[304] A disease in which deficient and ineffective surfactant plays a key and primary role is neonatal respiratory distress syndrome. Although the great majority of infants who develop this syndrome have phospholipid profiles on lung lavage or amniotic fluid analysis that accurately predict the immaturity of the lung, a recent study has suggested that in some, the syndrome may result from the presence of a protein inhibitor of surfactant function whose nature is as yet unidentified: in a study of 72 patients with RDS, Kankaanpaa and Hallman[305] identified 3 with a normal phospholipid profile but with a lung aspirate that showed a protein substance which inhibited the surface activity of lung effluent from normal neonates, suggesting the presence of a surfactant inhibitor. The role of altered surfactant metabolism and function in ARDS is less clear. Petty and his associates[306] examined pressure-volume curves and lung lavage fluid from the lungs of six patients who died from ARDS and compared the results with similar data from relatively normal lungs of patients who died of other causes: in the former group, the pressure-volume curves were shifted downward and to the right when volume was expressed as per cent predicted and per cent observed, and although the surface tension-lowering ability of the alveolar wash was preserved, the surface compressibility (an expression of the resistance of the surface film to compression) was increased.

In ARDS, the altered surfactant function is probably secondary to the basic insult, with exudation of protein-rich fluid into the alveolar air spaces. However, in the large study carried out by Hallman and colleagues,[307] it was suggested that a specific defect in phospholipid synthesis similar to that seen in the neonatal form of the disease may be present. These researchers obtained alveolar lavage fluid from 36 patients with ARDS and compared phospholipid profiles and surface activity with the lavage fluid from 128 patients with other respiratory diseases and from 12 healthy controls: they found that the lavage fluid from the patients with ARDS had lower lethicin-to-sphingomyelin ratios and a decreased content of phosphatidylglycerol; in addition, the lavage fluid showed poor surface-active characteristics. An alteration in surfactant almost certainly plays a role in the atelectasis associated with pulmonary thromboembolism:[304] ligation of either the right or left pulmonary artery results in a reduction in lung volume and a decrease in surface activity of the alveolar lavage fluid on the affected side. Although *acute* pulmonary artery occlusion actually stimulates surfactant secretion and transiently increases the pool size of alveolar surfactant on the affected side, prolonged occlusion presumably leads to depletion.[308]

In the dog, a lobe rendered atelectatic by bronchial ligation will show abnormalities of surface-active material within 24 hours;[309] re-expansion of the lobe up to 24 hours after ligation will restore surface-active properties to normal, but after that time the surface activity remains abnormal in both collapsed and re-expanded lobes. Oxygen toxicity also disrupts the surfactant system, both in susceptible animals[310, 311] and in humans; for example, two studies have indicated that lung compliance decreases after exposure to 100 per cent inspired oxygen in humans.[312, 313] However, a study of patients following open heart surgery indicated no alteration in pulmonary function.[314] Experimental studies in dogs with cardiopulmonary bypass showed a decrease in lung compliance, thought to be caused by atelectasis. Although light microscopy revealed no consistent differences in the number of granular pneumocytes in bypass and sham-operated dogs, inclusions in the type II cells were decreased in the former, suggesting early evidence of surfactant loss.[315, 316] The reports on effects on surfactant of lung reimplantation in dogs are conflicting, decreased surfactant having been reported in one study[317] and normal surfactant and lung stability in other similar experiments.[318] In the latter studies, total lung compliance decreased immediately after the procedure but returned to normal within 8 days.

Although the major clinical interest in surfactant relates to its underproduction and the resultant respiratory distress syndrome, the focus of attention has been extended by the finding that alveolar proteinosis is related to overproduction of osmiophilic material by the type II alveolar cells or the formation of an amount exceeding the capacity of the lungs to remove it.[319] Describing a surfactant inhibitor found in lung washings from patients with alveolar proteinosis, Kuhn and associates stated that the material had decreased surface activity despite a high content of phosphatidylcholine rich in palmitic acid.[320] Combining the use of antibody directed specifically against the apoprotein of surfactant and immunoperoxidase staining, Singh and associates have shown that the alveolar contents in pulmonary alveolar proteinosis are derived from type II cells and represent surfactant material; they speculate that the disease may be related to decreased macrophage clearance of surfactant debris.[321]

Although the use of positive end expiratory pressure has improved survival in infants with RDS and although the predictive value of amniotic fluid lecithin-to-sphingomyelin ratios and phosphatidylcholine measurements has made significant impact on mortality, the continued aim of many investigators has been the development of a surfactant replacement. The status of surfactant replacement therapy has recently been reviewed.[296, 322, 323] In both animal studies and the few clinical trials that have been carried out to date, natural surfactants recovered from calf or human amniotic fluid appear to be more effective than highly purified synthetic phospholipids. It is suggested that the 35,000-molecular-weight apoprotein is necessary for proper adsorption of the surfactant material to the alveolar surface and for dynamic spreadability of the surfactant layer from its deposition site in central airways to the alveolar surface.

Besides exhibiting the unique ability to decrease surface tension as lung volume decreases, surfactant imparts hysteresis to the lung's pressure:volume behavior. Thus, at any given lung volume, surface tension and therefore lung elastic recoil are greater during inflation than during deflation. It has recently been suggested that in addition to alteration in surface forces, lung hysteresis is due partly to a different sequence of recruitment and derecruitment of alveoli during inflation and deflation.[324, 325]

RESISTANCE OF THE AIRWAYS

The second major factor in the work of breathing is the force necessary to overcome the frictional resistance to air flow through the tracheobronchial tree. Resistance is the relationship of pressure to flow ($P/\dot{V}$) and can also be expressed as its reciprocal, conductance ($\dot{V}/P$). The pressure necessary to produce laminar flow through a tube is directly related to the length of the tube and the viscosity and flow rate of the gas and inversely related to the tube radius to the 4th power (r^4).

$$\text{Pressure required} \sim \frac{\text{Length} \times \text{Viscosity} \times \text{Flow}}{\text{Radius}^4}$$

It is apparent from this equation that airway radius is the dominant variable in determining resistance; a doubling of airway length would only double the pressure necessary to produce a given flow (i.e., double resistance), whereas a halving of radius would lead to a 16-fold increase in resistance. Under conditions of laminar flow, the flow rate is linearly related to pressure—that is, a doubling of pressure is required for a doubling of flow. However, with the development of turbulence and other nonlaminar flow regimes, the relationship becomes nonlinear such that a greater increase in pressure is required to produce a given increment in flow; in addition, with nonlaminar regimes, gas density begins to play a role, resistance decreasing with gases of low density (e.g., helium and oxygen).

$$\text{Pressure required} \sim \frac{(\text{Length} \times \text{Viscosity} \times \dot{V}) + (\text{Density} \times \dot{V}^2)}{\text{Radius}^4}$$

The importance of the added term depends on the type of flow regime. In normal individuals during quiet breathing through the mouth, the flow regime is almost laminar;[326] however, with breathing through the nose or through narrowed airways and during the increased flow rates of exercise, substantial turbulence may occur, resulting in an increasing proportion of the work of breathing going to overcoming resistance.

It has been shown that in normal subjects during quiet breathing nasal resistance constitutes up to two thirds of total airway resistance; it was found that the pressure/flow curve through the nose as well as across the pharynx, glottis, and larynx was nonlinear, indicating a nonlaminar regime.[327, 328]

As we measure it, total airway resistance represents the contribution of the resistances of the various levels of the airway from larynx and large cartilaginous airways down to respiratory bronchioles, added in series. Considerable confusion existed about the site of major airway resistance until the studies of Macklem and Mead[329] and of Hogg and his associates during the 1960s.[330] Using a retrograde catheter technique, these investigators partitioned the resistance in the airways below the larynx and showed that in normal subjects the majority of resistance is in large airways. The small resistance of smaller airways is related to their large cross-sectional area in the lung periphery. The low linear velocity of flow through peripheral airways also results in a more laminar flow regime whereas turbulent and orifice flow regimes occur in the larger airways and across the larynx. Recent studies of excised human lungs have questioned the original findings of Hogg and Macklem and their associates and have shown significantly higher peripheral resistance in normal lungs.[331] However, there is agreement that in disease the site of increased resistance is the small airways. The larynx also contributes substantially to total airway resistance, and movement of this structure probably accounts for the higher resistance during expiration.[332]

Airway caliber and therefore resistance is not a static phenomenon, being influenced by mechanical factors as well as by complex neurohumeral controls. Both intra- and extrathoracic airways respond to changes in lung volume and transpulmonary pressure, resistance increasing at low lung volume and in some individuals at very high lung volume.[518] A portion of the lung volume effect is reflexly mediated and is attenuated by prior administration of atropine.[518]

In addition to these passive forces that act on the conducting system and cause increase or decrease in resistance, there are active stimuli to both bronchodilation and bronchoconstriction. As discussed in the section dealing with the nerve supply of the lung (see page 154), airway caliber is under reflex control through afferent lung receptors and efferent autonomic cholinergic, adrenergic, and "purinergic" nerves. Local changes in gas tensions, either hypoxia[334] or hypercapnia,[335] can narrow airways; the resultant decrease in ventilation to areas of low PO_2 and high PCO_2 represents a compensatory mechanism that serves to promote a match between ventilation and perfusion; as such, it is analogous to, although less important than, hypoxic vasoconstriction.

In patients with pulmonary disease, increased airway resistance is the commonest cause of increased work of breathing. The processes that narrow airways and increase resistance are both acute and reversible and chronic and irreversible. They include reflex and humorally mediated smooth muscle constriction, degeneration of the supporting structures of both large and small airways, and peripheral airway obstruction by mucous plugging, inflammation, and scarring.

TISSUE RESISTANCE

During flow there is movement of the lungs and chest wall tissue, and, although their major impedance is elastic, they do provide a small amount of frictional resistance. This "tissue resistance" has been estimated to be between 5 and 40 per cent of total pulmonary resistance,[327, 336] but it has been suggested that this may be an overestimate.[329]

Collateral Ventilation

The interlobar drift of air in emphysematous lungs was first noted by Laennec.[337] Collateral air flow between lung units may be important in preserving gas exchange capacity and in matching ventilation and perfusion in the presence of airway obstruction. Acini beyond a completely obstructed airway can be ventilated through collateral channels; the effectiveness of this ventilation in maintaining alveolar gas tension depends on three variables. (1) The tidal volume of the collaterally ventilated space, which is related to the time constant of the space (resistance × compliance) and the respiratory frequency. (2) The completeness of gaseous diffusion between normally and collaterally ventilated units. (3) The gas tensions in the collaterally delivered tidal volume. This last factor critically depends upon the anatomic site of the collateral channels: If the obstructed unit is ventilated via a collateral respiratory bronchiole, the PO_2 will be higher than if collateral ventilation occurred from more distal parenchymal tissue in which inspired air has been in contact with capillaries and has undergone gas exchange.[338]

Recently, the factors that control collateral ventilation and collateral flow resistance have been the subject of a number of investigations that have stemmed largely from a methodology developed by Hilpert for the measurement of collateral flow resistance (Rcoll) in excised and intact lungs.[339, 340] In this method, gas is passed through a catheter that completely obstructs an airway, and the flow rate as well as the pressure within the obstructed segment is measured. The flow passes into the obstructed segment, inflates it, and exits via collateral channels. By relating the pressure to the flow within the obstructed segment, Rcoll can be calculated; then, by suddenly interrupting the flow, the rate of decrease in pressure in the obstructed segment can be used to calculate a time constant for the collateral channels. Woolcock and Macklem were the first to use a method similar to that of Hilpert's for measuring collateral flow resistance.[341] They showed that collateral resistance in the human lung was intermediate between that of the dog, whose collateral resistance is low, and the pig, whose collateral resistant is high—in fact, virtually infinite. In addition they studied the effects of Rcoll on lung volume, lung volume history, and age.

Following these studies performed in the early 1970s, a number of investigators have examined the effects on Rcoll of mechanical factors, pharmacologic agents, and pathologic events.[340] Collateral channels respond to alterations in inspired gas tension;[340] increasing the PCO_2 in inspired gas lowers collateral resistance, whereas the response is opposite with a decrease in inspired PO_2. It is probable that O_2 acts through its effect on the pulmonary vasculature: local hypoxemia will produce vasoconstriction and secondarily a decrease in local alveolar PCO_2 and an increase in Rcoll.

The effect on Rcoll of lung volume has been measured in animals[341] and in normal human volunteers in vivo.[342] Rcoll decreases with lung inflation in a manner similar to the decrease in airway resistance that occurs with lung inflation, and to a comparable degree. In normal lungs, however, collateral flow resistance at FRC is some 50 times greater than resistance to flow through the normal airways.[342] The effects of body position on regional Rcoll have been examined in dogs: Rcoll is increased in dependent lung regions, presumably as a result of the decrease in regional lung volume secondary to the pleural pressure gradient.[343] Collateral flow resistance also varies between lobes: Inners and colleagues found that in normal volunteers Rcoll was some five to six times higher in the middle lobe than in upper or lower lobes, and they hypothesized that this high collateral resistance may be an important factor in the pathophysiology of middle lobe syndrome.[344] Collateral flow resistance is increased after inhalation of an aerosol of histamine, an effect that is not blocked by vagotomy, suggesting a direct effect of histamine rather than a reflex action.[345] However, atropine by inhalation decreases baseline Rcoll, suggesting that there is some vagal influence on resting Rcoll.[340] Collateral flow resistance is also increased with pulmonary vascular congestion and pulmonary edema.[340] Cigarette smoke acutely increases Rcoll in excised dog lungs.[346] Gertner and his associates have shown that cigarette smoke can increase Rcoll in dog lungs *in vivo*, a response that is attenuated with a histamine blocker.[347] Using a similar preparation, these investigators also found that acute exposure of the lung periphery to 1.0 ppm ozone results in a biphasic increase in Rcoll that is partly mediated by a vagal reflex arc and partly by local histamine release.[348] It is interesting that the reflex component of the response diminishes with repeated exposure, in a manner similar to the progressive decline in the human symptomatic and physiologic response to ozone with repeated exposure (*see* further discussion in the chapter on Airways). Exposure to ozone also results in an enhancement in the response to nebulized histamine, reminiscent of the increased nonspecific airway reactivity seen in humans after ozone inhalation.[349]

Collateral flow resistance in the lung probably decreases with age. However, in a small group of normal subjects Terry and associates were unable to show a decreased Rcoll in older normal subjects *in vivo*.[350] In a study of human lungs post mortem, Rosenberg and Lyons were unable to demonstrate any collateral flow in the pediatric age group.[351]

Resistance to air flow through collateral channels is much lower in emphysematous than in normal lungs; in fact, in excised and *in vivo* emphysematous lungs, air flow resistance is much less through collateral channels than through regular conducting airways.[350, 352] This marked drop in collateral air flow resistance with even minor grades of emphysema may result from the formation of alveolar fenestrae secondary to destruction of alveolar walls. Such fenestrae offer less resistance to collateral flow than is provided by the other theoretic channels of collateral ventilation, the alveolar pores, canals of Lambert, or direct airway or acinar anastomoses.[352] Undoubtedly, the obliteration and plugging of multiple small airways in emphysema is largely responsible for the freer movement of air via alveolar fenestrae and collateral channels than via the conducting system itself.

The channels for collateral ventilation in the lung can be thought of as analogous to collateral perfusion channels in vascular beds. They represent an emergency backup system that allows more even distribution of ventilation in the presence of abnormalities in the conducting airways. It is also clear that collateral channels and collateral flow resistance are not passive and solely related to anatomy but are under complex neurohumeral control and are subject to the deleterious effects of cigarette smoke and atmospheric pollutants.

RESPIRATORY MUCUS AND MUCOUS RHEOLOGY

There has been a recent increase in interest in the role of respiratory mucus and mucociliary clearance as pulmonary defense mechanisms.[353-357] Respiratory mucus has three important roles: (1) in mucociliary clearance of particulate matter deposited within the respiratory tract; (2) as an antibacterial substance (respiratory mucus contains immunoglobulins; lactoferrin, which chelates iron necessary for the growth of some bacteria; and lysozyme, which destroys bacteria); and (3) as a humidifier of inspired air and as a preventative of excessive fluid loss from the airway surface by dint of its hydrophilic nature.[356] Mucociliary clearance is a complex function of the respiratory tract that involves interplay between the biochemical and physical characteristics of tracheobronchial secretions, the water and ion composition of the sol-phase of the secretions, respiratory ciliary motion, and the cough mechanism.

Normal respiratory mucus is produced by the submucosal tracheobronchial glands and the epithelial goblet cells; the proportion from each is not precisely known, but it has been estimated that in humans the volume of submucosal glands is some 40 times that of goblet cells.[108, 355] In normal subjects, the volume of cleared respiratory tract fluid has been estimated to range from 0.1 to 0.3 ml per kg of body weight, or up to about 10 ml per day.[355]

The precise definitions of mucus, tracheobronchial secretions, and sputum are sometimes confused. Mucus represents the products derived from secretion of glands and goblet cells, whereas tracheobronchial secretions include the mucus plus other fluid and solute derived from the alveolar surface and the circulation. Sputum is a pathologic substance consisting of bronchial mucus contaminated by saliva, transudated serum proteins, and inflammatory and desquamated epithelial cells.[355]

BIOCHEMICAL CHARACTERISTICS OF TRACHEOBRONCHIAL SECRETIONS

It has been difficult to characterize the biochemical composition of normal tracheobronchial secretions since they are not expectorated; by definition, sputum represents an increase in normal secretions and thus is pathologic.[354] Nevertheless, small quantities of normal respiratory secretions have been obtained by fiberoptic bronchoscopy and have been examined biochemically.[358-360] They can be divided into two portions—a glycoprotein fraction that gives respiratory mucus its characteristic viscoelastic and rheologic properties, and sol-phase proteins that are derived from both local production and transudation from the serum. The glycoproteins are the major agents responsible for the gelation of airway secretions; they contain single polypeptide chains that form 10 to 20 per cent of their molecular weight; numerous sugar residue side chains are present. The oligosaccharide side chains contain six different sugars: D-galactose, D-glucose, L-fructose, D-xylose, N-acetyl-D-glucosamine, and N-acetyl-D-galactosamine. The polypeptide core is synthesized in the rough endoplasmic reticulum and the carbohydrate side chains are attached to the protein in its passage through the Golgi apparatus of the mucus-secreting cell. Each side chain contains an average of 8 to 10 sugars.[362] The molecular weight of normal mucous glycoproteins is in the range of 3 to 7 million.[362] Intramolecular and intermolecular bonds, including disulfide linkages and ionic and sugar-sugar interactions, result in gelation of the mucus and account for its viscoelastic properties. The terminal portions of the sugar side chains contain sugar sequences that are blood group determinates; in addition, sialic acid residues on the side chains can bind to the hemagglutinins of influenza A and B and other myxoviruses.[363]

The protein and nonmucous glycoprotein content in the sol-phase of respiratory secretions has been characterized in sputum from patients and in bronchial lavage fluid from normal subjects.[107, 354, 359, 363] It has been difficult to quantify the amount of protein in airway secretions that is related to local production compared with that resulting from transudation from serum.[360] An estimate of local production can be obtained by assuming that the albumin content of tracheobronchial secretions is neither secreted nor locally produced and then correcting the concentrations of the other proteins for the content of albumin and the known plasma-lymph concentration ratio of the other molecules. Using these correction factors, it has been calculated that the quantity of IgG, IgA, transferrin, alpha-1-antitrypsin, and ceruloplasmin in bronchial secretions is greater than expected:[360] it was estimated that there was 37 per cent more IgG, 85 per cent more IgA, 45 per cent more transferrin, 15 per cent more alpha-1-antitrypsin, and 13 per cent more ceruloplasmin than should be present if transudation alone was the mechanism of their production. Neutral lipids, phospholipids, and glycolipids have been identified in secretions in both normal and diseased subjects. They can contribute up to one third of the total macromolecular material of normal airway mucus and can be increased in disease. The major source is probably alveolar surfactant, with contributions from lipid precursors of prostaglandins and from tissue fluid transudate and desquamated cells from the tracheobronchial tree. Their function in airway mucus is not known.[362]

The excess immunoglobulins are synthesized by plasma cells in the airway submucosa and released into the airway lumen. IgA forms a dimer that combines with a secretory component before it is released. The secretory component is synthesized in airway epithelial cells and is also secreted in an unbound form; it protects the IgA molecule from enzymatic digestion by proteolytic enzymes[363] and can be identified immunohistochemically in serous, mucous, and ciliated cells of bronchi, bronchioles, and tracheobronchial glands.[447] Although its function is primarily related to dimeric IgA, it has been suggested that it may also independently participate in the function of the mucociliary apparatus.[447] It has been estimated that there is eight to ten times the amount of IgA in airway secretions than would be expected from that associated with serum, using albumin as a marker, and twice as much alpha-1-antichymotrypsin.[107] Tracheobronchial secretions are also relatively enriched with lysozyme and lactoferrin; these are secreted by submucosal serous cells of the tracheobronchial glands, and both have antimicrobial properties.[363] Alpha-1-antitrypsin and alpha-1-antichymotrypsin are important in inhibiting neutral protease originating from leukocyte degeneration.[354]

Ninety-five to 98 per cent of the weight of normal mucus is water.[354] The electrolyte composition of the fluid phase of airway secretions is similar to that of serum but with important differences: for example, the relative concentration of chloride is significantly higher than in serum. Also, normal airway secretions appear to be hyperosmolar relative to plasma; this is presumably the result of constant evaporative water loss from the airway surface since the breathing of warmed, humidified air returns the osmolarity toward that of plasma. However, the chloride content remains higher than that of plasma and the sodium content becomes lower when breathing warm humidified air, supporting the concept of active chloride transport,[364] probably by airway epithelial cells.[16] Regional differences in airway surface ion composition have also been reported, suggesting local differences in ion transport.[365] Measurements of the true pH of tracheobronchial secretions have produced conflicting results:[354] some studies have found a pH of 6 to 6.7 in the trachea with more acid values in the bronchi; however, other studies have reported values of 7.4 to 8.2 in sputum.

CONTROL OF TRACHEOBRONCHIAL SECRETIONS

Tracheobronchial secretion is a two-phase fluid made up of a mucous fraction and a more liquid sol fraction. Studies in which the control of tracheobronchial secretions has been investigated can be divided into those examining the factors affecting secretion of mucous glycoproteins (which form the major structural component of the mucous phase) and those examining the secretion of water and ions in the sol phase.

Mucous Phase. A number of techniques have been developed to characterize the mechanisms that control the secretion of the mucous component. These include the insertion of a micropipette into individual gland ducts with analysis and quantification of the collected fluid,[366] the incorporation of tritium-labeled glucosamine into mucous glycoproteins in cultured human airway tissue,[367] the incorporation of labeled sulfate (^{35}S) into the luminal secretions of cultured airway epithelium,[368] and the quantification of hillocks on the airway surface after tantalum coating.[369, 370] The combined use of these techniques has yielded an increasingly clear picture of how mucous glycoprotein secretion is controlled.

Since atropine or vagal blockade decreases the basal secretion rate to approximately 60 per cent,[366, 369] normal secretion appears to be under a tonic cholinergic stimulation. There also appears to be both beta- and alpha-adrenergic stimulatory influences, and beta-blockade decreases basal secretions as well.[366, 369, 371] Adrenergic stimulation increases secretion from serous cells predominantly whereas beta-adrenergic stimulation chiefly increases mucous cell secretion. Cholinergic stimulation increases secretion from both cell types equally.[369] While a number of indirect effects on mucous secretion appear to act via the classic cholinergic and adrenergic reflexes, additional neural-humoral agents have direct effect. Hypoxia increases mucous gland secretion, apparently being subserved by carotid body and superior laryngeal nerve reflexes.[372] Stimulation of mechanoreceptors in the stomach increases mucous gland output as measured by the micropipette method.[373] Stimulation of the cough receptors in the trachea and bronchi with chemical agents increases tracheal mucous output via parasympathetic efferent pathways, an effect that also accompanies irritation of the nose, pharynx, or larynx. A wide variety of irritants such as ammonia, cigarette smoke, sulfur dioxide, and organic vapors stimulate mucous secretion. Many of the stimuli that elicit cough also result in enhanced mucous secretion, suggesting that these two defense mechanisms are linked.[370]

A long list of inflammatory mediators can stimulate airway mucous production: histamine is a relatively weak stimulator and acts via an H2 receptor; many of the prostaglandins increase mucous secretion although prostaglandin E decreases it; the leukotrienes, including LTC4, LTD4, and the HETEs, all stimulate mucous secretion, with LTD4 being the most potent.[367, 374] Vasoactive intestinal peptide (VIP) and the neurally released polypeptide substance P have also been shown to be effective respiratory mucous secretagogues.[370, 375]

Sol Phase. Optimal mucociliary clearance by respiratory tract cilia depends on a proper balance between the volume of the mucous layer and the more fluid and less viscid sol phase through which the rapid recovery stroke of the cilia occurs.[353] Increasing evidence supports the concept that water transport, and therefore the periciliary sol phase of tracheobronchial mucus, is linked to active ion transport across the epithelium.[376, 377] Evidence comes from studies in which Ussing chambers have been employed to measure both electric properties and ion transport across animal and human airway mucosa.[376, 378] In the trachea, an active sodium-potassium ATPase pump appears to be located on the basal lateral surface of the epithelial cells. This pump results in active exclusion of sodium at the basal lateral surface, with chloride being pumped into the cell and subsequently diffusing along with water down its electrochemical gradient across the apical epithelial cell surface into the lumen. Active sodium absorption at the mucosal surface has also been demonstrated.[378, 379] These active ion transport mechanisms result in an electrical potential difference across the airway epithelium, the lumen being approximately 30 millivolts negative relative to the submucosa.[379] A similar electrical potential difference has been demonstrated in normal humans by use of a recording electrode passed via a bronchoscope and referenced to a subcutaneous electrode; the potential difference was found to be 33 millivolts in the trachea of younger subjects, decreasing with age; the potential difference also decreased distally in the tracheobronchial tree to a lumen-negative value of 14 millivolts in segmental airways.[380]

There is evidence that this active transport mechanism is under neural-humoral control and that regional variations in transport exist. Pharmacologic alpha-adrenergic stimulation increases both the luminal movement of chloride and water and the submucosal movement of sodium, whereas beta-agonists increase only chloride secretion, and to a lesser extent.[371, 381] Acetylcholine, histamine, prostaglandins, theophylline, and cAMP also increase the active chloride transport.[376] Knowles and co-workers found that, unlike the case with the trachea, active sodium absorption is the dominant active ion flow in human bronchial epithelium and that chloride appears to be distributed passively; they found that with cholinergic stimulation there was net secretion of chloride in the bronchi and suggested that airways peripheral to the trachea ordinarily absorb sodium and water but can be made to secrete both substances with cholinergic stimulation.[378] The regional differences in active ion and water transport may have relevance in the coordination and control of the depth of the sol layer in the rapidly converging total cross-sectional area of airway lumen during the mouthward movement of tracheobronchial secretions.

PHYSICAL CHARACTERISTICS OF TRACHEOBRONCHIAL SECRETIONS

Adequate mucociliary clearance mechanisms depend not only on the quantity and biochemical composition of the mucous layer and the periciliary sol layer but also on the viscoelastic properties of the mucus. The rheologic properties of mucus cannot be described by measurements of viscosity alone. A true "newtonian" liquid has only viscosity and no elasticity, but respiratory mucus has characteristics of both a liquid and a solid and has been described as exhibiting "pseudoplastic behavior." This means that the shear rate or movement rate of mucus varies according to the shear stress; thus, the viscous characteristics of mucus are described as non-newtonian. Respiratory mucus also shows another unique physical-chemical characteristic known as thixotropy, which is a transient decrease in viscosity after exposure to high shear rates.[357, 382] The viscoelastic properties of mucus are related to a molecular-molecular interaction that results in gelation; the bonds that join the molecules into a gel matrix include covalent disulfide bonds, ionic bonds, hydrogen bonds, van der Waal's forces (which consist of weak bonds between methyl groups), and finally intermingling or entangling of the long molecules.[383]

The viscoelastic properties of airway mucus are best quantified by using oscillatory methods to establish dynamic stress-strain relationships; with these techniques, two parameters—the elastic modulus (also termed the storage modulus or G_1) and the dynamic viscosity related to frequency (also termed the loss modulus or G_{11})—can be determined.[382, 384, 385] Given a depth of mucus and periciliary sol layer and a constant ciliary beat frequency, mucous transport on ciliated surfaces relates in a complex fashion to both the elasticity and dynamic viscosity of mucus and sputum.[357] An optimal combination of elasticity and dynamic viscosity results in optimal mucous transportability; therefore, pathologic states theoretically can decrease mucociliary clearance by altering either of these properties.[357, 384, 385]

Despite accurate measurements of elasticity and dynamic viscosity, however, discrepancies between these physical characteristics and transport rate have been observed; an additional mechanical characteristic of bronchial mucus, "spinnability," has recently been described that may go some way toward explaining these discrepancies. Spinnability is the ability of mucus to stretch to a long thin thread. Puchelle and associates[386] have devised a method of quantifying the spinnability of bronchial mucus and have shown that this characteristic correlates closely with its transportability on a ciliated surface. It is interesting that spinnability has been extensively studied in mucus from the human cervix; the time of maximum spinnability for cervical mucus is also the time of maximum fertility when ciliated spermatozoa can move through highly spinnable mucus with the greatest of ease.[386]

Few data exist on the controlling mechanisms that optimize or disrupt tracheobronchial mucous elasticity and dynamic viscosity. The rate of secretion of mucous glycoprotein and periciliary fluid presumably influences these physical-chemical properties, but changes in the biochemical composition of the secreted mucus and the sol-phase proteins undoubtedly play a role as well. Vagal stimulation and methacholine inhalation tend to increase elasticity and dynamic viscosity at low stimulation frequencies and dose, whereas both viscoelastic characteristics decrease at higher frequencies and concentrations.[357, 387] Beta-adrenergic stimulation imparts a selective stimulation of mucous cells and leads to increased elasticity and dynamic viscosity; by contrast, alpha-adrenergic stimulation selectively stimulates serous cells and results in a more watery mucus.[357] The inhalation of prostaglandin F2α, histamine, or acetylcholine has been shown to produce alterations in the viscoelastic properties of mucus in normal subjects, but these agents also increase the transudation of serum proteins into the bronchial mucus, suggesting altered epithelial fluid permeability.[388]

The viscosity and elasticity of sputum vary considerably, not only from day to day but even during one day,[389] and viscosity increases with decreasing humidity.[390] Furthermore, purulent sputum is more viscous but less elastic than mucoid sputum,[389] and the decrease in viscoelasticity with time at room temperature is considerably more rapid in purulent than in mucoid samples. Slow freezing followed by rapid thawing does not seem to alter the viscoelastic properties of sputum and therefore can be employed when rheologic measurement is delayed after expectoration.[389] Studies in vitro[389, 391] and in vivo[392] have indicated that the viscosity can be decreased by the application of water-mist aerosol,[389] L-acetylcysteine, or dithiothreitol[393] and by the oral administration of guaithenacine, a glycerol ether of glycol.[392] Acetylcysteine directly affects glycoproteins, whereas the water mist and guaithenacine appear to increase the width of the sol mucous layer in which the cilia beat (see further on), thereby improving mucous mobility without appreciably changing sputum viscosity.

MUCOCILIARY TRANSPORT MECHANISM

The mucociliary apparatus consists of innumerable cilia that arise from the surface of the pseudostratified columnar epithelial cells and lie in a fluid "sol layer" deep to the less liquid mucous "gel layer." Cilia are present at all levels of the tracheobronchial tree down to and including the respiratory bronchioles. In each ciliated cell in the respiratory tract are about 200 cilia packed at the apex of the cell at a density of about 8 per square micrometer. The two major structural proteins that make up the cilia are tubulin and dynein. Tubulin is the major structural protein of the microtubules that form the longitudinal structural components of the cilia, whereas dynein (an enzyme with high specificity for ATPase) forms the so-called dynein arms that join the microtubules.

The best-accepted theory for the ciliary beating mechanism is the sliding microtubule hypothesis, similar to the sliding fiber theory of muscle contraction. Basically the dynein arms slide up and down adjacent tubules; since the microtubules are fixed in location, this sliding results in curvature of the cilia. The more rapid forward movement of the cilia is the effective stroke, whereas the slower movement through the less viscid sol phase is termed the recovery stroke. Nasal cilia drive secreted mucus downward and backward from the nasopharynx to the oropharynx, whereas the ciliated epithelial cells of the tracheobronchial tree propel mucus upward toward the oropharynx. The movement of the cilia in adjacent areas is synchronized, resulting in a so-called metachronal wave of fluid movement. The mucous blanket is probably not a continuous sheet but rather floating islands of mucus that gradually coalesce as the central airways are reached. The surface area on which the mucus lies converges about 2000-fold from small airways to the trachea, and thus some absorption of fluid must occur along the passage to accommodate this excess and prevent the plugging of central airways.[353] In the latter, a combination of increased numbers of ciliated cells, an increased length of individual cilia,[18] and increased ciliary beat frequency also contributes to more efficient clearing of secretions.

As proposed by the Lucas-Douglas model of bronchial mucous transport,[394, 395] the cilia normally lie in a bath of clear serous fluid of low viscosity; within this medium the cilia beat, propelling the mucus (gel layer) which floats on the surface of the liquid like a raft supported and propelled by many hands beneath it. During the rapid effective stroke, the cilia (which are equipped with tiny clawlike structures at their tips) probably extend about 1 μm into the mucous layer.[353, 357]

Considerable regional differences in mucociliary clearance rates and ciliary beat frequencies have been described. Studies in dogs,[396] humans,[397] and rats[398, 399] have shown a variation of up to 54-fold in mucociliary clearance rates from terminal bronchioles to the trachea. However, in one study in which the mucous clearance rate ranged from 0.4 mm per min in bronchioles to 20 mm per min in the trachea,[399] there was only a 3.7-fold variation in ciliary beat frequency, ranging from 400 per min in bronchioles to 1500 per min in the trachea; this suggests that factors other than ciliary beat frequency contribute to the regional variations in clearance rate. In one study,[400] epithelial cells were collected from the trachea and the main stem and basilar segmental bronchi of 30 patients during fiberoptic bronchoscopy; no difference could be detected between the trachea and more peripheral airways, the mean beat frequency of cilia being approximately 15 per sec at 37° C. In another study, the ciliary beat frequency was found to be lower in subsegmental airways than in the trachea and main stem bronchi;[401] however, still another study[402] showed a slight increase in ciliary beat frequency in more peripheral airways, a difference that could have been caused by the effect of local anesthesia on central airways. In the latter study of small groups of patients with chronic obstructive lung disease, asthma, lung cancer, and bronchiectasis, the mean beat frequency was 12.5 cycles per sec, with wide interindividual variation but good intraindividual reproductibility and no obvious abnormality of beat frequency.

In recent years, a number of techniques have been developed to measure mucociliary clearance in animals and humans:[403] (1) a radioaerosol technique in which radiolabeled, nonabsorbable particles or molecules are nebulized and inhaled into peripheral lung regions and their clearance rate from the lung measured with external counting devices;[404-406] (2) the monitoring of the movement of a single radioactive bolus or of radiopaque Teflon discs by fiberoptic bronchoscopy, external counting devices, or fluoroscopic techniques;[407-409] and (3) monitoring by roentgenographic techniques of the mouthward movement of the metallic dust powdered tantalum, following its insufflation.[410] The major advantage of the aerosol technique is that it measures mucociliary clearance from the entire ciliated airway surface. However, this method depends by necessity on the initial deposition pattern of the inhaled radioaerosol: even mild air flow obstruction can reduce peripheral deposition of inhaled radioaerosol, resulting in an erroneously fast calculated rate of clearance since label is preferentially deposited in central airways where mucociliary clearance is more rapid.[411] The other two techniques have the disadvantage that only central airway clearance is assessed; in addition, both are invasive since the tracer must be administered through a fiberoptic bronchoscope or an intra-airway catheter.[403] In one study in which whole lung clearance was measured with the radioaerosol technique and compared with central airway clearance techniques,[406] a remarkable correlation of the two was observed. It was concluded that the rate of movement of material from the peripheral to the central airways correlates well with central airway mucous velocity, and it was suggested that discoordination between central and peripheral clearance might occur with disease and be an important pathophysiologic mechanism.[406] A considerable variation in central airway mucous transport rates has been observed even when different techniques have been employed sequentially.[412] It has been suggested that the faster central airway transport rate observed with radiolabeled particles compared with Teflon discs is related to a stimulatory effect of local radiation on mucociliary clearance.[407] Simultaneous measurement of mucociliary clearance of particles averaging 3 microns, 110 microns, and 180 microns has shown no significant difference in clearance rates.[413]

As will be discussed in the Airways chapter,

disease states alter total lung and regional mucociliary clearance rates, but even in normal subjects pharmacologic and other factors influence clearance rates. The mechanism by which various interventions modulate the clearance rates is probably a complex interaction between ciliary beat frequency, the depth of the periciliary sol-phase, the quantity and viscoelastic properties of the airway mucus, and the state of dehydration. Beta-adrenergic agonists appear to enhance the mucociliary transport rates in normal subjects.[405, 414] Intravenous administration of atropine in dogs increases rather than decreases central airway mucociliary clearance rates.[415] In one study of perhaps more clinical relevance,[410] the clearance rate of insufflated tantalum was decreased in dogs with endotracheal tubes whether or not the cuff was inflated. In dogs, the use of high-frequency oscillatory ventilation has been shown to impair whole lung and central airway mucociliary clearance to a marked degree;[416] clearance improved immediately following cessation of the high-frequency oscillatory ventilation, suggesting that the effect was a functional disturbance rather than the production of a structural abnormality of the cilia or an alteration of the viscoelastic or biochemical characteristics of mucus.

In contrast to these results, King and associates[417] have shown that high-frequency chest wall oscillation results in enhanced central and peripheral mucociliary clearance; the discrepancy in the results obtained in these two studies[416, 417] is presumably related to the differential flow rates and air velocity rates in intrathoracic airways during inspiration and expiration when high frequency oscillatory ventilation is produced at the airway opening or at the chest wall. Such a mechanism has been invoked by Warwick[418] to explain the persistence of some mucociliary clearance in the complete absence of ciliary motility in patients with the dyskinetic ciliary syndromes.

Dehydration has been shown to decrease mucociliary clearance and rehydration to improve it,[419] whereas therapeutic levels of aspirin have been shown to cause a slight reduction in whole lung and tracheal mucociliary clearance rates in nonaspirin-sensitive normal subjects.[420] In a fascinating study, Smaldone and coworkers have shown that there is a disruption of the mucociliary clearance mechanisms at the site of flow limitation during forced expiration and cough; this resulted in deposition of inhaled irritants at the flow-limiting site, leading the investigators to speculate that such a mechanism could be responsible for the predominant central location of squamous cell carcinoma.[421]

COUGH

An important mechanism of respiratory defense and an adjuvant to the clearance of tracheobronchial secretions is cough. Cough can be initiated voluntarily or involuntarily and consists of an initial inspiratory maneuver followed by glottic closure. However, glottic closure is not essential for cough, and patients with tracheostomies can develop an effective cough mechanism.[422] Expiratory muscles then contract to increase pleural, abdominal, and alveolar pressures to levels of 100 or more mm Hg. The glottis is suddenly opened and expiratory flow begins, peaking in 30 to 50 milliseconds with flows at the mouth as high as 12 liters per sec. The initial high flow transients are contributed to both by a collapse of central airways with displacement of contained air mouthward and by bulk flow from the parenchyma. After about half a second and the expulsion of approximately 1 liter of air, expiratory flow stops due to glottic closure or expiratory muscle relaxation. During cough, expiratory flow limitation occurs by the same mechanism that limits maximal flow during forced expiratory maneuvers. An equal pressure point develops in the central airways where intrapleural and intra-airway pressure are the same; mouthward from this point, dynamic compression of the airways occurs. Cough may be repeated at lower lung volumes, resulting in progressive peripheral movement of the equal pressure point and progressive collapse of more and more of the intrathoracic airways. The marked collapse of intrathoracic airways leads to gas velocities that reach three quarters of the speed of sound at values of 1600 to 2400 cm per sec. These high air velocities produce enormous shear stress on the liquid layer lining the airways and move large amounts of mucus or other particulate debris proximally. Involuntary cough is initiated by stimulation of irritant receptors in the larynx, trachea, or large bronchi.

The receptors that mediate cough are thought to be fine, nonmyelinated nerve fibers that are present in an extensive network throughout the airway epithelium. Evidence that these fibers subserve the cough mechanism includes the observation that cough is stimulated with irritation of areas where these fibers are most numerous and the fact that single afferent fiber recordings of rapidly adapting receptors in the vagus nerve show a burst of activity when the epithelium is stimulated by events that stimulate cough. It is difficult to provoke cough by stimulating peripheral airways, suggesting that irritant receptor density is less in these locations. Although rapidly adapting receptors are present in the smaller airways, their stimulation may result in reflex hyperpnea rather than cough. Vagotomy abolishes or greatly reduces the cough reflex, indicating that nonvagal pathways must play a minor or no role in the reflex. The stimuli that provoke coughing can also provoke bronchoconstriction via the same reflex pathways. The narrowing of the airways that occurs with reflex bronchoconstriction could aid the cough mechanism by resulting in higher linear flow rates during the cough. In addition, it may stabilize the airway during the vigorous expiratory effort and high transmural pressures of coughing, as has been shown in large airways.[423]

Cough is most effective in clearing secretions from large airways but calculations suggest that some clearance can occur down to 20th generation airways. The greater the depth of the periciliary serous layer and the less viscous it is, the greater the effectiveness of cough. Theoretically, cough should be more effective when breathing gases of higher density than air since this increases turbulence and its contribution to clearance.[424]

THE PULMONARY VASCULAR SYSTEM

PULMONARY ARTERIAL AND VENOUS CIRCULATION

Morphology

The pulmonary trunk originates from the base of the right ventricle and extends cranially and slightly to the left for 4 to 5 cm, at which point it divides into the right and left main pulmonary arteries. The latter continues in more or less the same line as the pulmonary trunk until it reaches the hilum where it arches over the left main bronchus and divides into lobar branches. The right pulmonary artery arises at an angle to the axis of the pulmonary trunk and continues in a horizontal direction posterior to the aorta and superior vena cava and anterior to the right main bronchus.

Although the course of the main pulmonary arteries is fairly constant, the origin and branching pattern of lobar and segmental arteries shows considerable variation.[425] Despite this, the pulmonary arterial system is invariably related to the bronchial tree and divides with it, a branch always accompanying the appropriate bronchial division. In addition to these "conventional" branches, many "supernumerary" or accessory branches of the pulmonary artery arise at points other than corresponding

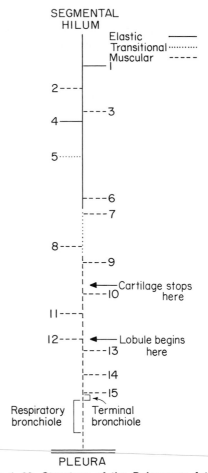

Figure 1–63. Structure of the Pulmonary Arteries. Diagrammatic representation (drawn to scale) of the full length of an anterior basal segmental artery. The structure of the artery is related to bronchial generations, and only conventional branches are included—those that accompany airways. (From Elliott FM, Reid L: Clin Radiol *16*:193, 1965.)

bronchial divisions and directly penetrate the lung parenchyma.[426] These supernumerary branches outnumber the conventional ones and originate throughout the length of the arterial tree, most frequently in a peripheral location. Thus, the branching ratio (average number of daughter branches emanating from one parent branch) increases as vessel size decreases; proximally, the ratio is 2.99, a value comparable to that of the conducting airways, and distally it rises to 3.59.[427] Detailed measurements of resin and gelatin casts of the human pulmonary arterial system have shown a linear relationship between Strahler order and the logarithm of both branch diameter and length.[427, 428] As with the conducting airways (*see* page 4), the number of Strahler orders has been estimated to be 17 down to branches 10 to 15 μm in diameter (Table 1–3).[427]

Histologically, precapillary pulmonary vessels can be conveniently divided into three morphologic types—elastic, muscular, and arteriolar. The number of generations of types of artery differs in various pathways. For example, in the anterior basal segmental artery (Fig. 1–63), elastic arteries stop at

Table 1–3. Integrated Data for the Total Pulmonary Arterial System with Revised Numbers of Branches for the Intermediate and Distal Zones

ORDER	NO. OF BRANCHES	DIAMETER (MM)	LENGTH (MM)
17	1.000	30.000	90.50
16	3.000	14.830	32.00
15	8.000	8.060	10.90
14	2.000×10^6	5.820	20.70
13	6.600×10^6	3.650	17.90
12	2.030×10^2	2.090	10.50
11	6.750×10^2	1.330	6.60
10	2.290×10^3	0.850	4.69
9	6.062×10^3	0.525	3.16
8	1.877×10^4	0.351	2.10
7	5.809×10^4	0.224	1.38
6	1.798×10^5	0.138	0.91
5	5.672×10^5	0.86	0.65
4	1.789×10^6	0.054	0.44
3	5.641×10^6	0.034	0.29
2	2.028×10^7	0.021	0.20
1	7.292×10^7	0.013	0.13

(From Horsfield K: Circ Res *42*:593, 1978. By permission of the American Heart Association, Inc.)

about the sixth order and are followed by two orders of transitional arteries coinciding with the end of the bronchial cartilage. Beyond this, the vessels are muscular in type.

Elastic arteries include the main pulmonary artery and its lobar, segmental, and subsegmental branches, extending roughly to the junction of bronchi and bronchioles. Histologically,[429] the large extrapulmonary vessels contain a multilayered latticework of elastic fibers similar to that seen in systemic vessels of equivalent size but which is fragmented, is more irregular in shape and size, and shows more intervening connective tissue (Fig. 1–64). Within the lung, the elastic artery laminae become more regular, with more or less prominent external and internal layers and a variable number of intervening layers. Despite their name, these vessels contain some muscle and are probably capable of active vasoconstriction.[430] As the vessels decrease in size, the number of laminae diminishes so that at a diameter of 1000 to 500 μm medial elastic tissue is lost altogether, leaving only well-developed internal and external laminae. The latter vessels constitute a transition between truly elastic and truly muscular arteries and are sometimes designated transitional.

The function of the elastic arteries is similar to that of the aorta: to provide a distensible but elastic reservoir for the ventricular ejection fraction. This distensibility has been found to undergo an age-related decrease,[431] and, although results of various studies have been conflicting, recent reports[431, 432] have failed to find either morphologic or chemical changes in elastin content that would explain this decrease; it has been suggested instead that physical changes in the constituents of the wall may be responsible.

Muscular arteries have an external diameter ranging from 50 to 70 μm and possess well-developed internal and external elastic laminae with an intervening variable number of circularly arranged smooth muscle cells (Fig. 1–64). Acinar vessels with recognizable arterial features and most supernumerary arterial branches are of this type. The number of smaller muscular arteries per unit of lung area decreases rapidly after birth and slowly thereafter into adulthood.[433]

Beyond a diameter of 70 to 80 μm, the small arteries gradually lose their medial smooth muscle to become *arterioles,* composed solely of a thin intima and a single elastic lamina that is continuous with the external elastic lamina of arteries. At this level, arterioles are histologically indistinguishable from pulmonary venules and can be identified only by special injection techniques or by the examination of serial sections. Within the acinus, arterioles continue to divide and accompany their respective branches of the respiratory tree. Although some continue to do this to the level of the alveolar sacs, many accessory branches arise that do not precisely follow the transitional airways.[434] These branches as well as those that terminate around the alveolar sacs break up to form the capillary network of the alveoli.

In general, pulmonary arterial and arteriolar vessels have a wide lumen and a relatively thin muscular media compared with systemic arteries of the same size. Morphometric measurements of medial thickness expressed as a percentage of external vessel diameter show a normal range of 3 to 7. No differences have been found between medial thickness of vessels of similar size in different parts of the same lung, including apical and basal regions.[435]

At all levels of the arterial system, the intima consists normally of a thin, unicellular endothelial layer and its adjacent basement membrane. With advancing age, however, alteration in this structure is common. Atherosclerosis, similar histologically and ultrastructurally to that seen in the systemic circulation,[436] is frequently present in individuals over 40 years of age; in one study, it was noted in 202 of 324 consecutive autopsies.[437] Its presence has been positively correlated with the degree of aortic atherosclerosis, pulmonary hypertension, and thromboembolism,[437] although in the absence of pulmonary hypertension or hyperlipidemia, it rarely exhibits the complicating features of systemic atheromas.[438] The atheromatous areas are almost always small and are most prominent near branch points in the larger elastic vessels.[438] Foci of intimal fibrosis without the features of atherosclerosis can also be found at all levels of the arterial tree, especially in the more peripheral muscular branches; their frequency and thickness increase with age, and in older individuals they occasionally comprise over 25 per cent of the total vessel diameter.[435] The fibrotic areas are often patchy in distribution and eccentrically located in the vessel wall, suggesting that they may represent foci of organized thrombi.[435] Ultrastructurally, the patches consist of collagen and a cellular population that is composed almost exclusively of smooth muscle cells, apparently derived from the media.[439]

Pericytes are found in alveolar capillaries and arterioles in intimate association with endothelial cells.[440, 441] They are rather uncommon and are located beneath the basement membrane near the luminal surface; ultrastructurally, they show fine, microfilament-containing cytoplasmic processes that extend toward and attach to the endothelial cell surface. The importance and precise function of these cells in the normal lung are not clear, but it has been suggested that they may act as either contractile or phagocytic elements.[440] A similar cell has been identified in precapillary arterioles beneath the internal elastic lamina but external to the endothelial basement membrane; it shows ultrastructural features of smooth muscle cells and has been termed an *intermediate cell* by Meyrick and Reid.[441, 442] Although its normal function is also unclear, these investigators have shown that in both hypoxic rats[442] and children with congenital heart

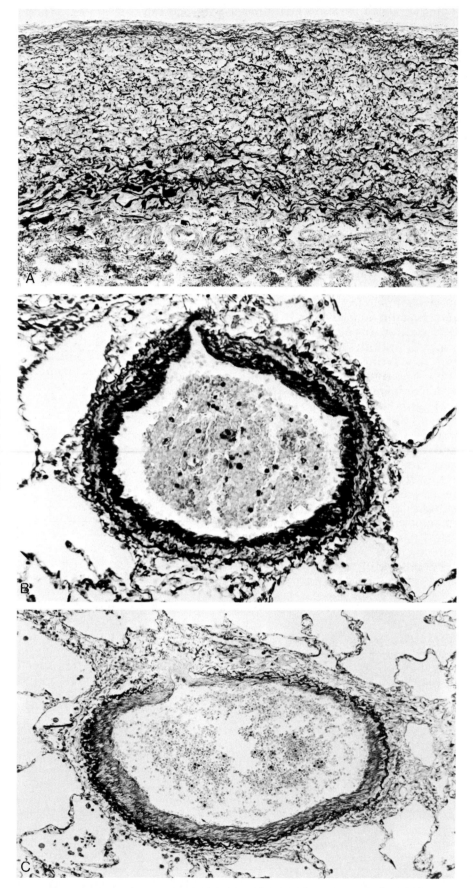

Figure 1–64. Histologic Characteristics of Pulmonary Vessels. *A*, Main pulmonary artery showing fragmented, multilayered elastic laminae. *B*, Muscular pulmonary artery with prominent internal and external elastic laminae and thin layer of medial smooth muscle. *C*, Pulmonary vein, showing mild intimal thickening and relatively indistinct elastic laminae. All micrographs are from a 60-year-old man with bronchogenic carcinoma. (Verhoeff–van Gieson; *A*, × 100; *B*, × 240; *C*, × 130.)

defects,[441] both pericytes and intermediate cells can develop into mature smooth muscle cells, a finding that may have significance in the pathogenesis of pulmonary hypertension.

The *pulmonary veins* arise from capillaries of the alveolar meshwork and from the capillary network of the pleura. The larger branches run within the interlobular septa and are thus separate from the pulmonary bronchoarterial pathways. Although their final course is somewhat variable, there are usually two superior and two inferior main pulmonary veins, the former draining the middle and upper lobes on the right side and the upper lobe on the left, and the latter the lower lobes. The right-sided veins course beneath the main pulmonary artery posterior to the superior vena cava and enter the left atrium separately; the left-sided veins pass anterior to the descending aorta and either enter the atrium separately as on the right or join within the pericardial cavity to enter the atrium as a common channel. Detailed analysis of resin casts of human pulmonary veins, classified by Strahler order, showed a 15-order system to the level of the superior and inferior veins (Table 1–4).[443] As with the conducting airways and pulmonary arteries, there is a roughly linear relationship between the order number and the logarithm of vessel diameter and length.[443] Histologically, smaller pulmonary venules are indistinguishable from arterioles. With increasing diameter, occasional smooth muscle cells and an elastic lamina become evident, and at a diameter of between 60 and 100 μm, they become recognizable as veins and enter the interlobular septa. Larger veins show a variable number of elastic laminae with interspersed small irregular bundles of smooth muscle cells and collagen. In contrast to arteries, there is no well-developed external elastic lamina; the adventitia and media blend together. With advancing age, fragmentation of the elastic laminae and focal intimal sclerosis similar to that seen in the arterial system are often found.

Table 1–4. Model of the Pulmonary Venous Tree

ORDER	NUMBER	DIAMETER (mm)	LENGTH (mm)	VOLUME (ml)
1	72,920,000	0.013	0.130	1.258
2	23,109,101	0.019	0.192	1.258
3	7,323,513	0.029	0.283	1.369
4	2,320,897	0.043	0.418	1.399
5	735,516	0.064	0.617	1.460
6	233,093	0.096	0.910	1.535
7	73,869	0.14	1.34	1.524
8	23,843	0.22	1.98	1.795
9	7,546	0.39	2.54	2.290
10	1,842	0.61	3.20	1.723
11	496	1.21	11.0	6.274
12	158	1.90	18.5	8.288
13	53	2.90	25.4	8.892
14	14	5.23	39.0	11.730
15	4	13.88	36.7	22.212
TOTALS	106,749,945		142.21	73.762

(From Horsfield K, Gordon WI: Lung *159*:216, 1981.)

The Pulmonary Endothelium

The pulmonary endothelium is of the nonfenestrated type and with minor variations is morphologically similar at all levels of the vascular tree.[444] The endothelial cell rests on a continuous basement membrane that is thought to be manufactured by the endothelial cell itself[444] and is fused to the epithelial basement membrane at the functional air-blood barrier of the alveolus. Although endothelial cells have been estimated to be the most common cell type in the lung (representing almost 35 to 40 per cent of all parenchymal cells),[137] they are relatively inconspicuous at the light microscopic level, being visible only as a series of small intraluminal bumps corresponding to their nuclei. The cells are rectangular or ovoid and are arranged in an interlocking mosaic.[445] Ultrastructurally, they posses scanty cytoplasm that exists mostly as thin, platelike processes measuring as little as 0.1 μm in thickness.[446] Cellular organelles, including Golgi apparatus, mitochondria, microtubules, Weibel-Palade bodies, and scanty endoplasmic reticulum are sparse and tend to be concentrated in a perinuclear location. The surface contains numerous, small, microvillus-like projections, which are present at all levels of the vascular system[446, 448] but are most prominent in veins and arteries. These greatly increase the cell surface area and, along with the pinocytotic vesicles (*see* further on), have been shown to stain immunochemically for angiotensin-converting enzyme (ACE),[449] implying a possible role in metabolic function. It has also been proposed that the irregularity and density of these projections could create turbulence of the cell-free plasma layer along the endothelial surface, resulting in slower flow and facilitating metabolite transfer between blood and endothelial cell.[448]

A prominent ultrastructural feature of the pulmonary endothelial cell is the presence of numerous small pits or vesicles (*caveolae intracellularis*) (Fig. 1–65). These are located in the thick, nongas-exchanging part of the cell, either at the luminal or abluminal surface or free in the cytoplasm.[450] The interior of many luminal surface vesicles is delimited by a thin membrane that appears to have a surrounding electron-dense rim, thought to function as a support.[450] Small electron-dense granules, considered to represent enzyme complexes responsible for various metabolic functions, can be seen at the bases of the vesicles attached to the limiting membrane. In support of a metabolic function, immunochemical and histochemical studies have localized both 5'-nucleotidase[450] and ACE[449] within the granules. However, other studies that have traced the uptake of substrates such as 5-hydroxytryptamine[451] have found no preferential localization within vesicles, and the relative importance of vesicular versus other plasma membrane enzymes in endothelial metabolism remains to be clarified. In addition to their metabolic activity, it is thought that the vesicles function as a transport medium for fluid and pro-

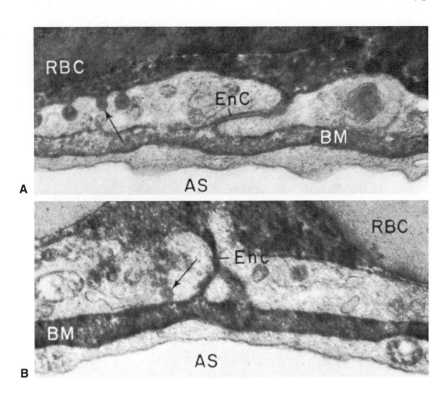

Figure 1–65. Endothelial Intercellular Cleft. Section of alveolar wall from the lung of a mouse sacrificed 90 sec after horseradish peroxidase injection. Reaction product in the capillary lumen (indicated by *RBC*) extends through the endothelial intercellular cleft (*EnC*) into the adjacent basement membrane (*BM*). In *A*, the staining of horseradish peroxidase is quite light, whereas in *B* the basement membrane is deeply stained. Reaction product is present in endothelial invaginations (caveolae intracellulari) on both the capillary side (*arrow in A*) and the alveolar side (*arrow in B*) of the cell. (TEM, × 46,000.) (From Schneeberger-Keeley EE, Karnovsky MJ: J Cell Biol *37*:781, 1968.)

teins between blood and interstitial tissues and across the air-blood barrier.[452, 453] The transport of specific compounds may depend on localized differences in the charges of different vesicles.[452]

Compared with the vesicular portion, the non-vesicular, gas-exchanging portion of the capillary endothelial cell has been found to have very few anionic binding sites.[159] Since red blood cells exhibit a negative surface charge, it has been suggested that this might lead to a slowing of blood flow in the region of the thin portion of the endothelium, thus facilitating gas transfer.[159]

Adjacent endothelial cells are joined by tight junctions,[445, 453] which by transmission electron microscopy appear as focal areas of fusion of the outer lamellae of adjacent cell membranes. For the most part, these are continuous although occasional in-

tercellular clefts measuring up to 4 nm are observed at the level of the alveolar capillaries (Fig. 1–66)[140, 452] As seen by freeze-fracture techniques, the junctions are less complex than those of the alveolar epithelium (Fig. 1–67): in addition to the presence of intercellular clefts and evidence provided by autoradiographic tracer studies, this suggests that the main site of solute impermeability in the air-blood barrier is the epithelium (Fig. 1–68).[454] The complexity of the endothelial junctions is variable, being greater in arterioles (which are felt to be relatively impermeable) and less in venules (which are thought to be the major site of vascular fluid leakage). As indicated by the number of connecting strands per junction, complexity has also been found to increase from the apex to the base of the lung; Yoneda has hypothesized that this reflects an

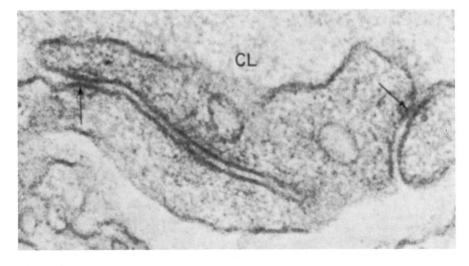

Figure 1–66. Endothelial Intercellular Cleft. A portion of a capillary lumen (*CL*) and two endothelial intercellular clefts can be seen. In the junction on the left (*arrow*) there is a distinct gap between the bounding unit membranes, whereas in the one on the right (*arrow*) details are obscured. (Uninjected mouse lung; TEM, × 140,000.) (From Schneeberger-Keeley EE, Karnovsky MJ: J Cell Biol *37*:781, 1968.)

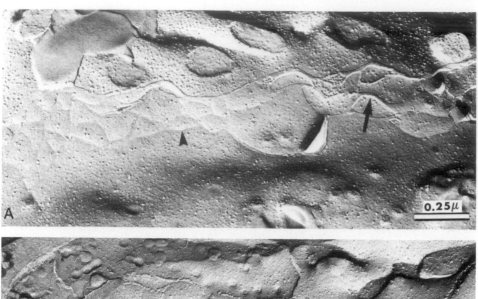

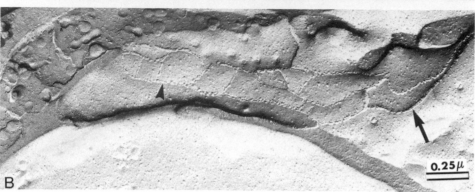

Figure 1–67. Epithelial and Endothelial Cell Junctions. *A,* An epithelial tight junction between a type I and a type II pneumocyte. On the ectoplasmic fracture face, the tight junction is a reticulum of furrows (*arrowhead*). On the protoplasmic fracture face, the tight junction is a reticulum of continuous fibers (*arrow*). *B,* An endothelial tight junction between two alveolar capillary endothelial cells. On ectoplasmic fracture faces, the tight junction is a reticulum of furrows containing particles (*arrowhead*). On the protoplasmic fracture face, the junctional complex consists of discontinuous particles (*arrow*). The differences in the complexity of the tight junction structure between endothelial and epithelial cells are believed to relate to the different permeability of these tissues. (Courtesy of Dr. David Walker, University of British Columbia, Vancouver.)

adaptation of pulmonary endothelium to regional differences in hydrostatic pressure.[455]

The endothelial cell is capable of division and normally replicates to replenish the endothelial surface at a rate of less than 1 per cent of the total endothelial population daily.[152] A rapid and marked increase in mitotic activity can occur in response to endothelial damage.[815]

Geometry and Dimensions of the Alveolar Capillary Network

Reports from Weibel's laboratory[10, 127] point out that the basic element of the *systemic* capillaries is a rather long, thin tube that may be connected at either end with other capillaries, thus forming a capillary network of fairly loose mesh. By contrast, the *pulmonary* capillaries form a dense network, enclosed in the alveolar wall (Fig. 1–69). The basic elements of this network, the capillary segments, fundamentally are shaped like short, cylindric tubes, modified at their bases in the form of wedges to allow each segment to join at either end with two adjacent segments (Fig. 1–70). In the great majority of instances three of these segments join, but junctures of four may easily occur. This results in an average angle of juncture of about 120 degrees. Thus the basic geometric structure of the capillary network is hexagonal, each mesh being surrounded, on average, by six segments. This two-dimensional

network on the alveolar facets becomes three-dimensional when three septal facets join, achieved by the rotation of the plane of juncture of three segments by approximately 90 degrees (Fig. 1–71).

Because of this rotation, each segment of the tripod lies in a different septal facet and therefore connects with the network within its facet. Thus the alveolar capillary network is continuous throughout many interalveolar facets. The extent of this continuity is unknown, but it may continue throughout pulmonary units such as lobules and possibly throughout segments.

Although convenient from a conceptual point of view, this description of capillary geometry is highly idealized. For example, in their study of latex cast replicas, Kendall and Eissman[1183] considered oval or circular capillary sheets to represent lung anatomy more accurately. In addition, the situation becomes more complicated when one considers the three-dimensional capillary and alveolar geometry under dynamic conditions. In these circumstances, Weibel and Bachofen[161] have pointed out that the shape of the various components of the alveolar septum can be affected by three mechanical factors, each of which can vary in the normal respiratory cycle: (1) tissue force due to tension on the interstitial connective tissue transmitted through the connective tissue of the visceral pleura; (2) capillary distending pressure; and (3) alveolar air-fluid surface forces. Scanning and transmission electron mi-

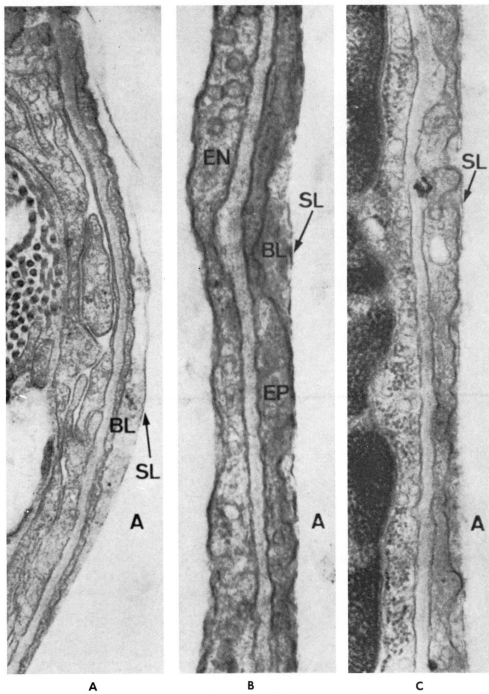

Figure 1–68. The Air-Blood Barrier. Three high-power magnifications show an extracellular duplex lining layer. Note the convexity of the surface in *A* and its flatness in *B* and *C*. These micrographs also demonstrate different appearances of the osmiophilic superficial layer (*SL*). *BL*, base layer; *EN*, capillary endothelial cell; *EP*, alveolar epithelial cell; *A*, alveolus. (TEM; *A*, × *49,200; B*, × 84,720; *C*, × 53,800.) (From Gill J, Weibel ER: Respir Physiol *8*:13, 1969.)

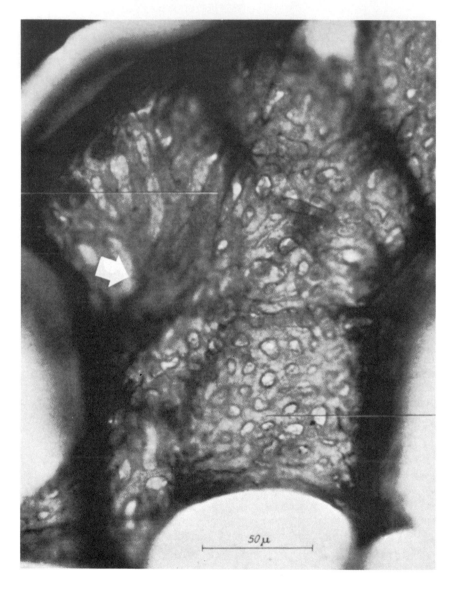

Figure 1–69. Alveolar Capillary Network.
Flat aspects of an interalveolar septum showing
the capillary network by staining of the capillary
basement membranes by PAS reaction. Fan-
shaped precapillary (*arrow*) leads into network.
(Human lung, × 580.) (From Weibel ER,
Gomez DM: Science *137*:577, 1962. Copyright
1962 by the American Association for the Advancement of Science.)

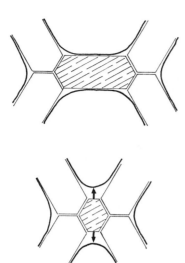

Figure 1–70. Alveolar Capillaries. Diagrammatic representation of the effect of smooth contour of capillary basement membrane on apparent diameter of short segments. (From Weibel ER: Morphometry of the Human Lung. New York, Academic Press, 1963.)

croscopic studies[161, 456] have demonstrated an irregularity of the alveolar surface produced by deep pleats or folds projecting into the inner portion of the septa within the capillary space, dividing it into intercommunicating chambers and giving the alveolus a crumpled appearance (Fig. 1–72). These folds are present in most alveoli at lower lung volumes, including tidal breathing, and tend to be obliterated at higher lung volumes as the alveolus expands. The alveolus has thus been likened to a nonelastic "doubled-walled paper bag"[456] that expands by unfolding its septal pleats rather than by stretching its wall. The folds often contain small pools of surface lining fluid at the alveolar surface, and their bases are usually adjacent to the thick portion of the interstitium (Fig. 1–73).

The precise forces leading to this arrangement are not clear. In addition to the mechanical factors, the contractile interstitial cells (*see* page 23) tend to be located at the bases of the folds and it is possible that they have an influence in the localization of the folds at these sites. Rosenquist and his colleagues have found an ordered structure to the connective tissue in these areas, with collagen and elastic tissue passing in a curved arrangement from one side of the septum to the other, suggesting a possible tethering effect of the connective tissue.[457]

Theoretically, the pleated arrangement has a number of important consequences. First is the tendency to isolate the thick portion of the interstitium to the interior of the septum and to leave the thin air-blood barrier exposed to the alveolar air, thus maximizing surface area contact between air and blood. Second, the pools of surface-active material within the folds may create localized areas of negative pressure concentrated at the thick portion of the septum; Weibel and Bachofen have hypoth-

esized that this may be of significance in determining the path of drainage of the small amount of fluid that normally leaks from alveolar capillaries into the interstitium.[161] Finally, it has been suggested that the intercapillary folds may act in a purely mechanical fashion to impede capillary blood flow; since the folds are greatest in extent in the more collapsed alveoli, this would have the effect of matching ventilation with perfusion.[456]

Weibel[10, 127] found that the external diameter of capillary segments in fresh lung averaged 8.6 μ; allowing 0.3 μ for the average thickness of the capillary endothelium, the average internal capillary diameter was estimated to be 8 μ. As Glazier and his colleagues have shown in rapidly frozen dog lungs, this value may vary substantially with both lung volume and capillary pressure.[458] The axial *length* of capillary segments ranged from 9 to 13 μ (average, 10.3). Weibel deduced that each alveolus is surrounded by about 1800 to 2000 capillary segments and that the total number of capillary segments in the entire lung shows a group average of about 280 billion. He estimated total capillary blood volume to be 140 ml; total capillary surface of the lung was 70 sq m, only slightly less than that of the alveolar surface. The volume of blood per alveolus was estimated at 4.7×10^{-7} ml and the capillary surface per alveolus 23.4×10^{-4} sq cm.

THE BRONCHIAL CIRCULATION

Anatomy

The existence of a systemic arterial supply to the lung was first described by Galen in the second century A.D.,[604] although in 1732 Ruysch claimed for himself the honor of discovering the bronchial

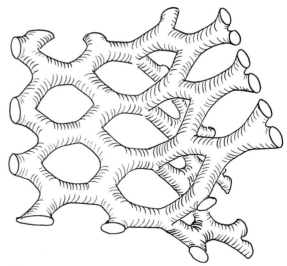

Figure 1–71. Alveolar Capillary Network. Schematic sketch of the capillary network at the juncture of three interalveolar septal facets showing continuity of network. (From Weibel ER: Morphometry of the Human Lung. New York, Academic Press, 1963.)

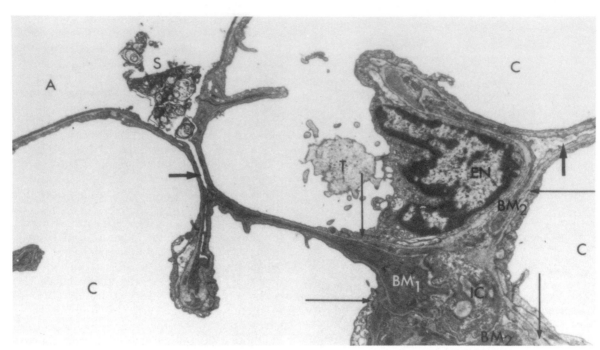

Figure 1–72. Alveolar Pleats or Folds. Folding of the thin portion of the air-blood tissue barrier over the thick portion, which appears to be shifted into the capillary lumen. Two collapsed alveolar lumina (*thick arrows*), one of which joins an open alveolus (*A*), are visible. The basement membranes (BM_1 and BM_2) of the two alveoli converge toward a contractile interstitial cell (*IC*) located at the thick portion of the barrier (the membrane portions seen at the bottom belong to the same collapsed alveolus as the one recognizable at the upper right). The alveolar and capillary basement membranes fuse with each other at the borders of the cell (*thin arrows*). *S*, Surfactant; *T*, thrombocytes; *EN*, endothelial cell; *C*, capillary. (Rat lung, fixation at 10 cm H_2O airway pressure. × 8600.) (From Assimacopoulos A, Guggenheim R, Kapanci Y: Lab Invest *34*:10, 1976. Copyright US-Canadian Division of IAP.)

arteries.[605] During the 19th century, the anatomy of the bronchial circulation was studied in considerable detail, and in 1908 its functional significance was first suggested by Reisseisen and Von Sommering as "die Vasa nutritiva der Lungen."[606] Despite the interest in the bronchial circulation at this time, no reference was made to the writings and drawings of Leonardo da Vinci, who some 300 years previously had clearly described the function of the bronchial circulation as the nutrient vessels of the lung.[607] During the early part of this century, extensive and detailed anatomic studies of the bronchial vasculature were carried out on human lungs post mortem using injection and casting techniques;[608-612] more recently, angiography has been employed for the same purpose.[613]

Human bronchial arteries normally arise directly from the aorta or the intercostobronchial trunk[614] and usually number from two to four.[608, 611, 615] The usual pattern consists of one bronchial artery on the right, originating from the third intercostal artery (the first right intercostal artery that arises directly from the aorta), and two on the left (arising directly from the aorta on its ventral aspect, usually opposite the fifth and sixth thoracic vertebrae). The average number of bronchial arteries per individual is 2.7, and there are invariably more on the left than on the right.[600, 601]

The extrapulmonary branches course to the hila where they form an intercommunicating circular arc around the main stem bronchi from which the true bronchial arteries radiate.[601] These vessels are situated within the peribronchial connective tissue, extending along the bronchial tree and branching with the airways; at least two divisions are present along each bronchus, one on each side of the bronchial wall. These branches have extensive horizontal intercommunications within the bronchial adventitia and also send twigs through the bronchial wall to form a similar intercommunicating capillary network in the submucosa. The arteries continue as far as the terminal bronchioles; with injection techniques, small arteriolar branches can be seen to extend to the alveolar ducts and occasionally even into the lung parenchyma around alveolar sacs.[601] Histologically, the larger arteries have a well-developed muscular media and a prominent internal elastic lamina. In addition, there is frequently a longitudinal intimal muscle layer that occasionally becomes quite voluminous and sometimes appears histologically to occlude the vascular lumen completely; it has been suggested by some[601] that this development is caused by stretching of the airways during normal respiration; others consider it to represent simply an age-related reparative change.[435]

In addition to providing a blood supply to the bronchial and bronchiolar walls, the bronchial arteries supply the loose peribronchial and perivascular connective tissue; the tracheal wall; the middle third of the esophagus; the visceral pleura over the mediastinal and diaphragmatic surfaces of the lungs

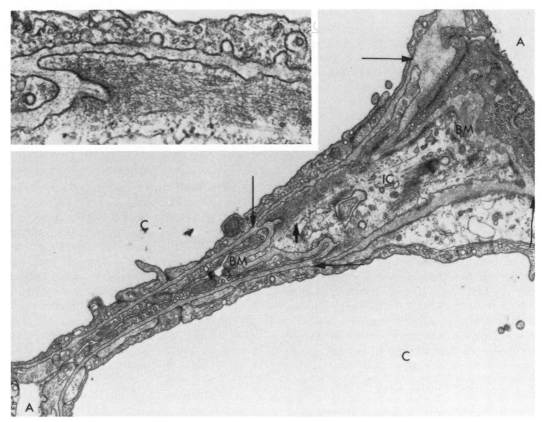

Figure 1–73. The Thick Portion of the Air-Blood Barrier. A contractile interstitial cell (*IC*) bridges across the capillary space (*C*). The basement membrane (*BM*) of the two adjacent alveoli (*A*) converges toward the cell and fuses with the capillary basement membrane at the borders of this cell (*thin arrows*). A high magnification of a bundle of microfilaments (*thick arrow*) is shown (inset). (Rat lung, fixation at 15 cm H$_2$O airway pressure. × 20,000; inset, × 67,000.) (From Assimacopoulos A, Guggenheim R, Kapanci Y: Lab Invest *34*:10, 1976. Copyright US-Canadian Division of IAP.)

(the visceral pleura over the lung convexities being supplied by pulmonary arteries); the paratracheal, carinal, hilar, and intrapulmonary lymph nodes and lymphoid tissue; the vagus and bronchopulmonary nerves; and sometimes the parietal layer of the pericardium and the thymus.[600] In addition, the vasa vasorum of the aortic arch, pulmonary arteries, and pulmonary veins is fed by branches of the bronchial arteries. Bronchial arteries sometimes anastomose with other systemic arteries, such as the coronaries.[616, 617]

The bronchial circulation is unique in that it has a dual venous drainage; a portion of the bronchial flow drains via the bronchial veins to the right side of the heart via the azygos and hemiazygos systems, whereas another portion forms extensive anastomoses with the pulmonary circulation at precapillary, capillary, and postcapillary sites and drains into the left atrium via the pulmonary veins.[618] This latter is the bronchopulmonary anastomotic flow, a subject recently reviewed by Murata and coworkers.[1160]

Bronchial arterial blood flow, first measured in 1931 by Berry and Daly using isolated perfused dog lungs,[619] was estimated to be about 1 per cent of cardiac output. A variety of techniques have since been used to measure flow, and it is not surprising that the results show considerable variability, even within the same species, with values ranging from less than 1 per cent to greater than 5 per cent of cardiac output. In more recent studies in which a modification of the radioactive microsphere technique has been employed on anesthetized dogs,[620] bronchial blood flow has been partitioned into parenchymal (anastomotic) and large airway fractions; it was shown that 55 per cent of the total bronchial blood flow goes to lung parenchyma and 45 per cent to the trachea and bronchi.

Because of the inacessibility of the bronchial vessels, very few measurements of human flow have been made. Measurements of bronchopulmonary anastomotic flow have been made in patients undergoing coronary artery bypass surgery, since during cross-clamping of the aorta bronchopulmonary anastomotic flow is the only blood returning to the left side of the heart: flow has been found to be highly variable, ranging from 1 per cent to almost 24 per cent of cardiac output; flow was increased in patients with pulmonary disease.[621]

Regulation and Nervous Control

Bronchial arterial blood flow has been shown to be directly related to changes in systemic pressure.[622, 623] An increase in systemic venous pressure or a decrease in left atrial pressure causes a decrease in bronchial venous drainage and preferential drainage to the left side of the heart, whereas the opposite occurs with elevation of the left atrial pressure and a decrease in systemic venous pressure.[622] The bronchial vasculature is compressed with increasing alveolar pressure[623, 624] and is also sensitive to changes in PO_2 and PCO_2, responding to acute changes in gas tensions differently than do either the pulmonary or systemic circulations.[625] Severe hypoxemia causes a significant increase in bronchovascular resistance; hypercapnia causes a decrease in bronchovascular resistance and an increase in bronchial blood flow. The bronchial vasculature has both parasympathetic and sympathetic innervation:[626] parasympathetic vagal stimulation causes vasodilatation whereas sympathetic stimulation results in vasoconstriction and a consequent reduction in bronchial blood flow.[627] It has also been shown that dogs have both alpha- and beta-adrenergic receptors:[628] alpha-receptors predominate and when stimulated result in vasoconstriction, whereas beta-receptors mediate vasodilatation.

Function

The bronchial vasculature may have several important functions although only a few have been examined in any depth. It may play an important role in the humidification and warming of inspired air;[629] anatomically, it is ideally suited for this function since it contains two venous plexuses, one lying superficially parallel to the bronchial epithelium and the second situated deep in the peribronchial connective tissue. These two plexuses are bridged by short venous radicles.[3, 630, 631] Recent studies in dogs have shown that the bronchial vasculature of the trachea and large airways is extremely sensitive to changes in inspired air temperature and humidity. Bronchial blood flow increases to more than twice its baseline value in response to the inhalation of cold air and up to ten times its baseline value in response to the inhalation of warm, dry air.[632] This increase in blood flow is not affected by vagotomy, alpha- or beta-adrenergic blockade, or the inhibition of prostaglandin synthesis.[633]

It has also been suggested by Pietra and associates that the bronchial circulation is important in the production of pulmonary edema and in the removal of excess edema fluid from the interstitial space.[631] Although it has long been known that the bronchial circulation contributes to the normal anatomic shunt, it also takes part in gas exchange:[634, 635] using the inert gas technique, Robertson and associates[636] have shown that only about 20 per cent of bronchial blood flow bypasses gas-exchanging units; thus, only 20 per cent of less than 1 per cent of the cardiac output is in fact "shunted" by this circulation.

The bronchial circulation also has the capacity to undergo marked increase in volume in many pulmonary and cardiac diseases. Flows of up to 25 per cent of cardiac output have been reported in patients undergoing cardiopulmonary bypass surgery. The circulation can also serve as an emergency backup system; for example, it is well known that the bronchial arteries maintain lung tissue integrity in areas where the pulmonary arteries are acutely or chronically occluded. In fact, over 100 years ago Virchow showed that pulmonary infarction rarely occurs after ligation of the main pulmonary artery because of collateral circulation entering the obstructed areas of lung.[637] The effects of acute pulmonary artery obstruction have been examined by several investigators, and it has been shown that a rapid increase in bronchial artery blood flow occurs that is maximal 2 weeks after embolization.[638]

The bronchial arteries also supply substrate and oxygen to airway smooth muscle and the specialized epithelial cells involved in mucociliary clearance and ion transport; however, their importance to these functions and the factors that regulate flow are largely unknown.

INTERVASCULAR ANASTOMOSES

Because of the lungs' dual blood supply, several combinations of intervascular anastomoses are theoretically possible. Employing histologic, functional, and corrosion cast techniques, many investigators have attempted to delineate and assess the extent and importance of these combinations; this subject has been reviewed in detail by Wagenvoort and Wagenvoort.[435]

Anastomoses between bronchial and pulmonary veins are undoubtedly the most frequent and, as indicated previously, represent the normal pathway for the bulk of bronchial and bronchiolar venous drainage. Bronchial artery–pulmonary artery anastomoses have been shown to occur in the normal lung, but their significance in terms of extent is debated; their number and size can increase appreciably in various disease states. Although investigated extensively, the existence of pulmonary arteriovenous anastomoses is uncertain; some studies find evidence for their presence and others do not. Arteriovenous anastomoses in the bronchial circulation have been noted but are uncommon. In the perinatal period, anastomotic channels from bronchial arteries to alveolar capillaries and from pulmonary arteries to the capillaries of bronchial walls and interstitial tissue can be readily identified; however, under normal circumstances these decrease dramatically in number or disappear altogether during infancy. In her study of normal lungs, Turner-Warwick could show no anastomoses between systemic and pulmonary arteries; however, in diseased lungs she observed subpleural and intrapleural anastomoses that appeared to represent enlargement of pre-existing channels, implying their normal existence.[603] Stocker and Malczak have demonstrated the presence of small arteries originating in the aorta and coursing in the pulmonary ligament to supply a portion of the medial, basal pleura; although normally these are not important in terms of flow, it has been suggested that their enlargement in diseased lung might be involved in the pathogenesis of pulmonary sequestration.

ROENTGENOLOGY OF THE VASCULAR SYSTEM

The *main pulmonary artery* originates in the mediastinum at the pulmonic valve and passes upward, backward, and to the left before bifurcating within the pericardium into the shorter left and longer right pulmonary arteries (Fig. 1–74). The *right pulmonary artery* courses to the right behind the ascending aorta before dividing behind the superior vena cava and in front of the right main bronchus into ascending (truncus anterior) and descending (interlobar) rami (Fig. 1–75). Although variable, the common pattern is for the ascending artery to subdivide into the segmental branches that supply the right upper lobe, whereas the descending branch ultimately contributes the segmental arteries to the middle and right lower lobes.[458] Jefferson

found that in 90 per cent of patients a portion of the posterior segment of the right upper lobe is supplied by a separate arterial branch that arises from the interlobar artery distal to the takeoff of the truncus anterior.[459] The first portion of the right interlobar artery is horizontal, interposed between the superior vena cava in front and the intermediate bronchus behind. It then turns sharply downward and backward, assuming a vertical orientation within the major fissure (thus its name) anterolateral to the intermediate and right lower lobe bronchi before giving off the segmental branches—one or two to the middle lobe and usually single branches to each of the five bronchopulmonary segments of the lower lobe.

The width of the interlobar artery can be a useful criterion in the assessment of diseases affecting the pulmonary vessels, and normal limits have been established. From a study of over 1000 normal adult American subjects, Chang found that in full inspiration the upper limit of the transverse diameter of the interlobar artery from its lateral aspect to the air column of the intermediate bronchus was 16 mm in men and 15 mm in women; these figures decreased by 1 to 3 mm in full expiration.[460] Simon's values for this measurement in normal middle-aged

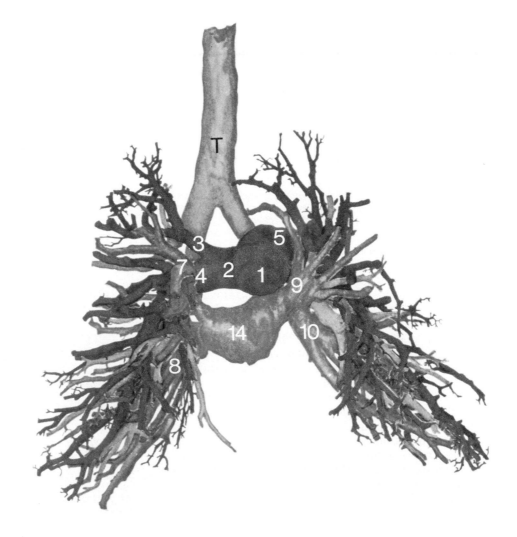

Figure 1–74. Anatomic Features of the Central Pulmonary Vasculature. (This illustration appears in color following page 314.) Anterior cast of the trachea (*T*), bronchi, pulmonary arteries, and pulmonary veins. The intricate relationship of these structures to one another is apparent. Note that the right (*7*) and the left (*9*) superior veins relate most closely to the anterior aspect of the upper hila whereas the right (*8*) and the left (*10*) inferior veins are situated posteromedial to the lower lobe bronchi. Numerical anatomic designations are used consistently throughout this section. *1*, Main pulmonary artery; *2*, right pulmonary artery; *3*, truncus anterior; *4*, right interlobar artery; *5*, left pulmonary artery; *7*, right superior pulmonary vein; *8*, right inferior pulmonary vein; *9*, left superior pulmonary vein; *10*, left inferior pulmonary vein; *14*, left atrium. (From Genereux GP: AJR *141*:1241, 1983.)

A third method for estimating changes in arterial caliber is the artery-bronchus index described by Wójtowicz.[464] In his study of 1200 tomograms of 250 normal subjects in the supine position, the ratio of the transverse diameter of a pulmonary artery to the contiguous bronchus viewed end-on in the perihilar area was independent of age, sex, and body build and provided a more objective assessment of disturbances in pressure and flow in the pulmonary circulation than was possible with direct measurement of the caliber of the artery itself. He found the normal mean value of the artery-bronchus index to be 1.30 immediately distal to the takeoff of the right upper lobe bronchus and 1.40 immediately beyond the origin of the left upper lobe bronchus. Our experience with this method is limited, but we feel that it may be useful in selected cases.

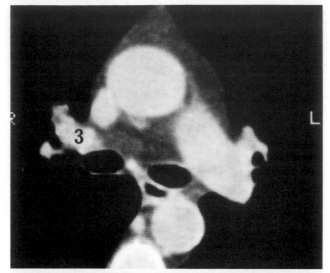

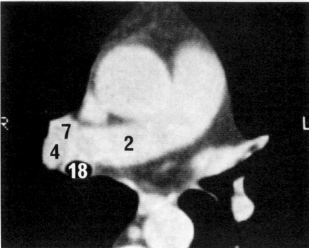

Figure 1–75. Anatomic Features of the Right Pulmonary Artery and Its Major Branches. The right pulmonary artery (2) divides within the pericardium into ascending (3) and descending (4) rami; the latter turns vertically at the hilum, lateral to the intermediate bronchus (18) and posterior to the right superior vein (7). Note that the interlobar artery is thus composed of a short horizontal limb and a longer, obliquely vertical part.

British adults averaged 13.9 mm but with a slightly higher maximal diameter of 19 mm.[461] This average figure compares favorably with the measurements obtained by Dr. Liu Yu-Qing of the Cardiovascular Institute of the Chinese Academy of Medical Sciences, Peking, in a 1957 study: the mean diameter of the right descending artery in 200 normal adult men was 13.28 mm and in 100 normal adult women, 12.68 mm.[462] Coussement and Gooding found that, in children, the diameter of the right interlobar artery could be related to the caliber of the trachea. In their study of chest roentgenograms of 112 normal children and 102 with left-to-right intracardiac shunts, they found that in the presence of a shunt the diameter of the right interlobar artery was always greater than that of the trachea; by contrast, in normal children the diameter was equal to or less than that of the trachea.[463]

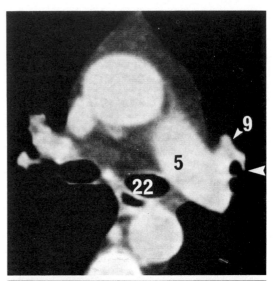

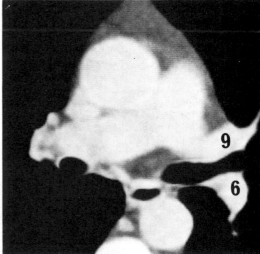

Figure 1–76. Anatomic Features of the Left Pulmonary Artery and Its Major Branches. The left pulmonary artery (5) passes over the left main bronchus (22), forming the interlobar (6) branch. The left superior vein (9) lies medial to the apicoposterior bronchus (*arrowhead*) before it passes into the mediastinum in front of the left upper/main bronchial continuum prior to its entrance into the top of the left atrium.

The higher *left pulmonary artery,* after passing over the left main bronchus, sometimes gives off a short ascending branch that subsequently divides into segmental branches to the upper lobe; more commonly, however, it continues directly into the vertically oriented left interlobar artery from which the segmental arteries to the upper and lower lobes arise directly.[458] The left interlobar artery lies posterolateral to the lower lobe bronchus (Fig. 1–76).

The course of the veins is remote from the bronchoarterial bundles, a relationship that commences in the lung periphery where the arterial system is in the center of the lobules and the venous system is located within the interlobular septa. This relationship persists, so that in all areas the arteries and their corresponding veins are separated by air-containing lung. Theoretically, this should permit distinction of artery from vein, particularly in the medial third of the lung where the continuity of the artery with its accompanying bronchus may be more readily distinguished and where the typical course of the larger veins on their way to the mediastinum can be recognized. However, in a pulmonary angiographic study of 50 patients in anteroposterior projection, the upper lobe artery and vein were superimposed in 40 to 50 per cent of subjects, the implication being that these vessels could not be distinguished on standard roentgenograms.[465]

Segmental veins from the right upper lobe coalesce to form the *right superior pulmonary vein* (Figs. 1–77 and 1–78), which descends medially into the mediastinum before attaching to the upper and posterior aspect of the left atrium as a superior confluence. Along its course caudad, this vessel is intimately associated from above downward with the anterior and posterior upper lobe segmental bronchi, the junction of the horizontal and vertical segments of the right interlobar pulmonary artery, and the anteromedial aspect of the middle lobe bronchus.[466] The *middle lobe vein,* after passing under the middle lobe bronchus, usually joins the left atrium at the base of the superior pulmonary venous confluence, although occasionally the three veins on the right (superior, middle, and inferior) remain separate.

On the left, the segmental veins from the upper lobe join to form the *left superior pulmonary vein* (Figs. 1–74 and 1–78), which, after uniting with the lingular vein, courses obliquely downward and medially into the mediastinum. Along its course caudad, this vessel lies medial to the apicoposterior bronchoarterial bundle, anterolateral to the left pulmonary artery, and, finally, anterior to the continuum formed by the left main and upper lobe bronchi.[466] It thus separates these airways from the left atrium before it inserts into this chamber.

The horizontally oriented lower lobe segmental veins on both sides coalesce medial to the lower lobe bronchi to form the *right* and *left inferior pulmonary veins;* as they attach to the left atrium medially, they form the inferior pulmonary venous confluences

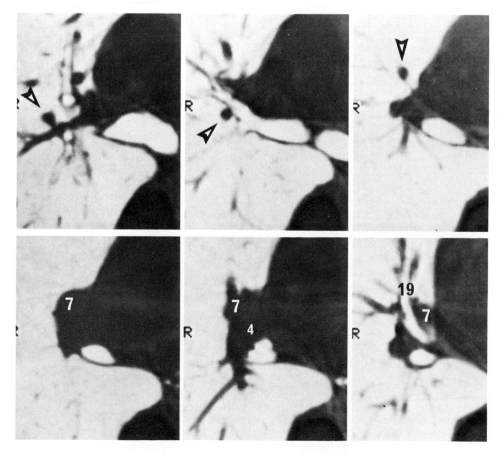

Figure 1–77. Right Superior Pulmonary Vein (RSPV). Sequential CT scans through the right hilum. The RSPV (*7*) is formed following the union of upper lobe segmental veins (*arrowhead*); so formed, it relates intimately to the horizontal limb of the interlobar artery (*4*) and the middle lobe bronchus (*19*) before entering the left atrium. The RSPV and the right interlobar artery form a typical "elephant head-and-trunk" configuration (middle frame, bottom).

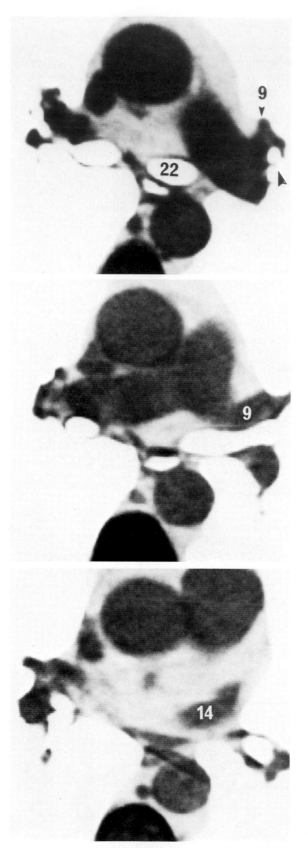

Figure 1–78. Left Superior Pulmonary Vein (LSPV). Sequential CT scans through the left hilum. The LSPV (*9*) is formed following union of the upper lobe segmental veins; it relates to the apicoposterior bronchus (*arrowhead*) before passing into the mediastinum in front of the left upper/main bronchial continuum (*22*) prior to its insertion into the superior portion of the left atrium (*14*).

(Fig. 1–79).[467, 468] The left inferior pulmonary vein and venous confluence are at the same level as or slightly higher than the right and slightly more posterior; this vein may join with the left superior vein to form a common chamber before entering the left atrium (Fig. 1–80). The normal superior and inferior venous confluences are sometimes prominent enough to simulate a mass on a lateral chest roentgenogram, particularly, but not exclusively on the right.

THE PULMONARY HILA

The term *hilum* is widely used in the roentgenographic literature in reference to the lungs, but the anatomic boundaries defining this area are vague.[467, 469–471] Some describe the hilum as lying immediately adjacent to the main bronchi, from the tracheal carina to the origin of the first lobar bronchus.[472] Consensus, however, seems to favor an imprecisely defined area between the mediastinum medially and the substance of the lung laterally, through which pass the bronchi, pulmonary and systemic arteries and veins, autonomic nerves, and lymph vessels and nodes.[469–471, 473–475] Consequently, we prefer to define the hila simply as those areas in the center of the thorax that connect the mediastinum to the lungs; since they are surrounded by aerated lung, they are visible on conventional chest roentgenograms. The anatomic structures rendering the hila visible are primarily the pulmonary arteries and veins, with lesser contributions from the bronchial walls, surrounding areolar and adipose tissue, and small lymph nodes.[474]

As viewed on a conventional posteroanterior roentgenogram, the hila can be divided into *upper* and *lower* components by an imaginary horizontal line transecting the junction of the upper lobe and intermediate bronchi on the right and the upper and lower lobe dichotomy on the left. The *right* upper hilar opacity relates to the ascending pulmonary artery (truncus anterior) and right superior pulmonary vein, whereas the lower hilar shadow is caused by the interlobar pulmonary artery and proximal right superior and inferior pulmonary veins. The major implication of this anatomic arrangement is that the undivided right pulmonary artery cannot form a part of the normal hilar vascular shadow[476] (as commonly suggested in the literature) since it lies more centrally in the mediastinum and thus does not relate to air-containing lung parenchyma.

The *left* upper hilar opacity results from the left pulmonary artery, proximal left interlobar artery, and left superior pulmonary vein; the lower hilar shadow relates to the interlobar artery and proximal left superior and inferior pulmonary veins.

There are four major roentgenographic techniques for examining the hila: (1) conventional roentgenograms in posteroanterior and lateral pro-

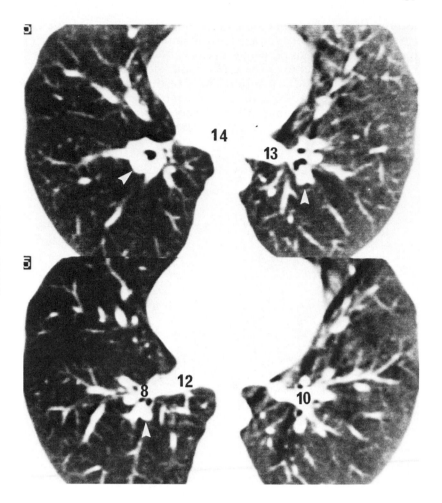

Figure 1–79. Right and Left Inferior Pulmonary Veins and Confluences. In contrast to the vertical orientation of the lower lobe arteries (*arrowheads*), the right (*12*) and left (*13*) pulmonary vein confluences, inferior pulmonary veins (*8, 10*), and their major branches are horizontally oriented in the lower lobes prior to their entry into the left atrium (*14*). The left inferior pulmonary vein is usually higher and more posterior than the right.

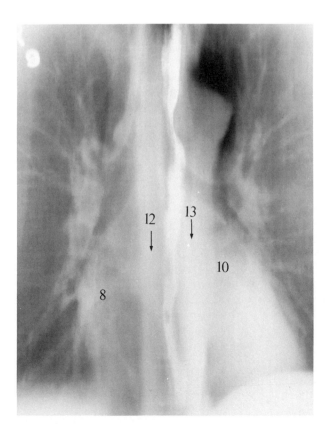

Figure 1–80. Inferior Pulmonary Veins. A conventional anteroposterior linear tomogram demonstrates the right (*8*) and left (*10*) inferior pulmonary veins and their respective confluences (*12, 13*).

jection, the method that suffices in the majority of cases; (2) conventional tomography in anteroposterior, oblique, and lateral projection; some observers regard this technique as the second line of investigation in cases in which close scrutiny of the hila is required; (3) computed tomography; and (4) magnetic resonance imaging. Each of these examinations possesses distinct advantages and disadvan-

tages; however, since they are all used to greater or lesser extent in clinical practice, we will describe the normal features of each in some (albeit repetitious) detail.

Assessment of the hila with any of these modes of examination requires a thorough understanding of normal anatomy, a subject that has been excellently reviewed by Vix and Klatte[477] and more

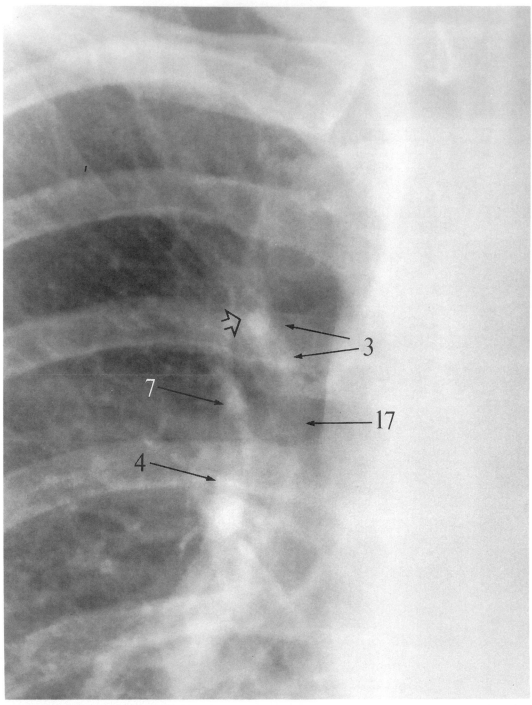

Figure 1–81. Right Upper Hilar Anatomy. A detail view of the right hilum from a conventional PA roentgenogram demonstrates the ascending (*3*) and descending (*4*) arteries. The right superior pulmonary vein (*7*) crosses the hilum obliquely to form the typical *V* configuration. The lumen of the right upper lobe bronchus (*17*) and of the end-on bronchus and the opaque artery (*open arrowhead*) of the anterior segment are shown.

recently by Proto and Speckman[478, 479] and by Müller and Webb.[1161]

CONVENTIONAL POSTEROANTERIOR AND LATERAL ROENTGENOGRAMS

In PA projection, the *right upper hilar opacity* relates to the ascending pulmonary artery and right superior pulmonary vein, including respective branches of each (Fig. 1–81). The end-on opacity and radiolucency, respectively, of the contiguous anterior (occasionally posterior) segmental artery and bronchus can be identified in the majority of normal subjects (in 80 per cent according to Fraser and his colleagues.[480] A short segment of the upper lobe bronchus, beneath the ascending right pulmonary artery, can sometimes be identified before it trifucates into the segmental branches serving the upper lobe.

The *lower portion of the right hilum* (Fig. 1–82) is formed by the vertically oriented interlobar artery, the right superior pulmonary vein superolaterally as it crosses the junction of the horizontal and vertical limbs of the interlobar artery, and the respective branches of these vessels. More inferiorly lies the horizontally oriented inferior pulmonary vein. The radiolucent lumen of the intermediate bronchus is invariably identified medial to the interlobar artery. Occasionally, segmental bronchi and arteries in the middle and lower lobes can be seen either in profile or end-on. Additional contributions to the normal roentgenographic density of the up-

per and lower hila are provided by small lymph nodes, fatty areolar tissue, and bronchial walls.

On the left, the *upper hilar opacity* is formed by the distal left pulmonary artery, the proximal portion of the left interlobar artery, its segmental arterial branches, and the left superior pulmonary vein and its major tributaries (Fig. 1–83). The proximal left pulmonary artery is almost always higher than the highest point of the right interlobar artery: in one series of 500 normal subjects, this feature was found in 97 per cent, the range of difference in the majority being 0.75 to 2.25 cm;[474] in 3 per cent the hila were at the same level, and in none was the right hilum higher than the left. As suggested by Simon, the reference point for the determination of this relationship is the point at which the right and left superior pulmonary veins cross their respective pulmonary arteries prior to entering the mediastinum.[461] The left superior hilum, unlike its counterpart on the right, is often partly or completely covered by mediastinal fat and pleura between the aortic arch and left pulmonary artery, or by a portion of the cardiac silhouette; therefore, it may be largely hidden from view (Fig. 1–84). The *lower portion of the left hilum* is formed by the distal interlobar artery, the lingular artery and vein, and more caudally the left inferior pulmonary vein (Fig. 1–85). The air columns of the left upper lobe bronchus and its superior and inferior (lingular) divisions, and the left lower lobe bronchus may be identified. As on the right, soft tissue elements contribute only slightly to the nor-

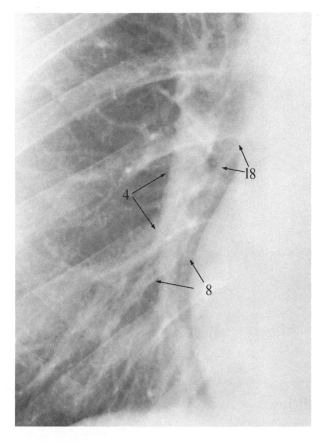

Figure 1–82. Right Lower Hilar Anatomy. On this detail view from a conventional PA roentgenogram, the interlobar (*4*) artery lies lateral to the intermediate bronchus (*18*). Note that this vessel dominates the roentgenographic anatomy of the lower hilum. The horizontally oriented inferior pulmonary vein (*8*) lies posteroinferior to the hilum.

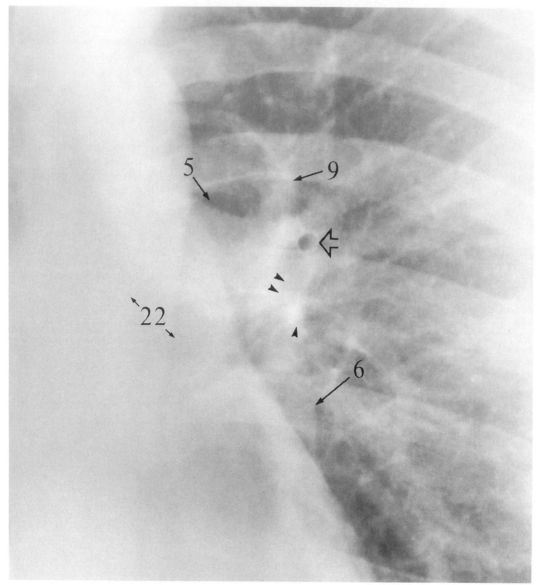

Figure 1–83. Left Upper Hilar Anatomy. A detail view of the left hilum from a PA chest roentgenogram shows the left pulmonary artery (*5*), the interlobar artery (*6*), and the left superior pulmonary vein (*9*). The left main bronchus (*22*) and its superior (*two arrowheads*) and inferior (*single arrowhead*) divisions are overlapped by the hilar vessels. The end-on bronchus and opaque artery (*single open arrowhead*) of the anterior segment are seen.

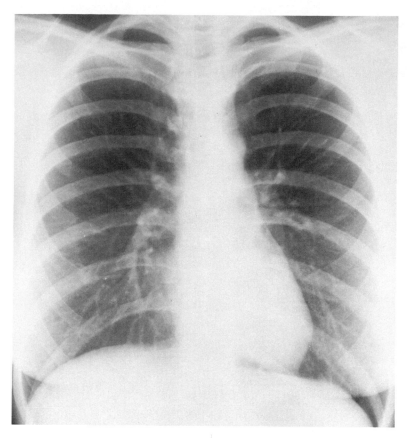

Figure 1–84. Hilar Anatomy Revealed by Conventional Posteroanterior Roentgenography. Note that the inferior portion of the hilum on the left may be overlapped by the cardiac silhouette; this is a normal feature in some subjects and should not be mistaken for bronchial displacement caused by minimal atelectasis of the left lower lobe.

mal roentgenographic hilar opacity. Frequently, the anterior segmental or lingular bronchoarterial bundle can be identified end-on in the upper hilum.

Certain normal variations caused by unusual prominence of the hilar vessels can be confused with hilar masses.[466] The majority of these *vascular pseudotumors* are caused by the large veins as they cross the hila on their way to the mediastinum. The right superior vein (Fig. 1–86), the left superior vein (Fig. 1–87), and the left superior or common venous confluence (Fig. 1–88) are the most frequent sources of these upper hilar pseudotumors. The right inferior venous confluence is a well-recognized cause of a pulmonary pseudotumor, particularly in patients with established postcapillary pulmonary hypertension due to left ventricular dysfunction or mitral valve disease (Fig. 1–89). The left pulmonary artery normally is oriented roughly in an anteroposterior plane as it enters the pleural space; occasionally, it courses more obliquely than usual, thus assuming an unusual prominence that creates an arterial hilar pseudotumor (Fig. 1–90).

The roentgenographic anatomy of the hila in *lateral projection* is complex since the right and left hilar components are to a large degree superimposed.[477–479] The carina is projected at the level of the 4th or 5th thoracic vertebra; however, vertebrae are sometimes difficult to count precisely on a lateral projection, and more useful landmarks are the left pulmonary artery or the proximal third of the intermediate stem line, structures that bear a close approximation to the tracheal bifurcation. Proto and Speckman[478] indicated that the air column of the normally more cephalad right upper lobe bronchus can be identified end-on in 50 per cent of subjects whereas that of the more caudad left upper lobe bronchus is seen in 77 per cent (Fig. 1–91). Occasionally, the uppermost radiolucency represents the right main bronchus and the lowermost radiolucency the left main bronchus, usually in asthenic individuals. The orifice of the right upper lobe bronchus is seldom as well circumscribed as that of the left: the former is not completely encircled by vessels, whereas the latter is surrounded by the left pulmonary artery above, the interlobar artery behind, and the mediastinal component of the left superior pulmonary vein in front. The right upper lobe bronchus is devoid of vascular envelopment on its posterior aspect so that aerated upper or lower lobe parenchyma normally abuts its wall. Consequently, clear identification of the right upper lobe bronchial lumen *en face* constitutes highly suggestive evidence that the airway is completely surrounded by soft tissue, most likely enlarged lymph nodes (Fig. 1–91).

The posterior wall of the right main and intermediate bronchi form the anatomic foundation for the *intermediate stem line*, a vertically oriented linear opacity measuring up to 3 mm in width (Fig. 1–91)[481] that according to Proto and Speckman[478] is visible in 95 per cent of individuals. The posterior wall of these two bronchi is rendered visible by air

Text continued on page 100

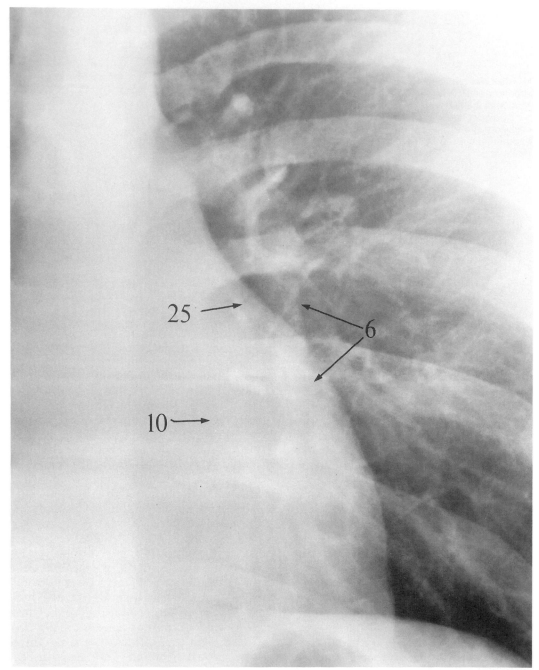

Figure 1–85. Left Inferior Hilar Anatomy. As revealed by a detail view of the left hilum from a posteroanterior roentgenogram, the interlobar artery (*6*) is situated posterolateral to the lower lobe bronchus (*25*). The obliquely oriented inferior pulmonary vein (*10*) is located posteromedial to the hilum.

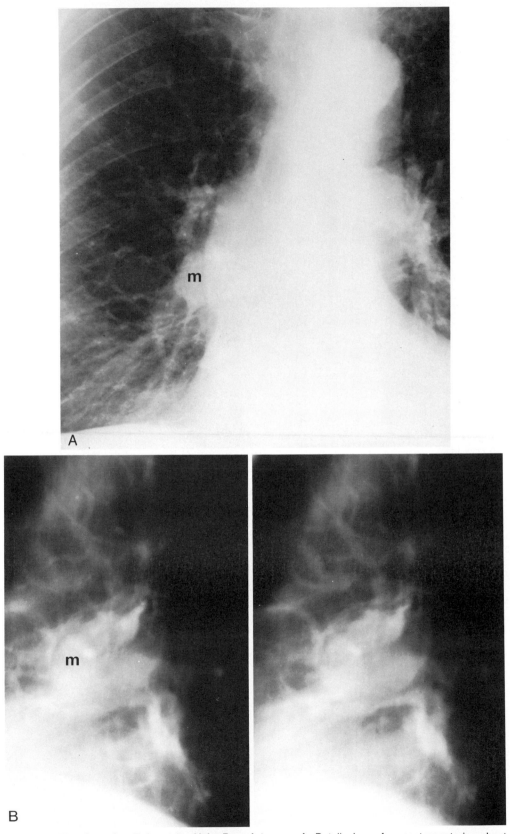

Figure 1–86. Right Hilar Superior Pulmonary Vein Pseudotumor. *A,* Detail view of a posteroanterior chest roentgenogram discloses an apparent right hilar mass (*m*). *B,* On conventional 55° right posterior oblique tomograms, the opacity (*m*) possesses the typical configuration of the right superior pulmonary vein.

Illustration continued on following page

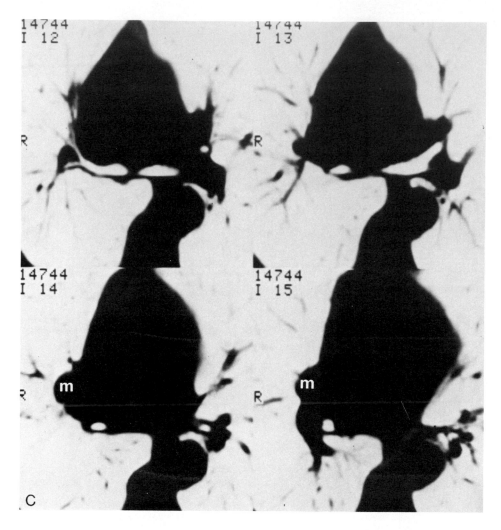

Figure 1–86 *Continued. C,* Unenhanced sequential CT scans through the right hilum show that the "mass" (*m*) results from a prominent right superior vein. On frame 15, note the typical "elephant head-and-trunk" configuration formed by the vein and vertical portion of the right descending artery. Compare with Figure 1–77. (From Genereux GP: AJR *141*:1241, 1983. © American Roentgen Ray Society.)

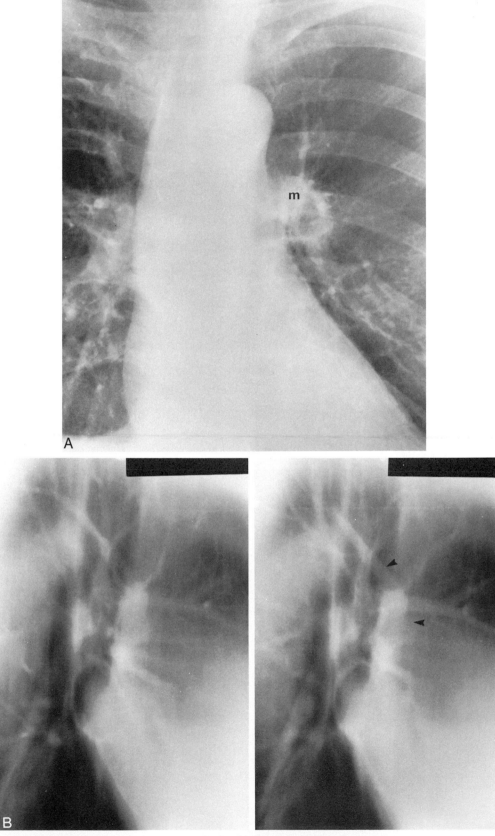

Figure 1–87. Left Hilar Superior Pulmonary Vein Pseudotumor. *A,* A detail view from a posteroanterior chest roentgenogram shows an elongated opacity (*m*) in the upper hilum. *B,* Conventional lateral linear tomograms through the hilum disclose the typical features of a prominent superior vein (*arrowheads*). Compare with Figure 1–78. (From Genereux GP: AJR *141*:1241, 1983. © American Roentgen Ray Society.)

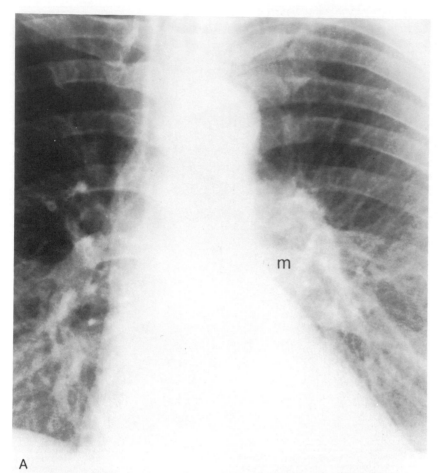

A

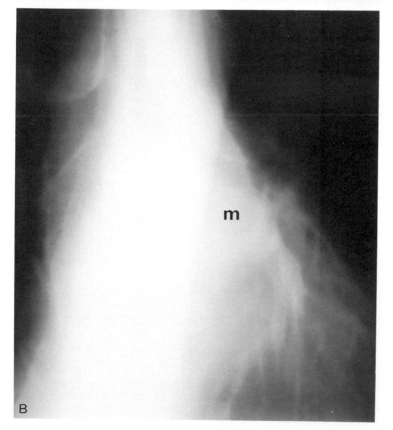

B

Figure 1–88. Prominent Left Common Venous Confluence as a Cause of Hilar Pseudotumor. *A*, A detail view of a posteroanterior chest roentgenogram discloses an unexplained opacity (*m*) beneath the left main bronchus. *B* and *C*, Anteroposterior and lateral conventional linear tomograms of the left hilum reveal the opacity (*m*) to represent a prominent left common venous confluence. *D*, Contrast-enhanced CT scans confirm this. Compare with Figures 1–74 and 1–79. (From Genereux GP: AJR *141*:1241, 1983. © American Roentgen Ray Society.)

Illustration continued on opposite page

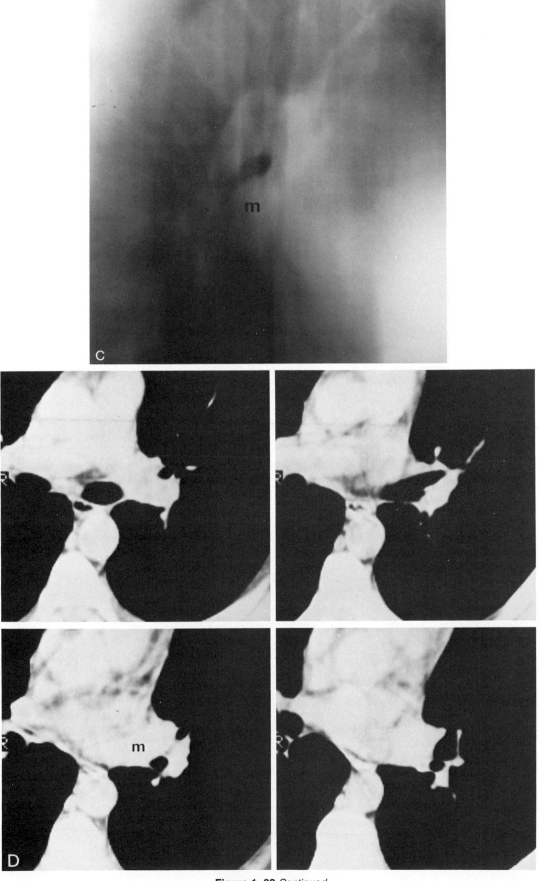

Figure 1–88 *Continued*

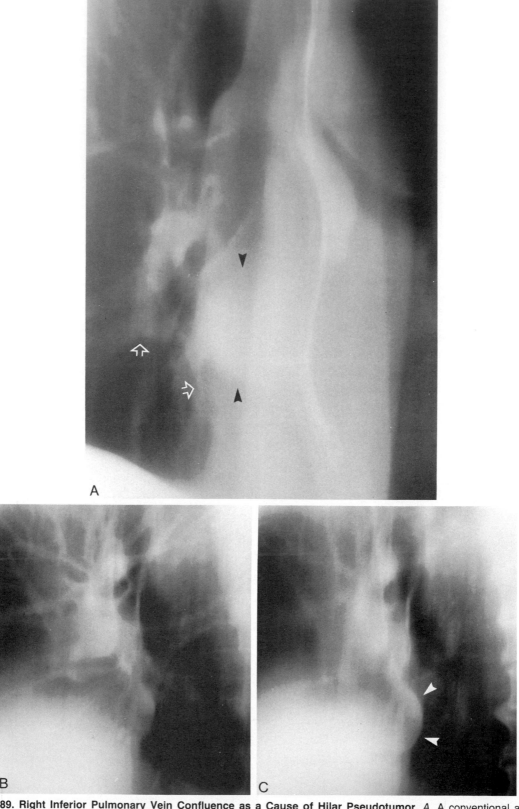

Figure 1–89. Right Inferior Pulmonary Vein Confluence as a Cause of Hilar Pseudotumor. *A*, A conventional anteroposterior linear tomogram through the carina with barium in the esophagus reveals an opacity (*arrowheads*) medial to the right lower lobe bronchus. Vessels can be seen to enter the inferior aspect of the shadow (*open arrows*). *B* and *C*, Conventional linear tomograms in lateral projection show the structure to represent a prominent right inferior pulmonary venous confluence (*arrowheads in C*).

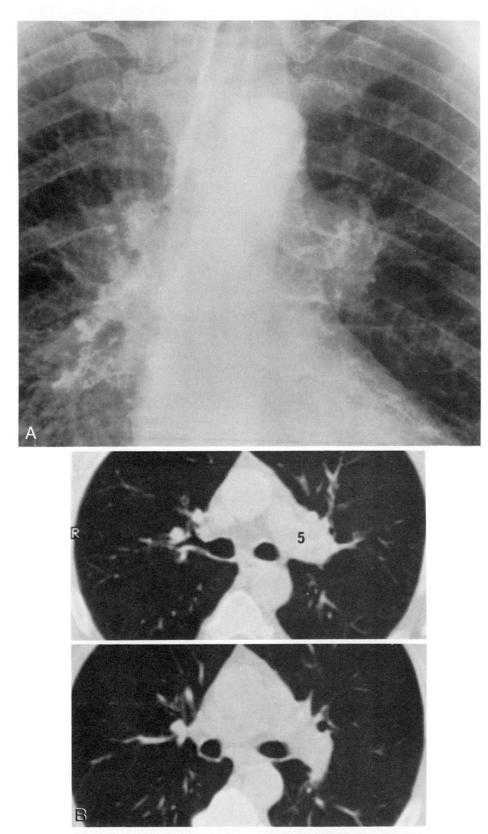

Figure 1–90. Prominent Left Pulmonary Artery as a Cause of Hilar Pseudotumor. *A,* A detail view of a posteroanterior chest roentgenogram discloses a prominent left hilum. *B,* CT scans through the carina reveal an obliquely directed, slightly enlarged left pulmonary artery (5) as the cause of the hilar prominence. Compare with Figure 1–76.

in their lumen in front and aerated lung parenchyma in the azygoesophageal recess behind. On a well-centered lateral projection, the line transects the mid or posterior third of the circular, radiolucent left upper lobe bronchus; it terminates caudally at the origin of the superior segmental bronchus of the right lower lobe, slightly proximal to or at the same level as the origin of the middle lobe bronchus anteriorly. We have not been able to identify the anterior wall of the intermediate bronchus, although Proto and Speckman reported this feature in 6 per cent of their cases.[478] We have no explanation for this discrepancy although it is difficult to understand how the anterior wall of the intermediate bronchus should be visible considering that it is closely abutted by the horizontal limb of the interlobar artery.

The physical characteristics that render the intermediate stem line visible are also operative to some extent on the left so that the posterior wall of the left main bronchus and the proximal portion of the left lower lobe bronchus may be profiled as the *left retrobronchial line* (Fig. 1–91).[482] This short, vertical linear opacity measures 3 mm or less in width and terminates caudally at the origin of the superior segmental bronchus of the left lower lobe. The distinction between the intermediate stem line and the left retrobronchial line is not difficult, bearing in mind that the former is both longer and more anteriorly located than the latter. Occasionally, a

convex, lenticular stripe can be identified in the anticipated location of the retrobronchial line, representing the *left retrobronchial stripe*: as shown on correlative conventional lateral roentgenographic and CT studies, behind this stripe is invariably located a gas-containing radiolucency (Fig. 1–92) representing gas within the esophagus; since the latter structure is closely applied to the left posterior tracheal wall and the posterior wall of the left main bronchus, the stripe represents the combined thickness of the anterior wall of the esophagus, mediastinal soft tissue, and the posterior wall of the left main bronchus. In essence, the left retrobronchial stripe is a mediastinal opacity, whereas the left retrobronchial line represents a portion of hilar anatomy. The anterior and posterior walls of the right lower lobe bronchus can be identified in 8 per cent of cases, whereas the arcuate configuration of the anterior wall of the left lower lobe bronchus, merging with the orifice of the left upper lobe bronchus, is visible in 43 per cent (Fig. 1–93).[478] Proto and Speckman were able to identify the middle lobe bronchus, the superior segmental bronchi, and the basilar bronchi in 4 per cent of their cases.[478, 479]

There has been much confusion concerning the nomenclature of the hilar vasculature, both in the recent literature and indeed in earlier editions of this textbook. A common misrepresentation has been to depict the right hilar opacity as the "right

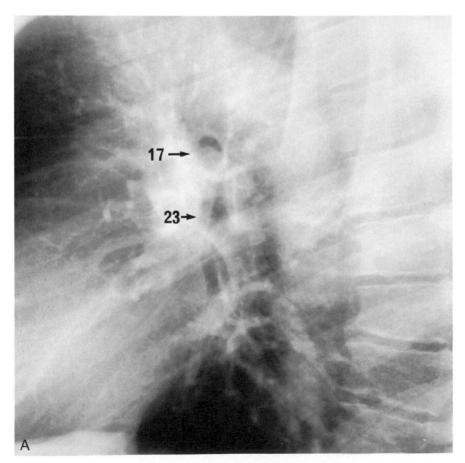

A

Figure 1–91. Hilar Anatomy Revealed by Conventional Lateral Roentgenograms. *A,* The end-on orifices of the right (*17*) and left (*23*) upper lobe bronchi can be easily identified. Although the left hilum is normally located cephalad to the right, the right upper lobe bronchus projects cephalad to its counterpart on the left.

Illustration continued on opposite page

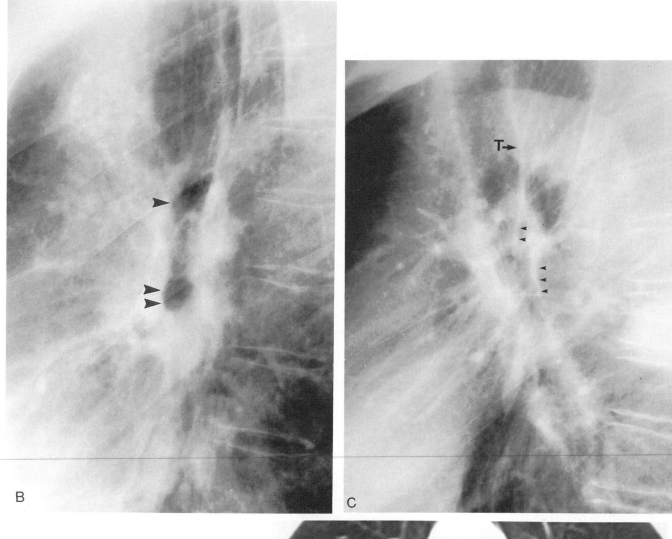

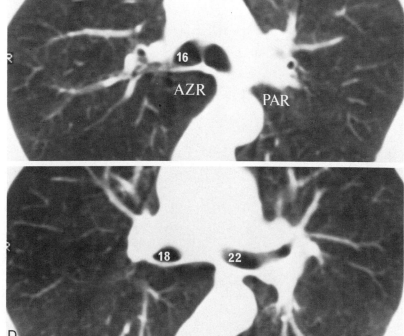

Figure 1–91 *Continued. B,* A detail view from a conventional lateral chest roentgenogram reveals exceptional clarity of the right (*arrowhead*) and left (*two arrowheads*) upper lobe bronchi. This appearance should suggest an excessive quantity of soft tissue surrounding the respective bronchial lumens, the most common cause of which is hilar node enlargement as in this patient with Hodgkin's disease. *C,* In another subject, a conventional lateral chest roentgenogram demonstrates the posterior tracheal stripe (*T*), intermediate stem line (*two arrowheads*), and left retrobronchial line (*three arrowheads*). On a true lateral view, the intermediate stem line may be straight or gently convex forward and characteristically bisects the orifice of the left upper lobe bronchus. *D,* CT scans through the carina (*top*) and 2 cm caudad (*bottom*) reveal the anatomic prerequisites underlying the features described in *C.* Aerated lung in the azygoesophageal recess (*AZR*) and the preaortic recess (*PAR*) abut the posterior wall of the right main (*16*) and intermediate (*18*) bronchi and the posterior wall of the left main bronchus (*22*), respectively. In essence, the intermediate stem line and the left retrobronchial line, representing the posterior wall of their respective bronchi, are rendered visible by an intrabronchial and intrapulmonary air envelope.

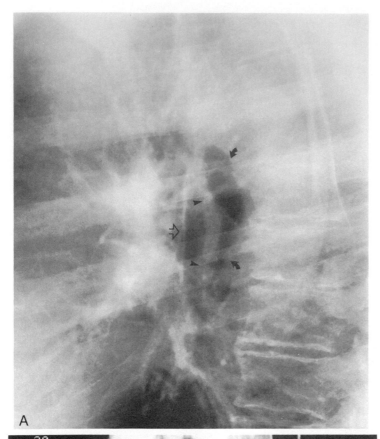

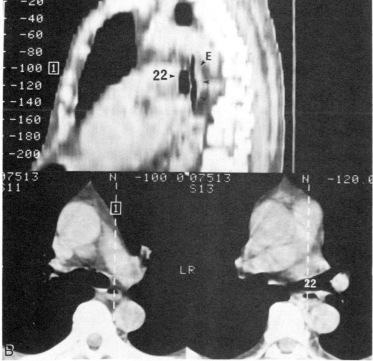

Figure 1–92. Left Retrobronchial Stripe. *A*, On this conventional lateral roentgenogram, there is a lenticular-shaped opacity (*arrowheads*), 3 to 4 mm thick, behind the intermediate stem line (*open arrow*), in the anticipated location of the left retrobronchial line. Note the similar-shaped radiolucency (*curved arrows*) posterior to the stripe. *B*, Sagittal CT reformation (*top*) and transverse CT scans (*bottom*) reveal the anatomic basis for the left retrobronchial stripe. Note that gas within the left main bronchus (*22*) and esophagus (*E*) allows for silhouetting of the mediastinal portion of the left main bronchus, mediastinal soft tissue, and anterior wall of the esophagus—the left retrobronchial stripe. Gas in the esophagus accounts for the radiolucency behind the stripe. (The supine position of the patient on the CT scan as opposed to the upright position on the conventional chest roentgenogram accounts for the fluid level in the esophagus in *B*.)

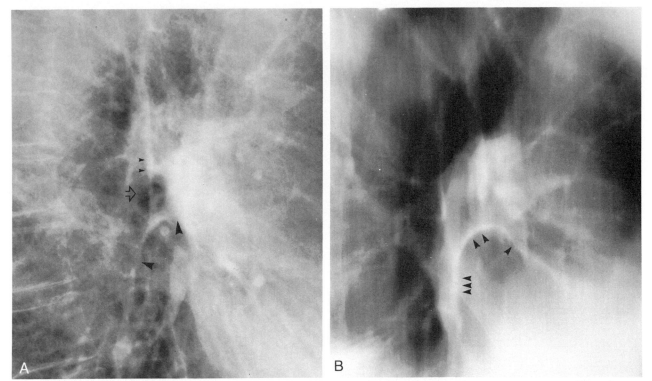

Figure 1–93. Hilar Anatomy in Lateral Projection. *A*, On a detail view from a lateral roentgenogram, there is a curvilinear (reversed comma-shaped) opacity (*large arrowheads*) anteroinferior to the end-on orifice of the distal left main or proximal left upper lobe bronchus (*open arrow*); this opacity represents, in succession, the inferior or anterior wall of the lingular bronchus, the left main bronchus, and the left lower lobe bronchus. The right-sided intermediate stem line (*small arrowheads*) bisects the bronchial lumen. *B*, A conventional lateral linear tomogram through the left hilum reveals the inferior wall of the lingula (*single arrowhead*), anterior wall of the left main bronchus (*two arrowheads*), and anterior wall of the left lower lobe bronchus (*three arrowheads*) as the three components of the line identified in *A*.

pulmonary artery." The right pulmonary artery, being an intramediastinal vessel and enveloped by other vessels or soft tissue elements, divides within the pericardium into ascending and descending (interlobar) branches; it is the latter that emerge from the mediastinum to comprise the true hilar arterial vessels. The right superior pulmonary vein abuts the anterior aspect of the right interlobar artery; consequently, the right hilar complex is composed of the superior vein anteriorly, the ascending and descending arteries posteriorly, and surrounding areolar and nodal tissue. Dilatation of the right superior pulmonary vein can produce a bulbous configuration of the anterior portion of the hilum, creating a vascular pseudotumor (Fig. 1–94). Conventional tomography is usually sufficient to identify the characteristic location and shape of this vessel, although contrast-enhanced CT or even angiography (Fig. 1–95) may be required occasionally for absolute distinction from a true hilar mass.

The major portion of the left hilar vasculature is visible behind the intermediate stem line. The top of the left pulmonary artery is seen in 96 per cent of subjects,[478, 479] usually as a sharply marginated opacity above and behind the radiolucency of the left upper lobe bronchus. Immediately posterior to this bronchus is the continuation of the left pulmonary artery, the interlobar artery. The left superior pulmonary vein, like its counterpart on

the right, is closely associated with the arterial vasculature of the hilum; however, this vein is not a contour-forming vessel on conventional lateral roentgenograms and thus cannot be identified. Prominence of the left common or superior pulmonary venous confluence can impinge upon and displace the left lower lobe bronchus superiorly and posteriorly both in normal subjects (Fig. 1–95) and when it becomes dilated as a result of postcapillary pulmonary hypertension.

The right and left inferior pulmonary veins are commonly imaged end-on as a result of their horizontal orientation, creating a nodular opacity below and behind the lower portion of the hila. Fortunately, vessels can usually be identified converging toward the opacity, permitting its distinction from a true parenchymal mass.

CONVENTIONAL TOMOGRAPHY

Some observers regard conventional linear or pluridirectional tomography as the first line of investigation whenever there is any doubt concerning the integrity of the hila,[483–485] although others prefer CT. If conventional tomography is to be performed, it is our opinion that a three-view study in anteroposterior, 55° posterior oblique, and lateral projection is required to delineate the anatomic features properly.[466] Consequently, in this section tomo-

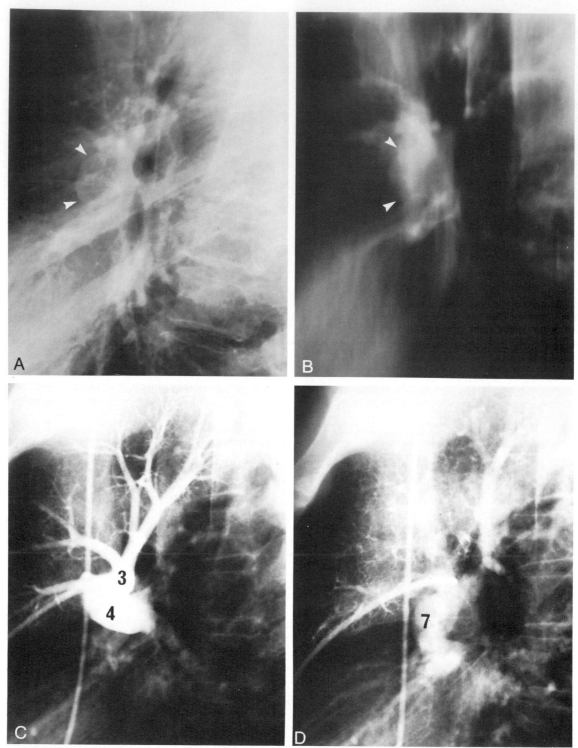

Figure 1–94. Venous Pseudotumor of the Right Hilum. A conventional lateral chest roentgenogram (*A*) and right lateral linear tomogram (*B*) suggest the presence of a small mass (*arrowheads*) in the right hilum. A selective distal right pulmonary angiogram in lateral projection during the arterial (*C*) and venous (*D*) phases shows that the hilar pseudotumor is caused by overlap of the right superior pulmonary vein (*7*) on the distal right artery (*3, 4*).

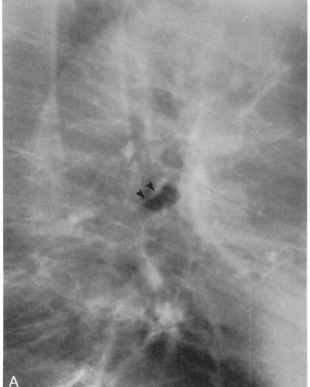

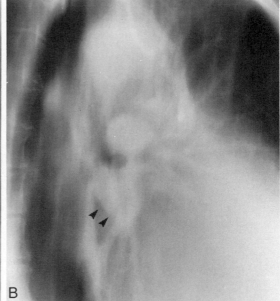

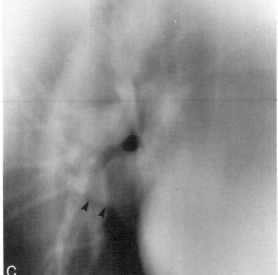

Figure 1–95. Venous Pseudotumor of the Left Hilum.
A, A detail view of a conventional lateral chest roentgenogram demonstrates displacement of the left main and lower lobe bronchi (*arrowheads*) superiorly and posteriorly by a contiguous soft tissue opacity. Conventional linear tomograms in 55° posterior oblique (*B*) and lateral (*C*) projections show that the bronchial displacement is related to a prominent venous confluence (*arrowheads*). This is a normal feature in some subjects and should not be mistaken for the bronchial displacement associated with left lower lobe atelectasis or postcapillary (venous) hypertension.

graphic anatomy is described in some detail; bronchographic and angiographic studies are illustrated to provide correlation with the tomographic features.

Anteroposterior Projection. The normal coronal tomogram at the level of the carina, with barium enhancement of the esophagus, is particularly appropriate for study of the trachea, right and left main bronchi, and the bronchi to the upper and lower lobes (Fig. 1–96). Commonly, the orifices of axial pathways of the segmental bronchi may also be seen. The extramediastinal portion of the right ascending pulmonary artery may be identified in front of and above the right upper lobe bronchus, whereas the right interlobar artery always appears lateral to the adjacent intermediate bronchus (Fig. 1–96).

The right superior pulmonary vein courses obliquely downward and medially from the upper lobe, crossing the interlobar artery and intermediate bronchus before entering the mediastinum (Fig. 1–96). A part of this vessel may be identified medial to the intermediate or middle lobe bronchus, provided there is sufficient intrusion of aerated middle lobe parenchyma in front of and below the vein. The horizontal lower lobe segmental veins coalesce behind, below, and medial to the right lower lobe bronchus. The right inferior venous confluence is usually lower and slightly more anterior than its counterpart on the left so that the two confluences usually are not in focus on the same tomogram.

The left pulmonary artery arches over the left main bronchus and proceeds backward and downward into the major fissure as the interlobar artery. Consequently, this vessel appears foreshortened and therefore is not optimally profiled, although the top of the vessel may be seen when aerated upper lobe parenchyma intrudes superiorly and

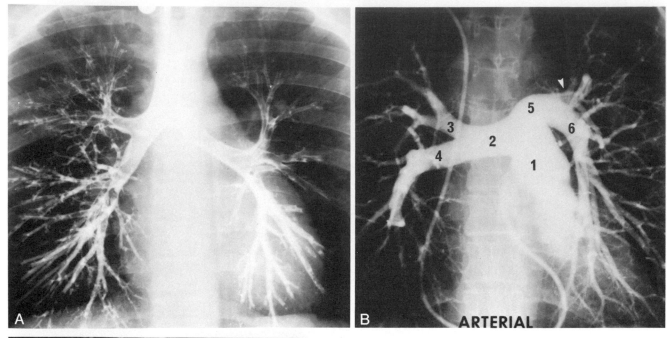

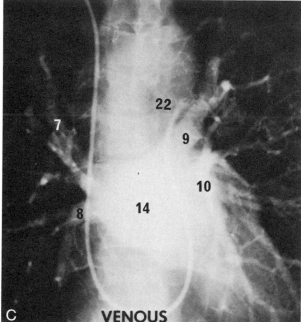

Figure 1–96. Normal Hilar Anatomy in Anteroposterior Projection. An anteroposterior tracheobronchogram (*A*) and anteroposterior angiogram during the arterial (*B*) and venous (*C*) phases for comparison of anatomic relationships. The main pulmonary artery (*1*) divides into shorter, higher left (*5*) and longer right (*2*) branches. In *B*, the right branch divides into ascending (*3*) and descending (*4*) arteries within the pericardium, behind the superior vena cava (note course of the catheter), before appearing as hilar vessels. The left pulmonary artery in this patient shows similar divisional features with relatively small ascending (*arrowhead*) and more prominent descending (*6*) branches. The venous phase of the angiogram (*C*) shows a close relationship between the right (*7*) and left (*9*) superior veins as they cross anterior to the hilar arterial vasculature. Note the typical course of the left superior vein in relation to the left main bronchus (*22*). On the right, three veins drain to the left atrium (*14*) whereas on the left, superior and inferior veins (*10*) join to form a common chamber before entering the atrium.

Illustration continued on opposite page

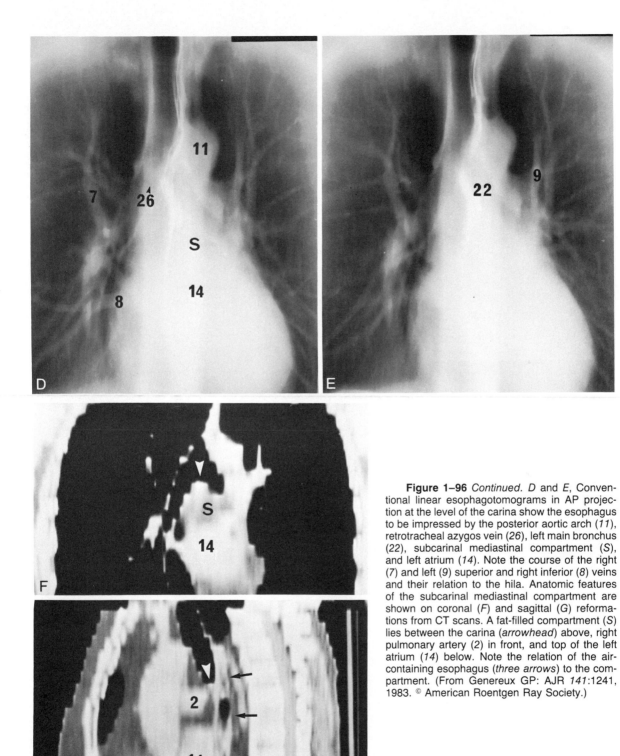

Figure 1–96 *Continued. D* and *E,* Conventional linear esophagotomograms in AP projection at the level of the carina show the esophagus to be impressed by the posterior aortic arch (*11*), retrotracheal azygos vein (*26*), left main bronchus (*22*), subcarinal mediastinal compartment (*S*), and left atrium (*14*). Note the course of the right (*7*) and left (*9*) superior and right inferior (*8*) veins and their relation to the hila. Anatomic features of the subcarinal mediastinal compartment are shown on coronal (*F*) and sagittal (*G*) reformations from CT scans. A fat-filled compartment (*S*) lies between the carina (*arrowhead*) above, right pulmonary artery (*2*) in front, and top of the left atrium (*14*) below. Note the relation of the air-containing esophagus (*three arrows*) to the compartment. (From Genereux GP: AJR *141*:1241, 1983. © American Roentgen Ray Society.)

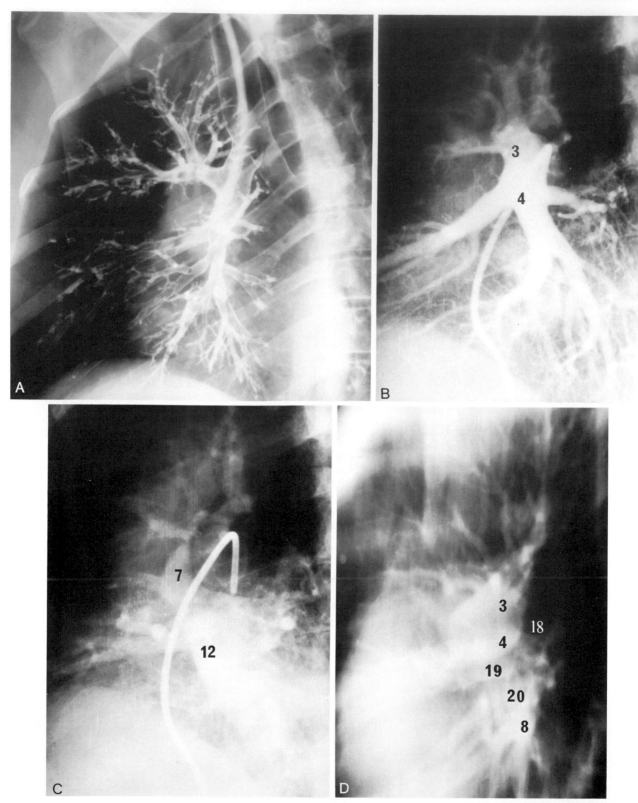

Figure 1–97. Normal Right Hilar Anatomy in 55° Posterior Oblique Projection. Right oblique projections of a right tracheobron-chogram (*A*) and a selective right pulmonary angiogram during the arterial (*B*) and venous (*C*) phases. The right superior vein (*7*) lies anterior to the ascending (*3*) and descending (interlobar) (*4*) pulmonary arteries. (The catheter is in the interlobar artery.) Venous confluence (*12*) entering the left atrium may be contour-forming beneath the middle lobe bronchus. *D* and *E*, Right posterior oblique tomograms of the right hilum demonstrate th egg- or comet-shaped hilar vascular complex to be framed by the right upper (*17*), intermediate (*18*), and middle lobe bronchi (*19*). Right ascending (*3*) and descending (*4*) pulmonary arteries surrounded by hilar areolar tissue account for the posterior opacity, whereas the right superior vein (*7*) provides the anterior contour. The right inferior vein (*8*) relates to the lower lobe bronchus (*20*). The end-on segmental middle lobe vein (*arrow*) is seen beneath the middle lobe bronchus. Right hilar width (*between asterisks*) and height (*between arrowheads*) can be measured.

Illustration continued on opposite page

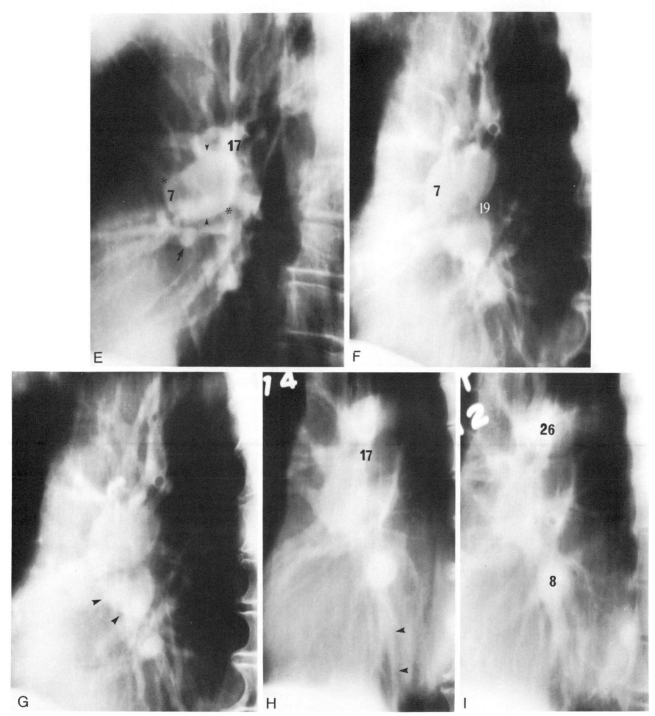

Figure 1–97 *Continued. F* and *G*, Right posterior oblique tomograms disclose an unexplained opacity (*arrowheads*) beneath the middle lobe bronchus (*19*). Continuity of the opacity with that of the superior vein (*7*) should suggest its vascular nature. The angiographic studies in *B* and *C* identify this structure as a prominent right superior venous confluence. *H* and *I*, Right oblique tomograms at different levels reveal a prominent distal azygos vein (*26*) passing over the right upper lobe bronchus (*17*). Typical elongated shape and position differentiate the vein from a true hilar mass. A linear opacity (*arrowheads*) extends from the end-on right inferior pulmonary vein (*8*) to the top of the right hemidiaphragm. This uncommon feature is thought to represent the intersublobar septum of the pulmonary ligament (*see* Figure 1–141 for illustration of a thickened pulmonary ligament). (From Genereux GP: AJR *141*:124, 1983. © American Roentgen Ray Society.)

medially (Fig. 1–96). More commonly, the superior margin of this artery is covered medially by mediastinal fat and laterally by pleura and aerated left upper lobe parenchyma; its smooth, superior contour defines the inferolateral boundary of the aortopulmonary window.

The left superior pulmonary vein passes anterior and medial to the apicoposterior segmental bronchus of the upper lobe, where it may be joined by the lingular vein lateral to the pulmonary artery; the left superior vein then passes in front of the junction of the left upper lobe and main bronchi before piercing the pericardium and entering the left atrium (Fig. 1–96). The segmental veins from the lower lobe join behind and medial to the lobar bronchus before entering the posterolateral aspect of the atrium. Prominence of the left superior venous confluence may impinge on the anteromedial wall of the left lower lobe bronchus, displacing it laterally and posteriorly.

From the aortic arch caudad to the left atrium, the barium-filled esophagus is imprinted successively by the right posterolateral wall of the aortic arch, the retrotracheal segment of the azygos vein, the left main bronchus or tracheal carina, the subcarinal mediastinal compartment, and the posterior wall of the left atrium (Fig. 1–96). The subcarinal mediastinal compartment is bordered by the tracheal carina above, the right pulmonary artery in front, and the top of the left atrium below; this fat-filled space is variable in depth and may be seen on some anteroposterior tomograms as a radiolucency between the left atrium and tracheal bifurcation, medial to the azygoesophageal interface (Fig. 1–96). In some patients, particularly the elderly, the esophagus may intrude beneath the aortic arch into the aortopulmonary window; commonly, air is trapped in a typical "V" or diamond-shaped configuration in this segment of the esophagus as its right and left walls are silhouetted by lower lobe parenchyma.

Fifty-Five-Degree Posterior Oblique Projection. On the right, the main, upper, intermediate, middle, and lower lobe bronchi are clearly seen, as well as the anterior segment of the upper lobe and the superior segment of the lower lobe (Fig. 1–97). Occasionally, other segmental bronchi can be identified. The posteromedial wall of the right main and intermediate bronchi, normally 3 mm or less in width,[481] terminates at the origin of the superior segmental bronchus of the lower lobe opposite the middle lobe bronchus. The right hilar vascular complex, framed by the upper, intermediate, and middle lobe bronchi, is composed of the proximal parts of the truncus anterior above and the interlobar artery below (Fig. 1–98) and the right superior pulmonary vein in front (Fig. 1–98). This vascular complex is egg- or comet-shaped, the "tail" of the comet being formed by the right superior vein before its shadow coalesces with that of the interlobar artery. Segmental arteries and veins can be

identified as such by following their branching pattern from the hilum or by observing the characteristic association of arteries with bronchial divisions. The angle formed by the inferior margin of the middle lobe bronchus and the anterior aspect of the lower lobe bronchus is sharp and usually devoid of soft tissue, although a part of the superior venous confluence may overlap, forming a soft tissue opacity (Fig. 1–98). The middle lobe vein may be identified end-on beneath the distal portion of the middle lobe bronchus before it coalesces with the right superior vein. The right inferior vein also is imaged end-on and consequently may appear as a nodular opacity lying in close proximity to the posterior wall of the lower lobe bronchus. The inferior pulmonary ligament is rarely identified as a thin curvilinear opacity extending caudad from the inferior vein to the top of the right hemidiaphragm (Fig. 1–98).

Measurements of the right hilar vascular shadow in the 55° oblique projection are taken in two planes:[466] its width is measured from the origin of the middle lobe bronchus to the widest anterior contour; the height of the hilum is measured from the inferior aspect of the anterior segmental bronchus of the right upper lobe to the superior margin of the midpart of the middle lobe bronchus. Normal right hilar measurements (range and mean) are given in Table 1–5.

On the left, the main bronchus, the superior and inferior divisions of the upper lobe bronchus, their segmental bronchi, and the lower lobe bronchus can be identified (Fig. 1–98). The truncated left pulmonary artery nestles atop the continuum formed by the upper surface of the left main and upper lobe bronchi; it continues upward and then sharply downward to form the interlobar artery, which can be seen as a soft tissue opacity paralleling the lower lobe bronchus (Fig. 1–98). Since this vessel also is foreshortened and viewed *en face*, optimal delineation should not be expected. The superior contour of the left pulmonary artery is smooth unless upper segmental arteries arise directly from its surface.

The left hilar vascular shadow can be measured in the left posterior oblique projection, its width being taken from the spur dividing the superior and inferior divisions of the upper lobe to the widest

Table 1–5. Normal Hilar Measurements in 55° Right and Left Posterior Oblique Projection

| HILUM | DIMENSIONS | |
	Width (mm)	Height (mm)
Right (n = 15)		
Range	26–35	28–43
Mean	33	36
Left (n = 15)		
Range	7–18	18–32
Mean	10	25

Thirty normal subjects (20 men and 10 women; mean ages, 56 and 53.3 years, respectively).

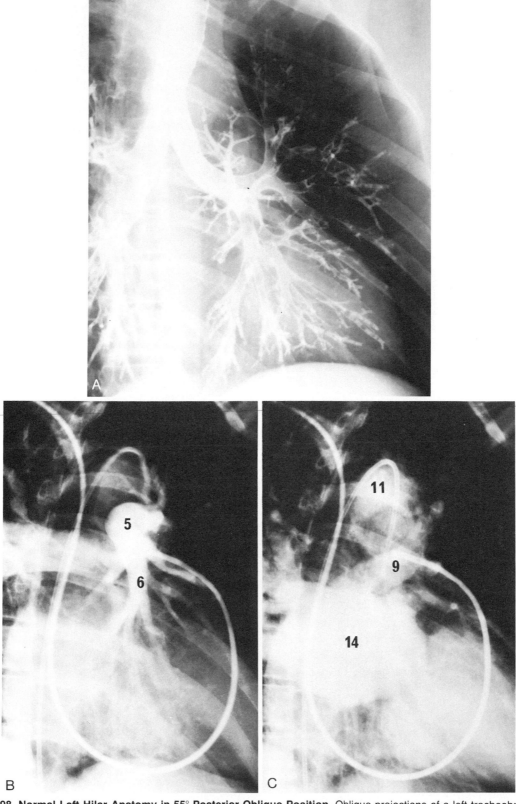

Figure 1–98. Normal Left Hilar Anatomy in 55° Posterior Oblique Position. Oblique projections of a left tracheobronchogram (*A*) and a selective left pulmonary angiogram during the arterial (*B*) and venous (*C*) phases. Before entering the left atrium (*14*), the superior pulmonary vein (*9*) is intimately related to the left pulmonary artery (*5*) and forms the anterior contour of the hilum. Contrast medium is present in the left interlobar artery (*6*) and aortic arch (*11*).

Illustration continued on following page

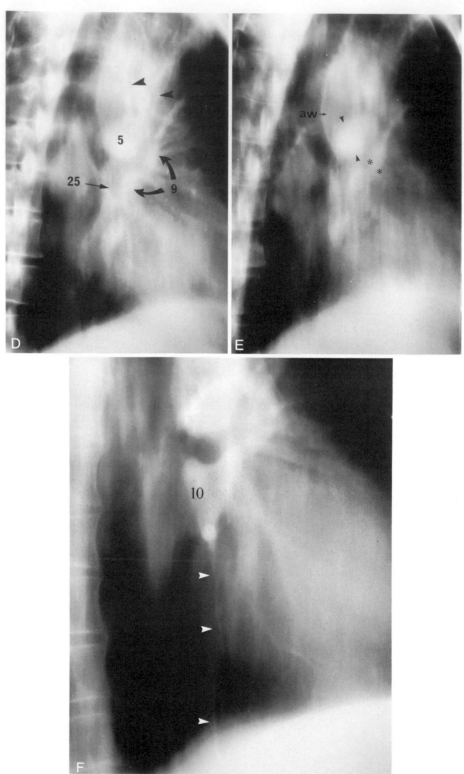

Figure 1–98 *Continued. D* and *E*, On left posterior oblique tomograms, the left pulmonary artery (*5*) has a smooth superior contour; upper lobe vessels (*large arrowheads*) originate from its superolateral surface. Note the course of the left superior vein (*9*) (*curved arrows*). The fat-filled, bowtie-shaped aortopulmonary window (*aw*) lies between the aortic arch and left pulmonary artery. Left inferior vein lies inferior to the lower lobe bronchus (*25*). Left hilar width (*between asterisks*) and height (*between small arrowheads*) can be measured. *F*, A left posterior oblique tomogram at a different level demonstrates a linear opacity (*arrowheads*) extending from the left inferior pulmonary vein (*10*) to the top of the left hemidiaphragm, representing the intersublobar septum of the pulmonary ligament. (From Genereux GP: AJR *141*:1241, 1983. © American Roentgen Ray Society.)

point along an arc described by the left superior vein; the height is measured from the top of the left pulmonary artery to the superior margin of the left upper lobe bronchus. The left hilar measurements (range and mean) are given in Table 1–5.

The "bowtie"-shaped aortopulmonary window, located between the top of the left pulmonary artery and the undersurface of the end-on or obliquely oriented aortic arch, is normally devoid of soft tissue elements other than fat (Fig. 1–98). The left superior vein can be followed along the anterior margin of the upper lobe airway to a point beneath the upper and lower lobe bronchi where it disappears into the mediastinum (Fig. 1–98). The left inferior vein is viewed end-on and may appear like a nodule or mass contiguous with the lower lobe bronchus. Like its counterpart on the right, the curvilinear shadow of the inferior pulmonary ligament can occasionally be identified beneath the inferior vein as it courses toward the left hemidiaphragm (Fig. 1–98). The left posterior oblique projection is often advantageous for evaluating the subcarinal component of the inferior azygoesophageal recess interface.

Lateral Projection. Roentgenographic anatomy of the right hilum in lateral projection (Fig. 1–99)

is similar to that in right posterior oblique projection, the main difference being that the lateral view elongates the interlobar artery and some of the segmental arteries and veins of the upper and lower lobes, whereas the oblique view tends to foreshorten these vessels. The lateral view depicts the posterior wall of the right main and intermediate bronchi to excellent advantage (Fig. 1–99).

The left lateral projection optimally profiles the left pulmonary artery and its major branch, the interlobar artery, as well as many of the segmental arteries and veins of the upper and lower lobes (Fig. 1–100). The left main bronchus is seen, including a short segment of the posterior wall silhouetted by lower lobe parenchyma; caudally, the posterior wall terminates at the origin of the superior segmental bronchus of the lower lobe (Fig. 1–100). The orifice of the left main or upper lobe bronchus viewed end-on, the inferior and anterior wall of the lingular and lower lobe bronchi, and the lower lobe bronchial lumen may be identified. Segmental bronchi to the upper lobe are not seen ideally in this view, although the apicoposterior bronchus often is well shown. The left superior vein forms the anterior convexity of the hilum, whereas the elongated

Text continued on page 118

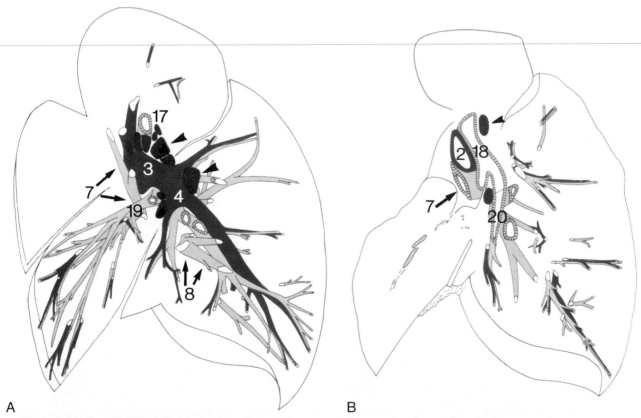

A   B

Figure 1–99. Normal Right Hilar Anatomy in Lateral Projection. (*A* and *B* appear in color following page 314.) *A*, and *B*, Sagittal drawings of the hilum from the medial aspect, depicting the hilar bronchi (*17, 18, 19, 20*), pulmonary arteries (*2, 3, 4*), and pulmonary veins (*7, 8*). Several small lymph nodes (*arrowheads*) are included in the illustration. The anterior contour of the right hilum is formed by the ascending (*3*) and the horizontal limb of the interlobar (*4*) pulmonary arteries; the hilum relates to the front of the intermediate bronchus (*18*) above and the superior pulmonary vein (*7*) below. The inferior pulmonary vein (*8*) relates to the lower lobe bronchi.

Illustration continued on following page

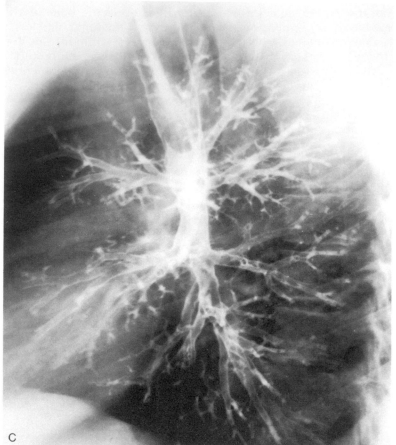

C

Figure 1–99 *Continued. C,* A right lateral tracheobronchogram and a selective right pulmonary angiogram during the arterial *(D)* and venous *(E)* phases show the right superior vein *(7)* to lie anterior to the ascending *(3)* and descending *(4)* pulmonary arteries. (The catheter is in the right pulmonary artery.) *F* and *G,* On right lateral xerotomograms, the posterior wall of the right main *(16)* and intermediate *(18)* bronchi unite to form the intermediate stem line, which terminates at the origin of the superior segmental bronchus *(21)* to the lower lobe *(20).* The right superior pulmonary vein *(7)* defines the anterior contour of the right hilum. (From Genereux GP: AJR *141*:1241, 1983.)

Illustration continued on opposite page

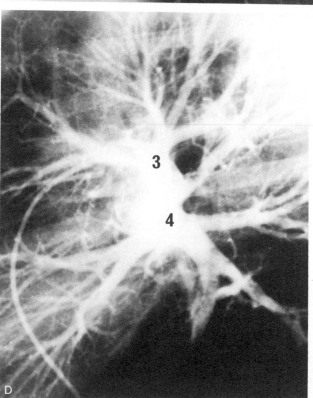

D

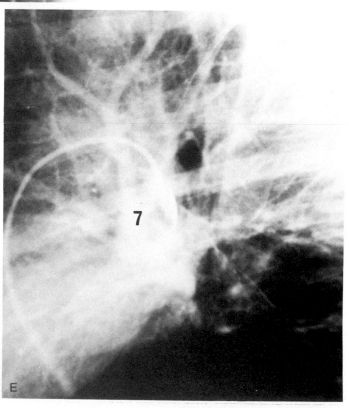

E

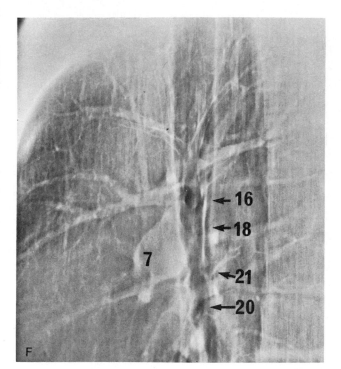

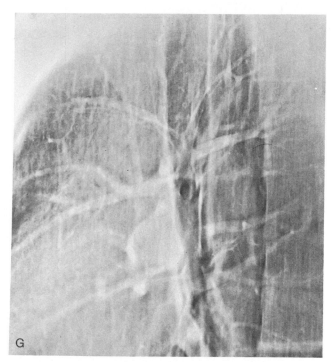

Figure 1–99 *Continued*

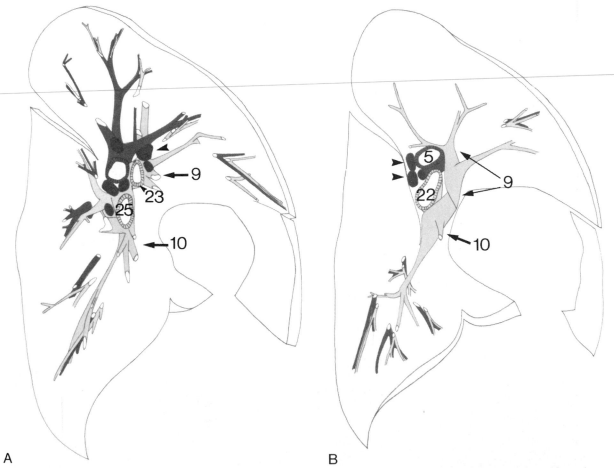

A

B

Figure 1–100. Normal Left Hilar Anatomy in Lateral Projection. (*A* and *B* appear in color following page 314.) *A* and *B*, Sagittal drawings of the left hilum from the medial aspect depict the hilar bronchi (*22, 25*), pulmonary artery (LPA) (*5*), and pulmonary veins (*9, 10*). Several small lymph nodes (*arrowheads*) are included. The entire anterior convexity of the left hilum relates to the superior pulmonary vein (*9*) in front of the left pulmonary artery (*5*) and left main bronchus (*22*). The relationship of the left inferior vein (*10*) to the left lower lobe bronchus (*25*) is shown.

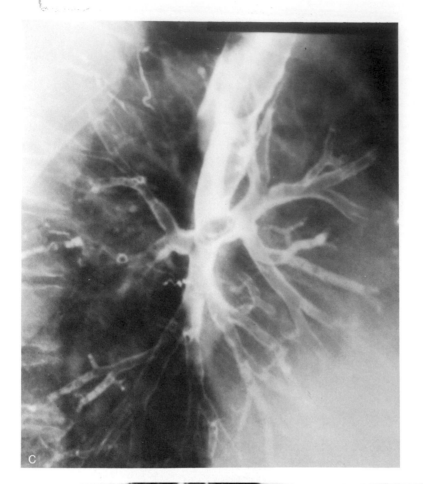

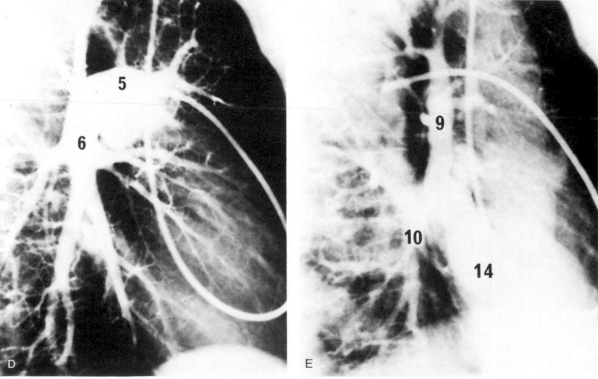

Figure 1–100 *Continued.* A lateral projection of a left tracheobronchogram (*C*) and a selective left pulmonary angiogram during the arterial (*D*) and venous (*E*) phases show that the superoposterior contour of the hilum is formed by the LPA (*5*) and proximal interlobar (*6*) artery. In this subject, the left superior (*9*) and inferior (*10*) veins coalesce to form a common chamber prior to entering the left atrium (*14*).

Illustration continued on following page

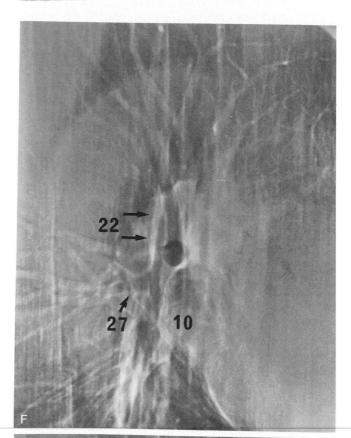

Figure 1–100 *Continued. F* and *G*, Left lateral xerotomograms demonstrate the posterior wall of the left main (22) and lower lobe bronchi terminating at the origin of the superior segmental bronchus (27) of the lower lobe (25). The anteroinferior walls of the lingular (24) and contiguous lower lobe bronchi are devoid of soft tissue. The circular lumen of the left upper lobe bronchus (23) is shown. The left superior (9) and inferior (10) pulmonary veins relate to the anterior hilum and the lower lobe bronchus, respectively. (From Genereux GP: AJR *141*:1241, 1983.)

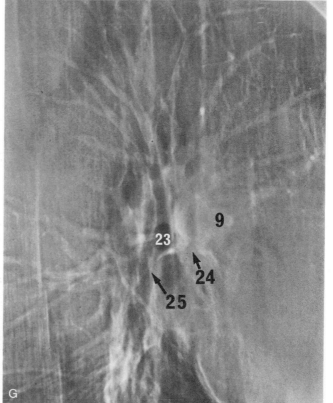

lower lobe veins can be followed to their termination at the left inferior venous confluence anterior and medial to the anterior wall of the lower lobe bronchus.

COMPUTED TOMOGRAPHY

CT is an ideal technique for imaging the hila. Although there is some dissenting opinion,[486] our feeling is that CT carries the hilar examination one step beyond that afforded by the conventional tomogram. It is of paramount importance that the radiologist pay meticulous attention to the examination technique. It is our opinion that noncontrast-enhanced scans suffice under most clinical circumstances, but if there is any uncertainty concerning an anatomic feature, the addition of contrast medium to the study generally serves to resolve most of the ambiguities. The patient should be examined in the supine position during suspended full inspiration. Ten- or 5-mm collimated scans with 10-mm spacing are generally adequate, although two or three additional "in between" scans may be needed to clarify any uncertain anatomic feature. The scans should always be viewed in continuity; although perhaps self-evident, this principle serves to diminish many of the well-known points of confusion that may arise from the viewing of an isolated scan. The study should be performed under radiologist supervision, viewed with multiple windows and levels, and recorded on hard copy film. There is no optimal set of viewing factors, but, in general, windows

in the 600- and 2000-HU range, adjusted to levels that yield the greatest subjective visual clarity for each, suffice under most clinical situations.

Anatomic features of the hila on CT are best described by a series of horizontal planes or levels through the tracheobronchial tree (Fig. 1–101).[487] In the description that follows, only the major anatomic features will be highlighted. In several recent reports,[487–491] the CT features of the normal and abnormal hilum have been described in considerable detail and the interested reader is referred to these for further information.

Level I (supracarinal trachea) (Fig. 1–101): On the *right*, the circular apical pulmonary artery lies medial to the radiolucent end-on apical bronchus; the apical pulmonary vein is situated lateral to this bronchoarterial bundle. On the *left*, the apicoposterior bronchus and artery are seen; the apical and anterior veins lie in front and medial to the bronchus and artery.

Level II (carina/right upper lobe bronchus) (Fig. 1–101): On the *right*, the upper lobe bronchus divides into the horizontally oriented anterior and posterior segmental bronchi. In front of the main bronchus and upper lobe bronchus is the ascending branch of the right pulmonary artery (Fig. 1–101); its anterior segmental branch parallels the bronchus medially or superiorly. The right superior pulmonary vein is invariably identified immediately lateral to the divisional point of the anterior and posterior segmental bronchi. In some patients, a small vein from the anterior and apical portion of the upper

Text continued on page 123

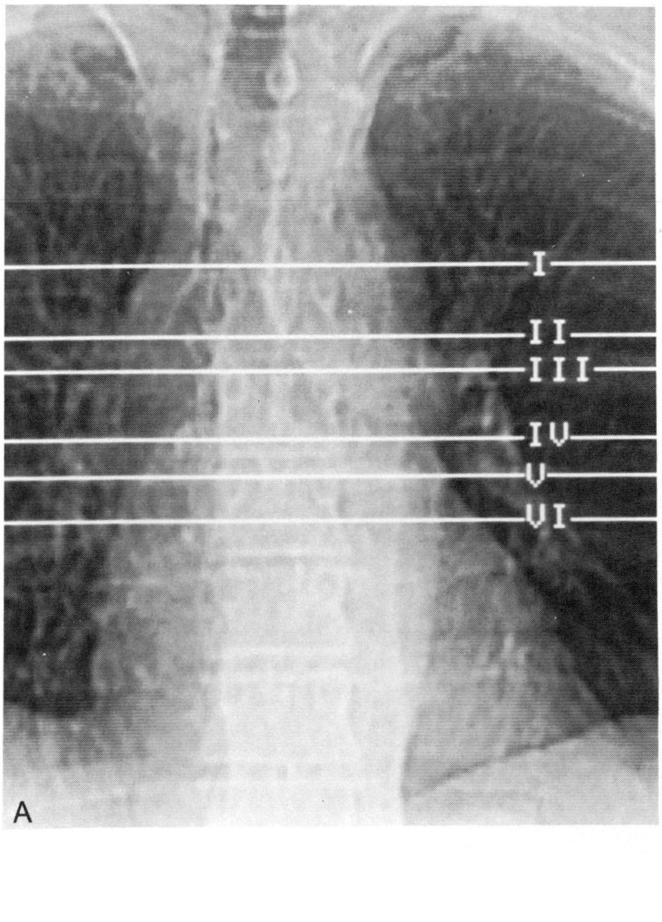

A

Figure 1–101. Normal CT Hilar Anatomy. *A,* On a scoutview of the thorax, the bars indicate the appropriate levels for *B* through *G.*

Illustration continued on opposite page

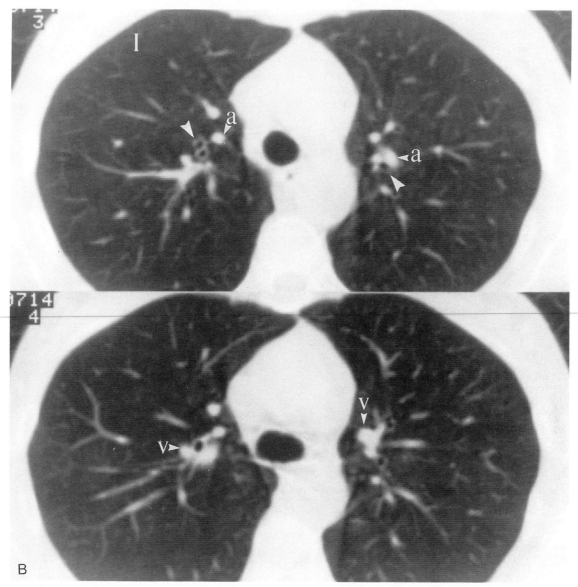

Figure 1–101 *Continued. B,* In *level I* (supracarinal trachea), the apical bronchus (*arrowhead*), artery (a), and vein (v) are depicted on the right, and the apicoposterior bronchus (*arrowhead*), artery (a), and vein (v) on the left.

Illustration continued on following page

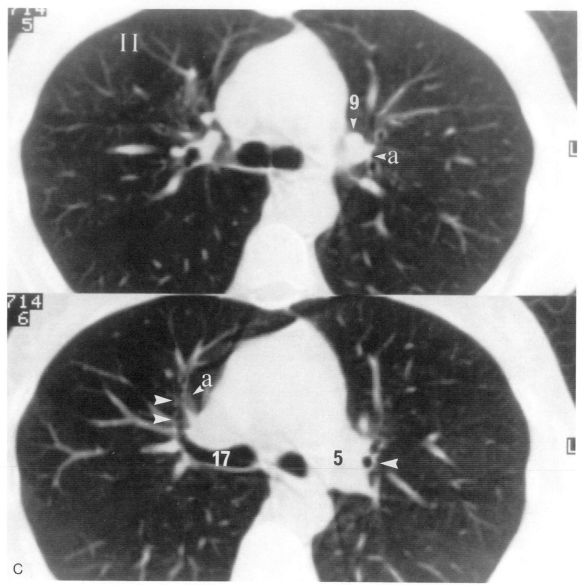

Figure 1–101 *Continued. C,* In *level II* (carina/right upper lobe bronchus), the upper lobe bronchus (*17*), anterior segmental bronchus (*two arrowheads*), and artery (*a*) are shown on the right; on the left, the apicoposterior bronchus (*arrowhead*) and artery (*a*) are stationed immediately lateral to the left pulmonary artery (*5*). The left superior pulmonary vein (*9*) is located anteromedial to the bronchoarterial bundle.

Illustration continued on opposite page

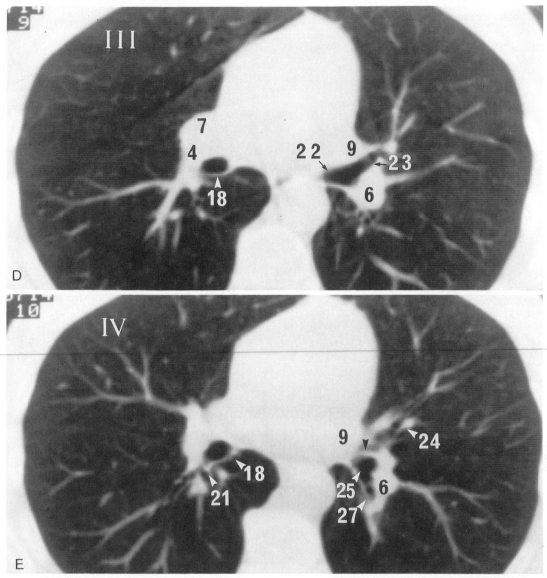

Figure 1–101 *Continued. D*, In *level III* (proximal intermediate bronchus/left upper lobe bronchus), on the right, the intermediate bronchus (*18*) is covered anteriorly and laterally by the interlobar artery (*4*). The RSPV (*7*) relates closely to the interlobar artery, creating a typical "elephant head-and-trunk" configuration. On the left, the distal main (*22*) and upper lobe (*23*) bronchial continuum is seen. Note the shallow indentation on the anterior and posterior wall of the upper lobe bronchus created by the mediastinal component of the left superior vein (*9*) and the proximal interlobar artery (*6*). *E*, In *level IV* (distal intermediate bronchus/lingular bronchus), the intermediate bronchus (*18*) and the superior segmental bronchus (*21*) of the lower lobe can be identified on the right, and the lingular bronchus (*24*) separated by the lingular spur (*arrowhead*) from the end-on orifice of the lower lobe bronchus (*25*) on the left. The superior segmental bronchus (*27*) lies posteriorly, the interlobar artery (*6*) posterolaterally, and the left superior pulmonary vein (*9*) anteromedially.

Illustration continued on following page

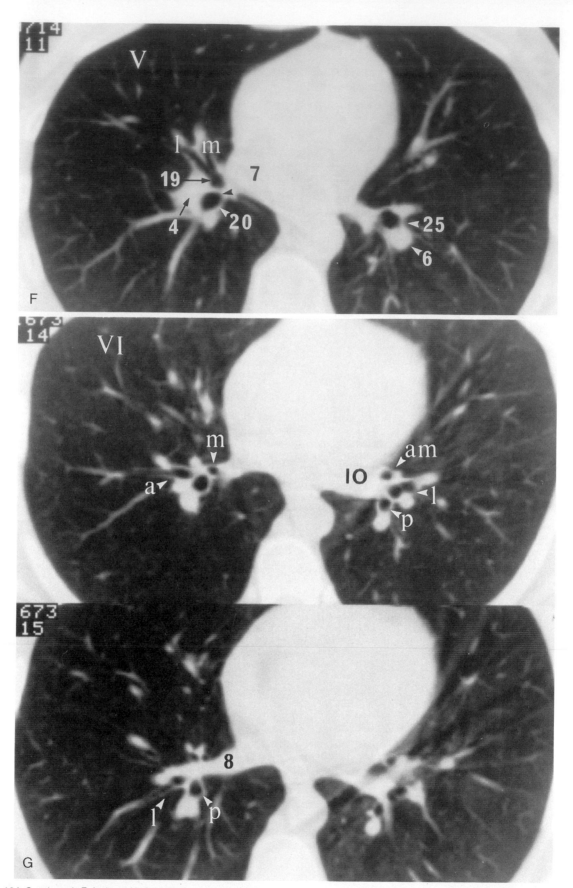

Figure 1–101 *Continued. F,* In *level V,* the middle lobe bronchus *(19)* divides into medial *(m)* and lateral *(l)* segmental bronchi. The lower lobe bronchus *(20)* is separated from the middle lobe bronchus by a distinct spur or carina *(arrowheads).* The RSPV *(7)* lies anteromedial to the middle lobe bronchus and the interlobar artery *(4)* anterolateral to the lower lobe bronchus. On the left, the interlobar artery *(6)* lies posterolateral to the lower lobe bronchus *(25). G,* In *level VI* (basilar lower lobe bronchi/inferior pulmonary veins), on the right, the medial *(m),* anterior *(a),* lateral *(l),* and posterior *(p)* segmental bronchi relate closely to the inferior pulmonary vein *(8).* On the left, the anteromedial *(am),* lateral *(l)* and posterior *(p)* segmental bronchi relate to the left inferior pulmonary vein *(10).*

lobe can be seen in front of the ascending artery. On the *left*, the circular apicoposterior bronchus and artery are stationed immediately lateral to the left pulmonary artery. The superior pulmonary vein is situated in front of and medial to the bronchus and artery.

Level III (proximal intermediate bronchus/left upper lobe bronchus) (Fig. 1–101): On the *right*, the intermediate bronchus is covered anteriorly by the horizontal limb of the interlobar artery and laterally by the vertical limb of the same vessel. The superior pulmonary vein abuts the junction between the horizontal and vertical components of the interlobar artery, creating a typical "elephant head-and-trunk" configuration (*see* Figure 1–77, page 85). On the *left*, the distal main and upper lobe bronchial continuum is seen. Frequently, the end-on radiolucency of the superior division of the upper lobe is demonstrated. The proximal portion of the interlobar artery forms a shallow indentation on the posterior aspect of the upper lobe bronchus. Partial volume-averaging through the left pulmonary artery as it crosses cephalad to the left main bronchus frequently causes a subtle "graying" to the normally radiolucent bronchial lumen. Medial to the interlobar artery, air in the superior segment of the left lower lobe may abut the posterior wall of the left main bronchus creating the CT "retrobronchial stripe."[482]

Level IV (distal intermediate bronchus/lingular bronchus) (Fig. 1–101): On the *right*, the anatomic features are similar to those of level III. On the *left*, the proximal portion of the lingular bronchus is separated from the end-on orifice of the lower lobe bronchus by the lingular spur. The superior segmental bronchus to the lower lobe arises posteriorly. The left interlobar artery is situated lateral to the carina or spur separating the lingular bronchus from the lower lobe bronchus. As it enters the mediastinum, the superior pulmonary vein is joined by the lingular vein in front of and medial to the lingular bronchus.

Level V (middle lobe bronchus) (Fig. 1–101): On the *right*, the horizontal middle lobe bronchus courses obliquely into the middle lobe where it divides after a centimeter or so into the medial and lateral segmental bronchi; behind, divided by a distinct carina or lateral spur, is the orifice of the lower lobe bronchus viewed end-on. The superior segmental bronchus to the lower lobe arises at or slightly superior to this level and passes posterolaterally for a few millimeters before dividing into two subsegmental bronchi. The vertical part of the interlobar artery is situated posterolateral to the middle lobe bronchus and anterolateral to the lower lobe bronchus as it enters lung parenchyma. The middle lobe artery or vein may be identified lateral to the middle lobe bronchus; the termination of the superior pulmonary vein is located anteromedial to this airway (*see* Figure 1–77, page 85). On the *left*, the end-on lumen of the lower lobe bronchus is

seen medial to the contiguous interlobar artery. Occasionally, a portion of the inferior pulmonary vein can be identified posteromedial to this bronchus.

Level VI (basilar lower lobe bronchi/inferior pulmonary veins) (Fig. 1–101): Segmental bronchi in the lower lobes are identified in 60 to 90 per cent of cases on the right and 30 to 80 per cent on the left.[491] On the *right*, the medial segmental bronchus, the first branch to be identified, is characteristically located in front of the horizontal inferior pulmonary vein. The anterior, lateral, and posterior basilar bronchi arise in succession to supply their respective segments. On the *left*, the anteromedial segmental bronchus is located anterior to the inferior pulmonary vein; the lateral and posterior segmental bronchi may be identified behind this vessel. A systematic evaluation of the anatomic relationships of the segmental bronchi, arteries, and veins of 107 right and 113 left lower lobes has recently been made by Jardin and Remy[1162] from CT scans of patients with normal chest roentgenograms.

MAGNETIC RESONANCE IMAGING

At the present time, the role that magnetic resonance imaging (MRI) will play in the study of the mediastinum and hila is uncertain, but preliminary reports have been encouraging. The physical principles underlying MRI are described in Chapter 2 (*see* page 332); in addition, the interested reader is referred to excellent reviews[492–495] and textbooks[496] for further discussion of this difficult topic.

MRI differs from computed tomography in several important aspects; firstly, flowing blood within the lumen of vessels provokes little or no signal and hence is perceived as a radiolucency on the MR scan (Fig. 1–102). This "flow-void" phenomenon[497–502] is therefore particularly advantageous in distinguishing a vessel from a mass (such as an enlarged lymph node) that is signal-provoking. Such distinction is often difficult or impossible on a noncontrast CT study, although the combination of contrast enhancement and dynamic scanning increases the sensitivity and specificity of the CT examination. Secondly, on both MRI and CT, the lumens of gas-containing bronchi are radiolucent; although both procedures are capable of clearly demonstrating the major airways, the superior resolution of CT permits routine demonstration of segmental and subsegmental bronchi whereas the identification of these smaller airways with MRI is possible in only about 30 per cent of cases.[503, 504] Thirdly, MRI is more adaptable in the display of sagittal and coronal planes without relying on the cumbersome maneuvers of patient positioning or reformatting of multiple transverse slices as is necessary with CT (Figs. 1–103 and 1–104).[505, 506] Lastly, characterization of normal and abnormal tissues within the mediastinum according to their

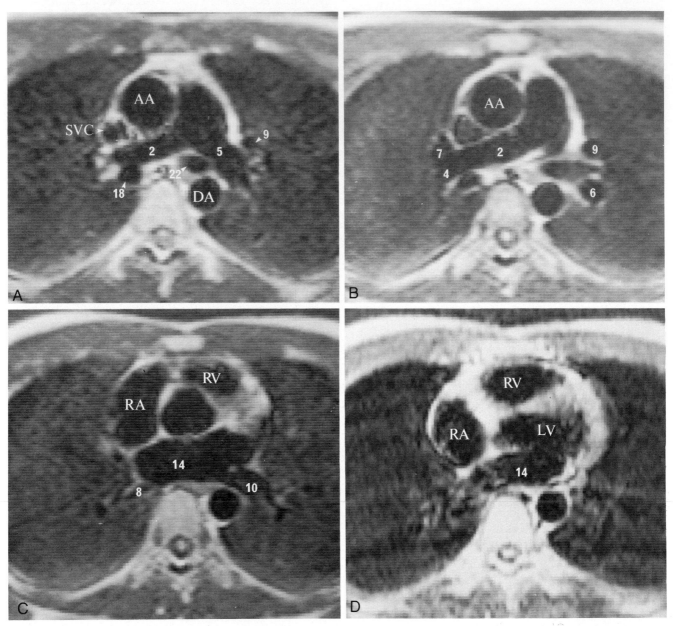

Figure 1–102. Anatomy of the Mediastinum and Hila on Axial Magnetic Resonance Images. Transverse SE 1163/40 scans from cephalad (*A*) to caudad (*D*) from a normal subject. Note that blood within vessels is lucent since flowing blood provokes little or no signal—the "flow-void" phenomenon. *AA*, ascending aorta; *DA*, descending aorta; *SVC*, superior vena cava; 9, left superior pulmonary vein; 7, right superior pulmonary vein; 2, right pulmonary artery; 5, left pulmonary artery; RB, right main bronchus; 22, left main bronchus; 6, left interlobar artery; 4, right interlobar artery; 18, intermediate bronchus; 14, left atrium; 10, left inferior pulmonary vein; 8, right inferior pulmonary vein; RA, right atrium; RV, right ventricle; LV, left ventricle. (Courtesy of Dr. David Li, University of British Columbia Hospital, Vancouver, B.C.)

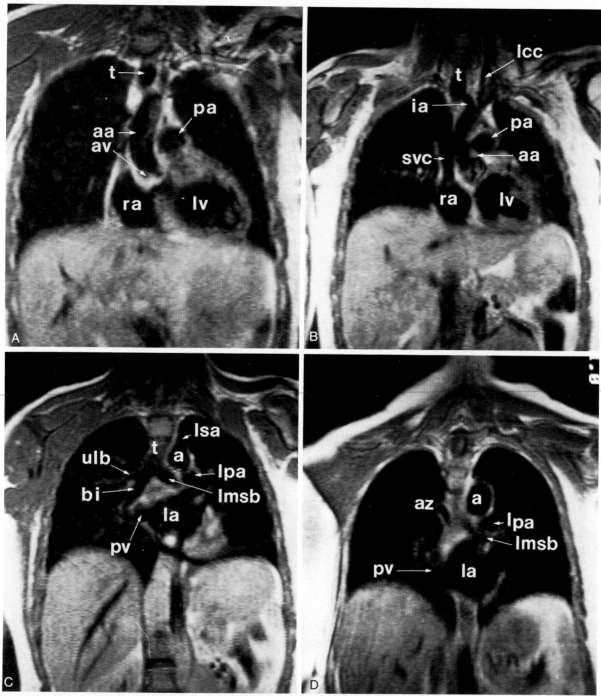

Figure 1–103. Anatomy of the Mediastinum and Hila on Coronal Magnetic Resonance Images. Normal coronal SE 1000/30 scans from anterior (*A*) to posterior (*D*). *aa*, Ascending aorta; *t*, trachea; *av*, aortic valves; *pa*, pulmonary artery; *ra*, right atrium; *lv*, left ventricle; *svc*, superior vena cava; *ta*, truncus anterior; *rpa*, right pulmonary artery; *lpa*, left pulmonary artery; *la*, left atrium; *ivc*, inferior vena cava; *lsa*, left subclavian artery; *ulb*, upper lobe bronchus; *bi*, intermediate bronchi; *rspv*, right superior pulmonary vein; *lspv*, left superior pulmonary vein; *lmsb*, left main bronchus; *16*, right main bronchus; *az*, azygos vein; *ia*, innominate artery; *lcc*, left common carotid artery. (From O'Donovan PB, Ross JS, Sivak SD, AJR *143*:1183, 1984. © American Roentgen Ray Society.)

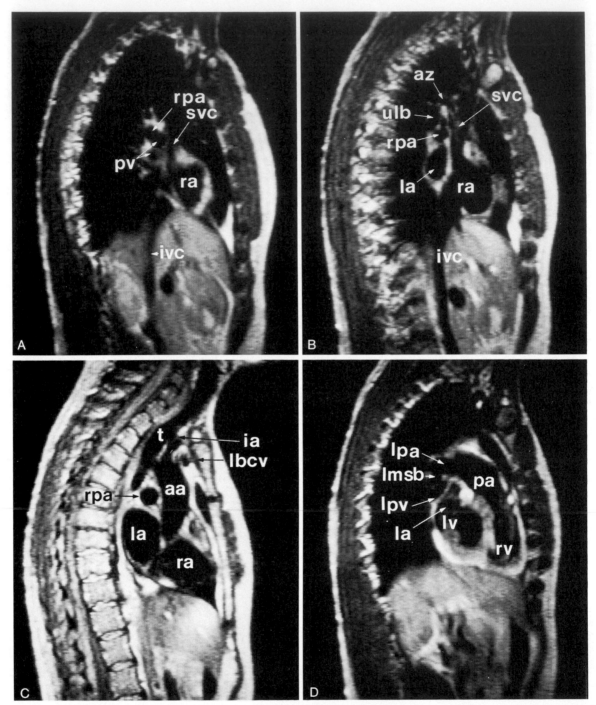

Figure 1–104. Anatomy of the Mediastinum and Hila on Sagittal Magnetic Resonance Images. Normal sagittal SE 1000/30 scans of the hila and mediastinum from right (*A*) to left (*D*). (*See* Figure 1–103 for appropriate anatomic designations). (From O'Donovan PB, Ross JS, Sivak SD, et al: AJR *143*:1183, 1984. © American Roentgen Ray Society.)

T1 (longitudinal) and T2 (transverse) relaxation times permits the distinction of cystic masses from fatty accumulations and solid tumors.[503, 507] In one report, these properties permitted the distinction of recurrent neoplasm from surrounding radiation fibrosis.[508]

According to Gamsu and his associates, the frequency with which normal structures of the mediastinum and hila are identified on MRI is as follows: aorta (100 per cent), central pulmonary arteries (100 per cent), arch arteries (100 per cent), mediastinal veins (100 per cent), lobar bronchi (100 per cent), one to three segmental bronchi (30 per cent), azygos vein or arch (50 per cent), hilar fat (50 per cent), and esophagus (20 per cent).[503] Normal lymph nodes as small as 5 to 10 mm in size can be seen in certain areas of the mediastinum, but CT is better suited for this purpose according to Dooms and his associates.[509]

FUNCTION OF THE VASCULAR SYSTEM

Perfusion of the Acinar Unit

Pulmonary blood volume (PBV) is defined as the volume of blood within the pulmonary arteries, pulmonary capillaries, pulmonary veins, and an indeterminate portion of the left atrium. When measured with a dye technique in 15 normal subjects, it ranged from 204 to 314 ml per sq m of body surface area (mean, 271 ml/m^2),[510] indicating that the amount of blood in the lungs at any one time is about 10 per cent of total blood volume. The capillary blood volume (Vc), which represents about 20 to 25 per cent of the PBV, is estimated to be 60 to 140 ml in the resting subject, increasing to 150 to 250 ml during exercise.[212, 510–514] These figures, largely calculated by measuring CO uptake by intracapillary erythrocytes, closely agree with estimates made by anatomic techniques.[515, 516] This may be interpreted as indicating that the capillary vascular bed, the surface area of which measures 70 to 100 sq m, is maximally distended during peak exercise.[514]

Various pressures modify the flow of blood through the capillaries. (1) *The mean intravascular pressure* is only 14 mm Hg in the pulmonary artery, despite the fact that it handles the same cardiac output as the systemic circulation. (2) *The transmural vascular pressure* for large extrapulmonary vessels and cardiac chambers is the intravascular or intracavitary pressure minus intrapleural pressure; for "extra-alveolar" intraparenchymal vessels, it is intravascular minus interstitial pressure; and for the "alveolar" vessels, it is intravascular minus alveolar pressure. (3) *The driving pressure* in the pulmonary circulation is the difference between arterial and pulmonary venous or left atrial pressures in the lower part of the lung and the difference between arterial and alveolar pressures in the upper part of the lung, in upright subjects at rest.

Although human capillary pressure cannot be measured directly, microvascular pressure has been measured in isolated perfused dog lungs by Bhattacharya and Staub.[1162] They found that the bulk of the resistance was in small vessels (70 per cent between arterioles 50 μm in diameter and venules 20 μm in diameter) and that 45 per cent was in the alveolar wall capillaries themselves. However, controversy exists as to the relative contributions of arterial, capillary, and venous resistance to total pulmonary vascular resistance (PVR). Hakim and his colleagues partitioned pulmonary vascular resistance into an arterial, venous and "middle" (capillary) compartment using a rapid occlusion technique in dogs. They found that the "capillary" compartment provides only approximately 16 per cent of total resistance, the rest being shared equally between arterial and venous compartments.[1163] Whatever the true capillary pressure, it must exceed left atrial pressure for flow to occur. A reasonable normal value is 9 cm H$_2$O, there being a gradient from the arteriolar to the venous end of the microvessels that is dependent on their resistance. Pulmonary "capillary" wedge pressure is thought to reflect pressure in large veins or the left atrium rather than in capillaries since during its measurement flow is transiently interrupted, thus any resistive pressure drop downstream from the point of occlusion is negated.

Since the colloidal osmotic pressure is thought to be 25 to 30 mm Hg, under normal resting conditions a considerable force keeps the alveoli dry; and even during maximal exercise, when cardiac output increases to 25 to 30 liters per min in healthy individuals, the hydrostatic pressure does not exceed the osmotic pressure.

The hemodynamics of the pulmonary circulation cannot be deduced on the basis of laws that relate to a rigid tubular system. Like the conducting system, the circulatory system is distensible; it branches and bends; it is subject to changing pressure on its walls and has a pressure at each end, either or both of which may vary in degree in certain circumstances. Flow is pulsatile but probably always laminar in small vessels and sometimes turbulent in larger ones. Viscosity is greater in the main vessels, but overall resistance to flow is mainly from arterioles and capillaries. When the left atrial pressure and transpulmonary (alveolar minus intrapleural) pressures are constant, an increase in pulmonary artery pressure causes vessels to distend (transmural pressure increase). As with the conducting system, doubling or halving the radius causes a 16-fold change in resistance; in this case, as cardiac output increases, vessels widen and closed capillaries open, leading to a fall in resistance.[517]

Part of this apparent decrease in resistance with increased flow and driving pressure may be due to the fact that the pulmonary vascular pressure/flow curve does not have a zero pressure intercept. Put simply, this means that a critical pulmonary artery pressure must be achieved before flow begins. Gra-

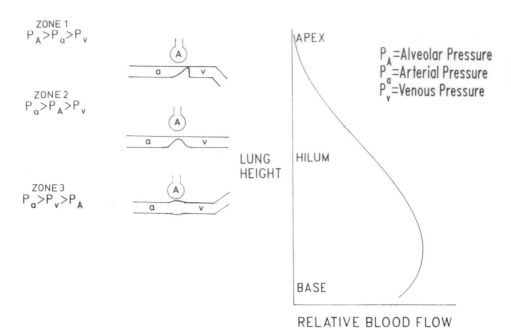

ZONE 1
$P_A > P_a > P_v$

ZONE 2
$P_a > P_A > P_v$

ZONE 3
$P_a > P_v > P_A$

LUNG HEIGHT

APEX

HILUM

BASE

RELATIVE BLOOD FLOW

P_A = Alveolar Pressure
P_a = Arterial Pressure
P_v = Venous Pressure

Figure 1–105. Regional Blood Flow in the Lung as Determined by the Relationship Between Alveolar (A), Pulmonary Arterial (a), and Pulmonary Venous (v) Pressures. At the apex, where pulmonary arterial and venous pressure may be subatmospheric, alveolar pressure will compress alveolar microvessels, increase resistance, and decrease flow (Zone 1). Lower in the lung, pulmonary arterial pressure exceeds alveolar pressure but alveolar pressure still exceeds the subatmospheric venous pressure and vessel caliber and flow depend on the difference between arterial and alveolar pressure (Zone 2). Nearer the base of the lung, arterial and venous pressure exceed alveolar pressure, dilating microvessels and further increasing flow (Zone 3). At the lung base (Zone 4), a region of decreased flow exists that cannot be simply explained by the relationship of Pa, PA, and Pv.

ham and her colleagues[1164] measured the critical opening pressure in canine lungs and pointed out the importance of taking this into account when calculating changes in pulmonary vascular resistance.

Factors Influencing Pulmonary Circulation

GRAVITY

Gravity has a major influence on the distribution of blood flow in the lung by altering regional vascular transmural pressures and therefore vascular diameters. The distribution of flow is largely governed by the relationship between arterial, alveolar, and venous pressures (Fig. 1–105). The zonal concept of gravity-dependent blood flow was developed by West and his colleagues[1165] and has recently been reviewed.[1166]

The lung measures approximately 30 cm from apex to base, and the hilum is positioned at about the midline. The pulmonary artery enters the lung at the hilum. Since a column of blood 15 cm high is equivalent to a column of mercury 11 mm high, in the erect subject gravity affects the intravascular pressure to the extent that systolic, diastolic, and mean pressures are reduced by 11 mm Hg at the apex and are increased by 11 mm Hg at the base. If pulmonary arterial pressure in the hilar vessels is taken as 20/9 mm Hg, it follows that pressure at the extreme apex will be 9/−2, while at the base, the pressure will be 31/20. Since the pulmonary veins enter the left atrium at approximately the same level, there also will be a similar and proportional variation in venous pressure.

These gravity-dependent changes in intravascular pressure result in regional differences in the capillary transmural pressure; since extraluminal

capillary pressure is 0 (atmospheric), apical vessels are virtually closed, at least during diastole, and in these regions the pulmonary vasculature acts as a Starling resistor in which the pertinent driving pressure is the difference between arterial and alveolar pressure (Zone 1) (Fig. 1–105). Further down the lung, pulmonary artery pressure exceeds alveolar pressure throughout the cardiac cycle, but alveolar pressure still exceeds venous pressure, resulting in a narrowing of capillaries at their downstream venous end (Zone 2). Finally, both arterial and venous pressures exceed alveolar pressure and the vasculature progressively dilates as the lung base is approached (Zone 3).

At the base of the lung, blood flow decreases once more—a phenomenon that has been termed Zone 4. This basilar increase in pulmonary vascular resistance has been observed in both intact dogs and humans,[518, 519] but at present there is no adequate explanation for it. Although it was originally postulated that the increased resistance at the base of the lung was caused by a decrease in the diameter of extra-alveolar vessels secondary to the gravity-dependent decrease in lung volume at the base, experiments in dogs relating regional vascular resistance and regional lung volume have cast doubt on this hypothesis.[518] Recent studies have shown a centrifugal decrease in regional blood flow from hilum to lung periphery, raising the possibility that the resistance of the longer precapillary pathways for blood flow at the apex and base may contribute to regional flow distribution in addition to the gravity-dependent changes in vascular pressures and dimensions. Nemery and his colleagues[519] showed a reduction in the extent of Zone 4 in humans by infusing the pulmonary vasodilator nitroprusside, suggesting a role for vascular tone in the flow reduction.

INTRAPLEURAL PRESSURE AND LUNG VOLUME

Macklin was the first to examine the effects of changes in lung volume on the capacity of the pulmonary vasculature.[336] The subsequent studies of Permutt and Howell[520, 521] showed that the pulmonary vasculature can be divided into two compartments, extra-alveolar and alveolar, based on their response to changes in lung volume.

The extra-alveolar compartment comprises the arteries and veins whose extraluminal pressure consists of pleural and/or interstitial pressure; they respond to such pressure by tending to dilate as lung volume increases. Alveolar vessels are microvessels that respond to alveolar pressure as their extraluminal pressure and they tend to be compressed as the lung is inflated. The interactions between these two compartments with change in lung volume make complex the resultant alterations in the distribution of the pulmonary blood volume and pulmonary vascular resistance. When pulmonary arterial pressure is held constant relative to alveolar pressure (constant zonal conditions), pulmonary vascular resistance initially falls with lung inflation but then rises at high lung volumes, presumably as a result of lengthening of extra-alveolar vessels.[522] When pulmonary artery pressure is not held constant relative to alveolar pressure, the effects on alveolar vessels predominate and PVR rises steeply with lung inflation.[523, 524]

It is possible to perfuse the lung slowly even when alveolar pressure substantially exceeds pulmonary artery pressure, due to the patency of the so-called "corner vessels;" these are microvessels situated at alveolar corners and, although anatomically they are alveolar vessels, functionally they are extra-alveolar.[525]

NEUROGENIC AND CHEMICAL EFFECTS

In addition to the pressure and volume changes that passively influence the pulmonary vasculature, neurogenic, humoral, blood gas, and chemistry changes can result in active vasomotion and modify the capillary circulation to acinar units. The alterations in vascular tone and diameter can occur generally throughout the lung or, more importantly on a regional basis, altering blood flow distribution and thus affecting regional ventilation-perfusion relationships. In addition, vasoconstriction or dilatation may occur upstream (arterial) or downstream (venous) from the gas-exchanging capillaries, resulting in varying relationships between regional blood volume and blood flow as well as modifying the hydrostatic pressure in the fluid-exchanging vessels.

Hypoxia has physiologically important effects on pulmonary vessels. The effect is predominantly local since the vasoconstrictor response is present in denervated lungs and indeed in excised perfused lungs.[526] The magnitude of hypoxia-induced pulmonary vasoconstriction is influenced by the initial tone, by the level of sympathetic stimulation, and by the amount of vascular smooth muscle.[527] Despite

its obvious importance in both the physiologic regulation of blood flow and the pathophysiology of pulmonary hypertensive states, the mechanism of hypoxic vasoconstriction has remained elusive. Most evidence suggests that it is the local alveolar PO_2 that provides the major stimulus, although mixed venous PO_2 may also influence the response.[528] The mystery lies in whether a locally released mediator or hypoxia itself is the important effector. Numerous mediators have been proposed, of which histamine has been the most persistent suspect;[527] however, recent studies that have examined the site of hypoxia and of histamine-induced pulmonary vasoconstriction have largely ruled out this substance as a mediator. Hypoxia causes increased resistance in capillary and precapillary vessels, whereas histamine acts predominantly on the venous side of the capillary bed.[529–531] In addition, in experimental animals, tissue histamine levels increase rather than decrease with prolonged hypoxia.[532] Postulated mechanisms for the direct effect of hypoxia on smooth muscle include alterations in membrane permeability to calcium, or direct effects on the energetics of the contractile process itself.[527]

Increased hydrogen ion concentration, whether induced by hypercapnia or metabolic acidosis, also produces pulmonary vasoconstriction by a separate mechanism and interacts with hypoxia in increasing pulmonary arterial pressure.[533, 534]

The pulmonary vessels receive a rich innervation from the pulmonary plexuses that are formed by a mingling of fibers from the sympathetic trunk and vagus. Appropriate staining techniques show both parasympathetic and catecholamine-containing fibers supplying vessels down to 30 μ in diameter, with relative sparsity on the venous side of the circulation.[535]

Although stimulation of sympathetic nerves in intact animals results in increased pulmonary vascular resistance and decreased compliance of large pulmonary vessels, little is known about afferent input that could produce such reflex changes.[535] Parenterally administered neurotransmitters have more pronounced effects on pulmonary vascular resistance: epinephrine, norepinephrine, serotonin, histamine, and prostaglandin F_2 vasoconstrict whereas beta-agonists and acetylcholine result in vasodilation.[536] Using the arterial and venous occlusion technique, serotonin, sympathetic stimulation, and prostaglandin F_2 have been shown to act predominantly on precapillary vessels whereas the vasoconstrictive effects of infused histamine and norepinephrine and of increased cerebrospinal fluid pressure act predominantly on venules.[529, 530]

Diffusion of Gas from Acinar Units to Red Blood Cells

DIFFUSION IN THE ACINAR UNIT

Diffusion of a gas occurs passively from an area of higher partial pressure of the gas to one of lower partial pressure. In a gaseous medium, a light gas diffuses faster than a heavier one. In a liquid or in tissue the rate of diffusion is largely dependent upon the solubility of the particular gas in that medium. Oxygen is slightly lighter than carbon dioxide and, therefore, diffuses more rapidly in acinar gas. In water and tissue, carbon dioxide is more soluble than oxygen, and diffuses through these media 20 times faster than does oxygen. Since both are able to diffuse many thousands of times more rapidly in a gaseous medium than in water or tissue, diffusion out of acini consists largely of getting through the alveolocapillary membrane and plasma and in and out of the red cell. Because diffusion through these structures is accomplished much more readily by carbon dioxide than by oxygen, outward diffusion of carbon dioxide never is a clinical problem, and further discussion need concern only the diffusion of oxygen.

Assuming a tidal volume of 450 ml and a dead space of 150 ml, 300 ml of fresh air and 150 ml of dead space alveolar air from the previous expiration enter the acinar units during each inspiration. Since the units already contain seven or eight times this volume (functional residual capacity), the "fresh" air that enters last may fill only the respiratory bronchioles and alveolar ducts. In the normal lung, however, because of the rapid diffusion of oxygen in a gaseous medium, complete mixing of this fresh air with intra-acinar gas is probably instantaneous. In obstructive emphysema, with the breakdown of alveolar septa and the creation of much larger air spaces, mixing may be delayed, and in these circumstances gaseous diffusion may limit the diffusing capacity.[537]

DIFFUSION ACROSS THE ALVEOLOCAPILLARY MEMBRANE

The membrane through which oxygen diffuses to reach plasma in capillaries is composed of (1) a surface-active liquid that lines the alveolar wall, (2) alveolar epithelial cells with attenuated cytoplasm, (3) basement membrane of the epithelial layer, (4) loose connective tissue, (5) basement membrane of the capillary endothelium, and (6) capillary endothelium. It is thought that diffusion takes place only through the lateral cytoplasmic extensions of the type I alveolar epithelial cells, and that the "blood-air pathway" in a normal lung is 0.36 to 2.5 μ thick.[2] Through this thin membrane, with a driving pressure of approximately 60 mm Hg (PO_2 of alveolar gas minus PO_2 of mixed venous blood [$100 - 40 = 60$ mm Hg]), under resting conditions oxygen almost fully saturates the blood in one third of the time taken by blood to traverse the pulmonary capillaries. During exercise, with increased cardiac output and pulmonary capillary blood volume, the transit time is reduced. Nevertheless, aided by the slightly higher PO_2 due to increased ventilation, the blood is virtually saturated by oxygen by the time it reaches the end of the capillary. With decreased

alveolar PO_2 (e.g., due to atmospheric conditions at high altitude, respiratory center depression, or neuromuscular disease), the driving pressure of oxygen is reduced; exercise under these conditions results in a shortened transit time which, together with the reduced driving pressure, may limit diffusion, so that the end capillary blood may be only partly oxygenated. Although the transit time is thought of in relation to capillaries only, it is probable that the process of diffusion starts in the arterioles which are the origin of capillaries, since their walls are in direct contact with alveolar air.[212, 538, 539]

In addition to the aforementioned factors that affect diffusion, the total area in which flowing blood comes in contact with ventilated acinar units influences the capacity for diffusion. This is exemplified by the decrease in diffusion that occurs after pneumonectomy,[540] and may be responsible in part for the decrease in diffusing capacity that occurs in emphysema, in which a considerable amount of the alveolocapillary membrane often is destroyed. The amount of *effective* alveolocapillary membrane usually is reduced because of mismatching of capillary circulation with acinar ventilation (see further on). Since this may be an inevitable accompaniment of diseases that thicken the alveolocapillary membrane, assessment of responsibility for diffusion impairment may be difficult.[541, 542]

Many diseases may involve the acinar unit in such a way as to interfere with diffusion (see Figure 1–106). In such cases the arterial oxygen saturation may be normal in patients at rest, despite significant reduction in diffusing capacity; however, exercise elicits hypoxemia because the transit time through capillaries is decreased.

INTRAVASCULAR DIFFUSION

The crossing of the alveolocapillary membrane by oxygen does not complete the process of diffusion, and it is probable that resistance to gas movement into red cells is often greater than that to gas movement from the alveoli into the blood.[543] This is due not to the distance to be traversed through plasma to the red cell but to the rate of reaction of oxygen molecules with red cell contents. Differences in the rate of gas exchange in the red cell, the final phase of diffusion, are not important in relation to normal lungs breathing air, but they play a significant role in diffusion impairment in states of low alveolar oxygen tension and in anemia.

MEASUREMENT OF DIFFUSING CAPACITY

The efficiency of the diffusion process for gas uptake by the lung can be quantified in individual subjects or patients by measuring the diffusing capacity. Measurement of the capacity for diffusion of oxygen is a very complicated and perhaps unreliable procedure. It is necessary to know the mixed venous PO_2 in order to determine the driving pressure of oxygen, and the rate of diffusion varies along the capillary as the driving pressure decreases while the P_{O_2} in capillary blood increases. Because of these problems, carbon monoxide generally is used to measure diffusion; it has a great affinity for hemoglobin and, therefore, only a minute quantity of a low concentration (0.3 per cent) is required. The diffusing capacity for carbon monoxide is the amount of this gas taken up per minute, divided by the difference between partial pressures of carbon monoxide in the alveolus and in capillary blood. Since there is no carbon monoxide in mixed venous blood, the amount of gas taken up is the difference between the carbon monoxide content of inspired and expired gas. The denominator of the equation is equal to the mean alveolar P_{CO}, which can be calculated from an end tidal sample; the mean capillary P_{CO} is so small that it can be ignored. Several techniques have been developed for using this gas; the advantages of particular methods have been discussed in detail by Bates and his colleagues.[540]

The three important variables that make up the overall diffusing capacity of the lung (D_L) are the alveolocapillary membrane diffusing capacity (D_m), the reaction rate of carbon monoxide with hemoglobin, and the pulmonary capillary blood volume (V_C). Since different inhaled oxygen concentrations affect the CO-hemoglobin reaction rate, the two other variables, D_m and V_C, can be separated by repeating the measurement with different FI_{O_2}s.[511] In theory this would allow further dissection of the various causes for a decreased D_{LCO}, summarized in Figure 1–106, but in fact this is rarely done in individual patients as a diagnostic test. Morphometric estimates of D_{LCO}, D_m, and V_C have been attempted recently, but unlike physiologic estimates that suggest that V_C and D_m are of equal importance, the results suggest that the capillary blood volume and the CO-hemoglobin reaction rate are the major diffusing-limiting steps.[544]

The D_m and V_C components of D_L both decrease with age, but the membrane component D_m decreases first.[1184]

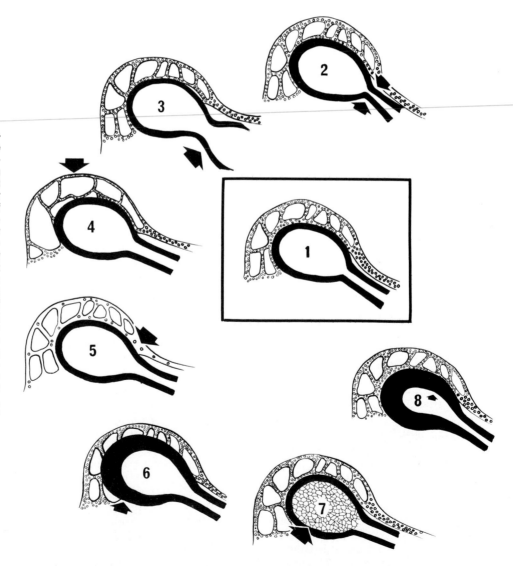

Figure 1–106. Pathophysiology of Diffusion Defect. The structure in the center of the diagram (1) is a normal air-containing acinar unit in which are depicted a conducting system, an alveolar cell lining, a normal amount of tissue between air space and capillary endothelium, and a capillary network containing a normal number of red blood cells. The acinar units around the periphery depict various mechanisms of diffusion defect: (2) obstruction to air entry; (3) dilatation and confluence of respiratory bronchioles (resulting in an increased pathway for diffusion, as in centrilobular emphysema); (4) loss of capillaries; (5) anemia; (6) increase in tissue between air space and capillary endothelium; (7) replacement of air in air space by edema, exudate, or blood; and (8) increase in alveolar lining cells.

Matching Capillary Blood Flow with Ventilation in the Acinus

Ideally, alveolar ventilation and alveolar perfusion should be uniform; i.e., each acinus should receive just the right amount of ventilation to oxygenate the hemoglobin completely and remove the carbon dioxide given off during gas exchange. This would mean that each of the 33,000 acini, with their 400 alveolar ducts and 8000 alveoli, would receive equal portions of the alveolar ventilation ($\dot{V}A$), which is estimated to average 4.5 liters per min, and the alveolar perfusion ($\dot{Q}$), which averages 5 liters per min. In other words, not only would the ratio of ventilation to perfusion ($\dot{V}A/\dot{Q}$) be 4.5:5 or 0.9 for each lung, but each acinar unit would have a $\dot{V}A/\dot{Q}$ ratio of 0.9 as well. Despite the fact that this is not true, even for the normal lung, the concept of an "ideal" $\dot{V}A/\dot{Q}$ ratio is useful as a point of reference in judging relationships between ventilation and perfusion within acini and the lung.[545] When the $\dot{V}A/\dot{Q}$ ratio is not ideal (i.e., other than 0.9), it is either because perfusion is reduced relative to ventilation (high $\dot{V}A/\dot{Q}$) or because ventilation is decreased relative to blood flow (low $\dot{V}A/\dot{Q}$).

Figure 1–107 shows the theoretic distribution of $\dot{V}A/\dot{Q}$ ratios in the lung, using a five-compartment model. The central unit (No. 3) corresponds to the "ideal" unit with a $\dot{V}A/\dot{Q}$ of 0.9. In this acinus, ventilation is sufficient to achieve an alveolar oxygen tension (PAO_2) of approximately 100 mm Hg. With unimpaired diffusion between alveolar gas and capillary blood, this results in a capillary oxygen tension (PcO_2) of 100 mm Hg in the blood leaving this unit, a level that is sufficient to achieve nearly 100 per cent saturation of the hemoglobin (20 ml O_2 per 100 ml of blood if the hemoglobin concentration is 15 grams per dl). The resulting $PACO_2$ and $PcCO_2$ is 40 mm Hg, which is sufficient to lower mixed venous carbon dioxide content from 53 to 48 ml per dl. Unit No. 1 represents the lowest possible $\dot{V}A/\dot{Q}$ region, amounting to 0, or true intrapulmonary shunt. Capillary blood emerges from such a unit with gas partial pressures and contents identical to those of mixed venous blood (i.e., $PcO_2 = 40$ mm Hg and $PcCO_2 = 46$ mm Hg in our example, for capillary contents of $O_2 = 13$ ml per dl and $CO_2 = 53$ ml per dl). Unit No. 2 has a $\dot{V}A/\dot{Q}$ ratio somewhere between 0.9 and 0, resulting in alveolar and capillary gas pressures and contents that are less than "ideal" for oxygen and more than "ideal" for carbon dioxide (i.e., $PcO_2 = 70$ mm Hg and $PcCO_2 = 44$ mm Hg in our example). Unit No. 5 represents true alveolar dead space, i.e., a region of lung that is ventilated but not perfused ($\dot{V}A/\dot{Q} = $ infinity). The ventilation to such a unit represents completely wasted ventilation since alveolar gas does not come in contact with capillary blood. Unit No. 4 has a $\dot{V}A/\dot{Q}$ ratio between 0.9 and infinity, resulting in alveolar and capillary partial pressures that are greater than "ideal" for oxygen and less than "ideal" for carbon dioxide (i.e.,

$PcO_2 = 130$ mm Hg and $PcCO_2 = 37$ mm Hg in our example).

Because of the shapes of the O_2 and CO_2 dissociation curves, $\dot{V}A/\dot{Q}$ mismatch has quite different effects on the efficiency of the lung to take up oxygen and remove carbon dioxide. As shown in Figure 1–108, the O_2 dissociation curve is flat above PO_2s of 70 or 80 mm Hg so that the overventilated unit (No. 4) cannot make up for the underventilated unit (No. 2) in terms of oxygen uptake. Although the elevated PO_2 in unit No. 4 results in a slight increase in the amount of dissolved oxygen in the capillary blood, hemoglobin is virtually 100 per cent saturated above a PO_2 of 100, and since dissolved oxygen can only increase by 0.0003 ml per dl of blood per mm Hg rise in PO_2, little gain is achieved by overventilating units.

For carbon dioxide removal, however, overventilated units can compensate for underventilated units: the CO_2 dissociation curve is virtually linear over the range of physiologic PCO_2 values, so that the lowered carbon dioxide content of blood from unit No. 4 can compensate for the greater than "ideal" content in unit No. 2.

When the blood from units 1, 2, 3, and 4 mix in the pulmonary veins and left atrium, the PaO_2 of this arterial blood will be less than the mean alveolar PO_2 of units 2, 3, and 4, whereas the $PaCO_2$ will be equal to the mean alveolar PCO_2. Put simply, $\dot{V}A/\dot{Q}$ mismatch decreases the efficiency of oxygen and carbon dioxide uptake and removal; in the case of oxygen, this results in a gradient between mean alveolar PO_2 and arterial PO_2 (A–a DO_2). $\dot{V}/\dot{Q}$ mismatch does not result in a gradient for carbon dioxide. If a disease process leads to the development of units with low $\dot{V}A/\dot{Q}$ ratios (No. 2) and to the development of areas of shunt (No. 1), arterial hypoxemia and hypercapnia will result. Since both a lowered PO_2 (indirectly) and an increased PCO_2 (directly) stimulate the respiratory center and increase ventilation, total alveolar ventilation will increase. The alveolar PO_2 in well-ventilated acinar units will rise while the PCO_2 in these units (No. 4) will fall. The excess carbon dioxide retained by blood circulating through the poorly ventilated units (Nos. 1 and 2) will be balanced by the supranormal output from the well-ventilated units. Comparison of the O_2 and CO_2 dissociation curves shows why this compensation can be accomplished for carbon dioxide but not for oxygen. Even if ventilation to an acinar unit is doubled and alveolar PO_2 rises to 130 mm Hg, the curve is so nearly horizontal in this range that a trivial increase in oxygen saturation is accomplished by this increase in PO_2.

Figure 1–107 is a simplified model that spans the entire range of possible $\dot{V}A/\dot{Q}$ ratios in five compartments. In fact, a continuous distribution of ratios is likely to exist, and even in the normal lung substantial regional variation in $\dot{V}A/\dot{Q}$ ratios has been demonstrated, largely in a gravity-dependent fashion. As discussed previously, the effect of gravity is to increase blood flow to the most dependent

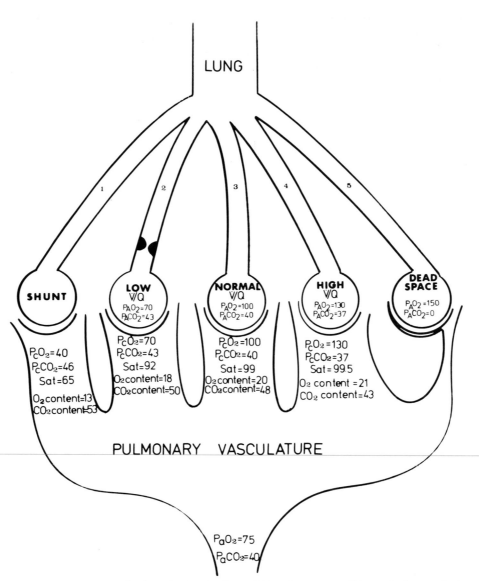

Figure 1–107. Theoretic Distribution of V̇A/Q̇ Ratios in the Lung. Although many possible ventilation: perfusion ratios can exist in a normal or diseased lung, these can be conveniently divided into five compartments. Unit 1 represents pure shunt, an area of lung with a ventilation: perfusion ratio of zero. Blood coming from such a unit will have gas tensions identical to those of mixed venous blood (P_{O_2} = 40 + P_{CO_2} = 46 in this example) and the P_{O_2} of blood from such units will be uninfluenced by changes in inspired O_2. Unit 2 represents a low V̇/Q̇ area in which there is insufficient ventilation to completely saturate hemoglobin or lower CO_2 content to normal arterial values. Unit 3 represents the perfect match of ventilation and perfusion, resulting in near 100 per cent saturation of hemoglobin and normal P_{CO_2}, whereas Unit 4 represents an overventilated (high V̇/Q̇) area. Blood from the high V̇/Q̇ area has a CO_2 content less than normal, which compensates for the higher than normal CO_2 content from Unit 2, but because of the shape of the O_2 dissociation curve, the overventilated unit cannot compensate for the underventilated unit with regard to O_2 transport. Unit 5 represents pure dead space in which the V̇/Q̇ ratio is infinity. Ventilation of such units is wasted and does not contribute to gas exchange. Note that although the mean P_{AO_2} of the ventilated units (2, 3, 4, and 5) is greater than 100, the P_{O_2} of the arterialized blood leaving the lung is 75. The V̇/Q̇ mismatch has resulted in an A–a gradient for O_2.

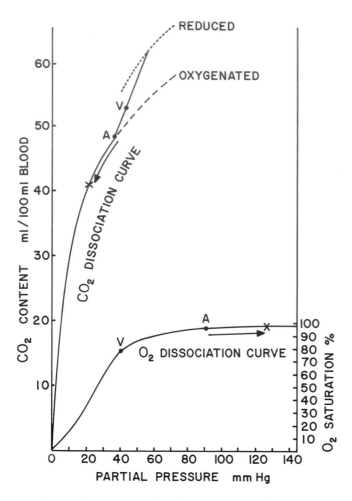

Figure 1–108. The Carbon Dioxide and Oxygen Dissociation Curves of Blood. The arrows (A → X) indicate the effect of doubling the ventilation on both CO_2 content and O_2 content (arterial oxygen saturation). The normal values for both arterial (A) and venous (V) oxygen and carbon dioxide are noted. It can be seen that, at any given P_{CO_2}, reduced blood can carry more carbon dioxide than oxygenated blood. *See* text.

portions of the lung—in the erect position to the lung base, in the supine posture to the posterior portion of the lung, and in the lateral decubitus position to the dependent lung. These changes in blood flow are the result of alterations in regional pulmonary vascular resistance secondary to gravity-dependent changes in intravascular hydrostatic pressure.[546] In upper lung regions, pulmonary arterial pressure is low relative to alveolar pressure, resulting in compression of the vessels and increased vascular resistance. Descending through the lung, pulmonary artery pressure increases relative to alveolar pressure, causing distention of the pulmonary vasculature and decreasing resistance. Finally, arterial and venous pressure exceed alveolar pressure, and blood flow continues to increase since pulmonary vessels are distended.

The regional distribution of ventilation is also modified by gravity.[547, 548] A gravity-dependent vertical gradient in pleural surface pressure results in alterations in regional lung volume:[549] in erect subjects pleural pressure at the lung apex (or anteriorly in the supine position) is more negative than at the base, and the local pleural pressure increases progressively (i.e., becomes less subatmospheric) as the base of the lung is approached. Since alveolar pressure is constant up and down the lung, this means that the local transpulmonary pressure varies in a gravity-dependent fashion. The local lung parenchyma responds to the local transpulmonary pressure along its pressure-volume curve, and, therefore, at the end of a quiet expiration, acinar units in upper lung regions are more distended and at a higher percentage of their TLC (total lung capacity) value than are the less well-distended units at the base of the lung. In experiments on dogs frozen intact in the erect (head up) position, Glazier and associates showed that at end-expiration the volume of an alveolus 25 cm from the lung apex was half the volume of an alveolus 5 cm from the apex.[550] The pleural pressure gradient averages about 0.25 cm H_2O per cm distance up and down the lung and has been shown to be relatively volume-independent;[549] that is, a similar gradient in pleural pressure exists when overall lung volume is at FRC (functional residual capacity), below FRC, or above FRC. Thus, at FRC, apical pleural pressure may be −7 cm H_2O and at the base +1 cm H_2O; at TLC, apical pleural pressure may be −37 cm H_2O and at the base −29 cm H_2O, a gradient of 8 cm H_2O at both lung volumes. Due to the curvilinear nature of the pressure-volume (PV) curve of the lung, the variation in regional lung volume is substantial at lower lung volumes, whereas near TLC, where the PV curve is relatively flat, the same gradient in applied pressures results in trivial differences in regional lung volume.[549]

Despite the considerable variation in end-expiratory pleural and transpulmonary pressure up and down the lung, the changes in pleural pressure (P) that occur during tidal breathing are similar at different vertical levels. Thus, because of the shape of the PV curve, upper lung units are less well ventilated per unit of lung volume than are acini at the lung base, which are on a steeper portion of their PV curve. In summary, the gravity-dependent pleural pressure gradient results in a regional variation in lung volume (V_o) and regional variation in ventilation ($\dot{V}/V_o$).

If the increase in $\dot{V}/V_o$ from apex to base were directly proportional to the increase in blood flow from apex to base, the $\dot{V}_A/\dot{Q}$ ratio would not vary. This is not the case, however, since the effect of gravity on regional perfusion is greater than the effect on regional ventilation, and thus blood flow and ventilation are slightly mismatched even in the normal lung. The details of regional ventilation and perfusion distribution and the resulting regional $\dot{V}_A/\dot{Q}$ ratios were described in the pioneering studies of Milic-Emili, West, and their colleagues.[547, 550–555] These investigators used external counters to measure the regional distribution of inhaled or intravenously infused inert radioactive gases to assess inter-regional ventilation, perfusion, and $\dot{V}_A/\dot{Q}$ distribution. Their studies showed that regional $\dot{V}_A/\dot{Q}$ ratios differ from "ideal" in normal subjects, and that during quiet breathing in the upright posture, the $\dot{V}_A/\dot{Q}$ ratio is between 2 and 3 at the lung apex, decreasing to between 0.5 and 1 at the lung base. The apex-to-base $\dot{V}_A/\dot{Q}$ mismatch disappears when the supine position is adopted, being replaced by an anterior-to-posterior gradient in regional ventilation, perfusion, and $\dot{V}_A/\dot{Q}$ ratios.[556]

At low lung volumes, ventilation to the lung bases in the upright position or posterior regions in the supine position does not follow the distribution suggested by regional pleural pressure, and it has been convincingly demonstrated by Engel and his associates that airway closure may occur in dependent lung regions during tidal breathing, even in normal subjects.[557] Airway size, like alveolar size, is dependent on regional transpulmonary pressure; with the relatively positive pressures at the lung base, closure of small airways can occur during a portion of the respiratory cycle. The overall lung volume at which airways in dependent lung regions first close is termed the "closing volume" and can be measured with the single breath nitrogen washout curve (*see* page 435). Since FRC decreases on assuming the supine posture while closing volume does not change, a greater number of dependent airways may close during supine tidal breathing, resulting in a paradoxic decrease in ventilation to dependent lung regions. Airway closure at the lung base results in a lower regional alveolar P_{O_2}, and this may secondarily influence regional perfusion by inducing hypoxic vasoconstriction. Prefaut and Engel found a preferential perfusion of nondependent lung regions in supine subjects with a high closing volume, an effect that was abolished by breathing an oxygen-enriched gas mixture.[558]

Although the distribution of ventilation during quiet breathing is dependent on regional lung compliance and applied pleural pressure, regional resistance can become important during the increased ventilation of exercise. Ventilation distribution becomes more uniform up and down the lung with increasing inspiratory flow rates, possibly because of variations in the regional time constant (the product of resistance and compliance): the time constant of a lung unit is a reflection of the rapidity of volume change that will occur in the unit in response to a step change in inflating or deflating pressure. Nondependent lung regions have a lower resistance owing to the higher regional lung volume and also a lower compliance because of the alinear pressure/volume curve; the product of a smaller resistance and a lower compliance produces a shorter time constant. During rapid respiratory cycling, this could influence regional ventilation distribution.[559] Alternatively, the more uniform distribution of ventilation during exercise could be contributed to by differences in applied pleural pressure up and down the lung as a result of recruitment of different inspiratory muscles during exercise.[559]

Inter-regional gas distribution can be altered with predominant rib cage or diaphragmatic breathing; slight differences in applied pleural pressure resulting from the different pattern of inspiratory muscle use are probably responsible for this effect.[560] During exercise the vertical gradient in perfusion also diminishes due to a slight elevation in pulmonary vascular pressures and this contributes to the decrease in gravity-dependent variations in $\dot{V}_A/\dot{Q}$ distribution.[561, 562] Most studies using radioactive gases have been designed to examine inter-regional variations in gas, blood flow, and $\dot{V}_A/\dot{Q}$ distribution, but it is evident that intraregional variations in $\dot{V}_A/\dot{Q}$ exist even in normal lungs and that during exercise intraregional mismatch may in fact increase.[563, 564]

With the development of lung disease, regional variations in ventilation, perfusion, and $\dot{V}_A/\dot{Q}$ ratios increase. In the normal lung, true intrapulmonary shunt (unit No. 1) probably does not occur, although some right-to-left flow through anatomic channels such as the thebesian vessels does take place. Any pathologic process in which alveolar air spaces are filled with transudate or exudate and in which perfusion persists results in a true shunt. Airway diseases that affect regional resistance and parenchymal diseases that change regional compliance can alter regional time constants and affect ventilation distribution. Abnormalities of the pulmonary vasculature, such as destruction of the capillary bed (as in emphysema) or obstruction of pulmonary vessels (as in thromboembolism), alter regional perfusion distribution; complete vascular obstruction, which may occur with pulmonary thromboembolic disease, converts affected regions of lung to dead space—ventilated but unperfused units (such as unit No. 5).

Measurement of Ventilation/Perfusion Mismatch

A number of methods are available to quantify $\dot{V}A/\dot{Q}$ mismatch, ranging from simple bedside calculations to more elaborate and invasive techniques. Calculation of the physiologic dead space using the Bohr equation provides a useful estimate of overventilated lung units. Ventilation of totally unperfused acinar units (No. 5) and the excess portion of ventilation of high $\dot{V}A/\dot{Q}$ units (No. 4) represent alveolar dead space; when the alveolar dead space ventilation is added to the anatomic dead space ventilation, the total is expressed as physiologic dead space. The ratio of physiologic dead space to tidal volume ($\dot{V}_D/\dot{V}_T$) can be calculated knowing arterial P_{CO_2} and mixed expired P_{CO_2}:

$$V_D/V_T = \frac{\text{Arterial } P_{CO_2} - \text{mixed expired } P_{CO_2}}{\text{Arterial } P_{CO_2}} \quad (1)$$

In this equation, arterial P_{CO_2} is reasonably assumed to reflect mean alveolar P_{CO_2}. With the advent of reliable, relatively low cost, rapid CO_2 analyzers, this calculation can be made easily, especially in the intensive care unit setting; it serves as an estimate of $\dot{V}A/\dot{Q}$ mismatch.

The most commonly used and easily calculated estimate of $\dot{V}A/\dot{Q}$ mismatch is the alveolar-arterial gradient for oxygen, P(A–a) O_2. Calculation of the P(A–a) O_2 requires knowledge of the mean alveolar P_{O_2}, which can be calculated using the alveolar air equation originally described by Fenn and colleagues:[565]

$$P_{AO_2} = P_{IO_2} - \frac{P_{ACO_2}}{R} + \left[P_{ACO_2} \cdot F_{IO_2} \cdot \frac{1-R}{R} \right] \quad (2)$$

where F_{IO_2} is the fractional concentration of oxygen in the inspired air and R is the respiratory exchange ratio (the ratio of CO_2 production to O_2 consumption).

In practice, calculation of R is somewhat cumbersome, requiring collection and analysis of expired gas; simplified methods to estimate P_{AO_2} have been advocated.[566] The alveolar air equation may be modified to the form:

$$P_{AO_2} = P_{EO_2} - \frac{P_{IO_2}(V_D/V_T)}{(1 - V_D/V_T)} \quad (3)$$

where P_{EO_2} is the partial pressure of oxygen in the expired gas and P_{IO_2} is the partial pressure of oxygen in the inspired gas. Using this equation, a single breath method for calculation of P_{AO_2} has been described, but the calculation still requires

analysis of carbon dioxide and oxygen tensions in expired air.[567]

The simplest and most often used form of the alveolar air equation is:

$$P_{AO_2} = P_{IO_2} - \frac{P_{aCO_2}}{R} \quad (4)$$

in which R is assumed to equal 0.8.

Since P_{aCO_2} is used for P_{ACO_2} in this equation, all that is required for calculation is knowledge of the arterial P_{CO_2} and F_{IO_2}. A comparison of P_{AO_2} that has been calculated, assuming a respiratory quotient of 0.8 and the measured value, suggests that equation (4) is adequate for clinical purposes.[1182]

Once the P_{AO_2} is calculated, the alveolar-arterial gradient for oxygen P(A-a)O_2 can be obtained by comparing P_{AO_2} with measured arterial P_{O_2}:

$$P(A\text{-}a)O_2 = P_{AO_2} - P_{aO_2} \quad (5)$$

Intrapulmonary shunt and $\dot{V}A/\dot{Q}$ mismatch are the major contributors to the P(A-a)O_2, although failure of diffusion equilibration of alveolar oxygen with capillary blood may contribute to the P(A-a)O_2 in three situations: (a) at extreme altitudes, (b) with very short red cell transit times through the lung, and (c) in certain lung diseases.

The calculation of P(A-a)O_2 as a measurement of shunt and $\dot{V}A/\dot{Q}$ mismatch has the disadvantage that it is influenced by the mixed venous P_{O_2} and inspired P_{O_2}. A given maldistribution of ventilation and perfusion will result in a different P_{aO_2} and calculated P(A-a)O_2 with changed mixed venous P_{O_2}. This is most easily understood with shunt: if 25 per cent of the cardiac output is shunted through a completely consolidated lung region, no gas transfer will occur and the shunted blood will have a P_{O_2} and P_{CO_2} equal to that of mixed venous blood; when this is added to blood coming from normally ventilated regions, arterial P_{O_2} will be decreased and arterial P_{CO_2} increased. The extent to which the shunted blood alters the arterial blood is determined by the gas tensions in mixed venous blood. With a very low cardiac output, mixed venous P_{O_2} and oxygen content can reach extremely low values, and a given shunt will be associated with much worse systemic hypoxemia than if the cardiac output were normal or increased. Thus, arterial P_{O_2} and the calculated P(A-a)O_2 can be influenced by mixed venous gas tensions and therefore do not purely reflect the gas-exchanging ability of the lung. A similar effect occurs with $\dot{V}A/\dot{Q}$ mismatch. In addition, the calculated P(A-a)O_2 is influenced by the P_{IO_2}, since a given degree of shunt or $\dot{V}A/\dot{Q}$ mismatch will produce a higher calculated P(A-a)O_2 as the P_{IO_2} is increased. Again the easiest example to consider is the situation in which $\dot{V}A/\dot{Q}$ is 0: if a patient is breathing room air and 35 per cent of the cardiac output is being shunted through a consolidated lobe resulting in a PaO_2 of 50 mm Hg (calculated $P(A-a)O_2 = 40$), the breathing of 100 per cent oxygen will increase arterial PO_2 only slightly by the addition of small amounts of dissolved oxygen in the normally ventilated areas. Thus, with 100 per cent oxygen, the PaO_2 might increase to only 80 mm Hg, with a resultant calculated $P(A-a)O_2$ of over 500!

Similarly, shifts of the oxygen dissociation curve due to changes in blood temperature or pH can influence the calculated $P(A-a)O_2$ without a true effect on the gas-exchanging ability of the lung.[568]

Calculations of venous admixture and shunt provide more accurate estimates of $\dot{V}A/\dot{Q}$ maldistribution and are less affected by mixed venous and inspired gas tension; however, they require a sample of mixed venous blood. The same equation is used for calculation of venous admixture and shunt:

$$\frac{\dot{Q}s}{\dot{Q}t} = \frac{C\dot{c}O_2 - CaO_2}{C\dot{c}O_2 - C\bar{v}O_2} \qquad (6)$$

where $\dot{Q}s/\dot{Q}t$ is the venous admixture ratio or shunt if 100 per cent oxygen is breathed, CcO_2 is the oxygen content of end-capillary blood, CaO_2 is the oxygen content of arterial blood, and $C\bar{v}O_2$ is the oxygen content of mixed venous blood; the equation assumes equilibration between alveolar and capillary PO_2. Ideal capillary PO_2 is calculated using the alveolar air equation (*see* equation 2). Content is calculated knowing the hemoglobin concentration and assuming that it is identical in venous, arterial, and capillary blood:

$$O_2 \text{ content (ml/100 blood)} =$$
$$(\text{Hgb, gm/dl} \times 1.39 \times \text{per cent saturation})$$
$$+ (PO_2 \times 0.003) \qquad (7)$$

where PO_2 is the PO_2 of capillary blood, arterial blood, or mixed venous blood; the first term in this equation is the oxygen content of hemoglobin, and the second term calculates dissolved oxygen.

When measurements for this calculation are obtained while the patient is breathing air or a gas mixture containing less than 100 per cent oxygen, the resulting ratio is the venous admixture which is an "as if" shunt, representing the amount of mixed venous blood that would have to be added to capillary blood in order to result in the observed arterial PO_2 and A-a gradient. As pointed out by West, both the venous admixture and the ratio of dead space to tidal volume (VD/VT) are unfortunately influenced by overall ventilation and blood flow and by the FIO_2.[569]

An additional shortcoming in use of $P(A-a)O_2$ and venous admixture as estimates of $\dot{V}A/\dot{Q}$ mismatch is the fact that both can be altered by diffusion impairment. Whether the partial pressure of capillary blood reaches the alveolar PO_2 during its transit through the pulmonary capillary depends on the red blood cell transit time and the driving pressure for diffusion—the difference between mixed venous and alveolar PO_2. In the normal lung at rest, red blood cell residence time in pulmonary capillaries approaches 1 sec, and the gradient between normal alveolar PO_2 and mixed venous PO_2 is sufficiently large to ensure complete equilibration. With the decreased red blood cell transit time that accompanies increased cardiac output, and especially with lowered PAO_2 secondary to increased altitude or hypoventilation, diffusion impairment may become important by contributing to the calculated $P(A-a)O_2$ and venous admixture.[570]

Only when pure oxygen is breathed for a time sufficient to wash nitrogen out of the lung completely can a measure be obtained of gas exchange uninfluenced by FIO_2 and $P\bar{v}O_2$. The calculation of shunt obtained using equation 6 gives an estimate of only one compartment in the $\dot{V}A/\dot{Q}$ spectrum.

In addition to giving limited information about the spectrum of $\dot{V}A/\dot{Q}$ mismatch, measurement of shunt with 100 per cent oxygen may in fact increase the intrapulmonary shunt. Dantzker and his associates have shown that regions with low $\dot{V}A/\dot{Q}$ ratios may be converted to regions of shunt when gas with higher oxygen partial pressures is breathed.[571] In a unit with a sufficiently low $\dot{V}A/\dot{Q}$, oxygen breathing can result in an oxygen uptake by pulmonary capillary blood that exceeds the oxygen delivered by alveolar ventilation. When a gas with a lower PO_2 is breathed, nitrogen, being very insoluble, serves to stabilize these units, preventing their collapse. The critical $\dot{V}A/\dot{Q}$ that results in alveolar instability is dependent on the $\dot{V}A/\dot{Q}$ ratio of the unit and the fraction of oxygen in the inspired gas.[571]

Measurement of regional ventilation/perfusion ratios using radioactive tracers has added greatly to our understanding of topographic $\dot{V}A/\dot{Q}$ distribution, but the techniques are basically insensitive in that only relatively large lung regions can be assessed with external counters, and probably of more importance in diseased lungs is intraregional, acinar-to-acinar $\dot{V}A/\dot{Q}$ mismatch. The advent of efficient gamma cameras has greatly simplified the qualitative and quantitative assessment of regional $\dot{V}A/\dot{Q}$ inhomogeneity.[572] Their greatest clinical use has been in the search for areas of alveolar dead space, ventilated but unperfused regions resulting from thromboembolic obstruction of large pulmonary vessels.

The most recent major advances in the measurement of $\dot{V}A/\dot{Q}$ mismatch came with the description by Wagner and his colleagues of a method to measure the "continuous" distribution of $\dot{V}A/\dot{Q}$ ratios in normal and diseased lungs.[573] The technique involves the intravenous infusion of up to 10 inert gases dissolved in saline; the gases used have a wide range of solubility in blood, and in their passage through the lung enter alveolar gas. The mixed expired and arterial concentration of each gas is measured by gas chromatography when a steady state is achieved; the retention and excretion of

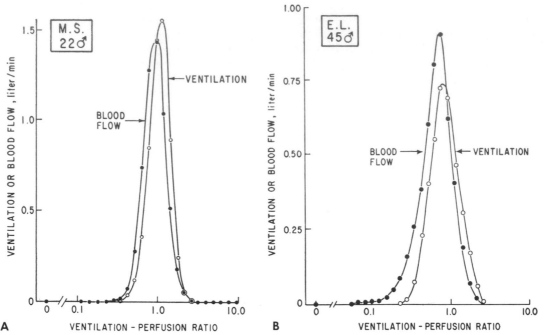

Figure 1–109. Distribution of Blood Flow and Ventilation in Relation to V̇/Q̇ Ratios. The distribution of blood flow and ventilation (vertical axis) to units with varying V̇/Q̇ ratios (horizontal axis) in a 22-year-old man (*A*) and a 45-year-old man (*B*). In both normal individuals, the bulk of the ventilation and perfusion is well matched, going to units with a V̇/Q̇ ratio near 1, and there is no shunt (V̇/Q̇ ratio = 0). In the older man a wider range of V̇/Q̇ ratios exists. (Reprinted from Wagner PD, Laravuso RB, Uhl RR, et al: J Clin Invest 54:54–68, 1974 by copyright permission of the American Society for Clinical Investigation and with the permission of the authors.)

each gas can then be calculated and plotted against solubility. From the plot, the distribution of blood flow and ventilation with respect to V̇A/Q̇ ratios can be calculated using a digital computer. The technique allows measurement of absolute shunt as well as alveolar dead space and also permits calculation of the proportion of perfusion and ventilation to a large number of normally distributed units of varying V̇A/Q̇ ratio.

The advantages of this technique are threefold: (1) it allows a multicompartmental description of the V̇A/Q̇ distribution rather than categorizing it into two or three compartments as do other techniques; (2) it is relatively noninvasive and does not require placement of a central venous line; and (3) no radioactive gases are used. An example of the results of this technique in a young and an older normal subject are shown in Figure 1–109. The disadvantage of the technique is that there is no unique solution to the retention and excretion curves. With simple disturbances, the method can adequately describe the V̇A/Q̇ relationships, but with complex derangements a number of interpretations of the data are possible.

Blood Gases and Acid-Base Balance

Blood Gases

The ability of the lung to perform its prime function—the exchange of oxygen and carbon dioxide—is readily determined from analysis of a sample of arterial blood. The oxygen carried can be meas-

ured as arterial oxygen saturation or as Po_2. (Arterial oxygen saturation = O_2 content/O_2 capacity [per cent].) Since each 1.0 gram of hemoglobin can combine with 1.34 ml of oxygen, the oxygen capacity of a subject with 15 grams of hemoglobin per dl of blood is approximately 20. The content is the amount of oxygen that the blood actually contains; this can be determined in a sample by extraction under anaerobic conditions. In a subject with normal lungs breathing air at sea level, this amounts to 19 ml (or slightly more) and, therefore, oxygen saturation is $19/20 \times 100$, or 95 per cent.

The Po_2 may be determined from the oxygen dissociation curve using arterial oxygen saturation, but this is not truly reliable because of the almost horizontal slope of the upper part of the curve (*see* Figure 1–108). The Po_2 can be measured directly by use of an electrode—which, as we have seen, is the only way of determining total oxygen carried by hemoglobin and plasma during the inhalation of 100 per cent oxygen.

In contrast to oxygen, which is carried almost entirely by hemoglobin, approximately 75 per cent of carbon dioxide is contained in plasma. In the resting subject, while mixed venous blood holds about 15 ml of oxygen per dl of blood at a Po_2 of 40 mm Hg and an oxygen saturation of 75 per cent, its carbon dioxide content is about 52 ml per dl of blood at a Pco_2 of 45 mm Hg. Although the red blood cell carries only 25 per cent of the carbon dioxide, it plays an essential role in the transport of this gas to the lungs; it contains the enzyme carbonic anhydrase, which rapidly hydrates the carbon dioxide passing through the erythrocyte membrane and converts it into carbonic acid, H ions, and bicarbonate ions. The bicarbonate ions (HCO_3) quickly permeate the cell membrane and enter the plasma in exchange for chloride ions; in this manner, as bicarbonate, most of the carbon dioxide from the tissues is carried by the blood. Since blood that contains reduced hemoglobin can carry more carbon dioxide than can fully oxygenated blood at the same PCO_2, the circumstances are ideal for the uptake of carbon dioxide in the tissues and for its unloading in the pulmonary capillaries when the hemoglobin has been reoxygenated (see Figure 1–108).

In anemia, no matter how severe, PO_2 is normal and hemoglobin is fully saturated, oxygen content and capacity being reduced. However, the small amount of oxygen taken up by the blood indicates the anemia and the resultant reduction in total oxygen transport to the tissues. When normal hemoglobin is replaced by methemoglobin, sulfhemoglobin, or carboxyhemoglobin, the PO_2 remains normal, although spectrophotometric analysis of the sample reveals reduced oxygen saturation.

Arterial hypoxemia may be due to one or more of four mechanisms—diffusion defect, true shunt, ventilation-perfusion inequality, or hypoventilation.

A diffusion defect results in hypoxemia if there is failure of equilibration of alveolar and capillary PO_2 in the brief transit of the red cell through the pulmonary capillary bed. There is continued controversy concerning the importance of this mechanism in the production of arterial hypoxemia in disease, but it is probable that failure of diffusive equilibration between alveolar gas and capillary blood contributes to the hypoxemia seen in emphysema, the increase in hypoxemia that occurs with exercise in patients with interstitial lung disease, the hypoxemia that develops in some individuals during severe exercise, and the hypoxemia of altitude. With exercise, the mechanism is probably a decrease in the red blood cell capillary transit time whereas at altitude it is related to a low alveolar PO_2. Since carbon dioxide is some 20 times more soluble than oxygen in water and the tissue membranes, equilibration times are more rapid, and diffusion limitation does not play a role in the genesis of carbon dioxide retention.

A true shunt of venous blood to systemic circulation may be due to congenital cardiac disease, arteriovenous aneurysm of the lung, or, in some diseases that affect the parenchyma, precapillary anastomosis of the pulmonary arteriole and venule. More commonly, intrapulmonary shunt is caused by pathologic processes that fill the alveolar air spaces with transudate or exudate, producing areas of lung that are unventilated but well perfused. This mechanism is the primary cause of hypoxemia in cardiogenic and noncardiogenic pulmonary edema and in other conditions characterized by air space consolidation, such as pneumonia. The shunted blood never comes in contact with acinar units, whether or not these are ventilated, and for this reason the PO_2 of the arterial blood cannot be raised to a normal value (approximately 600 mm Hg) during inhalation of 100 per cent oxygen. In fact, when the shunt handles 10 per cent or more of the cardiac output, the arterial PO_2 cannot rise above 400 mm Hg. All other mechanisms that produce hypoxemia can be fully corrected by the inspiration of 100 per cent oxygen, which replaces nitrogen in even the most poorly ventilated acini. In true shunt, the PCO_2 is usually normal or low, since additional ventilation removes more carbon dioxide from acini that are perfused and ventilated. The inability of this compensatory hyperventilation to improve uptake of oxygen significantly is apparent on study of the oxygen and carbon dioxide dissociation curves (see Figure 1–108). Doubling the ventilation decreases PCO_2 from 40 to 20 mm Hg and eliminates considerable amounts of carbon dioxide, whereas the increase in PO_2 that results from increase in ventilation insignificantly increases arterial-blood oxygen content and saturation.

$\dot{V}A/\dot{Q}$ inequality is the commonest cause of the hypoxemia that accompanies pulmonary diseases; chronic obstructive pulmonary disease, emphysema, asthma, and interstitial lung diseases are the clinical conditions most often associated with this physiologic disturbance. The capillary blood that perfuses underventilated acinar units is not fully saturated and does not release normal amounts of carbon dioxide since the gradient between the PCO_2 of blood and the acinus is reduced. However, because of the differences in the slopes of the dissociation curves, $\dot{V}/\dot{Q}$ mismatching tends to affect oxygen transport and arterial PO_2 to a greater extent than carbon dioxide transport and PCO_2. Hyperventilation of well-ventilated acini with consequent reduction in alveolar PCO_2 increases the blood-to-acinus gradient and eliminates more carbon dioxide from these areas. Consequently, in patients with $\dot{V}A/\dot{Q}$ inequality, PCO_2 may be low or normal. However, overventilation of these same units does not make up for the underventilated units in terms of oxygen uptake. The hypoxemia associated with $\dot{V}A/\dot{Q}$ inequality can be corrected by breathing 100 per cent oxygen since oxygen replaces nitrogen in even the most poorly ventilated areas. When carbon dioxide retention is also present, prolonged inhalation of high concentrations of oxygen increases the carbon dioxide concentration in the blood and may lead to confusion and coma. This additional retention of carbon dioxide during oxygen breathing is due in part to removal of the carotid body's hypoxic stimulus to ventilation and in part to an increase in physiologic dead space produced by a release of hypoxic vasoconstriction in low $\dot{V}/\dot{Q}$ areas.

Hypoxemia associated with a low inspired PO_2 occurs on ascending to altitude. This is usually of no clinical significance at moderate elevations, but the exponential decrease in PO_2 at higher altitudes can result in significant hypoxemia, especially if accompanied by pre-existing pulmonary disease.

If overall alveolar ventilation decreases, carbon dioxide retention occurs as well as alveolar hypoxia and resulting hypoxemia. The hypoxemia associated with hypoventilation does not produce an increased alveolar-arterial gradient for oxygen (A–a DO_2) and thus differs from that caused by diffusion defects, $\dot{V}A/\dot{Q}$ inequality, and shunt. Since hypoventilation often occurs in association with these gas exchange abnormalities, calculation of A–a DO_2 aids in separating the component of hypoxemia related to hypoventilation from that caused by gas exchange problems.

ACID-BASE BALANCE

Together with the analysis of arterial blood to determine PO_2 (or oxygen saturation)—which detects abnormality of the physiologic process and when combined with clinical information aids in diagnosis—determination of the H^+ (pH) concentration is of utmost importance. The highly complex acid-base state and its regulation have been reviewed in detail, and the interested reader desiring more comprehensive coverage is referred to these treatises.[574-580] The section that follows is a simplified account of disturbances in H^+ concentration, with particular reference to the commoner clinical states likely to be encountered by physicians interested in respiratory diseases.

Under normal conditions, values for H^+ concentration $[H^+]$, pH, bicarbonate concentration $[HCO_3^-]$, and PCO_2 remain within a relatively narrow range. In arterial blood, the $[H^+]$ may vary from 35 to 45 nM/liter, pH from 7.35 to 7.45, $[HCO_3^-]$ from 22 to 28 nM/liter, and PCO_2 from 35 to 45 mm Hg. Interpretation of disturbances of acid-base balance requires not only values of the various biochemical components but also knowledge of the clinical picture. For descriptive purposes it is simplest to consider disturbances of acid-base balance as physiologic derangements, defining acidosis as an abnormal condition or process that would decrease the pH or increase the $[H^+]$ of the blood if there were no secondary changes. Similarly, alkalosis can be defined as a process that tends to increase the pH or decrease the $[H^+]$ of the blood if there are no secondary changes. The terms *acidemia* and *alkalemia* are best restricted to situations in which arterial pH falls or rises, respectively.

Disturbances of acid-base balance can be further divided into those that are respiratory in origin and those that are primarily nonrespiratory (metabolic). Respiratory changes in the balance are due to overventilation or underventilation with excess removal or retention of carbon dioxide, which decreases or increases the total "carbonic acid pool" of the extracellular fluid. Nonrespiratory disturbances are the result of increase or decrease in noncarbonic acid or a loss or gain of bicarbonate by the extracellular fluid. Acidosis or alkalosis may be "simple," that is, purely respiratory or metabolic, or "mixed," reflecting physiologic disturbances that are both respiratory and nonrespiratory in nature, such as derangements of tissue perfusion and renal function, and the assimilation or loss of excessive acid or base through the gastrointestinal tract. The commonest type of "mixed" acidosis seen by the chest physician is that due to severe acute pulmonary edema, in which carbon dioxide retention and tissue hypoxia permit anaerobic glycolysis and the formation of lactic acid.

Compensatory Mechanisms. The range of blood $[H^+]$ compatible with life is about 20 to 160 nM/liter (pH 6.8 to 7.7). When the $[H^+]$ moves from the accepted normal range (38 to 42 nM/liter) the body's homeostatic mechanisms react to restore the balance. The type and magnitude of the mechanisms evoked depend on the degree of disturbance, its duration, and the type of imbalance (carbonic or noncarbonic). For adequate body function, it is more important to maintain near normality of $[H^+]$ than to maintain CO_2 or bicarbonate in the range found in health. In fact, regulation of acid-base balance is often reflected in abnormally high or low levels of carbon dioxide and bicarbonate in the extracellular fluid. Homeostatic mechanisms that operate in acid-base derangements include (1) buffering of the excess H^+ or HCO_3^- in intracellular and extracellular fluids, (2) compensatory increase or decrease in alveolar ventilation, and (3) renal response.

The buffer components in extracellular fluids are hemoglobin, plasma proteins, bicarbonate, and phosphate. In the blood itself, buffering is complete within a few minutes and is largely dependent on the bicarbonate and hemoglobin systems. The bicarbonate also moves from the interstitial fluid spaces into the blood in situations of H^+ excess; this may take 15 minutes to 2 hours.[580] Within the cells, buffering depends upon the presence of protein and phosphate radicals.

The respiratory compensatory mechanism is a result of $[H^+]$-induced stimulation of receptors in the central nervous system and the aortic and carotid bodies. Elimination or retention of carbon dioxide has been reported to take minutes to hours.

Shifts of H^+, K^+, and Na^+ from various tissues, particularly muscle, and carbonate from bone are somewhat slower in compensating for disturbances in acid-base balance, but quantitatively they are of great importance. The movement of H^+ into the cells is reflected in increased $[K^+]$ in the extracellular fluid.

The renal response to disturbances in acid-base balance may take up to 1 week for completion; in respiratory acidosis it is well developed in 48 hours and usually maximal within 5 days.[581] Renal compensation for alkalosis depends upon the rapidity of development of the alkalosis and, in chronic states, on the depletion of sodium, chloride, and potassium.

Respiratory Acidosis. Respiratory acidosis results from alveolar hypoventilation. Carbon dioxide retention develops as a result of $\dot{V}/\dot{Q}$ inequality (that is, regional hypoventilation of well-perfused areas in the lung) or generalized hypoventilation; in the latter, the lung parenchyma may be entirely normal but a neuromuscular defect limits movement of the thoracic cage. $\dot{V}/\dot{Q}$ abnormality is usually due to obstructive lung disease but may play a part in the pathophysiology of carbon dioxide retention in kyphoscoliosis and obesity. Generalized alveolar underventilation results from malfunction of the respiratory center or from injury or disease of the efferent neural pathway in the spinal cord, anterior horn cells, or peripheral nerves innervating the diaphragm and intercostal muscles. Myopathy or myositis, and extreme deformity of the thoracic cage, as in kyphoscoliosis, also may restrict alveolar ventilation.

Respiratory acidosis may be acute or chronic. The acute form occurs in severe status asthmaticus, acute respiratory center depression caused by drug intoxication, and rarely from neuromuscular disorders. Hypoventilation leading to chronic respiratory acidosis occurs in chronic bronchitis, emphysema, diseases in which the anterior horn cells are destroyed, and the muscular dystrophies. A rare cause of chronic respiratory failure is upper airway obstruction; this may be due to endotracheal cicatricial stenosis, functional obstruction associated with obesity, or tracheal tumor. Perhaps the commonest examples of respiratory acidosis are those due to acute infection or drug-precipitated acute respiratory center depression complicating chronic obstructive pulmonary disease in patients with compensated chronic respiratory acidosis.

Compensatory Mechanisms in Respiratory Acidosis. Sudden alveolar hypoventilation increases the P_{ACO_2} (partial pressure of alveolar CO_2) and hence the Pa_{CO_2} (partial pressure of arterial CO_2), forming carbonic acid and shifting the Henderson equation to the right ($H_2O + CO_2 \rightleftarrows H_2CO_3 \rightleftarrows H^+ + HCO_3^-$), thereby increasing both $[H^+]$ and HCO_3^-. The increased carbonic acid is buffered within a few minutes, chiefly by hemoglobin and plasma proteins. The degree of acid-base disturbance depends upon the extent of carbon dioxide retention and subsequent compensation. Ion shifts, lasting hours to days, occur between extracellular and intracellular fluids, especially in muscle and bone. H^+ ions penetrate cell membranes, allowing K^+ to escape and increasing extracellular potassium.

When carbon dioxide retention is prolonged there is a renal response, which also helps to keep $[H^+]$ within normal range. This mechanism is well developed by 48 hours and usually maximal within 5 days.[581] The kidney reacts to the acidosis by increasing its ability to reabsorb and generate HCO_3^-. The raised arterial P_{CO_2} apparently stimulates bicarbonate conservation; the raised P_{CO_2} in the renal tubule cells increases the formation of carbonic acid (H_2CO_3) and enhances renal intracellular $[H^+]$ and H^+ secretion; the augmented renal tubule H^+ secretion—resulting from carbonic acid dissociation—gives rise to *de novo* generation of HCO_3^- by the renal tubules. The end result of the compensatory HCO_3^- reabsorption and generation is increased excretion of Cl^- ions, with consequent hypochloremia.

Respiratory Alkalosis. Respiratory alkalosis results from hyperventilation. It is commonest in tension or anxiety states, in which circumstances it is usually acute and rarely prolonged. Some drugs (e.g., salicylic acid, paraldehyde, epinephrine, and progesterone) may cause hyperventilation by stimulating the respiratory center. Traumatic, infectious, or vascular lesions of the central nervous system may produce respiratory alkalosis. Fever and gram-negative bacteremia can induce hyperventilation, but if shock develops this is often rapidly balanced by lactic acidosis—the result of tissue hypoperfusion. Several pulmonary diseases are associated with mild respiratory alkalosis. In these circumstances, the stimuli to hyperventilation are probably a combination of hypoxemia and reflexes initiated in the lung parenchyma. Some of these pulmonary diseases are acute (e.g., asthma and pulmonary emboli) and others are chronic (e.g., granulomatous and fibrotic interstitial disorders that cause compensated respiratory alkalosis). Excessive artificial ventilation also may give rise to acute or chronic respiratory alkalosis.

Compensatory Mechanisms in Respiratory Alkalosis. Hyperventilation decreases P_{ACO_2} and hence Pa_{CO_2}: the decrease in arterial P_{CO_2} shifts the Henderson equation to the left ($H_2O + CO_2 \rightleftarrows H_2CO_3 \rightleftarrows H^+ + HCO_3^-$), and decreases both $[H^+]$ and $[HCO_3^-]$. H^+ moves from the intracellular fluid, where it is replaced by sodium and potassium, and increased amounts of lactic acid are produced in the tissues. This increase in lactic acid formation has been attributed to several factors, including intracellular alkalosis, hypocapnia (perhaps due to pyruvate carboxylase inhibition and subsequent increase in pyruvate and lactate), and tissue hypoxia.[582] The resultant decreased efficiency of oxygen delivery reflects both peripheral vasoconstriction and the reduced ability of hemoglobin to release oxygen. Buffering in the extracellular fluid and extracellular-intracellular ion shifts occur within minutes to hours.

Persistence of the alkalotic state evokes a renal response: the urinary excretion of H^+ decreases and that of HCO_3^- and K^+ increases.[583]

Metabolic Acidosis. Metabolic or nonrespiratory acidosis results from increased $[H^+]$ from noncarbonic acid or decreased $[HCO_3^-]$ in the extracellular fluid. The H^+ excess can result from ingestion or infusion of noncarbonic acid, excess acid metabolic products within the body, or decreased renal excretion of H^+.

Extraneous sources of noncarbonic acid include various drugs and toxic substances, including salicylates, paraldehyde, phenformin, methyl alcohol, ethylene glycol, ammonium chloride (NH_4Cl), and arginine and lysine hydrochloride. The acid-citrate-dextrose added to stored bank blood may cause metabolic acidosis, through anaerobic conversion of dextrose to lactic acid.[584]

Endogenous H^+ formation may result from the accumulation of large quantities of the keto acids—beta-hydroxybutyric acid and acetoacetic acid—in uncontrolled diabetes, starvation, and occasionally alcoholism. Lactic acid is the other major source of noncarbonic acid within the body: it is produced in tissue hypoxia and diffuses out of the cells in the un-ionized acid form, producing a temporary excess of noncarbonic acid in the extracellular fluid. Clinical situations in which lactic acid is produced include heavy muscular exercise and acute severe tissue hypoxemia or hypoperfusion secondary to arterial hypotension or high levels of circulating catecholamines. Lactic acid is formed also when oxygen supplies at the tissue level are reduced, as in severe hypocapnia, reflecting both the inability of hemoglobin to release oxygen in these circumstances and the vasoconstriction induced by low PCO_2. Lactic acid may play a major role in increasing the $[H^+]$ in acute pulmonary edema due to left ventricular failure, although in some instances there is a superimposed respiratory acidosis. In acute left ventricular failure with metabolic acidosis, lactic acid may be produced even in the absence of hypotension or clinical evidence of shock.[585, 586]

Hydration can cause acidosis by diluting the extracellular $[HCO_3^-]$ and thereby increasing $[H^+]$, but this minor degree of acidosis is rapidly corrected by compensatory hypocapnia.

In renal failure the deficiency in H^+ excretion is largely due to impaired ammonia secretion. In renal tubular acidosis, and sometimes in chronic pyelonephritis, a major difficulty appears to be inability to maintain the maximal H^+ gradient between renal tubule cells and the luminal fluid.[581] The loss of HCO_3^- or other conjugate base from the extracellular fluid, through the kidneys or gastrointestinal tract, increases the H^+ concentration; in the kidneys this occurs with the use of the carbonic anhydrase inhibitor acetazolamide (Diamox) and in the gastrointestinal tract it follows severe diarrhea or fistula.

Compensatory Mechanisms in Metabolic Acidosis. A rise in $[H^+]$ resulting from noncarbonic acid in the extracellular fluid elicits immediate buffering from hemoglobin, plasma proteins, bicarbonate, and phosphate. The Henderson equation shifts to the left, almost immediately decreasing $[HCO_3^-]$ and increasing carbonic acid (which is dissipated in the lungs as carbon dioxide). The action of the increased $[H^+]$, particularly on brain stem receptors but also on the peripheral aortic and carotid chemoreceptors, augments alveolar ventilation and rapidly eliminates carbon dioxide produced by the buffering of the excess H^+. Hyperventilation, which develops within minutes, depends

upon normality of the respiratory center and adequacy of ventilatory mechanics. The degree of compensatory hyperventilation reflects the severity of the metabolic acidosis, but it appears to be maximal when the PCO_2 reaches 12 mm Hg and $[H^+]$ is 80 nM/liter (pH 7.10). In these circumstances the limiting factor may be the muscular effort required over a prolonged period.[581] Delay in ventilatory response after rapid development of severe metabolic acidosis or its correction has been described in cholera, in which the fulminating diarrhea leads to hypovolemia and loss of base.[587] The reason for this delayed ventilatory response is not clear, but it probably relates to the relative lack of permeability of bicarbonate ions at the blood-brain barrier in contrast to molecular carbon dioxide.

Intracellular buffering, with the replacement by H^+ of K^+, Na^+, and Ca^{++} in tissues, including bone, is slower than extracellular buffering, but eventually more noncarbonic acid is buffered intracellularly than in the extracellular fluid;[588] carbonate $[CO_3^-]$ is released from bone and combines with some of the extra H^+ to form HCO_3^-.

As long as renal function is satisfactory there is a considerable adaptive increase in H^+ excretion, which may reach ten times normal; simultaneously, virtually all HCO_3^- filtered by the kidney is reabsorbed through the renal tubules. This compensatory mechanism, which operates for from hours to days, obviously cannot develop when the noncarbonic acid excess is due to renal failure.

Metabolic Alkalosis. Metabolic alkalosis results when the $[H^+]$ in extracellular fluid is decreased by loss of noncarbonic acid or increase in alkali. This disturbance of acid-base balance commonly develops in patients with chronic CO_2 retention who are receiving therapy for cardiac and respiratory failure. Therefore, some knowledge of the mechanisms involved is particularly pertinent to the specialist in pulmonary disease.

A common cause of metabolic alkalosis is the excessive loss of noncarbonic acid during severe, prolonged vomiting; the hydrochloric acid eliminated in this way depletes not only the H^+ in extracellular fluid but also chloride ions and fluid volume, both of which contribute to the alkalosis. The acute metabolic alkalosis that may result from excessive ingestion or infusion of alkali such as $NaHCO_3$ or $CaCo_3$ or trishydroxymethylamine methane (THAM) is readily reversed by increased urinary HCO_2^- excretion.

Patients who produce or are treated with large amounts of corticosteroid hormones retain Na^+ and HCO_3^-. The mechanism of the alkalosis that develops has not been clearly established but is known to depend on enhanced excretion of potassium.[589]

Undoubtedly, the commonest cause of metabolic alkalosis is the treatment of chronic carbon dioxide retention. As stated previously, in such patients the $[HCO_3]$ increases to compensate for the increased $[H^+]$. In most cases a decrease in chloride ions occurs in association with the increased renal acid excretion that compensates for the chronic respiratory acidosis. In such cases there may be cardiac as well as respiratory failure, and treatment will be directed toward correcting both decompensated states. If artificial ventilation is used to reduce the P_{CO_2} quickly, the patient is left with excess HCO_3^- and, therefore, with metabolic alkalosis. This will worsen if corticosteroids also are given. The diuretics and low sodium diet used in the treatment of heart failure deplete the body not only of Na^+ and Cl^- but also of extracellular fluid. As a result, the patient—originally in respiratory acidosis and perhaps still having carbon dioxide retention—now has an excess of HCO_3^- and a lack of Cl^- in a decreased extracellular fluid space, all factors that prolong the alkalosis. The renal attempt to regulate acid-base balance in the face of these difficult conditions is discussed further on.

Compensatory Mechanisms in Metabolic Alkalosis. An increased concentration of HCO_3^- is buffered in both extracellular and intracellular compartments. Lactic acid moves from the cells into the extracellular fluid, so that HCO_3^- and other conjugate bases are converted to the conjugate acids.

It is to be expected that the respiratory apparatus compensates for H^+ depletion or HCO^- excess by underventilation. This certainly occurs with alkalosis induced by sodium bicarbonate infusion, by THAM, and by ethacrynic acid.[590] Hypoventilation compensating for metabolic alkalosis also occurs following excessive and prolonged vomiting;[591] a P_{CO_2} of 60 mm Hg has been recorded in such circumstances in a patient whose pulmonary function was completely normal later.[591] Metabolic alkalosis resulting from thiazide diuretics and aldosterone apparently does not elicit compensatory underventilation.[581]

The renal response to acute metabolic alkalosis, which is prompt, is increased HCO_3^- excretion. If the cause of the alkalosis is not quickly corrected, however, compensation at the kidney level is complicated by such factors as the demand for renal Na^+ reabsorption and the Cl^- concentration in the extracellular fluid. As described earlier, some patients with chronic respiratory acidosis become depleted of Cl^- during therapy; in addition, the extracellular fluid volume decreases, requiring increased Na^+ reabsorption. What is called for in these circumstances is bicarbonate diuresis, but this is impossible because the unavailability of Cl^- and the strong stimulus for Na^+ reabsorption demand reabsorption of bicarbonate. To maintain electroneutrality, Na^+ reabsorption must be accompanied by reabsorption of an anion or excretion of the equivalent amount of cation. The cations available for excretion to enhance Na^+ reabsorption are H^+ and K^+. Under these circumstances of chronic metabolic alkalosis the urine is already rich in K^+ and H^+; should K^+ depletion supervene, even more H^+ will have to be excreted, further aggravating the metabolic state. The result of this complicated in-

teraction of multiple factors is the production of acid urine free of HCO_3^-; thus the kidney not only fails to excrete the excess alkali but reabsorbs it as it acidifies the urine. This situation can be corrected only by restoring the extracellular fluid volume and by providing Cl^-, K^+, and Na^+; this is readily accomplished by infusion of NaCl supplemented with K.[592]

Acid-Base Nomograms. Clinical information is indispensable for the correct interpretation of acid-base disturbances. Nevertheless, nomograms based on *in vivo* studies in humans and animals, delineating 95 per cent significance bands, may be very useful in determining whether the disturbance is "pure" or "mixed": significance bands in acid-base balance[593] define the range of acid-base values expected in 95 per cent of cases of a specific acid-base disorder. Values for P_{CO_2}, H^+, and HCO_3^- in response to acute[594, 595] and chronic[583, 596] hypoventilation and hyperventilation have been established. Unlike respiratory disorders, however, acute and chronic metabolic acid-base disturbances do not have clearly delineated significance bands. Arbus[597] has reviewed the data of metabolic acidosis and alkalosis.

The great variety of acid-base diagrams or nomograms suggested for clinical use[580, 597-599] plot either P_{CO_2} against H^+ (pH) or P_{CO_2} against HCO_3^-, with linear isopleths of the third component radiating from the origin. Figure 1–110, which depicts such a nomogram, shows 95 per cent significance bands for defining a single respiratory or metabolic acid-base disturbance. *Although values outside the bands almost certainly represent "mixed" disturbances, those within the bands do not necessarily represent a single disturbance.*[595]

Summary. The amount of oxygen carried by the arterial blood can be measured by determining its content per deciliter of blood and dividing this by the total amount of oxygen the same blood can carry when exposed to oxygen (oxygen capacity); this ratio is known as the arterial oxygen saturation. A more reliable method is to measure the P_{O_2} of arterial blood with an electrode.

Most of the carbon dioxide is carried in the plasma as bicarbonate. The red blood cell, however, contains carbonic anhydrase, an enzyme that converts carbon dioxide into carbonic acid, H ions, and bicarbonate, the last of which crosses the cell membrane in exchange for chloride ions. Blood that contains reduced hemoglobin can carry more carbon dioxide, an ideal circumstance for assimilating carbon dioxide in the tissues and releasing it in the lungs.

In diffuse infiltrative disease of the alveolar septa, arterial hypoxemia is due partly to $\dot{V}_A/\dot{Q}$ inequality and partly to diffusion defect and may be manifest only during exercise. Since carbon dioxide diffuses 20 times as readily as oxygen, in these diseases the diffusion defect is for oxygen only and the P_{CO_2} is normal or low.

A true or absolute shunt results in hypoxemia

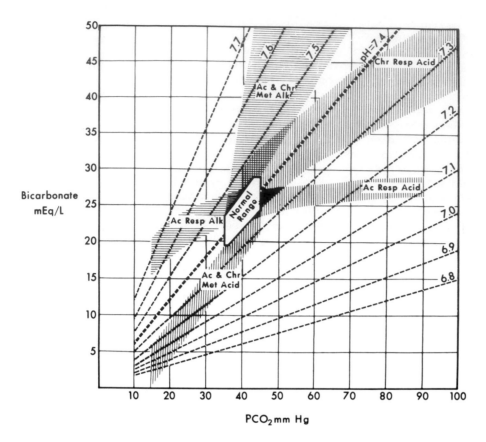

Figure 1–110. Acid-Base Nomogram. *In vivo* nomogram showing bands for defining a single respiratory or metabolic acid-base disturbance (From Arbus GS: Can Med Assoc J *109*:291, 1973.)

without carbon dioxide retention: patients with this condition hyperventilate and maintain low or normal levels of carbon dioxide. In chronic bronchitis and emphysema, hypoxemia is due mainly to $\dot{V}A/\dot{Q}$ abnormality; the PCO_2 is low, normal, or high, depending upon the patient's ability to hyperventilate and the amount of remaining functioning lung to compensate. Disease of the neuromuscular system or the respiratory center causes general hypoventilation and, therefore, hypoxemia and carbon dioxide retention. In the hypoventilation associated with obesity, the $\dot{V}A/\dot{Q}$ ratio at the lung bases appears to be grossly decreased; the unsaturation and carbon dioxide retention are corrected easily by the patients' taking a few deep breaths of even room air.

Measurement of the H^+ concentration of the arterial blood is an essential part of blood-gas analysis. Acute carbon dioxide retention is manifested by a rise in PCO_2 and a normal level of bicarbonate and, therefore, increase in H^+ concentration. Chronic carbon dioxide retention is accompanied by raised bicarbonate and normal H^+ concentrations. Similarly, a low PCO_2 with decreased H^+ indicates acute hyperventilation and, with normal H^+ concentration, chronic hyperventilation. Secondary hyperventilation and hypoventilation may be initiated by nonrespiratory acidosis or alkalosis. Respiratory and nonrespiratory acid-base disturbances may occur simultaneously and can be interpreted only with full knowledge of the clinical situation.

NONRESPIRATORY FUNCTIONS OF THE LUNG

Although the primary function of the lung is respiratory, it has become clear that it has several other functions, which may not ordinarily come to mind although they are of considerable importance to the maintenance of well-being. Our knowledge of this organ's metabolic functions has evolved largely as a by-product of studies to identify the physicochemical nature of surfactant,[260] studies that have revealed the lung's important role in lipid metabolism. Its nonrespiratory functions have been comprehensively reviewed by Heinemann and Fishman,[283] and in the paragraphs that follow we have borrowed freely from their 1969 report. Much of our knowledge is still fragmentary and speculative. Caution has been urged in extending to humans information obtained by research in animals,[639] and in making an overzealous interpretation of quantitative studies of lung metabolism using radioisotopes.[640]

The nonrespiratory functions of the lung encompass three general areas: metabolism, host defense mechanisms, and certain physical and other related functions.

Physical and Related Functions

The pulmonary capillary network is interposed between the systemic venous and arterial circulations and in normal circumstances receives the entire cardiac output. It thus has the capacity to act as a sieve, protecting the multiple vital organs on the systemic side of the circulation from various potentially harmful materials. Probably the most important of these is thrombus that originates in peripheral veins. One careful autopsy study by Freiman and his colleagues showed anatomic evidence of pulmonary thromboembolism in almost two thirds of 61 consecutive patients.[641] As these workers emphasized, their techniques probably provided a low estimate of the actual number of emboli reaching the lung, since effective thrombolysis might have been expected to remove many emboli without residual morphologic trace. Most such emboli are small and result in no significant damage, but it is clear that their potential for causing serious harm would be much greater in organs such as the heart or brain. Other less common substances that can be effectively sieved in the same manner include fat, bone marrow fragments, and occasionally exogenous material such as foreign substances injected by drug addicts.

Normally occurring tissue elements that are exceptionally large can also be filtered by the lungs. Fragments of placental trophoblast are frequently found in pulmonary capillaries in pregnant and postpartum women[642] and may be degraded in this location, at least in part. Megakaryocytes derived from bone marrow are also commonly seen within the lungs, in both fetuses and infants[643] as well as older individuals.[644, 645] They are more frequent in a hospital-based autopsy population, averaging 37 cells per cm^2 of lung tissue in one large study, but are also found in lesser numbers in previously healthy individuals who have died suddenly.[645] There is evidence that their numbers are especially increased in association with intravascular coagulation.[645-647] Studies of megakaryocytes in central venous and arterial blood have consistently shown significantly higher numbers in the former,[648-650] implying that they are indeed trapped within lung capillaries. Since it has also been shown that the number of platelets is greater in aortic than in pulmonary arterial blood,[650] these observations have suggested to several investigators that a substantial proportion of platelet production may normally occur within the lung,[648, 649, 651] possibly by purely physical fragmentation of megakaryocytes.[651] It has also been suggested that the lung may either remove or add leukocytes or platelets from or to the blood and thus partly regulate the normal blood level of these cells.[283]

The lungs also play a role in the excretion of volatile substances other than carbon dioxide, including acetone in diabetes and fasting, methylmercaptan and ammonia in liver cell failure, methanol of unknown source, allicin following garlic ingestion, a breakdown product of dimethyl sulfoxide (DMSO) that smells like garlic when applied to the skin, paraldehyde, and ethanol (a test used for determining the blood level of alcohol in automobile drivers).

Functions Involved in Host Defense

The contents of the pulmonary airways and air spaces are a direct extension of our environment, and the lungs possess a remarkable array of mechanisms to prevent damage from natural and manmade pollution.[194] It is important to realize that the phagocytic alveolar macrophages, whose capacity to engulf microorganisms and particles that penetrate to the respiratory portion of the lungs was described earlier, constitute the last line of defense, virtually all potentially pathogenic material being removed at a higher level in the tracheobronchial tree. Large particles impact on the surface of the lining membrane and are excreted on the mucociliary blanket. Very small particles (0.2 to 0.3 μ) remain suspended in air and are exhaled, rarely being deposited. Particles measuring 0.5 to 3 μ in diameter may penetrate to the respiratory portion of the lung, in which 90 per cent are deposited by gravity and are engulfed by alveolar macrophages that are excreted largely via the tracheobronchial tree.

The reaction to irritating or noxious gases is different. The first line of defense is cessation of ventilation; gases that do enter the conducting system are absorbed on the moist surface of the upper airways or are detoxified by chemical combination with a substance within the mucous blanket or elaborated by the lung as an antagonist or inhibitor.

Several noncellular enzymes and circulating chemical substances have a protective function, including lysozymes, lactoferrin, interferon, and, of course, surfactant. In addition, there are natural defense mechanisms against allergens entering the respiratory tract as particles or gases: IgG, IgA, and IgE are produced by plasma cells in the lamina propria and submucosa of the tracheobronchial tree; similarly, epithelial cells of the respiratory tract give rise to a secretory piece that combines with plasma IgA to form a specific immunoglobulin in airway secretions.[652] All these host defense mechanisms are adversely affected by hypoxia and hyperoxia, and by acidosis, cigarette smoke, corticosteroids, and various gases such as ozone. The importance of local as well as systemic host defense mechanisms in relation to opportunistic infection is considered in some detail in Chapter 6.

Metabolic Functions

The lungs are involved in the storage, transformation, degradation, and synthesis of a large variety of substances.[283] The presence in the lung of enzymes known to play a part in metabolic synthesis indicates their origin from lung tissue, but in most instances the specific site of synthesis within the lung is unknown. Studies of metabolic activity, including oxygen consumption, have identified intrapulmonary cells that contain the elements commonly associated with high metabolic activity[283, 653]—type II alveolar cells, Clara cells, alveolar macrophages, mast cells, and endothelial cells of the pulmonary vasculature. The first three were described previously, and it remains to discuss the activities of mast cells and vascular endothelial cells.

Mast cells are round-to-oval, medium-sized cells with centrally placed nuclei found throughout the lung in airway, alveolar, pleural, and interlobular interstitial tissue (see pages 16 and 23). Ultrastructurally, they contain numerous cytoplasmic granules with a variable but highly characteristic internal structure.[654] They are rich in heparin, histamine, slow-reacting substance (SRS), and several proteolytic and other enzymes. The number of mast cells in the lung appears to relate to the content of histamine, heparin, and SRS, but it is not known whether the mast cell synthesizes these chemical substances or simply stores them for release on demand.

The precise action and interaction of these substances in the human lung is not known, but it seems probable that they have specific activities. For example, histamine may play a role in anaphylactic shock; degranulation or rupture of mast cells, with consequent release of histamine, has been observed in guinea pigs.[655] Since heparin, an antithromboplastin and antithrombin agent, inhibits fibrin formation, probably one of its main roles within the lung is to promote hemofluidity. In addition, heparin inhibits hyaluronidase and has an antihistaminic effect. Its therapeutic efficacy in preventing bronchoconstriction in pulmonary thromboembolism has led to the suggestion that its role in the lung is to inhibit histamine released coincidentally from mast cells. The vast endothelial network of the pulmonary capillaries appears to serve not only as a barrier between blood and gas but also as a source of materials for fibrinolysis.[283] The lungs contain large amounts of plasmin activator and thrombokinase, the former converting plasminogen to plasmin and the latter converting the circulating precursor prothrombin to thrombin. Thrombin plays a key role in the conversion of fibrinogen to fibrin. Plasmin, which is an active proteolytic enzyme, dissolves fibrin.

It is apparent that this protective mechanism for preventing occlusion of the pulmonary vessels has limitations, in view of the development of pulmonary hypertension resulting from multiple small pulmonary emboli. Sometimes, following pulmonary manipulation in cardiac resuscitation or during pulmonary or open heart surgery, fibrinolysis becomes excessive, probably caused by the release of large amounts of plasmin activator into the circulation.

Reference has already been made to phospholipid synthesis by type II alveolar cells, and there is no question that the lungs are engaged in lipid metabolism. The presence of lipoprotein lipases within or on the surface of capillary endothelial cells indicates that the lungs have an enormous capacity for lipolysis. Lipids, especially long-chain fatty acids absorbed by the intestinal tract, enter the bloodstream as chylomicra (glycerides in stable emulsion), which pass up the thoracic duct and thence through the right side of the heart to the pulmonary vascular bed. The fatty acids released by hydrolysis of lipid ester bonds may be used by tissues, including the lung, both as a substrate for oxidative metabolism and for the formation of complex lipids. In addition, both in vivo and in vitro studies in animals have shown the lung's ability to synthesize protein[656] and glycoprotein.[657]

Other biologically active substances, about which even less is known, are stored, transformed, or synthesized in the lungs. Serotonin is metabolized to 5-hydroxyindoleacetic acid and may be taken up by platelets within the lung. Studies of isolated rat lung employing autoradiographic techniques have demonstrated significantly greater uptake of 5-hydroxytryptamine by capillary endothelium than by alveolar epithelium.[658] In cases of carcinoid tumors (see Chapter 8), the excessive serotonin scleroses the valves of the right side of the heart and may cause bronchoconstriction. The presence in lung tissue of enzymes known to be active in catecholamine synthesis and degradation suggests that the norepinephrine and epinephrine in the walls of bronchi and blood vessels may be produced and rendered inactive at these sites. Both E and F prostaglandins have been identified in lipid extracts of lungs from several mammalian species, including humans.[659] They appear to act directly on the muscle of bronchi and pulmonary vessels, prostaglandin E causing relaxation and F causing constriction; their physiologic effects may be altered by the enzyme prostaglandin dehydrogenase in lung tissue. Prostaglandins not only are synthesized and apparently extracted by the lung but also are released from pulmonary tissue. Results of studies of isolated guinea pig lungs[660] indicated that prostaglandin E was released in response to inflation and suggested that this substance may help maintain normal matching of ventilation and perfusion through pulmonary vasodilatation.

Human lung may be induced in vitro to release prostaglandin $F_{2\alpha}$ during anaphylaxis; this substance is considerably more abundant in lung parenchyma than in bronchial tissue. The mast cell itself does not appear to be a major source of prostaglandin.[661]

Angiotensin-converting enzyme (ACE), produced largely by endothelial cells, inactivates bradykinin, a powerful hypotensive and edematogenic substance, and simultaneously activates angiotensin II, an equally powerful pressor agent. In animals, ACE activity is inhibited by hypoxia; if this finding can be applied to humans, it may explain the systemic hypertension and pulmonary edema that sometimes occurs in lung disease associated with hypoxemia; it might also explain the rapid circulatory adaptation that occurs in the neonate with the first breath.[639]

Serum ACE levels are increased in a number of diseases, particularly sarcoidosis in which it appears to be secreted by the epithelioid cells of the granulomas; it is considered to reflect activity. Acute lung injury caused by a variety of means may produce a fall in serum ACE levels, a finding that may serve as a useful marker of such an event. Rats administered thiourea[662] initially manifest a rise in both serum and pleural fluid ACE coincident with a fall in lung ACE, lasting from 1 to 4 hours; subsequently, serum ACE levels fall, providing evidence for endothelial damage coincident with a reduction in 5-hydroxytryptamine uptake.[663, 664] These animal studies indicate that early and sensitive indices of lung damage may be at our disposal; although they are transitory, they occur in the absence of morphologic changes. In an *in vivo* study of rabbits in which normoxic controls were compared with animals with normobaric hyperoxia, Dobuler and coworkers showed that the latter group manifested an appreciable reduction in ACE activity after 16 hours and a decreased removal of 5-hydroxytryptamine at 24 hours.[664] This evidence for reduced metabolic activity was present when type I alveolar epithelial cells and capillary endothelial cells appeared morphologically normal.

Of great importance to the practicing physician is the realization that the pulmonary endothelial cell membrane can absorb a variety of circulating drugs without being engaged in any way in their active transport or metabolism.[665] The list of drugs that may accumulate in the pulmonary vascular bed includes, among others, most basic lipophilic amines.[665, 666] Studies in rats that have been rendered vitamin A-deficient have shown that uptake of these drugs may be enhanced, probably as a result of a decrease in pulmonary monoamine oxidase activity.[667]

DEVELOPMENT AND GROWTH OF THE LUNG

The growth and development of the lung has been divided into intrauterine and postnatal stages, although it is clear that the two overlap and that birth represents only one influence on the whole process. Intrauterine development has traditionally been divided into four periods: *embryonic, pseudoglandular, canalicular,* and *terminal sac.*[668] Some workers have questioned this scheme, suggesting either a simplification into three phases (embryonic, conducting, and respiratory)[669] or the addition of an intrauterine *alveolar* phase (*see* further on).[670] This subject has been discussed in greater detail in several monographs.[671, 672]

CONDUCTING AND TRANSITORY AIRWAYS AND ALVEOLI

Embryonic Period

The lung begins to develop at about 26 days of embryonic life as a ventral outpouching or diverticulum of the foregut near the junction of the occipital and cervical segments (Fig. 1–111A). The outpouching is lined by endodermal epithelium and is invested by splanchnic mesenchyme. During the next 2 to 3 days (26 to 28 days of intrauterine life), it gives rise to right and left lung buds which even at this early stage show a characteristic direction of growth, that on the right being directed caudally and that on the left more transversely (Figs. 1–111B and 1–111C). As the lung buds elongate, the respiratory portion of the gut becomes separated from the esophageal portion by lateral ingrowths of surrounding mesoderm that progressively meet to form the tracheoesophageal septum (Fig. 1–111D). By the end of another 2 days (28 to 30 days), the lung buds have elongated into primary lung sacs, and by days 32 to 34 the five lobar bronchi have appeared as monopodial outgrowths of the primary bronchi (Fig. 1–111D). Thus, by the end of the 5th week, the airways destined to become the five lobar bronchi have begun their development, a point marking the end of the embryonic period.[668]

Pseudoglandular Period

This period extends from the end of the 5th to the 16th week of gestation and is primarily concerned with the development of the bronchial tree. Following the appearance of the five lobar bronchi as outgrowths of the primary lung sacs, branching occurs quickly and more or less dichotomously. Between the 10th and 14th weeks, 65 to 75 per cent of all bronchial branching has occurred, and by the 16th week virtually all conducting airways are present. During this period, the airways are blind tubules lined by columnar or cuboidal epithelium—hence the term *pseudoglandular* (Fig. 1–112). Cartilage can be seen within the trachea as early as 7 weeks' gestation[673] and develops in the bronchi in a centrifugal direction thereafter. Although some authorities have found that all new foci of cartilage have appeared by 25 weeks,[673] others have documented evidence for their appearance into neonatal life.[674] Tracheobronchial gland development begins in the late pseudoglandular period and continues into the canalicular phase,[31, 675] so that by 25 weeks glands in the proximal airways have a prominent acinar appearance.

Canalicular Period

From the 16th to the 24th or 25th week of intrauterine life, the peripheral portion of the bronchial tree undergoes further development in the

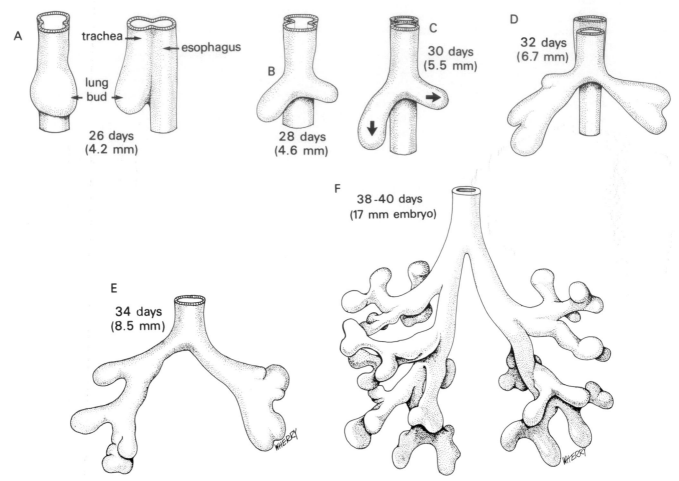

Figure 1–111. Development of the Human Lung. Diagrammatic representation of the development of human lung in the embryonic and pseudoglandular periods. *A* is depicted from the front and the side, all others from the front only. *See* text for description.

form of primitive canaliculi that represent early stages of the acinar airways. At the same time, the mesenchyme adjacent to the canaliculi becomes vascularized through ingrowth of capillaries.

Terminal Sac Period

By the 24th to 25th week, terminal thin-walled spaces with flattened epithelium, termed saccules, become visible at the ends of the canaliculi. This marks the beginning of the terminal sac period that is traditionally thought to last until birth. Acinar morphology is well developed, and by the 28th week of gestation several generations of respiratory bronchioles open into so-called transitional ducts, with several generations of saccules arising from them. Further development until birth consiasts largely of saccular proliferation and a corresponding decrease in and more organized vascularization of the mesenchyme. Alveolar development has been demonstrated as early as 30 weeks' gestation and in one study was uniformly present by 36 weeks.[670] It has thus been suggested that the final period of lung development, from 36 weeks to term, be designated the *alveolar phase*.[670]

Throughout the canalicular period, airway epithelium progressively decreases in height so that the entire acinar pathway is eventually lined by a cuboidal or flattened epithelium. At about 28 weeks, differentiation into type I and type II alveolar epithelial cells has begun and an occasional type II osmiophilic granule can be identified.[672] At this stage, a blood-gas barrier exists that is capable of permitting gas exchange. The earlier discussion on surfactant (*see* page 58) outlined the interaction between glucocorticoids and the morphology and function of alveolar type II cells and the changes that occur in the fatty acid pattern of pulmonary phospholipids, particularly dipalmitoyl lecithin. The rate of synthesis of the latter substance increases from about 34 weeks to term, at which point it is at its highest level; shortly after birth, it rapidly declines to normal adult levels.

Intraepithelial neuroendocrine cells develop first in the proximal airways and can be recognized as early as 8 to 10 weeks' gestation.[1167] Several types have been identified on the basis of ultrastructural differences in secretory granules and immunohistochemical characteristics,[67, 1167] but the significance of this is not known.

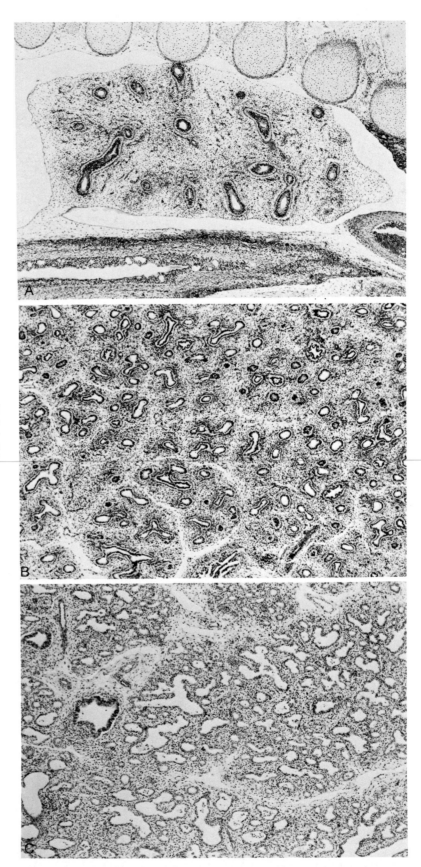

Figure 1–112. Developing Human Lung. *A,* Early pseudoglandular period showing occasional tubular channels within abundant mesenchyme. Thoracic vertebrae are at top. (× 40.) *B,* Late pseudoglandular period showing more numerous branching presumptive airways. (× 52.) *C,* Early canalicular period. (× 52.)

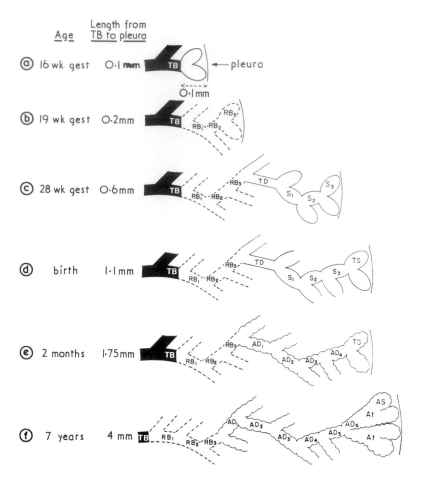

Figure 1–113. Development of the Acinus. Diagrammatic representation of the acinus at six stages of development. At all ages airway generations are drawn the same length so that increase in length represents an increase in generations. A given generation may be traced down the same vertical line, permitting remodeling in its structure to be followed. Actual increase in size is shown by the length from the terminal bronchiole (*TB*) to the pleura. *RB*, respiratory bronchiole; *TD* transitional duct; *S*, saccule; *TS* terminal saccule; *AD*, alveolar duct; *At*, atrium; *SA*, alveolar sac. (From Hislop A, Reid L: Thorax *29*:90, 1974.)

Postnatal Stage

Although there is variation in the structure of different acini,[672] the typical acinus at birth consists of three generations of respiratory bronchioles, one of transitional ducts, and three of saccules that end in a terminal saccule, all being the recognizable precursor components of an acinar unit (Fig. 1–113*D*; *see also* Fig. 1–29, page 29).[668, 676] During early postnatal development, acinar length increases and its components are remodeled, largely as a result of the appearance of true alveoli. Thus, terminal broncioles may be transformed into respiratory bronchioles and distal respiratory bronchioles into alveolar ducts. The saccules themselves probably develop into both alveolar ducts and sacs. Although there is little further true branching after birth, each terminal saccule may generate up to four additional alveolar sacs,[668] probably by budding. Alveoli themselves develop both peripherally in relation to the saccule and more centrally along the walls of the respiratory bronchioles and transitional ducts.

The extent of alveolar development at birth has been the subject of much debate, with the number of alveoli found by different investigators ranging from none to 70×10^6.[670, 672] Regardless of the number at birth, there is general consensus that the majority of alveoli appear during early childhood, probably up to 2 to 4 years of age,[677] and that they enlarge from childhood to adulthood. After

the age of 1 year, the male sex tends to have somewhat more alveoli than the female, an observation that correlates with a difference in lung volumes.[677] The age at which alveolar development is completed is also controversial, although it appears most likely that multiplication occurs until at least 8 years of age.[672] The average area of air-tissue interface increases from 3 to 4 m² at birth[670] to approximately 32 m² at 8 years and 75 m² in the adult, an increase that is related linearly to body surface area.[130] The total number of alveoli in adult lungs is generally accepted to be about 300 million,[130, 678] although studies by Thurlbeck in both children and adults[132, 677] showed considerable individual variation. One of these reported an estimated range of 212 to 605 million (mean, 375 million), with a significant relationship between alveolar number and body length.[132]

The acinus increases in length from early gestation to the age of 7 years (Fig. 1–113), at which time the respiratory zone appears adult; however, with increasing body size acini continue to lengthen and alveoli to enlarge until the adult acinus reaches a diameter of 6 to 10 mm.[206, 668] During this period, the conducting airways also increase in both length and diameter in proportion to body size.[672] Although evidence concerning the relative growth rate of different portions of the bronchial tree is conflicting, several studies have found that in children up to the age of 5 years, distal airway diameter increases disproportionately to proximal airway diameter.[672] This finding supports the observations that peripheral airways contribute a greater proportion of total airway resistance in young children than in adults, and that peripheral airway conductance increases significantly at about 5 years of age.[679]

The normal postnatal growth of the trachea has been described by Wailoo and Emery.[680] In the neonate, the configuration is funnel-shaped, the laryngeal end being wider than the carinal. A cylindric appearance gradually becomes evident with increasing age. The rate of growth in relation to crown-rump length appears to be greatest between 1 month and 4 years. Tracheal dimensions in relation to age and body height have been described by Griscom and Wohl.[1132]

THE VASCULAR SYSTEM

The pulmonary artery develops from the sixth aortic arch during the early embryonic period (Fig. 1–114). On both sides, the proximal part of the arch develops into the proximal segment of the right and left pulmonary arteries; however, on the right side the distal part loses its connection with the aortic arch whereas during intrauterine life the distal arch on the left maintains its connection with the aorta as the ductus arteriosus. Branches from both arches grow toward the developing lung buds and become incorporated with them in the future hila.

During embryonic and pseudoglandular periods, pulmonary arteries develop at approximately the same rate and in the same manner as the airways so that the majority of preacinar branches are pres-

ent by the end of the sixteenth week.[681] By 12 weeks, both conventional and supernumerary branches are in approximately the same proportion in the preacinar region as in the adult.[681] During the latter part of fetal life, the main feature of arterial development is an increase in vessel diameter and length. In the postnatal stage, there is a small continuing increase in the development of conventional branches until about age 18 months, related to the small increase in acinar airways that occurs during this period.[672] By contrast, a marked increase occurs in the supernumerary branches, corresponding to the prolific alveolar development of early childhood; this continues, although at a decreasing rate, until about 8 years of age.[682]

Histologically, the structure of the fetal arterial system differs considerably from that of the postnatal one, reflecting the different states of intravascular blood flow and pressure. The extrapulmonary arterial wall of the fetus closely resembles that of the aorta in thickness and structure, with multiple regular and thick medial elastic laminae. After birth, as intravascular pressure drops, wall thickness slowly decreases and the elastic laminae become swollen, fragmented, and fewer in number. This process is visible at about 4 months of age, and the final adult configuration is reached by about 2 years of age.[435]

Muscular arteries are not well developed in early fetal life; they contain only thin, poorly staining elastic laminae and muscle cells, but by the end of the canalicular period they are morphologically mature.[681] At this time, their lumens are small and their media quite thick, representing as much as 15 to 25 per cent of the total external diameter of the vessel,[435] again presumably related to the high pul-

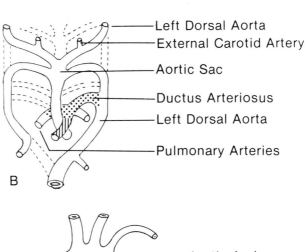

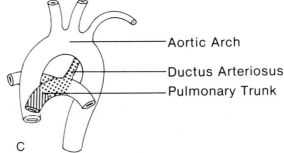

Figure 1–114. Development of the Pulmonary Arteries. A, Aortic arches (3, 4, and 6) and partly divided truncus arteriosus at 6 weeks. B, Aortic arches at 7 weeks; the parts of the dorsal aortas and aortic arches that normally disappear are indicated by the broken lines. C, Arterial arrangement at 8 weeks showing well-formed pulmonary trunk and main pulmonary arteries. (Modified from Moore KL: The Developing Human. 3rd ed. Philadelphia, WB Saunders, 1982.)

monary arterial pressure. By the second to third day after birth, there is a marked increase in luminal diameter and a corresponding medial thinning, a process that subsequently proceeds more gradually until an adult configuration is reached at about 18 months of age.[435]

In the embryonic stage, pulmonary venous blood drains via the splanchnic plexus into the primordia of the systemic venous system (including the cardinal and umbilico-vitelline veins) (Fig. 1–115). Subsequently, an outpouch of the sinoatrial region of the heart (termed the common pulmonary vein) extends toward and connects with that portion of the splanchnic plexus draining the lungs. Even-

tually, the common pulmonary vein is incorporated into the left atrial wall and the majority of the splanchnic-pulmonary connections are obliterated, leaving four independent pulmonary veins directly entering the left atrium.

In their study of fetal and infant lungs, Hislop and Reid injected the pulmonary veins with a radio-paque medium and described their drainage pattern and structure.[683] As in the preacinar arterial system, the postacinar drainage pattern was complete halfway through fetal life and the intra-acinar pattern developed during childhood. The pattern of growth in relation to the size and number of veins and their branching was generally similar to

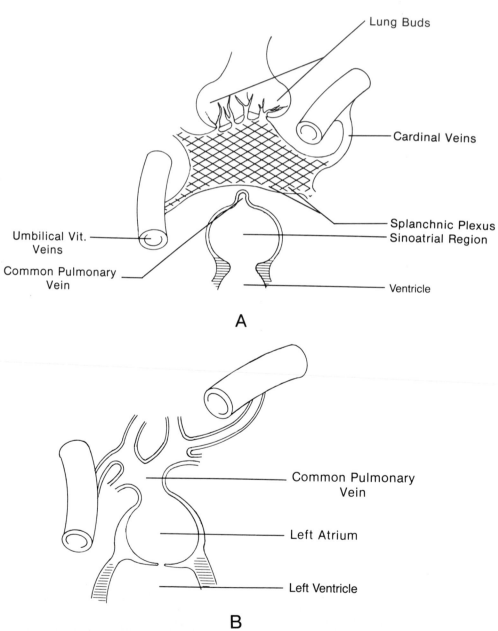

Figure 1–115. Development of the Pulmonary Veins. *A,* Lung buds draining via the splanchnic plexus into the umbilical and cardinal veins. Note the developing common pulmonary vein. *B,* Pulmonary veins, although still draining into the systemic circulation, now also communicate with the left atrium.

Illustration continued on opposite page

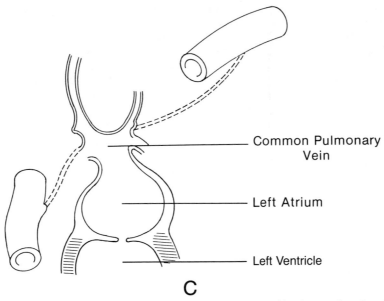

Common Pulmonary
Vein

Left Atrium

Left Ventricle

C

Figure 1–115 *Continued. C,* Primitive systemic connections disappear, resulting in complete flow into the left atrium.

that of the arteries. Histologically, in contrast to the pulmonary arteries, the veins are less muscular in the fetus than in the adult. Hislop and Reid could not find a measurable muscle layer in the walls of the veins before birth, although some small muscle fibers could be identified at 28 weeks' gestation.[683] The high resistance within the pulmonary arteries during fetal life may so limit the passage of blood to the venous circulation that venous pressure is too low to stimulate muscle development.

FACTORS INFLUENCING DEVELOPMENT AND GROWTH

The normal and abnormal factors that affect lung growth and development are not fully understood. Three that seem to have some importance are neural, hormonal, and local mesenchymal-epithelial interactions.[684] As previously discussed, the conducting airways develop by multiple sequential branchings of the bilateral lung buds. If the lung buds are removed from an animal in an early stage of development and then cultured, this branching process continues but only if the adjacent mesenchyme is included in the culture medium.[684] This mesenchymal supportive property has both general and highly specific properties: for example, embryonic mesenchyme from one species may have the ability to support branching in another species, but only if it is derived from the lung. On the other hand, significant differences exist between mesenchyme in the same lung—bronchial mesenchyme is able to induce treacheal epithelial branching whereas tracheal mesenchyme has an inhibitory effect on bronchial branching.[684] The factors responsible for this interaction are unknown; it is thought that cell surface interactions must somehow

be required,[684] and it is possible that production of locally active soluble factors also may be involved. Experimental evidence for both of these has been found in relation to functional maturation of the type II epithelial cell. Thus, in the rat the number of intercellular contacts between epithelial and mesenchymal cells increases as term and type II cell maturation approach.[685] In addition, the increase in surfactant production in fetal rat epithelial cells depends on glucocorticoid stimulation and has been shown to be mediated by a soluble substance produced by fetal lung fibroblasts.[686]

In addition to possible local biochemical control, tissue derived from mesenchyme may affect epithelial morphogenesis by purely physical means: Vaccaro and Brody have described two types of alveolar interstitial cell in the postnatal rat lung that develop early and may affect development in this manner.[687, 688] One has features characteristic of a myofibroblast; it is located at the tip of newly formed alveolar septa and ultrastructurally appears to be involved in the synthesis of elastin.[687] Emery has stated that this interstitial elastic tissue appears before actual alveolar development and hypothesizes that it may act as a kind of physical barrier around which the alveoli develop.[689] In support of this, it has been shown that neonatal rats administered β-aminopropionitrile (an inhibitor of lysyl oxidase, the enzyme necessary for elastin cross-linking) have significantly fewer and larger alveoli,[690, 691] suggesting that the elastic scaffold may be directly related to alveolar development. A second cell, termed the lipid-containing interstitial cell, occurs at the base of the alveolar septa and contains numerous lipid granules as well as fairly prominent microfilaments resembling actin.[688] It has been suggested that this cell, via its microfilaments, may have active contractile properties capable in some way of shaping the alveolar septum.[688] It is conceivable that the myofibroblastic interstitial cell just described could have a similar function.

Hutchins and his colleagues have suggested that purely physical factors may also be responsible for the characteristic dichotomous bronchial branching.[1185] They propose that as a bronchial bud grows, the mesenchyme, in direct opposition to its tip, becomes more and more compressed. At some point, the resistance to forward growth is great enough that this ceases and new branches develop in the region adjacent to the tip where the mesenchyme is not as compact. Physical abnormalities of the thoracic wall[1186] or intrathoracic structures may also place certain constraints on the potential for lung development and growth.

It is possible that the central nervous system plays an important role in normal lung development. Recent studies have documented pulmonary hypoplasia in animals subjected to intrauterine cervical or phrenic nerve injury.[692-694] It has been speculated that the effect is mediated by abnormalities of respiratory movement due to denervation.[692, 694]

The role of hormones in growth and development, although undoubtedly of significance, is for the most part poorly understood. Although histologic and morphometric differences between the lungs of men and women have not been identified,[670] it has been suggested that there may be a difference between the sexes in biochemical maturation, possibly related to differences in androgenic hormones.[695] Ultrastructural differences in the number of intercellular contacts between lung cells of male and female fetal rats provides some support for this hypothesis.[685] The influence of glucocorticoids and other hormones on the maturation of alveolar type II cells and on surfactant production has been best studied. The precise morphologic effects of other hormones, such as thyroxine and growth hormone, have not been well delineated.[672]

The effects on lung growth of bronchopulmonary or systemic disease acquired in childhood are not well understood. However, experimental evidence indicates that a variety of conditions such as viral infection,[696] starvation,[697] and ambient hypoxia[698] can have an important influence.

INNERVATION OF THE LUNG

The lung is innervated by fibers that travel in the vagus nerve and in nerves derived from the second to fifth thoracic ganglia of the sympathetic trunk. In addition, there is pharmacologic and morphologic evidence in both animals and humans for a nonadrenergic, noncholinergic, inhibitory efferent system (NAIS) of which the anatomic pathway has not been well defined.[701, 702] The vagus contains preganglionic, parasympathetic efferent fibers and afferent fibers from various lung receptors. The sympathetic fibers are largely postganglionic efferent in type, although in some animals there is physiologic evidence of an afferent component.[700] Small branches of the recurrent laryngeal nerve on the left side and of the vagus itself on the right are distributed directly to the trachea, where they form several plexuses that are most prominent on the posterior wall.[703] After giving off these branches, fibers from the vagus and sympathetic chain enter the hila, join with branches from the cardiac autonomic plexus, and form large posterior and smaller anterior plexuses in the peribronchovascular connective tissue. From these emanate multiple individual peribronchial and perivascular nerve fibers.

The subsequent course of these fibers within the human lung has been described in detail by Larsell and Dow,[704] by Gaylor,[705] and by Spencer and Leof;[706] the major part of the following description is taken from their studies. The nerves in the proximal airways number about four to five and are located in the peribronchial connective tissue, often in close association with bronchial arteries. They contain both thick and thin, myelinated and unmyelinated axons and are associated with groups of ganglion cells in which the vagal preganglionic fibers are believed to synapse. At numerous points along their course, they send out thick and thin fibers into the bronchial submucosa where they run as bronchial nerves. From these arise numerous thin, unmyelinated parasympathetic and sympathetic efferent fibers that terminate in bronchial muscle and mucous glands and around small blood vessels in the lamina propria and submucosa.

Thicker fibers thought to be largely of an afferent sensory type bypass the ganglia. They originate from receptors within the airway epithelium, the tracheobronchial smooth muscle, the lamina propria of the airways, the perichondrial region of large airways, the pulmonary parenchyma, and the pulmonary and bronchial arteries and veins.[704] Afferent receptors themselves have been divided into three functional groups on the basis of their distribution and physiologic response to various stimuli. The *irritant* or *cough receptors* are largely located in central airways, and their density decreases progressively as the smaller peripheral airways are approached.[1168] They are highly arborized myelinated nerve fibers with numerous free nerve endings that terminate in the airway epithelium immediately below cell junctions. The fibers are termed rapidly adapting stretch receptors, as well as cough or irritant receptors, because they show a brief burst of activity with lung inflation or deflation. They also respond to a wide variety of chemical and mechanical stimuli, including inhaled industrial pollutants, inflammatory mediators, and mechanical perturbations of the airway mucosa. Their stimulation results in a reflex bronchoconstriction, and their role is probably to inhibit inhalation of toxic material.[700, 707] Other fibers, also presumably of an afferent sensory type, have been identified at all levels of the conducting and transitory airways in relation to neuroepithelial bodies.[81] Their function and the precise course within the lung of the fibers seen in relation to them are not known.

The second major group of myelinated lung afferents traveling in the vagus nerve are from *stretch receptors*. Their nerve endings are found in the airway smooth muscle where they end in tendril-like structures closely applied to the surface of individual muscle cells. They are called slowly responding stretch receptors since they show prolonged discharge in response to lung inflation. They are responsible for sending information to the respiratory center regarding lung volume, and integration of their input results in offswitch activity in the respiratory center. There are also single and complex branching endings in the lamina propria that can detect changes in airway length and thus function as stretch receptors. Receptors are also present in the perichondrium of the larger airways that can sense changes in the curvature of the bronchial cartilages.[704]

The third type of lung afferent originates in the "J" or *juxtacapillary receptor*.[707–709] The nerve endings of these small, unmyelinated fibers are situated in lung parenchyma adjacent to alveolar walls and pulmonary capillaries. Although they have been thought to be sensitive to stretch of the capillaries and adjacent interstitial space, such as occurs with lung congestion or interstitial edema, recent studies in humans have questioned their significance.[710] Ultrastructurally, these fibers are associated with two types of nerve endings:[709] one contains many mitochondria and is thought to be consistent with a sensory function; the other contains numerous neurosecretory-like granules and is situated in close relationship to type II alveolar epithelial cells. Hung and his colleagues consider this to be morphologic evidence for a possible neural control of surfactant secretion.[709] Similar nonmyelinated fibers, termed "C" fibers, have been demonstrated in the airway smooth muscle.

As indicated, the efferent innervation of the lung includes preganglionic fibers from vagal nuclei, which descend in the vagus to synapse with postganglionic neurons in the ganglia around the airways, and postganglionic fibers from the cervical sympathetic ganglia, which enter the lung at the hilum. Postganglionic cholinergic efferent fibers supply the mucous glands of the large airways and also send fibers that stimulate goblet cell secretion; stimulation of these nerves increases glandular secretion by the submucosal glands and stimulates goblet cell discharge. Vagal efferent fibers also supply airway smooth muscle and pulmonary vascular smooth muscle; stimulation of these cholinergic fibers causes airway smooth muscle contraction and airway narrowing and vascular smooth muscle relaxation and pulmonary vasodilatation. All these cholinergic effects are blocked by atropine.

The major innervation of postganglionic adrenergic fibers is pulmonary and bronchial vascular smooth muscle; in some animals, bronchial smooth muscle is also supplied. Adrenergic stimulation results in constriction of the pulmonary and bronchial vessels, although it causes bronchodilatation in animals with innervation of the airway smooth muscle.[711] Whether adrenergic nerve fibers exist in the human lung is controversial; some studies[1169] have identified them while others[712, 713] have not. Despite this, radioligand labeling and autoradiographic studies have shown that airway smooth muscle fibers possess numerous adrenergic (largely beta-2) receptors.[714] The density of these receptors increases as peripheral airways are approached. Alveolar walls also contain numerous beta-receptors, but it has not been established whether these are related to the alveolar wall epithelium or to pulmonary capillary endothelium.[715] These noninnervated adrenergic receptors respond to circulating catecholamines and are the reason that therapeutically administered aerosols of beta-adrenergic agonists are so effective in relaxing smooth muscle. The density of beta-receptors on airway smooth muscle is very much greater than that of alpha-receptors, which explains why noradrenaline, which normally stimulates both, has a predominant bronchodilating action.[715] Similar studies that have examined the density of cholinergic receptors in airway smooth muscle have shown that these decrease in peripheral airways (in contrast to the increase in adrenergic receptors).

The third component of the autonomic nervous system, the so-called nonadrenergic inhibitory system (NAIS), has only recently been demonstrated.[716, 1170] Initially it was studied *in vitro* using electrical field stimulation of isolated airway smooth muscle, but subsequently it has been shown to function *in vivo* in guinea pigs and cats.[717, 718] In the cat, the effectiveness of stimulation in terms of bronchial smooth muscle relaxation is equipotent to that of adrenergic stimulation, and in the guinea pig NAIS is the major bronchodilator system.[719] There is still controversy concerning the nature of the mediator released by nonadrenergic inhibitory neurons; the balance of evidence suggests that vasoactive intestinal polypeptide (VIP) is the neurotransmitter.[720-722] In the gut, where the nonadrenergic inhibitory system was first demonstrated, its absence leads to Hirschsprung's disease, while deficiency of the NAIS in the esophagus may be important in the pathogenesis of achalasia. The importance of NAIS in the lung and possible alterations in its function in disease are still matters of some controversy. It has been suggested that a defect in this system may be important in the production of nonspecific bronchial hyperreactivity, a characteristic feature of asthma and other airway diseases. Against its importance, however, is the recent demonstration that in comparison with beta-agonists, it is relatively ineffective in producing airway smooth muscle relaxation in excised human bronchi.[723]

The nerves to the pulmonary arteries run in the perivascular adventitia and consist largely of a plexus of thin fibers that interconnects extensively with the peribronchial nerves. Ganglion cells are not seen, and the fibers are thought to be primarily sympathetic in type and to provide arterial motor innervation. They continue along the arterial tree at least as far as parenchymal arterioles. In addition to these thin fibers, a number of thicker fibers extend to the adventitial-medial junction of the larger arteries and end in a series of tortuous branchings. Their structure and location have led to speculation that they are sensory in type and that they function as baroreceptors; support for this hypothesis has been provided by physiologic studies that have shown a reflex pulmonary arterial vasoconstriction brought about by balloon distention of lobar pulmonary arteries.[724]

Although some nerve fibers in the large pulmonary veins end in the adventitia in a manner similar to those of the major pulmonary arteries and possibly possess a similar baroreceptor function, the majority extend into the inner media where they form a complex subendothelial network. Because of this location, it has been suggested that they may function as chemoreceptors. Other nerves continue as a plexus within the interlobular septa around the venous radicles and eventually end in the deeper layers of the visceral pleura. The bronchial arteries contain a prominent nerve plexus at the medial-adventitial junction, presumably consisting of efferent supply to the smooth muscles of these vessels; this plexus also sends numerous branches to the bronchial mucous glands.

Collections of tissue resembling paraganglionic tissue of the carotid body have been described in association with both the extrapulmonary and intrapulmonary vasculature. One of these, the glomus pulmonale,[725] is situated in the adventitia of the main pulmonary artery adjacent to the aorta. Because of its location, the suggestion has been made that it may function as a receptor for pulmonary arterial oxygen or carbon dioxide. However, Becker has shown that the vascular supply of the glomus pulmonale originates in the left coronary artery, making it an unlikely candidate for this purpose.[77]

Korn and his colleagues have described small, intrapulmonary tumors that bear a close relationship to small blood vessels and that possess cytologic and histologic similarity to typical carotid body tumors.[727] They called these tumors "chemodectomas" and speculated that they might derive from cells that normally possess an intrapulmonary chemoreceptor function. However, subsequent ultrastructural study of these tumors has failed to show the characteristics of paraganglionic tissue,[728] and physiologic studies have revealed no convincing evidence of intrapulmonary chemoreceptor function;[707] the nature of such structures is therefore in doubt.

THE PLEURA

MORPHOLOGY

The pleural space is enclosed by the visceral pleura, which covers the lungs, and by the parietal pleura, which lines the chest wall, diaphragm, and mediastinum. The two join at the hila. Although they may come into intimate contact locally, the left and right pleural spaces are normally separate. Pleural morphology, especially as it relates to function, has been described in detail by Wang.[818]

The Visceral Pleura

The visceral pleura is a thin but strong membranous structure that overlies and is loosely attached to the lobular limiting membrane. It has been divided into three layers: the superficial endopleura, the chief layer, and the juxtaparenchymal vascular layer.[1] Although there is variability in the development of each of these in different regions of the thorax, the overall appearance is similar.[819]

The *endopleura* is composed of a continuous layer of mesothelial cells and a delicate underlying network of irregularly arranged collagen and elastic fibers.

The *chief layer* (*external elastic lamina*) is primarily responsible for pleural mechanical stability and consists of dense collagenous and elastic tissue. Whereas the elastic tissue is arranged in a more or less haphazard manner, the collagen fibers are grouped into well-developed bundles the orientation of which varies in different regions.[1] The thickness of the connective tissue elements also varies,[819] and it has been suggested that these local differences are the result of variations in pleural stress during the respiratory cycle.[4, 819] Chemical analysis of the collagen in this region has shown it to be predominantly type I.[1171]

The *vascular* (*interstitial*) *layer* lies beneath the chief layer and consists of loose connective tissue in which lymphatic channels, veins, arteries, and numerous capillaries are situated. It is continuous with the interstitial tissue of the interlobular septa and directly overlies the lobular limiting membrane (*internal elastic lamina*). The latter is a thin, elastic-collagen layer that encases almost all lung parenchyma and separates alveoli from the pleura, interlobular septa, and bronchovascular bundles. Collagenous connections are present between the pleural chief layer and the limiting membrane, but the two are only loosely attached and may be readily separated in the connective tissue plane of the vascular layer. In appropriate circumstances, liquid or gas readily accumulates in this region.

The Mesothelial Cell

Mesothelial cells form a continuous layer over the whole of the visceral and parietal pleural surfaces. Their shape and size are variable. Normally they are inconspicuous at the light microscopic level, each measuring from 16 to 42 μm in diameter and only 7 μm in thickness.[818] Their diameter varies directly with transpulmonary pressure, the cells becoming more flattened as the lung expands.[818] However, regional differences in size at the same transpulmonary pressure are also apparent, at least in animals in which a bumpy or flattened appearance has been correlated with the composition of the underlying connective tissue (Fig. 1–116).[820] Mesothelial cells are easily stimulated and show reactive changes in a variety of conditions, occasionally to a degree at which cytologic or histologic

differentiation from a malignant neoplasm is difficult. When stimulated, individual cells enlarge, become cuboidal or columnar in shape, and develop large nuclei with prominent nucleoli.

Ultrastructurally (Fig. 1–117), mesothelial cells are joined by tight junctions and occasionally by desmosomes.[818] Within the cytoplasm are moderately abundant mitochondria, microtubules, endoplasmic reticulum, dense bodies, and an occasional Golgi apparatus. A thin basal lamina is usually present and pinocytotic vesicles are visible on both luminal and basal aspects. The cell surface is characterized by microvilli whose number ranges from only a few to more than 600 per cell (Figs. 1–116

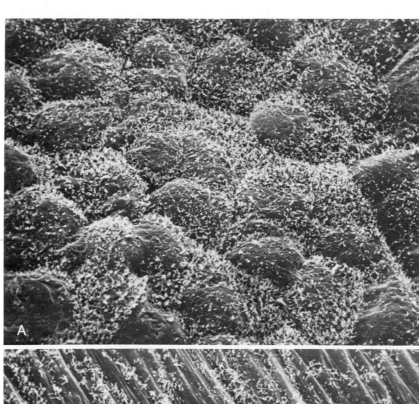

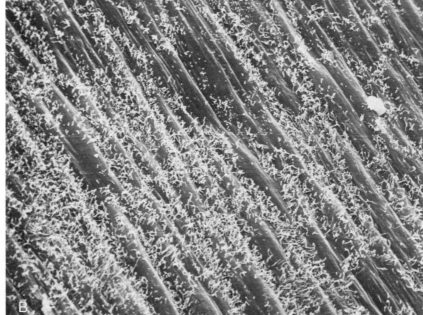

Figure 1–116. Mesothelial Cells. *A*, Note the bumpy appearance, usually indicative of loose and fatty subpleural connective tissue. (Rabbit mediastinal parietal pleura; SEM, × 1950.) *B*, A flattened appearance, implying a more rigid substructure. Note the numerous microvilli in both illustrations. (Rabbit intercostal parietal pleura; SEM, × 1650.) (Courtesy of Dr. Nai-San Wang, McGill University, Montreal.)

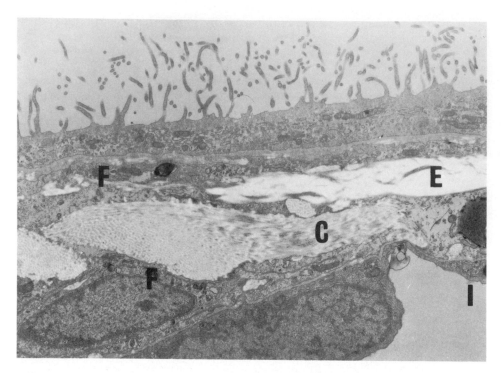

Figure 1–117. Ultrastructure of Mesothelial Cells. Rabbit visceral pleura, showing fibroblasts (*F*), elastic (*E*) and collagen (C) fibers, type I pneumocyte (*I*), and surface mesothelial cell with numerous elongated microvilli. (× 12,600.) (from Wang N-S: Am Rev Respir Dis *110*:623, 1974.)

and 1–117);[818] they tend to be more numerous on the visceral than on the parietal pleura. They are typically long and thin, measuring about 0.1 μm in diameter and up to 3 μm in length. Fine strands approximately 150 Å in diameter emanate from the surface glycocalyx and extend between microvilli;[821] it has been suggested that fluid trapped in compartments formed by these strands and by the microvilli protects the mesothelial cells from the potential trauma of normal pleural movement.[821]

Presumably by means of their microvilli and pinocytotic vesicles, mesothelial cells are responsible at least in part for regulating the composition and amount of pleural fluid. It is not certain whether they actively synthesize substances found in the fluid or simply transport them from underlying connective tissue cells or blood.[818] However, there is evidence that they may have the ability to produce components of the submesothelial connective tissue itself,[822] suggesting that they may in addition be capable of direct contribution to the pleural fluid. Mesothelial cells have also been shown to produce prostaglandins[818] and to possess fibrinolytic activity,[823] the latter feature possibly being important in decreasing the frequency and extent of fibrous adhesions following pleural injury. Although the mechanism of repair of damaged mesothelium is controversial, recent investigations suggest that this occurs by hyperplasia and migration of mesothelial cells from both the periphery of an area of injury and across fibrin bridges from the opposite pleural surface.[824, 825] It has also been proposed that submesothelial mesenchymal cells can proliferate and differentiate into mesothelial cells as part of the reparative process.[1172]

The origin of the blood supply of the visceral pleura is debated. According to some observers,[1, 4, 733] it derives from the pulmonary artery, except for the hilar region and part of the mediastinal and interlobar regions. Others have stated that, although this situation pertains in dogs, cats, and monkeys, in species with a thick pleura (humans, sheep, horses, cows, and pigs) the main blood supply to the visceral pleura is from the bronchial arteries.[630, 734] Regardless of the origin of the arterial supply, however, venous drainage is via the pulmonary veins.[735]

ROENTGENOLOGY

The combined thickness of the parietal and visceral pleural layers over the convexity of the lungs and over the diaphragmatic and mediastinal surfaces is insufficient to render these layers roentgenographically visible in the normal human subject. The diaphragmatic and mediastinal pleura, when uniformly thickened, is never visible, its water density precluding roentgenographic separation from contiguous diaphragm and mediastinum; by contrast, local thickening as from pleural plaques of asbestos-related disease can be identified because of the alteration they produce in the normally smooth contour of the diaphragm. Over the convexity of the lungs, even slight thickening (1 to 2 mm, for example) can be appreciated because of the greater density of contiguous ribs.

In the interlobar regions, contiguous layers of visceral pleura are roentgenographically visible because of the presence of air-containing lung on both sides. Interlobar fissures become visible when the x-ray beam passes tangentially along their surfaces;

these are of value in the assessment of disease of the pulmonary lobes that form them. Much of our knowledge of the incidence of roentgenographic identification of normal and accessory fissures has been supplied by Felson.[737]

Fissures

NORMAL INTERLOBAR FISSURES

Fissures form the contact surfaces between pulmonary lobes. Their depth varies from complete lobar separation to a superficial slit no more than 1 to 2 cm deep in the lung surface. The depth of interlobar fissures is important: the less complete a fissure line, the larger the bridge of lung parenchyma connecting two contiguous lobes. Such parenchymal bridges provide a ready pathway for collateral air drift or for the spread of disease to another lobe, creating roentgenographic signs that may give rise to erroneous conclusions. In their study of 100 fixed and inflated lung specimens (50 right and 50 left), Raasch and his colleagues[738] found considerable variation in the frequency with which the three fissures were complete. An incomplete fissure (fusion) was found between the right lower and upper lobes in 70 per cent of cases (Fig. 1–118) but between the right lower and middle lobes in only 47 per cent; in addition, fusion between the lower and upper lobes (Fig. 1–118) was commonly more extensive than between the lower and middle lobes. In the left lung, fusion between the lower and upper lobes was somewhat less frequent than on the right: 40 per cent of Raasch and associates' cases showed an incomplete fissure between the left lower lobe and the superior part of the upper lobe, and 46 per cent between the lower lobe and lingula. Incompleteness of the minor fissure was far more common than in any portion of either major fissure: of the 50 right lungs examined, extensive fusion was present in 88 per cent of cases, especially medially; thus, fusion is more common and usually more extensive between the middle and upper lobe (across the minor fissure) than between the middle and lower lobe (across the major fissure).

Yamashita[826] examined 270 fixed and inflated lungs (140 right and 130 left) for completeness of the fissures between the upper and lower lobes on the two sides. On the right, a complete major fissure was seen in 28.6 per cent, an incidence almost identical to that obtained by Raasch and his colleagues;[738] in an additional 30 per cent, the incompleteness was only minimal. In 21 per cent of patients, fusion was present in over half the surface between the two lobes. Yamashita observed very little fusion between the upper and lower lobes in the central portion of the right lung, most of it occurring superomedially. On the left, 26.9 per cent showed complete fissures, an incidence considerably lower than that found by Raasch and associates; the remainder showed incompleteness that ranged from very minor to almost complete. In the Ya-

mashita study,[826] 22.1 per cent of 140 right lungs possessed a complete interlobar fissure between the middle and upper lobes, whereas in 0.7 per cent there was no fissure at all; in 77.2 per cent of cases, fissural incompleteness ranged from slight to that occupying two thirds of the surface area between the two lobes. In all instances of incompleteness, the fusion extended to and involved the perihilar parenchyma.

The *oblique (major) fissures*, which separate the upper (and on the right, the middle lobe) from the lower lobes, begin at or about the level of the fifth thoracic vertebra and extend obliquely downward and forward, roughly paralleling the sixth rib, ending at the diaphragm a few centimeters behind the anterior pleural gutter (Fig. 1–119). According to Yamashita,[826] the top of the left lower lobe is usually higher than that of the right, the right major fissure being at the same level as the left in only 23 per cent of cases. The proportion of upper and lower lobes that contact the posterior chest wall is 1 to 4 and 1 to 5 for the right and left lungs respectively.

Some variation exists in the orientation of the right and left major fissures. In the study by Raasch and his colleagues,[738] the anterior surface of the right lower lobe was seen to be divided into upper and lower parts by an interfissural crest that separated the area of contact with the upper lobe from the area of contact with the middle lobe. The upper part of this surface almost always faced slightly laterally (Fig. 1–119) and was usually concave; the lower part also faced somewhat laterally (in over 80 per cent of cases) but was convex rather than concave. The orientation of the left major fissure was somewhat different: whereas the upper part of the fissural surface almost always faced laterally and was usually concave (as on the right), the lower part usually faced medially although its surface was generally convex. Thus, the lateral orientation of the upper half of the fissure and the medial orientation of the lower half created a twisted appearance similar to that of a propellor, a feature that was not observed on the right side. In a study of 100 consecutive CT scans of adults, Proto and Ball[827] concurred with Raasch and his associates that the upper part of each major fissure is oriented with its lateral aspect posterior to its medial aspect (lateral facing). However, in the lower part of the thorax, these investigators found that the lateral aspect of both the right and left major fissures was normally anterior to the medial aspect (medial facing) (Fig. 1–119); at the level of the carina, the lateral and medial aspects of the fissure were in the coronal plane.

Not infrequently, a triangular opacity is present at the lower end of the major fissures, its base contiguous with the diaphragm and its apex tapering cephalad into the fissure. Gale and Greif[1173] identified such an opacity in 39 of 212 CT scans, and showed it to be composed entirely of fat.

The *horizontal (minor) fissure* separates the an-

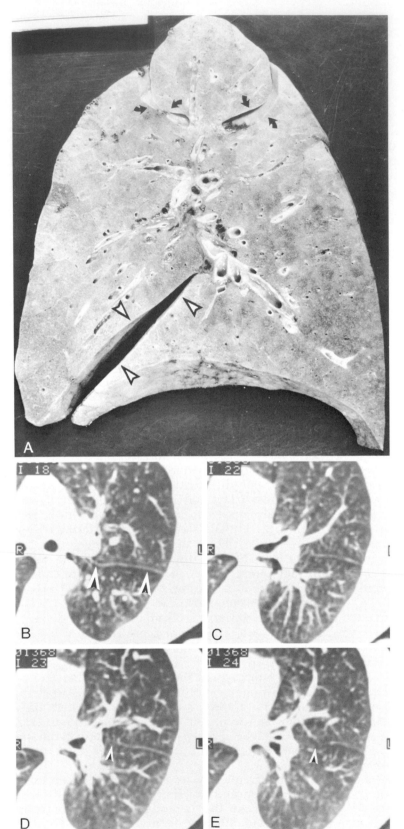

Figure 1–118. Incomplete Pleural Fissures. *A*, sagittal section of an inflated postmortem right lung specimen demonstrates the lower portion of the major fissure (*arrowheads*) to be complete. However, note the complete absence of the upper portion of the major fissure and the entirety of the minor fissure at this level. An azygos lobe fissure (*arrows*) is present at the top of the lung. *B–E*, Sequential 5-mm-thick CT scans with 10 mm spacing demonstrate the left major fissure to be complete (*large arrowheads*) at the level of the proximal left interlobar artery but to be incomplete (*small arrowheads*) adjacent to the hilum.

Illustration continued on opposite page

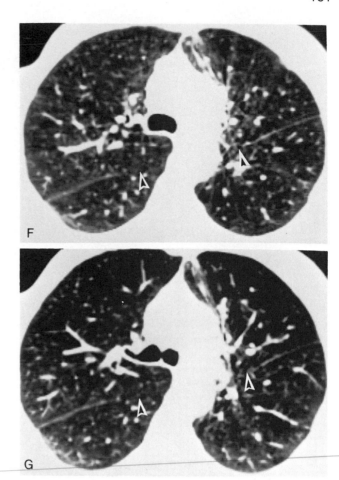

Figure 1–118. *Continued.* In another patient, CT scans (5 mm thick; 10 mm spacing) at two levels (*F* and *G*) demonstrate incomplete fissures bilaterally (*arrowheads*) between the upper and lower lobes. Such incompleteness permits collateral ventilation between the upper and lower lobes and is typically situated medially.

terior segment of the right upper lobe from the middle lobe and lies roughly horizontal at about the level of the fourth rib anteriorly. Raasch and his associates found considerable variation in its orientation, the anterior aspect generally being lower than the posterior and the lateral part lower than the medial.[738]

The incidence and completeness of identification of the pleural fissures on conventional roentgenograms is highly variable. This is not difficult to understand considering the curved orientation of the fissures and the fact that the major fissures are almost always oriented slightly away from the coronal plane; as a result, the major fissures are seldom seen along their entirety on lateral chest roentgenograms. This variable orientation of the fissural plane implies that the x-ray beam on a lateral chest roentgenogram is most apt to be tangent to the anterolateral aspect of the major fissures in the lower thorax and the middle or posterolateral surface in the upper thorax. In their study of 300 normal lateral roentgenograms, Proto and Speckman identified a major fissure along its entire length in only 2 per cent of cases, although they could see part of one or both major fissures in the other 98 per cent.[828] Similarly, they were able to identify the entirety of the minor fissure in only 6 per cent of the 300 roentgenograms and part of the fissure in

only 44 per cent. Other reports of the roentgenographic identification of the minor fissure in normal subjects vary: Felson[739] saw it in 56 per cent, Ritter and Eyband[740] in 70 per cent, and Simon[461] in over 80 per cent. Anatomically, the minor fissure rarely reaches the mediastinum and then only in its anterior portion; despite this, one of the more constant relationships noted by Felson on PA roentgenograms was the fissure's medial termination (or projected termination) at the lateral margin of the interlobar pulmonary artery. A fissure line or interface that projects medial to this point is almost invariably a downward displaced major fissure, providing certain evidence of volume loss in the right lower lobe.

On a lateral chest roentgenogram, the posterior extent of the minor fissure is sometimes projected behind the hilum and right major fissure (Fig. 1–120). The probable explanation for this seeming roentgenologic paradox relates to the undulating course of the major and minor fissures so that in lateral projection the x-ray beam images different areas of each. For instance, the lateral segment of the middle lobe, covered by the posterolateral aspect of the minor fissure, normally resides behind a coronal plane through the hila; it is this particular contour of the minor fissure that can be identified in some patients (Fig. 1–120). If the medial contour

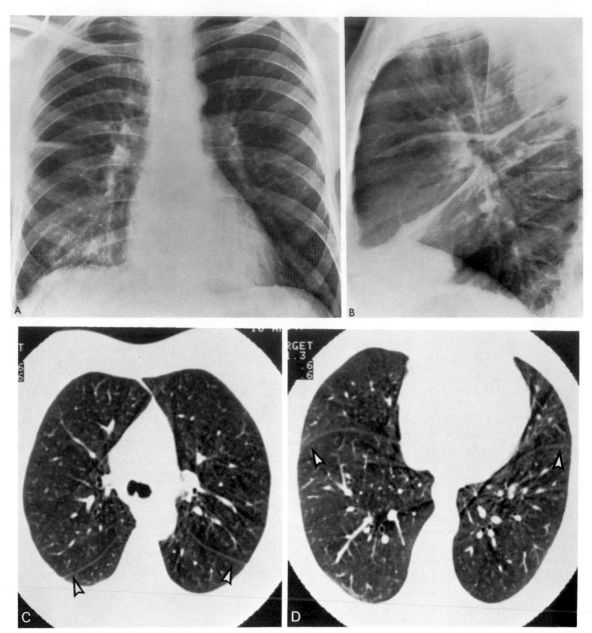

Figure 1–119. Interlobar Fissures, Right Lung. The presence of minimal interlobar effusion renders the fissures clearly visible in posteroanterior (*A*) and lateral (*B*) roentgenograms. *C*, A CT scan through the upper thorax reveals the lateral portion of the right and left major fissures (*arrowheads*) to be situated posterior to the anteromedial portion of the fissure, so-called "lateral facing." *D*, A CT scan through the lower thorax shows that the lateral portion of the major fissures (*arrowheads*) is located anterior to the anteromedial aspect of the major fissures, so-called "medial facing."

of the major fissure is simultaneously displayed, the anatomic conditions that explain the apparent discrepancy just described are more readily understood.

The superolateral portion of the major fissures was studied by Proto and Ball on conventional PA chest roentgenograms of 1068 normal patients ranging in age from 18 to 70 years.[827] In 14 per cent of cases, they identified a curving shadow in the upper hemithorax that appeared as either a curvilinear opacity or a curving edge; the latter configuration, observed in the great majority of cases, consisted of a ground-glass opacity laterally

and a radiolucency medially (Fig. 1–121); a curving line was seen in only a small percentage of cases. These two appearances, whether on the right or left, approached the lateral chest wall in proximity to the sixth posterior rib. These contours were seen on the right side alone in 4 per cent, on the left alone in 6 per cent, and bilaterally in 4 per cent. When bilateral, the left contour almost always extended slightly higher than the right, occasionally reaching the fourth posterior rib. With the help of correlative postmortem and CT studies, Proto and Ball[829] showed that the curving line appearance resulted from orientation of the superolateral por-

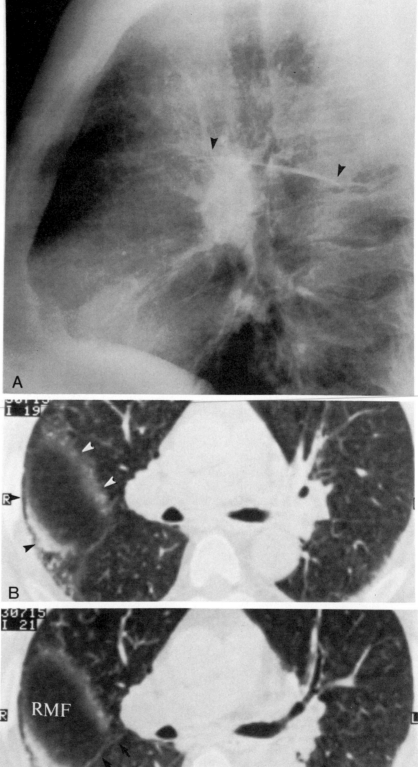

Figure 1–120. Position of the Minor Fissure Relative to the Hilum in Lateral Projection. *A*, A conventional lateral chest roentgenogram discloses a horizontal curvilinear stripe (*arrowheads*) representing a thickened minor fissure. Note that is this patient the fissure extends well behind the right hilum, overlapping the disc space at T6–7. *B* and *C*, CT scans at the level of the intermediate bronchus reveal an oval lucency representing the dome of the minor fissure (*RMF*). The fissure is slightly thickened owing to pleural effusion (*arrowheads*). Scans show that the component of the minor fissure that is seen behind the hilum relates to the posterolateral aspect of the middle lobe. A small portion of the right major fissure (*arrows*) is shown. If the medial portion of the major fissure and the lateral component of the minor fissure are arranged so that both are tangential to the x-ray beam, the posterior portion of the minor fissure will be depicted behind the medial aspect of the major fissure.

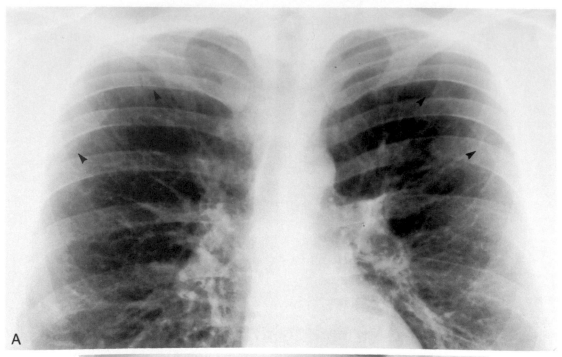

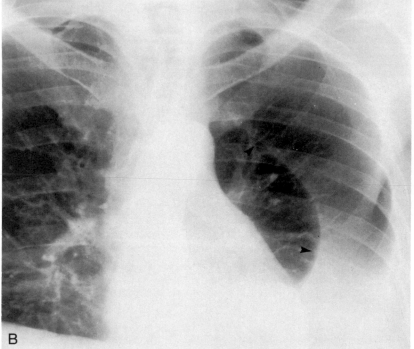

Figure 1–121. Superolateral Major Fissures. *A,* A detail view of a conventional posteroanterior chest roentgenogram in a normal, young adult man. A curvilinear edge (*arrowheads*) with a ground-glass opacity laterally can be identified bilaterally, representing the superolateral aspect of the major fissures. The left fissure is slightly higher than the right. *B,* A view of the left lung from a conventional posteroanterior chest roentgenogram in a patient with pleural effusion shows the superolateral aspect of the left major fissure (*arrowheads*) to be accentuated by the interlobar effusion.

Illustration continued on opposite page

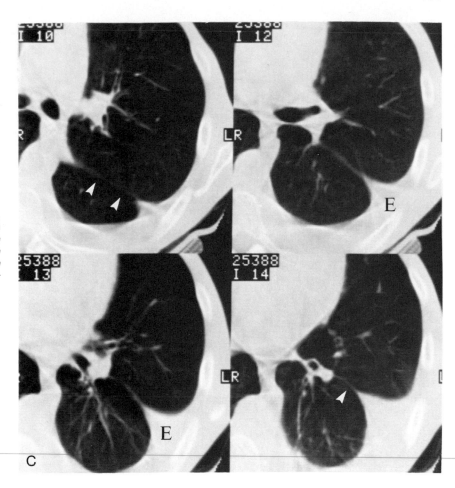

Figure 1–121. *Continued.* In this patient, CT scans (*C*) show a small part of the effusion (*E*) intruding into the lateral aspect of the major fissure (*arrowheads*), accounting for the enhanced visibility. It is emphasized that the appearance in *B* does *not* represent an incomplete fissure.

tion of the major fissure tangential to the x-ray beam, whereas the curving edge configuration was attributed to extrapleural fat intruding into the major fissure superolaterally (Fig. 1–121).

The pleural fissures can often be seen on CT scans. Marks and Kuhns[830] identified the fissures as avascular zones in 20 (84 per cent) of 23 consecutive scans; on 21 per cent of the axial images, a "ground-glass" band was identified within the zone of hypovascularity, considered by these investigators to be caused by partial volume averaging of the pleural fissure with the adjacent lung. On the basis of 100 consecutive CT scans of adults, Proto and Ball[827] observed three different manifestations of the right and left major fissures—in decreasing order of frequency, lucent bands, lines, and dense bands (Fig. 1–122). Depending on the level of the scan (upper, middle, or lower thorax), the lucent band form was seen in 60 to 73 per cent of cases on the right and 58 to 74 per cent on the left. The linear manifestation was identified at the three levels in 1 to 10 per cent on the right and 1 to 20 per cent on the left. Dense bands were the least common presentation, being identified in up to 4 per cent on the right and up to 6 per cent on the left. The varying appearance of the major fissures was considered by Proto and Ball to be related to the plane of the fissure on the cross-sectional image.[827] Thus, a per-

pendicular fissure (such as in the upper thorax) is likely to produce a linear configuration, whereas a more oblique orientation causes a well-defined, dense (ground-glass) band. If the upper part of the major fissure is not quite perpendicular to the cross-sectional image, the smaller vessels at the periphery of the lobes on both sides of the fissure tend to cause the fissure to be displayed as a relatively avascular lucent band.

The minor fissure and the plane of the CT scan are more or less tangential to one another, resulting in a lucent area relatively devoid of vessels when compared with the same region in the left lung; this appearance was identified by Proto and Ball[827] in 52 per cent of their patients. We have occasionally identified the minor fissure as a ground-glass opacity, presumably as a result of fortuituous sectioning through the precise plane of the fissure. The lucent area is generally seen on only one or two scans, usually at the level of the intermediate bronchus. In 44 per cent of cases, the lucent area is triangular in shape, its apex at the hilum; in 8 per cent, it is round or oval (Fig. 1–122), a shape considered by Proto and Ball to be caused by the domelike configuration of the minor fissure.

In a review of the CT scans of 50 patients (26 men, 24 women) ranging in age from 14 to 68

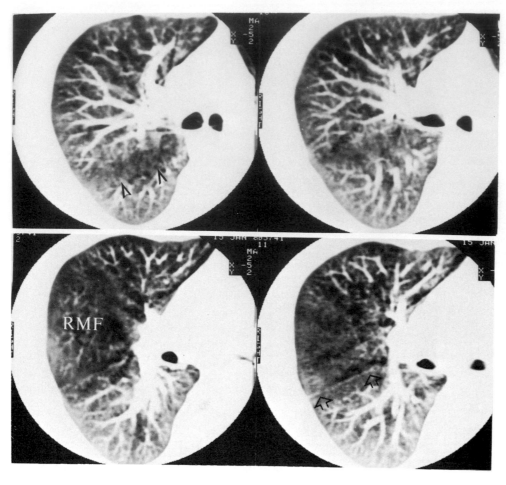

Figure 1–122. CT Appearance of Major and Minor Fissures. Sequential CT scans (10 mm thick; 10-mm spacing) demonstrate the right major fissure as either a lucent band (*arrowheads*) or a thin line (*open arrow*). The broad, triangular lucency (the right midlung window) identifies the apex of the minor fissure (*RMF*).

years, Goodman and his coworkers[831] identified a focal vascular deficiency in the right midlung that they termed the *right midlung window*. This deficiency was seen on the right in 46 patients (92 per cent) and on the left in three (6 per cent); 92 per cent of the right midlung windows were located at the level of the intermediate bronchus. Goodman and his associates[831] observed that the midlung window corresponded to the minor fissure and attributed the difference between the right and left lungs to the arrangement of arteries: on the right, the truncus anterior branch of the pulmonary artery enters the hilum where it courses cephalad to supply the right upper lobe; the interlobar artery gives rise to the middle lobe branch at the level of the minor fissure and then continues caudally to supply the lower lobe. Consequently, the region lateral to the bronchus intermedius is normally devoid of major vessels and hence is perceived as an area of diminished vascularity. By contrast, the left pulmonary artery possesses divisional characteristics different from the right and displays a more even spatial distribution of major pulmonary vessels within the upper lobe (including the lingula). The uncommon occurrence of a left minor fissure separating the anterior segment of the upper lobe from the lingula could obviously account for a left midlung window (Fig. 1–123).

THE PULMONARY LIGAMENT

The inferior pulmonary ligament (more properly called the pulmonary ligament since there is no superior component) consists of a double layer of pleura that drapes caudally from the lung hilum, tethering the medial aspect of the lower lobe to the mediastinum and diaphragm.[832–835] The ligament is formed by the mediastinal (parietal) pleura as it reflects over the main bronchi and pulmonary arteries and veins onto the surface of the lung as the visceral pleura (Fig. 1–124). Although the anterior and posterior layers of this pleural reflection are excluded from one another at the hilum, apposition is possible caudal to the inferior pulmonary vein (rarely cephalad to the pulmonary vein), thus forming the pulmonary ligament. The ligament can terminate in a free falciform border anywhere between the inferior pulmonary vein and the superior aspect of the hemidiaphragm (*incomplete* form), or it can extend inferiorly and cover a portion of the medial aspect of the hemidiaphragm (*complete* form). Thus, the pulmonary ligament divides the mediastinal pleural space below the hilum into either complete or incomplete anterior and posterior compartments. The bare area of mediastinum thus created contains a network of connective tissue, small bronchial veins, lymphatics, and lymph nodes.

Several observers[832–835] have proposed that the pulmonary ligament consists of two components—a small peak that represents the mediastinal attachment and a long component, or septum, termed the intersublobar septum, that divides the medial from the posterior basal lung segments. The left pulmonary ligament is closely related to the esophagus and is bordered posteriorly by the descending aorta; the shorter, right ligament can be situated anywhere along an arc that extends from the inferior vena cava anteriorly to the azygos vein posteriorly.

The right and left pulmonary ligaments are never seen on conventional posteroanterior or lateral chest roentgenograms but can occasionally be identified on 55° oblique hilar tomograms (Fig. 1–125) and frequently on CT; in Rost and Proto's series of 129 normal adult patients,[833] CT revealed the left ligament in 67.4 per cent, the right ligament in 37.2 per cent, both ligaments in 27.1 per cent (Fig. 1–125), and neither in 22.4 per cent. In another CT study of 50 subjects,[835] the right ligament alone was identified in 26 per cent, and the left in 30 per cent, both in 32 per cent, and neither in 12 per cent. Cooper and his colleagues[834] studied 55 men and 45 women with an age range of 14 to 78 years and found that one ligament was visible on CT in 42 per cent of patients but that both were identified in only 8 per cent; the left ligament was seen more frequently than the right (38 per cent versus 12 per cent). In their study, the incidence of CT detection of the ligament was neither age- nor gender-dependent.

The CT appearance of the ligament is variable but usually consists of a small peak or pyramid on the mediastinal surface that represents the ligament, and a thin linear opacity that extends from the apex of the peak to the lung, marking the intersublobar septum. Rost and Proto[833] noted that the ligament is most evident on scans obtained at or just above the level of the hemidiaphragm, although Godwin and his colleagues[835] stated that the long linear opacities in this location more likely represent the diaphragmatic component of the ligament rather than the intersublobar septum. In 92 per cent of cases, the course of the ligament on both sides is obliquely posterior.[833] Ordinarily, the right ligament is seen at a level slightly higher than the left, and both ligaments can be appreciated on only one or two slices of a series.

The function of the pulmonary ligament is unknown although it undoubtedly serves as an anchor for the lower lobe in resisting torsion. However, Rabinowitz and his colleagues[832] noted that the ligament plays an important role in modifying the roentgenographic appearance of pneumothorax, lower lobe atelectasis, and medial pleural effusion. Pathologic involvement of the pulmonary ligament by tumors, cysts, varicosities,[833] and fat (Fig. 1–126) has been described.[832] The subject of

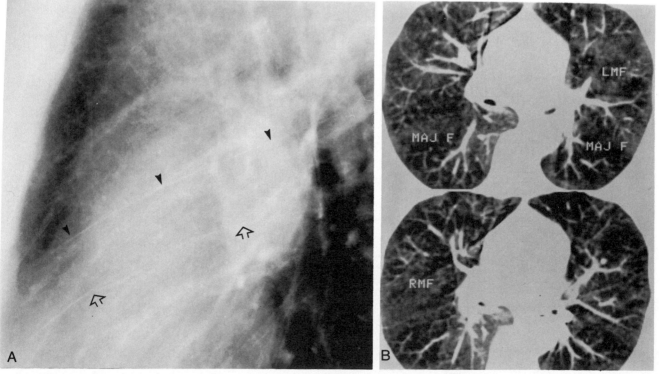

Figure 1–123. Left Minor Fissure. *A,* A conventional lateral chest roentgenogram of a normal adult woman demonstrates two thin curvilinear opacities. The left minor fissure (*arrowheads*) is typically higher than the right (*open arrows*). *B,* CT scans through the left hilum slow a left midlung window representing the dome of the left minor fissure (*LMF*). The major fissures (*MAJ F*) and a small portion of the right minor fissure (*RMF*) are also seen.

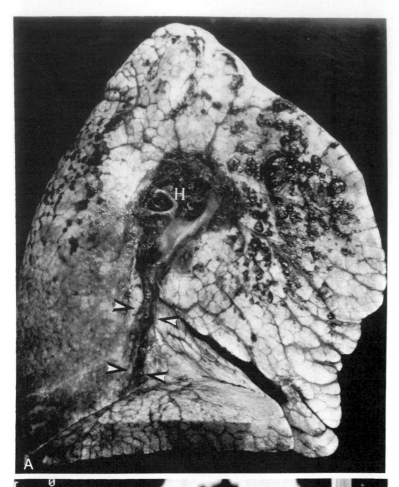

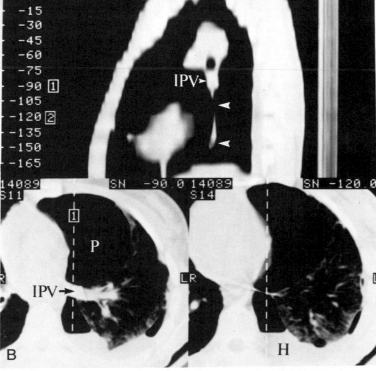

Figure 1–124. The Pulmonary Ligament. *A*, As seen on an inflated postmortem specimen of the left lung viewed from the mediastinal aspect, the mediastinal (parietal) pleura reflects over the hilum superiorly, anteriorly, and posteriorly; caudally these pleural layers are more closely apposed to comprise the pulmonary ligament (*arrowheads*). In *B* are a reformatted CT scan (*top*) and representative transverse images (*bottom*) through the plane of the left inferior pulmonary vein (*IPV*) and 3 cm caudally in a patient with a spontaneous hydropneumothorax (*H* and *P*). Note that the vertically oriented intersublobar septum (*arrowheads*) divides the mediastinal pleural space into anterior and posterior compartments.

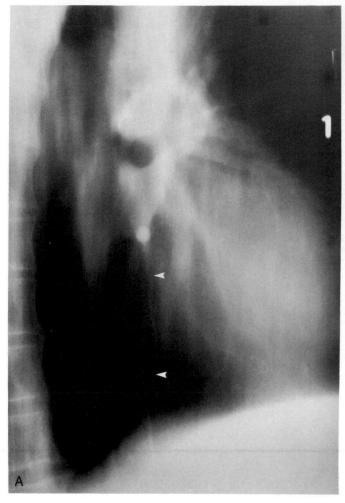

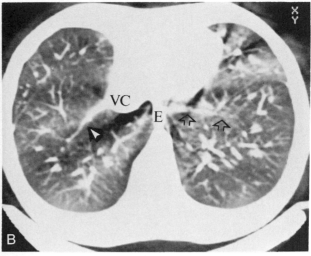

Figure 1–125. The Pulmonary Ligament. *A,* A 55° left posterior oblique conventional linear tomogram shows a thin, vertically oriented opacity (*arrowheads*) extending from the inferior pulmonary vein to the top of the left hemidiaphragm, representing the left intersublobar septum of the pulmonary ligament. *B,* A CT scan through the lower thorax of a different patient (with atopic asthma) demonstrates the right (*closed arrow*) and the left (*open arrows*) intersublobar septa of the pulmonary ligaments. The left ligament and septum relate closely to the esophagus (*E*) whereas on the right the septum and ligament are closely aligned to the inferior vena cava (*VC*).

gas collections within the ligament is controversial; some investigators[836-838] consider that air can dissect into the mediastinum from the lung between the leaves of the ligament, creating a typical triangular radiolucency in the lower hemithorax on a PA roentgenogram. However, this hypothesis has been challenged: Friedman[839] described two patients and Godwin and his associates[840] an additional four in whom conventional PA and lateral roentgenograms revealed a radiolucency conforming to the shape of the pulmonary ligament in one or other hemithorax; long fluid levels, inconsistent with the normal anatomic location of the ligament, were identified in three of the six subjects. CT analysis of the gas collections showed quite clearly that they were located either between pleural layers in front of or behind the ligaments or within the mediastinum outside the parietal pleura altogether. We have examined one patient in whom a CT scan demonstrated air within the right pulmonary ligament following an open lung biopsy (Fig. 1–126); however, convincing evidence that the gas accumulation resided within the ligament was lacking on conventional roentgenograms.

Accessory Fissures

Any segment of lung may be partly or completely separated from adjacent segments by an accessory pleural fissure. The anatomic incidence is much higher than is generally appreciated, amounting to about 50 per cent of lungs, according to von Hayek.[1] These fissures vary in their degree of development, from superficial slits in the lung surface not more than 1 or 2 cm deep to complete fissures that extend all the way to the hilum. Most are of little more than academic interest roentgenologically.

When well developed, however, their recognition is important for three reasons: (1) the segment they subtend may be the only site of disease whose spread is prevented by the fissure; (2) a fissure in a specific anatomic location, such as between the superior and basal segments of the right lower lobe, can be mistaken for the minor fissure between upper and middle lobes and thus create confusion in interpretation; and 3) accessory fissures are important components of plate atelectasis (*see* page 635).

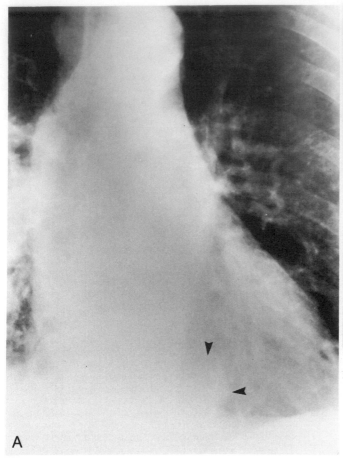

A

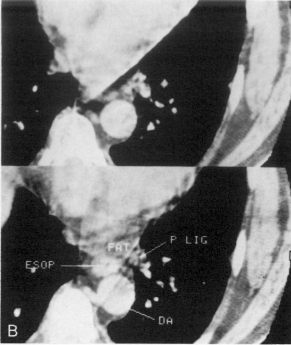

B

Figure 1–126. Pathologic Features of the Pulmonary Ligament. *A*, A detail view from a posteroanterior chest roentgenogram of a middle-aged man discloses a vague retrocardiac opacity (*arrowheads*). *B*, CT scans through the lower thorax reveal mediastinal fat extending into the apex of the pulmonary ligament (*P LIG*) as the cause of the unexplained opacity. Note the relationship of the ligament to the esophagus (*ESOP*) and the descending aorta (*DA*).

Illustration continued on opposite page

AZYGOS FISSURE

Perhaps the best known of the accessory fissures, although of no known pathologic significance, is the azygos fissure (the mesoazygos), which is created by downward invagination of the azygos vein through the apical portion of the right upper lobe (Figs. 1–127 and 1–128). The familiar curvilinear shadow extends obliquely across the upper portion of the right lung and terminates in the "tear drop" shadow caused by the vein itself at a variable distance above the right hilum. It is formed by four pleural layers (two parietal and two visceral) since the azygos vein runs outside the parietal pleura and thus invaginates four layers in its downward course. Felson states that this fissure is visible in 0.4 per cent of chest roentgenograms.[737] Fisher has noted a decided male preponderance of azygos fissures, of the order of 2 to 1: of 100 consecutive cases of azygos lobe, 68 were men.[742] Postmus and his colleagues[1174] have recently described a familial incidence of the anomaly: of 12 members of one family, 5 had an azygos fissure. The mode of inheritance is probably autosomal dominant.

In a CT study of 11 patients with an azygos lobe, considerable alteration was observed in contour of the right side of the mediastinum and in the relation of lung to the superior vena cava and

trachea.[743] In the presence of an azygos lobe, the azygos arch occupies a more cephalad position than normal, and the axis of the superior vena cava becomes oriented toward the left. Lung tissue within the azygos lobe intrudes into the pretracheal and retrotracheal mediastinum, contacting the anterior wall and most of the posterior wall of the trachea in the majority of patients. Similarly, lateral displacement of the azygos vein permits lung to intrude posterior to the superior vena cava, permitting identification of the posterior wall of this structure on lateral chest roentgenograms.

Although the bronchial supply of the azygos lobe is variable, either the apical or anterior subsegmental branch of the apical bronchus is always present.[744] Larger lobes may contain both these subsegments or the apical subsegments of the apical and posterior segmental bronchi. The importance of the anomaly roentgenologically (in addition to the reasons previously stated) lies in the failure of the apical pleural surfaces to separate when pneumothorax is present.

INFERIOR ACCESSORY FISSURE

This accessory fissure is of variable depth and separates the medial basal segment from the remainder of the lower lobe; when complete, the

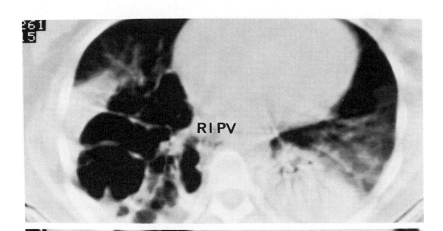

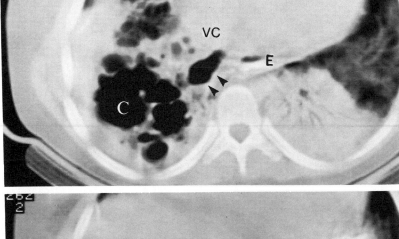

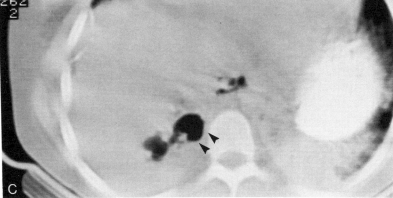

Figure 1–126 *Continued. C*, CT scans through the lower lobes of a different patient with traumatic lung cysts (*C*) reveal a collection of gas (*arrowheads*) within the intersublobar septum and ligament caudal to the right inferior pulmonary vein (*RIPV*). This lucency was indistinguishable from the cystic spaces within the lung on conventional posteroanterior and lateral chest roentgenograms. *VC*, inferior vena cava; *E*, esophagus.

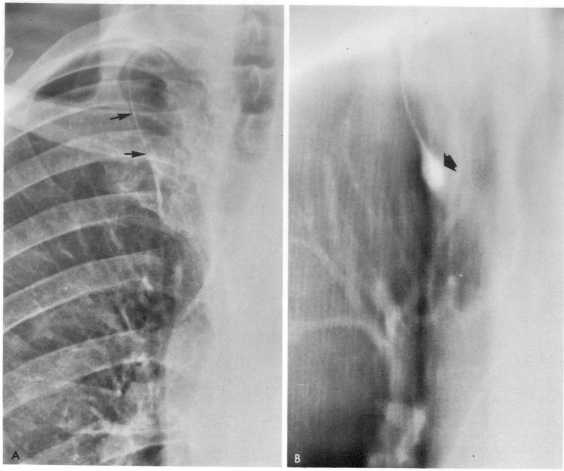

Figure 1–127. Accessory Fissure of the Azygos Vein. *A,* On a standard roentgenogram is posteroanterior projection, the fissure can be identified as a curvilinear shadow (*arrows*) extending obliquely across the upper portion of the right lung, its lower end some distance above the right hilum. *B,* A tomographic section with the patient in the supine position permits better perception of the teardrop shadow of the vein (*arrow*) because of distention.

isolated lung is termed the inferior accessory or retrocardiac lobe. On the diaphragmatic surface of the lung, the fissure extends laterally from near the pulmonary ligament and then makes a convex arc forward to join the major fissure. On conventional roentgenograms, the fissure line extends superiorly and slightly medially from the inner third of the right or left hemidiaphragm. As with all normal and accessory fissures, consolidation in contiguous lung parenchyma provides a sharp interface between diseased and normal lung parenchyma.

This anomalous fissure is a fairly common anatomic finding: von Hayek[1] found it in 30 per cent of lungs, and Schaffner[745] is said to have seen it in 45 per cent of 210 lungs studied at necropsy. Its incidence roentgenographically depends to some extent on the mode of examination: Rigler and Ericksen[746] found it in 41 (8.2 per cent) of 500 roentgenograms, 33 times on the right, 5 times on the left, and 3 times bilaterally; by contrast, in a prospective study by Godwin and Tarver[747] of 50 patients examined by both conventional chest roentgenography and CT, the latter mode permitted identification of eight inferior accessory fissures (16

per cent); of these only two were also visible on chest roentgenograms. On the other hand, conventional roentgenograms showed three fissures that were not visible on CT, so that the overall incidence in this series of 50 patients was 22 per cent.

SUPERIOR ACCESSORY FISSURE

This fissure separates the superior segment from the basal segments of the lower lobes, more commonly on the right (Fig. 1–129). It varies in length and depth from a complete fissure to a subtle notch. Since this fissure commonly lies horizontally at the same level as the minor fissure, the two may be confused on a frontal roentgenogram, although their separate anatomic positions may be clearly established on lateral or oblique roentgenography.

LEFT MINOR FISSURE

This fissure separates the lingula from the rest of the left upper lobe, and in almost all cases the usual segmental anatomy of the left lung is preserved. Boyden[748] observed the fissure in 8 per cent

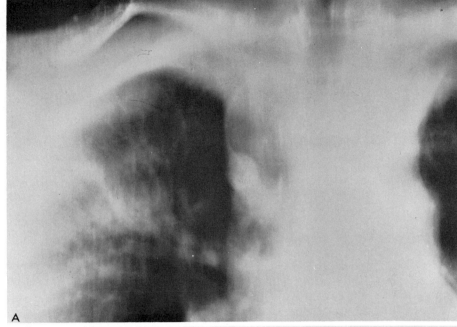

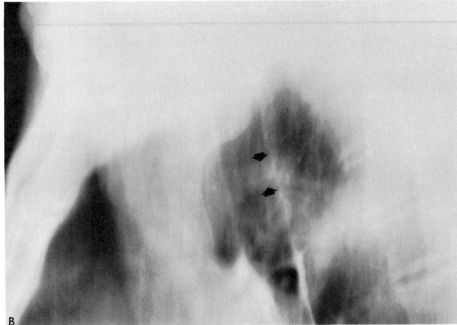

Figure 1–128. Accessory Fissure of the Azygos Vein (in Congestive Heart Failure). *A,* A tomographic section of the upper thorax in antero-posterior projection, supine position, reveals a slightly distended azygos vein at the lower end of a thickened fissure. The patient was in cardiac decompensation. *B,* In lateral projection, the shadow of the vein (*arrows*) can be seen lying in a horizontal plane extending anteriorly to the shadow of the brachiocephalic vessels. In *B,* note the interface caused by the insertion of a tongue of lung behind the posterior wall of the superior vena cava.

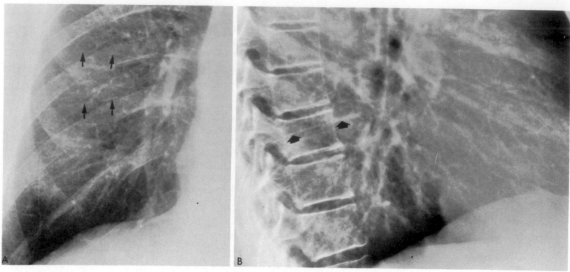

Figure 1–129. Accessory Fissure Between the Superior and Basal Segments of the Right Lower Lobe. *A,* In a posteroanterior projection of the lower half of the right lung two horizontal fissures can be identified, the superior (*upper arrows*) representing the normal minor fissure and the inferior (*lower arrows*) representing an accessory fissure between the superior and basal bronchopulmonary segments of the right lower lobe. *B,* In lateral projection, the accessory fissure is well seen (*arrows*).

of 100 specimens, none of which had any derangement of segmental anatomy. Austin[1175] identified the fissure on 32 (1.6 per cent) of 2000 consecutive PA and lateral chest roentgenograms of normal subjects; its position was usually more cephalad than the right minor fissure, and its lateral end usually superior to its medial end.

A vertical line shadow has been reported in the lower lung regions of some infants and children; this is termed the "vertical fissure line."[749-751] The line is visible on frontal projections of the thorax; it extends from the lateral portion of the diaphragmatic dome upward and slightly medially, roughly parallel to the thoracic wall, and terminates at the level of the horizontal fissure. It has been identified in both lungs but more often in the right. Several theories have been postulated to explain this fissure line; most of the evidence indicates that it represents the lower portion of the major fissure, thrown into profile by alteration in position of the middle and lower lobes. How or why this positional change occurs is not clear, but the major importance of the line lies in its recognition as such and in its differentiation from the visceral pleural line in pneumothorax. It seems likely that, ultimately, the line will prove to be similar to the phenomenon seen in the chest roentgenograms of adults when partial collapse of the lower lobe has caused downward and medial displacement of the major fissure, rendering it visible in profile in frontal projection.

PHYSIOLOGY

The visceral and parietal pleura form smooth membranes that facilitate the movement of the lungs within the pleural space, chiefly as the result of secretion and absorption of pleural fluid. The material that follows on pressures within the pleural cavity and the formation and absorption of pleural fluid is only a brief summary of these complex subjects, and the reader interested in acquiring additional information is directed to the excellent reviews by Agostoni and colleagues[759] and Black.[752]

Pressures

Pressure within the pleural cavity is generated by the difference between the elastic forces of the chest wall and of the lungs. At functional residual capacity (FRC) the lung tends to recoil inward while the chest wall and the rib cage tend to recoil outward. Even at the end of a maximal expiration (RV), the lungs continue to recoil inward; the relaxed position of a normal lung is only achieved after removal from the chest or with pneumothorax "minimal volume." By contrast, the chest wall's resting position is at about 55 per cent of vital capacity or 70 per cent of total lung capacity; below this volume the chest wall has a tendency to expand whereas above this volume it tends to recoil toward its resting position. At FRC the outward recoil of the chest wall and the inward recoil of the lung generate a pleural pressure of about -5 cm H_2O. However, the pleural pressure is not uniform through the pleural cavity, being more negative at the apex than at the base, with a gradient of about 0.2 cm H_2O per centimeter of vertical height. The gradient is gravity dependent, being reversed in subjects in the head down position and altered to an anterior/posterior gradient in patients in the supine position.

The effects of this gradient have been demonstrated by Milic-Emili and others,[547] who have shown that the upper lung zones are more expanded than the lower in subjects in the upright position at all lung volumes other than total lung capacity. The lower lung zones expand more than the upper during inspiration, and this is reflected by the greater ventilation of the lower zones in healthy, young, erect subjects. Regional volume behavior of the lung has been compared to that of an easily extensible coiled spring.[547] If the spring is held at its upper end so that it is acted upon only by the force of gravity, the coils will be further apart at the upper than at the lower end: this is analogous to the greater alveolar volume in the upper than in the lower lung zones. If the spring is lengthened by applying a weight at the bottom, the distances between coils will increase until they are equal: the change in distance between the coils is greater at the lower end, corresponding to the greater change in volume at the bottom of the lung.

Fluid Formation and Absorption

According to Yamada,[753] the amount of pleural fluid in normal humans ranges from less than 1 ml (the majority) to 20 ml. He was able to aspirate some fluid in about 30 per cent of a group of healthy soldiers at rest and in about 70 per cent of them after exercise. Müller and Löfstedt,[754] who performed thoracentesis on some of their patients following roentgenographic demonstration of up to 15 ml of pleural fluid in 15 of 120 healthy subjects, found that the smallest amount of fluid identified by their special roentgenographic technique (*see* page 322) was 3 to 5 ml. The volume of liquid in a single pleural space in humans is approximately 2 ml,[755] and it has been calculated[756] that the pleural fluid in dogs and rabbits totals 2.5 ml and 1.0 ml, respectively. Human pleural fluid is reported to have an average protein concentration of 1.77 grams per dl (range, 1.38 to 3.35)[753] and to contain sodium, potassium, and calcium concentrations similar to those of interstitial fluid. The pleural fluid in dogs, cats, and mice averages approximately 10 μ thick over most of the costal region,[757] and it is thicker (probably more than 100 μ) in the region of the lobar margins.

In normal humans, transudation and absorption of fluid within the pleural cavity follow the Starling equation and depend upon a combination of hydrostatic, colloid osmotic, and tissue pressures. The tissue pressures are not known, but knowledge of the first two suggest that, in health, fluid is formed at the parietal pleura and absorbed at the visceral pleura (Fig. 1–130). The net hydrostatic pressure that forces fluid out of the parietal pleura results from the hydrostatic pressure in systemic capillaries that supply the parietal pleura (30 cm H_2O) and the pleural pressure (−5 cm H_2O at functional residual capacity). Thus, the net hydrostatic drive is 35 cm H_2O pressure. The colloid osmotic pressure in the systemic capillaries is 34 cm

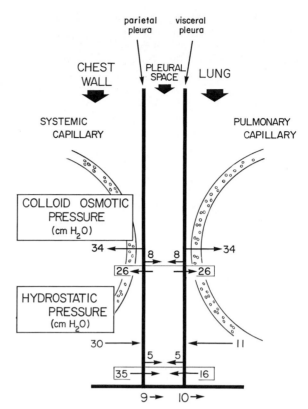

Figure 1–130. Diagrammatic Representation of the Pressures Involved in the Formation and Absorption of Pleural Fluid. *See* text for description.

H_2O, and that of the pleura[758] approximately 8 cm H_2O, yielding a net drive of 26 cm colloid osmotic pressure from the pleural space to the capillaries of the parietal pleura. The balance of these forces (35 − 26 cm = 9 cm H_2O) is directed from the parietal pleura to the pleural cavity. The visceral pleura, other than over the mediastinal surfaces, is supplied by pulmonary artery capillaries, whose hydrostatic pressure is approximately 11 cm H_2O. Other pressures remain roughly constant. Thus, the net hydrostatic pressure from visceral pleura toward pleural cavity is 16 cm H_2O (11 + 5 cm). The osmotic colloid pressures remain constant, with a pressure of 26 cm away from the pleural cavity. The new effect of these forces is a drive of 10 cm H_2O (26 − 16 cm) toward the visceral pleural capillaries.

This discussion of the forces governing formation and absorption of pleural fluid is an oversimplification, since it ignores tissue pressures, the permeability of the mesothelial layer, and pressures within the lymphatics through which excess fluid will be absorbed. However, the estimate of the forces that act on pleural fluid is supported by the findings of Agostoni and associates[759] that the visceral pleura of the dog absorbs saline at a pressure related to these forces.

As has been noted, in health the pleural fluid has a low protein content,[753, 760, 761] permitting fluid formation by the parietal pleural capillaries and its absorption by the visceral pleural capillaries according to Starling's principles. When the protein concentration of pleural fluid rises sufficiently, the effect of colloid osmotic pressure in visceral pleural capillaries is reduced to negligible proportions, and the only route of absorption of pleural fluid is by bulk flow via the lymphatics.[762, 763] Nearly all lymphatic absorption takes place in the parietal pleura.[764] Communication between lymphatics and the pleural cavity appears to be through temporary dehiscence of adjoining mesothelial cells, which occurs when the pleura is stretched. Since parietal pleural lymphatic vessels pass through the diaphragm and intercostal muscles, movement of the chest wall might increase lymphatic flow and the speed of absorption from the pleural space—this has been shown to occur in unanesthetized dogs.[763] Stewart[760] found that in humans the rate of absorption of fluid high in protein falls significantly during the night, and he postulated that the decreased rate and depth of respiration during sleep might account for this.

It is apparent that abnormal amounts of fluid may accumulate when hydrostatic pressure or capillary permeability is increased or colloid osmotic pressure is decreased. Increased hydrostatic pressure causes the pleural effusion that occurs in heart failure, and increased capillary permeability is responsible in inflammatory and neoplastic disease of the pleura. The *site* of accumulation of fluid depends upon hydrostatic forces and, to some extent, capillary attraction between the lung and the thoracic wall.

THE LYMPHATIC SYSTEM

LYMPHATICS OF THE LUNGS AND PLEURA

Although the entire cardiac output passes through the lungs, which have a rich lymphatic supply, lymphatic flow from them is small compared with that which drains the systemic circulation. Pleural lymphatics are variable in size and number as well as in their overall anatomic distribution. They course within the vascular layer where they form a plexus of broad channels roughly following the pleural lobular boundaries. Between these channels and joining with them are smaller intercommunicating and blindly ending tributaries that ramify over the pleural surface. Branches occasionally dip into the immediate subpleural lung parenchyma, form a short loop, and then return to the pleural surface. This network is much more prominent in neonatal than in adult lungs, in which larger channels tend to show a much more random nonlobular distribution.[765] The lymphatic network runs over the whole of the pleural surface, although it is much better developed over the lower than the upper lobes (Fig. 1–131); it drains eventually into the medial aspect of the lung near the hilum where

it anastomoses with the lymphatics of the parenchymal plexus.

Within the lung, lymphatic channels form two major pathways, one in the bronchoarterial and the other in the interlobular septal connective tissue. In both, lymph flows centripetally toward the hilum (Fig. 1–122), eventually reaching the bronchial and mediastinal lymph nodes. Anastomotic channels connect the interlobular perivenous lymphatics with those in the bronchoarterial sheath; they are up to 4 cm long and usually lie approximately midway between the hilum and the periphery of the lung. (Distention of these communicating lymphatics and edema in their surrounding connective tissue result in Kerley A lines; similar processes in the interlobular lymphatics and connective tissue result in Kerley B lines). Anastomotic channels also connect the bronchoarterial and pleural plexuses;[3, 765, 766] although fluid from the pleural cavity theoretically can reach the hilum through these connecting lymphatics,[765] it has been argued that the presence of lymphatic valves directed toward the pleural surface would effectively preclude significant flow in this direction.[3]

Although lymphatic capillaries have not been identified within alveolar interstitial tissue (the bronchoarterial lymphatics begin in the region of the distal respiratory bronchioles),[767] they may be seen in intimate apposition to alveolar air spaces next to interlobular, pleural, peribronchial, and perivascular connective tissue. These channels have been termed "juxta-alveolar" lymphatics by Lauweryns,[768] because of their close topographic and possible functional relationship to the alveolar lumen, even though they are not part of the interalveolar septa themselves.

Morphologically, the lymphatics can be divided into capillaries and collecting channels.[767] In the normal lung, both are relatively inconspicuous under the light microscope and appear only as small spaces lined by a single layer of flattened endothelial cells. Occasionally, the presence of scattered mural smooth muscle cells or valves marks the presence of a collecting duct. Extensive ultrastructural investigations have been carried out by Lauweryns and associates.[767] The capillary endothelium rests on a discontinuous basement membrane that can be entirely absent for considerable lengths. In some areas the endothelial cells are joined by intercellular junctions, but in others they are entirely free, leaving significant gaps in vascular integrity. Perilymphatic collagen fibers and fine filaments are in close contact with endothelial cells and basement membrane and have been regarded as a tethering mechanism that keeps the capillaries open. These features—endothelial and basement membrane discontinuities and connective tissue anchoring system—appear to be ideal for the provision of easy and continuous access of interstitial fluid to the capillary lumen.

Lymphatic endothelial cells are large and possess central nuclei surrounded by flattened cytoplasmic processes. Many irregular cytoplasmic protrusions extend into the lumen and into the perilymphatic connective tissue. The cytoplasm itself contains inconspicuous mitochondria, endoplasmic reticulum, occasional pinocytotic vesicles, and lysosomes. In addition, there are fairly numerous microfilaments, some of which are thought to constitute an actin-like contractile system that possibly regulates the opening or closing of intercellular gaps.[767] Ultrastructurally, the larger collecting channels differ from the capillaries by having a continuous basement membrane and a more regular endothelium.

Numerous valves 1 to 2 mm apart direct lymph flow in both pleural and intrapulmonary lymphatics. They consist of a connective tissue core covered by a continuous layer of endothelium and apparently are firmly attached to the adjacent connective tissue.[767] Although they appear to be bicuspid in two-dimensional histologic sections, stereomicroscopic studies have shown most to be monocuspid. They have been compared with a funnel in shape; as Lauweryns and Baert have noted,[767] they are well adapted to unidirectional flow since they cannot be inverted but can be easily occluded by flow in an abnormal direction.

The pulmonary lymphatic vessels help clear interstitial fluid from the lungs and remove foreign particles and antigens that have reached the alveoli.[769, 770] Warren and Drinker showed in anesthetized dogs that cessation of ventilation abruptly diminishes flow in mediastinal lymphatics draining lung lymph.[769] The flow of lymph through pulmonary lymphatic channels may depend on a "pumping" action of ventilation,[769, 771] and Fleischner[772] postulated that the "butterfly" pattern of pulmonary edema may be caused by the greater ventilatory excursion of the periphery (cortex) than of the central portion (medulla) of the lung, thereby facilitating clearance of edema fluid from peripheral zones. Hendin and Greenspan[766] studied 15 adult human lungs removed at necropsy in an attempt to assess the influence of ventilation on the movement of contrast medium within pulmonary lymphatics. Ethiodized oil injected into pleural lymphatics filled the deep pulmonary lymphatics; subsequently, when a fixed inflation pressure was maintained, flow did not occur within the lymphatics. Forward flow occurred only during ventilation and appeared to depend on the lung volume at the time the lymphatics were filled. When contrast medium was injected with lung volume maintained at functional residual capacity, forward flow occurred within the lymphatics; by contrast, when filling was obtained at a lung volume of 70 per cent total lung capacity, ventilation resulted in no forward movement of contrast medium within lymphatics. Hendin and Greenspan suggested that this difference is best

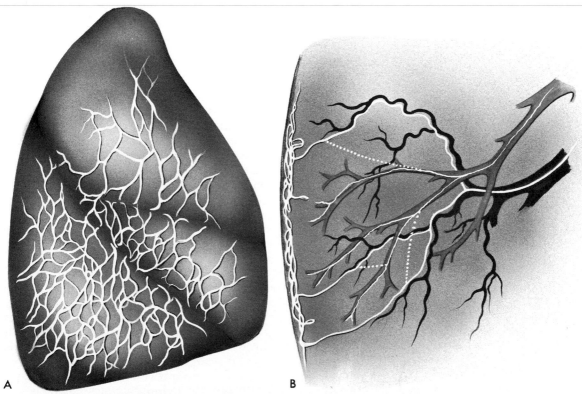

Figure 1–131. The Lymphatic Drainage of the Pleura and Lungs. *A,* A drawing of the lateral aspect of the right lung shows the pleural lymphatics to be much more numerous over the lower half of the lung than over the upper. *B,* In a coronal section through the midportion of the lung, lymphatic channels from the pleura enter the lung at the interlobular septa and extend medially to the hilum along venous radicles (*dark-shaded vessels*); lymphatic channels originating in the peripheral parenchyma extend medially in the bronchovascular bundles (*light-shaded vessels*). Communicating lymphatics (*dotted lines*) extend between the peribronchial and perivenous lymphatics.

explained on the basis of the smaller volume of parenchymal lymphatic segments at high rather than at low lung volumes, reducing the influence of subsequent ventilation. They concluded that ventilatory pumping of lymphatics occurs in the living human lung. It was not determined which lymphatic channels are "pumped."

One year later Hendin,[773] employing similar techniques on six fresh postmortem human lungs, found that the ethiodized oil flowed toward the hilum in all deep lymphatics when lung volume was increased from FRC to 80 per cent total lung capacity (TLC). In four lungs, one or more deep lymphatic segments virtually emptied at 80 per cent TLC, suggesting that ventilation-related constriction of deep lymphatic segments may contribute to pulmonary lymph flow during life.

In many mammals, including human beings, the lung contains abundant lymphoid tissue, often in relation to lymphatic channels. Collections in the vicinity of airways, termed "bronchus-associated lymphoid tissue" by Bienenstock and colleagues[112] have been discussed previously (see page 15). Lymphoid aggregates are also frequently seen within the visceral pleura. Occasionally, intraparenchymal lymphoid nodules are present that resemble lymph nodes and that are large enough to be visualized macroscopically and roentgenographically.[775, 1187] Trapnell found these in 5 of 28 lungs in which he could outline the deep lymphatic channels.[774] It has been suggested that these may represent foci of hyperplastic lymphoid tissue in the interlobular connective tissue.[1187]

THE THORACIC DUCT AND RIGHT LYMPHATIC DUCT

Knowledge of the anatomy of the thoracic duct and the right lymphatic duct is important for a number of reasons. Perhaps the major abnormality to which the thoracic duct is subject is traumatic rupture, and here the roentgenographic manifestations differ according to the anatomic location of the injury. By contrast, the right lymphatic duct seldom is injured, but knowledge of its anatomy is important because it drains the bulk of lymph from both lungs (except for the apical portion of the left lung, which drains into the thoracic duct).[769]

The radiologic anatomy of the *thoracic duct* has been described in detail by Rosenberger and Abrams[776] on the basis of 390 sequential lymphangiograms. It originates at the junction of two lumbar lymphatic trunks, the initial prominent confluence being the cisterna chyli on the anterior aspect of the vertebral column from T12 to L2. (In a similar study by Fuchs and Galeazzi, in 13 per cent of 336 lymphangiograms the cisterna chyli was at the level of T10.[777]) The thoracic duct, which is a continuation of the cisterna chyli, enters the thorax through the aortic hiatus of the diaphragm. In the majority of subjects it lies to the right of the aorta and follows its course cephalad; thus, in the lower portion of the thorax it lies roughly in the midline of the vertebral column or slightly to one side. In patients with a markedly tortuous aorta the duct lies to the left of the spine. At roughly the level of the carina, the duct crosses the left main stem bronchus and runs cephalad in a plane parallel to the left lateral wall of the trachea and slightly posterior to it. In Rosenberger and Abrams' study[776] the distance between the left tracheal wall and the thoracic duct on posteroanterior roentgenograms did not exceed 10 mm in normal subjects, a diameter greater than this indicating lateral displacement by a mediastinal mass. The duct leaves the thorax between the esophagus and left subclavian artery and runs posterior to the left innominate vein; much of the cephalic one third (the cervical portion) is supraclavicular. It joins the venous system most commonly by emptying into the internal jugular vein and sometimes into the subclavian, innominate, and external jugular veins.

In the normal subjects studied by Rosenberger and Abrams[776] the diameter of the thoracic duct ranged widely, from 1 to 7 mm, and thus could not be used as a single determinant of obstruction. Valves were identified within the duct in 84 per cent of cases, primarily in the upper two thirds; a maximum of 13 valves were found. Rosenberger and Abrams also observed several congenital variations in the thoracic duct.

The roentgenologic anatomy of the *right lymphatic duct* has been poorly documented since this vessel cannot be suitably opacified. As described by Abramson,[778] this duct is an inconstant channel: the three trunks—the right jugular, right subclavian, and right mediastinal—often open separately into the jugular, subclavian, and innominate veins, respectively. Unfortunately, collecting lymph from the right lymphatic duct can be exceedingly difficult, because it may consist of multiple fine vessels or a network instead of a single channel. This anatomic peculiarity hampered studies of the lymphatics in experimental disease states until 1959, when Leeds and his colleagues[779] described a simple, reliable method for collecting lymph from the multichannel right lymphatic duct in dogs. By creating an artificial chamber from the external jugular vein near the entrance of the multiple small lymphatic vessels, they collected all lymph flowing through these channels without interfering with blood flow through the vein. Since developing this ingenious technique these investigators have reported several studies in dogs, determining the role of the lymphatics in acute and chronic pulmonary edema[780-782] and following irradiation of the lungs;[783] the conclusions derived from these studies are discussed in appropriate sections of this book.

LYMPH NODES OF THE MEDIASTINUM

A thorough knowledge of the pulmonary and pleural lymphatic system, as described in the previous section, is obviously important to the physician in the understanding of the pathophysiologic mechanisms underlying many pleuropulmonary diseases such as pulmonary edema and pleural effusion. However, lymphatics *per se* are not visible roentgenographically, whereas the intrathoracic repository of the pleuropulmonary conduits, the hilar and mediastinal lymph nodes, are discernible, particularly when enlarged. Indeed, involvement of the hilar and mediastinal lymph nodes is a common and often diagnostically important feature of disease arising within the thorax; furthermore, individual patterns of lymph node involvement can supply an important clue to the origin or nature of diseases originating both within and outside the thorax.

Although lymph nodes are widely distributed throughout the mediastinum, the number of normal nodes has not been well studied. Beck and Beattie reported that the average number of mediastinal lymph nodes in five autopsied patients was 64; 80 per cent were situated in relation to the trachea, carina, and main bronchi.[784] On the other hand, the general organization of mediastinal and hilar lymph nodes has been thoroughly described by several observers, and various classifications have been proposed, including those of Rouvière,[785] Heitzman,[786, 787] Yamashita,[788] and the Subcommittee on Anatomic Definitions of the American Thoracic Society Committee on Lung Cancer Staging and Reporting.[789] The multiplicity of schemes is eloquent testimony to the difficulty that both anatomists and radiologists have had in wrestling with the problem of lymph node classification.

In most individuals, the majority of mediastinal nodes relate to the right and left innominate veins, the anterior and anterolateral aspects of the trachea, the circumference of the main bronchi, and beneath and to the left of the aortic arch. In earlier editions of this textbook, the anatomy of mediastinal lymph nodes was divided into the three major compartments: anterior, middle, and posterior; however, since certain lymph node chains reside in more than one compartment and since lymphatic drainage from the lungs to these nodes is intricate and only generally predictable, this approach will be abandoned for a more practical description.

According to Leigh and Weens,[790] intrathoracic lymph nodes are composed of *parietal* and *visceral* components; the former reside outside the parietal pleura in extramediastinal tissue where they drain the thoracic wall and other extrathoracic structures, whereas the latter are located within the mediastinum between the pleural membranes and are concerned particularly with the drainage of the intrathoracic tissues.

The Parietal Lymph Nodes

The parietal lymph nodes are divided into three groups.

1. The *anterior parietal* or *internal mammary* nodes are located in the upper thorax behind the anterior intercostal spaces bilaterally, either medial or lateral to the internal mammary vessels (Fig. 1–132). They receive afferent channels from the upper anterior abdominal wall, anterior thoracic wall, anterior portion of the diaphragm, and the medial portion of the breasts. These lymph nodes communicate with the visceral group of the anterior mediastinal nodes and the cervical nodes; their main efferent channel is the right lymphatic duct or thoracic duct.

2. The *posterior parietal* lymph nodes relate to the rib heads in the posterior intercostal spaces (*intercostal nodes*) and to the vertebrae (*juxtavertebral nodes*) (Fig. 1–133). Both groups drain the intercostal spaces, parietal pleura, and vertebral column. They communicate with other posterior mediastinal lymph nodes that relate to the descending aorta and the esophagus. Efferent channels drain to the thoracic duct in the upper thorax and to the cisterna chyli in the lower thoracic area.

3. The *diaphragmatic* lymph nodes (Fig. 1–134) are composed of the *anterior* (*prepericardiac*) group that is located immediately behind the xiphoid and to the right and left of the pericardium anteriorly; the *middle* (*juxtaphrenic*) group that is located in relation to the phrenic nerves as they meet the diaphragm; and the *posterior* (*retrocrural*) nodes that reside behind the right and left crura of the diaphragm. The diaphragmatic nodes drain the diaphragm and the anterosuperior portion of the liver.

The Visceral Lymph Nodes

The visceral lymph nodes are also divided into three chains.

1. The *anterosuperior mediastinal* (*prevascular*) nodes are congregated along the anterior aspect of the superior vena cava, right and left innominate veins, and ascending aorta (Fig. 1–135). A few nodes are situated posterior to the sternum in the lower thorax while a similar number reside behind the manubrium anterior to the thymus. These nodes drain most of the structures in the anterior mediastinum, including the pericardium, thymus, thyroid, diaphragmatic and mediastinal pleura, part of the heart, and the anterior portion of the hila. Efferent channels drain into the right lymphatic or thoracic duct.

2. The *posterior mediastinal* lymph nodes (Fig. 1–136) are located around the esophagus (*periesophageal nodes*) and along the anterior and lateral aspects of the descending aorta (*periaortic*

Text continued on page 187

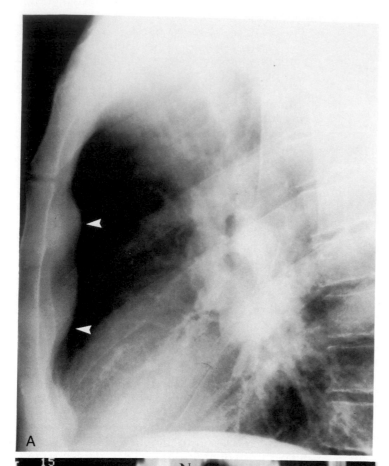

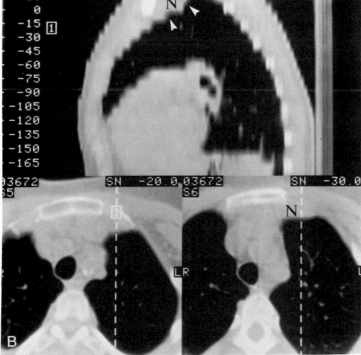

Figure 1–132. Enlargement of Internal Mammary Lymph Nodes. *A,* A detail view from a conventional lateral chest roentgenogram reveals a smooth, lobulated, homogeneous soft tissue opacity (*arrowheads*) in the retrosternal area caused by enlargement of the anterior parietal (internal mammary) lymph nodes. No abnormality was discernible on a conventional posteroanterior projection. The patient is a middle-aged man with Hodgkin's disease. In *B* are a reformatted sagittal CT scan (*top*) and corresponding transverse images (*bottom*) of a patient with metastatic breast adenocarcinoma. Note the typical semilunar configuration (*arrowheads*) of the enlarged internal mammary nodes (*N*).

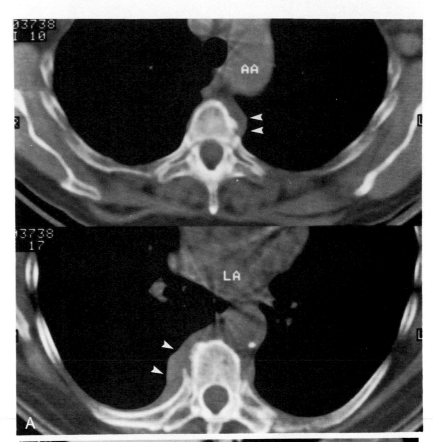

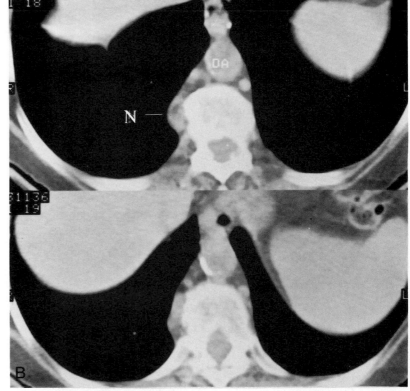

Figure 1–133. Enlargement of Posterior Parietal Lymph Nodes. *A*, Transverse CT scans through the aortic arch (*AA, top*) and left atrium (*LA, bottom*) show lobulated masses related primarily to the costovertebral junctions (*arrowheads*). These features represent enlargement of the posterior parietal (intercostal) nodes in this patient with Hodgkin's disease. *B*, CT scans through the lower thorax of a patient with non-Hodgkin's lymphoma show enlargement of the juxtavertebral nodes (*N*). DA, descending aorta.

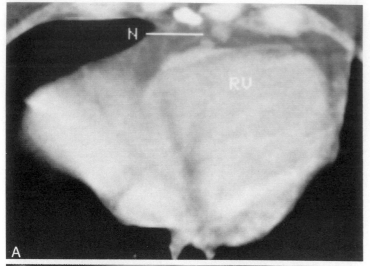

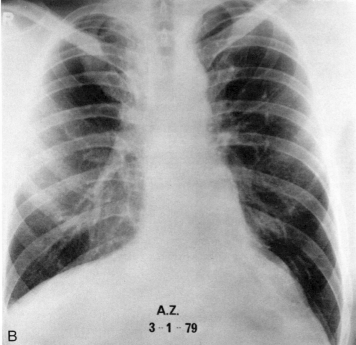

Figure 1–134. Enlargement of Diaphragmatic Lymph Nodes. *A,* In this CT scan, the anterior (preparacardiac) group is located immediately behind the xiphoid and anterior to the right ventricle (*RV*) and the pericardium. There is only slight enlargement of the nodes (*N*) in this young patient with Hodgkin's disease; even massive involvement of this group is sometimes undetectable by conventional roentgenographic means. *B,* A posteroanterior chest roentgenogram of a 26-year-old man with Hodgkin's disease reveals the cardiophrenic angles to be blunted and the right and left hemidiaphragms to be abnormally contoured, suggesting enlargement of the right and left preparacardiac chains of nodes. However, distinction from prominent epicardial fat pads cannot be determined with certainty without a CT scan. *C,* A CT scan of the patient depicted in *B* confirms the presence of enlarged nodes (*N*) anterior and lateral to the right ventricle (*RV*). Note that the enlarged nodes and the heart are isodense.

Illustration continued on opposite page

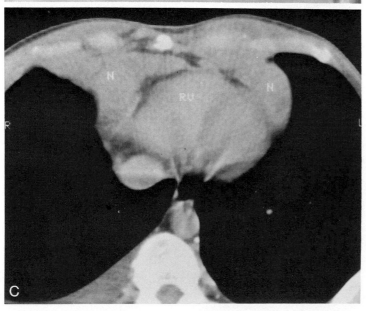

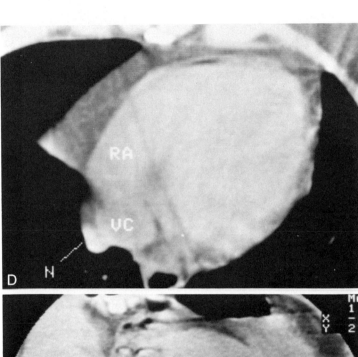

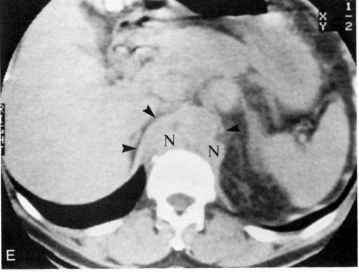

Figure 1–134 *Continued.* *D,* In a 40-year-old man with histiocytic lymphoma, a CT scan through the lower thorax reveals enlargement of the middle (juxtaphrenic) nodes (*N*). Note the relationship of this nodal group to the inferior vena cava (*VC*) and right atrium (*RA*). *E,* Posterior (retrocrural) lymph node enlargement (*N*) is present on the CT scan of this 60-year-old man with metastatic adenocarcinoma of the left kidney. The crura (*arrowheads*) are displaced laterally by the enlarged nodes.

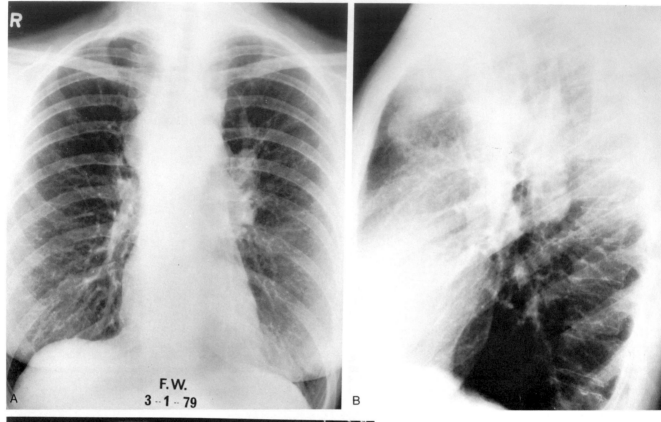

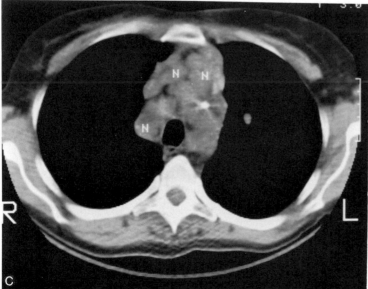

Figure 1–135. Enlargement of the Anterior (Prevascular) Group of Mediastinal Nodes. Conventional posteroanterior (*A*) and lateral (*B*) roentgenograms show a widened and lobulated contour to the upper mediastinal silhouette, best appreciated on the frontal projection. *C*, A CT scan through the superior mediastinum confirms the presence of the enlarged nodes (*N*) and reveals their intimate relationship to the great vessels. The patient is a middle-aged woman with metastatic pulmonary carcinoma.

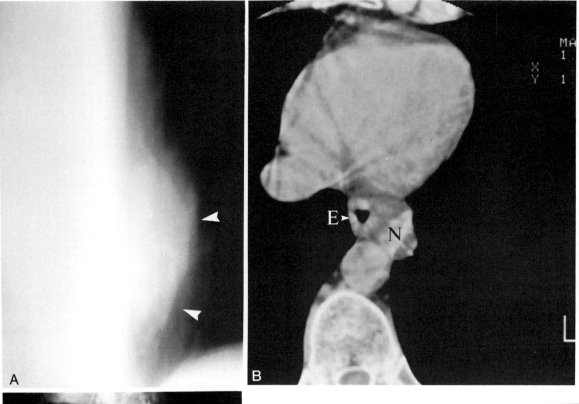

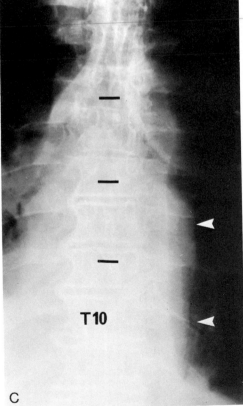

Figure 1–136. Enlargement of Posterior Mediastinal Lymph Nodes. *A*, A conventional anteroposterior tomogram through the posterior mediastinum reveals a soft tissue opacity (*arrowheads*) with extrapleural characteristics that obliterates a portion of the para-aortic line. Note that the paraspinal line is intact. *B*, A CT scan confirms the presence of node enlargement in a periesophageal node (*N*) (the patient had metastatic carcinoma from the lower esophagus). The esophagus (*E*) is distended with air. *C*, An anteroposterior view of the thoracic spine of a patient with periaortic mediastinal lymphoma and pleural effusion reveals slight lobulation of the descending aorta (*arrowheads*). The mediastinum was studied by CT at the levels indicated by the bars.

Illustration continued on following page

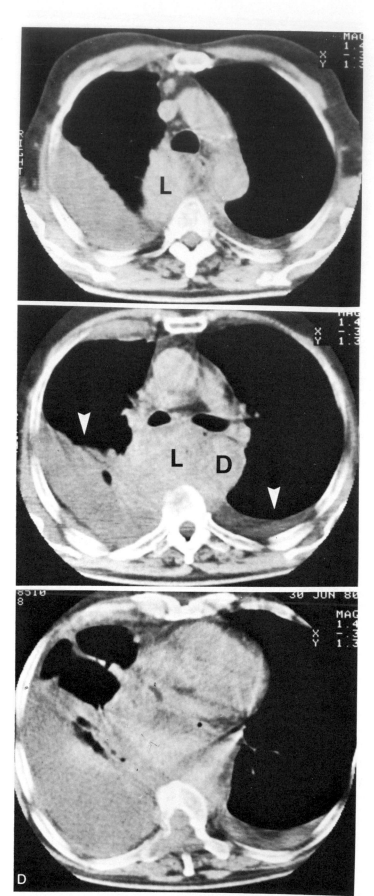

Figure 1–136 *Continued. D*, Unenhanced scans show that the descending aorta (*D*) is isodense with and enveloped by extensive posterior mediastinal lymphoma (*L*), representing massive enlargement of the periaortic nodes. Bilateral pleural effusions are present (*arrowheads*). (*C* and *D* from Genereux GP: AJR *141*:141, 1983. © American Roentgen Ray Society.)

nodes); they are most numerous in the lower portion of the thorax. Their afferent channels arise from the posterior portion of the diaphragm, the pericardium, the esophagus, and directly from the lower lobes of the lungs via the right and left inferior pulmonary ligaments. They communicate with the tracheobronchial nodes, particularly the subcarinal group, and drain chiefly via the thoracic duct.

3. The third and most important member of the visceral nodes is the *tracheobronchial* group. The *paratracheal* lymph nodes (Fig. 1–137) are located in front and to the right and left of the trachea; occasionally, a retrotracheal component is present. The right paratracheal chain is usually the best developed; its lowermost member, the azygos node, is situated medial to the azygos vein arch in the pretracheal mediastinal fat. These lymph nodes receive afferent channels from the bronchopulmonary and tracheal bifurcation

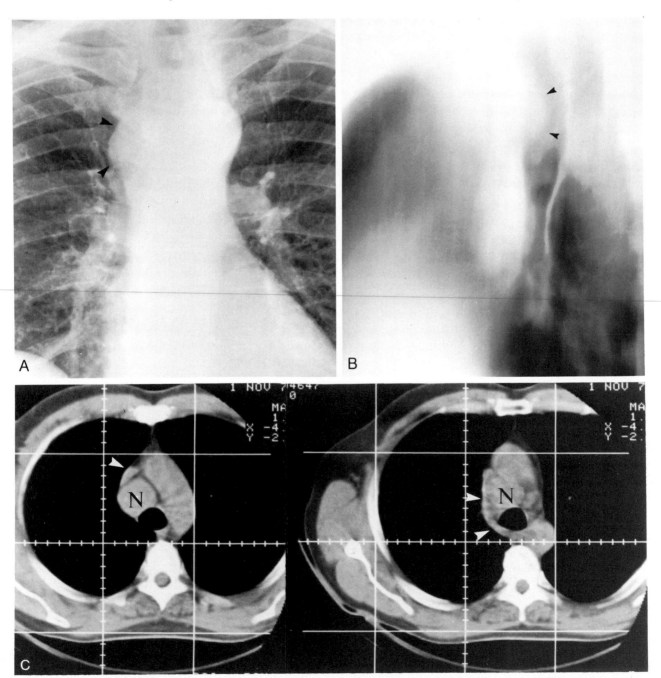

Figure 1–137. Enlargement of the Paratracheal Nodes. A posteroanterior chest roentgenogram (*A*) and conventional lateral tomogram (*B*) reveal an abnormal contour of the mediastinum (*arrowheads*) in the right tracheobronchial angle. Note that the posterior boundary of the mass on the lateral tomogram (*arrowheads*) does not extend behind an imagined coronal plane through the trachea as would be anticipated with enlargement of the azygos vein. *C*, CT scans in this patient reveal the mass to be an enlarged azygos lymph node (*N*) caused by metastatic anaplastic carcinoma from the lung. The superior vena cava (*arrowhead*) is displaced anteriorly and the azygos vein (*two arrowheads*) laterally.

nodes, the trachea, the esophagus, and directly from the right and left lungs without diversion through the bronchopulmonary or tracheal bifurcation nodes. Direct communication also exists with the anterior and posterior visceral mediastinal nodes. The efferent channels are the right lymphatic and thoracic ducts. The lymph nodes of the *tracheal bifurcation*, or carina (Fig. 1–138), are situated in the precarinal and subcarinal fatty compartments, as well as around the circumference of the right and left main bronchi. On the left, the nodes that are located in mediastinal fat between the left pulmonary artery and aortic arch are usually designated *aortopulmonary window* nodes (Fig. 1–139); these are arranged into medial, lateral (subpleural), and superior compartments and merge above with the left prevascular chain. Carinal lymph nodes receive afferent drainage from the bronchopulmonary nodes, anterior and posterior mediastinal nodes, heart, pericardium, esophagus, and lungs. Efferent drainage is to the paratracheal group, particularly the right-sided component. The *bronchopulmonary* or *hilar* lymph nodes (Fig. 1–140) are numerous but are normally too small to be detected by conventional or CT studies (*see* further on). They are located around the bronchi and vessels, particularly at their points of division. They receive afferent channels from all lobes of the lungs; their efferent drainage is to the carinal and paratracheal nodes. Lymph nodes located within the right and left inferior pulmonary ligaments (Fig. 1–141) are often included as components of the lower hilar lymph node chain.

Imaging Methods in the Evaluation of Mediastinal and Hilar Lymph Nodes

Posteroanterior and lateral chest roentgenograms suffice for the identification of gross hilar and mediastinal lymph node enlargement. However, lesser degrees of enlargement in both areas are more appropriately evaluated by CT. We feel that conventional linear tomography should be restricted to evaluation of the right paratracheal and subcarinal regions and the aortopulmonary window; consensus holds that CT is the preferred method for study of mediastinal nodes.[791-794] Although several investigators prefer conventional tomography over CT in the evaluation of pulmonary hila,[791, 793-799] and while we agree that conventional tomography is adequate for *screening* purposes, we believe that as radiologists become more familiar with hilar anatomy in the transverse plane they will find that CT is at least as sensitive and specific as linear tomography, a view recently supported by Glazer and his colleagues.[800]

One of the most important advances that CT has made in the investigation of thoracic disease is the ability to image such structures as small mediastinal lymph nodes (Fig. 1–142). Although conventional tomography can demonstrate gross lymph node enlargement, it suffers from being unable to distinguish the variable tissue densities within the mediastinum, especially fat and soft tissue. Since adipose tissue is so ubiquitous within the mediastinum and is usually abundant, pathologically enlarged lymph nodes ranging in diameter from 20 to 30 mm can be completely enveloped by fat and therefore invisible on conventional studies. Both CT and magnetic resonance imaging easily resolve this difficulty; and as a consequence, emphasis in the following discussion will be on the CT depiction of mediastinal lymph nodes.

The reported range in size of normal lymph nodes visible on a CT scan varies considerably. Rea and his colleagues[801] have stated that normal mediastinal lymph nodes are not visible, whereas Baron and his associates[802] reported that nodes are normal if less than 10 mm in diameter and abnormal if greater than 20 mm; measurements ranging from 10 to 20 mm were considered indeterminate. Osborne and his colleagues[791] suggested that a lymph node was normal if it measured less than 7 mm in diameter, whereas others have increased this figure to 11 mm[792, 803, 804] and 15 mm.[797] Schnyder and Gamsu[805] limited their evaluation to the pretracheal space and indicated that lymph nodes larger than 10 to 11 mm in diameter were suspicious whereas those larger than 15 mm should be considered abnormal. Shevland,[806] Underwood,[807] Mitzer,[793] Hirleman,[794] and their respective colleagues provided no data concerning the size criterion of normality in patients undergoing staging for pulmonary carcinoma.

Genereux and Howie[808] carried out a combined autopsy and CT study that was designed to evaluate the size, number, and location of normal mediastinal lymph nodes. These researchers divided the mediastinum into four zones that related to the left innominate vein, the pretracheal space and right tracheobronchial angle, the precarinal/subcarinal compartment, and the aortopulmonary window. These divisions, designated zones I to IV, were chosen to conform to areas that are most accessible to cervical mediastinoscopy or parasternal mediastinotomy.

ZONE I: RETROINNOMINATE SPACE

The left innominate vein courses downward and to the right in front of the innominate artery to join the right innominate vein to form the superior vena cava. It separates anterior and posterior compartments, but since the sometimes speckled pattern of the normal adult thymus in the anterior compartment[809] can be confused with small anterosuperior mediastinal lymph nodes, the investigators chose to exclude the anterior compartment from consideration. The posterior compartment or retroinnominate space is bounded anteriorly by the

Text continued on page 194

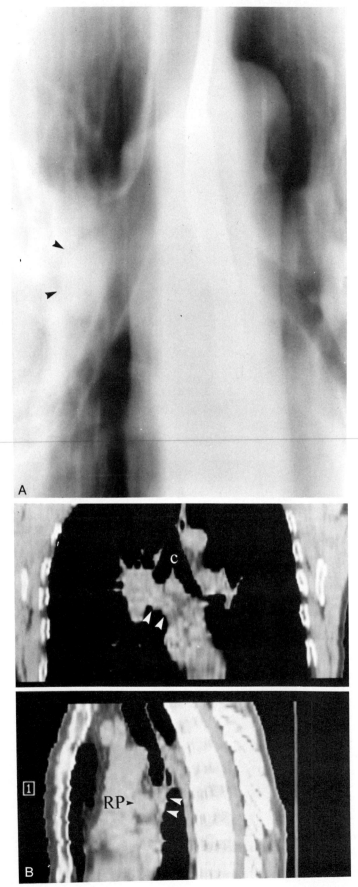

Figure 1–138. Enlargement of the Tracheal Bifurcation Nodes. *A,* A conventional anteroposterior tomogram with barium in the esophagus shows no convincing mediastinal abnormality (55-year-old man with a partly occluding right upper lobe pulmonary carcinoma). The opacity contiguous with the intermediate bronchus is an enlarged hilar lymph node (*arrowheads*). *B,* Coronal (*top*) and sagittal (*bottom*) CT reformations through the carina (*C*) reveal lymph node enlargement (*arrowheads*) in the precarinal/subcarinal compartment of the superior azygoesophageal recess. Note that these nodes lie above and behind the right pulmonary artery (*RP*). Enlargement of the precarinal lymph nodes is commonly undetectable by conventional roentgenographic means; deformity of the barium-enhanced esophagus implies an abnormality in the subcarinal component.

Illustration continued on following page

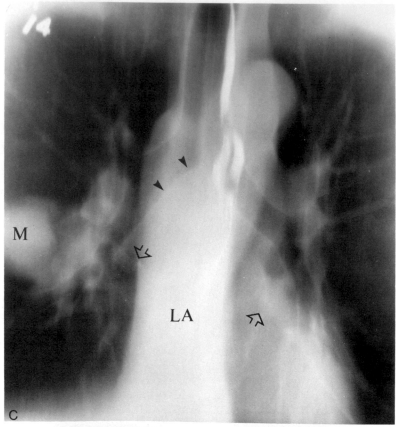

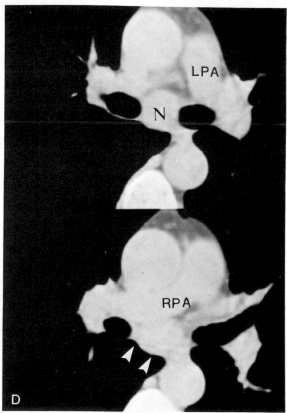

Figure 1–138 *Continued. C,* A conventional anteroposterior tomogram in another patient with primary carcinoma of the middle lobe (*M*) reveals a soft tissue opacity above the insertion of the inferior pulmonary veins (*open arrows*) into the left atrium (*LA*), compression and displacement of the barium-filled esophagus to the left, and minimal upward displacement of the right main bronchus (*arrowheads*), constituting the important features of subcarinal lymph node enlargement. *D,* CT scans through the carina (*top*) and 2 cm caudad (*bottom*) show the abnormal mass in the patient depicted in *C* to be enlarged nodes (*N*) in the precarinal/subcarinal compartment. Note that the normal concavity of the azygoesophageal recess interface at this level has been obliterated by the convex nodal mass (*arrowheads*). *RPA,* right pulmonary artery; *LPA,* left pulmonary artery. (*C* from Genereux GP: AJR *141*:141, 1983. © American Roentgen Ray Society.)

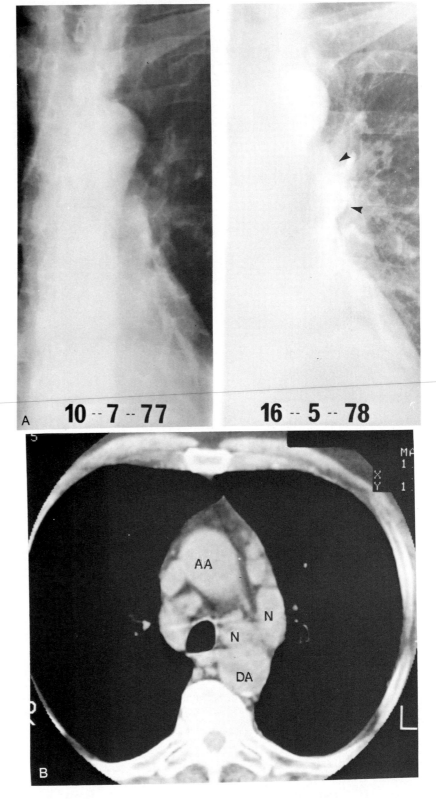

Figure 1–139. Enlargement of the Aortopulmonary Nodes. *A*, Detail views of the left hilar region from posteroanterior chest roentgenograms before (*left*) and after (*right*) involvement of the aortopulmonary lymph nodes by Hodgkin's disease in a middle-aged man. Note the typical lobulated contour (*arrowheads*) between the aortic arch and main pulmonary artery. *B*, A CT scan confirms the presence of numerous enlarged nodes (*N*) in the aortopulmonary window. *AA*, ascending aorta; *DA*, descending aorta.

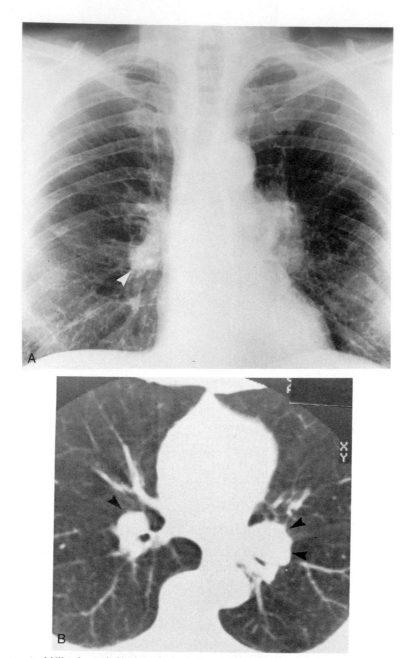

Figure 1–140. Enlargement of Hilar Lymph Nodes. *A*, A posteroanterior chest roentgenogram in this middle-aged man reveals an enlarged, lobulated left hilum; the right inferior hilum shows a focal increase in density (*arrowhead*). These features are consistent with bilateral hilar node enlargement. *B*, A transverse CT scan through the lower hila confirms the presence of bilateral node enlargement (*arrowheads*). Metastatic small cell carcinoma of the lung.

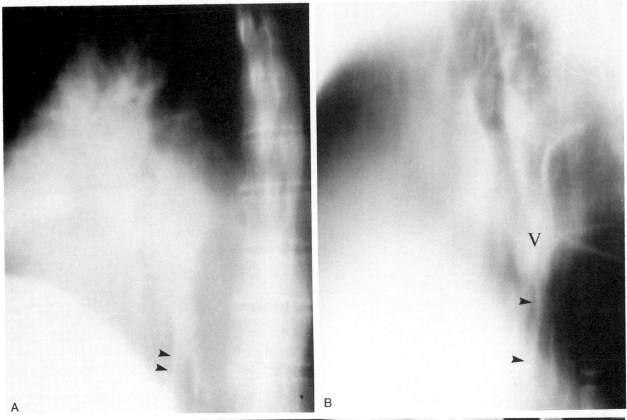

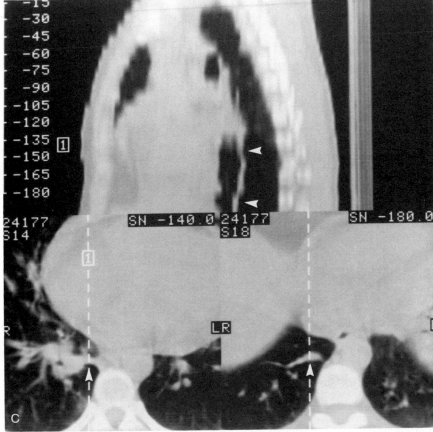

Figure 1–141. Enlargement of Nodes in the Right Pulmonary Ligament. Conventional right 55° oblique (A) and right lateral (B) tomograms reveal an abnormal vertically oriented linear opacity (*arrowheads*) extending from the inferior pulmonary vein (V) to the diaphragm. The appearance is consistent with a thickened intersublobar septum of the pulmonary ligament. C, A reformatted sagittal CT scan (*top*) and representative transverse scans (*bottom*) confirm the presence of thickening of the interlobar septum of the right pulmonary ligament (*arrowheads*). Metastatic pulmonary carcinoma; the primary tumor resided in the right upper hilum.

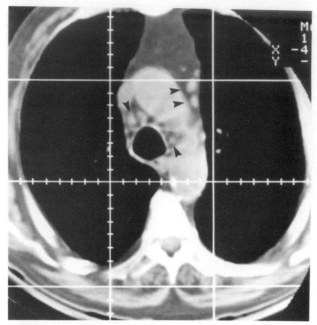

Figure 1–142. CT Depiction of Lymph Nodes of Normal Size in the Pretracheal Space, Aortopulmonary Window, and Anterosuperior Mediastinum. Individual lymph nodes as small as 5 to 10 mm (*arrowheads*) are readily discernible. Patient is a 60-year-old man with chronic bronchitis. (*See* Figures 1–143 to 1–146 for description of these anatomic compartments.)

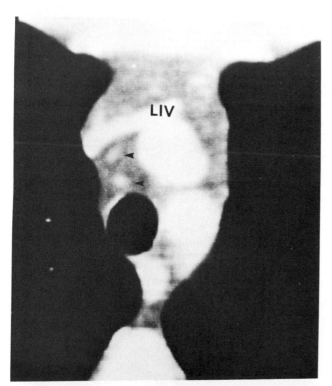

Figure 1–143. The Retroinnominate Space (Zone I). The left innominate vein (*LIV*) divides the superior mediastinum into an anterior and a posterior compartment; the latter, the retroinnominate space, constitutes the primary area of interest. Two small lymph nodes (*arrowheads*) are depicted in the illustration. (From Genereux GP, Howie JL: AJR *142*:1095, 1984. © American Roentgen Ray Society.)

left innominate vein, posteriorly by the trachea, medially by the innominate artery, and laterally by the pleura (Fig. 1–143).

ZONE II: PRETRACHEAL SPACE

This space or compartment is bounded anteriorly by the superior vena cava, posteriorly by the trachea, medially by the ascending aorta, and laterally by the distal portion of the azygos vein arch (Fig. 1–144).

The pretracheal-retrocaval space was studied in detail by Schnyder and Gamsu in 127 normal subjects.[805] Its surface area increased in size with mediastinal adiposity and subject age, and to a lesser extent with elongation of the thoracic aorta; in patients aged 20 to 35 years, the surface area was 146.5 mm^2, a value that more than doubled, to 313.7 mm^2, in patients over 66 years of age.

In the 127 patients in the Schnyder and Gamsu study, a total of 160 lymph nodes were counted with a mean diameter of 5.5 mm ($\pm$ 2.8 mm SD). The average diameter increased from 4.8 mm in patients aged 20 to 35 years to 6.6 mm in patients over 66 years of age. Only 3 of the 160 lymph nodes were larger than 11 mm, and the investigators concluded that nodes larger than 10 to 11 mm should be viewed with extreme suspicion, and that nodes larger than 15 mm should be considered definitely abnormal.

ZONE III: PRECARINAL/SUBCARINAL COMPARTMENT

This compartment is formed by two intercommunicating areas that are partly separated by the right pulmonary artery. One is the *precarinal* space, bounded by the ascending aorta anteriorly, the carina posteriorly, the left pulmonary artery on the left, the truncus anterior on the right, the pretracheal space superiorly, and the right pulmonary artery inferiorly (Fig. 1–145). The precarinal space merges imperceptibly with the aortopulmonary window on the left and the pretracheal space above and to the right. The other is the *subcarinal* space, bounded by the ascending aorta anteriorly, the esophagus posteriorly, the right and left lower lobe mediastinal pleura laterally, the right pulmonary artery superiorly, and the top of the left atrium inferiorly (Fig. 1–145).

ZONE IV: AORTOPULMONARY WINDOW

The boundaries of this space are the aortic arch superiorly, the left pulmonary artery inferiorly, the ascending aorta anteriorly, the descending aorta (at a distance) posteriorly, the left main bronchus inferomedially, and the left upper lobe mediastinal pleura laterally (Fig. 1–146)

Attention to CT imaging technique, preferably under radiologist supervision, is essential for proper evaluation of both the mediastinum and hila. Scans

Text continued on page 199

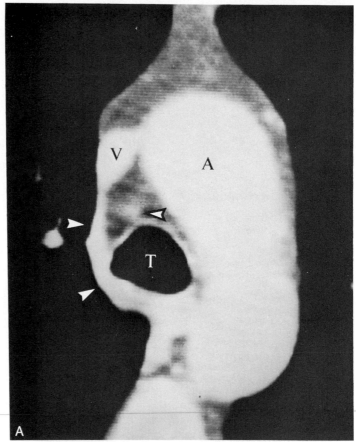

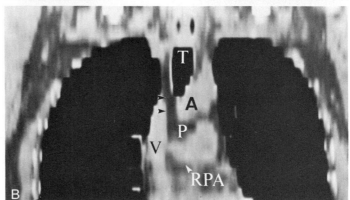

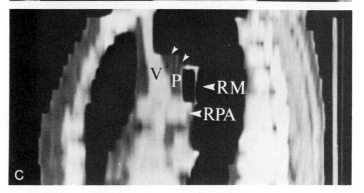

Figure 1–144. The Pretracheal Space (Zone II). *A,* On a CT scan, the triangular pretracheal space is bordered by the ascending aorta (*A*), trachea (*T*), azygos arch (*two arrowheads*), and superior vena cava (*V*). A single lymph node of normal size (*arrowhead*) is shown. Coronal (*B*) and sagittal (*C*) reformations depict the relation of the pretracheal space (*arrowheads*) to the vena cava (*V*) and trachea (*T*). The pretracheal space merges below with fat in the precarinal space (*P*) anterior to the right main bronchus (*RM*) and above the right pulmonary artery (*RPA*). (From Genereux GP, Howie JL: AJR *142*:1095, 1984. © American Roentgen Ray Society.)

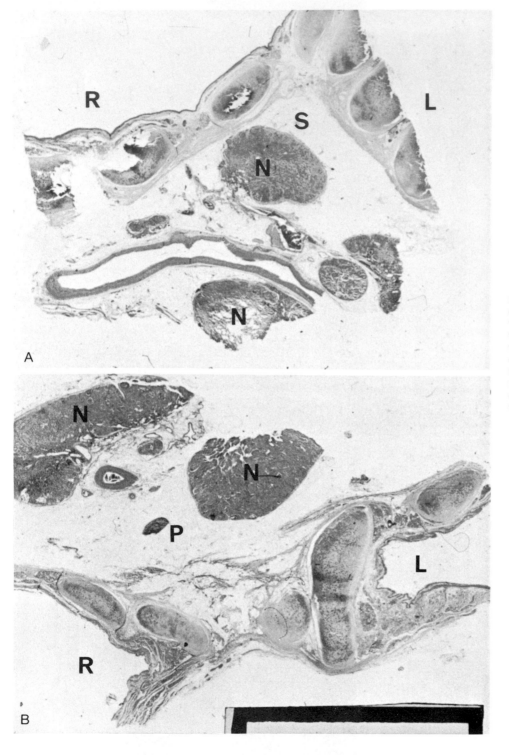

Illustration continued on
opposite page

Figure 1–145. The Precarinal/Subcarinal Compartment (Zone III). Coronal (*A*) and transverse (*B*) anatomic sections through the carina from two autopsied patients show the location of normal-sized lymph nodes (*N*) in the subcarinal (*S*) and precarinal (*P*) fat. *R*, right main bronchus; *L*, left main bronchus. Centimeter scale is depicted in *B*.

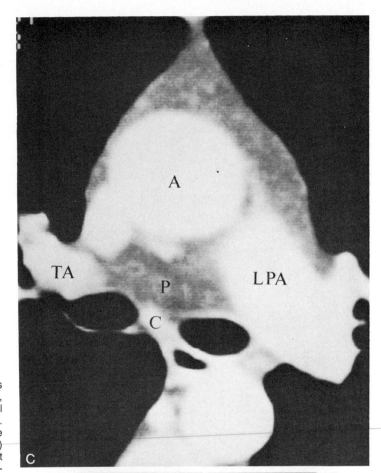

Figure 1–145 *Continued*. *C*, A transverse scan shows that the left pulmonary artery (*LPA*), ascending aorta (*A*), carina (*C*), and truncus anterior (*TA*) enclose the precarinal (*P*) area. No lymph nodes are identified in this patient. Coronal (*D*) and sagittal (*E*) CT reformations demonstrate the anatomic features of the percarinal (*P*) and subcarinal (*S*) compartments. This fat-containing area relates to the left atrium (*LA*), right pulmonary artery (*RPA*), esophagus (*arrowheads*), carina (*C*), and ascending aorta (*A*). (From Genereux GP, Howie JL: AJR *142*:1095, 1984. © American Roentgen Ray Society.)

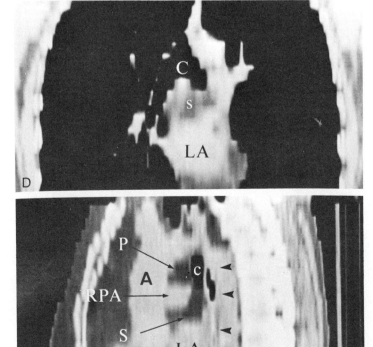

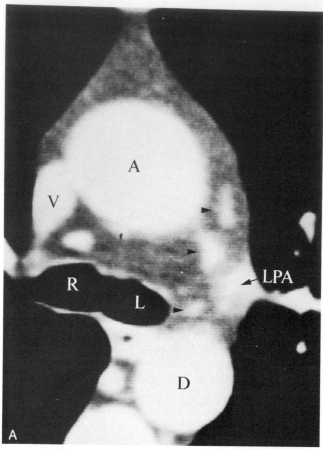

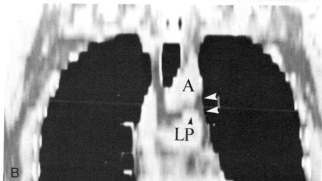

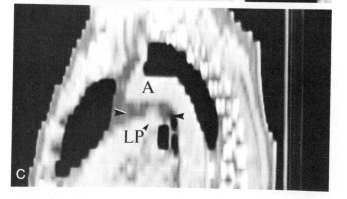

Figure 1–146. The Aortopulmonary Window (Zone IV). *A,* A transverse CT scan through the aortopulmonary window reveals medial, lateral, and superior groups of lymph nodes (*arrowheads*). The space lies beneath the aortic arch (*A*) and above the top of the left pulmonary artery (*LPA*). Partial volume averaging through the top of the left pulmonary artery may be confused with lymph nodes. Ascending aorta (*A*), descending aorta (*D*), superior vena cava (*V*), and right (*R*) and left (*L*) main bronchi are shown. Note continuity with precarinal space in front of the main bronchi. Coronal (*B*) and sagittal (*C*) CT reformations demonstrate the anatomic features of the aortopulmonary window (*arrowheads*). *A,* aortic arch; *LP,* left pulmonary artery. (From Genereux GP, Howie JL: AJR *142*:1095, 1984. © American Roentgen Ray Society.)

should initially by obtained without contrast medium enhancement, using 5 or 10 mm collimation, 10 mm apart, from the suprasternal notch to the top of the diaphragm in the supine position during suspended full inspiration. The images may be viewed using a minimal magnification factor (e.g., 1.5×) and lymph nodes counted and measured, the latter with the addition of superimposed grid scale. A window width of 500 or 600 Hounsfield units (HU) with the window level adjusted to yield the greatest subjective visual clarity (commonly in the +50 to −75 HU range) is appropriate. It is our feeling that most clinical problems can be resolved using this methodology, but the addition of dynamic CT scans following a bolus injection of intravenous contrast medium (e.g., four rapid-sequence scans at each level of interest; 4.8 sec scan time; 1.4 sec interscan delay) has been recommended in difficult situations.[810]

The CT criteria by which a lymph node may be identified consist of a round or oval structure of soft tissue density, with or without central or eccentric radiolucent fat, in a location that does not conform to vascular or neural elements. The presence of mediastinal fat greatly facilitates the CT depiction of lymph nodes, a capability not present on conventional tomography. Foci of calcification or lymphangiographic contrast medium can serve as a more obvious marker for lymph node identification.

The size of normal mediastinal lymph nodes in 12 cadavers in the Genereux and Howie study[808] is detailed in Table 1–6. The average size in the four zones was 12.6 × 8.3 mm (length × width), corresponding closely to the measurements from the CT portion of the study (see further on). However, lymph nodes were identified at autopsy that were clearly larger than any CT measurement in this or previous studies.[791, 792, 797, 802, 803, 805, 806] The probable explanation for this discrepancy is the tendency for lymph nodes to be oriented vertically along their long axis; thus, the transverse plane of the CT scan generally records the width (short axis) and not the length (long axis) of most lymph nodes. On the other hand, the pathologist logically measures the greatest dimension, which is usually the length.

The relevant CT data pertaining to lymph node size in the Genereux and Howie study[808] are detailed in Table 1–7 and Figure 1–147. In zone I, there

Table 1–6. Normal Mediastinal Lymph Nodes at Autopsy

ZONE	NUMBER OF PATIENTS	NORMAL SIZE (LENGTH × WIDTH) (mm)	
		Mean	*Range*
I	4*	6.2 × 3.5	8 × 3
II	12	13.3 × 9.2	30 × 5
III	12	20.0 × 13.9	30 × 7
IV	12	11.2 × 6.6	15 × 4

*Eight patients had nonencapsulated lymphoid tissue that could not be measured. (From Genereux GP, Howie JL: Am J Roentgenol *142*:1095, 1984.)

Table 1–7. Size of Normal Mediastinal Lymph Nodes by Zone

LYMPH NODE SIZE (mm)	NUMBER OF LYMPH NODES				TOTAL NODES	% NODES BY SIZE
	I	II	III	IV		
16–20	0	0	1	1	2	0.9
11–15	0	3	2	5	10	4.4
6–10	5	29	34	30	98	43.5
1–5	67	26	4	18	115	51.1

(From Genereux GP, Howie JL: Am J Roentgenol *142*:1095, 1984.)

were no lymph nodes larger than 10 mm in transverse diameter, and 93 per cent were smaller than 6 mm. In zones II, III, and IV, lymph nodes less than 11 mm in diameter accounted for 95, 93, and 89 per cent, respectively. No lymph node in any zone exceeded 20 mm in diameter, although 2.4 per cent of nodes in zone III and 1.8 per cent in zone IV measured 16 to 20 mm. *Of the 225 lymph nodes from all zones, 94.6 per cent were smaller than 11 mm, 4.4 per cent were 11 to 15 mm in diameter, and 0.9 per cent measured 16 to 20 mm.*

There was a distinct tendency for lymph nodes to vary in size according to their location within the mediastinum (Table 1–8 and Fig. 1–138). For example, in zone I only 7 per cent of nodes measured more than 5 mm in diameter, whereas in zones II, III, and IV, 55, 90, and 67 per cent of nodes, respectively, were larger than 5 mm. Consequently, whereas a lymph node measuring 11 to 15 mm is an appropriate size for zones II to IV, it is an inappropriate dimension for zone I.

Schnyder and Gamsu[805] found that in the pretracheal space, lymph nodes were visible in 88 per cent of normal subjects and were multiple in 30 per cent. These findings correspond very closely with the zone II data in the Genereux and Howie study in which nodes were identified in 87 per cent of patients and were multiple in 41 per cent (Table 1–8 and Fig. 1–148). Zones III and IV were the most

Table 1–8. Number of Normal Mediastinal Lymph Nodes by Zone

NUMBER OF LYMPH NODES PER CT SLICE	NUMBER OF PATIENTS BY ZONE				TOTAL ZONES	% ZONES BY NUMBER OF NODES
	I	II	III	IV		
6	0	0	0	1	1	0.6
5	0	0	0	0	0	
4	2	2	1	1	6	3.8
3	8	4	0	7	19	12.2
2	13	10	13	8	44	28.2
1	14	18	11	7	50	32.0
0	2	5	14	15	36	23.0
Total zones	39	39	39	39	156	
Total nodes	72	58	41	54		
Average number of nodes per zone	1.8	1.5	1.0	1.4		

(From Genereux GP, Howie JL: Am J Roentgenol *142*:1095, 1984.)

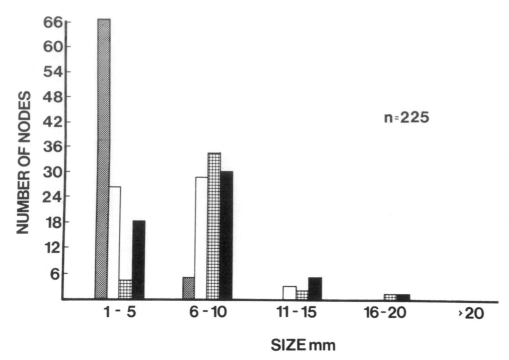

n=225

common areas in which no lymphoid tissue was detected on CT, in 35.8 and 38.5 per cent of patients, respectively. These results are at variance with the findings at autopsy where 100 per cent of patients had lymph nodes in zones II, III, and IV; this discrepancy is most likely related to the technique of CT examination (10 mm collimation, single slice selection for analysis) that can create apparent "gaps" in lymph node continuity. The autopsy material, however, involved dissection of the entire area, thus eliminating the potential error inherent in the CT methodology. In clinical practice, lymph nodes larger than 15 mm would not likely be overlooked with the CT scanning technique described earlier because of both partial volume averaging and multiple slices.

In 1959, in an attempt to define the anatomic extent or stage of (lung) cancer more precisely, the American Joint Committee (AJC) for Cancer Staging and End Results Reporting adopted the Tumor–Nodal involvement–Metastasis (TNM) system.[811] In 1985, the American Thoracic Society (ATS)[789] expressed the opinion that the AJC classification was inadequate because it failed to provide a detailed description of the anatomic limits of particular lymph node locations or nodal stations. The ATS group recommended that the terms "mediastinal" and "hilar" be dropped because of a lack of clinical-anatomic specificity and replaced with carefully defined "nodal stations." Further, they recommended that the nodal map should be based upon relationships to major anatomic structures

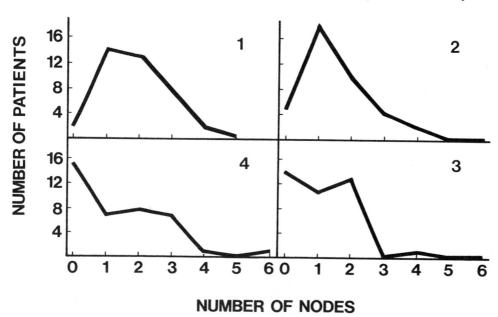

that the surgeon could identify at mediastinoscopy or the radiologist could see on standard roentgenograms or CT scans. The major anatomic structures that the mediastinoscopist can identify include (on the right side) the innominate artery, trachea, azygos vein, right main bronchus, origin of the right upper lobe bronchus, and carina, and (on the left side) the aorta, left pulmonary artery, ligamentum arteriosum, and left main bronchus. Based upon the identification of these major anatomic structures, carefully defined lymph node stations were defined (Table 1–9 and Fig. 1–149). Glazer and his colleagues[1176] have recently suggested the CT demonstration of calcified mediastinal lymph nodes can act as a guide to the ATS classification.

Using the comprehensive ATS scheme, Glazer and his associates[804] carried out a CT study of the number and size of normal mediastinal lymph nodes at 11 intrathoracic nodal stations, measuring both the short and long axis diameters in the transverse plane. The results of their findings in 31 men

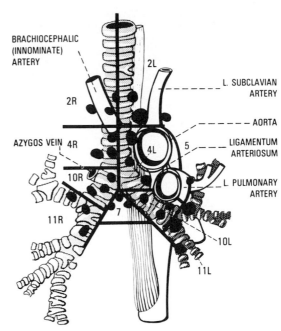

Figure 1–149. American Thoracic Society Map of Regional Pulmonary Nodes. *See* text. (From Tisi GM, Friedman PJ, Peters RM, et al: Am Rev Respir Dis *127*:659, 1983.)

aged 21 to 75 years (mean, 50.3 years) and 25 women aged 18 to 82 years (mean, 50.8 years) are given in Table 1–10. The largest nodes were in the subcarinal and right tracheobronchial regions where the mean short axis measurement for nodal station 7 was 6.2 mm and for station 10R, 5.9 mm. Upper paratracheal nodes (station 2) were smaller than lower paratracheal (station 4) or tracheobronchial nodes (station 10), a finding that was emphasized in the earlier Genereux and Howie study.[808] Glazer and his colleagues also found that there were more nodes in station 4 than in stations 2 and 10. Finally, these researchers indicated that the threshold size for nodal enlargement depended upon the particular station under scrutiny: in the upper paratracheal region (station 2), the value of the short axis measurement above which a lymph node was considered enlarged was found to be 7 mm, whereas for nodes residing in the lower paratracheal region (station 4) or around the carina (stations 7 and 10), the figure was 10 to 11 mm. The data comparing the frequency of lymph nodes less than 11 mm in diameter by location in Glazer and associates' study[804] and the Genereux and Howie report[808] are in close agreement (Table 1–11).

In an earlier report, Glazer and his coworkers[812] evaluated the mediastinum preoperatively in 60 patients with non–small cell carcinoma; 49 of the 60 had thorough surgical-pathologic sampling of mediastinal nodes. Nodes were measured in long and short axes on the transverse images, and their nodal cross-sectional area was calculated from the product of these diameters. Nodes larger than 100 mm² in cross-sectional area were considered to be enlarged. Using the area-size criterion, preoperative staging of the 49 patients resulted in a 95 per cent

Table 1–9. American Thoracic Society Definitions of Regional Nodal Stations

X	**Supraclavicular nodes**
2R	**Right upper paratracheal nodes:** nodes to the right of the midline of the trachea, between the intersection of the caudal margin of the innominate artery with the trachea and the apex of the lung
2L	**Left upper paratracheal nodes:** nodes to the left of the midline of the trachea, between the top of the aortic arch and apex of the lung
4R	**Right lower paratracheal nodes:** nodes to the right of the midline of the trachea, between the cephalic border of the azygos vein and the intersection of the caudal margin of the brachiocephalic artery with the right side of the trachea
4L	**Left lower paratracheal nodes:** nodes to the left of the midline of the trachea, between the top of the aortic arch and the level of the carina, medial to the ligamentum arteriosum
5	**Aortopulmonary nodes:** subaortic and para-aortic nodes, lateral to the ligamentum arteriosum or the aorta or left pulmonary artery, proximal to the first branch of the left pulmonary artery
6	**Anterior mediastinal nodes:** nodes anterior to the ascending aorta or the innominate artery
7	**Subcarinal nodes:** nodes arising caudal to the carina of the trachea but not associated with the lower lobe bronchi or arteries within the lung
8	**Paraesophageal nodes:** nodes dorsal to the posterior wall of the trachea and to the right or left of the midline of the esophagus
9	**Right or left pulmonary ligament nodes:** nodes within the right or left pulmonary ligament
10R	**Right tracheobronchial nodes:** nodes to the right of the midline of the trachea, from the level of the cephalic border of the azygos vein to the origin of the right upper lobe bronchus
10L	**Left peribronchial nodes:** nodes to the left of the midline of the trachea, between the carina and the left upper lobe bronchus, medial to the ligamentum arteriosum
11	**Intrapulmonary nodes:** nodes removed in the right or left lung specimen plus those distal to the main stem bronchi or secondary carina

(Modified from Tisi GM, Friedman PJ, Peters RM, et al.: Am Rev Respir Dis *127*:659, 1983.)

Table 1–10. Number and Size of Normal Mediastinal Lymph Nodes in 56 Patients

STATION	NUMBER OF PATIENTS WITH VISIBLE NODES	NUMBER		NODES MAXIMUM NUMBER	SHORTEST DIAMETER (mm)	
		Mean	(±SD)		Mean	(±SD)
2R	53	2.1	1.3	6	3.5	1.3
2L	42	1.9	1.6	6	3.3	1.6
4R	56	3.2	2.0	10	5.0	2.0
4L	47	2.1	1.6	7	4.7	1.9
5	33	1.2	1.1	3	4.7	2.1
6	48	4.8	3.5	12	4.1	1.7
7	53	1.7	1.1	6	6.2	2.2
8R	32	1.0	1.1	4	4.4	2.6
8L	25	0.8	1.21	6	3.8	1.7
10R	56	2.8	1.3	7	5.9	2.1
10L	39	1.0	0.8	3	4.0	1.2

(Modified after Glazer GM, Gross BH, Quint LE, et al: Am J Roentgenol 144:261, 1985.)

sensitivity and a 64 per cent specificity; the overall accuracy of CT was 78 per cent, the positive predictive accuracy was 67 per cent, and the negative predictive accuracy was 95 per cent. Using receiver operating characteristic (ROC) curve analysis, Glazer and his associates[812] suggested that the optimal size criterion for the diagnosis of malignant mediastinal node enlargement is 10 to 15 mm (short axis measurement).

The recent advent of magnetic resonance imaging (MRI) has raised the possibility that this modality may prove superior to CT in the evaluation of hilar and mediastinal structures. Using a lymph node size criterion of 16 mm or more as abnormal, Heelan and his colleagues[813] carried out a preoperative blind comparison of MRI and CT in 20 patients with pulmonary neoplasms, noting specifically involvement of hilar and mediastinal structures. Pathologically, 10 of the 20 had positive and 10 had negative findings of neoplastic involvement of the mediastinum. False-positive interpretations were made on three CT scans and five MR scans; there were no false-negative scans with either modality. Both CT and MRI identified all 10 patients with an abnormal mediastinum; of the 10 patients with a normal mediastinum, 7 of 10 on CT and 5

of 10 on MR were correctly stated as being negative. The sensitivity of both CT and MRI was 100 per cent whereas the specificity for these two modalities was only 70 and 50 per cent, respectively. Accuracy comparison between the two imaging techniques was 85 per cent (CT) and 75 per cent (MRI). Heelan and his associates[813] concluded that although the sensitivity of the two imaging techniques was identical, specificity was slightly better for CT, probably as a result of the poor spatial resolution of current MRI.

Webb and his associates[814] compared the findings of MRI, CT, and surgery in 33 patients being staged for pulmonary carcinoma. In 29 of the 33 patients, CT and MRI provided identical interpretations of lymph nodes being normal (less than 10 mm), suspicious (10 to 15 mm), or abnormal (greater than 15 mm). MRI and CT interpretations differed in four instances, and pathologic correlation was available in three of these: in one patient, CT suggested a subcarinal mass (differentation from the left atrium was not possible) whereas MRI clearly defined the true neoplastic nature of the mass. In two other patients, the superior resolution of CT permitted the identification of two or more discrete, normal-sized lymph nodes, whereas the impression on MRI was of a single, large abnormal mass. Webb and his colleagues[814] also suggested that it may be possible to distinguish lymph nodes that are involved or uninvolved by neoplasm by measuring their T1 value, although they cautioned that the T1 values of normal nodes (generally less than abnormal nodes) were possibly influenced through partial volume averaging from the very low T1 value of mediastinal fat.

At present, several conclusions can be drawn from these two studies: (1) Both CT and MRI are capable of defining normal and abnormal lymph nodes, but the superior resolution of CT is better suited for the identification and separation of small (usually normal) lymph nodes. (2) MR images are better for distinguishing mediastinal nodes from vascular structures, even when the CT is contrast-enhanced. (3) Whereas the sensitivity of CT and MRI is comparable in the mediastinum, the speci-

Table 1–11. Comparison of Frequency of Lymph Nodes Less than 11 mm in Diameter by Location in Two Studies

ZONE OR STATION	GENEREUX & HOWIE*	GLAZER & ASSOCIATES†
Retroinnominate (I) ATS 4R	72/72 (100%)	54/54 (100%)
Pretracheal (II) ATS 10R	55/58 (94.8%)	54/55 (98%)
Precarinal/Sub-carinal (III) ATS 4L, 7, 10L	38/41 (92.6%)	138/139 (99.2%)
Aortopulmonary (IV) ATS 5	213/225 (94.6%)	33/33 (100%)

*Data from Genereux GP, Howie JL: Am J Roentgenol 142:1095, 1984.
†Data from Glazer GM, Gross BH, Quint LE, et al: Am J Roentgenol 144:261, 1985.

ficity of CT is greater, probably as a result of inferior MRI resolution. And (4), it may be possible in the future to distinguish normal from abnormal lymph nodes on MRI by their T1 characteristics.

LYMPH NODES OF THE HILA

On CT, normal lymph nodes in the hila are inconspicuous and are not demonstrable as separate units. Sone and his colleagues[810] studied the anatomic location of hilar lymph nodes in relation to the bronchi and pulmonary vessels on the basis of transverse scans of four cadavers (two showed moderately enlarged hilar and mediastinal lymph nodes caused respectively by malignant lymphoma and anthracosis); patients were also studied in a clinical setting using dynamic CT scans (25 ml contrast medium; 4 rapid-sequence scans at each level of interest; 4.8 sec scan time with 1.4 sec interscan delay). They found that the lymph nodes in the right hilum could be divided into four principal groups (right upper lobe, descending right pulmonary artery, middle lobe, and lower lobe) and in the left hilum into three main groups (left upper lobe, descending pulmonary artery, and lower lobe). Most hilar lymph nodes are situated along the bronchi in close relation to pulmonary vessels; according to Sone and his associates,[810] it is this close proximity of lymph nodes to the hilar vessels (themselves often imaged end-on) that renders the noncontrast-enhanced study difficult to interpret; they suggest that a contrast-enhanced CT scan is indispensable for the precise determination of suspected hilar node enlargement.

LYMPHATIC DRAINAGE OF THE LUNGS

The location of enlarged lymph nodes within the mediastinum may be important in determining the intrapulmonary site of origin of infections or neoplasms. Much of our knowledge of patterns of regional lymph node drainage from the lung derives from Rouvière's treatise on the anatomy of the human lymphatic system, published in 1938, which was based on necropsy studies of 200 fetuses, neonates, and children.[843] Many of his observations have since been confirmed.[447, 842] Rouvière subdivided the lungs into three main drainage areas—the superior, middle, and inferior—without correspondence to pulmonary lobes.

On the Right Side

On the right side, in the superior area, lymph drains directly into the paratracheal and upper bronchopulmonary nodes. The middle zone drains directly into the paratracheal nodes, the bifurcation nodes, and the central group of bronchopulmonary nodes. The inferior zone drains into the inferior bronchopulmonary and bifurcation nodes and the posterior mediastinal chain. Thus, on the right side, all the lymph drains eventually via the right lymphatic duct.

On the Left Side

Rouvière[843] stated that, in the left superior area, lymph drains both into the prevascular group of anterior mediastinal nodes and directly into the left paratracheal nodes. The middle zone drains mainly via the bifurcation and central group of bronchopulmonary nodes and partly directly into the left paratracheal group. The inferior zone drains into the bifurcation and inferior bronchopulmonary nodes and into the posterior mediastinal chain. Thus, according to Rouvière, the superior portion and part of the middle zone drain via the left paratracheal nodes into the thoracic duct, and lymph drainage from the remainder of the left lung empties eventually into the right lymphatic duct.

The "crossover" phenomenon was long thought to be of diagnostic and therapeutic importance in diseases originating in the middle or lower portion of the left lung, but recent investigations have cast some doubt on the validity of the phenomenon in adults. For example, in a study of 1000 consecutive necropsies, Klingenberg[844] found 17 cases of primary carcinoma of the left lung, only one of which had heterolateral prescalene node metastases; unfortunately, the sites of origin in the left lung were not stated. Similarly Baird[845] performed bilateral prescalene node biopsies in 218 patients, 110 of whom had pulmonary carcinoma; the direction of lymphatic spread within the mediastinum was cephalad and usually ipsilateral, irrespective of the location of the primary growth. Contralateral spread was uncommon and about equally frequent from either lung.

On the strength of these observations, it is reasonable to conclude that prescalene node biopsies should always be performed first on the same side as the pulmonary disease; should this prove negative, contralateral biopsy *occasionally* may be productive.

THE MEDIASTINUM

The mediastinum constitutes a compartmented septum or partition that divides the thorax vertically. Considerable controversy has raged over the years concerning the most practical and informative method of dividing the mediastinum into compartments. To place the matter in proper perspective, we will describe several of the methods that have received support, ending with a decision as to which method we feel possesses the greatest merit. Irrespective of the method that the individual radiologist may choose, the essential foundation for any classification is a thorough understanding of gross mediastinal anatomy, since all pathologic classifications ultimately relate to a statistical weighing of possibilities based on the anatomy of each particular area or compartment. Interested readers may find some enjoyment in perusing a historical review of mediastinal classifications by Leszczynski and Pawlicka.[846]

Mediastinal Compartments

THE TRADITIONAL METHOD

Classic anatomy divides the mediastinum into superior and inferior compartments by an imaginary line extending from the sternal angle to the fourth intervertebral disc; the inferior compartment is further subdivided into prevascular or anterior, cardiovascular or middle, and postvascular or posterior compartments.[847] This has undoubtedly been the most popular and generally accepted classification of the mediastinum over the years. Since each compartment contains anatomic structures almost unique to it, many of the afflictions to which the mediastinum is subject tend to occur *predominantly* in one or other compartment. A modification of this classification, employed by us in the second edition of this book, is the exclusion of the superior compartment since it contains structures that are for the most part continuous with the compartments below; thus, its separation serves little diagnostic purpose.

In this modification of the traditional classification, the *anterior mediastinal compartment* is bounded anteriorly by the sternum and posteriorly by the pericardium, aorta, and brachiocephalic vessels. It is narrowest anteriorly where the pleura of the right and left upper lobe converge to form the anterior junction line (*see* further on); it broadens posterosuperiorly in an apex-down triangular configuration to form the anterior mediastinal triangle. The anterior mediastinum contains the thymus gland or its remnants, branches of the internal mammary artery and vein, lymph nodes, the inferior sternopericardial ligament, and variable amounts of fat.

The *middle mediastinal compartment* contains the pericardium and its contents, the ascending and transverse portions of the aorta, the superior and inferior vena cava, the brachiocephalic arteries and veins, the phrenic nerves and upper portion of the vagus nerves, the trachea and main bronchi and their contiguous lymph nodes, and the pulmonary arteries and veins.

The *posterior mediastinal compartment* is bounded anteriorly by the pericardium and the vertical part of the diaphragm, laterally by the mediastinal pleura, and posteriorly by the bodies of the thoracic vertebrae (although for practical purposes, the paravertebral gutters are included). It contains the descending thoracic aorta, esophagus, thoracic duct, azygos and hemiazygos veins, autonomic nerves, fat, and lymph nodes.

Heitzman feels that this classification contains certain deficiencies and limitations because it is insufficiently based on roentgenologic anatomy, minimizes detailed anatomic analysis, and has virtually no application to the gross pathologic diagnosis of mediastinal lesions.[467]

THE ZYLAK METHOD

This approach[848] favors the concept of the mediastinum being divided into three longitudinal compartments—anterior, middle, and posterior—extending uninterruptedly from the level of the thoracic inlet to the diaphragm. It seems to us that the divisions and contents of these compartments as described by Zylak and his colleagues are very little different from those in the modified traditional method.

THE FELSON METHOD

The three mediastinal compartments employed by Felson[739] are derived purely from the lateral chest roentgenogram and bear little relationship to "anatomic" descriptions. Two vertically oriented lines drawn or visualized on a lateral roentgenogram establish three compartments as follows: a line traced upward from the diaphragm to the thoracic inlet along the back of the heart and in front of the trachea separates the anterior from the middle mediastinal compartment. A second line connects a point on each thoracic vertebral body 1 cm behind its anterior margin, thereby dividing the middle from the posterior compartment. Thus, all lesions in the posterior compartment are situated in the paravertebral gutters and invariably make contact with the posteromedial thoracic wall.

THE NAIDICH METHOD

Naidich and his associates[849] have recommended that the mediastinum be partitioned by structure rather than boundary, based upon the densitometric capability of computed tomography to distinguish fat, soft tissue, calcium, and water density structures. We feel that there is considerable merit to this approach since there is little question that thorough analysis of mediastinal anatomy and pathology can only be achieved by CT (or MRI). Using CT, normal fat or fatty masses can be clearly and easily distinguished from all other structures, both normal and abnormal, in the mediastinum. Similarly, water-density masses and various acquired and congenital vascular abnormalities are usually easily recognized, particularly when the CT study is performed with contrast medium enhancement.

THE HEITZMAN METHOD

Heitzman[467] credits the original description of this classification to Tillier (quoted by Leszczynski and Pawlicka[846]). It deviates widely from the three-compartment mediastinum of the other three methods, and includes seven separate anatomic regions.

(1) *The thoracic inlet*: a region with a narrow cephalocaudad dimension marking the cervicothoracic junction and lying immediately above and below a transverse plane through the first rib.

(2) *The anterior mediastinum*: a region extending from the thoracic inlet to the diaphragm in front of the heart, ascending aorta, and superior vena cava.

The remaining five subdivisions reside behind the anterior mediastinum and depend on the relationship of anatomic structures to the arches of the aorta and azygos vein.

(3) *The supra-aortic area*: the region above the aortic arch.

(4) *The infra-aortic area*: the region below the aortic arch.

(5) *The supra-azygos area*: the region above the azygos arch.

(6) *The infra-azygos area*: the region below the azygos arch.

(7) *The hila*: the regions containing major bronchi, blood vessels, and lymph nodes in a connective tissue sheath that is continuous with the infra-aortic and infra-azygos areas.

Heitzman justifies the logic of this classification by pointing to the approximately equal size of the areas on the right and left sides of the mediastinum separated by the major vascular channel. Further, he states that the aortic and azygos arches actually serve as functional anatomic boundaries in certain disease states such as the limitation of the spread of localized mediastinal abscesses.

The second edition of this book employed the traditional method of compartmentalizing the mediastinum, and we still feel that this method is a reasonable approach, particularly when combined with CT. However, upon deliberation we have decided that the Heitzman method possesses more merit from both anatomic and functional points of view, and we have decided to adopt it in this edition in relation to conventional roentgenographic studies.

The descriptions that follow of the normal anatomy of the mediastinal compartments have been derived from several sources to which reference will be made in the appropriate sections. However, the bulk of the material, including the classification, has come from the superb treatises on the mediastinum by Heitzman[467] and by Proto and his colleagues.[850, 851] More recent descriptions of mediastinal analysis, with emphasis on CT, have been published by Woodring and Daniel[1177] and by Chasen and his colleagues.[1178] Since it would be needlessly repetitious for us to describe mediastinal morphology and roentgenology in the detail that these investigators have already done so well, we will describe only those features that are essential for a reasonable understanding of the mediastinum and its diseases.

THE THORACIC INLET

The thoracic inlet, or cervicomediastinal continuum, represents the junction between structures at the base of the neck and those of the thorax. It parallels the first rib and thus is higher posteriorly than anteriorly. Utilizing this fact of anatomy, Felson[852] has pointed out that an opacity on a PA chest roentgenogram that is effaced on its superior aspect and that projects at or below the level of the clavicles must be situated anteriorly, whereas one that projects above the clavicles is retrotracheal and posteriorly situated. From front to back, structures occupying the thoracic inlet include the upper portion of the thymus gland, the right and left innominate veins (which join behind the right side of the manubrium to form the superior vena cava), the common carotid arteries (lying immediately anterior to the subclavian arteries and medial to the subclavian veins), the trachea (situated either in the midline or slightly to the right or left immediately behind the great vessels), the esophagus (located behind the trachea and in front of the spine), and the recurrent laryngeal nerves on either side of the esophagus. The lower trunk of the brachial plexus is situated immediately behind the subclavian artery in relation to the first rib; the vagus and phrenic nerves enter the thorax in front of the subclavian arteries and behind the great veins. The thoracic duct is situated along the left side of the esophagus from which point it arches anteriorly to terminate at the junction of the left internal jugular and subclavian veins.

The spread of disease processes from the neck into the mediastinum (and vice versa) occurs through precise anatomic pathways termed by Oliphant and his colleagues[853] the cervicothoracic continuum. A fascial envelope, the *deep cervical fascia*, surrounds the deep structures of the neck and divides into three layers that define distinct compartments: (1) The posterior layer (*prevertebral fascia*) delineates the prevertebral space that extends from the occipital bone to the thorax where it becomes continuous with the anterior longitudinal ligament of the spine. Pathologic processes within the prevertebral space of the neck (e.g., an abscess secondary to infectious spondylitis) can extend caudally to the thoracic inlet but usually not below this point because of merging of the prevertebral fascia with the anterior longitudinal ligament of the thoracic spine. (2) The middle layer (*pretracheal fascia*) lies anterior to the trachea and extends inferiorly from the thyroid gland into the thorax where it blends with the fascia that surrounds the aorta and pericardium. The pretracheal fascia anteriorly, the prevertebral fascia posteriorly, and the carotid sheaths laterally define the *visceral compartment* of the cervicothoracic continuum; it contains the pharynx, larynx, trachea, and esophagus and is continuous with the mediastinum across the thoracic inlet. Pathologic processes arising in this compartment (such as retropharyngeal abscess) can readily spread inferiorly into the mediastinum; similarly, various abnormalities originating in the mediastinum (such as abscess or hemorrhage) can extend upward into the neck. (3) At the level of the thyroid gland, the anterior layer of the deep cervical fascia forms the suprasternal space, enclosing the salivary gland, the mastoid process, and the mandible. Infections arising from these structures can enter the suprahyoid space but are generally confined there by the fascial planes and seldom extend into the mediastinum. However, it is by this route that goiters extend from the neck inferiorly to become retrosternal; occasionally, goiters grow into the mediastinum posteriorly rather than anteriorly, descending along the perivisceral fascia around the trachea and esophagus; this type is almost invariably right-sided and is confined to the supra-azygos area.

THE ANTERIOR MEDIASTINAL COMPARTMENT

The anatomic boundaries and constituents of this compartment were described earlier, and in this section we will discuss the normal thymus gland and a number of important aspects of roentgenologic anatomy.

THE NORMAL THYMUS GLAND

The thymus gland is located in the anterosuperior portion of the mediastinum and extends from a point above the manubrium to the fourth costal cartilage. Posteriorly, it relates to and is molded by the trachea, left innominate vein, aortic arch and its branches, and the pericardium covering the ascending aorta and main pulmonary artery. The normal thymus is a bilobed structure[467] in keeping with its embryologic derivation from the bilateral third pharyngeal pouches. Septa divide the two thymic lobes into irregular lobules, a feature that is particularly evident in younger individuals; as the gland undergoes involution and fatty replacement with age, lobulation becomes less apparent.

In an extensive CT study of the normal thymus gland of 154 subjects, Baron and his colleagues[854] found the following:

(1) *The gland.* The thymus was recognized in 100 per cent of patients under age 30 years, in 73 per cent of patients between the ages of 30 and 49 years, and in 17 per cent of patients over 49 years of age. The maximum thymic size was observed in individuals between 12 and 19 years of age, regression occurring between 20 and 60 years and usually associated with fatty replacement of the parenchyma; by the age of 60 years, the thymus was found to weigh 50 per cent less than at age 19 years.

(2) *Shape.* Sixty-two per cent of normal glands showed an arrowhead configuration, while 32 per cent had separate right and left lobes (Fig. 1–150). The shape of the separate lobes was highly variable,

being ovoid, elliptic, triangular, or semilunar. In 6 per cent of cases, only a right or left lobe was identified. In a comparison CT study of the thymic morphology in 309 normal subjects and 23 patients with clinically or surgically proved thymic abnormality, Francis and his colleagues[1131] found that thymic shape reliably separates normal from abnormal glands; specifically, they found that multilobularity was never a feature of the normal gland at any age but was seen only in patients with thymic abnormality.

(3) *Size.* The left lobe was almost invariably larger than the right. The CT width (long axis or anteroposterior dimension of a lobe) tended to decrease in older patients, although this was not statistically significant; the mean width of the right and left lobes in the 6 to 19 year old group was 20 mm (± 5.5 mm SD) and 33 mm (± 1.1 mm SD), respectively, and in the 40 to 49 year old group it was 14 mm (± 6.6 mm SD) and 19 mm (± 7.6 mm SD), respectively. By contrast, the thickness (short axis or transverse dimension of a lobe) displayed a statistically significant decrease between the 6 to 19 year old and 40 to 49 year old comparison groups; the thickness of the right and left lobes in these two age categories was 10 mm (± 3.9 mm SD) and 11 mm (± 4.0 mm SD), and 6 mm (± 2.3 mm SD) and 6 mm (± 2.0 mm SD), respectively.

(4) *Density.* Baron and his colleagues[854] found that the CT attenuation values of the thymus decreased with age: under 19 years of age, the gland was isodense, being equal to or higher than the chest wall musculature; in the majority of patients over 40 years of age, thymic density approached that of fat (Fig. 1–150). It has recently been suggested that magnetic resonance imaging may permit more accurate assessment of the thymus gland than CT: in a study of the MR characteristics of the normal thymus in 18 patients ranging in age from 5 to 77 years and without thymic or other mediastinal pathology, de Geer and his associates[1130] found the thymus to be visible in all patients regardless of age and to differ from subcutaneous fat in hydrogen density (the average thymus-to-fat hydrogen density ratio was 0.60). Although the T1 relaxation times of the thymus were much longer than those of fat in patients under 30 years of age, this difference decreased with age. The thymus appeared thicker on MR images than on CT scans in patients older than 20 years. It was suggested by these workers that MR may be better than CT in distinguishing between thymus replaced by fat and mediastinal fat itself.

On conventional roentgenograms of the chest, the thymus is visible only in infants and young children in whom it fills much of the anterior mediastinal space. Although CT has shown that the thymus attains its maximum weight in people between 12 and 19 years of age,[854] it is inconstantly visible roentgenographically after the age of 2 or 3 years, an apparent paradox explained by the fact that the body is also growing and that the ratio of

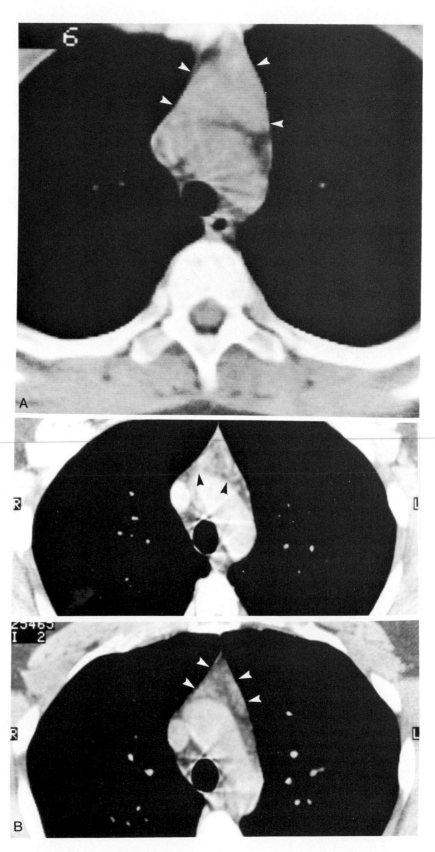

Figure 1–150. The Normal Thymus Gland.
A, A CT scan through the superior mediastinum of a normal 15-year-old boy reveals a triangular opacity (*arrowheads*), the apex of which points forward while the base abuts the great vessels. CT density is equivalent to that of the chest wall musculature. *B*, CT scans through the superior mediastinum of an elderly man disclose a thymus gland (*arrowheads*) composed of isolated nodular opacities and intervening fat (compare the CT density of the gland with the subcutaneous fat).

Illustration continued on following page

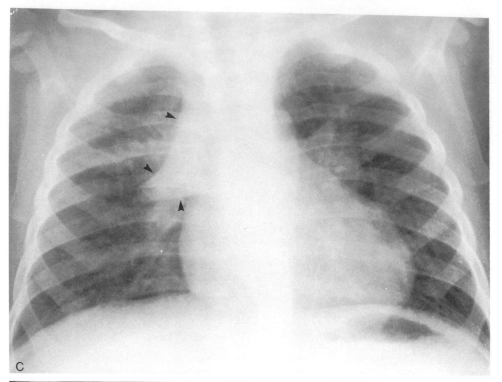

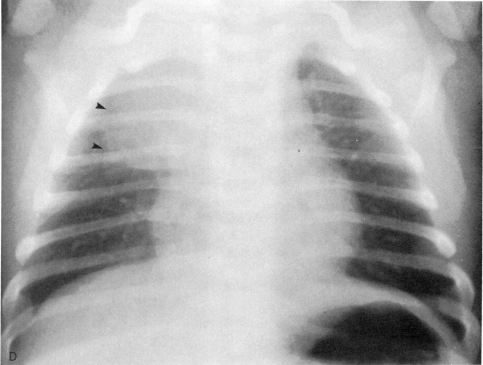

Figure 1–150 *Continued. C*, A chest roentgenogram of a normal infant in anteroposterior projection shows a triangular opacity (*arrowheads*) projecting into the right lung, simulating the sail of a boat (the *sail sign*). *D*, An anteroposterior chest roentgenogram in another infant shows gentle undulations (*arrowheads*) along the contour of the opacity caused by impression from the anterior ribs (the *thymic wave sign*).

thymic weight to body weight decreases with age. In addition to its location, three roentgenographic signs aid identification of the normal thymus gland: the *thymic notch sign* consists of an indentation in the thymic contour at the junction of the thymus and the heart, either unilaterally or bilaterally; the *sail sign* is a triangular opacity of thymic tissue that projects to the right or left (or sometimes both), and is present in only 5 per cent of infants;[855] and the *thymic wave sign* is a rippled or undulating contour of the thymic border caused by anterior rib indentation (Fig. 1–150).

Roentgenographic Anatomy of the Anterior Mediastinum

The anteromedial portions of the right and left lungs and their pleura contact the mediastinum in the retrosternal area to form the *anterior junctional anatomy*,[850] composed of the superior recesses, the anterior junction line, and the inferior recesses. All three components show a typical although variable appearance that largely depends upon the quantity of mediastinal fat and the degree of lung inflation.

THE SUPERIOR RECESSES

As viewed on a posteroanterior roentgenogram, the superior recesses are formed by contact of lung with the retromanubrial mediastinum; typically they marginate a V-shaped area, the *anterior mediastinal triangle,* the apex of which points caudally (Fig. 1–151). It has been stated that the right and left boundaries of this triangle are formed by the innominate veins,[467] but based upon correlative CT

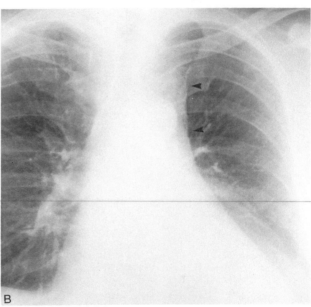

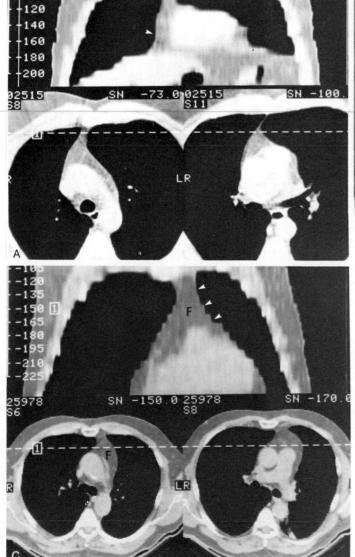

Figure 1–151. Anterior Junction Anatomy. *A,* A coronal CT reformation (*top*) and appropriate transverse images (*bottom*) reveal the superior (*upper arrowheads*) and inferior (*lower arrowhead*) recesses of the anterior junction anatomy. The superior recesses, composed of mediastinal fat, relate closely to the innominate veins. The anterior junction line (*large arrowhead*) separates the superior and inferior recesses. *B* is a detail view from a conventional posteroanterior chest roentgenogram of a middle-aged man with left lower lobe atelectasis caused by an obstructing pulmonary carcinoma. The left superior recess and contiguous fat in the anterior, superior mediastinal triangle (*arrowheads*) are displaced to the left. *C,* A coronal CT reformation (*top*) and representative transverse images (*bottom*) reveal the displacement to the left of the mediastinal fat (*F*) in the anterior mediastinal triangle (*arrowheads*).

Illustration continued on following page

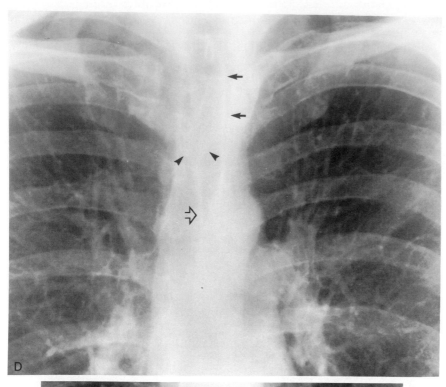

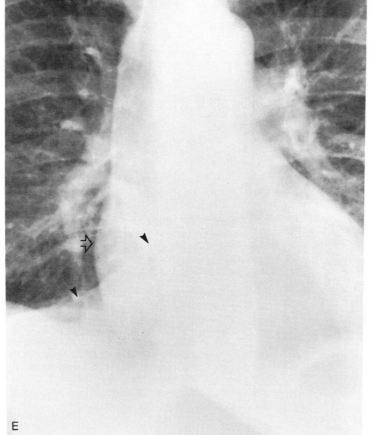

Figure 1–151 *Continued. D,* A posteroanterior chest roentgenogram of a normal adult man shows the anterior mediastinal triangle (*small arrowheads*) and anterior junction line (*open arrow*). Note that the posterior junction line, also shown (*arrows*), extends above the medial border of the clavicles. Inferiorly it terminates at the aortic arch. *E,* In another patient, a detail view of the heart from a conventional posteroanterior chest roentgenogram demonstrates a curvilinear opacity (*arrowheads*) that is projected over the lower margin of the right atrium (*arrow*) and contiguous hemidiaphragm. This opacity represents the caudal portion of the right inferior recess. Occasionally a similar feature can be seen overlying the left side of the heart.

scans, we tend to agree with Proto and his colleagues[850] that each superior recess usually marginates retromanubrial mediastinal fat in front of or contiguous with the innominate veins rather than the veins themselves. Displacement of the superior recesses to the right has been described as a secondary sign of right lower lobe atelectasis[856] caused by intrusion of hyperinflated left upper lobe into the right hemithorax (see Fig. 1–141). We have also seen displacement of the anterior mediastinal triangle into the left hemithorax in association with left lower lobe atelectasis.

THE ANTERIOR JUNCTION LINE (ANTERIOR MEDIASTINAL LINE)

As the two lungs approximate anteromedially, they are separated by four layers of pleura and a variable quantity of intervening mediastinal adipose tissue, thus forming a septum of variable thickness. As seen on CT, this creates a curvilinear opacity that courses vertically from front to back, angling to the right or to the left, and ranging in thickness from 1 to more than 3 mm. On a posteroanterior chest roentgenogram, the anterior junction line typically is oriented obliquely from upper right to lower left behind the sternum; cephalad, it begins at the apex of the anterior mediastinal triangle and continues caudally for several centimeters before terminating at the apex of the inferior recess. Since the septum dividing the two lungs is variable in thickness, the resulting opacity may be either a line (see Fig. 1–141) or a stripe; if the former, Mach band formation contributes strongly to the visibility of the line.

THE INFERIOR RECESSES

Inferiorly, the anteromedial portions of the right and left lungs are further separated from one another by the heart and adjacent mediastinal fat; consequently, these lung surfaces in contact with the lower anterior mediastinum form interfaces that marginate an inverted V-shaped area termed by Proto and his colleagues the inferior recesses (Fig. 1–151). On a lateral chest roentgenogram, the inferior recesses cannot be identified since they are not profiled; however, their posterior contour may be portrayed as components of the right and left cardiac incisuras, to be described further on.

In essence, the anterior junctional anatomy is composed of two opposing triangular soft tissue opacities superiorly and inferiorly, separated by an oblique line or stripe constituting the anterior junction line.

THE RETROSTERNAL STRIPE, PARASTERNAL STRIPE, AND CARDIAC INCISURA

On a true lateral roentgenogram of the chest, the relationship between the back of the sternum and the two lungs is normally intimate, creating little or no discernible shadow.[467] However, lung may be excluded from this close contact by mediastinal fat, creating a vertical retrosternal opacity, the retrosternal stripe (Fig. 1–152).[857] Jemelin and associates[858] studied this stripe on lateral chest roentgenograms in 153 normal subjects and found that its thickness averaged 2.67 mm (SD 1.38); the maximum width was 6.8 mm (3 SD greater than mean). These measurements can occasionally be of value in the assessment of the upper half of the retrosternal shadow but seldom of the lower half because of wide variation in the retrosternal line.

According to Proto and Speckman,[857] the lung can also contact the upper two thirds of the anterior chest wall, either to the right or left of the midline, thus outlining the parasternal areas and creating the parasternal stripe (Fig. 1–152). This stripe is particularly prominent when there is indentation of the anterior surface of the lung by costal cartilages and ribs, creating a lobulated contour; as expected, each lobulation is centered at the level of an anterior rib. A lobulated contour also can be caused by enlargement of the internal mammary lymph nodes, tortuosity of the internal mammary arteries associated with coarctation of the aorta, and extrapleural hematomas associated with multiple anterior rib fractures; in such cases, differential diagnosis is of obvious importance.

On the left side, as the sternum is followed inferiorly, the lung is normally excluded from the anteromedial chest wall by the cardiac apex or the epicardial fat pad or both. This deficiency has been named by anatomists the cardiac incisura; the interface between the cardiac incisura and contiguous left lung has a variable appearance, including straight, angular, or rounded (Fig. 1–152).

On the right side, lung may profile the lower third of the right anteromedial wall of the chest unless the right cardiophrenic angle fat pad causes separation as on the left (a common occurrence in our experience).

On a lateral projection, the superior limit of the anterior mediastinum behind the manubrium sometimes causes confusion in roentgenologic interpretation because of a smooth, homogeneous opacity that indents the lungs, simulating an anterior mediastinal mass. In a roentgenographic-morphologic correlative study of adult cadavers frozen in the erect position and sectioned in horizontal and sagittal planes, Whalen and his colleagues[859] suggested that this slightly undulating interface is related to a composite of normal anatomic structures, the subclavian arteries causing the superior and posterior indentation and the innominate veins the inferior and anterior indentation. These indentations were called the vascular incisura analogous to its counterpart in the lower thorax adjacent to the heart. Whalen and his associates cautioned that the first costochondral junctions can cause an opacity similar to that formed by the venous indentation; although others have concurred in this interpretation,[857] in our experience the so-called venous vas-

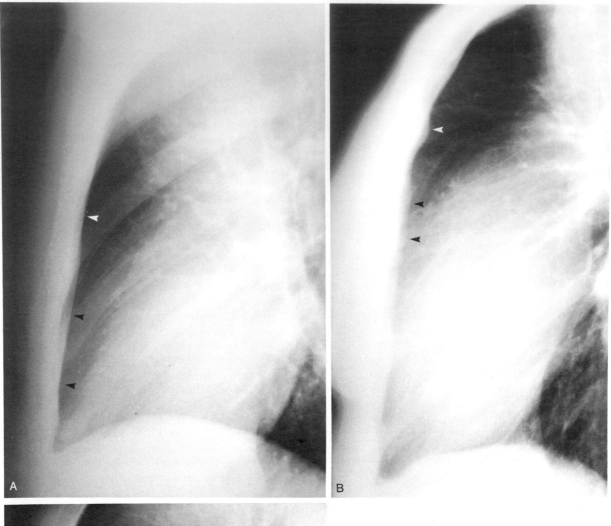

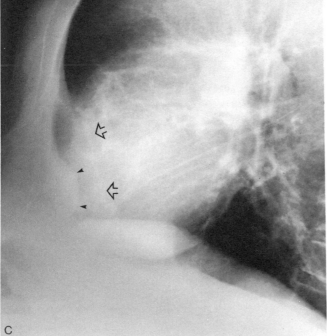

Figure 1–152. Lateral Roentgenographic Anatomy of the Anterior Mediastinum. *A,* A detail view from a lateral chest roentgenogram shows a vertical retrosternal opacity that constitutes the *retrosternal stripe (arrowheads).* The stripe is formed as retrosternal mediastinal fat excludes coalition of the anteromedial portion of the right and left lungs in the anterior mediastinum. *B,* In another patient, a closeup view of a lateral chest roentgenogram discloses an undulating stripe (the *parasternal stripe*) *(arrowheads)* in which lobulation can be seen to relate to the anterior ribs. *C,* In a third patient, a conventional lateral chest roentgenogram reveals a rounded opacity *(arrowheads)* overlying the anteroinferior aspect of the cardiac silhouette (the *cardiac incisura*); a second curvilinear opacity *(open arrows)* is seen behind the incisura.

Illustration continued on opposite page

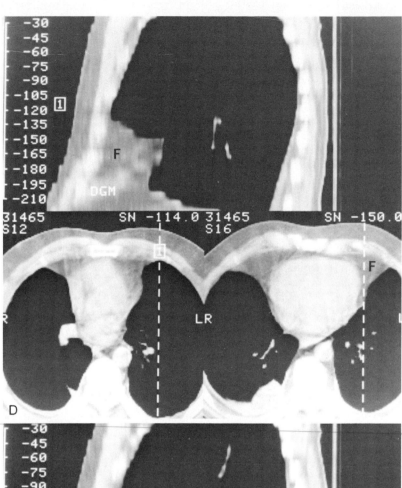

Figure 1–152 *Continued. D,* A sagittal CT reformation slightly to the left of the cardiac apex (*above*) and appropriate transverse images (*below*) show that the more posterior opacity in Part *C* is formed by paracardiac mediastinal fat (*F*) contiguous with the cardiac apex. Note that the opacity relates to the epicardial fat pad and not to the cardiac apex. *DGM,* diaphragm. *E,* Similar features on CT were demonstrated on the right, accounting for the second, more anterior, shadow.

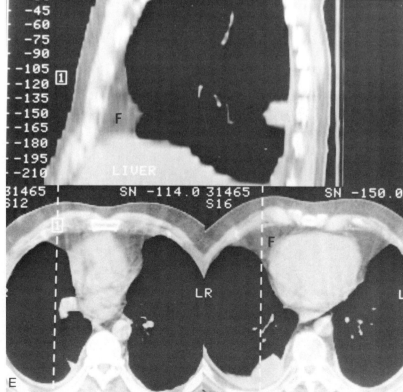

cular incisura is more commonly related to mediastinal fat surrounding the left innominate vein than to the vein itself (Fig. 1–153).

The Supra-aortic Area

This compartment comprises that portion of the left side of the mediastinum extending from the aortic arch to the thoracic inlet, behind the anterior mediastinum. Structures included within this area are the left subclavian artery, the left wall of the trachea, the left superior intercostal vein, and mediastinal fat. On a lateral roentgenogram of the chest, the area bounded by the posterior wall of the trachea, the top of the aortic arch, and the anterior surface of the thoracic vertebral bodies constitutes the *supra-aortic triangle*.

Left Subclavian Artery

The left subclavian artery arises from the aorta behind the left common carotid artery, passing upward and lateral to the trachea in contact with the left mediastinal pleura. It thus forms an interface with the superomedial left upper lobe that can be identified on a posteroanterior roentgenogram as an arcuate opacity (concave laterally) extending from the aortic arch to a point at or just above the medial end of the clavicle (Fig. 1–154). At this point, the vessel relates posteriorly to the scalenus anterior muscle where its roentgenographic visibility depends on the depth of the groove it creates in the apical portion of the left lung. On a lateral roentgenogram, posteromedial lung can intrude above the aortic arch and in so doing may reveal

either the posterior third or two thirds of the aortic arch (in 73 per cent of cases); the area of obscuration between the outline of the ascending aorta and the aortic arch represents the sites of origin of the innominate artery, the left common carotid artery, and the left subclavian artery.[857] Unlike the left subclavian artery, which is frequently abutted by left upper lobe parenchyma, the innominate artery and the left common carotid artery are commonly enveloped by mediastinal fat and are therefore unlikely to be contour-forming. Consequently, on a lateral chest roentgenogram the posterior margin of the left subclavian artery may be identified through the posterior portion of the tracheal air column as a relatively straight opacity coursing obliquely upward toward the neck (Fig. 1–154). The posterior margin of the innominate artery/right subclavian artery complex merges with the posterior wall of the right innominate vein/superior vena cava complex to form a typical sigmoid-shaped interface (Fig. 1–154).[857]

The opacity of an aberrant *right subclavian artery* can occasionally be identified on posteroanterior and lateral roentgenograms of the chest. In a study in which conventional roentgenograms were correlated with great vessel angiograms of 12 patients with aberrant right subclavian arteries,[860] an oblique opacity ascending from left to right from the superior margin of the aortic arch could be identified in seven patients on the conventional roentgenogram; in two cases, the lateral projection revealed a round shadow contiguous with the superior margin of the aortic arch overlying the tracheal air column. These features should indicate further investigation by barium study of the esophagus in which the

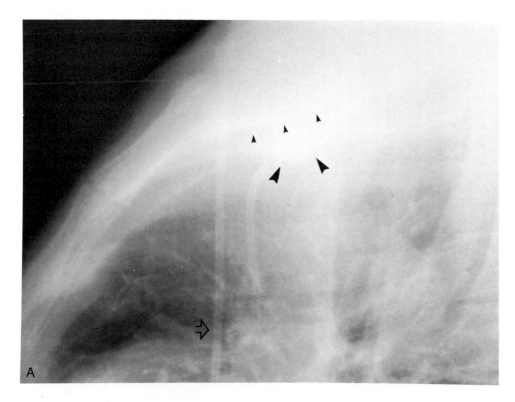

A

Figure 1–153. The Vascular Incisura. *A,* A detail view of the retromanubrial superior mediastinum from a conventional lateral chest roentgenogram reveals an undulating opacity that appears to relate to the left innominate vein (*arrowheads*); a second, shallow opacity (*small arrowheads*) is located more cephalad. A catheter is in the left innominate vein; a longer catheter (*arrow*) lies outside the thorax.

Illustration continued on opposite page

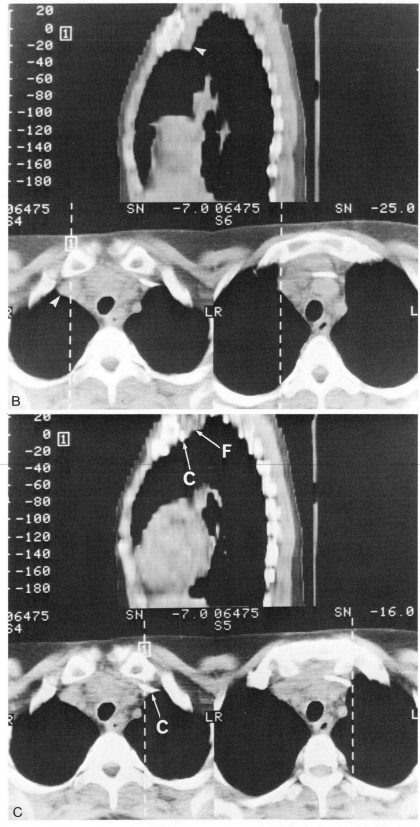

Figure 1–153 *Continued.* Sagittal CT reformations (*top*) with representative transverse images (*bottom*) through the right (*B*) and left (*C*) innominate veins show that the lower opacity in *A* relates to the right vein and surrounding fat (*arrowheads*). Note that the shallow upper opacity in *A* is caused by mediastinal fat (*F*) in front and above the left innominate vein. Catheter (*C*) in vein is white in the illustration.

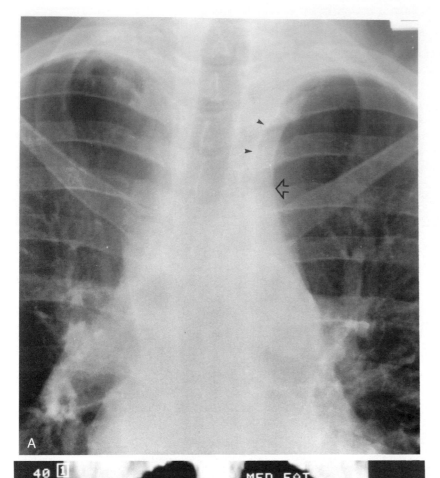

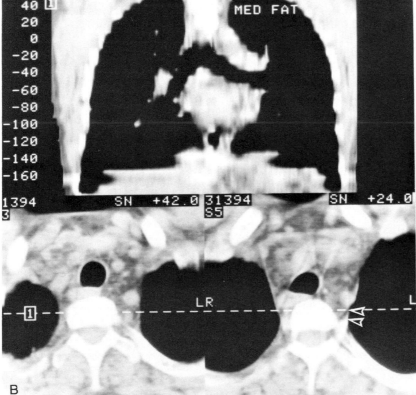

Figure 1–154. The Supra-aortic Area. *A,* A detail view from a posteroanterior chest roentgenogram reveals two curvilinear interfaces that extend superiorly and laterally from the aortic arch and trachea. The medially positioned interface (*arrowheads*) represents lung abutting the posterior mediastinum; because it is *concave,* it is illuminated by a positive Mach band. By contrast, the more lateral opacity (*arrow*) is created by the left subclavian artery and is a *convex* surface; consequently, it is highlighted by a negative Mach band. Coronal CT reformations with transverse images through the superior mediastinum posteriorly (*B*) and at the level of the left subclavian artery (*C*) show that the more medial curvilinear opacity in *A*—the *left superior paraspinal line*—is formed by the concave interface (in the transverse plane) formed by lung and mediastinal fat (*MED FAT*) (*arrowheads*). On the other hand, the left subclavian artery (*LSA*) possesses a convex shape in the transverse plane (*arrowheads*) as it abuts the lung. *D,* A conventional lateral chest roentgenogram reveals a relatively straight opacity (*arrowheads*) that courses through the tracheal air column (*T*), representing the left subclavian artery.

Illustration continued on opposite page

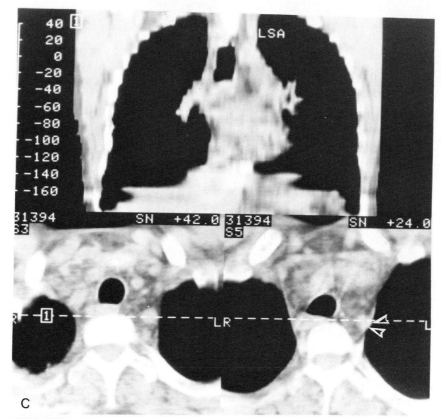

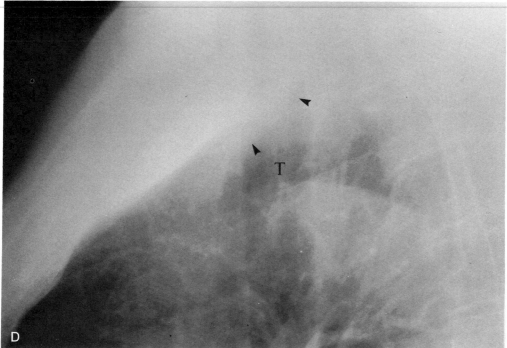

Figure 1–154 *Continued*

Illustration continued on following page

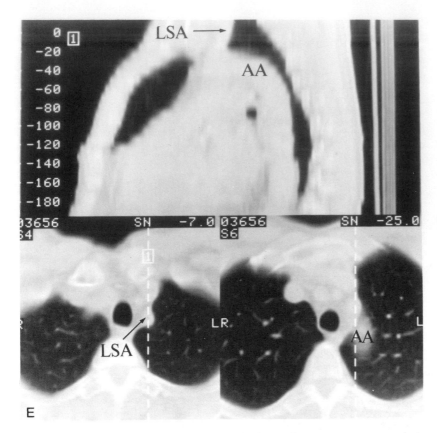

Figure 1–154 *Continued. E*, A sagittal CT reformation (*top*) with appropriate transverse images (*bottom*) demonstrates the contour-forming left subclavian artery (*LSA*) as it courses toward the apex of the thorax above the aortic arch (*AA*).

aberrant artery causes an oblique indentation on the posterior wall of that structure.

LEFT SUPERIOR INTERCOSTAL VEIN

Venous blood from the first left intercostal space drains into the left supreme intercostal vein, whereas that from the second, third, and fourth intercostal spaces drains into a common vessel, the *left superior intercostal vein*. In approximately 75 per cent of subjects,[467] as the vessel descends along the spine it communicates with the accessory hemiazygos vein. At T3 or T4, the vein arches forward adjacent to the aortic arch to empty into the posterior aspect of the left innominate vein.

According to Ball and Proto,[861] three components of the left superior intercostal vein can sometimes be identified roentgenographically, the "aortic nipple," the paraspinal portion, and the retroaortic portion. The aortic nipple consists of a rounded protuberance adjacent to the aortic arch, created by the vein seen end-on as it passes anteriorly adjacent to the aortic knob before entering the left innominate vein. The incidence with which it is viewed on posteroanterior roentgenograms of erect normal subjects ranges from 1.4 per cent in the 500 cases studied by Friedman and associates[862] to 9.5 per cent of the 469 cases examined by Ball and Proto;[861] the euphemistic designation aortic nipple was given this opacity by McDonald and his colleagues[863] who identified it in 4 per cent of the cases they studied. In normal subjects in the erect position, the nipple

ranges in size from a small protuberance to a maximum diameter of 4.5 mm.[862] As expected, the vein dilates and becomes more prominent in the supine position and with the Mueller maneuver; it can be seen to best advantage on supine tomography. According to Ball and Proto,[861] the position of the nipple in relation to the aortic arch can vary from superomedial to inferolateral (Fig. 1–155). A variety of disease states that result in increased flow or pressure (or both) within the systemic venous system can cause the vein to dilate, comprising a useful roentgenographic sign analogous to the abnormal distention of the azygos vein in the presence of systemic venous hypertension.

As the paraspinal portion of the left superior intercostal vein turns anteriorly at the level of T3 or T4, it may abut aerated lung that delineates the top of the left paraspinal line (*see* further on), thus forming an interface that is roentgenographically visible.[864] In our experience, however, it is more common for the vein to be surrounded by mediastinal fat and buried deep within the mediastinum, so that its presence is only indirectly related to the cephalad portion of the paraspinal interface.

The third roentgenographic portrayal of the left superior intercostal vein, the retroaortic portion, was first described by Ball and Proto.[861] As the vein courses anteriorly from the spine to the aorta, it can contact aerated left lung behind the aorta, thus creating an interface that projects through the aortic knob. This interface can angle upward, downward, or horizontally, the last creating a squared-off appearance to the aortic arch (Fig. 1–155).

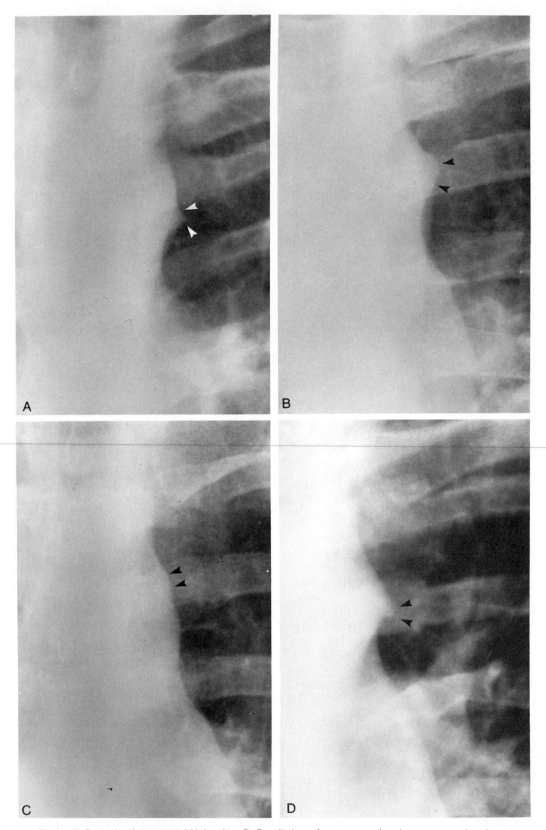

Figure 1–155. The Left Superior Intercostal Vein. *A* to *D*, Detail views from conventional posteroanterior chest roentgenograms of four normal adult patients show variations of the "aortic nipple" (*arrowheads*) representing the left superior intercostal vein as it passes anteriorly adjacent to the aortic knob; note that its position can vary from superomedial to inferolateral. In the upright position, the vein appears as a small protuberance along the lateral contour of the aortic arch.

Illustration continued on following page

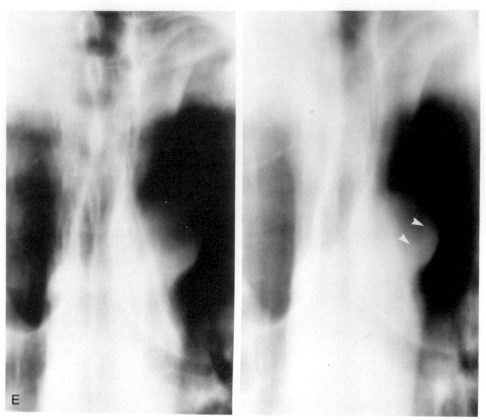

Figure 1–155 *Continued. E,* Conventional linear tomograms in AP projection through the aortic arch discloses a squared-off appearance (*arrowheads*) of the vein (the *retroaortic component*) as it courses anteriorly from the spine.

OTHER STRUCTURES

The left lateral wall of the trachea is rarely visible on a posteroanterior chest roentgenogram because of contiguity of the left subclavian artery and mediastinal fat. Similarly, the esophagus, which typically lies immediately posterior to the trachea on its left side, seldom creates a distinct interface with the left lung unless it is distended with gas; in the latter circumstance, a vertical stripe is created constituting the *left superior esophagopleural stripe.* Occasionally, the opacity of the left paraspinal line above the aortic arch (Fig. 1–154) can be seen medial to the interface formed by the left subclavian artery.

The posterior junction line is described in the section on the supra-azygos area.

The Infra-aortic Area

This compartment of the left side of the mediastinum extends from the aortic arch above to the diaphragm below and from the anterior mediastinal space in front to the paravertebral region behind. The contour of the mediastinum cephalad from the diaphragm includes the left ventricle, the left atrial appendage (seldom if ever identifiable as a separate opacity in normal subjects), the left border of the main pulmonary artery, the pleural reflection from the aorta downward onto the main pulmonary ar-

tery, and the aortic knob. General characteristics of the cardiac silhouette are described later. In this section we describe the paraspinal lines, the preaortic recess, and the inferior reflections of pleura off the aortic knob.

THE AORTOPULMONARY WINDOW AND AORTIC-PULMONARY LINE

The aortopulmonary window consists of a space situated between the arch of the aorta and left pulmonary artery and occupied largely by mediastinal fat; its lateral boundary is the mediastinal pleura and visceral pleura over the left lung, thus creating the aortopulmonary window interface. Within this space are situated fat, the ligament of the ductus arteriosus, the left recurrent laryngeal nerve, and lymph nodes. Its boundaries were described in the section on mediastinal lymph nodes (*see* page 194).

On a frontal chest roentgenogram, the patterns of pleural reflection in the vicinity of the aortic knob, left pulmonary artery, left hilum, and left heart border have been described by Blank and Castellino,[865] by Keats,[80] and by Heitzman and his colleagues.[866] In their study of 278 normal subjects, Blank and Castellino described two predominant patterns of pleural configuration, which they labeled reflection "A" and reflection "B." In more than 50 per cent of their cases, the contour was seen as a continuous opacity with a sharp left border extending caudad from the aortic arch to the level of the left main bronchus, usually as a smooth prolongation of the left heart border (reflection A). Five contour subdivisions were observed in this group.[867] It appears that the lower portion of reflection A is related to the main pulmonary artery, itself separated from the pleura by fat and connective tissue; this interface almost invariably projects through the aortic knob and represents the *aortic-pulmonary line* or stripe described by Keats (Fig. 1–156).[80] Computed tomographic correlation indicates that the interface is formed largely by mediastinal fat residing in front and to the left of the transverse portion of the aortic arch, anterolateral to the left pulmonary artery (Fig. 1–156). Displacement of this interface laterally, particularly as revealed by sequential roentgenograms, should suggest the possibility of mediastinal pathology (Fig. 1–156). To test the accuracy of PA and lateral roentgenograms in the assessment of aortopulmonary window pathology, Jolles and his colleagues[1188] recently carried out a retrospective study of 80 patients for whom conventional PA and lateral roentgenograms and CT images were available for review; in all patients CT revealed convincing evidence of abnormality in the aortopulmonary window. In 39 patients (49 per cent), there was no detectable abnormality in the window on the conventional roentgenograms, and in 8 patients (10 per cent) the findings were equivocal. Major contributing factors to this low detectability were the size and, more importantly, the location of lesions within the window.

In 38 per cent of Blank and Castellino's cases,[865] no continuous border opacity was seen; the pleura over the left margin of the aortic arch simply extended inferiorly and merged with the superior margin of the left pulmonary artery (reflection B).

The Posterior Pleural Reflections

The reflection of the pleura off the posterior thoracic wall, the anatomic basis for the paraspinal lines, has long intrigued anatomists and radiologists. The left paraspinal line is illustrated in the 1928 edition of the textbook by Schinz and his associates[868] as a line resulting from a pleural reflection. Subsequently, in 1942, on the strength of correlative anatomic-radiologic studies, Lachman[869] suggested that the posterior mediastinal boundaries of the lung and pleura were such that they appeared in the lower thoracic region as longitudinal linear opacities closely paralleling the lateral borders of the vertebrae. Lachman and others[869-874] postulated that the line is produced by the tangential x-ray projection of the pleura, lying in a sagittal plane, against aerated lung. Garland[872] introduced the term "linear thoracic paraspinal shadow" and suggested that it might be related to enlargement of the hemiazygos venous system. Heitzman[874] recently reaffirmed that the line represents the visceral and parietal pleura reflected off the posteromedial chest wall in a sagittal plane, and that it is seen because it represents an interface between highly radiolucent lung and mediastinal fat. There is universal agreement[868-874] that the right paraspinal line is seen less often than the left because the two pleural membranes on the right cross obliquely in front of the vertebrae, thus rendering their orientation inappropriate for the creation of a tangential interface.

Paramount to an understanding of the right and left pleural reflections is a knowledge of the distribution of normal mediastinal fat. Since the advent of CT, it has become increasingly clear that fat is a ubiquitous tissue within the mediastinum of the adult (fat is absent or small in amount in childhood), enveloping all of the important structures to some extent. Unfortunately, anatomy textbooks pay little attention to the distribution and quantity of mediastinal fat; indeed, most anatomic illustrations depict structures with the fat carefully removed. The quantity and location of mediastinal fat vary considerably depending on the habitus, nutritional state and age of the patient, the shape of the thorax, and the integrity and position of the vascular structures.[875] Fat normally accumulates in the superior, anterior, and lower posterior mediastinum (Fig. 1–157). Above the level of the aortic arch, the retroesophageal prevertebral space is usually devoid of fat, so the right and left upper lobe pleura can approximate, forming the posterior junction line. The quantity of fat around the esophagus tends to increase at the aortic arch, but below this point the paraesophageal and para-aortic fat diminish, only to increase again in the posterior mediastinum above the diaphragm. The lower thoracic aorta may be prespinal and completely surrounded by mediastinal fat, hence forming no contour with the lung. Above the aortic arch, the quantity of fat lateral to the vertebral bodies is usually symmetric, although below this level the left side almost always has more than the right, provided the aorta descends in the left para- or prespinal location (Fig. 1–157). If the aorta descends on the right, the opposite pertains. Rarely, paravertebral fat is present only on the right or is completely absent.

In the left hemithorax, the pleura reflects off the posterior chest wall and passes forward for a few centimeters in an anteroposterior plane before deviating over the posterior and lateral wall of the descending aorta; in the transverse plane, the shape of this interface between the retroaortic, paravertebral lung and the mediastinum is usually concave although at a lower level it may be either straight or slightly convex. The descending aorta normally deviates anteromedially and lies in a more central position before it exits through the aortic hiatus; in so doing, it may lose its contour-forming left border. As the aging aorta unfolds and protrudes into the left hemithorax, fat is deposited posteriorly, medially, and anteromedially to it (Fig. 1–158).

Text continued on page 226

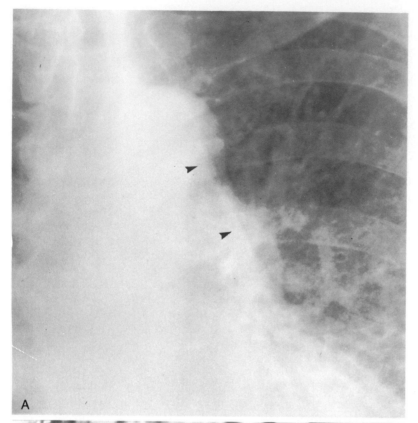

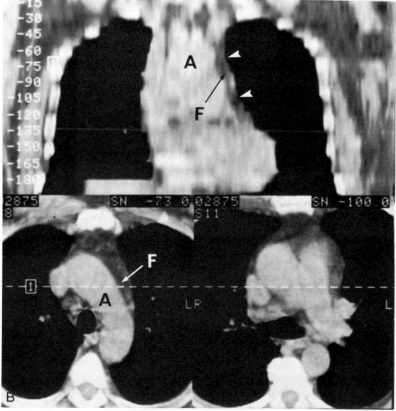

Figure 1–156. The Infra-aortic Area. *A,* A detail view from a conventional posteroanterior chest roentgenogram discloses a sharply defined interface that extends caudally from the aortic arch to the level of the left main bronchus (*arrowheads*), defining the *aortopulmonary line* or *interface. B,* A coronal CT reformation (*top*) and representative transverse images (*bottom*) show that the interface (*arrowheads*) represents air-containing lung abutting normal mediastinal fat (*F*) between the aortic arch (*A*) and the upper hilum. Detail views from posteroanterior chest roentgenograms of a middle-aged woman with Hodgkin's disease and rheumatoid arthritis before (*C*) and several months after (*D*) institution of corticosteroid therapy for the joint disease show an increasingly lobulated configuration in the contour of the aortopulmonary interface (*arrowheads*). *E,* Sequential CT scans reveal normal (albeit abundant) mediastinal fat (*F*) as the cause of the lobulated contour; this unusual fat deposition presumably relates to the corticosteroid therapy.

Illustration continued on opposite page

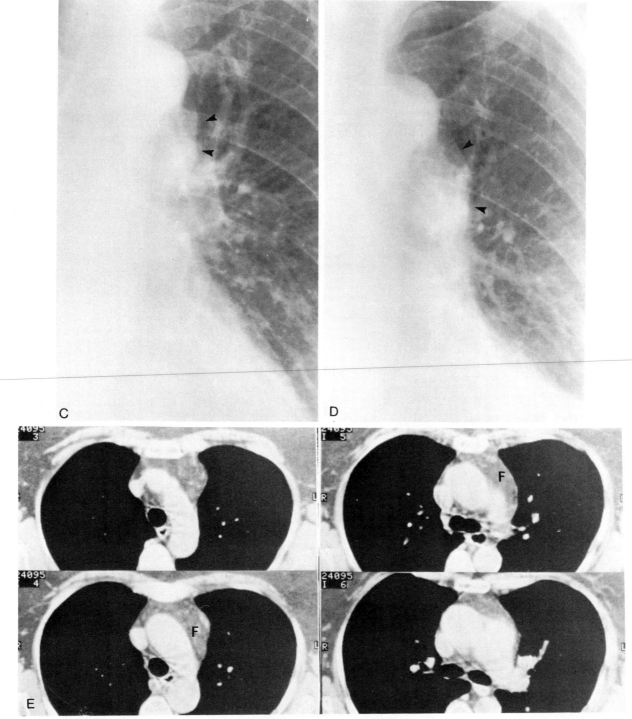

Figure 1–156 *Continued*

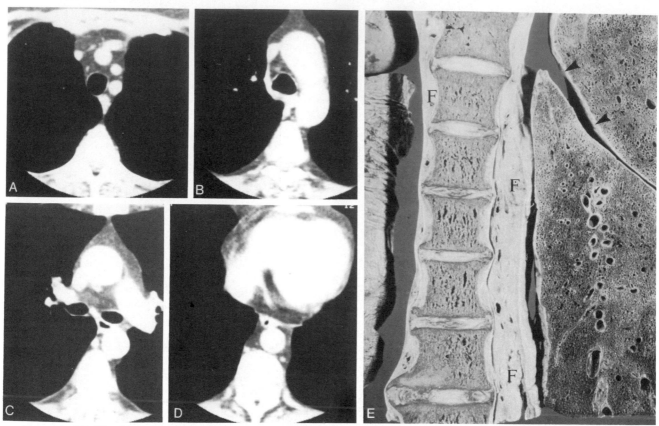

Figure 1–157. The Posterior Pleural Reflections. Representative CT scans through the superior mediastinum (*A*), aortic arch (*B*), left pulmonary artery (*C*), and left ventricle (*D*), reveal the normal locations of fat within the mediastinum. The major fat deposits in the adult are in the superior, anterior, and lower posterior mediastinum. Above the aortic arch, the retroesophageal prevertebral space is commonly devoid of fat. The quantity of fat around the esophagus tends to increase at the aortic arch, but below this point the paraesophageal and para-aortic fat diminishes, increasing again in the posterior mediastinum above the diaphragm. *E,* In a coronal anatomic section through the midthoracic vertebrae, the quantity of posterior mediastinal fat (*F*) to the right and left of the vertebrae at the level of the aortic arch (medial border of the left major fissure) (*arrowheads*) is equal; below this level, paravertebral fat is much more prominent on the left. (*A* to *D* from Genereux GP: AJR *141*:141, 1983, © American Roentgen Ray Society; *E* from Heitzman ER: The Mediastinum; Radiologic Correlations with Anatomy and Pathology. St. Louis, CV Mosby, 1977, pp 33–66.)

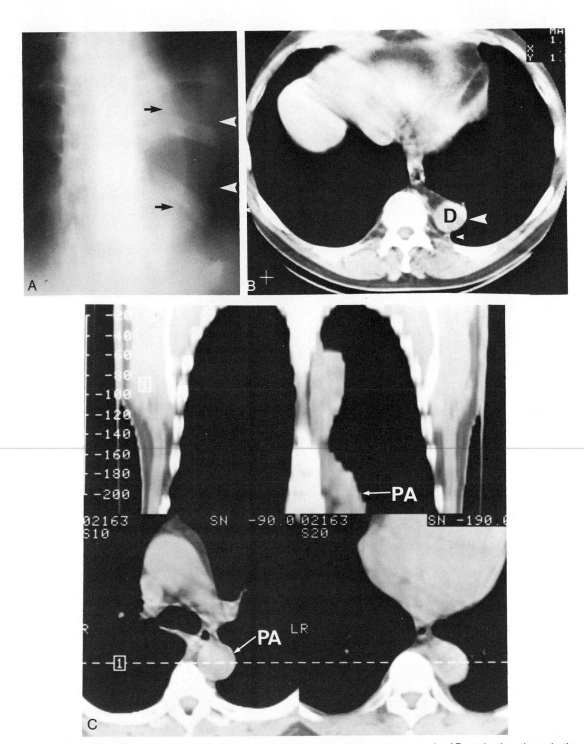

Figure 1–158. The Posterior Pleural Reflections. *A,* A conventional linear tomogram in AP projection through the posterior mediastinum shows the left paraspinal line (*arrows*) to be displaced laterally, closely paralleling the course of the elongated descending aorta (*arrowheads*). *B,* An unenhanced transverse CT scan through the lower thorax reveals posterior and lateral displacement of the descending aorta (*D*); the quantity of fat medial to the aorta is increased. The concave interface between lung and mediastinum behind the aorta (*small arrowhead*) is situated medial to the outer edge of the convex descending aorta (*arrowhead*). Coronal CT reformations (*top*) and appropriate axial images (*bottom*) through the descending aorta (*C*) and immediately posterior to it (*D*) permit correlation with the linear tomogram in *A*: note that in AP projection the paraspinal (*PS*) and para-aortic (*PA*) lines are both convex toward the lung whereas in the transverse plane their true shape is concave and convex respectively, accounting for the positive and negative Mach band enhancement that characterizes these interfaces. (*A* and *B* from Genereux GP: AJR *141*:141, 1983. © American Roentgen Ray Society.)

Illustration continued on following page

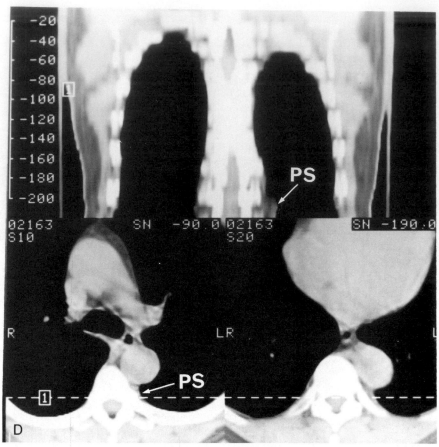

Figure 1–158 *Continued*

On the right side, the pleura continues in a posteromedial orientation and is often inseparable from the cortex of the contiguous vertebral bodies; above and below the azygos arch, it usually intrudes medially into the supra- and infra-azygos recesses.

In a study of eight normal subjects (5 men and 3 women, age range of 53 to 74 years) in which conventional linear tomography, computed tomography, and photodensitometry were employed (Fig. 1–159), Genereux[875] clarified the nature of the right and left posterior pleural reflections. The right and left paraspinal lines are about 1 mm wide and appear as linear opacities on an anteroposterior thoracic spine film or conventional tomogram. The left line extends from the top or middle of the aortic arch to the level of the ninth to twelfth thoracic vertebrae, depending on the degree of lung inflation (Fig. 1–159). When mediastinal fat is abundant, the line may be visible above the aortic arch, projected through the arch as a smooth curvilinear opacity that extends over the apex of the lung medial to the left subclavian artery (*see* Fig. 1–154). The left line tends to parallel the lateral margin of the vertebral bodies and can lie anywhere medial to the interface formed by the lung and the descending aorta, although commonly its position is midway between the spine and aorta. The lateral relationship of the descending aorta to the left paraspinal line exists throughout most of its course, although as the aorta declines toward the midline inferiorly it tends to overlap the paraspinal line. Rarely, the left paraspinal line can project outside the plane of the descending aorta, causing the latter to disappear from view.[875] The lung-aorta interface is marginated by a 1 mm black line, a feature that serves to distinguish it from the left paraspinal line.

The right paraspinal line is seen less often than the left and usually extends for only two or four vertebral segments at the T8 to T12 level before it merges below with the right crus of the diaphragm. Normally, the right line lies within a few millimeters of the vertebrae, reflecting the lesser quantity of paravertebral fat on the right side.

The traditional explanation for the visibility of the left paraspinal line holds that as the visceral and parietal pleura reflect off the posteromedial chest wall, they become oriented in a plane tangential to the x-ray beam in a frontal projection, thus creating an image.[869-874] Conversely, the failure to see a right paraspinal line has been explained on the basis that the two layers of pleura cross obliquely in front of the vertebrae, thereby rendering their orientation less conducive to imaging. Implicit to this theory is the assumption that the pleural layers are actually visible, i.e., they are interposed between two naturally high-contrast tissues, mediastinal fat and aerated lung. However, this hypothesis suffers from certain discrepancies, as we have pointed out:[838]

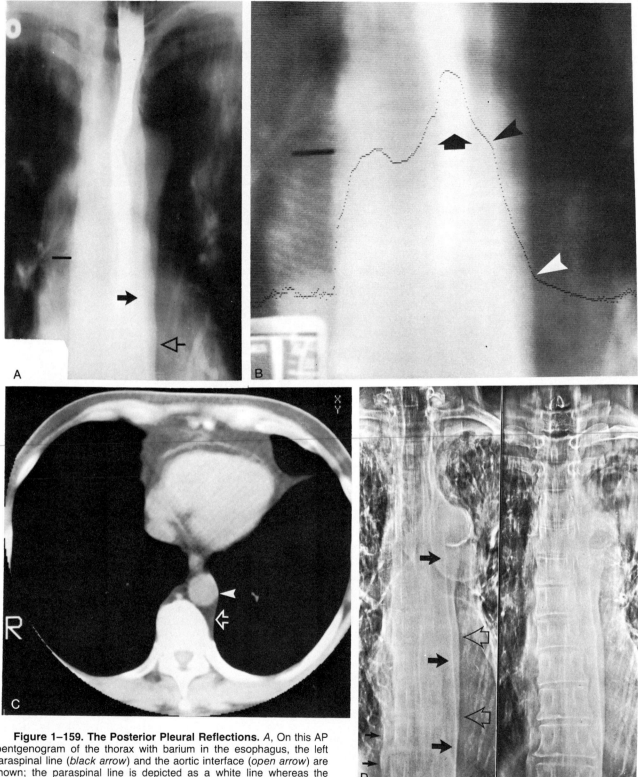

Figure 1–159. The Posterior Pleural Reflections. *A,* On this AP roentgenogram of the thorax with barium in the esophagus, the left paraspinal line (*black arrow*) and the aortic interface (*open arrow*) are shown; the paraspinal line is depicted as a white line whereas the aortic interface is enhanced by a black line. *B,* Photodensitometric analysis of the lines depicted in *A* at the level of the horizontal bar reveals a broad positive plateau over the spine and a focal peak (*broad arrow*) through the barium in the esophagus. There is no similar deflection over the left paraspinal line (*black arrowhead*) or aortic line (*white arrowhead*). These lines are Mach bands that are related to the shape of the lung-mediastinal interface rather than to the composition of tissue interposed between the lung and mediastinum. *C,* A transverse CT scan through the posterior mediastinum at the level of the bar depicted in *A* shows that the paraspinal line (*arrow*) relates to the *concave* interface between the lung and posterior mediastinum behind the aorta; by contrast, the aortic line is caused by the *convex* shape of the descending aorta (*arrowhead*) as it abuts the lung. *D,* Anteroposterior xerotomograms through the carina (*left*) and 2 cm posterior to the carina (*right*) reveal the 1-mm white, left paraspinal line (*large solid arrows*) extending from the midaortic arch to a point opposite T12, paralleling the vertebrae. Superiorly, the line is medial to the lateral wall of the descending aorta, the latter margined by a 1-mm black line (*open arrows*); inferiorly, the lines converge. Both lines disappear when opaque paper is placed adjacent to them, proving their optical properties as Mach bands. A right paraspinal line (*small arrows*) is seen in the lower hemithorax.

Illustration continued on following page

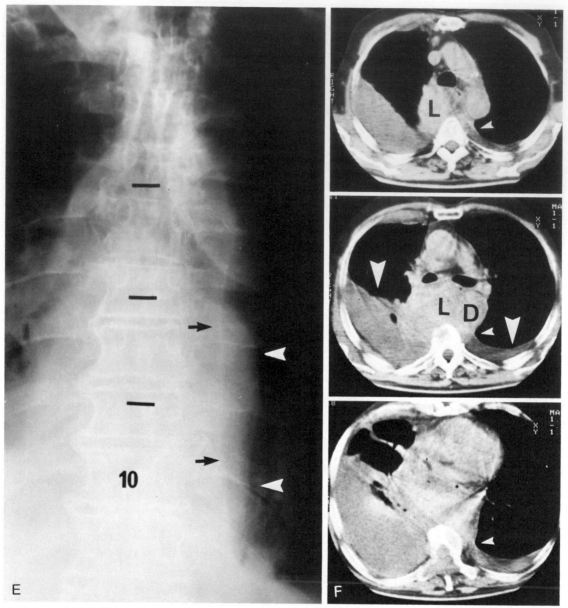

Figure 1–159 *Continued. E,* An anteroposterior roentgenogram of the thoracic spine demonstrates an apparently normal, white, left paraspinal line (*arrows*) medial to the descending aorta (*arrowheads*). *F,* Transverse CT scans at the level of the bars in *E* show that the descending aorta (*D*) is isodense with and enveloped by extensive posterior mediastinal lymphoma (*L*). Bilateral pleural effusions are present (*large arrowheads*). Note that the interface formed by the left lung and pleural effusion (*small arrowheads*) is concave in the supine position, accounting for a white line simulating a normal paraspinal line.

(1) The width of the paraspinal line observed roentgenographically is about 1 mm whereas the actual anatomic width of the visceral and parietal pleura is only approximately 0.4 mm; even with the interposition of a thin layer of normal pleural fluid, the total width probably does not exceed 0.5 mm.

(2) The theory does not adequately explain why there is not a reversal in the perceived appearance of the interface formed by the lung abutting the left posterior mediastinum when the descending aorta is enveloped by fat; in this circumstance, the descending aorta is marginated by a black line rather than a white line. Since the physical conditions (lung–pleura–mediastinal fat) traditionally employed to explain the visibility of the left paraspinal line are the same as around the aorta (pleura interposed between the lung and mediastinal fat), the interface delineating the descending aorta should appear as a white line rather than a black line, a feature that in our experience is never seen nor have we seen published illustrations in support of this hypothesis.

(3) Photodensitometric analysis through the paraspinal and para-aortic lines indicates that there is no density increase or decrease corresponding to these respective interfaces (Fig. 1–159).

(4) If the traditional explanation is correct, a small posterior pleural effusion should spread the

pleural membranes apart and should be perceived as a noticeably thickened paraspinal line or stripe analogous to the situation in which a small pericardial effusion may be visible on a lateral chest roentgenogram.[876] This feature has never been seen in our material nor have we seen published illustrations in support of this appearance; on the contrary, Trackler and Brinker[877] have shown that small pleural effusions simply cause the line to move laterally rather than to appear as a stripe (Fig. 1–159).

These and other arguments[875] lead to the conclusion that the paraspinal and para-aortic lines are Mach bands or edge-enhancing phenomena created by the retina in response to strong differences in transmitted illumination. Mach band formation is optimum when differences in transmitted light are created by structures whose surfaces are oriented at angles of less than 90° (i.e., concave or convex surfaces).[878] These two prerequisites are met in the posterior mediastinum (and indeed, elsewhere within the thorax) by the interfaces formed by the lung and mediastinum and the lung and descending aorta. The former is usually concave so that the eye enhances this interface by forming a positive (white) Mach band; the latter is convex, and consequently a negative (black) Mach band marginates its surface. In essence, it is the *true shape* of the lung-mediastinal interface (as viewed in the transverse plane) that defines the physical conditions for the visual perception of the paraspinal and para-aortic lines and *not* the tissue composition of this interface.

THE PREAORTIC RECESS

The left lower lobe can intrude anterior to the descending aorta and medial to the esophagus into the preaortic space (or recess), forming with the soft tissues of the mediastinum an interface known as the *preaortic line*.[866] Anatomically, the left-sided recess is analogous to the azygoesophageal recess on the right (*see* further on), although there are noteworthy differences; in keeping with the nomenclature of the azygoesophageal recess, we feel that the left-sided features are properly termed the *preaortic recess* and the medial contact of the lungs with the mediastinum, the *preaortic recess interface*.

The preaortic recess extends from the aortic arch above to the left hemidiaphragm below. Usually, only a small amount of lower lobe lung parenchyma invaginates into the preaortic region, creating a much narrower and smaller recess than its equivalent on the right. Occasionally, however, in patients with emphysema or kyphosis (for example), the depth of the preaortic recess (and azygoesophageal recess) can increase greatly, permitting recognition of both recess interfaces simultaneously (*see* Fig. 1–171D, page 247). The left pulmonary artery passes over the left main bronchus and then extends backward and downward into the interlobar fissure; in so doing, particularly when the depth of the aortopulmonary window is diminished, the artery

can "close" the cephalad portion of the recess so that it extends only from the inferior border of the interlobar artery to the diaphragm. Furthermore, the left inferior pulmonary vein and venous confluence can divide the preaortic recess into superior and inferior compartments (*see* Fig. 1–171B, page 246); more often, however, the recess can be identified as a shallow convex-medial, straight, or concave-medial interface (*see* Figs. 1–171C and 1–172B, pages 247 and 250). If gas is present in the proximal and middle portion of the infra-aortic esophagus, the interface will be depicted as the *left inferior esophagopleural stripe*.

The Supra-azygos Area

The supra-azygos area is that portion of the right side of the mediastinum that extends cephalad from the azygos arch to the thoracic inlet; it is separated from the infra-azygos area by the azygos vein and arch, an important landmark in roentgenologic interpretation.

The *azygos vein* originates in the upper lumbar region at the level of the renal veins as the continuation of the right subcostal vein or as an extension of the right ascending lumbar vein. It ascends into the thorax in the aortic hiatus medial to the right crus of the diaphragm.[879] In the thorax, the vein pursues a somewhat variable course and can be situated in front, to the right, or rarely to the left of the lower eight thoracic vertebrae (Fig. 1–160); it is joined at the T8 or T9 level by the hemiazygos vein ascending on the left. At the T4 or T5 level, the azygos vein arches anteriorly and slightly inferiorly and relates intimately to the lateral wall of the esophagus and the right posterior surface of the trachea. It then turns laterally for a short distance before proceeding anteriorly once again, passing over the right main bronchus and truncus anterior and lateral to the right inferior tracheal wall; it finally inserts into the back of the superior vena cava (Fig. 1–160). Along its course, the vein receives tributaries from the 5th to 11th intercostal veins on the right, the right subcostal vein, the right superior intercostal vein (that terminates in the azygos vein as it passes forward from the spine at the T4 or T5 level), the right bronchial veins, and the superior and inferior hemiazygos veins.

The *superior hemiazygos vein* begins at the vertebral end of the fourth left intercostal space as the continuation of the fourth posterior intercostal vein; the upper part is often connected to the left superior intercostal vein. It courses downward and forward in relation to T4 and then descends in close relationship to the left side of the descending aorta as far as the eighth thoracic vertebra. It then bends abruptly to the right and crosses behind the aorta to terminate in the azygos vein.

The *inferior hemiazygos vein* originates from the posterior aspect of the left renal vein or as a continuation of the left subcostal vein or left ascending lumbar vein. The hemiazygos vein enters the thorax

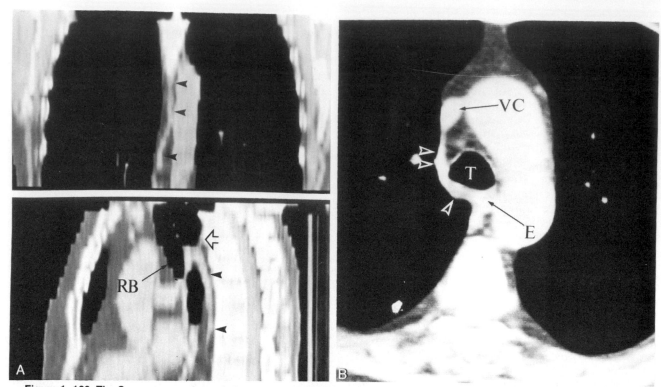

Figure 1–160. The Supra-azygos Area. *A,* Coronal (*top*) and sagittal (*bottom*) CT reformations demonstrate the course of the azygos vein (*arrowheads*). The azygos arch receives the right superior intercostal vein (*arrow*) and turns forward slightly above the plane of the right upper lobe bronchus (*RB*). *B,* A CT scan identifies the transverse course of the azygos vein. Note that before entering the superior vena cava (*VC*), it relates closely to the esophagus (*E*), the right posterior tracheal wall (*T*) (*arrowhead*), and the right upper lobe bronchus (*double arrowheads*).

medial to the left crus of the diaphragm and behind the descending aorta; it ascends anterolateral to the vertebral column; at the level of T8 or T9 it turns abruptly to the right and joins the azygos vein.

THE TRACHEAL INTERFACES

The trachea is normally bordered on its right lateral aspect by pleura covering the right upper lobe, and to a variable extent on its anterior and posterior aspects as well. Contact of the right lung in the supra-azygos area with the right lateral wall of the trachea creates a thin stripe of water density usually visible on frontal chest roentgenograms, designated the *right tracheal stripe* (Fig. 1–161). The stripe is formed by the right wall of the trachea, contiguous parietal and visceral pleura, and intervening areolar tissue. Occasionally, a variable quantity of mediastinal fat envelops the anterolateral surface of the trachea, creating the *right paratracheal line*[467] or *right paratracheal stripe* (Fig. 1–161).[880] Considerable variation exists in the incidence with which the right tracheal stripe or line is identified on posteroanterior roentgenograms; Felson identified it in 63 per cent of patients,[739] Heitzman in 82 per cent,[467] and Savoca and his colleagues in 94 per cent of 1259 normal subjects.[880] In the last-named series, the maximum width of the stripe was 4 mm, a measurement whose significance has been questioned by Heitzman in view of the variation in the

amount of tissue that separates the lung and trachea.[467] The thickness of the stripe must be measured above the level of the azygos vein; an increase in width on serial films is a more important sign of abnormality than is a single static measurement. Rarely, the left upper lobe abuts the left lateral wall of the trachea; since the left subclavian artery and contiguous mediastinal fat usually relate to the left side of the trachea, a *left paratracheal stripe* is seldom seen.

The *posterior tracheal stripe*, originally designated the *posterior tracheal band* by Bachman and Teixidor,[881] is a vertically oriented opacity formed by the posterior wall of the trachea in contact with right upper lobe parenchyma that inserts into the retrotracheal space. On well-exposed lateral roentgenograms of the chest, this stripe is frequently seen for the entire length of visible trachea and is often continuous inferiorly with the line or stripe formed by the posterior wall of the right main and intermediate bronchi (Fig. 1–162). Descriptions of the precise nature of the anatomic structures that make up the posterior tracheal stripe have been somewhat confusing: some investigators[882-884] consider that the stripe is formed by the combined thickness of the posterior tracheal wall and the esophagus; however, Palayew[885] has suggested, and Proto and Speckman have concurred,[828] that either retrotracheal soft tissue (Fig. 1–162) or the anterior esophageal wall related to a small amount of intraesophageal gas

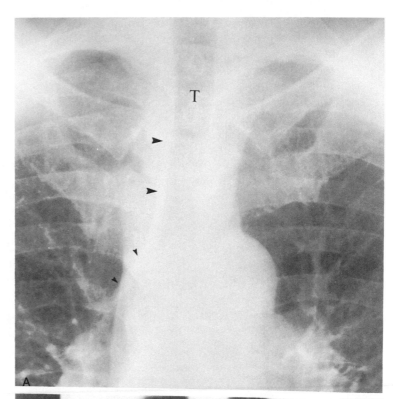

Figure 1–161. The Right Tracheal Interfaces.
A, A detail view from a PA chest roentgenogram shows a vertically oriented 2-mm linear opacity (*large arrowheads*) that parallels the tracheal air column (*T*) and is designated the *right tracheal stripe*. The ovoid opacity in the right tracheobronchial angle (*small arrowheads*) represents the third portion of the azygos arch as the vein passes over the right main and upper lobe bronchi. *B*, A coronal CT reformation (*top*) and transverse images (*bottom*) through the mid and lower trachea (*T*) show minimal areolar tissue between the tracheal wall and the lung (*arrowheads*). The linear opacity identified in *A* is caused primarily by the width of the tracheal wall.

Illustration continued on following page

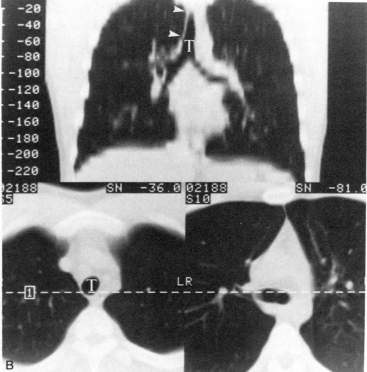

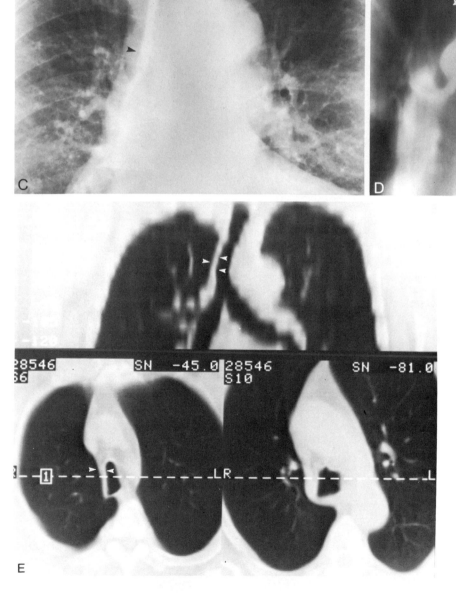

Figure 1–161 *Continued. C,* In another patient, detail views from a conventional PA chest roentgenogram and *D,* an anteroposterior linear tomogram show a tracheal stripe that measures 4 to 5 mm in diameter (*arrowheads*). *E,* A coronal CT reformation (*top*) with appropriate transverse scans (*bottom*) through the mid and lower trachea of this patient reveals a small amount of intervening fat between the tracheal wall and aerated right upper lobe parenchyma (*between arrowheads*). Since the amount of mediastinal fat is highly variable, quantitative values for the width of the stripe should not be relied upon as the sole determinant of abnormality; an increase in the width on serial films is a more important sign of abnormality.

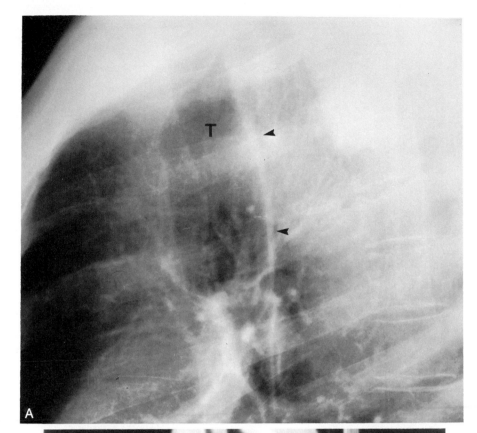

Figure 1–162. The Posterior Tracheal Interface. *A*, A conventional lateral chest roentgenogram demonstrates a 4-mm wide stripe (*arrowheads*) that parallels the air column of the trachea (*T*), the *posterior tracheal stripe. B*, A sagittal CT reformation (*top*) and transverse images (*bottom*) through the trachea (*T*) at the level of the aortic arch show that the stripe is caused by the posterior wall of the trachea itself (*arrowheads*). Note that in this patient, the esophagus (*E*) is not contour forming in lateral projection and thus does not contribute to the stripe.

Illustration continued on following page

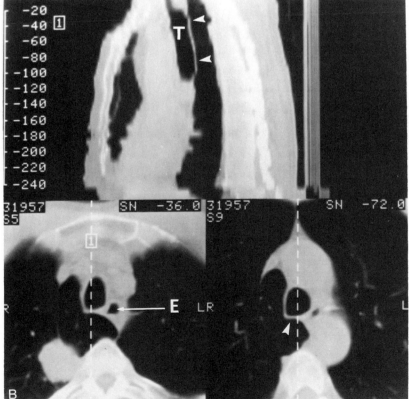

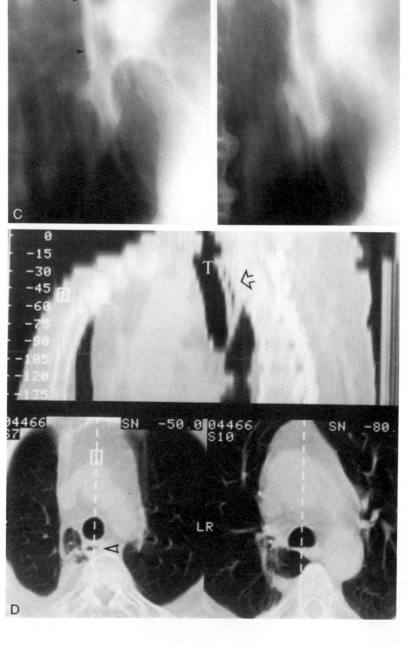

Figure 1–162 *Continued. C*, Detail views from conventional linear tomograms in lateral projection disclose a stripe 5 mm in width that extends along the entire length of the tracheal air column (*T*) (*arrow*) and intermediate stem line (*arrowheads*). *D,* A sagittal CT reformation (*top*) and transverse images (*bottom*) show that the linear opacity identified in *C* is caused by a combination of the posterior tracheal wall, mediastinal soft tissue, and gas-containing esophagus (*arrowhead*), thus constituting the *tracheoesophageal stripe* (*arrow*). A CT scan is needed to distinguish the two appearances with certainty.

(or both) could account for the stripe. Thus, according to the latter researchers, the soft tissue stripe behind the tracheal air column should be considered as either a *posterior tracheal stripe* or a *tracheoesophageal stripe* (Fig. 1–162), the former being composed of the posterior tracheal wall and any surrounding mediastinal tissue and the latter by the posterior tracheal wall, the anterior esophageal wall (the lumen containing a small amount of air), and any surrounding mediastinal tissue (Fig. 1–162). As a consequence of the variability in the amount of retrotracheal soft tissue, the position of the esophagus, and the amount of gas within the esophageal lumen, the tracheoesophageal stripe ranges in thickness from 1 to 5.5 mm (mean, 2 mm).[828] Palayew[885] has recommended that the upper limits of normal width for the posterior tracheal stripe be 2 to 3 mm. Distinction between the two varieties of stripes is possible only occasionally on conventional roentgenograms, but the tracheoesophageal stripe can be identified as such if a thin vertical radiolucency of fat separates the soft tissue stripe of the trachea from the esophagus, or if the stripe courses through the level of the azygos arch.[828] The incidence of visibility of the posterior tracheal stripe in the Palayew series was slightly less than 50 per cent, similar to that found by Proto and Speckman. The only certain way of distinguishing the two is by computed tomography.

To the best of our knowledge, Figley[886] was the first to draw attention to the importance of this stripe and its relationship to esophageal pathology, a relationship that has been substantiated by several other groups.[881-884] There is general agreement that a posterior tracheal stripe or tracheoesophageal stripe that measures more than 5 mm in width should be considered abnormal, most commonly as a manifestation of primary or recurrent esophageal carcinoma. Regardless of the accuracy of this measurement, it is certain that computed tomography is necessary to clarify the nature of the stripe in any individual case.

In a CT study of 100 normal subjects in which the trachea and its surrounding tissues were studied at the level of the sternal notch and 2 cm caudad, Kittredge[1179] found that the average thickness of the stripe was 8.4 mm ($\pm$ 3.8 mm SD), whereas at a CT level 2 cm below the sternal notch the posterolateral tracheal stripe had an average thickness of 6.4 mm ($\pm$ 1.8 mm SD).

THE POSTERIOR JUNCTION ANATOMY

The apices of the right and left upper lobes contact the mediastinum behind the esophagus anterior to the first and second vertebral bodies. In so doing, they create a V-shaped triangular opacity that constitutes the *posterior mediastinal triangle*; marginating this triangular configuration are the *right* and *left superior recesses* (Fig. 1–163). Caudally, the lungs intrude deeper into a prespinal location posterior to the esophagus and anterior to the third through fifth vertebral bodies where they form a pleural apposition that, along with any intervening mediastinal tissue, forms the *posterior junction line* (Fig. 1–163). On a posteroanterior roentgenogram, the posterior junction line usually projects through the air column of the trachea; it may be straight or slightly concave to the right. When intervening mediastinal tissue is abundant or a narrowed retroesophageal space precludes lung apposition, the posterior junction line can appear as a distinct stripe (Fig. 1–163).[851]

Below the posterior junction line, the lungs are excluded from the midline by the forward arching of the right and left superior intercostal veins and by the posterior portion of the azygos arch on the right and the aortic arch on the left. This divergence defines an inverted V-shaped opacity that, analogous to the situation superiorly, is marginated by the *right* and *left inferior recesses*. The right inferior recess is usually longer and extends more caudad than the left, reflecting the more caudal location of the azygos arch than the aortic arch.

THE RIGHT AND LEFT SUPERIOR ESOPHAGEAL STRIPES

Proto and Lane[887] identified air in the esophagus on the posteroanterior roentgenogram of the chest in 36 per cent of 200 normal subjects and in approximately 50 per cent of 200 patients with abnormal chest roentgenograms. The commonest site for esophageal air to be identified relates to the aortic arch, and in decreasing order of frequency includes that portion of the esophagus immediately below, above, and medial to the arch. The posteromedial portion of the upper lobe abuts the lateral wall of the esophagus on the right side whereas the posteromedial portion of the left upper lobe may or may not show a similar relationship, depending upon the position of the esophagus, the depth of the retroesophageal mediastinum, and the quantity of mediastinal fat. When gas is present within the upper esophagus, a vertically oriented soft tissue stripe may be identifiable on the right side or left side or both, provided the inner and outer margins of both esophageal walls are tangential to the x-ray beam. Originally designated the *esophagopleural stripe* by Cimmino,[888, 889] this stripe was renamed the *esophageal stripe* by Proto and Lane[887] and by Heitzman,[874] negating the contribution of the paper-thin pleura (Fig. 1–164).

In its most typical configuration, the right esophageal wall courses obliquely from upper right to lower left and is usually convex along its inner border. The left esophageal wall runs parallel to the right, although the two may diverge superiorly and inferiorly in relation to the superior and inferior recesses of the posterior junction.

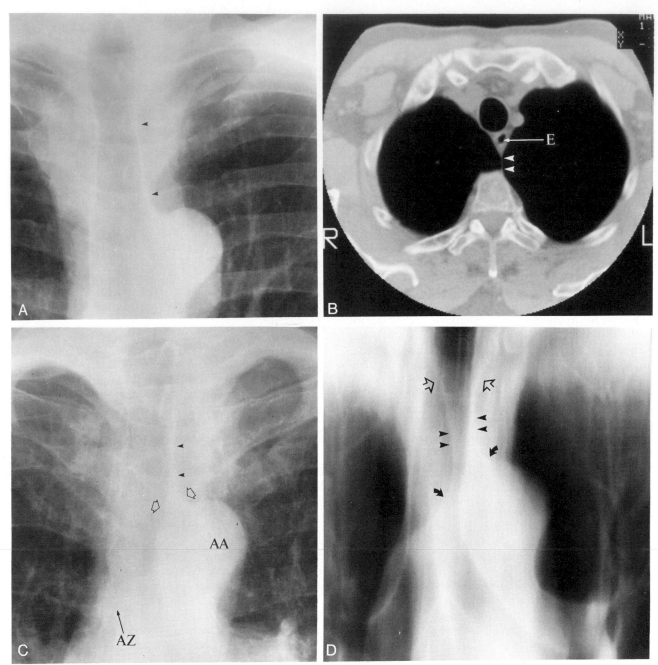

Figure 1–163. Posterior Junction Anatomy. *A,* A detail view of the superior mediastinum from a conventional PA chest roentgenogram demonstrates a thin linear opacity called the *posterior junction line (arrowheads).* It courses obliquely from above downward, slightly to the left of the midline, and relates to thoracic vertebrae 3 to 5. *B,* On a transverse CT scan through the posterior mediastinum above the aortic arch, the right and left upper lobes can be seen to be almost contiguous with one another behind the esophagus (*E*), separated only by a small amount of mediastinal soft tissue and four layers of pleura (*arrowheads*). *C,* In a different patient, a detail view from a posteroanterior chest roentgenogram demonstrates a somewhat thicker posterior junction line (*arrowheads*), which terminates inferiorly in a triangular opacity whose apex points cephalad and whose base abuts the aortic arch (*AA*). The right and left interfaces (*arrows*) are designated the *right* and *left inferior recesses.* The right recess extends caudally to cover the azygos arch (*AZ*) whereas the shorter left recess terminates on the medial aspect of the aortic arch. *D,* A conventional linear tomogram in AP projection reveals a thick stripe (*arrowheads*) or septum that connects the superior (*open arrows*) and inferior (*closed arrows*) recesses. This manifestation is caused by a narrow retrotracheal space or increased mediastinal fat or both.

Illustration continued on opposite page

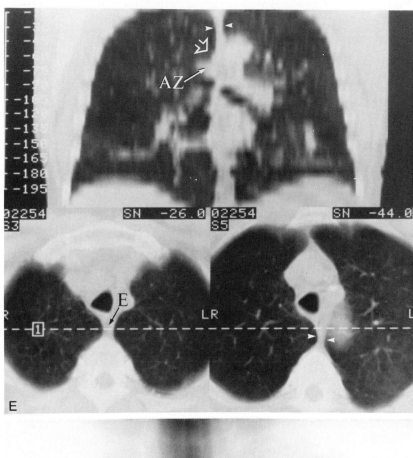

Figure 1–163 *Continued. E,* On a different patient, a coronal CT reformation (*top*) with appropriate transverse images (*bottom*) shows the upper lobes behind the esophagus (*E*) to be separated by a thick septum (*arrowheads*) composed of posterior mediastinal fat, the esophagus, and four layers of pleura; the right inferior recess (*arrow*) extends to the azygos vein arch (*AZ*). *F,* A conventional linear tomogram in AP projection through the posterior mediastinum demonstrates the three components of the posterior junction anatomy: (1) the right and left superior recesses (*small arrowheads above*) separated by the superior, posterior triangle (*SM*); (2) the posterior junction line (*large arrowheads*); and (3) the right and left inferior recesses (*small arrowheads below*) separated by the inferior, posterior mediastinal triangle (*IM*).

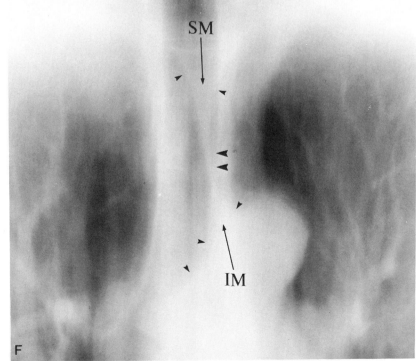

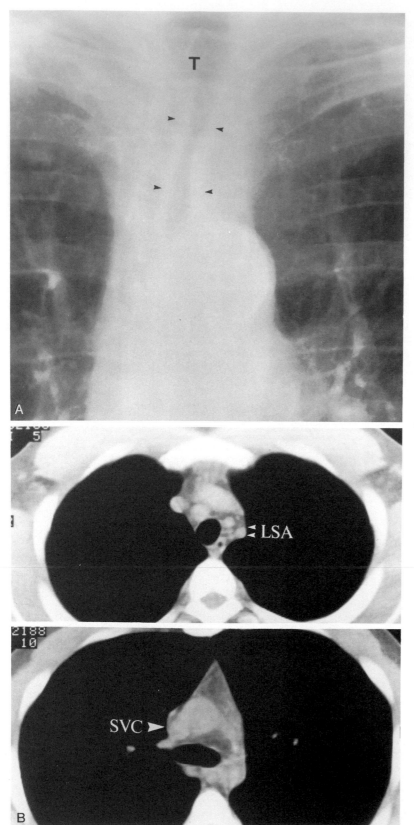

Figure 1–164. The Superior Esophageal Stripes. *A,* A detail view from a conventional posteroanterior chest roentgenogram shows two vertical stripes (*arrowheads*) projected through the tracheal air column (*T*). The linear opacities represent the right and left walls of the gas-distended esophagus, designated the *right* and *left superior esophagopleural* or *esophageal stripes. B,* CT scans through the superior mediastinum show the right and left esophageal wall (*arrowheads*) separated by a small amount of gas within the esophageal lumen (*EL*). Aerated lung in the right and left upper lobes abuts mediastinal fat and the lateral esophageal wall, accounting for the linear opacities seen in *A.*

THE AZYGOS ARCH

At the level of the aortic arch, the azygos vein is composed of three parts, posterior (paraesophageal), middle (retrotracheal), and anterior (right tracheobronchial angle). Heitzman has described in some detail the configuration as seen on anteroposterior tomograms.[874] The *posterior* part is abutted by right upper or lower lobe parenchyma laterally and the esophagus medially. The posterior turn of the azygos vein merges above with that of the right inferior recess and below with the pleura in the cephalad portion of the azygoesophageal recess. The *middle* or retrotracheal component is seen through the air column of the trachea as an opacity that is angled slightly downward and to the right; it merges laterally with the oval or elliptic shadow of the *anterior* component viewed end-on as it passes forward in the tracheobronchial angle. Depending upon the distention of the vessel and the depth of the supra-azygos and infra-azygos recesses, the vein may be identified on a lateral chest roentgenogram or conventional lateral tomogram (Fig. 1–165) as a retrotracheal elongated opacity as it passes forward over the right main bronchus. This appearance should not be mistaken for a mass such as enlarged lymph nodes.

In a tomographic study of 78 adult subjects in the supine position, Austin and Thorsen identified the retrotracheal part of the normal azygos vein in 38 (49 per cent).[891] Five distinct patterns were found, depending chiefly on the course of the inferior margin of the arch: (1) the inferior margin crossed posterior to the right main bronchus, the superior margin being retrotracheal (compare item 5); (2) the inferior margin passed posterior to the left main bronchus; (3) the inferior margin was not identified but the retrotracheal superior margin was well seen; (4) the inferior margin crossed at the carina; and (5) both the inferior and superior margins of the arch crossed posterior to the proximal part of the right main bronchus.

Mensuration of the anterior portion of the azygos vein is important in some diseases, notably portal hypertension, obstruction of the superior vena cava, and systemic venous hypertension. The only segment that can be measured accurately on conventional roentgenograms is the point at which the vein is viewed roughly tangentially in the right tracheobronchial angle as it enters the superior vena cava. In this location, it often is visible as a slightly flattened elliptic opacity (Fig. 1–166). Fleischner and Udis[1180] measured the vein from its outer border to the contiguous air column of the right main bronchus on erect posteroanterior roentgenograms and recorded a maximal transverse diameter of 6

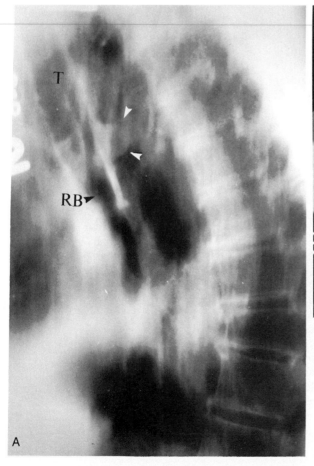

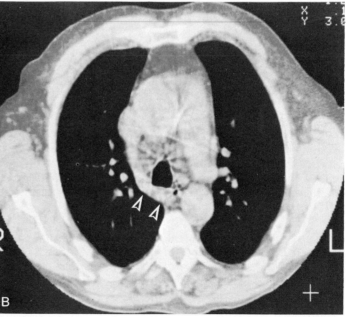

Figure 1–165. The Azygos Vein: Retrotracheal Component. *A*, conventional lateral tomogram through the trachea (*T*) reveals a rounded opacity (*arrowheads*) above the right upper lobe bronchus (*RB*), representing the retrotracheal component of the azygos arch. Its location and shape serve to differentiate this presentation from enlarged lymph nodes. *B*, A CT scan at the level of the azygos arch demonstrates the retrotracheal component (*arrowheads*) abutted by aerated right upper lobe, accounting for the visibility of the vein in this location.

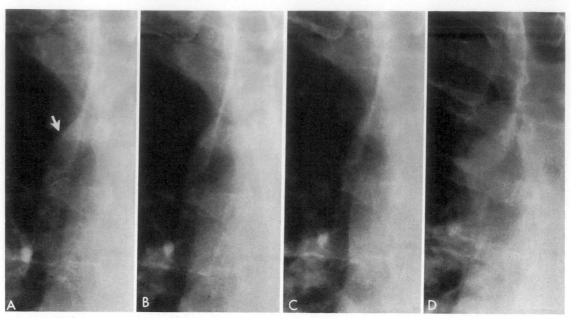

Figure 1–166. Physiologic Variations in Azygos Vein Diameter. Detail views of the region of the right tracheobronchial angle from four posteroanterior roentgenograms of a healthy 30-year-old man showing the variations in size of the azygos vein caused by changes in intrathoracic pressure. *A*, At full inspiration with sustained Mueller maneuver, vein diameter 13 mm (*arrow*); *B*, at full inspiration, maintained with glottis open, vein diameter 7 mm; *C*, at full inspiration with sustained Valsalva maneuver, vein diameter 3 mm; *D*, at full expiration with sustained Mueller maneuver, vein diameter 17 mm. *See* text for discussion.

mm. In a study of the roentgenograms of 100 men and 100 nonpregnant women, Keats and his associates[892] found an average diameter of 4.9 mm (range, 3 to 7 mm) in the men and 4.8 mm (range, 3 to 7 mm) in the women. These values are lower than those recorded by other workers: for example, Felson[739, 893] states that a transverse diameter of 10 mm may be normal, and we have observed the same diameter in many normal subjects. In fact, one of our radiology residents, a healthy 30-year-old man who had a screening chest roentgenogram exposed while he tried to inspire beyond TLC with the glottis open, had an azygos vein diameter of 13 mm (Fig. 1–166). Review of his previous roentgenograms exposed in the usual manner showed the vein diameter to be approximately 7 mm, indicating that the increased venous return occasioned by the modified Mueller maneuver was responsible for the distention.

During the 1970s, for all subjects 30 years of age or over, we routinely performed posteroanterior chest roentgenography at both full inspiration and maximal expiration; this showed great variation in the size of the azygos vein shadow, being larger on inspiration than on expiration in some patients and vice versa in others (Fig. 1–167). Since these included a majority of subjects with no suspicion of pulmonary or cardiovascular disease, it is clear that variation in azygos vein diameter is related to intrathoracic pressure phenomena: when the vein is smaller on inspiration than on expiration, the patient is probably involuntarily performing the Valsalva maneuver when asked to hold his or her

breath for exposure of the inspiration film, whereas a subject with a larger vein diameter on the inspiratory film is presumably holding his or her breath with the glottis open.

Of considerable interest in the report of Keats and his associates[892] was the wide range of measurements and increased average size of the azygos vein observed in 100 pregnant women. The minimal diameter was 3 mm, but the maximal diameter was 15 mm and the average, 7.14 mm. This normal effect of pregnancy, undoubtedly related to hypervolemia, should be borne in mind when considering the differential diagnosis of azygos vein enlargement.

Determination of the azygos vein's maximal diameter under various conditions of transthoracic pressure requires further study; meanwhile, it is reasonable to adopt the following general rules. In the majority of normal subjects in the erect position, the azygos vein diameter is 7 mm or less; a diameter of 7 to 10 mm is seen sometimes and is almost always within the normal range; a diameter exceeding 10 mm should be regarded as pathologic except in pregnant women and in unusual circumstances of maximal negative intrapleural pressure (as in our resident). Vascular distention caused by change in body position from erect to recumbent increases the vein's diameter (Fig. 1–168). Doyle and his associates,[894] using a tomographic technique with a shortened focus-film distance, measured the maximal diameter of 40 healthy subjects in the supine position and plotted this against several parameters, including age, sex, weight, height, and body surface

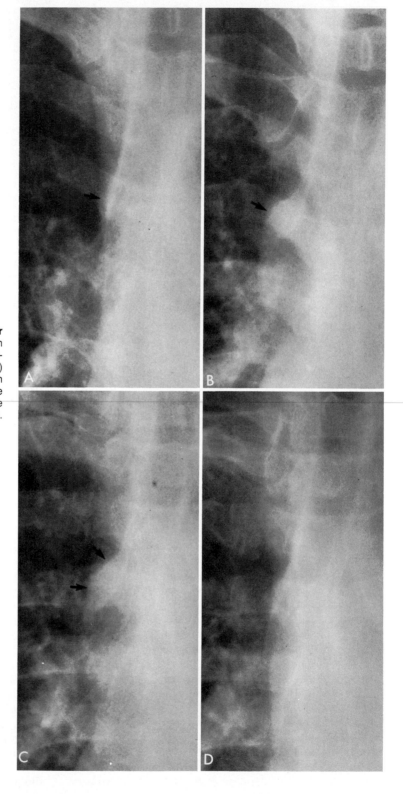

Figure 1–167. Variation in Azygos Vein Diameter from Inspiration to Expiration. Detail view of the region of the right tracheobronchial angle from two normal subjects in the erect position, in maximal inspiration (*TLC*) and full expiration (*RV*). In *A* and *B* the azygos vein (*arrow*) is smaller on inspiration than on expiration, the more common appearance. In *C* (*arrows*) and *D* the azygos vein is larger on inspiration than on expiration. *See* text for discussion.

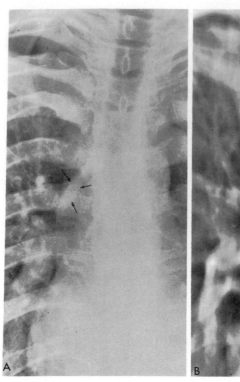
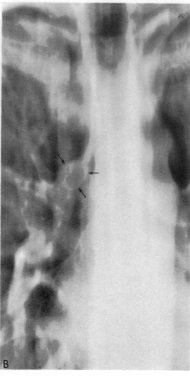

Figure 1–168. Effect of Body Position on Azygos Vein Diameter. *A,* A roentgenogram in the erect position shows the azygos vein as an elliptic shadow projected in the right tracheobronchial angle (*arrows*). *B,* In the same subject, a tomographic section of the midmediastinum in the supine position demonstrates a much larger vein shadow (*arrows*) owing to distention brought about by the supine body position.

area. The only significant correlation was with body weight. Standardization of the diameters to a body weight of 64 kg yielded a mean azygos vein diameter of 14.2 mm; the diameter exceeded 16 mm in only eight subjects. It seems reasonable to employ these figures to indicate normality or otherwise in patients whose roentgenograms must be obtained in a supine position at the bedside.

THE VASCULAR PEDICLE

In an extensive review of the superior mediastinal vascular interfaces, Milne and his associates[895] pointed out that a large portion of the mediastinal opacity on both posteroanterior and anteroposterior chest roentgenograms is caused by the great systemic vessels, and that the heart may be considered to be "hanging" from these vessels; this concept prompted these workers to call this structure *the vascular pedicle.* On the frontal chest roentgenogram, the vascular pedicle extends from the thoracic inlet to the top of the heart. On the right, its boundary is formed by the right innominate vein above and the superior vena cava below. The left border of the pedicle is formed by the left subclavian artery above the aortic arch. In essence, the right side of the pedicle is situated anteriorly and is entirely venous whereas the left side lies more posteriorly and is arterial (Fig. 1–169). Milne and his coworkers measured the width of the vascular pedicle on PA (or AP) chest roentgenograms from the point at which the superior vena cava crosses the right main

bronchus to the point at which the left subclavian artery arises from the aortic arch (Fig. 1–169). Using these landmarks in 83 normal subjects, it was determined that the mean value was 48 mm (± 5 mm SD). As anticipated, there was considerable difference in the width between sthenic and asthenic subjects, and it was concluded that 95 per cent of people will fall within two standard deviations of the mean (38 to 58 mm).

The azygos vein was seen in 70 of the 84 normal subjects (84 per cent), possessing a mean dimension of 5.14 mm (± 1.36 mm SD); no significant difference was detected between the 36 men and 34 women used in the assessment. Pistolesi and his associates[896] and Milne and his colleagues[897] applied the concept of the vascular pedicle width and the azygos vein width in the assessment of the hemodynamic status of the systemic circulation in 61 patients with cardiac disease and correlated these features with total blood volume. It was shown that there was a highly significant linear correlation between the width of the vascular pedicle and total blood volume (r = 0.80, p<0.001). In patients with dilated neck veins, vascular pedicle width was greater than 62 mm, a measurement that correlated strongly (r = 0.93, p<0.0001) with a change in total blood volume (0.5 cm change in pedicle width = 1.0 liter change in blood volume). By contrast, the correlation between the azygos vein width and total blood volume was poor (r = 0.50, p<0.01), although the correlation between vein width and mean right atrial pressure was stronger (r = 0.74, p<0.001).

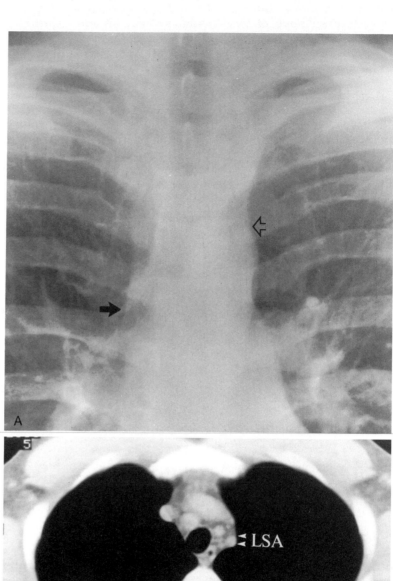

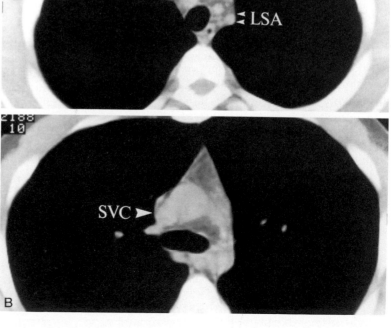

Figure 1–169. The Normal Vascular Pedicle.
A, A detail view from a conventional posteroanterior roentgenogram demonstrates the points for measuring the width of the vascular pedicle (VPW). The right (venous) border of the VPW is the point at which the superior vena cava crosses the right main bronchus (*closed arrow*), whereas the left border is the point of takeoff of the left subclavian artery from the aorta (*open arrow*). The VPW is measured from the superior vena cava to a perpendicular line extended caudally from the left subclavian artery. *B*, A CT scan through the superior mediastinum at the level of the superior vena cava (*SVC*) (*single arrowhead*) and left subclavian artery (*LSA*) (*arrowheads*) show that the right border is entirely venous and the left border entirely arterial.

In an attempt to differentiate between physiologic and pathologic intravascular and extravascular causes for widening of the vascular pedicle, Milne and his associates[897] correlated the width of the pedicle with visibility of the right tracheal stripe and the azygos vein on the posteroanterior roentgenograms of 158 patients. The widened pedicle was attributed to intravascular causes in 108 patients and to vascular bleeding or inappropriate infusion through malpositioned subclavian lines in 50 patients. An increase in systemic blood volume (or the supine position) resulted in a combination of widening of the vascular pedicle to the right and dilatation of the azygos vein (Fig. 1–170); the tracheal stripe and azygos vein were visible in 77 to 100 per cent of patients in this group. By contrast, extravascular causes of widening of the mediastinal silhouette (e.g., aortic trauma or extravasation of blood or saline) resulted in widening of the pedicle to either the left or right of the midline (depending upon the specific etiology), obliteration of the tracheal stripe, and loss of visibility of the azygos vein. Of 40 patients with post-traumatic bleeding into the vascular pedicle and in 10 patients with inadvertent extravascular infusion into the pedicle, visibility of the tracheal stripe and azygos vein ranged from zero to 15.4 per cent.

The Infra-azygos Area

THE AZYGOESOPHAGEAL RECESS

As previously described, the azygos vein ascends in the posterior mediastinum in relation to the right side or front of the vertebral column. The esophagus is usually located slightly anterior and to the left of the vein in the prevertebral region although they are sometimes in contact. Between the esophagus and the azygos vein is a small space into which the right lower lobe parenchyma may intrude to a variable degree. Termed by anatomists the *crista pulmonis* and by Heitzman and his colleagues[898, 899] the *azygoesophageal recess*, this space is highly variable in depth, depending largely upon the degree of lung inflation and the position of the descending aorta. The recess slopes obliquely from above downward so that the superior component is located posterior to the inferior; consequently, in some subjects the anterior aspect of the azygoesophageal recess can be divided by the right inferior pulmonary vein into well-defined superior and inferior divisions (Fig. 1–171).

The azygoesophageal recess is frequently identified on well-penetrated posteroanterior roentgenograms as an interface that extends from the diaphragm below to the level of the azygos arch above. Its right side is sharply delineated by aerated right lower lobe parenchyma, but its left side is usually of unit density because of contiguity of the azygos vein, esophagus, aorta, and surrounding posterior mediastinal connective tissue. Viewed from above downward on a frontal chest roentgenogram, the configuration of the azygoesophageal recess interface is variable: typically, it presents as a continuous shallow or deep arc concave to the right (Fig. 1–171); however, sometimes this continuity is interrupted by the right inferior pulmonary vein and venous confluence, giving rise to a shallow figure 3 configuration (concave to the right both superiorly and inferiorly and interrupted in the middle by a venous part convex to the right). As emphasized by Heitzman,[467] concavity of the superior aspect of the azygoesophageal recess interface is the rule, and any deviation should raise the suspicion of pathology. However, in young adults, a straight or slightly dextroconvex interface can be a normal CT variant.[900]

Occasionally, the anterior interface of the azygoesophageal recess can be identified on a lateral chest roentgenogram as a discontinuous or continuous serpentine linear opacity that extends from the end-on orifice of the left upper lobe bronchus above to the posterior margin of the inferior vena cava below. Continuity of the line is frequently interrupted in its midportion as the right inferior pulmonary venous confluence is formed; the latter creates a distinct convex posterior bulge in the contour. The upper part of the interface is located approximately 10 to 20 mm in front of the left lower lobe bronchus, its surface being marginated by a faint positive Mach band; on the other hand, the lower component above the hemidiaphragm is usually accentuated by a negative Mach band. Correlation of conventional lateral roentgenograms and CT scans suggests that the contour is formed in succession from above downward by lung in the anterior portion of the azygoesophageal recess abutting the posterior wall of the right main bronchus, the mediastinum medial to the intermediate bronchus, the right posterior surface of the left atrium, the posterior margin of the right inferior pulmonary vein, and caudally, the inferior vena cava, right atrium, or mediastinal soft tissue adjacent to the coronary sinus (Fig. 1–171).

If gas is present in a distended esophagus, the combined thickness of the right esophageal wall and contiguous pleura can create a vertically oriented linear opacity or stripe known as the *right inferior esophagopleural stripe* (Fig. 1–172). Although there is a potential for the left lung to abut the left wall of the esophagus, it is normally excluded by paraesophageal fat and the descending aorta; when intruding lung does make contact with the gas-distended esophagus, a *left inferior esophagopleural stripe* may be formed (Fig. 1–172). If the right and left lower lobe pleura meet behind the esophagus (an uncommon situation), a *posteroinferior junction line* may be identified (Fig. 1–173).

Text continued on page 252

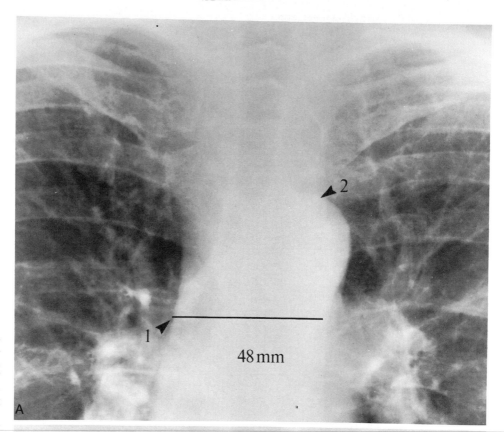

Figure 1–170. The Abnormal Vascular Pedicle. *A,* A detail view from a conventional posteroanterior chest roentgenogram reveals a vascular pedicle width of 48 mm. (VPW is measured from point 1 to a perpendicular dropped from point 2—*see* Figure 1–169.) *B,* Following the onset of congestive heart failure, the vascular pedicle width has increased to 72 mm (compare the size of the upper lobe vasculature in the two illustrations). Most of the increase in the VPW is caused by distention of the superior vena cava.

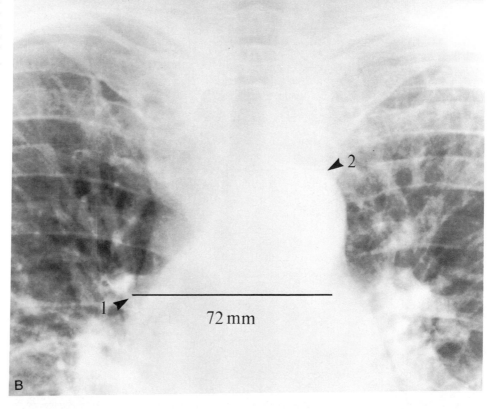

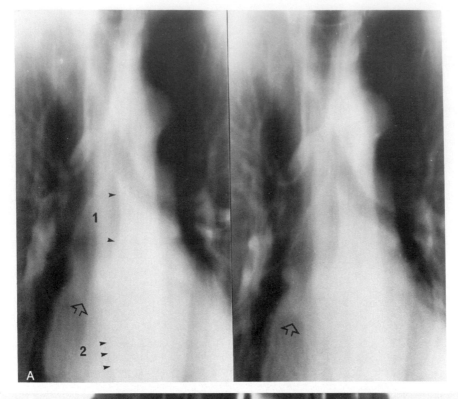

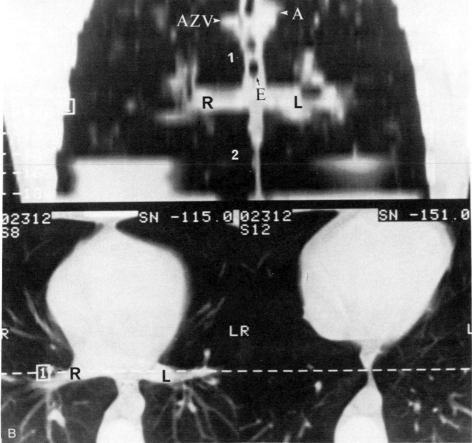

Figure 1–171. The Infra-azygos Area. *A,* Conventional linear tomograms in AP projection, 1 cm behind (*left*) and through the right inferior pulmonary venous confluence (*right*) (*arrow*), show the configuration of the *azygoesophageal recess (arrowheads).* In some subjects, the venous confluence serves to divide the anterior portion of the azygoesophageal recess into superior (*1*) and inferior (*2*) components. *B,* A coronal CT reformation (*top*) and representative transverse images (*bottom*) through the right (*R*) and left (*L*) inferior pulmonary veins demonstrate how these veins compartmentalize the azygoesophageal recess into superior (*1*) and inferior (*2*) components. The azygos vein (*AZV*) covers the cephalad portion of the azygoesophageal recess. A small amount of gas is present in the infra-azygos portion of the esophagus (*E*). The *preaortic recess* on the left, beneath the aortic arch (*A*), shows similar features.

Illustration continued on opposite page

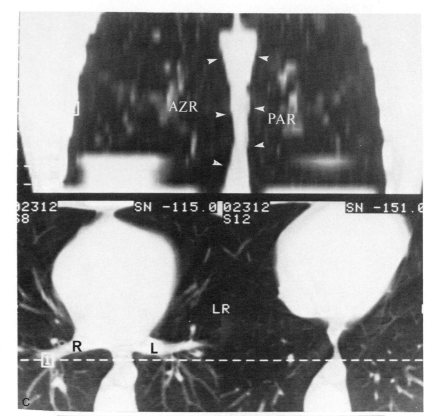

Figure 1–171 *Continued. C,* A coronal CT reformation (*top*) and representative transverse images (*bottom*) approximately 1 cm behind the right (*R*) and left (*L*) inferior pulmonary veins reveal the more usual configuration of the azygoesophageal recess (*arrowheads*) (concave to the right) and the preaortic recess (*PAR*) (*arrowheads*).

D, In a detail view from a conventional PA chest roentgenogram of a middle-aged man with miliary tuberculosis, the concave, deep azygoesophageal recess (*open arrows*) and the straight preaortic recess (*closed arrows*) are shown. The cephalad portion of these two recesses is the azygos arch (*AZV*) and the aortic arch (*AA*), respectively.

Illustration continued on following page

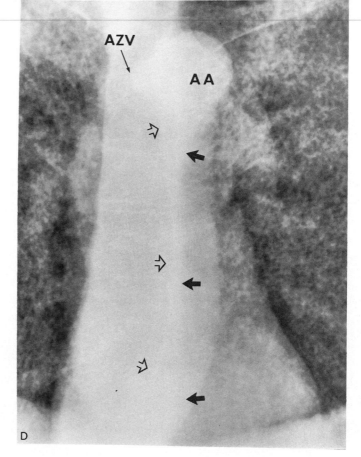

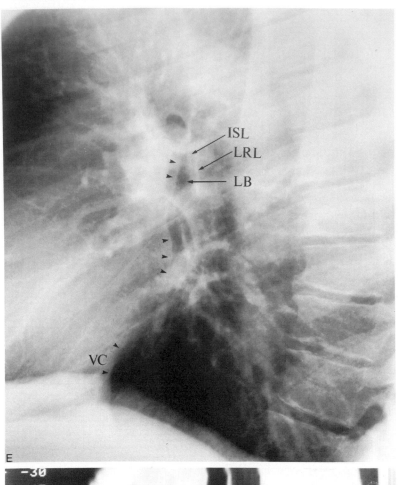

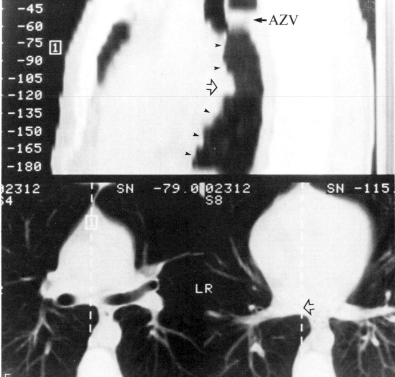

Figure 1–171 *Continued. E,* A detail view from a conventional lateral chest roentgenogram reveals a linear opacity (*two small arrowheads*) that transects the left upper lobe bronchus (*LB*); more caudally this interface possesses a convex posterior component (*three small arrowheads*). Still further caudally, the line is interrupted, only to be perceived again above the right hemidiaphragm at the level of the inferior vena cava (*VC*). These latter features are formed by lung in the anterior portion of the azygoesophageal recess. The intermediate stem line (*ISL*) and the left retrobronchial line (*LRL*) are also shown.

F, A sagittal CT reformation (*top*) and representative transverse images (*bottom*) from the patient shown in *E* demonstrate the typical shape of the anterior margin of the azygoesophageal recess (*arrowheads*). The roof of this space is the azygos vein arch (*AZV*). Note the posterior convex protuberance (*arrow*) in the contour that identifies the confluence of the right inferior pulmonary vein.

Illustration continued on opposite page

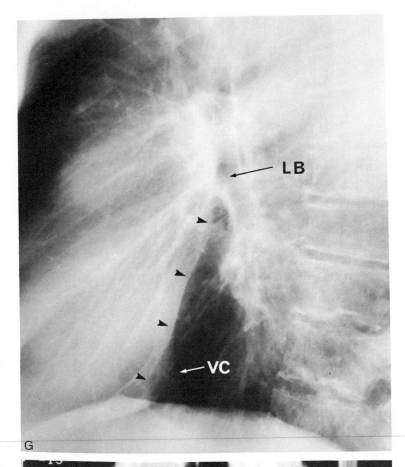

Figure 1–171 *Continued. G,* A detail view from a conventional lateral chest roentgenogram of another patient shows a continuous serpentine opacity (*arrowheads*) that extends from a point slightly anterior to the left upper lobe bronchus (*LB*) to a point anterior to the contour of the inferior vena cava (*VC*) below. *H,* A sagittal CT reformation (*top*) and representative transverse images (*bottom*) reveal the typical shape of the anterior margin of the azygoesophageal recess (*arrowheads*). (*See* text for the precise anatomic structures forming the contour.)

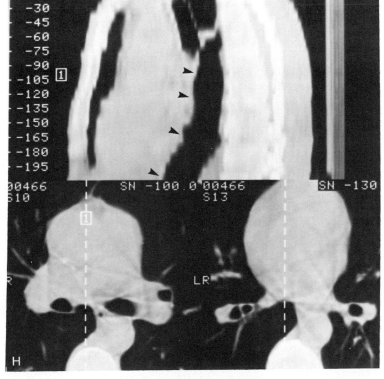

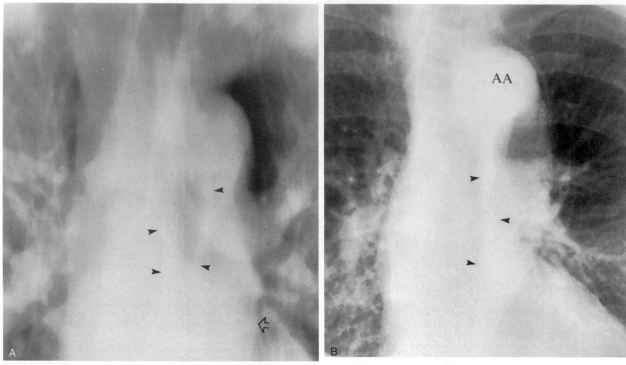

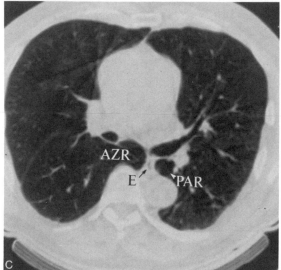

Figure 1–172. The Inferior Esophagopleural Stripes. *A,* An antero-posterior linear tomogram through the carina reveals two curvilinear opacities (*arrowheads*) that extend from the infra-aortic region caudally. The opacities converge distally at the level of the left ventricle. Moderate unfolding of the thoracic aorta is present (*arrow*). The linear opacities represent the right and left wall of the gas-distended esophagus. *B,* A detail view from a posteroanterior chest roentgenogram discloses a single thick stripe (*arrowheads*) that extends caudally from the aortic arch (*AA*). The stripe represents the nondistended esophagus behind the heart, abutted by right and left lower lobe parenchyma in the azygoesophageal and preaortic recesses, respectively. *C,* A transverse CT scan through the carina shows the deep intrusion of the right lower lobe across the midline into the azygoesophageal recess (*AZR*). On the left, the lower lobe has expanded into the preaortic recess (*PAR*) behind the left main bronchus and in front of the descending aorta. The two lungs are separated by the septum created by the esophagus (*E*), mediastinal areolar tissue, and four layers of pleura.

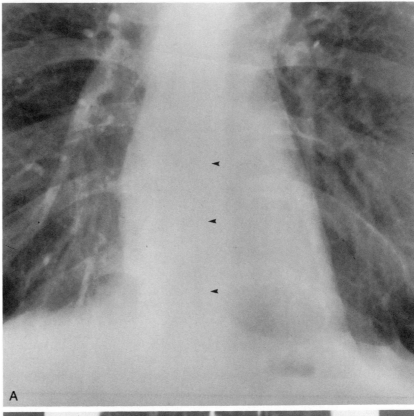

Figure 1–173. The Inferior Posterior Junction Line. *A*, A closeup from a posteroanterior chest roentgenogram reveals a thin, white linear opacity (*arrowheads*) behind the heart. *B*, A coronal CT reformation (*top*) with representative transverse images (*bottom*) shows a thin septum (*arrowheads*) behind the esophagus (*E*), representing apposition of the right and left lower lobes and pleura in front of the vertebrae, forming the inferior posterior junction line. The situation is analogous to that of the superior posterior junction line.

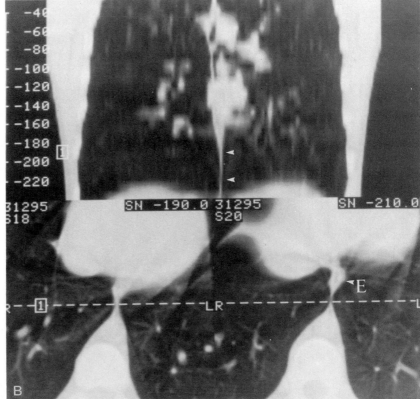

THE HEART

It is beyond the scope of this book to discuss the roentgenology of the heart in detail. However, it is important to recognize that certain deviations in the normal roentgen anatomy of the cardiovascular silhouette may give rise to confusion.

In a frontal roentgenogram of the normal chest (see Figure 1–194, page 287), the position of the heart in relation to the midline of the thorax depends largely upon the patient's build. Assuming roentgenographic exposure with lungs fully inflated, in asthenic patients the heart shadow is almost exactly midline in position, projecting only slightly more to the left; in those of stockier build it lies a little more to the left of midline (in the range of three quarters to one quarter).[461] A study of 500 healthy adults[739] showed the following variations in the heart's position relative to the midline: in 87.5 per cent, a small-to-moderate segment of the heart projected to the right of the spine; in 7 per cent, the heart extended to the right almost as far as to the left of the spine; in 0.2 per cent (one subject), it extended more to the right than to the left; in 3.3 per cent, the right border of the heart and spine coincided; and in about 2 per cent the right heart border was projected over the spine (a common finding in patients with pectus excavatum).

In normal subjects, the transverse diameter of the heart measured on standard teleroentgenograms is usually in the range of 11.5 to 15.5 cm;[461] it is less than 11.5 cm in approximately 5 per cent, and only rarely exceeds 15.5 cm (in very heavy subjects of stocky build, often manual laborers). The custom of trying to assess cardiac size by relating it to the transverse diameter of the chest, i.e., cardiothoracic ratio, is inaccurate. Although 50 per cent is widely accepted as the upper limit of normal for this ratio, in fact it exceeds 50 per cent in at least 10 per cent of normal subjects.[461] This ratio is especially fallacious in patients who have a small heart. As pointed out by Simon,[461] in a person with an 8 cm transverse cardiac diameter in a 24 cm thorax, the heart would have to enlarge 4 cm before the cardiothoracic ratio reached the mythic 50 per cent. In our view, it is preferable to evaluate cardiac size subjectively on the basis of experience; alternatively, it is reasonable to assume that a heart whose transverse diameter exceeds 15.5 to 16 cm is enlarged until proved otherwise.

Chiefly as a result of the influence of systole and diastole, both the size and contour of the heart may vary from one examination to another, even when all examinations are made with an identical degree of lung inflation. In one study, in 324 patients for whom posteroanterior roentgenograms were obtained in both systole and diastole (through electrocardiographic monitoring),[901] the change in transverse cardiac diameter was 0.3 cm or less in 52 per cent, 0.4 to 0.9 cm in 41 per cent, and 1.0 to 1.7 cm in 7 per cent. An addendum to this report states that the researchers had observed a cardiac diameter increase of 2.0 cm or more from systole to diastole in only 5 of about 1500 patients. In another study of 200 normal subjects, the maximal difference in transverse cardiac diameter on successive examinations was 2 cm (in one patient only) and the group average was 0.5 cm.[461]

When the influence of systole and diastole is controlled (by exposure of 1 sec or longer), the major influences on cardiac size and contour are threefold. (1) *The height of the diaphragm*, which in turn is influenced by the degree of pulmonary inflation: the lower the position of the diaphragm, the longer and therefore narrower is the cardiovascular silhouette. (2) *Intrathoracic pressure*, which influences not only cardiac size but also the appearance of the pulmonary vascular pattern. (3) *Body position*: assuming equality of all other factors, the heart is broader when a subject is recumbent than when he or she is erect. The physiologic and roentgenographic effects of variation in intrathoracic pressure and body position are discussed later in this chapter.

Standardization of all these influences is essential for accurate comparison of heart size on roentgenograms taken at different times. Methods of standardization vary but could well include the criteria enumerated here. The patient should be in the erect position in posteroanterior projection; at a standard 6 ft (or 10 ft) film focus distance; with the lungs inflated to TLC (or some other easily reproducible level of lung inflation, measured by spirometry); at a known intrathoracic pressure (preferably atmospheric, attained by suspending respiration with glottis open and specifically without a Valsalva maneuver); and with a radiation exposure of 1 sec or longer. Obviously the time required for such an examination renders it impractical for routine use. These parameters are outlined to stress the importance of their control for accurate comparison of heart size on successive examinations.

Physiologic accumulations of fatty tissue are common in the cardiophrenic recesses bilaterally and produce an obtuse angular configuration of the inferior mediastinum at its junction with the diaphragm. Their density may be slightly less than that of the heart, allowing identification through them of the approximate position of the cardiac borders. These pleuropericardial fat shadows should not be misinterpreted as cardiac enlargement or as mediastinal or diaphragmatic masses of possible importance; however, as stated earlier, the bilateral cardiophrenic regions contain parietal lymph nodes of the middle mediastinal chain, whose enlargement in patients with lymphoma may simulate pleuropericardial fat.[902]

THE CONTROL OF BREATHING

The main purpose of breathing is to achieve and maintain alveolar and arterial blood gas hemostasis so that the oxygen demands of the organism are met, and the metabolic byproduct, carbon dioxide, is exhaled. The respiratory control system can be divided broadly into (1) afferent inputs to a central respiratory controller, (2) the controller and its central integration, (3) outputs from the respiratory center, and finally (4) the effectors of the output, the respiratory muscles. In this section we will consider each component separately and examine how higher centers, exercise, added loads, altered blood gas tensions, and sleep influence the reflex and voluntary control of ventilation.

The whole area of control of breathing has received considerable attention recently, and the interested reader would benefit from these excellent reviews.[903-909] Figure 1–174 is an overview of the respiratory control systems.

The Inputs

The major inputs from the periphery to the central regulator of respiration feed back information about arterial blood gas tensions, lung mechanics, and respiratory muscle function. The peripheral and central chemoreceptors respond to alterations in arterial PO_2, PCO_2 and hydrogen ion concentration; afferents from receptors in the respiratory tract and lungs are influenced by lung mechanics; and afferents from muscle spindles and tendon organs in the respiratory muscles close the loop by monitoring the effectiveness of contraction of the peripheral effector system.

PERIPHERAL CHEMORECEPTORS

The anatomy and physiology of the peripheral chemoreceptors have been extensively reviewed,[910, 911] and the following material has been excerpted from these reviews. The carotid body is the major peripheral chemoreceptor, the aortic body being of minor importance.[912] The carotid body develops with the third branchial arch and can be recognized in the human embryo as early as 6 weeks of gestation. The most distinctive cell in the carotid body, and perhaps the one that serves as the chemoreceptor, is the glomus cell, a cell that is derived from neural crest ectoderm and that contains abundant catecholamines and indole-amines. Sensory neurons traveling in the glossopharyngeal and carotid sinus nerves terminate on glomus cells within the carotid body, and their axons ascend in the glossopharyngeal nerve to nerve bodies in the glossopharyngeal sensory ganglia. The glomus cells contain abundant dopamine as well as norepinephrine, 5-hydroxytryptamine, and acetylcholine. Hypoxia increases dopamine release and synthesis by glomus cells, and it is probable that in some way they act as the chemoreceptive transducers, stimulating postsynaptic afferent nerve endings by release of mediators. In normal subjects, the carotid bodies constitute less than 1 millionth of total body weight, yet the organ

has an enormous blood supply, receiving up to 2 liters per minute per 100 grams of tissue (more than 40 times the flow/gm to the brain). This enormous blood supply results in a virtually unchanged PO_2 in the blood's passage through the carotid body.

In the presence of chronic hypoxia, the carotid body enlarges as a result of hypertrophy and hyperplasia of glomus cells as well as a proliferation of blood vessels and connective tissue elements; in such circumstances the organ can reach eight times its normal size. Enlargement of the carotid bodies also occurs in pulmonary disease associated with chronic hypoxemia; some infants who die of sudden death syndrome (SIDS) have been noted to have enlarged carotid bodies, although in another group of SIDS patients, carotid bodies were smaller than normal. People who live continuously at high altitudes not only have enlarged carotid bodies but also an increased incidence of carotid body tumor.

The receptor activity from the carotid body can be measured by recording afferent nerve impulses in the whole carotid sinus nerve before it joins the glossopharyngeal nerve or by splitting out individual afferent fibers and recording their response characteristics. There is always some afferent activity from the carotid body, even with very high PO_2s, and the firing frequency increases progressively as the PO_2 is lowered, increasing steeply below a PO_2 of 200. The firing frequency in the carotid chemoreceptor nerves is increased not only by hypoxia but separately by hypercapnia and changes in pH. The hypoxic and hypercapnic responses are additive in that both stimuli together result in enhanced response. In addition to the steady state responses of the chemoreceptor, enhanced firing appears to accompany rapid swings in arterial PO_2 and PCO_2, suggesting that the rate of change of arterial blood gas tensions is as important a stimulus as the average levels. In humans at rest, there are substantial swings in arterial PO_2 and PCO_2 related to the ventilatory and cardiac cycles; these swings tend to increase during exercise, hence rates of change of arterial PO_2 and PCO_2 may be important in the regulation of exercise ventilation.[910, 911]

The carotid body receives sympathetic and parasympathetic efferent input. Stimulation of either causes increased chemoreceptor activity, which may be produced by redistribution of blood flow within the receptor. Stimulation of the carotid body receptors by hypoxia, hypercapnia, and acidosis results in increased ventilation. Stimulation of the carotid body also causes an increase in bronchomotor tone, systemic blood pressure, and pulmonary vascular resistance, as well as a generalized increase in catecholamine secretion; during sleep, it may cause arousal.[913] In the absence of the peripheral chemoreceptors, hypoxic ventilatory response is abolished, and, in fact, hypoxemia may cause ventilatory depression. Under the circumstances, however, 85 per cent of the ventilatory response to CO_2 is preserved.[909]

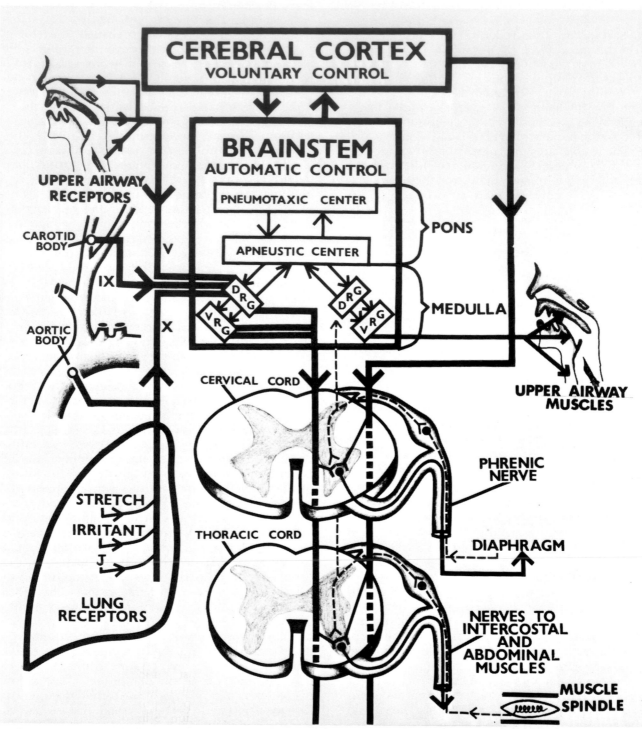

Figure 1–174. The Respiratory Control System. The central respiratory control is shared by voluntary (cerebral) and automatic (brain stem) centers. The efferent fibers from each run in distinct spinal cord pathways, as depicted on the left side of the coronally sectioned spinal cord (right side of drawing). A variety of interconnections exist between the cortex and the different components of the brain stem. Afferent fibers ascending the fifth (V), ninth (IX), and tenth (X) cranial nerves from upper airway receptors, peripheral chemoreceptors, and lung receptors connect with the ipsilateral dorsal respiratory group of neurons (*DRG*). In addition, afferents from Golgi tendon organs in the diaphragm and intercostal muscle spindles travel in the phrenic and intercostal nerves and reach the anterior horn cells as well as ascending to the DRG via the dorsal columns. Respiratory neurons in the DRG are connected with those in the ventral respiratory group (*VRG*) from which the descending neural output originates. The efferent fibers cross in the brain stem and supply the upper airway muscles via cranial nerves as well as descending in the cord to supply the diaphragm, intercostal, accessory, and expiratory muscles.

CENTRAL CHEMORECEPTORS

The exact location and structure of the central chemoreceptors has not yet been established. Three areas in the ventrolateral surface of the medulla oblongata, some 200 to 500 microns below the surface, respond to alterations in the cerebrospinal fluid and extracellular hydrogen ion concentration, resulting in increased ventilation. The exact cells involved in this transduction and their connections to the dorsal and ventral respiratory neurons that generate the respiratory rhythm have not yet been fully elucidated.[914] The pertinent stimulus for these receptors is the hydrogen ion concentration of brain extracellular fluid. Since the blood-brain barrier is not freely permeable to hydrogen ion or bicarbonate ion but is permeable to carbon dioxide, hypercapnic acidosis is a more powerful stimulus to central chemoreceptors than is metabolic acidosis. With the increased circulating hydrogen ion associated with metabolic acidosis, there is stimulation of the peripheral chemoreceptors and an increase in ventilation and decrease in P_{CO_2}; there can actually be a paradoxic decrease in cerebrospinal fluid (CSF) hydrogen ion concentration despite the blood metabolic acidosis. The higher CSF pH tends to attenuate the central ventilatory response to metabolic acidosis changes. Similarly, the acute ventilatory response to hypoxia from stimulation of peripheral chemoreceptors is partly offset by the resulting hypocapnic alkalosis. With time, the changes in CSF pH occur as hydrogen ion equilibrates across the blood-brain barrier over a period of hours. Thus, if the acidosis is prolonged, there is a progressive fall in CSF pH to more acid levels, resulting in progressive stimulation of ventilation so that arterial P_{CO_2} continues to decrease as metabolic acidosis is sustained. The exact mechanism by which CSF hydrogen ion concentration is regulated remains controversial, and both passive and active transporting mechanisms have been suggested.[909]

RECEPTORS IN THE RESPIRATORY TRACT AND LUNGS

There is afferent input to the respiratory center from receptors at all levels in the respiratory tract, carried by the fifth, ninth, and tenth cranial nerves. Nasal receptors, which travel in the trigeminal nerve, are responsible for sneezing, reflex bronchodilation, and increased respiratory tract production of mucus; they may be important in initiating the diving reflex. When stimulated, rapidly adapting fibers in the nasopharynx result in bronchodilatation and increased secretion of mucus; these receptors, whose afferent fibers are carried in the glossopharyngeal nerve, also may be important in modulating the ventilatory response to carbon dioxide and have been shown to result in inhibition of diaphragmatic contraction when stimulated by the passage of cold air through the nasopharynx.[915-917]

The larynx is richly supplied with afferent nerve endings, which are carried in both the superior laryngeal and recurrent laryngeal nerves; superficial receptors in this region, situated in both the epithelium and submucosa, initiate coughing, apnea, expiratory efforts, bronchoconstriction, and laryngeal constriction, and when stimulated cause increased airway mucous secretion. The laryngeal receptors also appear to respond to changes in transmural pressure, upper airway air flow, and contraction of the upper airway muscles.[915, 918] These mechanoreceptor reflexes are important in maintaining upper airway patency during the increased transmural pressure swings associated with upper airway obstruction.

The tracheobronchial receptors have been the most thoroughly studied and include irritant, stretch, and J receptors. Irritant receptors are also termed rapidly adapting stretch or cough receptors; they are most densely located in the large airways around the carina. The receptors themselves are probably represented by the intraepithelial nerve fiber network that extends throughout the epithelium, ending in free nerve endings just below the epithelial tight junctions. These receptors respond to mechanical as well as nonspecific chemical irritation by substances such as ammonia, sulfur dioxide, cigarette smoke, and possibly carbon dioxide. Histamine is a potent stimulator of irritant receptors, probably acting both directly and indirectly in producing bronchoconstriction. Stimulation of irritant receptors produces cough, increased mucous production, and rapid shallow breathing, chiefly by shortening the expiratory duration. Irritant receptor stimulation has been implicated in the bronchoconstriction associated with asthma and in alterations of breathing pattern seen in patients with chronic airway disease and COPD.

Pulmonary stretch receptors are also termed slowly adapting stretch receptors; they are situated within airway smooth muscle. They are responsible for the well-known Hering-Breuer reflex and are concentrated in the trachea and large airways; 40 per cent are situated in extrapulmonary airways. Stretch receptors respond by increasing their firing frequency with lung inflation or with increases in transpulmonary pressure. They have a low threshold, and in animal studies most fire within the tidal volume range; airway smooth muscle constriction increases their responsiveness.

The last group of intrapulmonary afferents are the so-called "J" receptors, abbreviated from juxtapulmonary capillary receptors. These are small, nonmyelinated, slowly conducting fibers that respond to microembolization of the pulmonary circulation, pulmonary edema, irritant gases such as ammonia, volatile anesthetics such as halothane, and the administration of drugs such as phenyl diguanide and capsaicin. These receptors, which are located largely in the periphery of the lung in close proximity to pulmonary capillaries, respiratory bronchioles, and alveolar ducts, probably play little role in the normal control of breathing, but in the presence of pulmonary pathology such as pneumonia and pulmonary congestion, their firing frequency may increase, resulting in reflex rapid shallow breathing, laryngeal constriction, hypotension, and bradycardia. Unlike most of the other airway receptors, their stimulation does not appear to enhance airway mucous secretion.[915]

RESPIRATORY MUSCLE AFFERENTS

The last major peripheral input to the respiratory center is provided by respiratory muscle receptors. This is the least understood of the peripheral inputs to the respiratory center and has recently been reviewed by Duron.[920]

The major striated muscle receptors are Golgi tendon organs and muscle spindles. In the diaphragm, the chief sensory organ appears to be the Golgi tendon apparatus, muscle spindles being rare. The Golgi tendon apparatus consists of numerous free nerve endings entwined in the tendinous fibers of muscle origins where they serve as stretch receptors. Their input into the primary efferent alpha motor neurons at the spinal level and the importance of central projections of these afferents are still unknown. The muscle spindle, a more complex receptor, predominates in the intercostal muscles, both inspiratory and expiratory, as well as in the accessory muscles of respiration. These organs, similar to those found in other skeletal muscle, consist of a spindle, in which an intrafusal muscle fiber is innervated by sensory nerve endings, and a gamma motor efferent. Stimulation of the afferent intrafusal fiber results in the classic gamma loop excitation by alpha motor neurons of extrafusal muscle fibers in the same spinal cord segment (intrasegmental reflex). Extrasegmental reflexes that presumably originate in the muscle spindles have also been demonstrated by electrical stimulation of afferents in the central cut end of intercostal nerves, resulting in contraction of adjacent intercostal muscles. In addition, an intercostal-diaphragmatic reflex has been identified by experiments in which stimulation of the central cut end of lower thoracic intercostal nerves causes reflex excitation of phrenic motor neurons. The precise role of these afferents and their influence on the central respiratory controller is unknown, but a number of studies suggest that they may be important. Cutting the dorsal cervical and thoracic roots can lead to temporary respiratory muscle paralysis in both animals and humans, and stimulation of splanchnic or muscle afferents produced by the trauma of upper abdominal surgery depresses diaphragmatic activity.[920-923]

The Central Controller

Central control of respiratory rhythm and pattern can originate in the voluntary cortical centers or brain stem automatic centers or both. Automatic breathing originates from a highly complex accumulation of interconnected nerve cell groups situated in the brain stem. The most rostral of these centers is the so-called pneumotaxic center (PNC) which is situated within the pons and is now believed to be important in influencing the timing of the inspiratory cut-off by providing tonic input to pattern generators located at other sites. Thus, cells in the PNC may modulate the respiratory response to stimuli such as hypercapnia, hypoxia, and lung inflation.[904, 923, 924]

Immediately caudal to the PNC near the pontomedullary border lies the apneustic center (APC). Apneusis is the cessation of rhythmic breathing due to prolonged inspiratory activity. Little is known about the APC, but damage to it results in inactivation of the inspiratory cutoff switch and the production of apneusis when vagal input is also abolished. Transection of the brain stem between the medulla and the pons so that signals from the PNC and APC are removed does not abolish respiratory rhythmicity, and the current view is that the medulla alone is capable of generating a primary respiratory rhythm, the PNC and the APC being modulators of the timing mechanism. However, the rhythm generated from the isolated medulla is slower and of a more gasping nature than that developed when the PNC and the APC are intact. It is possible that multiple rhythm generators exist within the brain stem and that they only function as pacemakers after ablation of higher order centers—a situation analogous to that of the heart in which Purkinje fibers and the A-V node serve as backup to the S-A node.

Within the medulla the respiratory neurons are grouped in two distinct areas: (1) the dorsal respiratory group (DRG) comprising two bilateral aggregations of neurons located near the nucleus of the tractus solitarius and consisting almost exclusively of inspiratory cells, and (2) the ventral respiratory group (VRG), which lies close to the nucleus ambiguus and the nucleus retroambigualis and contains both inspiratory and expiratory cells. The DRG appears to play an important role in the regulation of respiration, since it is the site of primary projection of numerous afferent fibers that travel in the fifth, ninth, and tenth cranial nerves from sensors originating in the upper airway and lungs as well as the peripheral chemoreceptor. It is also probable that it is the site of projection of proprioceptive afferents from the respiratory muscles and the chest wall. It is thought that the DRG is the primary site of rhythm generation, with the axons originating from this accumulation of cells projecting to and descending in the contralateral spinal cord and serving as the principal respiratory rhythmic drive to anterior horn cells that innervate the diaphragm and inspiratory intercostals. Cells from the DRG also project to stimulate cells in the VRG, which does not appear to have inherent respiratory rhythmicity or sensory input from peripheral or central chemo- and mechanoreceptors. The axons from the VRG cross and descend in the spinal cord to innervate anterior horn cells in the cervical and thoracic cord, which project to the intercostal inspiratory and expiratory muscles as well as to the abdominal and accessory muscles of respiration. Neurons in the VRG also project via the ipsilateral ninth, tenth, and twelfth nerves to the upper airways, where they innervate the laryngeal, genioglossal, geniohyoid, and other muscles. These muscles receive rhythmic respiratory input and are important in maintaining upper airway patency.

The beginning of neural inspiration in the brain stem is initiated by an abrupt termination of inhibition of inspiratory neurons. Thus, there is a sudden onset of inspiratory motor neuron activity followed by a slowly augmenting ramp of increasing activity that is terminated by a sudden switchoff. The switchoff is followed by a resurgence of a lesser degree of inspiratory activity, termed the postinspiratory inspiratory activity or PIIA. The PIIA is insufficient to prolong inspiration but serves to brake the rate of exhalation and in some instances may be important in setting functional residual capacity (FRC) at a higher level than the static recoil of the lung and chest would otherwise dictate. The neurons responsible for the PIIA may be different from those responsible for the main inspiratory ramp of activity. Following cessation of PIIA, there is neural "quiet" unless expiratory neurons are recruited. Expiratory neurons are not stimulated until after the PIIA ceases and are usually recruited only with increased ventilatory drive. The more the ventilatory drive, the shorter the PIIA and the greater the expiratory neuronal discharge.[925]

The pattern of central drive is altered depending upon the stimulus. For instance, hypoxia exerts a stronger action on inspiratory activity than does hypercapnia, which exerts a stronger action on expiratory muscles when matched for the same level of ventilation. The output to muscles controlling the upper airway is influenced more by peripheral than by central chemoreceptors, and stretch receptor–induced inspiration is accomplished preferentially by inspiratory intercostals rather than the diaphragm. The onset of stimulation of intercostal muscles occurs slightly later than phrenic motor neuron discharge during quiet breathing, although with increased ventilatory drive this difference in timing is lost.

The act of breathing involves control not only of the major pumping muscles of the respiratory system, the diaphragm and intercostals, but also the muscles of the larynx, pharynx, tongue, and face, which control patency of the upper airway. The pattern of recruitment of the muscles that control upper airway caliber differs strikingly from that of the main inspiratory muscles. Their onset of stimulation is in very early inspiration, and their peak activity coincides with peak inspiratory flow rather than volume. Thus, their activity is in phase with flow-related negative pressure in the upper airway, and their contraction counteracts the tendency for the negative pressure to narrow the airway. Laryngeal abductor activation occurs early in expiration and, along with PIIA, brakes expiration. The rate of rise of central inspiratory activity and therefore the discharge rate down the phrenic and intercostal nerves is dependent upon the intensity of the afferent inputs that are integrated in the central integrator. The offswitch that terminates the ramp of inspiratory activity is influenced by the input of pulmonary stretch receptors from the vagus.[926]

Although most of our knowledge of central respiratory control involves the automatic brain stem controlling mechanisms, it is clear that the cerebral cortex can influence brain stem mechanisms or bypass them completely to accomplish behavior-related respiratory activity like speech, cough, defecation, micturition, singing, and so on. During voluntary activity such as speech, requirements for tone or loudness may override chemical and mechanical inputs. For instance, during speech the response to inhaled carbon dioxide is markedly depressed and the sensation of dyspnea diminished when compared with similar CO_2 levels occurring without speech.[927] The classic concept that a basic respiratory rhythm is generated in the brain stem and only modulated by chemoreceptor and other inputs must be questioned, since it appears that the respiratory rhythmicity itself is dependent on input. Both high-frequency oscillatory ventilation and CO_2 removal from venous blood by means of an extracorporeal circuit result in central apnea and cessation of respiratory rhythm generation. This occurs despite mean levels of arterial P_{CO_2} that would normally be associated with substantial neural output. It has been suggested that the ventilation-related fluctuations in arterial P_{O_2} and P_{CO_2} represent one of the inputs that generates central respiratory rhythmicity, since both extracorporeal CO_2 removal and high-frequency oscillatory ventilation abolish these fluctuations.[928, 929]

The Outputs

Knowledge about the central respiratory controller can only be obtained in animals and humans by altering inputs and observing changes in output. The three input variables that have been employed most commonly include alterations in the concentration of inhaled O_2 and CO_2, which stimulate peripheral and central chemoreceptors; added resistive or elastic loads that stimulate muscle and lung mechanoreceptors; and exercise.

By measuring respiratory center output at various levels of stimulation by these inputs, an assessment of respiratory center integrity can be made. As will be discussed in more detail in Chapter 3, major difficulties exist in extrapolating from the measured outputs back to neuronal drive, since most tests of output are some steps removed from the actual neural output. The most fundamental outputs are minute ventilation and its components, tidal volume (VT), and respiratory frequency (F). Minute ventilation can also be divided into mean inspiratory flow (VT/Ti) and the ratio of inspiratory time over total respiratory cycle time (Ti/Ttot). It has been proposed that VT/Ti reflects the neural drive while Ti/Ttot is a measure of central timing mechanisms, and these methods of respiratory pattern analysis have gained wide acceptance.[930]

The study of respiratory pattern has been hampered until recently by the necessity of using a mouthpiece and nose-clip, which in themselves can alter the breathing pattern in conscious subjects.[931] With methods such as a head mask or, more recently, the respiratory inductance plethysmograph, breathing patterns can be monitored in a more natural state, and with this technique input-dependent differences in pattern have been observed:[932-935] with CO_2, for instance, breathing frequency increases less and tidal volume more than at matched ventilation stimulated by exercise.[935]

The most commonly employed inputs by which respiratory control is assessed are increasing levels of inhaled CO_2 and decreasing levels of inhaled O_2. The methods by which hypoxic and hypercapnic ventilatory response curves are generated is described fully in Chapter 3. Briefly, in normal subjects progressive hypercapnia produces a linear increase in ventilation, but the slope of the curve can vary widely between individuals. With progressive hypoxemia, a parabolic curve of ventilation against PO_2 is generated, with little increase in ventilation until PO_2 falls to between 50 and 60 mm Hg; the curve can become linear by plotting ventilation against arterial O_2 saturation. There is also wide variability between individuals in the response to progressive hypoxemia. The CO_2 response curve largely reflects the integrity of central chemoreceptor activity.

There is a marked genetic influence in chemosensitivity to CO_2 and O_2. Studies in which monozygotic and dizygotic twins are compared have shown not only a genetic influence on the slopes of the hypoxic and hypercapnic ventilatory response curves but also on the pattern of breathing in response to hypoxemia; no genetic influence was observed on the ability to detect added resistive loads.[936-939]

The ventilatory response curves to CO_2 and O_2 are influenced by various drugs and extraneous factors. Ethanol decreases ventilatory response to CO_2 but not O_2, an effect that is abolished by naloxone, suggesting ethanol-induced endorphin release.[90] Almitrine increases peripheral chemoreceptor responsiveness to hypoxia but has little effect on CO_2 sensitivity or on resting ventilation.[941] Aminophylline increases the slope of the ventilatory response curve to hypoxia and in some studies to hypercapnia.[942] In normal volunteers, semistarva-

tion has been shown to produce decreased ventilatory response to hypoxia but not to hypercapnia.[943] Propranolol and other beta-blockers have little influence on ventilatory response to CO_2.[944-946] Halothane markedly decreases the ventilatory response to hypoxia at both sedative and anesthetic levels, although it has little influence on the response to hypercapnia.[947] As discussed later, sleep has an important influence on the control of breathing, decreasing ventilatory response to CO_2 and hypoxia.

Genetic or acquired alterations in ventilatory response curves to hypoxia and hypercapnia can have profound influences in disease states and may govern the ability of normal subjects to perform various functions. It has been postulated that the genetically determined ventilatory drives to hypoxia and hypercapnia influence the pattern and course of chronic obstructive pulmonary disease (COPD): patients with genetically determined brisk responses to CO_2 and O_2 tend to maintain blood gas tensions near normal despite significant airway obstruction (pink puffers), whereas those with depressed ventilatory responses tend to hypoventilate (blue bloaters).[948] The hypothesis is supported by familial studies which show that unobstructed relatives of patients with hypercapnic COPD have significantly decreased hypoxic ventilatory response curves when compared with relatives of patients with similar degrees of airflow obstruction but without hypercapnia. It is interesting that the hypercapnic ventilatory drive in relatives does not separate hypercapnic from nonhypercapnic COPD patients despite the fact that there is considerable genetic influence on the hypercapnic response curve.[949]

Inherited ventilatory drives can also influence exercise capacities in normal individuals. Trained endurance athletes have a significantly reduced ventilatory drive to hypoxemia and hypercapnia when compared with normal controls, whereas similarly fit, successful high-altitude mountain climbers have significantly increased hypercapnic and hypoxic drive when compared with distance runners.[950, 951] Whether these athletes have genetically determined ventilatory response curves that facilitate their performance or altered responses secondary to their conditioning programs remains controversial. A study which examined the effect of short-term exercise on ventilatory response to CO_2 showed no change, suggesting that it is the genetic influences that preselect athletes.[952]

Although it is clear that the major receptor mediating hypercapnic hyperpnea is the central chemoreceptor, there has been a continuing search for, and controversy regarding, the possibility of upper airway or intrapulmonary CO_2 receptors that might contribute to hypercapnic ventilatory responses. Ventilatory responses are lower when breathing is carried out through the nose rather than mouth, especially when the air is cold.[917, 953] Evidence for intrapulmonary CO_2 receptors that enhance ventilatory response to CO_2 has been provided by studies in which, during separate perfusion of the systemic and pulmonary circuits, increased ventilation is observed with increased pulmonary CO_2 tensions at constant systemic PCO_2.[954] In seeming contradiction, others have suggested that pulmonary receptors may attenuate CO_2 responses since the blocking of airway slowly adapting stretch receptors with inhaled local anesthetic agents or by blockade of the vagus nerve results in enhanced ventilatory response to CO_2.[1189]

Control of Ventilation During Exercise

The study of the control of ventilation during exercise is a large and controversial topic and will be touched on only briefly. Excellent reviews have been published recently.[955, 956]

The precise control of arterial gas tensions during exercise, when O_2 consumption and CO_2 production can reach 20 times their resting levels, is an impressive phenomenon indeed. The mechanisms by which this control is achieved remain a fascinating but elusive study. There appear to be at least four phases in the ventilatory response to exercise. *Phase one* is an abrupt increase in ventilation that coincides with the start of exercise and may in fact precede it if the subject is cued to the time of beginning of exercise. This increase in ventilation occurs prior to any alterations in the gas tensions of mixed venous blood and has in the past been termed the "neurogenic component" of the ventilatory response. The difficulty has been in determining what neurogenic sensation mediates the responses, although muscle spindles in the exercising muscles are likely important. The carotid body chemoreceptors are not responsible for this early phase since there is preservation of phase one hyperpnea in patients with resected carotid bodies. *Phase two* of the hypercapnic response to exercise begins some 10 or 15 seconds following the onset, coincident with alterations in blood gas tensions in mixed venous blood. The carotid bodies have some role in this phase since there is a lag in the ventilatory response in patients without carotid bodies; however, the ultimate level of ventilation achieved is not different. *Phase three* represents the steady state response to exercise and is closely linked to CO_2 production. Finally, with heavy exercise—*phase four*—a further increase in ventilation occurs coincident with the metabolic production of lactic acid. This stage in progressive exercise is termed the anaerobic threshold, and at this point ventilation becomes uncoupled from metabolic CO_2 production. This final lactic acidosis–induced hyperpnea is mediated by peripheral chemoreceptors. An additional component of the hyperpnea of heavy exercise is related to increasing body temperature, and in some normal subjects a decrease in arterial PO_2 at extremely high work rates may be an additional stimulus. This paradoxic increase in the alveolar-arterial oxygen tension gradient is thought to be caused by O_2 diffusion limitation secondary to the rapid red cell pulmonary capillary transit times.

It is apparent that the tight control of ventilation during exercise cannot be totally accounted for by known neural, chemoreceptor, and humoral inputs; although all appear to play a role in the total ventilatory response to exercise, their importance and integration during the various phases of the response remain a mystery.[955, 956] It is interesting that breathing 100 per cent oxygen during exercise can prolong exercise capacity in normal subjects and patients with COPD. This may be related to the recent demonstration that breathing 100 per cent oxygen during exercise results in significantly less catecholamine release, peripheral lactate production, and heart rate response.[957] The fact that hypoxia and exercise are additive in their effect on ventilation, even at levels of arterial PO_2 that do not normally stimulate peripheral chemoreceptors, indicates that in some way exercise may increase chemoreceptor responsiveness to hypoxemia. It has been suggested that stimulation of some peripheral muscle chemoreceptors by low oxygen tension enhances the chemoreceptor response.[958]

Compensation for Added Ventilatory Loads

The impedance that the inspiratory muscles must overcome consists of three components: a resistive load related to the friction of air flow through the tracheobronchial tree, an elastic load related to the stretching of the lung and chest wall, and a trivial inertial load related to the acceleration of inspired air.

Small changes in upper airway caliber and alterations in body position produce rapid fluctuation in the resistive and elastic loads against which the respiratory muscles must shorten. The decrease in tidal volume and ventilation that would occur with an added elastic or resistive load can be calculated by the ratio of initial to added impedance. Studies in humans have shown that the decrease in tidal volume that occurs with such added loads is less than would be expected on a purely mechanical basis. This discrepancy indicates that some compensatory mechanisms are brought into play during loaded breathing to protect tidal volume and acinar ventilation.

The *first* of these compensatory mechanisms is related to the basic mechanical properties of skeletal muscle. The force generated by skeletal muscle is related to its velocity of shortening. An unloaded muscle will shorten rapidly and produce little force, but with an added load shortening is slowed and force generation increased, tending to counteract the expected decrease in tidal volume. The *second* mechanism of load compensation involves reflexes initiated by mechanoreceptors in the lung and chest wall, and the pulmonary stretch receptors are especially important in this regard. With an added elastic or resistive load, inspiration is slowed, and because of the adaptive nature of pulmonary stretch receptors, their level of activity at any volume during inspiration is decreased; this results in prolonged inspiration, tending to increase tidal volume back toward control levels.[959] Upper airway receptors also respond to the increases in transmural pressure that occur with added external resistive loads and, by causing reflex stimulation of upper airway muscles, aid in compensation.[918, 919] Muscle spindles represent a *third* mechanism by which load compensation is accomplished. As discussed, they are largely confined to the intercostals, being rare in the diaphragm. The muscle spindles contain intrafusal fibers that regulate the spindles' stretch and contract in concert with the extrafusal fibers that move the rib cage. Muscle spindle afferent activity increases whenever contraction of the extrafusal fibers is hindered, increasing the alpha motor neuron activity via the gamma loop segmental reflex and thus enhancing the activity of the intercostal muscles. The final load compensation is initiated when central and peripheral chemoreceptors detect changes in the arterial blood gas composition.[959] There is a greater response to a given increase in resistance when it is produced by bronchoconstriction with methylcholine than by added external resistance, suggesting that mechanical and irritant receptors enhance the response elicited from muscle afferents.[960]

Closely tied to the topic of load detection and compensation is respiratory sensation and the symptom of dyspnea. Dyspnea should be distinguished from hyperventilation or hyperpnea and is the unpleasant awareness of breathing and respiratory distress, signaled by proprioceptive information from the lungs and chest wall. Normal breathing is an automatic, unconscious motor act. The mechanism by which the sensation of breathing reaches the conscious level and respiratory effect engenders the sensation of dyspnea is poorly understood. The afferent inputs that could result in such a sensation include information from peripheral and central chemoreceptors, lung afferents, or receptors in the chest wall and respiratory muscles. The fact that most patients with dyspnea do not have sufficient alterations in blood gas tensions to stimulate ventilation is strong evidence against chemoreceptor activation as a major contributor. The discomfort of breath-holding can be relieved by breathing a gas mixture that results in further deterioration of blood gas tensions, suggesting that some stimulus related to the act of breathing itself rather than arterial PO_2 and PCO_2 is important in the generation of the dyspneic sensation. Lung receptors do not subserve conscious respiratory sensation since dyspnea persists after vagal blockade. Although upper airway receptors contribute to load compensation, they are not important for load detection since inhaled local anesthetics cause no change in the ability to sense added elastic loads.[961]

Strong support for the role of muscle receptors

and afferents as the origin of respiratory sensation was provided by studies showing that respiratory muscle paralysis induced by curare completely abolishes the sensation of dyspnea.[962] Chest wall vibration impairs the respiratory sensation of volume, suggesting that muscle spindles are sensory organs.[963] The balance of evidence suggests that dyspnea occurs when afferent input from respiratory muscles in some way signals an inappropriateness of the central neurogenic drive to breathe and the resulting displacement of the lung and chest wall.[964] By measuring the effects of different flow rates, lung volumes, and timing on the ability to detect added loads, Killian and associates[965] concluded that it is the relationship between flow and pressure early in inspiration that is the major signal for load detection and the sensation of dyspnea. Load detection was not influenced by increased ventilation during exercise or CO_2 breathing.[966] When the load is sufficiently high, normal subjects can distinguish between a resistive and an elastic load because of the different time sequence in the major impedance.[967] The ability to detect added resistive loads is quantitative using the Weber fraction; this fraction consists of the ratio of the added load first detected over the initial load; it remains constant over a wide range of baseline resistance values. The sensitivity of load detection decreases at very low and very high baseline resistances; probably some signal related to the phase difference or delay between respiratory motor neuron output and rate of change of volume input from muscle receptors indicates the mechanical inappropriateness that, when severe, is interpreted centrally as dyspnea.[968, 969]

Control of Upper Airway Muscles

With the current recognition of the importance of obstructive sleep apnea, respiratory center control of upper airway muscles that are important in maintaining airway patency, especially during sleep, has received considerable attention. Numerous muscles of the pharynx, hypopharynx, larynx, and tongue, including the genioglossals, the tensor palatini, the medial pterygoids, the thyrocricoid, and posterior cricoarytenoids, receive respiratory-related rhythmic neurogenic input.[970] As discussed, stimulation of upper airway muscles occurs earlier in the respiratory cycle than that of the diaphragm and intercostals, coinciding with the period of peak inspiratory flow and presumably peak negative upper airway pressure. Hypercapnia and hypoxia increase neural drive to upper airway muscles, although the relationship between phrenic output and hypoglossal output is not linear, the latter increasing steeply at higher drives.[971] The increased drive to upper airway muscles in response to hypoxia and hypercapnia may not relate only to increased input from central or peripheral chemoreceptors, since blockade of pulmonary stretch receptors impairs upper airway muscle contraction during hypoxia and hypercapnia.[972] The genioglossal muscles may be especially important in maintaining upper airway patency during sleep, and ingestion of alcohol results in selective reduction in genioglossal electromyographic activity in normal subjects.[973, 974]

Control of Breathing During Sleep

Alterations in the regulation of respiration that occur during sleep have been the subject of considerable recent interest and review.[970, 975, 976] Breathing is controlled by two essentially separate control-integrating mechanisms, the automatic or metabolic control system and the voluntary or behavioral control system. The major purpose of the metabolic system is to maintain acid-base and oxygen homeostasis, whereas the behavioral system is involved in such activities as speech and singing, in which the respiratory system is used for nonrespiratory purposes. During wakefulness, control of breathing is constantly being shared by the automatic and behavioral systems, but during sleep the automatic metabolic control predominates, at least during slow-wave sleep. Absence of the volitional control of breathing results in respiratory apraxia, whereas absence of autonomic control results in Ondine's curse.[977]

The profound influences that sleep has on the various aspects of the control of breathing are summarized in Table 1–12. Resting ventilation is decreased during slow-wave sleep, with both tidal volume and frequency being less than during wakefulness.[978] During rapid eye movement (REM) sleep, resting ventilation varies as a result of marked irregularity of the breathing pattern, but on the whole hyperventilation rather than hypoventilation is the rule. The hypoventilation of slow-wave sleep is associated with a slight rise in arterial P_{CO_2} and fall in arterial P_{O_2}, and during REM there is considerable fluctuation in arterial blood gas tensions. During stages 1 and 2 of slow-wave sleep, periodic breathing reminiscent of Cheyne-Stokes respiration may occur, changing to a regular pattern during the deeper stages (3 and 4) of slow-wave sleep. The pattern of breathing during REM sleep is characterized as irregular rather than periodic: although the mean tidal volume decreases and frequency increases, the characteristic feature is marked breath-to-breath variability. During slow-wave sleep the metabolic control system appears to dominate respiratory control, but during REM sleep a dissociation occurs between metabolic demands and ventilatory responses. Intercostal and upper airway muscles, which are normally more involved in postural and behavioral activities, are depressed during slow-wave sleep and profoundly depressed during REM sleep when there appears to be central inhibition of gamma loop neurons; this occurs in the respiratory muscles as well as in skeletal muscle

Table 1–12. Effects of Sleep on Breathing

	SLOW-WAVE SLEEP	REM SLEEP
Alveolar ventilation	Decreased due to $\downarrow V_T$ and $\downarrow F$	Variable
Arterial P_{CO_2}	$\downarrow$ 4–6 mm Hg	Variable
Arterial P_{O_2}	$\downarrow$ 4–8 mm Hg	Variable
Breathing pattern	Stages 1 and 2 periodic	Irregular
	Stages 3 and 4 regular	$\uparrow$ F plus $\downarrow V_T$
Diaphragmatic contraction	No change	No change
Intercostal contraction	$\downarrow$	$\downarrow\downarrow$
Upper airway muscle contraction	$\downarrow$	$\downarrow\downarrow$
Ventilatory response to CO_2	$\downarrow$	$\downarrow\downarrow$
Ventilatory response to hypoxemia	$\downarrow$	$\downarrow\downarrow$
Response to lung afferents	$\downarrow$	$\downarrow\downarrow$
Response to respiratory muscle afferents	$\downarrow$	$\downarrow\downarrow$

generally. The diaphragm, which is virtually devoid of muscle spindles, is immune from this flaccidity so that during REM sleep maintenance of ventilation is dependent on diaphragmatic activity.

The responsiveness of the respiratory control mechanisms to afferent inputs is also profoundly altered during sleep: for example, responsiveness to hypercapnia is decreased during slow-wave sleep and further decreased during REM sleep.[979, 980] Although less certain, it has been suggested in recent studies that hypoxic responses are also depressed in both stages of sleep, more profoundly during REM.[981, 982] The respiratory centers also appear to ignore afferent input from other sources during sleep: pulmonary stretch and irritant receptor discharge, as well as muscle spindle input, are less effective in increasing ventilation and effecting load compensation during sleep. The profound changes that occur during REM sleep make this period one of special vulnerability for patients with abnormalities of the respiratory control system or of the lungs and airways.

The influence of sleep on control of ventilation is not confined to the period of sleep itself: it has recently been shown in normal subjects that sleep deprivation for 24 hours results in decreased ventilatory responses to carbon dioxide and oxygen. Such an alteration in respiratory control resulting from sleep deprivation could have importance in hospitalized patients whose sleep is disturbed and in patients with sleep apnea syndromes.[983] Respiratory dysrhythmia is common during sleep and is related to prolonged circulation times, increased receptor gain, and decreased receptor damping. Hypoxic drive is usually the source of respiratory cycling, since damping is poor as a result of the alinearity of the hypoxic response curve and the low O_2 stores.

THE RESPIRATORY MUSCLES

The respiratory muscles are divided into four distinct groups with different functions and mechanisms of action—the upper airway muscles, the diaphragm, the intercostal and accessory muscles, and the abdominal muscles.[984-986]

Although respiratory neural input into upper airway muscles has been known for some time, interest in this area has increased recently because of the relationship between the dysfunction of these muscles and obstructive sleep apnea.[984] The genioglossal and geniohyoid muscles, as well as the muscles of the larynx and pharynx, display electromyographic (EMG) activity related to the respiratory cycle.[974, 984] Apparently upper airway receptors in the hypopharynx and larynx respond to increased negative pressure and result in a reflex increase in activity of the upper airway muscles. The afferent limb of this reflex is carried in the superior laryngeal and the ninth and tenth cranial nerves.[987, 988] There is a further recruitment of these muscles with increased neural output generated by hypoxia and hypercapnia.[971, 989, 990] These muscles contract simultaneously with the inspiratory muscles, although EMG activity starts somewhat earlier and peaks during maximal inspiratory flow. When phrenic nerve discharge is out of phase with upper airway muscle contraction, there is a tendency for increased resistance of the upper airways or for complete closure.[991] Such incoordination of inspiratory action between the upper airway muscles and the diaphragm could account for the obstruction that develops in patients with electrical pacers of the phrenic nerve.[992] The upper airway muscles are more sensitive than the other respiratory muscles to depression by sleep, anesthesia,[991] partial paralysis with curare,[993] and alcohol consumption.[974] This probably explains the increased tendency for upper airway obstruction that occurs during sleep, anesthesia, and sedation.

The diaphragm is the principal muscle of inspiration. It probably acts alone during quiet breathing, with the intercostal and accessory muscles being recruited only when the demand for ventilation increases. However, there is some tonic inspiratory muscle activity in the intercostal muscles in the upright posture, which prevents paradoxic inward movement of the rib cage with diaphragmatic descent. During REM sleep, anesthesia, or high spinal cord section, this tonic activity is absent and paradoxic inward motion of the chest wall occurs with inspiration.[994] The intercostal muscles include the internal (expiratory) and external (inspiratory) intercostals. The major accessory muscles are the scalenes, the sternomastoids, and the trapezoids, but at high levels of inspiratory activity when these muscles come into play, they are probably assisted by other muscles of the thoracic cage, particularly the back muscles. The abdominal muscles include the rectus and transverse abdominis and the external and internal obliques. They, along with the internal intercostals, are generally regarded as expiratory muscles, but as we shall see the abdominal muscles show tonic activation in the upright posture and may play an active role in inspiration.[995] In healthy individuals, expiration is largely passive, with expiratory muscle activity becoming manifest only when the minute ventilation exceeds about 50 per cent of the maximal voluntary ventilation.[996]

THE DIAPHRAGM

Development

The precursor of the diaphragm is first noted in human embryos of 3 weeks' gestation as a mesodermal ridge, termed the "septum transversum," that originates between the stalk of the yolk sac and the pericardial cavity (Fig. 1–175). It extends dorsally to divide the coelomic cavity incompletely, leaving two large dorsolateral intracoelomic openings, the pericardioperitoneal canals. The developing lung buds expand within the cranial portion of these canals and burrow into the mesenchyme of the dorsolateral body wall. In the process, the mesenchyme is partially eroded except for a midline portion that eventually forms a mesentery for the esophagus and in which develop the diaphragmatic crura. The pericardioperitoneal canals are eventually divided into definitive thoracic and abdominal cavities by mesenchymal folds, the pleuroperitoneal membranes; by the sixth to seventh week, these have grown anteriorly and medially to fuse with the esophageal mesentery and the septum transversum. During the third month, there is further extension of the developing lungs into the lateral body walls, at which time a further layer of body wall tissue is split off and incorporated into the peripheral portion of the diaphragm. The definitive diaphragm is thus derived from four structures (Fig. 1–175): (1) the septum transversum, which corresponds to the adult central tendon; (2) the two pleuroperitoneal membranes, which are thought to represent only a very small portion of the mature diaphragm; (3) the esophageal mesentery with incorporated crura; and (4) the body wall component, which corresponds to the majority of the mature muscular portion.

This rather complex development can result in a variety of diaphragmatic anomalies, including failure of formation or fusion of the various diaphragmatic components (resulting in complete or partial absence of the diaphragm or in posterolateral [foramen of Bochdalek] hernia), incomplete muscularization of the lateral or anterior body wall segments (causing eventration of the diaphragm, or anterior [foramen of Morgagni] hernia) and defects of the septum transversum (pericardioperitoneal

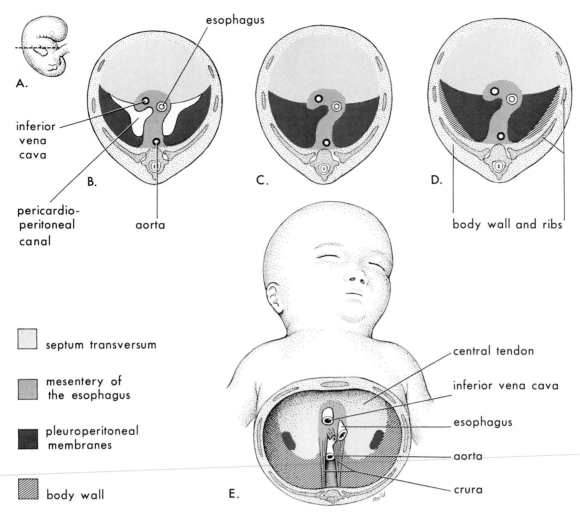

Figure 1–175. Drawings illustrating development of the diaphragm. *A,* Sketch of a lateral view of an embryo at the end of the fifth week (*actual size*) indicating the level of section. *B* to *E* show the diaphragm as viewed from below. *B,* Transverse section showing the unfused pleuroperitoneal membranes. *C,* Similar section at the end of the sixth week after fusion of the pleuroperitoneal membranes with the other two diaphragmatic components. *D,* Transverse section through a 12 week embryo after ingrowth of the fourth diaphragmatic component from the body wall. *E,* View of the diaphragm of a newborn infant, indicating the probable embryologic origin of its components. (From Moore KL: The Developing Human. 3rd ed. Philadelphia, WB Saunders, 1982.)

communication). These defects are discussed in more detail in the chapter on the diaphragm (Volume 4).

Morphology

The diaphragm is a musculotendinous sheet separating the thoracic and abdominal cavities (Fig. 1–176). The central tendon is a broad sheet of decussating fibers, in shape similar to a broad-bladed boomerang, the point of the boomerang being directed toward the sternum and the concavity toward the spine. The costal muscle fibers arise anteriorly from the xiphoid process and around the convexity of the thorax from ribs 7 to 12; posteriorly, the crural fibers arise from the lateral margins of the first, second, and third lumbar vertebrae on the right side, and from the first and second lumbar vertebrae on the left. These fibers converge toward the central tendon and are inserted into it

nearly perpendicular to its margin. The muscle fibers are of variable length, from 5 cm anteriorly at the sternal origin to 14 cm posterolaterally where they originate from the ninth, tenth, and eleventh ribs.[1] Von Hayek[1] pointed out that the greatest respiratory excursion occurs in the posterolateral portion of the hemidiaphragms where the muscle fibers are longest. The muscle fibers that compose the sternal attachment and those that arise from the seventh rib are separated bilaterally by triangular spaces poor in muscular and tendinous tissue, which may subsequently be the site of herniation or eventration (*see* further on).

Recent evidence suggests that the diaphragm is in fact two distinct muscles with separate nervous and vascular supply as well as function.[997] The costal portion of the diaphragm is mechanically in series with the intercostal and accessory muscles, and its contraction results in both descent of the diaphragm

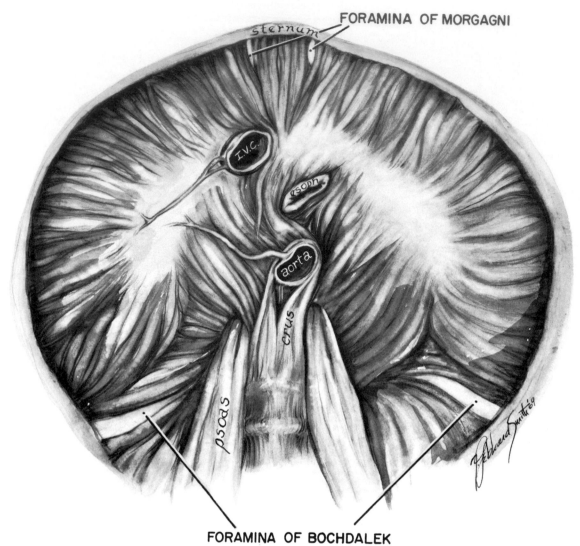

FORAMINA OF MORGAGNI

FORAMINA OF BOCHDALEK

Figure 1–176. Anatomy of the Normal Diaphragm Viewed from Below. *See* text.

and elevation of the rib cage; by contrast, the crural portion is in parallel with the diaphragm, and its contraction results in descent of the diaphragm without elevation of the rib cage (Fig. 1–177).[997]

Like other mammalian skeletal muscles, the human diaphragm is composed of three types of muscle fibers, each with specific physiologic features and corresponding histochemical profiles;[998, 1000] all fibers within individual motor units are of the same type. The three types of muscle fibers are known as (1) slow-twitch oxidative fatigue-resistant units (type 1), (2) fast-twitch oxidative glycolytic fatigue-resistant units (type 2a), and (3) fast-twitch glycolytic fatiguable units (type 2b). In the normal human diaphragm, type 1 represents approximately 50 per cent of muscle fibers, whereas type 2a represents about 20 per cent and type 2b about 30 per cent; these percentages could conceivably change with atrophy or training of the respiratory muscles.[1001, 1002] It is likely that the diaphragm behaves like other skeletal muscles, and that slow-twitch motor units are recruited during low intensity contractions, such as in sustained or quiet breathing, and that fast-twitch units, both fatigue-resistant and fatigue-susceptible, play a greater role with increasing respiratory activity.

The relative proportion of the different types of motor unit fibers present in the diaphragm may be of great importance in the pathogenesis of muscle fatigue and ventilatory failure (*see* further on). A paucity of slow-twitch oxidative fibers in premature infants[1003] may explain their poor tolerance to respiratory loads and their susceptibility to ventilatory failure. The discovery that the red muscle fibers (consisting largely of slow-twitch units) of mature guinea pigs can increase in number with exercise training[1004] and decrease with detraining[1005] indicates that the proportion of fiber types is not static. Sufficiently rapid atrophy of fatigue-resistant fibers could explain the extreme susceptibility of patients being weaned from artificial ventilation and also offer some hope for efforts being made to restore strength and endurance with respiratory muscle training. The weight of the diaphragm appears to be closely related to body weight,[1008] although there is evidence that in some disease states, such as emphysema, there may be a loss of muscle with resultant decreased weight that is independent of any change in body weight itself.[1008, 1009]

Microscopically (Fig. 1–178), the muscular portion comprises multiple muscle fascicles of variable size containing individual muscle fibers with differing ultrastructural and functional characteristics.[1006] In addition to numerous blood vessels, there is also an extensive intradiaphragmatic lymphatic network (see further on).

BLOOD SUPPLY

The diaphragm receives its blood supply from the phrenic and intercostal arteries and from branches of the internal thoracic (mammary) arteries. Small phrenic branches generally arise directly from the lower part of the thoracic aorta, and sometimes from the renal arteries. They are distributed to the posterior part of the upper surface of the diaphragm and anastomose with the musculophrenic and pericardiophrenic arteries. The latter two arteries are separate branches from the internal thoracic arteries and approach the diaphragm from a more anterior position.[1010] The internal mammary and phrenic arteries anastomose to form an arterial circle around the central tendon. This circle gives off branches which form an arcade; a second arterial circle is formed by the intercostals around the insertion of the diaphragm. This diversity of blood supply may be an important factor in the diaphragm's resistance to fatigue.[1011]

Scanning electron microscopic studies have shown individual myofibers to be surrounded by 8 to 10 blood vessels (Fig. 1–178), with an extensive capillary network in close topographic relationship with each myofiber. This intimate arrangement of capillaries and myofibers facilitates diffusion of gases, nutrients, and metabolites along the surface of the sarcolemma. The diaphragm has an abundant blood supply and, in contrast to limb skeletal muscle, there is no evidence for blood flow limitation on contractile effort. In fact, the increasing demand for oxygen by the working diaphragm is largely supplied by augmenting the blood flow rather than by increasing the extraction of oxygen from the blood.[1012]

LYMPHATIC DRAINAGE

An extensive intradiaphragmatic lymphatic network drains via collecting vessels into mediastinal channels and removes fluid, cells, and foreign materials from the diaphragm and from the pleural and peritoneal cavities.[1006] A single layer of mesothelial cells, continuous with the cells lining the wall of the chest and abdominal cavities, covers the peritoneal and pleural surfaces of the diaphragm. These mesothelial cells rest on a loose connective tissue layer containing a rich plexus of lymphatic

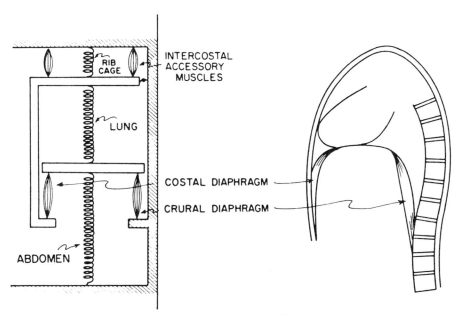

Figure 1–177. A Mechanical Model of the Inspiratory Musculature. The bar into which the crural and costal portions of the diaphragm insert represents the central tendon of the diaphragm. The inverted L-shaped structure represents the rib cage. The springs represent the elastic properties of rib cage, lung, and abdomen. The hatched area represents the bony skeleton. The costal and crural portions of the diaphragm are arranged mechanically in parallel. When in parallel, the force applied is the sum of the forces generated by the two muscles, but the displacement (volume change) is equal to the displacement of either muscle. The costal part of the diaphragm is in parallel with the intercostal and accessory muscles whereas the crural part is in series. When in series, the displacements of the two muscles can be added while the forces are not summed. The drawing on the right represents a more anatomically realistic illustration of the diaphragm showing separation of costal and crural parts. (From Macklem PT, Macklem DM, De Troyer A: J Appl Physiol 55:547, 1983.)

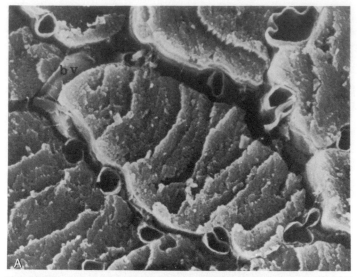

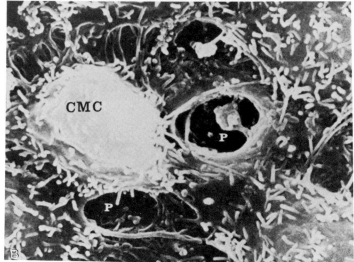

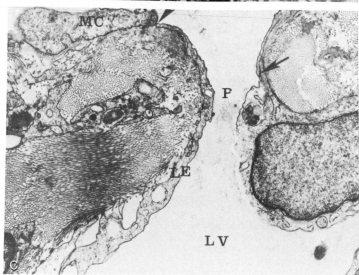

Figure 1–178. Morphologic Characteristics of the Diaphragm. *A,* A low-power scanning electron micrograph depicting a cross section of myofibers surrounded by numerous blood vessels (*bv*). (× 3000.) *B,* This electron micrograph shows the cuboidal cells (*CMC*) and the pores (*P*) that are formed between several adjoining cells. (× 8950.) *C,* A thin section of the diaphragm taken from an area of a pore (*P*) in the surface of the diaphragm. Portions of the mesothelial cells (*MC*) appear in the upper right and left areas of the micrograph. The lymphatic endothelial cells (*LE*) extend onto the peritoneal surface to form intercellular junctions (*arrows*) with the surface mesothelial cells. The close contact between the two cell types provides a direct passageway between the peritoneal cavity and the underlying lymphatic vessels (*LV*). (× 16,200.) (From Leak LV, Rahil K: Am Rev Respir Dis *119*(Suppl):8, 1979.)

channels. On the peritoneal surface, small pores 4 to 12 microns in diameter have been demonstrated between mesothelial cells (Fig. 1–178); these appear to provide direct communication between the peritoneal cavity and lymphatic spaces.[1006, 1007] Both particulate and cellular material have been shown to concentrate around and apparently enter these pores,[1006] thus providing a direct pathway for the transport of intraperitoneal neoplastic cells or fluid into the mediastinum or pleural space.

NERVE SUPPLY

The phrenic nerve is the sole motor nerve supply to the diaphragm. It arises chiefly from the fourth cervical nerve but also receives contributions from the third and fifth. At the level of the diaphragm each phrenic nerve gives off a few fine branches, which are distributed to the parietal pleura above and the parietal peritoneum below the central part of the diaphragm. They then divide into three motor branches, the anterior or sternal branch, the anterolateral branch, and the posterior branch, which supplies the crural part of the diaphragm. As we shall see in the discussion of the respiratory pump, this branch distribution probably has a significant functional correlation in humans: as shown by De Troyer and associates in the dog,[997] the costal and crural parts of the diaphragm can be separately stimulated, the costal branch increasing and the crural branch decreasing the dimensions of the lower rib cage. De Troyer and coworkers[1013] have also produced evidence that, in most individuals, hemidiaphragmatic and intercostal muscle activity has a predominantly contralateral cortical representation; for example, in patients with acute hemiplegia secondary to a cerebrovascular accident, diaphragmatic and intercostal electromyograms usually show a striking reduction in activity on the side of the paresis. In a minority of patients, however, innervation of the diaphragm appears to be bilaterally symmetric. The conduction velocity in the phrenic nerve is high, reaching a maximum of 78 meters per second; also, the innervation is dense, each nerve fiber subserving a low number of motor units—an anatomic arrangement that is usually seen in muscles performing precise movements, such as those of the eye. The intercostal motor neurons are located between T1 and T12 in the spinal cord and reach the intercostal muscles via the intercostal nerves. Abdominal motor neurons are located between T11 and L1.[1014]

A contracting diaphragm can also be sensed,[1015, 1016] with most people experiencing a "squeezing" sensation in the lower chest with breath-holding. This phenomenon is not abolished by spinal lesions or spinal anesthesia below the level of the C3 to C5 anterior horn cells, but it is eliminated by transection of the cord at the C3 level and by curarization;[1016, 1017] it appears that the afferent limb for this sensation lies in the ninth or tenth cranial nerve.

ROENTGENOLOGY

Roentgenographic Height of the Normal Diaphragm

A definitive study of the height of the hemidiaphragms on roentgenograms of normal adults was reported by Lennon and Simon[736] in 1965. These authors assessed frontal roentgenograms of the chest of 500 normal adults, 250 of each sex, over 21 years of age. In 94 per cent, the level of the cupola of the right hemidiaphragm was projected in a plane ranging from the anterior end of the fifth rib to the sixth anterior interspace; 41 per cent were at the level of the sixth rib anteriorly; and only 4 per cent were at or below the level of the seventh rib. Generally speaking, the height of the right dome was higher in women, in subjects of heavy build, and in those over the age of 40 years.

Relationship between the Height of the Right and Left Hemidiaphragms

The tendency for the plane of the right diaphragmatic dome to be about half an interspace higher than the left is well recognized, but in 9 per cent of 500 normal subjects examined by Felson,[739] both were at the same height or the left was higher than the right. Similarly, in the 114 healthy young men studied by Young and Simon,[1018] the left hemidiaphragm was higher than the right in 12 per cent. Although half the subjects of the 9 per cent reported by Felson had gaseous distention of the stomach or colon—a potential cause of left hemidiaphragmatic elevation—this was not observed in those reported by Young and Simon. In 2 per cent of Felson's 500 cases the right hemidiaphragm was more than 3 cm higher than the left.

It is a common error for students of roentgenology to ascribe elevation of the right hemidiaphragm to the mass of the liver beneath it. To these and other interested readers we recommend Wittenborg and Aviad's report[1019] of their investigation or organ influence on normal diaphragmatic posture in 60 children with anomalous organ positions. They found that the apex of the heart normally lies on the same side as the lower hemidiaphragm and that this relationship is maintained in the majority of cases of congenital malposition of thoracic and abdominal viscera. They also observed that the closer to normal the development of the heart into right and left sides, the more constant and clearly defined were disparate hemidiaphragmatic heights. The relationship of diaphragmatic height to cardiac anomalies is stated as follows: "In the presence of clear-cut inequalities in height of the hemidiaphragms (and absence of complicating pulmonary or neuromuscular disease) the odd-shaped cardiac silhouette may take on more meaning with the knowledge that, in all probability, the apex of the systemic or functional left ventricle is projected over the lower hemidiaphragm, irrespective of whether it be right or left and irrespective of the presence of anomalous positions of other organs."[1019]

Thus it is clear that the lower position of one hemidiaphragmatic dome relates to the contiguous mass of the left side of the heart.

Range of Diaphragmatic Excursion of Respiration

In a study of 114 young healthy men for whom inspiratory and expiratory roentgenograms were available, Young and Simon[1018] found unequal movement of the two hemidiaphragmatic domes to be common. Considering differences measured to 1 mm, movements were equal in only 10 subjects, being greater on the right in 73 (never by more than 1.9 cm) and greater on the left in 31 (exceeding 1.4 cm in only one case). These results are at variance with the earlier findings of Simon and his colleagues in older subjects,[1020] but agree with those obtained by Alexander[1021] and Schmidt.[1022] In a study of inspiratory-expiratory roentgenograms of 350 subjects aged 30 to 80 years without evidence of respiratory disease, we found the mean excursions of the right and left hemidiaphragms to be 3.3 cm and 3.5 cm, respectively (unpublished data), somewhat less than those observed by others. However, none of the subjects had been trained to perform the expiratory maneuver, which no doubt limited their degree of diaphragmatic excursion.

In their study of 114 healthy young men, Young and Simon[1018] found a range of diaphragmatic excursion of from 0.8 to 8.1 cm; it was 5 to 7 cm in 57 (50 per cent) and less than 3 cm in 16 persons (14 per cent). These investigators emphasized that diaphragmatic excursion of less than 3 cm is not necessarily abnormal, which has been our experience also. In fact, they found no relationship between diaphragmatic movement and vital capacity: some patients with mean diaphragmatic excursions of less than 3 cm had a vital capacity of over 5 liters. In our study of 350 subjects (unpublished data), we found no age-related differences in diaphragmatic excursion, and height and weight appeared to exert no significant influences, although diaphragmatic movement averaged 0.5 cm less in women than in men.

Physiologic Variations in Diaphragmatic Contour

Scalloping of the diaphragm, in which the normally smooth contour is replaced by smooth, arcuate elevations, is relatively uncommon (Fig. 1–179); Felson[739] observed it in only 5.5 per cent of 500 normal subjects. In the majority it was confined to the right side, and in only a small percentage was it bilateral. The significance of this pattern is not known.

In some subjects, muscle slips originating from the lateral and posterolateral ribs can be identified

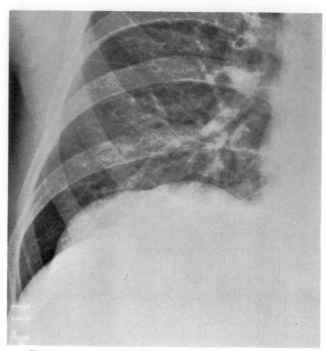

Figure 1–179. Scalloping of the Diaphragm. A roentgenogram of the right hemidiaphragm reveals two smooth arcuate elevations disturbing the normally smooth contour of the dome, a finding of no known significance.

as short, meniscus-shaped shadows along the lateral half of both hemidiaphragms; these are produced by exceptionally low descent of the diaphragm during inspiration. Although such appearances are common in association with severe pulmonary overinflation (Fig. 1–180), as in asthma or emphysema, they may occur in the normal state, particularly in healthy young men; in the absence of supportive evidence they should not be interpreted as a sign of air trapping.

Local "eventration" may occur anywhere in the diaphragm but is seen most commonly in the anteromedial quadrant on the right. This finding possesses no known significance.

THE RESPIRATORY PUMP

During the last decade, physiologists have recognized the importance of respiratory muscle function, to the extent that muscle weakness and fatigue are now considered to be an important determinant of ventilatory failure in almost all instances. The muscles of ventilation are striated and generally behave much as do other muscles of the body.[1023, 1024] They differ in that they are under voluntary as well as automatic control and, in contrast to the inertial loads facing most other skeletal muscle, the respiratory muscles must principally overcome resistive and elastic loads.[996] The diaphragm plays the major role in breathing, but, unlike muscles that are subcutaneous in position, its function cannot be measured directly because of its inaccessibility, at least in humans. This necessitates the use of a variety of indirect means of measurement, all of which have certain limitations. In the following sections we shall consider the components of the respiratory pump machinery under the headings of contractile mechanism and energy sources.

CONTRACTILE MECHANISM

When the diaphragm contracts, it not only pushes down on the abdominal viscera and displaces the abdominal wall outward, but it also lifts and expands the chest cage because of rib articulation and its insertion onto the lower ribs. The increased abdominal pressure (Pab) occasioned by the descent of the diaphragm also contributes to the upward and outward displacement of the thorax. If the abdominal muscles are contracted during inspiration, abdominal pressure increases, descent of the diaphragm is restricted, and rib cage movement is accentuated. At the end of a quiet expiration, the diaphragm is relaxed, and pleural (Ppl) and abdominal (Pab) pressures are equal. On inspiration, intrapleural pressure becomes more negative and abdominal pressure more positive, i.e., transdiaphragmatic pressure difference (delta Pdi) increases. Normally this pressure difference exceeds 25 cm H_2O at a position of maximum inspiration. When the abdominal muscles are relaxed, as they tend to be with quiet breathing in the supine position, this increase in pressure causes protrusion of the abdominal wall. The abdominal and accessory muscles also act as fixators or positioning muscles, which adjust the configuration of the rib cage and abdomen in such a way as to optimize the efficiency of the diaphragm.[996] This is particularly evident in the upright position, especially during exercise when abdominal muscle contraction tends to lengthen the diaphragmatic muscle fibers. Because of the length-tension relationship of skeletal muscle, the longer fibers can generate more tension for a given neuronal drive.[1025] Abdominal expiratory muscles can also aid inspiration by decreasing the

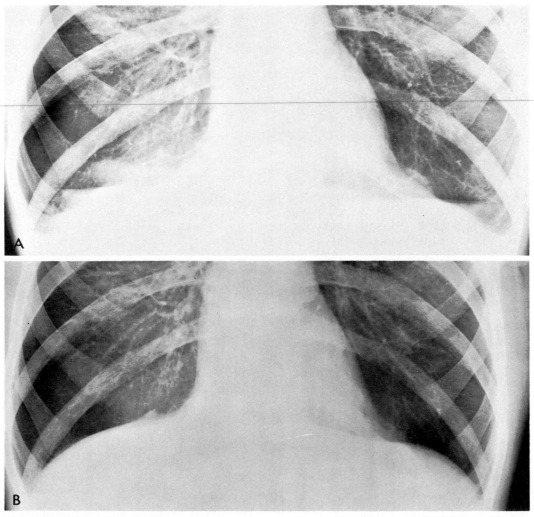

Figure 1–180. Diaphragmatic Muscle Slips. Inspiratory (A) and expiratory (B) roentgenograms of the lower half of the thorax of a patient with severe emphysema reveal short, meniscus-shaped shadows extending laterally from each hemidiaphragm. These muscle slips are prominent on full inspiration and disappear on expiration.

end expiratory lung volume below the relaxed volume of the rib cage and abdomen, and then suddenly relaxing at the onset of inspiration. The sudden descent of the diaphragm along its passive length-tension curve represents an energy-independent inspiratory contribution. This strategy is employed by normal subjects in the hyperpnea of CO_2 rebreathing and exercise[1014] and in patients with bilateral diaphragmatic paralysis.[1026] The maneuver is effective in the upright and lateral decubitus postures but ineffective in the supine position, probably accounting for the characteristic increase in dyspnea noted by patients with bilateral diaphragmatic paralysis when they assume the supine posture.[1026]

The force generated by the contracting diaphragm is a function of the muscle fiber length and the mechanical advantage of the muscle. Like all skeletal muscles, the diaphragmatic fibers have a characteristic length-tension relationship. Thus, at a specific optimal length at which maximal cross-bridging between actin and myosin fibers occurs, maximal force can be generated with a given stimulation. As the fibers are lengthened or shortened beyond this point, the tension generated by a given stimulus is decreased. Recent studies in the dog have shown that diaphragmatic muscle fibers are at nearly optimal length at functional residual capacity.[1027]

The force and transdiaphragmatic pressure generated by the diaphragmatic muscle in contraction is also related to the mechanical advantage of the muscle; for a curved, domed muscle such as the diaphragm, this is related to the radius of curvature. The greater the curvature (the smaller the radius of curvature) the more pressure is generated for a given tension in the diaphragm (law of Laplace). It was formerly thought that this was an important determinant of diaphragmatic muscular function: with a decrease in lung volume and elevation of the diaphragm, the radius of curvature was thought to decrease, whereas with increasing lung volume and descent of the diaphragm, the radius of curvature was thought to increase. However, recent studies suggest that the Laplace relationship may not be such an important determinant of diaphragmatic function, since the radiologically determined radius of curvature of the diaphragm does not change with lung volume.[1028] In contrast to the mechanical advantage given to the diaphragm by abdominal muscle contraction, hyperinflation of the lung decreases the efficiency of the diaphragm as a muscle by shortening muscle fiber length. This situation obviously applies chiefly to patients with obstructive lung disease,[1029] but it has also been shown to be true for normal volunteers breathing at high lung volumes.[1030, 1031]

The other determinant of diaphragmatic contractility is the respiratory neurogram, the rate of stimulation of the muscle. Diaphragmatic force is maximum in humans when the phrenic nerve is stimulated at a frequency of 100 Hertz (Hz); it is reduced to 94 per cent maximum at 50 Hz, 70 per cent maximum at 20 Hz, and 25 per cent maximum at 10 Hz.[1031] Strength of the muscle is assessed as the degree of response to maximal stimulation and varies with the length of the muscle at the time of excitation; endurance depends on the force and duration of contraction.

ENERGY SOURCES

The energy sources of respiratory muscles are oxygen, stored glycogen and protein, and the nutrients extracted from the circulation; as already discussed, the abundant blood supply to the diaphragm does not appear to represent a limiting factor in O_2 supply even under maximal demand.[1032] However, when oxygen transport to the tissues is impaired by a reduction in cardiac output or by severe hypoxemia or anemia, a critical shortage of O_2 for effective diaphragmatic activity may occur, and the body's homeostatic mechanism may be faced with the predicament of deciding which vital organs or tissues should be deprived.[1029]

Experimental studies in dogs[1032] have shown that the diaphragm derives approximately one half its energy requirement from oxidation of carbohydrate and the remainder from lipid substances in the blood. The diaphragm is extremely resistant to anaerobic metabolism,[1032] producing lactic acid only when severely hypoxic—as may occur in severe pulmonary edema with hyperventilation, low lung compliance, arterial hypoxemia, and reduced cardiac output.[1029]

RESPIRATORY MUSCLE FATIGUE

Ultimately, all patients with ventilatory respiratory failure develop inadequate contraction of respiratory muscles. The three major factors that can lead to failure of adequate inspiratory muscle function are decreased neuronal drive, weakness of the respiratory muscle, and fatigue of the muscle. In fact, the last two of these are essentially similar in that the muscles eventually reach a point where the demand placed on them exceeds their capacity to generate force and hence pressure. However, in the case of weakness the primary problem is a decrease in the muscles' ability to generate force against normal loads, whereas in the case of fatigue the major problem is a failure of force generation by a normally functioning muscle against increased load.[1033] A failure of central drive with resulting ventilatory respiratory failure occurs in central neurogenic hypoventilation or drug overdosage. Failure related to weakness is seen in neuromuscular disease, such as myasthenia gravis or muscular dystrophy, whereas fatigue of the respiratory muscles is the common final pathway in the majority of patients with respiratory failure related to the increased work of breathing.

There has been much recent interest in the

study of respiratory muscle fatigue.[994, 1034, 1035] The respiratory muscles are the most fatigue-resistant muscles in the body: for example, when intravenous curare was administered in a dose sufficient to completely abolish hand-grip and head-raising, diaphragmatic strength was decreased to only 42 per cent of the control value.[993, 1036] In humans, the critical transdiaphragmatic pressure required for fatigue is approximately 40 per cent maximum,[1037] but the time that it takes a muscle to fatigue depends not only on the power that it has to generate its strength but also on the energy stores it has and the energy supplies that are delivered to it. The power output depends upon the compliance and resistance of the respiratory system, whereas strength is related to lung volume, atrophy, and nutritional status. The factors that determine energy availability for the respiratory muscles include the oxygen content of the arterial blood supplying the muscles, the respiratory muscle blood flow, substrate concentration in the blood, and the energy stores in the muscle.[1034] All these factors can be altered with disease.

The muscle mass of the diaphragm depends upon the nutritional status and lean body weight;[1038] COPD, especially when accompanied by weight loss, is associated with atrophy of the respiratory muscles, especially type 2 fibers.[1039] The resting oxygen consumption of the respiratory muscles normally ranges from 1 to 3 per cent of total oxygen consumption and can increase markedly in the presence of cardiorespiratory disease, reaching as high as 25 per cent of total oxygen consumption.[1040] Normal subjects breathing a hypoxic gas mixture have a marked and significant decrease in the time to reach respiratory muscle fatigue during loaded breathing.[1041]

Recognition of the importance of muscle fatigue in respiratory failure has stimulated an interest in detecting the weakened muscle before the development of hypercapnia. In the relaxed and supine state, most healthy humans have predominant abdominal rather than rib cage motion,[1042] a finding that correlates with breathing with the diaphragm as opposed to the intercostal muscles.[1043] By contrast, normal subjects fatigued from breathing against resistance[1044] exhibit an interesting sequence of clinical manifestations that correlates with electromyographic evidence of muscle fatigue and the onset of respiratory acidosis. Such individuals are first noted to have very shallow and rapid breathing; this is followed by paradoxic movement of the abdominal wall, the exhausted and flaccid diaphragm being sucked in by the negative intrapleural pressure created by rib cage expansion. In some patients, alternation between rib cage and abdominal breathing (respiratory alternans) is observed, a presumed homeostatic maneuver that permits resting of one group of muscles while the other works.[1045] These signs of diaphragmatic weakness are best detected with the patient in the supine position; the hand should be placed on the abdominal wall to exclude the possibility that the indrawing is caused by contraction of abdominal muscles. Although we are not aware of any clinical or roentgenographic studies of diaphragmatic movement aimed specifically at detecting diaphragmatic fatigue or paralysis, a recent report[1046] indicates that percussion of the level of the diaphragm is not a valid physical sign.

Respiratory muscle strength can be measured by assessing the inspiratory and expiratory pressures at the mouth.[1047] This test requires patient cooperation and is open to error if the facial muscles are weakened and allow air leak; also, the external intercostal and accessory muscles of respiration contribute to the results. Magnetometry or respiratory inductance plethysmography can be used as an objective means of determining movement of the diaphragm; the dimensions of the rib cage and abdomen are measured simultaneously and separately during the respiratory cycle.[1048]

The diaphragmatic electromyogram (EMGdi), employing either esophageal or surface electrodes, can be used as an index of respiratory motoneuron drive.[1000, 1029, 1049, 1050] In normal subjects, changes in inspiratory muscle pressure and ventilation have been shown to be proportionate to changes in inspiratory neural drive as assessed by EMGdi.[1050] Like random noise, the EMG is made up of a whole spectrum of frequencies. Serial measurements of patients who suffer diaphragmatic fatigue show a shift in the power spectrum, with low-frequency components increasing and those of high frequency decreasing. This shift of the high/low ratio precedes clinical evidence of fatigue and blood gas abnormalities and may therefore represent an important early warning sign.[1051, 1052]

Perhaps the most effective means of identifying fatigue of the diaphragm is the measurement of transdiaphragmatic pressure (Pdi), accomplished by recording pressures in balloons placed in both the esphagus and stomach. Gastric and esophageal pressure devices and EMG have recently been incorporated into a single catheter.[1053] If the diaphragm has become completely flaccid as a result of muscle fatigue and the patient does not contract his or her abdominal muscles, Pdi undergoes no change in full inspiration, the negative pleural pressure (Ppl) inducing a negative abdominal pressure (Pab). However, when the diaphragm is not completely flaccid, this method of assessing diaphragmatic function may not be reliable since simultaneous contraction of the diaphragm and other inspiratory muscles results in a change in abdominal pressure that depends not only on the relative strength of contraction of the two muscle groups combined[1054] but also on the degree of abdominal muscle relaxation. Studies in normal subjects have shown that during both slow and forced inspiratory maneuvers there is a considerable intersubject variation, with some individuals showing a natural tendency to low Pdi values.[1055, 1056] Recently, tests have been designed to measure respiratory muscle endurance as opposed to strength, and these may prove to be more relevant to the assessment of the eventual development of respiratory muscle fatigue and ventilatory failure.[1057]

Two types of fatigue occur in skeletal muscle—low and high frequency: high-frequency fatigue is a failure of force generation at high-stimulation frequencies; it is fatigue that recovers rapidly following cessation of the exhaustive work load. By studying diaphragmatic tension generation with different frequencies of phrenic nerve stimulation in the neck, Aubier and associates[1058] found that high-frequency fatigue recovered within 10 minutes of the exhaustive exercise, whereas low-frequency fatigue (20 Hz) was still present (30 per cent of control levels) even 30 minutes after the exercise. Low-frequency fatigue may be related to some impairment of the excitation contraction coupling and not simply to a depletion of muscle energy stores.[994, 1058]

The prompt recognition of inspiratory muscle weakness is of the greatest importance since it clearly indicates impending ventilatory failure and death; a period of muscle rest on a ventilator and treatment of the underlying causes of the weakness may produce complete recovery. This is perhaps most obvious in patients in cardiogenic shock in whom diversion of oxygen away from the respiratory muscles to other vital organs may be life-saving.[1059] Although by no means a substitute for mechanical ventilation in this situation, the recent demonstration that aminophylline or isoproterenol therapy improves diaphragmatic contractility[1060-1062] raises the possibility that still other and more powerful medications will be discovered that reduce or abolish muscle fatigue. It is also encouraging that, in animals, training increases the slow-twitch fibers that are concerned with diaphragmatic endurance;[1001, 1004] this finding appears to be reflected in the reported improvement in exercise performance produced by inspiratory muscle training in patients with chronic air flow limitation.[1063]

THE CHEST WALL

The structures of the thoracic wall, both soft tissue and osseous, form a complex of shadows on roentgenograms of the chest that may be important to roentgenographic analysis, and a working knowledge of their normal anatomy and variations is indispensable.

Soft Tissues

On frontal roentgenograms of the thorax (see Figure 1–194, page 287) the soft tissues, consisting of the skin, subcutaneous fat, and muscles, usually are distinguishable over the shoulders and along the thoracic wall. On successive examinations, a decrease or increase in their extent may constitute a valuable sign of loss or gain in weight.

The pectoral muscles form the anterior axillary fold, a structure that normally is visible in both male and female patients, curving smoothly downward and medially from the axilla to the rib cage. In men, particularly those with heavy muscular development, the inferior border of the pectoralis major muscle may be seen as a downward extension of the anterior axillary fold, passing obliquely across the middle portion of both lungs. In women, this shadow is obscured by the breasts, whose presence and size must be taken into consideration in assessing the density of the lower lung zones. Congenital absence of the pectoralis muscle is rare.[1064]

In many cases the shadow of the sternomastoid muscle is visible as a density whose lateral margin parallels the spine in the medial third of the lung apices; it curves downward and laterally to blend with the companion shadow on the superior aspect of each clavicle. The latter shadow, which is 2 to 3 mm thick, parallels the superior aspect of the clavicle; it is formed by the skin and subcutaneous tissue overlying the clavicles and is rendered visible roentgenologically by the supraclavicular fossae and the tangential direction in which the x-ray beam strikes the clavicles.

The frequency of identification of the companion shadows of the clavicles varies: in healthy subjects with no demonstrable physical abnormality they may be bilaterally symmetric, seen more clearly on one side than the other, well on one side and not on the other, or invisible on both sides. Absence of a companion shadow on one side may suggest enlargement of supraclavicular lymph nodes or some other pathologic process such as edema, but one must exercise caution in interpreting such asymmetry as significant without confirmatory signs.

Sometimes, the floor of the supraclavicular fossa can be identified as a saucer-shaped opacity projected behind the clavicle, running laterally from the sternomastoid shadow.[1070] In one series of frontal roentgenograms of 500 randomly selected patients,[1070] the fossa was identified on at least one side in 29 per cent. Although it can occasionally present as a roughly horizontal opacity suggesting a fluid level, its true nature can be readily discerned by simply following the line out laterally beyond the chest wall. The suprasternal fossa, consisting of a depression on the skin surface of the neck between the sternal heads of the sternocleidomastoid muscles, can also be infrequently identified on posteroanterior roentgenograms. It is roughly U- or V-shaped and projects immediately above the manubrium of the sternum; it is seen most frequently in cachectic or very thin individuals and in patients with severe chronic obstructive lung disease.[1071] It can occasionally simulate a fluid level in the esophagus.

Bones

In the absence of pulmonary or pleural disease, deformity of the spine, or congenital anomalies of the ribs themselves, the rib cage should be symmetric. Both the upper and lower borders of the ribs should be sharply defined except in the middle and lower thoracic regions; here, the thin flanges created by the vascular sulci on the inferior aspects of the ribs posteriorly are viewed *en face*, creating a less distinct inferior margin. In some cases the inferior aspects of the ribs posteriorly within 2 or 3 cm of their tubercles may show local superficial indentations; these should not be mistaken for pathologic rib notching, which is situated more laterally near the midclavicular line in cases of increased collateral circulation through the intercostal vessels (as in coarctation of the aorta).

Calcification of the rib cartilages is common and probably never of pathologic significance. (It has been pointed out by King[1068] that the term "calcification" as applied to costal cartilages is a misnomer, since this is true ossification. Despite the validity of the observation, however, it is difficult to overcome common usage and we shall continue to use "calcification" here.)

The first rib cartilage usually is the first to calcify, often shortly after the age of 20 years. In a roentgenographic study of 100 adults, 60 of whom were male and 40 female, Sanders[1069] observed fairly consistent differences in the pattern of costal calcification in the two sexes: in men, the upper and lower borders of the cartilage become calcified first, extending in continuity with the end of the rib; calcification of the central area follows. By contrast, calcification in women tends to occur first in a central location, in the form of either a solid tongue or as two parallel lines extending into the cartilage from the end of the rib (Fig. 1–181). These findings have been confirmed by Navani and associates,[1072] who studied the chest roentgenograms of 1000 patients aged 10 to 95 years. "Marginal" calcification appeared in 69.8 per cent of males and 11.3 per cent of females, whereas predominantly "central" calcification was observed in 12.0 per cent of males and 76.2 per cent of females; a mixed type of calcification was observed in approximately 7 per cent of both sexes. The relation between age and costal cartilage calcification varied. In males, any calcification was uncommon under the age of 20, and marginal calcification increased from 3.3 per cent in these young adults to 89.3 per cent in men aged 60 years and over. By contrast, central calcification was observed in 45.2 per cent of females under the age of 20 and increased to 88.4 per cent in patients 60 years of age and over. Both Navani and colleagues[1072] and Felson[739] state that in about 95 per cent of cases the sex of adult patients can be determined from the pattern of calcium deposition in the ribs. Furthermore, in Sanders'[1069] study all five women with a "male pattern" of calcification

had undergone pelvic surgery. Sanders suggested that the pattern of costal cartilage calcification may be under hormonal control, whereas Vastine and his colleagues,[1073] who found a strikingly similar pattern of costal cartilage calcification in a pair of homozygotic twins, concluded that such calcification is determined primarily by genetic influences.

Thin, smooth shadows of water density that parallel the ribs and measure 1 to 2 mm in diameter project adjacent to the inferior and inferolateral margins of the first and second ribs and to the axillary portions of the lower ribs. These "companion shadows" (Fig. 1–182) are caused by visualization in tangential projection of parietal pleura and the soft tissues immediately external to the pleura and should not be interpreted as local pleural thickening. In his 1936 anatomic-roentgenographic study, Zawadowski[1074] demonstrated that the shadows are caused by a combination of muscle, fascia, and adipose tissue between the rib and the parietal pleura. More recently, Gluck and his colleagues[1075] showed that the bulk of these "companion shadows" is due to fat (Fig. 1–183). The latter investigators measured the thickness of soft tissue shadows accompanying the second, third, and fourth ribs on posteroanterior roentgenograms of 22 obese patients and 22 subjects of normal weight and showed a statistically significant difference. (For example, the mean thickness of the accompanying shadow of the second rib was 2.7 mm and 2.2 mm in obese males and females, respectively, compared with 1.8 mm and 0.7 mm in those of normal weight.) In addition, they measured the thickness of the companion shadows in eight obese patients before and after weight reduction: the mean value decreased significantly (p < 0.001), from almost 3.0 mm before dieting to approximately 1.2 mm afterward. Vix[1076] has since shown by pathologic-roentgenologic correlation that extrapleural fat is most abundant over the fourth to eighth ribs posterolaterally and that it relates chiefly to the ribs rather than to the interspaces.

In 300 normal subjects in whom the companion shadows were specifically sought by Felson[739] they were seen adjacent to the first rib in 35 per cent and to the second rib in 31 per cent. In approximately half the cases the shadows were bilateral; when unilateral, they were more commonly on the right side. Companion shadows adjacent to the axillary portions of the lower ribs were seen more often (in 75 per cent of 700 normal subjects).

Congenital anomalies of the ribs are relatively uncommon; supernumerary ribs (Fig. 1–184) arising from the seventh cervical vertebra were identified in 1.5 per cent of 350 normal subjects examined by Felson;[739] nearly all were bilateral but many had developed asymmetrically. An extreme example has been reported by Foley and Whitehouse.[1077] A 35-year old Caucasian male, admitted to the hospital for complaints unrelated to the thorax, was found to have 15 pairs of thoracic ribs arising from 15

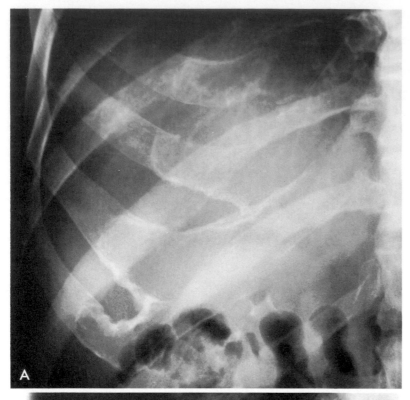

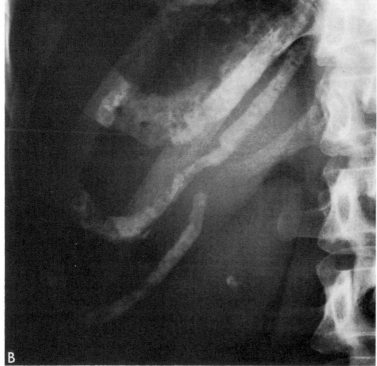

Figure 1–181. Patterns of Rib Cartilage Calcification in Men and Women. *A,* Marginal calcification in a man. *B.* Central calcification in a woman. *See* text.

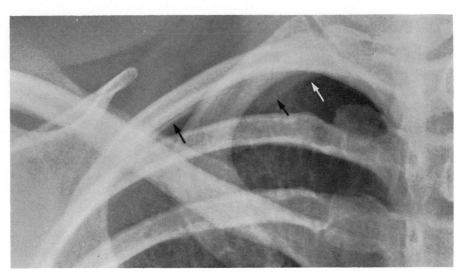

Figure 1–182. Companion Shadows of the Ribs. A magnified view of the apex of the right hemithorax reveals thin smooth shadows of water density lying roughly parallel to the inferior surfaces of the first and second ribs (*arrows*). These companion shadows are caused by perception in tangential projection of a combination of parietal and visceral pleura and the soft tissues immediately external to the pleura.

thoracic vertebrae; he had seven cervical and five lumbar vertebrae, several showing congenital anomalies. All the ribs were well developed and roughly symmetric. (The height of the patient is not recorded!) Other anomalies, such as hypoplasia of the first rib (observed by Felson in 1.2 per cent of 350 normal subjects[739]), bifid or splayed anterior ribs, and, rarely, local fusion of ribs usually are important only in that they may give rise to an erroneous interpretation of abnormal lung density.

Intrathoracic rib is a rare congenital anomaly. Only 12 examples had been reported by 1969,[1083] and two cases have been reported since then.[1084, 1085] This anomaly, which is an innocuous intrathoracic structure, consists of an accessory rib that arises within the bony thorax, more commonly on the right, either from the anterior surface of a rib or from a contiguous vertebral body; it usually extends downward and slightly laterally to end at or near the diaphragm. This pattern may vary. For exam-

ple, in one patient the supernumerary rib originated from the posterior portion of the left third rib and extended through lung substance to join the anterior portion of the left second rib;[1083] this "transthoracic rib" occasioned no symptoms. An even rarer abnormality is an anomalous rib arising from the right side of the last sacral vertebra—a pelvic rib.[1086]

Occasionally, the inferior aspect of the clavicles has an irregular notch or indentation 2 to 3 cm from the sternal articulation; its size and shape are varied, from a superficial saucer-shaped defect to a deep notch 2 cm wide by 1.0 to 1.5 cm deep. These *rhomboid fossae* (Fig. 1–185) give rise to the costoclavicular or rhomboid ligaments that radiate downward to bind the clavicles to the first rib.[1064, 1078] The incidence varies from 10 per cent of clavicles studied anatomically[1079] to 0.59 per cent of 10,000 photofluorograms.[1080] Of the latter cases, 39 were unilateral and 20 bilateral.

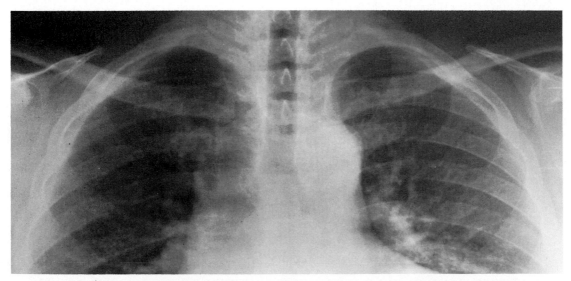

Figure 1–183. Companion Shadows of the Ribs in an Obese Subject. A view of the upper portion of the thorax from a posteroanterior roentgenogram of an exceptionally obese man reveals unusually wide companion shadows caused by accumulation of fat.

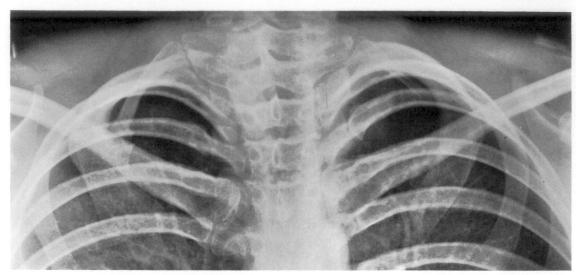

Figure 1–184. Cervical Ribs. Bilateral supernumerary ribs arise from the seventh cervical vertebra. The right rib is longer than the left and shows a synchondrosis with the medial aspect of the first rib.

A tiny foramen may be seen occasionally near the superior aspect of the center of the clavicle, either unilaterally or bilaterally. This foramen permits passage of the middle supraclavicular nerve and is said to be present in 6 per cent of dry skeletal specimens.[1064]

A congenital anomaly infrequently seen in the Western Hemisphere is the *coracoclavicular joint,* a true synovial joint between the coracoid process of the scapula and a bony process extending inferiorly from the clavicle.[1081] These joints are genetically determined anatomic variants, which Cockshott states are seen more frequently in Asia than in Europe and Africa;[1081] there is an unusually high incidence in people from southern China. Although these joints are subject to osteophyte formation with age, they do not give rise to symptoms or disability. Other anatomic variants of no clinical significance are sharply circumscribed lucencies in the body of the scapula surrounded by a thin layer of cortical bone;[1082] these are usually multiple and do not occasion symptoms; they most likely represent areas of incomplete bone formation during maturation.

The normal *thoracic spine* is straight in frontal projection and gently concave anteriorly in lateral projection. Its roentgenographic density in lateral projection decreases uniformly from above downward, and any deviation from this should arouse suspicion of intrathoracic disease.

The lateral and superior borders of the *manubrium* are the only portions of the sternum visible on frontal projections of the thorax, although the whole of the sternum should be clearly seen tangentially in lateral roentgenograms. Goodman and his colleagues[1087] studied the normal CT anatomy of the sternum in 35 patients. They found that the body of the sternum was ovoid-to-rectangular in shape and usually possessed sharp cortical margins. In the manubrium, part of the posterior cortical margin was unsharp and irregular in 34 of 35 patients, and part of the anterior cortical margin was indistinct in 20 of the 35 patients. This potential abnormality could be eradicated by angulating the CT gantry to a position more nearly perpendicular to the manubrium, the definition of these cortical margins being rendered sharp by this maneuver.

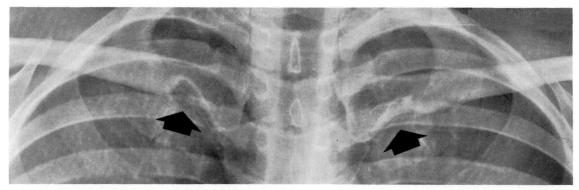

Figure 1–185. Rhomboid Fossae. An irregular notch or indentation is present in the inferior aspect of both clavicles approximately 2 cm from their sternal end (*arrows*). These fossae give origin to the costoclavicular or rhomboid ligaments.

THE NORMAL CHEST ROENTGENOGRAM

As the preceding sections have shown, the lungs are composed of an almost incredible complex of tissues, each of which separately has a unique function but all of which together perform the act of respiration. The morphologist can examine each tissue and pronounce on its normal or abnormal characteristics. In many ways, through the application of special techniques such as computed tomography and angiography, the roentgenologist similarly can assess individual components of the lungs, although his or her methods are necessarily more gross. However, the bulk of the chest roentgenograms that the diagnostician must interpret are plain films, taken without contrast media, and therefore he or she is dealing with a summation of relatively low contrast objects forming a complex group of roentgenographic shadows of varied definition and density. The composition of the lungs in relation to their "density"* and to their roentgenographic pattern has received insufficient attention in the literature, and in this section an attempt is made to clarify some of these issues.

Normal Lung Density

It is readily apparent that the "roentgenographic density" of the lungs is the result of the absorptive powers of each of its component parts—gas, blood, and tissue. Although precise figures for the contributions of blood and tissue vary somewhat depending upon whether results are obtained by anatomic or physiologic methods, data have been compiled that allow a reasonable approximation.

If we apply the *average* figures for total maximal tissue volume, derived from anatomic and physiologic estimates, and the predicted total lung capacity (6500 ml)[1088] of a 20-year-old man 170 cm high, the *average density* of lung is 740 g:7240 ml,† or 0.10 g per ml.

This figure, of course, represents the density of a structure whose composite parts are uniformly distributed, a situation which hardly pertains in the lung. Some of the roentgenographic density of lung is contributed by the major blood vessels, which are visible as homogeneous tapering structures with a density of 1.0 g per ml. Since the average density of lung is only 0.10, a considerable portion of lung tissue must possess a density *less* than this to compensate for the relatively high density of the visible blood vessels. Obviously a high proportion of air must be contained in such tissue—logically, the lung parenchyma or respiratory portion of the lung.

Weibel[515] estimated that the lung parenchyma comprises 90 per cent of total lung volume. Using a point-counting technique, he measured the volumetric proportion of the three components of lung parenchyma: *air* accounted for 92 per cent, and *tissue and capillary blood* for 8.0 per cent (including interstitium, endothelial and epithelial cells, vessel walls, and blood). On the basis of Weibel's figures and again assuming a total lung volume of 7240 ml, the parenchymal component is approximately 6500 ml (90 per cent of 7240 ml), 500 ml of which consist of tissue and blood (8 per cent of 6500 ml). Thus, *the density of lung parenchyma at total lung capacity is 0.08* (500 grams: 6500 ml). *It follows that in a chest roentgenogram all the tissue visible in the peripheral 2 cm of the lung or between vascular shadows has a density of 0.08 g per ml.*

Rhodes and his colleagues[1133] have developed a technique to measure regional values of vascular and extravascular lung density using positron emission and transmission tomography. Quantitative values of lung density in the transverse plane were obtained by recording transmission scans during the exposure of a ring source of positron-emitting germanium/gallium-68, which encircles the subject in the plane of the scan. Values of blood density were obtained by scanning in the emission mode following the labeling of the subjects' red blood cells with a quantity of ^{11}C-carbon monoxide inhaled as a bolus. Subtraction of the normalized blood volume scan from the normalized lung density (transmission) scan provided for regional values of extravascular lung density (Fig. 1–186). Measurements of lung density made on five normal adults in the supine position resulted in a mean density of 0.29 g per ml for a region in the caudal part of the lung (range, 0.26 to 0.32 g per ml).

The density of lung parenchyma has been measured by CT by several groups.[1134-1138] Lung density is determined primarily by the relative proportions of blood, gas, extravascular fluid, and pulmonary tissue.[1134, 1135] Fluctuations in these four variables can have a profound effect on CT density measurements. For example, local or general excess or deficiency in one or more of these components can be readily identified on a CT scan by either an increase or decrease in attenuation, respectively. However, CT densitometry is incapable of distinguishing an increase in capillary blood volume from minimal interstitial edema or mild interstitial pneumonitis;[1137, 1140] similarly, a decrease in attenuation

---

*In this context, the word "density" applies to the *weight of tissue per volume*, or specific gravity (for comparative purposes, the figures for lung tissue may be related to the density of soft tissue as equivalent to water at 1.0 g per ml and to the density of air as zero). It should not be confused with "roentgenographic density," which is a measure of the blackening of film caused by a reduction in silver emulsion by the incident roentgen beam. The greater the amount of radiation passing through the body, the denser the blackening of the roentgenogram; thus, since the tissue density of bone is greater than that of lung, transmission of roentgen rays through bone is less, so that bones appear relatively white in comparison to the blackness of lung. Therefore, *roentgenographic density is dependent upon "tissue" density*, at least in adequately exposed chest roentgenograms.

†The ratio of total weight (740 g, with a volume of 740 ml) to total volume (6500 ml + 740 ml).

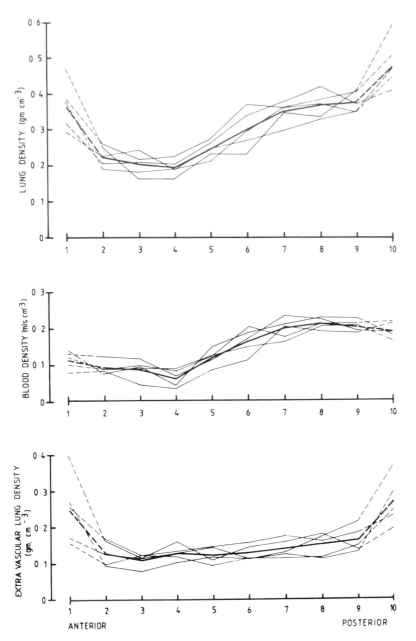

Figure 1–186. Relationship Between CT Attenuation, Lung Density, Blood Density, and Extravascular Lung Water Density. Anteroposterior profiles of lung density, blood density, and extravascular lung water density in five normal subjects (mean values are denoted by the heavy line) obtained from a 1.7-cm-wide strip in the region of interest through the caudal scan of the right lung. Note that there is a definite gradient for lung and blood density whereas the extravascular lung density gradient is negligible down the lung. (From Rhodes CG, Wollmer P, Fazio F, et al: J Comp Assist Tomogr 5:783, 1981.)

caused by emphysema (increased gas, decreased blood flow) or thromboembolism (decreased blood flow) cannot be reliably distinguished on the basis of CT densitometry alone.[1140]

The measurement of lung density with CT is based on an approximately linear relationship that exists between the attenuation of an x-ray beam of 65 Kev (about 120 kVp) and the density of materials of low atomic number (ranging from air to water).[1133, 1134] Attenuation on a CT scan is commonly expressed in terms of the Hounsfield unit (HU) scale in which water is 0 HU and air is -1000 HU. Hedlund and coworkers[1134, 1135] recommend that the relationship between the physical density (weight of tissue per unit volume) and the Hounsfield scale could be emphasized by converting to a "scaled CT quotient" by adding 1000 to the HU value. Using this formulation, CT quotient values

that range from air to water are approximately equal to physical density in mg/cc (Fig. 1–187).[1134, 1135] For example, a CT density reading of -825 HU (approximate value for normal lung at total lung capacity)[1137] represents a scaled CT quotient of 175 or a density equivalent of 175 mg per cc. The validity of this concept has been confirmed by Hedlund and his associates[1134, 1135] by scanning phantom materials of known density, and by measuring tissue density in experimental animals on CT scans and gravitometrically. In the latter instance, CT density was recorded from scans of intact frozen dog thoraces and was compared with the gravitometric measurement of the same volume of lung (1 cm thick frozen slices) at the level of the scan: the CT estimate of lung density in a single slice was within 4 per cent of the gravitometric measurement.

Rosenblum and his colleagues[1089, 1136] measured

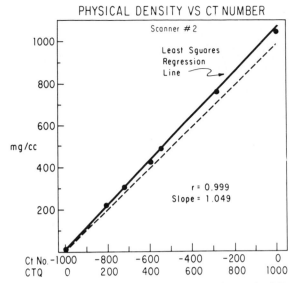

Figure 1–187. Plot of Physical Density (mg/cc) of Standard Materials, CT Density in Hounsfield Units, and CTQ Values. The solid line is the best-fitted line base on least-squares regression analysis. The dashed line shows perfect identity. (From Fullerton G, Haus AG, Properzio WS, et al [eds]: Proc SPIE 347:174, 1982.)

the mean density of the periphery of the lungs in a group of normal subjects over the age of 10 years in two phases of respiration—quiet respiration and breath-holding at full inspiration. The average parenchymal density for the 44 individuals studied during quiet respiration was −754 HU with a standard deviation of 53 HU. The average parenchymal density for the 19 individuals who were studied during inspiratory breath-holding was −813 HU (±37 HU SD). Overall, the lung density of the breath-holding subjects was significantly less than that of the population studied during quiet breathing, the average difference being 68 HU. Although the lungs of the children below the age of 10 years were denser than those of the adults (attributable to less air within the lungs of the children), parenchymal density did not show any marked change with advancing age once adulthood was reached.

Genereux[1137] studied 22 normal patients (9 men and 13 women) with a mean age of 39.3 years (range, 11 to 84 years) and determined that the total mean density of the right lung was −821 HU (±35 HU SD). Wegener and his associates[1138] reported a mean lung density of −840 HU, whereas Goddard and his colleagues[1139] indicated that 79 per cent (15 of 19 subjects) of their normal patients measured between —820 and −860 HU, the majority being in the —820 to −840 HU range.

In these studies, the average parenchymal density recorded during inspiratory breath-holding corresponds to a physical density of roughly 160 to 187 mg per cc (1000 plus CT density measurement), which is more than double the figure of 80 mg per cc that we estimated. The reasons for this discrepancy are not entirely clear, although Rosenblum

and his associates[1089, 1136] suggested that it may be attributable to the fact that their subjects were not able to maintain full inspiration for the 18 second scan.

An attenuation coefficient gradient is normally present between the nondependent and dependent portions of the lung in the supine, prone, and lateral decubitus positions,[1133-1138] attributable primarily to the influence of gravity on blood flow. Rhodes and his colleagues[1133] showed that the anteroposterior gradient for both lung and blood density is pronounced whereas that for extravascular lung water is small (Fig. 1–186). In Rosenblum and associates' study, the average difference between the nondependent and dependent lung parenchyma in the subjects studied during quiet respiration was 112 HU (± 47 HU SD); for the 19 individuals studied during inspiratory breath-holding, the average density gradient was 71 HU (± 35 HU SD).

Genereux[1137] studied the attenuation coefficient gradients at full inspiration, choosing for analysis scans through the aortic arch, the carina, and immediately above the dome of the right hemidiaphragm. Each scan was viewed under 1.3 magnification at a window width of 300 or 500 HU, the level being adjusted for greatest visual clarity (usually between −650 and −850 HU). He delineated a cursor region of interest in the form of a box corresponding to an area of 0.25 cm² or 0.37 cm² (medium or large body calibration), each enclosing 35 voxels (Fig. 1–188). An anterior and posterior peripheral (subpleural) zone was arbitrarily designated the "CT cortex" while two additional areas 2 to 3 cm more centrally were chosen to represent the "CT medulla" (Fig. 1–189). Region-of-interest

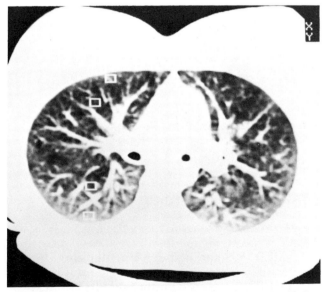

Figure 1–188. Methodology for Attenuation Coefficient Density Evaluation. ROI boxes indicate peripheral and central and anterior and posterior areas in the right lung from which attenuation values are recorded. ROI areas ranged from 0.25 cm² to 0.37 cm² depending on scanner calibration; each contains 35 voxels. (From Genereux GP: J Can Assoc Radiol 36:88, 1985.)

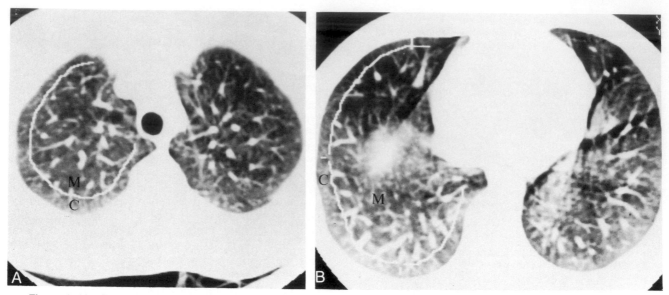

Figure 1–189. The CT Cortex and Medulla. CT scans through the upper lobes (*A*) and lower lobes (*B*) with trace ball delineating the boundaries of the cortex (*C*) and medulla (*M*). The posterior cortex is visually wider than the anterior cortex, apparently as a result of gravitational distention of vessels in the dependent portion of the lung. (From Genereux GP: J Can Assoc Radiol *36*:88, 1985.)

attenuation coefficient measurements were recorded and the values from each scan level were analyzed in the following fashion:

(1) $C^a - C^p$

(2) $M^a - M^p$

(3) $C^a - M^a$

(4) $C^p - M^p$

(5) $\dfrac{C^a + M^a}{2} = AMLD$

(6) $\dfrac{C^p + M^p}{2} + PMLD$

(7) $\dfrac{AMLD_A + PMLD_A}{2} = TMLD_{A\ or\ C\ or\ D}$

(8) $\dfrac{AMLD + PMLD}{2}$ at $A + C + D$

$= TMLD_R$

where

C^a = anterior cortex
C^p = posterior cortex
M^a = anterior medulla
M^p = posterior medulla
AMLD = anterior mean lung density
PMLD = posterior mean lung density
$AMLD_A$ = anterior mean lung density, arch
$PMLD_A$ = posterior mean lung density, arch
$TMLD_A$ = total mean lung density, arch
$TMLD_R$ = total mean lung density, right lung
A = aortic arch
C = carina
D = diaphragm

Using these formulas, Table 1–13 lists the mean anterior and posterior cortical and medullary attenuation densities, the mean anterior and posterior lung densities, the total mean lung density for each scan and for the entire right lung, and the anteroposterior gradients. It can be seen that anterior mean lung density became more negative toward the base while the posterior mean lung density became more positive caudally, resulting in an increasing anteroposterior gradient between the apical and basal scans (Fig. 1–190*A*). Accordingly, the gradient at the aortic arch was 36 HU whereas at

Table 1–13. Attenuation Coefficient Values for GE CT/T 8800 Scanner

	ANTERIOR CORTEX MEDULLA		POSTERIOR CORTEX MEDULLA
Arch	824(49) 841(41) $AMLD_A$833(44)		779(55) 815(49) $PMLD_A$797(51)
		$TMLD_A$815(46) AP GRAD 36(22)	
Carina	850(25) 860(24) $AMLD_C$855(23)		769(59) 812(54) $PMLD_C$790(55)
		$TMLD_C$822(37) AP GRAD 65(42)	
Diaphragm	866(22) 872(16) $AMLD_D$869(17)		753(50) 809(45) $PMLD_D$781(46)
		$TMLD_D$825(27) AP GRAD 88(44)	
		$TMLD_R$821(35)	

AP GRAD = Anteroposterior gradient (AMLD − PMLD) at each level. See text for other definitions.

Values were taken from 22 normal patients and were recorded in Hounsfield units (negative sign deleted) with one standard deviation (parentheses). (From Genereux GP: J Can Assoc Radiol *36*:88, 1985.)

the diaphragm it was 88 HU. The range of both anterior and posterior mean lung densities was greatest at the arch; however, down the lung the range narrowed more anteriorly than it did posteriorly.

The mean cortical density was always more negative anteriorly than posteriorly, a feature that was also present in the medulla (Fig. 1–190B). At the aortic arch, the anteroposterior gradient for the cortex was 45 HU and at the base of the lung, 113 HU. The increasing cortical gradient was shared jointly by a decrease in the anterior and an increase in the posterior density between the top and bottom of the lung. However, the former changed more than the latter, so that the mean anterior cortical measurement decreased by 42 HU down the lung whereas the mean posterior cortical value increased by 26 HU. Similarly, the anteroposterior gradient for the medulla increased from top to bottom, from 26 HU at the arch to 60 HU at the base. However, between the apex and base, although the mean anterior medullary density showed a shift to the

right (increasingly negative, similar to the cortex) amounting to 31 HU, the mean posterior medullary value increased by only 6 HU. The corticomedullary difference narrowed anteriorly and widened posteriorly between the top and bottom of the lung (Fig. 1–190B). The total mean lung density changed only slightly down the lung, being some 10 HU lower at the base (−825 HU) than at the aortic arch (−815 HU). The total mean lung density for the entire right lung was −821 HU (± 35 HU SD).

The increasing attenuation coefficient gradient between the nondependent and dependent portions of the lung on the apical and basal scan is caused more by a decrease in the anterior than by an increase in the posterior density, although a shift clearly occurs in both directions. Thus, the difference between the anterior mean lung density at the arch (−833 HU) and the diaphragm (−869 HU) is 36 HU, whereas the difference in posterior mean lung density at the same levels amounts to only 16 HU (Table 1–13). This tendency for the anterior value to shift more than the posterior is magnified

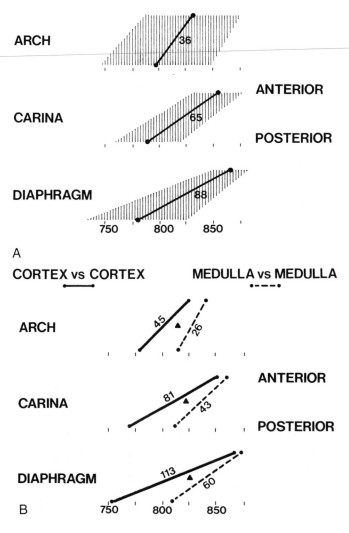

Figure 1–190. Normal CT Lung Attenuation Gradients. *A,* The graft depicts the anterior mean lung density (*AMLD*) and the posterior mean lung density (*PMLD*), anteriorly and posteriorly, at the arch, carina, and diaphragm (*see* text). The gradient between AMLD and PMLD increases down the lung owing to a shift in anterior and posterior values toward increasing negativity and positivity, respectively. The anterior values show greater displacement than the posterior figures. The values along the X-axis represent attenuation coefficient in Hounsfield units (negative sign omitted). Shaded area represents one standard deviation. *B,* The graph compares the intercortical and intermedullary gradients, anteriorly and posteriorly, at the arch, carina, and diaphragm. The anterior cortex, anterior medulla, and posterior cortex show a definite shift down the lung; posterior medulla is virtually fixed at the three levels, being 6 HU lower at the base than it is at the top of the lung. Total mean lung density per slice (solid triangle) decreases by 10 HU between the arch and the diaphragm. Values along the X-axis represent the attenuation coefficient in Hounsfield units (negative sign omitted). (From Genereux GP: J Can Assoc Radiol 36:88, 1985.)

when the mean cortical and medullary gradients are analyzed: whereas the density of the posterior cortex changes by 26 HU between the arch and diaphragm, the posterior medulla alters by only 6 HU; thus, at each level the cortical and medullary gradients do not parallel one another as might be intuitively anticipated considering the dominant impact that gravity has on pulmonary blood flow.

In erect subjects, estimates of regional vascular pressure and blood flow at the apex of the lung have suggested that both are low as a result of gravity but that each increases linearly down the lung. This concept implies that in supine individuals, CT density of the anterior cortex should be more negative than that in the anterior medulla, but in fact precisely the reverse is true: anterior cortical values are always less negative (more positive) than are those in the anterior medulla. Posteriorly, however, the recorded densities are in accordance with predictions based upon gravity-dependence of blood flow, cortical values always exceeding those of the medulla.

If the extravascular tissue volume is assumed constant, the overall roentgenographic density of lung (average, 0.1 g/ml) equals the ratio of its blood and gas content. The blood content can be further subdivided into a capillary component, which creates the *background density* of the lung parenchyma (0.08 g/ml), and a large vessel component, which creates the *visible lung markings* (density, 1.0 g/ml). Figures for *total capillary blood volume* vary according to the measurement technique. Physiologic techniques have yielded estimates, in the resting subject, of 60 to 100 ml,[212, 511–513] whereas anatomic studies have indicated a volume of 150 to 200 ml.[515, 516] Piiper and colleagues,[1142] who subdivided total pulmonary blood volume in the dog into its three vascular components, estimated 27 per cent to be in the arteries, 38 per cent in capillaries, and 35 per cent in veins. If these percentages can be extended to the human lung, the average of 390 ml for total pulmonary blood volume can be broken down to indicate a *capillary volume of 150 ml and a large vessel volume of 240 ml.* Although somewhat higher than the figures quoted earlier in this chapter in the discussion on physiology of acinar perfusion, a capillary blood volume of 150 ml probably represents an acceptable average of the figures obtained by anatomic and physiologic techniques of measurement.

It is important to appreciate the distinction between capillary and visible vessel components of the lung, in their separate contributions to lung density. For example, variation in total *capillary* blood volume probably is difficult, if not impossible, to appreciate subjectively on plain roentgenograms of the chest (although this can be accomplished objectively by roentgen densitometry; *see* Chapter 2). Although an increase in capillary blood volume is known to occur in ventricular septal defect[1090] and in atrial septal defect,[1091] without concomitant alteration in lung volumes,[1092] it is doubtful whether the increase in lung density that must result from this increased capillary volume can be appreciated roentgenographically, except by densitometry. In such situations, roentgenologic assessment of vascular plethora (pleonemia) must be based on increase in the size and number of visible pulmonary vessels, both arterial and venous.

These statements apply only to conditions in which perfusion is *uniformly* altered throughout the lungs—for example, in the pleonemia that accompanies intracardiac left-to-right shunt (Fig. 1–191*A*) or in the oligemia of diffuse emphysema (Fig. 1–191*B*). When reduction in blood flow is local, as with lobar emphysema (Fig. 1–191*C*) or occasionally with massive pulmonary embolism (Westermark's sign[1093]), alteration in density in the involved area of lung is the result of reduction in *both* capillary blood volume (background density) *and* visible vascular shadows. Such alteration of background lung density is an exceedingly valuable roentgenologic sign and is referred to repeatedly throughout this book.

Alteration in Lung Density

In any clinical situation, alteration in roentgenographic lung density may be due to one of three mechanisms or a combination thereof.

PHYSIOLOGIC MECHANISMS

A frequently observed physiologic variation in lung density with which every roentgenologist is familiar is the change that may occur from one examination to another in the same subject, depending upon depth of inspiration. Such variation is readily explained by comparing the contributions of the three components of the lung to its density. For example, again consider a 20-year-old man, 170 cm in height, and assume that pulmonary blood volume and tissue volume are reasonably constant at different degrees of lung inflation. According to the tables of normal values constructed by Goldman and Becklake,[1088] predicted lung volumes for such a subject will be: total lung capacity, 6.5 liters; functional residual capacity, 3.4 liters; and residual volume, 1.5 liters. Assuming a total maximal tissue volume of 740 ml, average lung density at total lung capacity is 0.10; at functional residual capacity, density is almost double (0.18); and at residual volume it is more than treble (0.33) (Fig. 1–192). Thus it is clear that, assuming total pulmonary blood volume to be constant at different degrees of lung inflation, *lung density is inversely proportional to the amount of contained gas.*

PHYSICAL (OR TECHNICAL) MECHANISMS

Symmetry of roentgenographic density of the two lungs in a normal subject depends upon proper

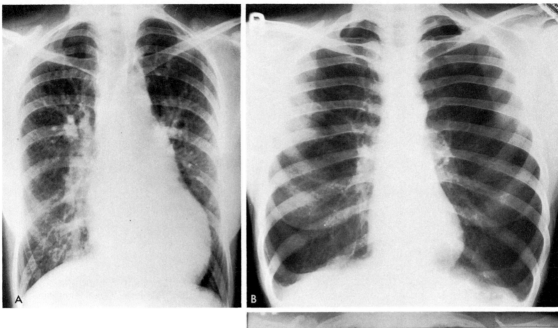

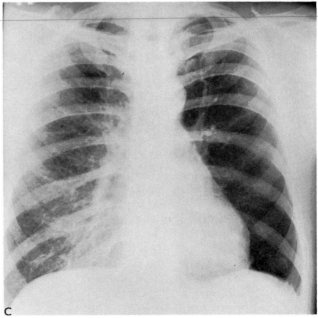

Figure 1–191. Alteration in Lung Density Owing to Abnormalities of Perfusion. Generalized pleonemia, as seen in patent ductus arteriosus (*A*), and diffuse oligemia, as in generalized emphysema (*B*), are evidenced by an increase or decrease, respectively, in the size of the major pulmonary vessels rather than by discernible alteration in background lung density. *C,* When alteration in blood flow is local as in unilateral emphysema (Swyer-James syndrome), reduction in density is apparent because of a decrease in *both* capillary blood volume (background density) and visible vascular shadows.

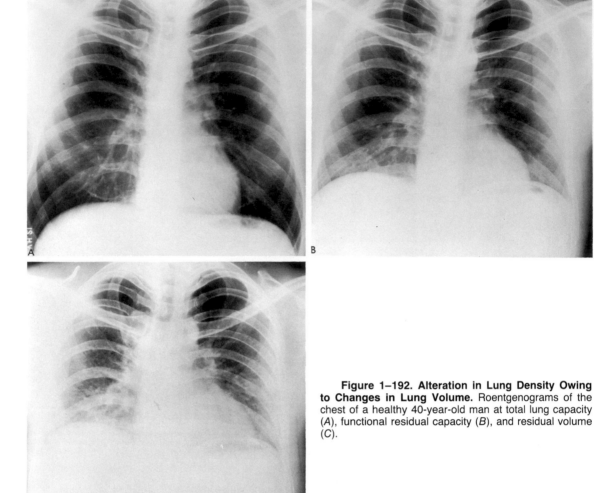

Figure 1–192. Alteration in Lung Density Owing to Changes in Lung Volume. Roentgenograms of the chest of a healthy 40-year-old man at total lung capacity (*A*), functional residual capacity (*B*), and residual volume (*C*).

positioning for roentgenography. If the patient is rotated as little as 2 or 3 degrees, the density of the lung closer to the film will be uniformly *greater* than that of the other lung (Fig. 1–193); conversely, the lung that is farthest away from the film will be uniformly blacker, creating a unilateral hyperlucent hemithorax that can sometimes make differential diagnosis difficult. In previous editions of this book, we have submitted that this effect is produced by the greater thickness of thoracic wall musculature through which the x-ray beam must pass when a patient is rotated to one side, a logical conclusion that was unsubstantiated until confirmed by an ingenious study carried out by Joseph and associates.[1094] In a radiographic study of phantoms, these researchers showed that 80 per cent of the increase in unilateral film blackening resulting from rotation is caused by asymmetric absorption of the primary x-ray beam, with the remaining 20 per cent being due to scatter radiation. Measurements of chest wall thickness showed that the x-ray beam traversed less

tissue on the side of increased film blackening (or conversely more tissue on the side of increased opacity), owing chiefly to the pectoral muscles. It is of some interest that these workers regarded our statement as erroneous concerning the side of increased blackening in relation to the side to which the patient was rotated; in fact, our statement is correct and is not in any way at variance with their findings, a minor paradox that is readily attributable to semantics. Since rotation to the right or to the left means different things to different people (is it rotation into the right anterior oblique or left posterior oblique?), it is clearly preferable to relate the increased opacity or increased lucency to the side that is closest to or farthest removed from the film, respectively. To reiterate, *the density of the hemithorax closer to the film will be uniformly greater than that of the contralateral hemithorax; conversely, the hemithorax farthest removed from the film will be uniformly blacker than that of the other hemithorax.* A similar effect is produced by incorrect centering of the x-ray beam.

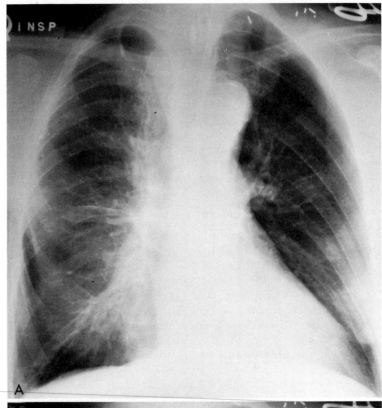

Figure 1–193. Alteration in Lung Density Owing to Improper Positioning. *A,* A roentgenogram of the chest in posteroanterior projection was exposed with the patient rotated slightly into the right anterior oblique position, producing an overall increase in density of the right lung compared with the left. In *B,* positioning has been corrected and the asymmetry has disappeared.

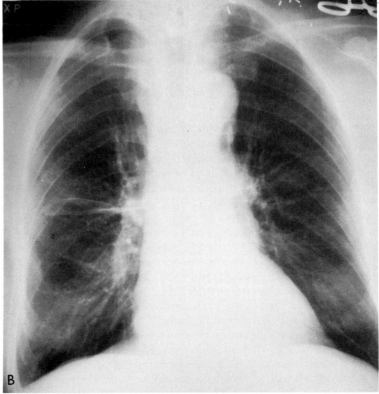

Provided the patient is not rotated and the x-ray beam is properly centered, any discrepancy in the density of the two lungs must be interpreted as being pathologic. The etiology varies from such benign conditions as scoliosis or congenital absence of the pectoral muscles to more potentially significant diseases such as Swyer-James syndrome; this differential diagnosis is described briefly in the following section but in considerably more detail in Chapter 4.

PATHOLOGIC MECHANISMS

Excluding from consideration the contribution to roentgenographic density from the soft tissues of the thoracic wall, and provided physiologic and physical causes can be excluded, variation in lung density is always due to increase or decrease in one or more of the three elements—air, blood, and tissue. As discussed in the Introduction, change in density seldom is produced by alteration in one component to the exclusion of the others. Examples of such "pure" alteration are the reduction in density (increased translucency) produced by pulmonary embolism without infarction (Westermark's sign), in which there is reduction in blood volume but little change in gas or tissue volume; or diffuse pulmonary inflammation, such as in sarcoidosis, in which there is increase in extravascular tissue volume but little change in gas or blood volume. In the majority of clinical situations, change in density, whether increased or decreased, local or diffuse, is the result of change in all three components. The contribution of each component is discussed in detail in the appropriate sections.

The Pulmonary Markings

Roentgenologists must have a thorough knowledge of the pattern of linear markings throughout the normal lung. Unfortunately, such knowledge cannot be gained through didactic teaching; it requires exposure to thousands of normal chest roentgenograms to acquire the experience—perhaps, more, the art—to be able to distinguish normal from abnormal. It requires not only familiarity with the distribution and pattern of branching of these markings (described in the section on roentgen anatomy), but also an awareness of normal caliber, extent of normal roentgenologic visibility, and changes that may occur in different phases of respiration and in various body positions. There are two main reasons for needing such knowledge: (1) a change in the caliber of arteries and veins constitutes one of the most valuable roentgenologic signs of pulmonary venous and pulmonary arterial hypertension, and (2) a redistribution of vessels, with consequent modification of the number of roentgenologically visible markings, may constitute the major evidence for pulmonary collapse or previous pulmonary resection.

The linear markings are created by a complex bundle of structures that are intimately related to one another in their passage through the lungs (Figs. 1–194 and 1–195). These structures are the pulmonary arteries, bronchial arteries, bronchi, nerves, and the lymphatic channels and lymphoid collections. All these structures are connected, at least proximal to the arterioles, by a cuff of loose areolar tissue. The arterial bundles fan outward from both hila, tapering gradually as they proceed distally. In the normal state they are visible up to about 1 to 2 cm from the visceral pleural surface over the convexity of the lung, at which point lung structure becomes totally acinar and the lung markings invisible (the lung parenchyma).

As indicated in the section dealing with the pulmonary vascular tree, the anatomic remoteness of the pulmonary veins from the arteries often renders their distinction possible roentgenographically. In the region of the pulmonary ligaments, especially, these vessels should be readily distinguishable, since the pulmonary veins in the lower lung zones lie almost horizontally and on a lower plane than the arteries. Simon[1141] pointed out that a horizontal line drawn across a posteroanterior roentgenogram of the chest at a midpoint between the apex and diaphragm separates the pulmonary artery complex in the hila (at or above this line) and the veins (below the line). A pulmonary angiographic study of 50 subjects[465] showed superimposition of the upper lobe pulmonary artery and vein in almost half the subjects. Thus it is probable that in roughly half of all patients the upper lobe arteries and veins cannot be distinguished on plain roentgenograms of the chest in posteroanterior projection. When the vessels can be identified separately, the veins that drain the upper lobes always project lateral to their respective arteries—a relationship particularly valuable in the right hilar region, in which the superior pulmonary vein forms the lateral aspect of the hilum superiorly and thus produces the upper limb of its concave configuration (Fig. 1–194). Flattening of this concavity is evidence of collapse of the right upper lobe or, in the presence of pulmonary venous hypertension, indicates dilatation of the upper lobe vein.[1095]

The posteroanterior chest roentgenogram of a normal erect subject invariably shows some discrepancy in size of the linear markings in the upper lung zones compared with the lower, owing to less perfusion of the former. In erect subjects, hydrostatic pressure increases pulmonary blood flow progressively from apex to base, a unit volume of lung at the base of the thorax having four to eight times the blood flow of a similar volume at the apex.[553] In recumbent subjects, absence of the influence of gravity renders this discrepancy in vascular size minimal. In an angiographic study of the pulmonary vascular bed,[465] the mean pulmonary vein diameter at the level of the main pulmonary artery was 7 mm in recumbent subjects and 4 mm in erect

Text continued on page 291

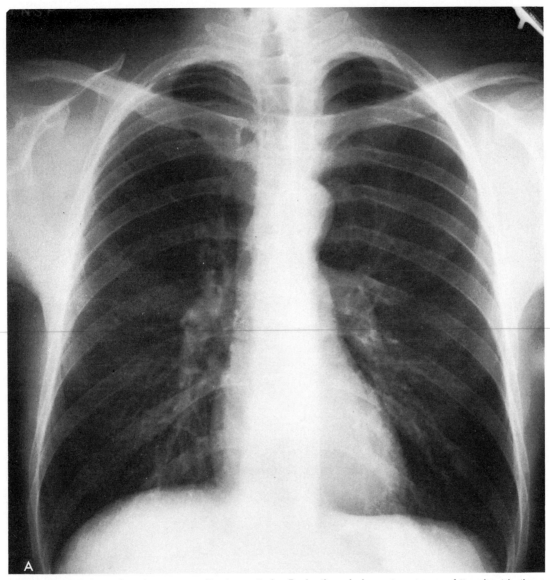

Figure 1–194. Normal Chest Roentgenogram, Posteroanterior Projection. *A,* A roentgenogram of the chest in the erect position of an asymptomatic 26-year-old man.

Illustration continued on following page

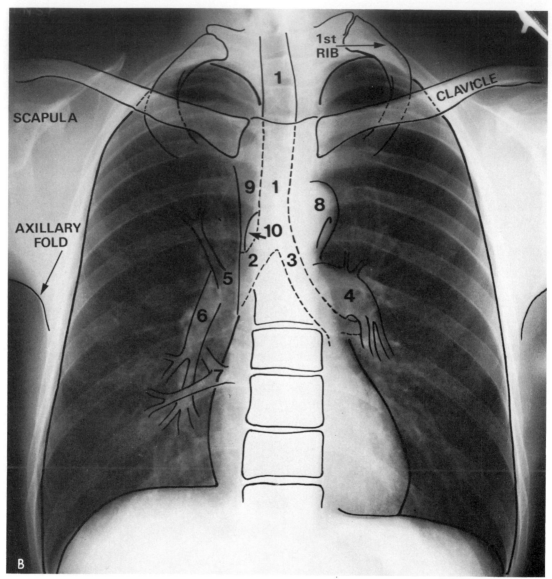

Figure 1–194 *Continued. B,* A diagrammatic overlay shows the normal anatomic structures numbered or labeled: (*1*) trachea; (*2*) right main bronchus; (*3*) left main bronchus; (*4*) left pulmonary artery; (*5*) right upper lobe pulmonary vein; (*6*) right interlobar artery; (*7*) right lower and middle lobe vein; (*8*) aortic knob; and (*9*) superior vena cava.

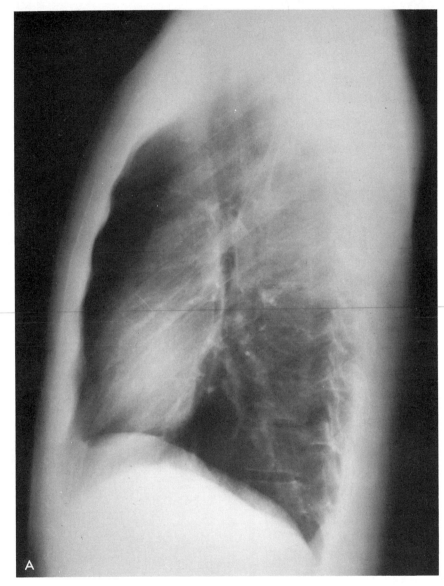

Figure 1–195. Normal Chest Roentgenogram, Lateral Projection. *A,* A roentgenogram of the chest in the erect position of an asymptomatic 26-year-old man.

Illustration continued on following page

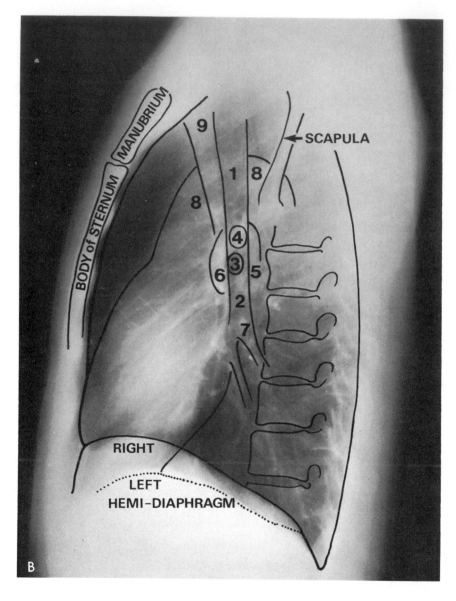

Figure 1–195 *Continued. B,* A diagrammatic overlay shows the normal anatomic structures numbered or labeled: (*1*) tracheal air column; (*2*) right intermediate bronchus; (*3*) left upper lobe bronchus; (*4*) right upper lobe bronchus; (*5*) left interlobar artery; (*6*) right interlobar artery; (*7*) confluence of pulmonary veins; (*8*) aortic arch; and (*9*) brachiocephalic vessels.

ones. Since the roentgenograms from which these measurements were taken were exposed at a 40 inch target film distance, these diameters will be considerably smaller on standard chest roentgenograms exposed at 6 or 10 ft. The caliber of the upper lobe vessels in supine patients is influenced also by the recumbency-induced increase in pulmonary blood volume, which is said to amount to about 30 per cent.[1096] Thus the gravitational advantage enjoyed by the upper lobes in the supine position may make the upper lobe vasculature look quite different on such films than it does on films made in the erect position, a discrepancy that must not be misinterpreted as evidence of disease (Figure 1–196).

Estimates by various investigators of the relative physiologic blood flow to the two lungs have yielded conflicting figures. Dollery and his associates,[1099] using lung scanning techniques with [15]oxygen-labeled carbon dioxide, found significantly greater blood flow through the left than the right upper zone. In contrast, Friedman and associates,[1100] in a study using intravenously injected ^{131}I-MAA (macroaggregated albumin), showed slightly greater average distribution of blood flow to the right lung than to the left—as might be expected in view of the larger size of the right lung. These latter results concur with those obtained by Chen and his colleagues,[1101] who used ^{131}I-MAA and monitored each complete lung area by anterior and posterior scanning. Thus the evidence favors slightly greater blood flow in all zones of the right lung than the left.

Complex interrelationships between transthoracic pressure and pulmonary blood flow occur during inspiration and expiration and during the Valsalva or Mueller maneuvers.* During inspiration the blood volume increases in the pulmonary arteries and veins and decreases in the capillaries.[1102] This change in volume has been documented roentgenographically by Chang,[460] who measured the right descending pulmonary artery in more than 1000 subjects and found the caliber consistently larger during inspiration than during expiration in normal subjects, the range of difference being 1 to 3 mm. He found these measurements particularly helpful in assessing pulmonary hypertension, in which the inspiratory-expiratory ratio is reversed—a point also emphasized by Rigler.[1103]

Use of the Valsalva and Mueller maneuvers to produce increase and decrease, respectively, in intra-alveolar pressure has important but limited application in roentgen diagnosis.[1104] In 1944

Westermark[1105] suggested that increasing the intra-alveolar pressure might prove valuable in differentiating certain diseases of the lungs roentgenographically. He considered that increasing the intra-alveolar pressure reduced the size of congested vessels in pulmonary venous engorgement and "pushed" edema fluid from the air spaces and interstitium back into the vascular tree, thus allowing differentiation of congestion from an infectious process in which this phenomenon did not occur. Although it possesses interesting theoretic possibilities, this technique has proved of little practical value in our experience, although the institution of positive end expiratory pressure (PEEP) ventilation in patients with pulmonary edema can result in remarkably rapid reduction in the amount of water in the lungs. The Valsalva maneuver may be used to advantage in another context—differentiation of vascular and solid lesions within the thorax.[1103, 1104] Vascular structures are reduced in size when intra-alveolar pressure is increased, whereas solid lesions remain unchanged. The method is of particular value in the differentiation of an azygos vein from an enlarged azygos lymph node (Fig. 1–197), or a pulmonary arteriovenous fistula from a solid mass. It is important that high intrathoracic pressure be maintained for several seconds in order for hemodynamic effects of sufficient magnitude to occur to be roentgenographically visible. Tomography may be used to advantage during these maneuvers.[1106]

These examples of the use of the Valsalva and Mueller maneuvers indicate a trend increasingly emphasized in recent years—the application of physiologic principles to roentgen diagnosis. Knowledge of pathophysiology has played a major role in the roentgenologic study of the cardiovascular system for many years, but probably has not received the attention it deserves in pulmonary diseases. A major stimulus to its more frequent application was given by Rigler[1103] in 1959, in his classic paper entitled "Functional Roentgen Diagnosis: Anatomical Image—Physiological Interpretation." Repeated reference is made throughout this book to the ways in which physiologic events can be used to aid in roentgenologic diagnosis of pulmonary disease.

PERCEPTION IN CHEST ROENTGENOLOGY

Observer Error

The roentgenologic diagnosis of chest disease begins with *identification* of an abnormality on a roentgenogram: that which is not *seen* cannot be appreciated. These statements may appear self-evident, but they express an observation that deserves constant re-emphasis. The gain in confidence in ability to *interpret* changes apparent roentgenographically must not be mistaken by roentgenologists for an improvement in the accuracy with which they see them in the first place. Many studies

---

*The Valsalva maneuver consists of forced expiration against a closed glottis, and the Mueller maneuver consists of inspiration against a closed glottis. For proper hemodynamic effect, pressures of plus and minus 40 to 50 cm H_2O, respectively, should be maintained for 7 to 10 seconds. For roentgenograms to be comparable, both maneuvers should be performed at the same degree of lung inflation, preferably at the end of a quiet inspiration.

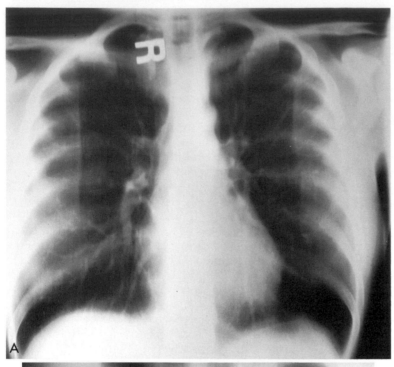

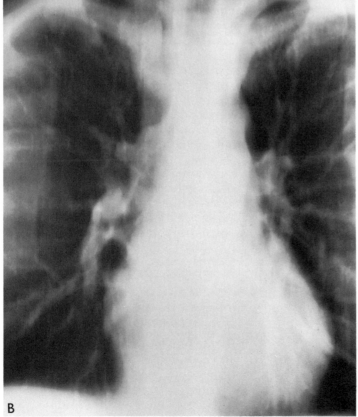

Figure 1–196. Effect on Pulmonary Vasculature of Change in Body Position. Tomographic sections through the midportion of both lungs in the erect (*A*) and supine (*B*) positions reveal a significant difference in the size of the vascular channels. In the supine roentgenogram, not only are the upper lobe arteries and veins more prominent than in the erect study but the overall "grayness" of the upper zones is greater, indicating increased capillary perfusion. Note the difference in the size of the azygos vein in the two studies.

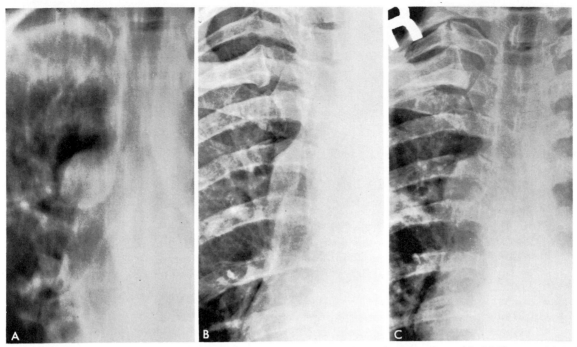

Figure 1–197. Valve of Valsalva and Mueller Procedures in Distinguishing the Vascular or Solid Nature of Intrathoracic Lesions. *A,* A tomographic section of the midmediastinum reveals a well-defined circular shadow situated in the right tracheobronchial angle; differential diagnosis includes an enlarged azygos lymph node or a markedly dilated azygos vein. *B,* A roentgenogram of the same area in the erect position during the Valsalva procedure reveals a marked reduction in the size of the shadow. *C,* A similar projection during the Mueller procedure shows a considerable increase in the size of the shadow compared with *B*. Subsequent angiographic studies proved the shadow to be a markedly dilated azygos vein associated with infradiaphragmatic interruption of the inferior vena cava.

of the accuracy of diagnostic procedures, notably those by Garland[1107, 1108] and by Garland and Cochrane,[1109] have revealed an astonishingly high incidence of both intraobserver* and interobserver† error among experienced roentgenologists. For example, in one series[1107] the interpreters missed almost one third of roentgenologically positive minifilms and overread about 1 per cent of negative films; in another series[1108] based only on positive roentgenograms, interobserver error ranged from 9 to 24 per cent and intraobserver error from 3 to 31 per cent. Since these figures are derived from studies by competent, experienced observers, it is clear that no roentgenologist should be lulled into a false sense of security concerning his or her competence to "see" a lesion: confidence should be continually modified by studied scientific reserve.

A report by Felson and associates[1110] describing the influence of multiple readings on the detection and evaluation of roentgenographic abnormalities in coal workers' pneumoconiosis revealed a truly astonishing level of interobserver disagreement. Three groups of "readers" were employed: group A was composed of radiologists or other physicians residing in the mining areas being studied; group B contained 24 radiologists, with considerable ex-

perience with pneumoconiosis, from three departments of radiology; and group C comprised seven radiologists with extensive experience in pneumoconiosis roentgen interpretation. The A and B readers agreed in approximately 75 per cent of their readings. However, excluding roentgenograms interpreted as normal by both groups of readers (leaving roughly 17,000 roentgenograms), one reader disagreed with the other in 82.2 per cent of cases and agreed in only 17.7 per cent! Agreement between readers in groups A and C was even worse: of 14,369 readings, there was disagreement in three quarters (75.3 per cent); in fact, in only 10.1 per cent did both A and C readers agree that the chest was normal. Comparison between the B and C group readings showed lower levels of disagreement than between the other two, but even here the results were rather discouraging: in 14,594 cases, there was 70 per cent agreement and 30 per cent disagreement between the two groups. Felson and his colleagues suggested four possible factors responsible for the low level of observer agreement: (1) roentgenograms of poor technical quality; (2) a basic lack of experience with the pneumoconiosis classification systems employed; (3) a general lack of familiarity with the roentgen manifestations of coal workers' pneumoconiosis; and (4) inherent factors of interobserver disagreement, as discussed in the preceding paragraphs.

The reasons for observer error are both subjective and objective and are highly complex; every

*Inconsistent observations made by one roentgenologist on two separate readings of the same roentgenograms.

†Inconsistent observations made by two or more roentgenologists on the same roentgenograms.

physician concerned with the interpretation of chest roentgenograms must become thoroughly familiar with the physical and physiologic principles of perception, so that errors are kept to a minimum. Some of the more important of these principles are outlined here, but the reader is urged to review more extensive works on the subject, particularly those by Tuddenham[1111-1114] and Garland[1107] and Riebel's discussion on use of the eyes in roentgenologic diagnosis.[1115]

A roentgenogram can be inspected in two ways, each of which may be usefully employed in different situations. *Directed search* is a method whereby a specific pattern of inspection is carried out, commonly along such lines as thoracic and extrathoracic soft tissues, bony thorax, mediastinum, diaphragm, pleura, and, finally, the lungs themselves, the latter usually by individual inspection and comparison of the zones of the two lungs from apex to base. Such a method *must* be employed by roentgenologists-in-training, for it is only through the exercise of this routine during thousands of examinations that the *pattern* of the normal chest can be recognized. The alternative method of inspection is *free global search*, in which the roentgenogram is scanned without a preconceived orderly pattern. This technique is recommended by Tuddenham,[1111] who found some objective evidence of its being the scanning method employed by the majority of expert roentgenologists; our experience supports this. However, we consider that discovery of an abnormality during free-search scanning must be followed by an orderly pattern of inspection so that other, less obvious abnormalities are not overlooked.

In a recent study of the influence of viewing time and visual search on the interpretation of chest roentgenograms, Kundel and Nodine[116] showed ten radiologists a series of ten normal and ten abnormal roentgenograms under two viewing conditions—(1) a 0.2 sec flash, and (2) unlimited viewing time. The overall accuracy of the flash viewing was surprisingly high (70 per cent true positives) considering that no search was possible; as expected, performance improved with free search (97 per cent true positives). The researchers concluded that their results supported the hypothesis that "Visual search begins with a global response that establishes content, detects gross deviations from normal, and organizes subsequent foveal checking fixations to conduct a detailed examination of ambiguities; the total search strategy then consists of an ordered sequence of interspersed global and checking fixations."

Of a somewhat different character was the study carried out by Carmody and his colleagues[1120] in which a number of chest films were inspected for the presence of lung nodules by five radiologists under two viewing conditions—segmented search, in which films were divided into six sections and viewed piecemeal, and global search, in which the complete film was presented and viewed in its en-

tirety. Nodules varied in edge gradient from sharp to fuzzy. As might be expected, nodules with sharper edges were identified faster, more frequently, and with higher confidence than nodules with less sharp edges, regardless of the method of viewing. Segmented search did not increase the probability of nodule detection; rather, it led to an increase in the number of false-positives, resulting in lower overall performance when compared with global search.

The excellent work by Kundel and his colleagues at Temple University on visual search patterns and strategies during the viewing of chest roentgenograms has contributed valuable information to this important topic,[1117-1119] and the interested reader is directed to their publications as well as those referred to previously.

It is important to view every chest roentgenogram from a distance of at least 6 to 8 ft, or through diminishing lenses. The reasons are twofold: (1) the slight nuances of density variation between similar zones of the two lungs can be better appreciated at a distance than from the traditional viewing position, and (2) the visibility of shadows with ill-defined margins is significantly improved by minification. The physiologic mechanisms underlying this improved visibility have been explained by Tuddenham.[1111] The perception of a roentgenologic shadow in the lungs depends largely upon the gradation of density at the border of the lesion or its sharpness of definition. At standard viewing distance the retina more readily appreciates a lesion whose borders are sharply defined than one whose borders are indistinct. Since such appreciation is dependent upon the visual angle which the border of the lesion subtends at the observer's retina, increased viewing distance (or the use of a diminishing lens), by reducing this visual angle, enhances appreciation of a lesion with indistinct borders. A practical demonstration of this principle was provided by Newell and Garneau[1121] through roentgenography of multiple lucite discs whose borders had been beveled at increasing angles from the perpendicular. Discs with margins perpendicular to the x-ray beam showed no variation in degree of perceptibility with distance of viewing, whereas perception of the beveled discs improved significantly with minification.

A more recent study at the University of New Mexico[1122] investigated the performance of observers in detecting solitary lung nodules 1.0 and 1.5 cm in diameter at viewing distances of 1.5, 3, 6, and 16 feet. There was no difference in observer accuracy in the detection of 1.5 cm nodules at the three closest viewing distances but a deterioration of about 30 per cent at 16 feet. By contrast, observer performance for the detection of 1.0 cm nodules improved as the viewing distance increased from 1.5 to 3 feet, then decreased at the two longer viewing distances. Further, a study of visual system transfer function and optimal viewing distance for radiologists[1123] showed that roentgenologic viewing at a fixed distance increased the risk of failure to detect abnormalities. These results support the contention that in clinical situations multiple viewing distances are desirable. Thus, the practical application of this basic physiologic principle of viewing to everyday roentgenography cannot be overstressed.[1111]

Since perception of a roentgen image depends upon the rate of change in illumination across the retina corresponding to the border of the roentgen shadow (the retinal illumination gradient[1111]), *magnification* logically should reduce perception by increasing the distance across the retina over which a given change in illumination occurs. Although this is true for many intrapulmonary lesions whose borders are indistinct, magnification may aid in the perception of small shadows of relatively high contrast, in much the same manner as it improves the visibility of trabeculae in bone. We find magnification of value in assessing diffuse diseases of the lung in which numerous densities of relatively high contrast are crowded so closely together as to be almost indistinguishable with standard viewing; a classic example is provided by the tiny calcific shadows of alveolar microlithiasis (*see* Fig. 2–2, page 320).

In general, therefore, *minification*—either by distance viewing or through the use of diminishing lenses should be employed at some time in every roentgenographic examination of the chest; *magnification* is of value only when small shadows of relatively high contrast and sharp definition are difficult to separate visually at a standard viewing distance.

As a further means of reducing the frequency of "missing" lesions roentgenologically, the mechanism of *double viewing* has been advocated by several investigators, notably Tuddenham[1111] and Garland.[1107] The latter considered that dual interpretation, by the same observer on two occasions or by two different observers, decreases by at least one third the number of positive films missed. (It is important, of course, that the interpretation given on the first reading should not be known at the second.) We cannot dispute the improvement in diagnostic accuracy to be expected from dual interpretation of every roentgenographic examination of the chest, but the practicality of employing the method routinely in large radiology departments staggers the imagination. Two compromise solutions are suggested: (1) a second reading of all films first interpreted as negative; and (2) a more universal adoption of personal viewing by referring physicians of the roentgenograms of their patients. Many chest physicians and surgeons become highly competent in roentgen interpretation as a result of many years of personal viewing; if this is carried out in consultation with the roentgenologist, the "second look" may reveal abnormalities missed on the first interpretation.

In a survey conducted by Berkson and his associates[1124] at the Mayo Clinic, diagnostic accuracy improved only slightly with the use of stereoscopic roentgenograms. Of 500 chest examinations (98 positive and 402 negative) reviewed by nine readers (five roentgenologists and four chest specialists), the incidence of false-negatives was 18.5 per cent and of false-positives 3.4 per cent when single posteroanterior roentgenograms were viewed. The averages were reduced only to 14.9 per cent and 2.5 per cent, respectively, when stereoscopic roentgenograms were reviewed at a second interpretation. This report originated from an institution in which stereoscopy is an advanced art; what amounts to a relatively low gain in diagnostic accuracy in experienced hands would undoubtedly be even less in centers in which stereoscopy is little used.

Threshold Visibility

In a study reported by Newell and Garneau[1121] in 1951 in which lucite discs were employed as test objects, it was found that a structure of unit density must be at least 3 mm in thickness to be roentgenographically visible. Further, it was observed that this *threshold visibility* applied only if the margins of the lucite discs were parallel to the plane of the roentgen beam—visibility diminished progressively as the margins were increasingly beveled. In 1963, Spratt and his associates[1125] found that roentgenologists could locate the shadows of lucite balls regularly only if the balls were at least 1 to 2 cm in diameter; balls 0.6 cm in diameter could be located only when projected over intercostal spaces, and those as small as 0.3 cm could be identified only in retrospect. The difference between the 3 mm measurement of Newell and Garneau and the larger figures reported by Spratt and his colleagues lies in the character of the *border* of the shadow: the 3 mm measurement applies only to lesions whose borders are sharply defined, and lesions with indistinctly defined or beveled margins (such as a sphere) must be greater than 3 mm in diameter to be roentgenographically visible. Some support is lent these observations by roentgenologic-pathologic studies which have shown that most solitary tumors are not identifiable roentgenologically until their diameter exceeds 6 mm,[1125] and that a cancer less than 1.0 cm in diameter is seldom identified by standard roentgenographic methods.[1126]

These limits of visibility apply, of course, to individual shadows within the lung rather than to multiple diffuse nodular opacities produced, for example, by miliary tuberculosis. In the latter instance, the question of summation of images is raised, and, although we are not able to enter into a discussion of the pros and cons of summation as a roentgenographic effect, we consider that the proposals put forward by Resink[1127] possess considerable merit. Resink suggests that wide distribution of a large number of small lesions throughout the lungs allows visibility of individual deposits only when they are *not* summated and that when summation does occur the appreciation of individual deposits is lost through blurring. (It should be noted that concepts of the effects of summation are conflicting; for example, Newell and Garneau[1121] state that objects of subliminal absorption may be brought above threshold by summation of their shadows.)

Certain objective reasons for missing lesions during roentgenologic interpretation have been clarified by studies in which postmortem roentgenography of the chest has been correlated with subsequent morphologic study of the lungs.[1128, 1129] In one such study[1128] of more than 300 cadavers, the lesions most often missed roentgenologically were small calcified or uncalcified nodules 3 mm or slightly more in diameter in the region of the pleura or subpleural parenchyma. Many metastatic nodules measuring up to 1 cm in diameter were not identified. In 4 of the 300 cases, lesions measuring 2 to 5 cm in diameter that were discovered on roentgenography of the removed lungs were not visible even in retrospect in films taken with the lungs *in situ*. These investigators describe two areas within the thorax in which it is difficult to project a lesion so that it is related to air-containing parenchyma without a superimposed confusion of overlying bones and major blood vessels: over the convexity of the lungs in close proximity to the pleura and rib cage, and in the paramediastinal regions, where the shadows of the aorta, heart, and spine are quite dense. Lesions in close proximity to the diaphragm probably come within the same category. Clearly, it is important to be aware of these relatively "blind" areas in the thorax and to pay particular attention to them in the development of a scanning routine.

Another area of particular importance in the interpretation of chest roentgenograms comprises all the structures outside the limits of the thorax. The importance to diagnosis of such abnormalities as hepatomegaly or splenomegaly, calcification in these organs, displacement or alteration in the contour of the gastric air bubble, and calcification within the thoracic soft tissues cannot be overstressed. Finally, we have been repeatedly impressed by the information to be gained from thorough inspection of the "corners and borders" of roentgenograms. In most departments the name and age of the patient is inscribed thereon by photographic imprinting, particulars which should be noted for definite identification; similarly, an appreciation of dextrocardia or transposition of the thoracic and abdominal viscera may depend upon the position of the "right" or "left" marker.

Psychologic Aspects of Roentgenologic Interpretation

This subject is all too often neglected. Three aspects will be considered briefly, and the reader is referred to more complete discussions of this important topic.[1107, 1111, 1115]

READER FATIGUE

The recent enormous increase in the use of roentgenologic services has resulted in a significant increase in the number of examinations each roentgenologist may be required to report. The inevitable result is "reader fatigue." No experienced roentgenologist denies the diminution in visual and mental acuity that develops during the day when the workload necessitates a heavy reporting schedule. The degree of susceptibility varies, but fatigue eventually affects all to a point at which lack of efficiency accrues to the detriment of the patient. Each individual must set his or her own standards, but two mechanisms can be employed to reduce reader fatigue to a minimum: frequent "rest periods" away from the viewbox and the establishment of a reasonable maximal number of examinations to be reported each day.

PHYSICAL ASPECTS

The atmosphere in which reporting is carried out deserves more attention than it is usually given. Quiet surroundings, away from distracting influences, are most desirable for necessary thought and reflection. Viewing facilities should be optimal. Garland[1107] points out that the illuminator probably is the least expensive and yet one of the most important pieces of apparatus in any department of roentgenology; yet, all too often, insufficient attention is paid to such aspects as light intensity and background illumination, an observation recently confirmed in a very convincing way by Alter and his colleagues.[1181] Riebel's work[1115] on the use of eyes in roentgenology deserves attention in this regard. The necessity for comfort and convenience of viewing and dictation requires no comment.

INTANGIBLE FACTORS

Intimately linked with the complex causes of observer error are several abstract phenomena that inevitably confront all roentgenologists but that defy adequate explanation. A typical example is the variation with which the same examination may be reported from one day to another: a roentgenogram of the chest (often in the troublesome borderland between normal and abnormal) may be pronounced normal on Monday morning and be interpreted by the same observer as showing "diffuse reticular disease" on Friday afternoon! It is a moot point whether fatigue is the dominant influence in these intraobserver disagreements; rather, they may be more realistically ascribed to a "state of mind" that is continually fluctuating and represents an intangible influence on one's approach to a problem. Intraobserver disagreements are bound to occur, but every radiologist must constantly strive to reduce their incidence by effecting the most efficient system of roentgenographic perception of which he or she is capable.

REFERENCES

1. von Hayek H: The Human Lung. New York, Hafner Publishing Company, 1960.
2. Nagaishi C: Functional Anatomy and Histology of the Lung. Baltimore, University Park Press, 1972.
3. Miller WS: The Lung. Springfield, IL, Charles C Thomas, 1937.
4. Krahl VE: Anatomy of the mammalian lung. *In* Fenn WO, Rahn H (eds): Handbook of Physiology. Section 3, Respiration. Vol 1. Washington, DC, American Physiological Society, 1964, pp 213–284.
5. Gail DB, Lenfant CJM: State of the art. Cells of the lung: Biology and clinical implications. Am Rev Respir Dis *127*:366, 1983.
6. Horsfield K, Cumming G: Morphology of the bronchial tree in man. J Appl Physiol *24*:373, 1968.
7. Strahler AN: Equilibrium theory of erosional slopes approached by frequency distribution analysis. Am J Sci *248*:673, 1950.
8. Cumming G, Horsfield K, Harding LK, et al: Biological branching systems with special reference to the lung airways. Bull Physiopathol Resp *7*:31, 1971.
9. Cumming G: Airway morphology and its consequences. Bull Physiopathol Resp *8*:527, 1972.
10. Weibel ER: Morphometry of the Human Lung. New York, Academic Press, 1963.
11. Thurlbeck A, Horsfield K: Branching angles in the bronchial tree related to order of branching. Resp Physiol *41*:173, 1980.
12. Phalen RF, Yeh HC, Schum GM, et al: Application of an idealized model to morphometry of the mammalian tracheobronchial tree. Anat Rec *190*:167, 1978.
13. Breeze RG, Wheeldon EB: The cells of the pulmonary airways. State of the art. Am Rev Respir Dis *116*:705, 1977.
14. McDowell EM, Barrett LA, Harris CC: The respiratory epithelium. 1. Human bronchus. J Natl Cancer Inst *61*:539, 1978.
15. Rhodin JAG: The ciliated cell. Ultrastructure and function of the human tracheal mucosa. Am Rev Respir Dis *93*:1, 1966.
16. Nathanson I, Nadel JA: Movement of electrolytes and fluid across airways. Lung *162*:125, 1984.
17. Watson JHL, Brinkman GL: Electron microscopy of the epithelial cells of normal and bronchitic human bronchus. Am Rev Respir Dis *90*:851, 1964.
18. Serafini SM, Michaelson ED: Length and distribution of cilia in human and canine airways. Bull Eur Physiopathol Resp *13*:551, 1977.
19. Kilburn KH: A hypothesis for pulmonary clearance and its implications. Am Rev Respir Dis *98*:449, 1968.
20. Respiratory Tract Mucus. *In* Ciba Foundation Symposium 54 (New Series). New York, Excerpta Medica, Elsevier/North-Holland, 1978.
21. Kuhn C: Ciliated and Clara cells. *In* Bouhuys A (ed): Lung Cells in Disease. New York, Elsevier/North-Holland Biomedical Press, 1976, p 91.
22. Satir P: How cilia move. Sci Am *231*:45, 1974.
23. Gibbons IR: Studies on the protein components of cilia from *Tetrahymena pyriformis*. Proc Natl Acad Sci *50*:1002, 1963.
24. Jeffrey PK, Reid L: New observations of rat airway epithelium: A quantitative and electron microscopic study. J Anat *120*:295, 1975.
25. McDowell EM, Barrett LA, Harris CC, et al: Abnormal cilia in human bronchial epithelium. Arch Pathol Lab Med *100*:429, 1976.
26. Ailsby RL, Ghadially FN: Atypical cilia in human bronchial mucosa. J Pathol *109*:75, 1973.
27. Lungarella G, Fonzi L, Ermini G: Abnormalities of bronchial cilia in patients with chronic bronchitis. An ultrastructural and quantitative analysis. Lung *161*:147, 1983.
28. Wisseman CL, Simel DL, Spock A, et al: The prevalence of abnormal cilia in normal pediatric lungs. Arch Pathol Lab Med *105*:552, 1981.
29. Fox B, Bull TB, Makey AR, et al: The significance of ultrastructural abnormalities of human cilia. Chest *80*:796, 1981.
30. Ebert RV, Terracio MJ: The bronchiolar epithelium in cigarette smokers. Observations with the scanning electron microscope. Am Rev Respir Dis *111*:4, 1975.
31. Bucher U, Reid L: Development of the mucus-secreting elements in human lung. Thorax *16*:219, 1961.
32. Tos M: Mucous elements in the airways. Acta Otolaryngol *82*:249, 1976.
33. McDowell EM, Combs JW, Newkirk C: Changes in secretory cells of hamster tracheal epithelium in response to acute sublethal injury: A quantitative study. Exp Lung Res *4*:227, 1983.
34. Lumsden AB, McLean A, Lamb D: Goblet and Clara cells of human distal airways: Evidence for smoking-induced changes in their members. Thorax *39*:844, 1984.
35. Adler KB, Hardwick DH, Craighead JE: Porcine tracheal goblet cell ultrastructure: A three-dimensional reconstruction. Exp Lung Res *3*:69, 1982.
36. Korhonen LK, Holopainen E, Paavolainen M: Some histochemical characteristics of tracheobronchial tree and pulmonary neoplasms. Acta Histochem [Suppl] (Jena) *32*:57, 1969.
37. Marsan C, Cava E, Roujeau J, et al: Cytochemical and histochemical characterization of epithelial mucins in human bronchi. Acta Cytol *22*:562, 1978.
38. Spicer SS, Schulte BA, Chakrin LW: Ultrastructural and histochemical observations of respiratory epithelium and gland. Exp Lung Res *4*:137, 1983.
39. Tamai S: Basal cells of the human bronchiole. Acta Pathol Jpn *33*:123, 1983.
40. Lane BP, Gordon R: Regeneration of rat tracheal epithelium after mechanical injury: I. The relationship between mitotic activity and cellular differentiation. Proc Soc Exp Biol Med *145*:1139, 1974.
41. Blenkinsopp WK: Proliferation of respiratory tract epithelium in the rat. Exp Cell Res *46*:144, 1967.
42. Gordon RE, Lane BP: Ciliated cell differentiation in regenerating rat tracheal epithelium. Lung *162*:233, 1984.
43. Wynne JW, Ramphal R, Hood CI: Tracheal mucosal damage after aspiration. A scanning electron microscope study. Am Rev Respir Dis *124*:728, 1981.
44. Kölliker A: Zur Kentniss des Baues der Lunge des Menschen. Verh Physik Med Ges Wurzburg *16*:1, 1881.
44a. Clara M: Zur Histobiologie des Bronchalepithels. Z Mirrosk Anat Forsch *41*:321, 1937.
45. Plopper CG: Comparative morphologic features of bronchiolar epithelial cells. The Clara cell. Am Rev Respir Dis *128*:S37, 1983.
46. Widdicombe JG, Pack RJ: The Clara cell. Eur J Respir Dis *63*:202, 1982.
47. Cutz E, Conen PE: Ultrastructure and cytochemistry of Clara cells. Am J Pathol *62*:127, 1971.
48. Plopper CG, Hill LH, Mariassy AT: Ultrastructure of the nonciliated bronchiolar epithelial (Clara) cell of mammalian lung. III. A study of man with comparison of 15 mammalian species. Exp Lung Res *1*:171, 1980.
49. Azzopardi A, Thurlbeck WM: The histochemistry of the nonciliated bronchiolar epithelial cell. Am Rev Respir Dis *99*:516, 1969.
50. Niden AH: Bronchiolar and large alveolar cell in pulmonary phospholipid metabolism. Science *158*:1323, 1967.
51. Ebert RV, Kronenberg RS, Terracio MJ: Study of the surface secretion of the bronchiole using radioautography. Am Rev Respir Dis *114*:567, 1976.
52. Yoneda K: Pilocarpine stimulation of the bronchiolar Clara cell secretion. Lab Invest *37*:447, 1977.
53. Gil J, Weibel ER: Extracellular lining of bronchioles after perfusion-fixation of rat lungs for electron microscopy. Anat Rec *169*:185, 1971.
54. Mahvi D, Bank H, Harley R: Morphology of a naphthalene-induced bronchiolar lesion. Am J Pathol *86*:559, 1977.
55. Yoneda K: Ultrastructural localization of phospholipases in the Clara cell of the rat bronchiole. Am J Pathol *93*:745, 1978.
56. Evans MJ, Cabral-Anderson LJ, Freeman G: Role of the Clara cell in renewal of the bronchiolar epithelium. Lab Invest *38*:648, 1978.
57. Castleman WL, Dungworth DL, Schwartz LW, et al: Acute respiratory bronchiolitis. An ultrastructural and autoradiographic study of epithelial cell injury and renewal in rhesus monkeys exposed to ozone. Am J Pathol *98*:811, 1980.
58. Mooren HWD, Kramps JA, Franken C, et al: Localisation of a low-molecular-weight bronchial protease inhibitor in the peripheral human lung. Thorax *38*:180, 1983.
59. Fröhlich F: Die "Helle Zelle" der Bronchialschleimhaut und ihre Beziehungen zum Problem der Chemoreceptoren. Frankfurter Zeitsch Pathol *60*:34, 1946.
60. Feyrter F: Zur Pathologie des argyrophilen Helle-Zellen-Organes im Bronchialbaum des Menschen. Virchows Arch *325*:723, 1954.
61. Pack RJ, Widdicombe JG: Amine-containing cells of the lung. Eur J Respir Dis *65*:559, 1984.

62. Becker KL, Gazdar AF (eds): The Endocrine Lung in Health and Disease. Philadelphia, WB Saunders, 1984.
63. Cutz E: Neuroendocrine cells of the lung. An overview of morphologic characteristics and development. Exp Lung Res 3:185, 1982.
64. Tateishi R: Distribution of argyrophil cells in adult human lungs. Arch Pathol 96:198, 1973.
65. McDougall J: Endocrine-like cells in the terminal bronchioles and saccules of human fetal lung: An ultrastructural study. Thorax 33:43, 1978.
66. Stahlman MT, Gray ME: Ontogeny of neuroendocrine cells in human fetal lung. I. An electron microscopic study. Lab Invest 51:449, 1984.
67. Hage E: Electron microscopic identification of several types of endocrine cells in the bronchial epithelium of human foetuses. Z Zellforsch 141:401, 1973.
68. Marchevsky AM, Keller S, Fogel JR, et al: Quantitative studies of argyrophilic APUD cells in airways. The effects of sensitization and anaphylactic shock. Am Rev Respir Dis 129:477, 1984.
69. Editorial: The endocrine lung. Lab Invest 48:507, 1983.
70. Pearse AGE, Takor TT: Embryology of the diffuse neuroendocrine system and its relationship to the common peptides. Fed Proc 38:2288, 1979.
71. Hage E: Amine-handling properties of APUD-cells in the bronchial epithelium of human foetuses and in the epithelium of the main bronchi of human adults. Acta Pathol Microbiol Scand 81:64, 1973.
72. Pearse AGE: The cytochemistry and ultrastructure of polypeptide hormone-producing cells of the APUD series and the embryologic, physiologic and pathologic implications of the concept. J Histochem Cytochem 17:303, 1969.
73. Sidhu GS: The endodermal origin of digestive and respiratory tract APUD cells. Am J Pathol 96:5, 1979.
74. Bosman FT, Louwerens J-WK: APUD cells in teratomas. Am J Pathol 104:174, 1981.
75. Keith IM, Will JA: Hypoxia and the neonatal rabbit lung: Neuroendocrine cell numbers, 5-HT fluorescence intensity, and the relationship to arterial thickness. Thorax 36:767, 1981.
76. Moosavi H, Smith P, Heath D: The Feyrter cell in hypoxia. Thorax 28:729, 1973.
77. Becker AE: The glomera in the region of the heart and great vessels. A microscopic-anatomical study. Pathol Eur 1:410, 1966.
78. Taylor W: Pulmonary argyrophil cells at high altitude. J Pathol 122:137, 1977.
79. Lauweryns JM, Peuskens JC: Neuro-epithelial bodies (neuroreceptor or secretory organs?) in human infant bronchial and bronchiolar epithelium. Anat Rec 172:471, 1972.
80. Keats TE: The aortic-pulmonary mediastinal stripe. Am J Roentgenol 116:107, 1972.
81. Lauweryns JM, Cokelaere M, Theunynck P: Neuro-epithelial bodies in the respiratory mucosa of various mammals. A light optical, histochemical and ultrastructural investigation. Z Zellforsch 135:569, 1972.
82. Lauweryns JM, Goddeeris P: Neuroepithelial bodies in the human child and adult lung. Am Rev Respir Dis 111:469, 1975.
83. Lauweryns JM, Cokelaere M, Theunynck P: Serotonin producing neuroepithelial bodies in rabbit respiratory mucosa. Science 180:410, 1973.
84. Lauweryns JM, Cokelaere M: Hypoxia-sensitive neuro-epithelial bodies and intrapulmonary secretory neuroreceptors, modulated by the CNS. Z Zellforsch 145:521, 1973.
85. Wang N-S, Chen M-F, Schraufnagel DE, et al: The cumulative scanning electron microscopic changes in baby mouse lungs following prenatal and postnatal exposures to nicotine. J Pathol 144:89, 1984.
86. Kleinerman J, Marchevsky A: Quantitative studies of argyrophilic APUD cells in airways. 2. The effects of transplacental diethylnitrosamine. Rev Respir Dis 126:152, 1982.
87. Kawanami O, Bassett F, Ferrans VJ, et al: Pulmonary Langerhans' cells in patients with fibrotic lung disorders. Lab Invest 44:227, 1981.
88. Lamb D, Lumsden A: Intraepithelial mast cells in human airway epithelium: Evidence for smoking-induced changes in their frequency. Thorax 37:334, 1982.
89. Monkhouse WS, Whimster WF: An account of the longitudinal mucosal corrugations of the human tracheo-bronchial tree, with observations on those of some animals. J Anat 122:681, 1976.
90. Vanpeperstraete F: The cartilaginous skeleton of the bronchial tree. Adv Anat Embryol Cell Biol 48:1, 1974.
91. Hakansson CH, Mercke U, Sonesson B, et al: Functional anatomy of the musculature of the trachea. Acta Morphol Neerl-Scand 14:291, 1976.
92. Wailoo M, Emery JL: Structure of the membranous trachea in children. Acta Anat 106:254, 1980.
93. Matsuba K, Thurlbeck WM: A morphometric study of bronchial and bronchiolar walls in children. Am Rev Respir Dis 105:908, 1972.
94. Stephens NL, Kroeger EA: Ultrastructure, biophysics, and biochemistry of airway smooth muscle. In Nadel JA (ed): Physiology and Pharmacology of the Airways. New York, Marcel Dekker, 1980, p 81.
95. Watts CF, Clagett OT, McDonald JR: Lipoma of the bronchus: Discussion of benign neoplasms and report of a case of endobronchial lipoma. J Thorac Surg 15:132, 1946.
96. Whimster WF, Lord P, Biles B: Tracheobronchial gland profiles in four segmental airways. Am Rev Respir Dis 129:985, 1984.
97. Thurlbeck WM, Benjamin B, Reid L: Development and distribution of mucous glands in the foetal human trachea. Br J Dis Chest 55:54, 1961.
98. Tos M: Anatomy of the tracheal mucous glands in man. Arch Otolaryngol 92:132, 1970.
99. Meyrick B, Sturgess JM, Reid L: A reconstruction of the duct system and secretory tubules of the human bronchial submucosal gland. Thorax 24:729, 1969.
100. Meyrick B, Reid L: Ultrastructure of cells in the human bronchial submucosal glands. J Anat 107:281, 1970.
101. Matsuba K, Takizawa T, Thurlbeck WM: Oncocytes in human bronchial mucous glands. Thorax 27:181, 1972.
102. Poitiers W De, Lord PW, Biles B, et al: Bronchial gland histochemistry in lungs removed for cancer. Thorax 35:546, 1980.
103. Lamb D, Reid L: Histochemical types of acidic glycoprotein produced by mucous cells of the tracheobronchial glands in man. J Pathol 98:213, 1969.
104. Reid L: Evaluation of model systems for study of airway epithelium, cilia, and mucus. Arch Intern Med 126:428, 1970.
105. Brandtzaeg P: Mucosal and glandular distribution of immunoglobulin components: Differential localization of free and bound SC in secretory epithelial cells. J Immun 112:1553, 1974.
106. Mooren HWD, Meyer CJLM, Kramps JA, et al: Ultrastructural localization of the low molecular weight protease inhibitor in human bronchial glands. J Histochem Cytochem 30:1130, 1982.
107. Wiggins J, Hill SL, Stockley RA: Lung secretion sol-phase proteins: Comparison of sputum with secretions obtained by direct sampling. Thorax 38:102, 1983.
108. Reid L: Measurement of the bronchial mucous gland layer: A diagnostic yardstick in chronic bronchitis. Thorax 15:132, 1960.
109. Dunnill MS, Massarella GR, Anderson JA: A comparison of the quantitative anatomy of the bronchi in normal subjects, in status asthmaticus, in chronic bronchitis, and in emphysema. Thorax 24:176, 1969.
110. Douglas AN: Quantitative study of bronchial mucous gland enlargement. Thorax 35:198, 1980.
111. Kaltreider HB: Expression of immune mechanisms in the lung. Am Rev Respir Dis 113:347, 1976.
112. Bienenstock J, Clancy RL, Perey, DYE: Bronchus-associated lymphoid tissue (BALT): Its relationship to mucosal immunity. In Kirkpatrick CH, Reynolds HY (eds): Immunologic and Infectious Reactions in the Lung. New York, Marcel Dekker, 1976, p 29.
113. Emery JL, Dinsdale F: The postnatal development of lymphoreticular aggregates and lymph nodes in infants' lungs. J Clin Pathol 26:539, 1973.
114. Chamberlain DW, Nopajaroonsri C, Simon GT: Ultrastructure of the pulmonary lymphoid tissue. Am Rev Respir Dis 108:621, 1973.
115. Macklin CC: Pulmonary sumps, dust accumulations, alveolar fluid and lymph vessels. Acta Anat 23:1, 1955.
116. Bienenstock J, Befus AD, McDermott M: Mucosal immunity. Monogr Allergy 16:1, 1980.
117. Soutar CA: Distribution of plasma cells and other cells containing immunoglobulin in the respiratory tract of normal man and class of immunoglobulin contained therein. Thorax 31:158, 1976.
118. Brinkman GL: The mast cell in normal bronchus and lung. J Ultrastruct Res 23:115, 1968.
119. Gold WM, Meyers GL, Dain DS, et al: Changes in airway mast cells and histamine caused by antigen aerosol in allergic dogs. J Appl Physiol 43:271, 1977.
120. Guerzon GM, Pare PD, Michoud M-C, et al: The number and distribution of mast cells in monkey lungs. Am Rev Respir Dis 119:59, 1979.
121. Pump KK: Morphology of the acinus of the human lung. Dis Chest 56:126, 1969.
122. Boyden EA: The structure of the pulmonary acinus in a child of six years and eight months. Am J Anat 132:275, 1971.
123. Schreider JP, Raabe OG: Structure of the human respiratory acinus. Am J Anat 162:221, 1981.
124. Hansen JE, Ampaya EP, Bryant GH, et al: Branching pattern of airways and air spaces of a single human terminal bronchiole. J Appl Pathol 38:983, 1975.
125. Parker H, Horsfield K, Cumming G: Morphology of distal airways in the human lung. J Appl Pathol 31:386, 1971.
126. Whimster WF: The microanatomy of the alveolar duct system. Thorax 25:141, 1970.

127. Weibel ER, Gomez DM: Architecture of the human lung. Science 137:577, 1962.
128. Elze C, Hennig A: Die inspiratorische Vergröberung von Volumen and innerer Oberfläche der menschlichen Lunge. Z Anat Entwicklung 119:457, 1956.
129. Thompson DW: On Growth and Form. Cambridge, England, University Press, 1942, p 948.
130. Dunnill MS: Postnatal growth of the lung. Thorax 17:329, 1962.
131. Dunnill MS: Evaluation of a simple method of sampling the lung for quantitative histological analysis. Thorax 19:443, 1964.
132. Angus GE, Thurlbeck WM: Number of alveoli in the human lung. J Appl Physiol 32:483, 1972.
133. Thurlbeck WM: The internal surface area of nonemphysematous lungs. Am Rev Respir Dis 95:765, 1967.
134. Dormans JAMA: The alveolar type III cell. Lung 163:327–335, 1985.
135. Weibel ER: Morphological basis of alveolar-capillary gas exchange. Physiol Rev 53:419, 1973.
136. Kuhn C III: Cytochemistry of pulmonary alveolar epithelial cells. Am J Pathol 53:809, 1968.
137. Crapo JD, Barry BE, Gehr P, et al: Cell number and cell characteristics of the normal human lung. Am Rev Respir Dis 125:332, 1982.
138. Weibel ER, Gehr P, Haies D, et al: The cell population of the normal lung. In Bouhuys A (ed): Lung Cells in Disease. 1976, p 3.
139. Bartels H: The air-blood barrier in the human lung: A freeze-fracture study. Cell Tissue Res 198:269, 1979.
140. Schneeberger EE: Barrier function of intercellular junctions in adult and fetal lungs. In Fishman AP, Renkin EM (eds): Pulmonary Edema. Bethesda, MD, American Physiological Society, 1979, p 21.
141. Bartels H, Oestern H-J, Voss-Wermbter G: Communicating-occluding junction complexes in the alveolar epithelium: A freeze-fracture study. Am Rev Respir Dis 121:1017, 1980.
142. Schneeberger EE: The integrity of the air-blood barrier. In Brain JD, Proctor DF, Reid LM (eds): Respiratory Defense Mechanisms. New York, Marcel Dekker, 1977, p 687.
143. Brody AR, Kelleher PC, Craighead JE: A mechanism of exudation through intact alveolar epithelial cells in the lungs of cytomegalovirus-infected mice. Lab Invest 39:281, 1978.
144. Heppleston AG, Young AE: Uptake of inert particulate matter by alveolar cells: An ultrastructural study. J Pathol 111:159, 1973.
145. Suzuki Y, Churg J, Ono T: Phagocytic activity of the alveolar epithelial cells in pulmonary asbestosis. Am J Pathol 69:373, 1972.
146. Brody AR, Hill LH, Stirewalt WS, Adler KB: Actin-containing microfilaments of pulmonary epithelial cells provide a mechanism for translocating asbestos to the interstitium. Chest 83(Suppl):11S, 1983.
147. Sorokin SP: A morphologic and cytochemical study on the great alveolar cell. J Histochem Cytochem 14:884, 1966.
148. Kikkawa Y, Smith F: Biology of disease. Cellular and biochemical aspects of pulmonary surfactant in health and disease. Lab Invest 49:122, 1983.
149. Rooney SA: Function of type II cell lamellar inclusions in surfactant production. In Bouhuys A (ed): Lung Cells in Disease. New York, North-Holland Biomedical Press, 1976, p 147.
150. Ahmed A, Chiswick ML: Origin of osmophilic inclusion bodies in type II pneumocytes. J Pathol 113:161, 1974.
151. Johnson NF: Release of lamellar bodies from alveolar type 2 cells. Thorax 35:192, 1980.
152. Crystal RG: Biochemical processes in the normal lung. In Bouhuys A (ed): Lung Cells in Disease. New York, North-Holland Biomedical Press, 1976, p 17.
153. Evans MJ, Cabral LJ, Stephens RJ, et al: Renewal of alveolar epithelium in the rat following exposure to NO_2. Am J Pathol 70:175, 1973.
154. Kapanci Y, Weibel ER, Kaplan HT, et al: Pathogenesis and reversibility of the pulmonary lesions of oxygen toxicity in monkeys. II. Ultrastructural and morphometric studies. Lab Invest 20:101, 1969.
155. Adamson IYR, Bowden DH: Origin of ciliated alveolar epithelial cells in bleomycin-induced lung injury. Am J Pathol 87:569, 1977.
156. Huang TW, Carlson JR, Bray TM, et al: 3-Methylindole-induced pulmonary injury in goats. Am J Pathol 87:647, 1977.
157. Ryan SF, Bell AL Jr, Barrett CR Jr: Experimental acute alveolar injury in the dog. Am J Pathol 82:353, 1976.
158. Mason RJ, Williams MC, Widdicombe JH: Secretion and fluid transport by alveolar type II epithelial cells. Chest 81:61S, 1982.
159. Simionescu D, Simionescu M: Differentiated distribution of the cell surface charge on the alveolar-capillary unit. Characteristic paucity of anionic sites on the air-blood barrier. Microvasc Res 25:85, 1983.
160. Koffler D, Sandson J, Carr R, et al: Immunologic studies concerning the pulmonary lesions in Goodpasture's syndrome. Am J Pathol 54:293, 1969.
161. Weibel ER, Bachofen H: Structural design of the alveolar septum and fluid exchange. In Fishman AP, Renkin EM (eds): Pulmonary Edema. Bethesda, MD, American Physiological Society, 1979, p 1.

162. Fishman AP: Pulmonary edema: The water-exchanging function of the lung. Circulation 46:390, 1972.
163. Raghu G, Striker LJ, Hudson LD, et al: Extracellular matrix in normal and fibrotic human lungs. Am Rev Respir Dis 131:281, 1985.
164. Madri JA, Furthmayr H: Collagen polymorphism in the lung. An immunochemical study of pulmonary fibrosis. Hum Pathol 11:353, 1980.
165. Torikata C, Villiger B, Kuhn C III, et al: Ultrastructural distribution of fibronectin in normal and fibrotic human lung. Lab Invest 52:399, 1985.
166. Takaro T, Gaddy LR, Parra S: Thin alveolar epithelial partitions across connective tissue gaps in the alveolar wall of the human lung. Ultrastructural observations. Am Rev Respir Dis 126:326, 1982.
167. Kapanci Y, Assimacopoulos A, Irle C, et al: "Contractile interstitial cells" in pulmonary alveolar septa: A possible regulator of ventilation/perfusion ratio? J Cell Biol 60:375, 1974.
168. Fox B, Bull TB, Guz A: Mast cells in the human alveolar wall: An electron microscopic study. J Clin Pathol 34:1333, 1981.
169. Kawanami O, Ferrans VJ, Fulmer JD, et al: Ultrastructure of pulmonary mast cells in patients with fibrotic lung disorders. Lab Invest 40:717, 1979.
170. Williams A, Heath D, Kay JM, et al: Lung mast cells in rats exposed to acute hypoxia, and chronic hypoxia with recovery. Thorax 32:287, 1977.
171. Haas F, Bergofsky EH: Role of the mast cell in the pulmonary pressor response to hypoxia. J Clin Invest 51:3154, 1972.
172. Heath D, Trueman T, Sukonthamarn P: Pulmonary mast cells in mitral stenosis. Cardiovasc Res 3:467, 1969.
173. Brain JD, Sorokin SP, Godleski JJ: Quantification, origin, and fate of pulmonary macrophages. In Brain JD, Proctor DF, Reid LM (eds): Respiratory Defense Mechanisms. New York, Marcel Dekker, 1977, p 849.
174. Quan SG, Golde DW: Surface morphology of the human alveolar macrophage. Exp Cell Res 109:71, 1977.
175. Pratt SA, Smith MH, Ladman AJ, et al: The ultrastructure of alveolar macrophages from human cigarette smokers and nonsmokers. Lab Invest 24:331, 1971.
176. Hocking WG, Golde DW: The pulmonary-alveolar macrophage (first of two parts). N Engl J Med 301:580, 1979.
176a. Hocking WG, Golde DW: The pulmonary-alveolar macrophage (second of two parts). N Engl J Med 301:639, 1979.
177. Brody AR, Craighead JE: Cytoplasmic inclusions in pulmonary macrophages of cigarette smokers. Lab Invest 32:125, 1975.
178. Plowman PN, Flemans RJ: Human pulmonary macrophages: The relationship of smoking to the presence of sea blue granules and surfactant turnover. J Clin Pathol 33:738, 1980.
179. Matulionis DH, Traurig HH: In situ response of lung macrophages and hydrolase activities to cigarette smoke. Lab Invest 37:314, 1977.
180. Lasser A: The mononuclear phagocytic system: A review. Hum Pathol 14:108, 1983.
181. Johnson KJ, Ward PA, Striker G, et al: A study of the origin of pulmonary macrophages using the Chediak-Higashi marker. Am J Pathol 101:365, 1980.
182. Golde DW, Finley RN, Cline MJ: The pulmonary macrophage in acute leukemia. N Engl J Med 290:875, 1974.
183. Lin H-S, Kuhn C III, Chen D-M: Effects of hydrocortisone acetate on pulmonary alveolar macrophage colony-forming cells. Am Rev Respir Dis 125:712, 1982.
184. Adamson IYR, Bowden DH: Role of monocytes and interstitial cells in the generation of alveolar macrophages. II. Kinetic studies after carbon loading. Lab Invest 42:518, 1980.
185. Green GM: Lung defense mechanisms. Med Clin North Am 57:547, 1973.
186. Morgan TE: Pulmonary surfactant. N Engl J Med 284:1185, 1971.
187. Sanders CL, Jackson TA, Adee RR, et al: Distribution of inhaled metal oxide particles in pulmonary alveoli. Arch Intern Med 127:1085, 1971.
188. Kennedy JR, Elliott AM: Cigarette smoke: The effect of residue on mitochondrial structure. Science 168:1097, 1970.
189. Green GM, Carolin D: The depressant effect of cigarette smoke on the in vitro antibacterial activity of alveolar macrophages. N Engl J Med 276:421, 1967.
190. Normann SJ, Sorkin E (eds): Macrophages and Natural Killer Cells. Regulation and Function. New York, Plenum Press, 1982.
191. Villiger B, Broekelmann T, Kelley D, et al: Bronchoalveolar fibronectin in smokers and nonsmokers. Am Rev Respir Dis 124:652, 1981.
192. Eckert H, Lux M, Lachmann B: The role of alveolar macrophages in surfactant turnover. An experimental study with metabolite VIII of bromhexine (Ambroxol). Lung 161:213, 1983.
193. Brain JD: Free cells in the lungs. Arch Intern Med 126:477, 1970.
194. Green GM: The J. Burns Amberson Lecture. In defense of the lung. Am Rev Respir Dis 102:691, 1970.
195. Gupta PK, Frost JK, Geddes S, et al: Morphological identification

of alpha-1-antitrypsin in pulmonary macrophages. Hum Pathol 10:345, 1979.

196. Hsueh W: Prostaglandin biosynthesis in pulmonary macrophages. Am J Pathol 97:137, 1979.

197. Martin TR, Altman LC, Albert RK, et al: Leukotriene B₄ production by the human alveolar macrophage: A potential mechanism for amplifying inflammation in the lung. Am Rev Respir Dis 129:106, 1984.

198. Wyatt JP, Fischer VW, Sweet HC: The pathomorphology of the emphysema complex. Am Rev Respir Dis 89:533, 1964.

199. Heitzman ER, Markarian B, Berger I, et al: The secondary pulmonary lobule: A practical concept for interpretation of chest radiographs. I. Roentgen anatomy of the normal secondary pulmonary lobule. Radiology 93:507, 1969.

200. Heitzman ER, Markarian B, Berger I, et al: The secondary pulmonary lobule: A practical concept for interpretation of chest radiographs. II. Application of the anatomic concept to an understanding of roentgen pattern in disease states. Radiology 93:513, 1969.

201. Raskin SP, Herman PG: Interacinar pathways in the human lung. Am Rev Respir Dis 111:489, 1975.

202. Pump KK: The morphology of the finer branches of the bronchial tree of the human lung. Dis Chest 46:379, 1964.

203. Raskin SP: The pulmonary acinus. Historical notes. Radiology 144:31, 1982.

204. Loeschcke H: Die Morphologie des normalen und emphysemetösen Acinus der Lunge. Beitr Z Pathol Anat 68:213, 1921.

205. Gamsu G, Thurlbeck WM, Macklem PT, et al: Roentgenographic appearance of the human pulmonary acinus. Invest Radiol 6:171, 1971.

206. Osborne DRS, Effmann EL, Hedlund LW: Postnatal growth and size of the pulmonary acinus and secondary lobule in man. Am J Roentgenol 140:449, 1983.

207. Aschoff L: Lectures on Pathology. New York, Hoeber, 1924, pp 53–57.

208. Twining EW: In Shanks SC, Kerley P (eds): A Textbook of X-Ray Diagnosis. Vol II. Philadelphia, WB Saunders, 1951, p 208–209.

209. Lui YM, Taylor JR, Zylak CJ: Roentgen-anatomical correlation in the individual human pulmonary acinus. Radiology 109:1973.

210. Ziskind MM, Weill H, Payzant AR: The recognition and significance of acinus-filling processes of the lungs. Am Rev Respir Dis 87:551, 1963.

211. Ziskind MM, Weill H, Buechner HA, et al: Recognition of distinctive radiologic patterns in diffuse pulmonary disease. Arch Intern Med 114:108, 1964.

212. Staub NC: The interdependence of pulmonary structure and function. Anesthesiology 24:831, 1963.

213. Pump KK: The circulation in the peripheral parts of the human lung. Dis Chest 49:119, 1966.

214. Loosli CG: Interalveolar communications in normal and in pathologic mammalian lungs. Review of the literature. Arch Pathol 24:743, 1937.

215. Parra SC, Gaddy LR, Takaro T: Ultrastructural studies of canine interalveolar pores (of Kohn). Lab Invest 38:8, 1978.

216. Desplechain C, Foliguet B, Barrat E, et al: Les pores de Kohn des alveoles pulmonaires (the pores of Kohn in pulmonary alveoli). Bull Eur Physiopathol Resp 19:59, 1983.

217. Takaro T, Price HP, Parra SC: Ultrastructural studies of apertures in the interalveolar septum of the adult human lung. Am Rev Respir Dis 119:425, 1979.

218. Boatman ES, Martin HB: Electron microscopy of the alveolar pores of Kohn. Am Rev Respir Dis 88:779, 1963.

219. Gil J, Weibel ER: Improvements in demonstration of lining layer of lung alveoli by electron microscopy. Resp Physiol 8:13, 1969.

220. Lindskog GE: Collateral respiration in the normal and diseases lung. Yale J Biol Med 23:311, 1950–51.

221. Martin HB: The effect of aging on the alveolar pores of Kohn in the dog. Am Rev Respir Dis 88:773, 1963.

222. Pump KK: Fenestrae in the alveolar membrane of the human lung. Chest 65:431, 1974.

223. Lambert MW: Accessory bronchiole-alveolar communications. J Pathol Bacteriol 70:311, 1955.

224. Duguid JB, Lambert MW: The pathogenesis of coal miner's pneumoconiosis. J Pathol Bacteriol 88:389, 1964.

225. Krahl VE: Microscopic anatomy of the lungs. Am Rev Respir Dis 80:24, 1959.

226. Boyden EA: Notes on the development of the lung in infancy and early childhood. Am J Anat 121:749, 1967.

227. Martin HB: Respiratory bronchioles as the pathway for collateral ventilation. J Appl Physiol 21:1443, 1966.

228. Henderson R, Horsfield K, Cumming G: Intersegmental collateral ventilation in the human lung. Resp Physiol 6:128, 1969.

229. Anderson JB, Jespersen W: Demonstration of intersegmental respiratory bronchioles in normal human lungs. Eur J Respir Dis 61:337, 1980.

230. Jackson CL, Huber JF: Correlated applied anatomy of the bronchial tree and lungs with system of nomenclature. Dis Chest 9:319, 1943.

231. Brock RC: The nomenclature of broncho-pulmonary anatomy. An international nomenclature accepted by the Thoracic Society. Thorax 5:222, 1950.

232. Boyden EA: Segmental Anatomy of the Lungs. New York, McGraw-Hill, 1955.

233. Kittredge RD: Computed tomography of the trachea: A review. CT 5:44, 1981.

234. Gamsu G, Webb WR: Computed tomography of the trachea: Normal and abnormal. Am J Roentgenol 139:321, 1982.

235. Breatnach E, Abbott GC, Fraser RG: Dimensions of the normal human trachea. Am J Roentgenol 141:903, 1984.

236. Griscom NT, Wohl MEB: Tracheal size and shape: Effects of change in intraluminal pressure. Radiology 149:27, 1983.

237. Alavi SM, Keats TE, O'Brien WM: The angle of tracheal bifurcation: Its normal mensuration. Am J Roentgenol 108:546, 1970.

238. Haskin PH, Goodman LR: Normal tracheal bifurcation angle: A reassessment. Am J Radiol 139:879, 1982.

239. Cleveland RH: Symmetry of bronchial angles in children. Radiology 133:89, 1979.

240. Fraser RG: Measurements of the caliber of human bronchi in three phases of respiration by cinebronchography. J Can Assoc Radiol 12:102, 1961.

241. Merendino KA, Kiriluk LB: Human measurements involved in tracheobronchial resection and reconstruction procedures; Report of case of bronchial adenoma. Surgery 35:590, 1954.

242. Jesseph JE, Merendino KA: The dimensional interrelationships of the major components of the human tracheobronchial tree. Surg Gynecol Obstet 105:210, 1957.

243. Boyden EA, Hartmann JF: An analysis of variations in the bronchopulmonary segments of the left upper lobes of fifty lungs. Am J Anat 79:321, 1946.

244. Boyden EA, Scannell JG: An analysis of variations in the bronchovascular pattern of the right upper lobe of fifty lungs. Am J Anat 82:27, 1948.

245. Scannell JG: A study of variations of the bronchopulmonary segments in the left upper lobe. J Thorac Surg 16:530, 1947.

246. Scannell JG, Boyden EA: A study of variations of the bronchopulmonary segments of the right upper lobe. J Thorac Surg 17:232, 1948.

247. Scannell JG: An anatomic approach to segmental resection. J Thorac Surg 18:64, 1949.

248. Smith FR, Boyden EA: An analysis of variations of the segmental bronchi of the right lower lobe of fifty injected lungs. J Thorac Surg 18:195, 1949.

249. Boyden EA, Hamre CJ: An analysis of variations in the bronchovascular patterns of the middle lobe in fifty dissected and twenty injected lungs. J Thorac Surg 21:172, 1951.

250. Bloomer WE, Liebow AA, Hales MB: Surgical Anatomy of the Bronchovascular Segments. Springfield IL, Charles C Thomas, 1960.

251. Nelson S: Personal communication, 1965.

252. Engel LA, Macklem PT: Gas mixing and distribution in the lung. Int Rev Physiol Respir Physiol 14:37, 1977.

253. Engel LA, Paiva M: Analyses of sequential filling and emptying of the lung. Resp Physiol 45:309, 1981.

254. Paiva M, Engel LA: The anatomical basis for the sloping N₂ plateau. Resp Physiol 44:325, 1981.

255. Mead J: Mechanical properties of lungs. Physiol Rev 41:281, 1961.

256. Martin JG, Habib M, Engle LA: Inspiratory muscle activity during induced hyperinflation. Resp Physiol 39:303, 1980.

257. Leith DE, Mead J: Mechanisms determining residual volume of the lungs in normal subjects. J Appl Physiol 23:221, 1967.

258. Pierce JA, Ebert RV: Fibrous network of the lung and its change with age. Thorax 20:469, 1965.

259. Oderr C: Architecture of the lung parenchyma: Studies with a specially designed x-ray microscope. Am Rev Respir Dis 90:401, 1964.

260. von Neergaard K: Neue Auffassungen uber einen Grundbegriff der Atemmechanik: Die Retraktionskraft der Lunge, abhängig von der Oberflächenspannung in den Alveolen. Z Ges Exp Med 66:373, 1929.

261. Macklin CC: The pulmonary alveolar mucoid film and pneumocytes. Lancet 1:1099, 1954.

262. Dermer GB: A method for the visualization of pulmonary surfactant in the light microscope. Arch Intern Med 127:415, 1971.

263. Brooks RE: Ultrastructural evidence for a noncellular lining layer of lung alveoli. A critical review. Arch Intern Med 127:426, 1971.

264. Finley TN, Pratt SA, Ladman AJ, et al: Morphological and lipid analysis of the alveolar lining material in dog lung. J Lipid Res 9:357, 1968.

265. Kikkawa Y, Motoyama EK, Cook CD: The ultrastructure of the lung of lambs: The relation of osmiophilic inclusions and alveolar lining

layer to fetal maturation and experimentally produced respiratory distress. Am J Pathol 47:877, 1965.

266. Balis JU, Conen PE: Fine structure of alveolar lining layer. Fed Proc 26:406, 1967.

267. Kikkawa Y: Morphology of alveolar lining layer. Anat Rec 167:389, 1970.

268. Manabe T: Freeze-fracture study of alveolar lining layer in adult rat lungs. J Ultrastruct Res 69:86, 1979.

269. Kuhn C III, Finke EH: The topography of the pulmonary alveolus: Scanning electron microscopy using different fixations. J Ultrastruct Res 38:161, 1972.

270. Scarpelli EM: Lung surfactant: Dynamic properties, metabolic pathways and possible significance in the pathogenesis of the respiratory distress syndrome. Bull NY Acad Med 44:431, 1968.

271. Kikkawa Y, Smith F: Cellular and biochemical aspects of pulmonary surfactant in health and disease. Lab Invest 49:122, 1983.

272. Jalowayski AA, Giammona ST: The interaction of bacteria with pulmonary surfactant. Am Rev Respir Dis 105:236, 1972.

273. Klaus MH, Clements JA, Havel RJ: Composition of surface-active material isolated from beef lung. Proc Natl Acad Sci USA 47:1858, 1961.

274. King RJ: Pulmonary surfactant. J Appl Physiol 53:1, 1982.

275. Shelley SA, Balis JU, Paciga JE, et al: Biochemical composition of adult human lung surfactant. Lung 160:195, 1982.

276. King RJ, Macbeth MC: Physicochemical properties of dipalmitoyl phosphatidylcholine after interaction with an apolipoprotein of pulmonary surfactant. Biochim Biophys Acta 557:86, 1979.

277. Tsilibary EC, Williams MC: Actin and secretion of surfactant. J Histochem Cytochem 31:1298, 1983.

278. Clements JA: Comparative lipid chemistry of lungs. Arch Intern Med 127:387, 1971.

279. Clements JA: Pulmonary surfactant. Am Rev Respir Dis 101:984, 1970.

280. Scarpelli EM: The Surfactant System of the Lung. Philadelphia, Lea & Febiger, 1968.

281. Brumley GW, Chernick V, Hodson WA, et al: Correlations of mechanical stability, morphology, pulmonary surfactant and phospholipid content in the developing lamb lung. J Clin Invest 46:863, 1967.

282. Brumley GW: Lung development and lecithin metabolism. Arch Intern Med 127:413, 1971.

283. Heinemann HO, Fishman AP: Nonrespiratory functions of mammalian lung. Physiol Rev 49:1, 1969.

284. Avery ME: The J. Burns Amberson Lecture. In pursuit of understanding the first breath. Am Rev Respir Dis 100:295, 1969.

285. Beppu OS, Clements JA, Georke J: Phosphatidylglycerol-deficient lung surfactant has normal properties. J Appl Physiol 55:496, 1983.

286. Gluck L, Kulovich MV, Borer RC, et al: The interpretation and significance of the lecithin/sphingomyelin ratio in amniotic fluid. Am J Obstet Gynecol 120:142, 1974.

287. Avery ME: Pharmacological approaches to the acceleration of fetal lung maturation. Br Med Bull 31:13, 1975.

288. Oyarzun MJ, Clements JA: Control of lung surfactant by ventilation adrenergic mediators and prostaglandins in the rabbit. Am Rev Respir Dis 117:879, 1978.

289. Massaro D, Clerch L, Massaro GD: Surfactant secretion: Evidence that cholinergic stimulation of secretion is indirect. Am J Physiol 243:C39, 1982.

290. Massaro GD, Massaro D: Morphologic evidence that large inflations of the lung stimulate secretion of surfactant. Am Rev Respir Dis 127:235, 1983.

291. Massaro D, Clerch L, Temple D, et al: Surfactant deficiency in rats without a decreased amount of extracellular surfactant. J Clin Invest 71:1536, 1983.

292. Corbet A, Cregan J, Frink J, et al: Distention-produced phospholipid secretion in postmortem in situ lungs of newborn rabbits. Inhibition by specific beta-adrenergic blockade. Am Rev Respir Dis 128:695, 1983.

293. Kunc L, Kuncova M, Holusa R, et al: Physical properties and biochemistry of lung surfactant following vagotomy. Respiration 35:192, 1978.

294. Schurch S: Surface tension at low lung volumes. Dependence on time and alveolar size. Resp. Physiol 48:339, 1982.

295. Albert RK, Lakshminarayan S, Hildebrandt J, et al: Increased surface tension favors pulmonary edema formation in anesthetized dogs' lungs. J Clin Invest 63:115, 1979.

296. Notter RH, Shapiro DL: Lung surfactant in an era of replacement therapy. Pediatrics 68:781, 1981.

297. Hills BA: What is the true role of surfactant in the lung? Thorax 36:1, 1981.

298. Hills BA: Contact-angle hysteresis induced by pulmonary surfactants. J Appl Physiol 54:420, 1983.

299. Hills BA, Butler BD, Barrow RE: Boundary lubrication imparted by pleural surfactants and their identification. J Appl Physiol 53:463, 1982.

300. Gardner DE, Pfitzer EA, Christian RT, et al: Loss of protective factor for alveolar macrophages when exposed to ozone. Arch Intern Med 127:1078, 1971.

301. LaForce FM, Kelly WJ, Huber GL: Inactivation of staphylococci by alveolar macrophages with preliminary observations on the importance of alveolar lining material. Am Rev Respir Dis 108:784, 1973.

302. Juers JA, Rogers RM, McCurdy JB, et al: Enhancement of bactericidal capacity of alveolar macrophages by human alveolar lining material. J Clin Invest 58:271, 1976.

303. Schwartz LW, Christman CA: Alveolar macrophage migration. Influence of lung lining material and acute lung insult. Am Rev Respir Dis 120:429, 1979.

304. Smith FB: Role of the pulmonary surfactant system in lung diseases of adults. NY State J Med 83:851, 1983.

305. Kankaanpaa K, Hallman M: Respiratory distress syndrome in very low birth weight infants with occasionally normal surfactant phospholipids. Eur J Pediatr 139:31, 1982.

306. Petty TL, Silvers GW, Paul GW, et al: Abnormalities in lung elastic properties and surfactant function in adult respiratory distress syndrome. Chest 75:571, 1979.

307. Hallman M, Spragg R, Harrell JH, et al: Evidence of lung surfactant abnormality in respiratory failure. Study of bronchoalveolar lavage phospholipids, surface activity, phospholipase activity and plasma myoinositol. J Clin Invest 70:673, 1982.

308. Baritussio A, Clements JA: Acute effects of pulmonary artery occlusion on the pool of alveolar surfactant. Resp Physiol 43:323, 1981.

309. Sutnick AI, Soloff LA, Sethi RS: Influence of alveolar collapse upon surface activity of lung extracts. Dis Chest 53:257, 1968.

310. Morgan TE, Finley TN, Huber GL, et al: Alterations in pulmonary surface active lipids during exposure to increased oxygen tension. J Clin Invest 44:1737, 1965.

311. Clements JA, Fisher HK: The oxygen dilemma. N Engl J Med 282:976, 1970.

312. Burger EJ Jr, Mead J: Static properties of lungs after oxygen exposure. J Appl Physiol 27:191, 1969.

313. Barber RE, Lee J, Hamilton WK: Oxygen toxicity in man. A prospective study in patients with irreversible brain damage. N Engl J Med 283:1478, 1970.

314. Singer MM, Wright F, Stanley LK, et al: Oxygen toxicity in man. A prospective study in patients after open-heart surgery. N Engl J Med 283:1473, 1970.

315. Sobonya RE, Kleinerman J, Primiano F, et al: Pulmonary changes in cardiopulmonary bypass: Short-term effects on granular pneumocytes. Chest 61:154, 1972.

316. Balis JU, Cox WD, Pifarré R, et al: The role of pulmonary hypoperfusion and hypoxia in the postperfusion lung syndrome. Ann Thorac Surg 8:263, 1969.

317. Trimble AS, Kim J-P, Bharadwaj B, et al: Changes in alveolar surfactant after lung reimplantation. J Thorac Cardiovasc Surg 52:271, 1966.

318. Lincoln JCR, Barnes ND, Gould T, et al: Pulmonary mechanics and surfactant measurement in canine lungs following reimplantation. Thorax 25:180, 1970.

319. Heppleston AG, Young AE: Alveolar lipo-proteinosis: An ultrastructural comparison of the experimental and human forms. J Pathol 107:107, 1972.

320. Kuhn C, Györkey F, Levine BE, et al: Pulmonary alveolar proteinosis: A study using enzyme histochemistry, electron microscopy, and surface tension measurement. Lab Invest 15:492, 1966.

321. Singh G, Katyal SL, Bedrossian CW, et al: Pulmonary alveolar proteinosis. Staining for surfactant apoprotein in alveolar proteinosis and in conditions simulating it. Chest 83:82, 1983.

322. Taeusch HW, Clements J, Benson B: Exogenous surfactant for human lung disease. Am Rev Respir Dis 128:791, 1983.

323. Robertson B: Surfactant substitution; Experimental models and clinical applications. Lung 158:57, 1980.

324. Smaldone GC, Mitzner W, Itoh H: Role of alveolar recruitment in lung inflation; Influence on pressure-volume hysteresis. J Appl Physiol 55:1321, 1983.

325. Nielson D, Olsen DB: The role of alveolar recruitment and decruitment in pressure-volume hysteresis in lungs. Resp Physiol 32:63, 1978.

326. Lisboa C, Ross WRD, Jardim J, et al: Pulmonary pressure-flow curves measured by a data-averaging circuit. J Appl Physiol 47:621, 1979.

327. Ferris BG, Mead J, Opie LH: Partitioning of respiratory flow resistance in man. J Appl Physiol 19:653, 1964.

328. Anch AM, Remmers JE, Bunce H: III. Supraglottic airway resistance in normal subjects and patients with occlusive sleep apnea. J Appl Physiol 53:1158, 1982.

329. Macklem PT, Mead J: Resistance of central and peripheral airways measured by a retrogade catheter. J Appl Physiol 22:395, 1967.

330. Hogg JC, Macklem PT, Thurlbeck WM: Site and nature of airway obstruction in chronic obstructive lung disease. N Engl J Med 273:1355, 1963.

331. Van Brabandt H, Cauberghs M, Verbeken E, et al: Partitioning of pulmonary impedance in excised human and canine lungs. J Appl Physiol 55:1733, 1983.

332. England SJ, Bartlett D Jr, Daubenspeck JA: Influence of human vocal cord movements on airflow resistance during eupnea. J Appl Physiol 52:773, 1982.

333. Vincet NJ, Knudson R, Leith DE, et al: Factors influencing pulmonary resistance. J Appl Physiol 29:236, 1970.

334. Saunders NA, Betts MF, Pengelly LD, et al: Changes in lung mechanics induced by acute isocapnic hypoxia. J Appl Physiol 42:413, 1977.

335. Widdicombe JH, Gashi AA, Basbaum CB, et al: Structural changes associated with fluid absorption by dog tracheal epithelium. Exp Lung Res 10:57, 1986.

336. Macklin CC: Evidences of increase in the capacity of pulmonary arteries and veins of dogs, cats and rabbits during inflation of the freshly excised lung. Rev Can Biol 5:199, 1946.

337. Laennec RTH: A treatise on the Diseases of the Chest. New York, Hafner, 1962, p 81.

338. Macklem PT: Airway obstruction and collateral ventilation. Physiol Rev 51:368, 1971.

339. Hilpert P: Collaterale Ventilationhabilitations-schrift aus der Medizinischen (thesis). Tübingen, Germany, Tübingen Universitätklinik, 1970.

340. Menkes HA, Traystman RJ: Collateral ventilation, lung disease. In Murray J (ed): Lung Disease—State of the Art. New York, American Lung Association, 1978, p 87.

341. Woolcock AJ, Macklem PT: Mechanical factors influencing collateral ventilation in human, dog, and pig lungs. J Appl Physiol 30:99, 1971.

342. Inners CR, Terry PB, Traystman RJ, et al: Effects of lung volume on collateral and airways resistance in man. J Appl Physiol 46:67, 1979.

343. Batra G, Traystman R, Rudnick H, et al: Effects of body position and cholinergic blockade on mechanics of collateral ventilation. J Appl Physiol 50:358, 1981.

344. Inners CR, Terry PB, Traystman RJ, et al: Collateral ventilation and the middle lobe syndrome. Am Rev Respir Dis 118:305, 1978.

345. Kaplan J, Smaldone GC, Menkes HA, et al: Response to collateral channels to histamine. Lack of vagal effect. J Appl Physiol 51:1314, 1981.

346. Nakamura M, Hildebrandt J: Cigarette smoke acutely increases collateral resistance in excised dog lobes. J Appl Physiol 56:166, 1984.

347. Gertner A, Bromberger B, Traystman R, et al: Histamine and pulmonary responses to cigarette smoke in the periphery of the lung. J Appl Physiol 53:582, 1982.

348. Gertner A, Bromberger-Barnea B, Dannenberg AM, et al: Responses of the lung periphery to 1.0 ppm ozone. J Appl Physiol 55:770, 1983.

349. Gertner A, Bromberger-Barnea B, Traystman R, et al: Effects of ozone on peripheral lung reactivity. J Appl Physiol 55:777, 1983.

350. Terry PB, Traystman RJ, Newball HH, et al: Collateral ventilation in man. N Engl J Med 298:10, 1978.

351. Rosenberg DE, Lyons HA: Collateral ventilation in excised human lungs. Respiration 37:125, 1979.

352. Hogg JC, Macklem PT, Thurlbeck WM: The resistance of collateral channels in excised human lungs. J Clin Invest 48:421, 1969.

353. Sleigh MA: The nature and action of respiratory tract cilia. In Brain JD, Proctor DF, Reid LM (eds): Respiratory Defense Mechanisms—Part I. Lung Biology in Health and Disease. Vol 5. New York, Marcel Dekker, 1977, pp 247–288.

354. Lopez-Vidriero MT, Das I, Reid LM: Airway secretion: Source, biochemical and rheological properties. In Brain JD, Proctor DF, Reid LM (eds): Respiratory Defense Mechanisms— Part I. Lung Biology in Health and Disease. Vol 5. New York, Marcel Dekker, 1977, pp 389–356.

355. Keal EE: Physiological and pharmacological control of airway secretion. In Brain JD, Proctor DF, Reid LM (eds): Respiratory Defense Mechanisms—Part I. Lung Biology in Health and Disease. Vol 5. New York, Marcel Dekker, 1977, pp 357–401.

356. Gallagher JT, Richardson PS: Respiratory mucus: Structure, metabolism and control of secretion. In Chantler EN, Elder JJB, Elstein M (eds): Mucus in Health and Disease. #2, Advances in Experimental Medicine and Biology. New York, Plenum Press, 1982, pp 335–350.

357. King M: Mucus and mucociliary clearance. Basics Resp Dis 11:1, 1982.

358. Williams IP, Hall RL, Miller RJ, et al: Analyses of human tracheo-bronchial mucus from healthy subjects. Eur J Respir Dis 63:510, 1982.

359. Low RB, Davis GS, Giancola MS: Biochemical analyses of bronchoalveolar lavage fluids of healthy human volunteer smokers and nonsmokers. Am Rev Respir Dis 118:863, 1978.

360. Szabo S, Barbu Z, Lakatos L, et al: Local production of proteins in normal human bronchial secretion. Respiration 39:172, 1980.

361. Brown DT, Marriott C, Beeson MF, et al: Isolation and partial characterization of a rheologically active glycoprotein fraction from pooled human sputum. Am Rev Respir Dis 124:285, 1981.

362. Lopez-Vidriero MT: Airway mucus production and composition. Chest 80:799, 1981.

363. Boat TF, Cheng PW: Biochemistry of airway mucus secretions. Fed Proc 39:3067, 1980.

364. Man SFP, Adams GK III, Proctor DF: Effects of temperature, relative humidity and mode of breathing on canine airway secretions. J Appl Physiol 46:205, 1979.

365. Boucher RC, Stutts MJ, Bromberg PA, et al: Regional differences in airway surface liquid composition. J Appl Physiol 50:613, 1981.

366. Ueki I, German VF, Nadel JA: Micropipette measurement of airway submucosal gland secretion—autonomic effects. Am Rev Respir Dis 121:351, 1980.

367. Shelhamer JH, Marom Z, Sun F, et al: The effects of arachnoids and leukotrienes on the release of mucus from human airways. Chest 81:36S, 1982.

368. Nadel JA, Davis B: Parasympathetic and sympathetic regulation of secretion from submucosal glands in airways. Fed Proc 39:3075, 1980.

369. Nadel JA: New approaches to regulation of fluid secretion in airways. Chest 80:849, 1981.

370. Nadel JD, Davis B, Phipps RG: Control of mucus secretion and ion transport in airways. Annu Rev Physiol 41:369, 1979.

371. Phipps RJ, Nadel JA, Davis B: Effect of alpha-adrenergic stimulation on mucus secretion and on ion transport in cat trachea in vitro. Am Rev Respir Dis 121:359, 1980.

372. Davis B, Chinn R, Gold J, et al: Hypoxemia reflexly increases secretion from tracheal submucosal glands in dogs. J Appl Physiol 52:1416, 1982.

373. German VF, Corrales R, Ueki IF, et al: Reflex stimulation of tracheal mucus gland secretion by gastric irritation in cats. J Appl Physiol 52:1153, 1982.

374. Marom Z, Shelhamer JH, Bach MK, et al: Slow-reacting substances, leukotrienes C4 and D4, increase the release of mucus from human airways in vitro. Am Rev Respir Dis 126:449, 1982.

375. Peatfield AC, Barnes PJ, Bratcher C, et al: Vasoactive intestinal peptide stimulates tracheal submucosal gland secretion in ferret. Am Rev Respir Dis 128:89, 1983.

376. Widdicombe JH, Welsh MJ: Ion transport by dog tracheal epithelium. Fed Proc 39:3062, 1980.

377. Widdicombe JH, Ueki IF, Bruderman I, et al: The effects of sodium substitution and ouabain on ion transport by dog tracheal epithelium. Am Rev Respir Dis 120:385, 1979.

378. Knowles MR, Murray GF, Shallal JA, et al: Ion transport in excised human bronchi and its neurohumoral control. Chest 81:11S, 1982.

379. Olver RE, Davis B, Marin MG, et al: Active transport of NA+ and Cl− across canine tracheal epithelium in vitro. Am Rev Respir Dis 112:811, 1975.

380. Knowles MR, Buntin WH, Bromberg PA, et al: Measurements of transepithelial electric potential differences in the trachea and bronchi of human subjects in vivo. Am Rev Respir Dis 126:108, 1982.

381. Davis B, Marin MG, Yee JW, et al: Effect of terbutaline on movement of Cl− and Na+ across the trachea of the dog in vitro. Am Rev Respir Dis 120:547, 1979.

382. Marriott C: The viscoelastic nature of mucus secretion. Chest 80 (6 Suppl):804, 1981.

383. Lofdahl C-G, Odeblad E: Biophysical variables relating to viscoelastic properties of mucus secretions, with special reference to NMR methods for viscosity measurement. Eur J Respir Dis 61:113, 1980.

384. Giordano AM, Holsclaw D, Litt M: Mucus rheology and mucociliary clearance; Normal physiologic state. Am Rev Respir Dis 118:245, 1978.

385. King M: Viscoelastic properties of airway mucus. Fed Proc 39:3080, 1980.

386. Puchelle E, Zahm JM, Duvivier C: Spinnability of bronchial mucus. Relationship with viscoelasticity and mucous transport and properties. Biorheology 20:239, 1983.

387. King M, Cohen C, Viires N: Influence of vagal tone on rheology and transportability of canine tracheal mucus. Am Rev Respir Dis 120:1215, 1979.

388. Lopez-Vidriero MT, Das I, Smith AP, et al: Bronchial secretion from normal human airways after inhalation of prostaglandin F2, acetylcholine, histamine, and citric acid. Thorax 32:734, 1977.

389. Adler K, Wooten O, Philippoff W, et al: Physical properties of

sputum. III. Rheologic variability and intrinsic relationships. Am Rev Respir Dis 106:86, 1972.

390. Richards JH, Marriott C: Effect of relative humidity on the rheologic properties of bronchial mucus. Am Rev Respir Dis 109:484, 1974.

391. Dulfano MJ, Adler K, Wooten O: Physical properties of sputum. IV. Effects of 100 per cent humidity and water mist. Am Rev Respir Dis 107:130, 1973.

392. Thomson ML, Pavia D, McNicol MW: A preliminary study of the effect of guaiphenesin on mucociliary clearance from the human lung. Thorax 28:742, 1973.

393. Barton AD, Lourenço RV: Bronchial secretions and mucociliary clearance. Arch Intern Med 131:140, 1973.

394. Litt M: Mucus rheology. Relevance to mucociliary clearance. Arch Intern Med 126:417, 1970.

395. Lucas AM, Douglas LC: Direction of flow of nasal mucus. Proc Soc Exp Biol Med 31:320, 1934.

396. Asmundsson T, Kilburn KH: Mucociliary clearance rates at various levels in dog lungs. Am Rev Respir Dis 102:388, 1970.

397. Morrow PE, Gibb FR, Gazioglu KN: A study of particulate clearance from the human lungs. Am Rev Respir Dis 96:1209, 1967.

398. Ceesay SM, Melville GN, Mills JL, et al: Comparative observations of mucus transport velocity in health and disease. Respiration 44:184, 1983.

399. van As A: Regional variations in mucus clearance in normal and in bronchitic mammalian airways. In Chantler EN, Elder JB, Elstein M (eds): Mucus in Health and Disease. #2, Advances in Experimental Medicine and Biology. New York, Plenum Press, 1982, p 417.

400. Yager JA, Ellman H, Dulfano MJ: Human ciliary beat frequency at three levels of the tracheobronchial tree. Am Rev Respir Dis 121:661, 1980.

401. Rutland J, Griffin WM, Cole PJ: Human ciliary beat frequency in epithelium from intrathoracic and extrathoracic airways. Am Rev Respir Dis 125:100, 1982.

402. Konietzko N, Nakhosteen JA, Mizera W, et al: Ciliary beat frequency of biopsy samples taken from persons with various lung diseases. Chest 80:855, 1981.

403. Clarke SW, Pavia D: Lung mucus production and mucociliary clearance: Methods of assessment. Br J Clin Pharmacol 9:537, 1980.

404. Pavia D, Sutton PP, Agnew JE, et al: Measurement of bronchial mucociliary clearance. Eur J Respir Dis 64(Suppl 127):41, 1983.

405. Foster WM, Langenback EG, Bersofsky EH: Lung mucociliary function in man: Interdependence of bronchial and tracheal mucus transport velocities with lung clearance in bronchial asthma and healthy subjects. Ann Occup Hyg 26:277, 1982.

406. Yeates DB, Pitt BR, Spektor DM, et al: Coordination of mucociliary transport in human trachea and intrapulmonary airways. J Appl Physiol 51:1057, 1981.

407. Ahmed T, Januszkiewicz AJ, Landa JF, et al: Effect of local radioactivity on tracheal mucous velocity of sheep. Am Rev Respir Dis 120:567, 1979.

408. Chopra SK, Taplin GB, Simmons DH, et al: Measurement of mucociliary transport velocity in the intact mucosa. Chest 71:155, 1977.

409. Toomes H, Vogt-Moykopf I, Heller WD, et al: Measurement of mucociliary clearance in smokers and nonsmokers using a bronchoscopic video-technical method. Lung 159:27, 1981.

410. Forbes AR, Gamsu G: Lung mucociliary clearance after anesthesia with spontaneous and controlled ventilation. Am Rev Respir Dis 120:857, 1979.

411. Agnew JE, Bateman JR, Watts M, et al: The importance of aerosol penetration for lung mucociliary clearance studies. Chest 80(6 Suppl):843, 1981.

412. Wolff RK, Muggenburg BA: Comparison of two methods of measuring tracheal mucous velocity in anesthetized beagle dogs. Am Rev Respir Dis 120:137, 1979.

413. Connolly TP, Noujaim AA, Man SFP: Simultaneous canine tracheal transport of different particles. Am Rev Respir Dis 118:965, 1978.

414. Mossberg B, Strandbert K, Camner P: Stimulatory effect of beta-adrenergic drugs on mucociliary transport. Scand J Respir Dis (Suppl) 101:71, 1977.

415. Chopra SK: Effect of atropine on mucociliary transport velocity in anesthetized dogs. Am Rev Respir Dis 118:367, 1978.

416. McEvoy RD, Davies NJ, Hedenstierna G, et al: Lung mucociliary transport during high-frequency ventilation. Am Rev Respir Dis 126:452, 1982.

417. King M, Phillips DM, Gross D, et al: Enhanced tracheal mucus clearance with high frequency chest wall compression. Am Rev Respir Dis 128:511, 1983.

418. Warwick WJ: Mechanisms of mucus transport. Eur J Respir Dis 64:162, 1983.

419. Chopra SK, Taplin GV, Simmons DH, et al: Effects of hydration and physical therapy on tracheal transport velocity. Am Rev Respir Dis 115:1009, 1977.

420. Gerrity TR, Cotromanes E, Garrard CS, et al: The effect of aspirin on lung mucociliary clearance. N Engl J Med 308:139, 1983.

421. Smaldone GC, Itoh H, Swift DL, et al: Effect of flow-limiting segments and cough on particle deposition and mucociliary clearance in the lung. Am Rev Respir Dis 120:747, 1979.

422. Leith DE: In Lenfant C, Brain JD, Proctor DF, et al (eds): Respiratory Defense Mechanisms—Part II. Lung Biology in Health and Disease. Vol 5. New York, Marcel Dekker, 1977, p 545.

423. Widdicombe JG: Mechanisms of cough and regulation. Eur J Respir Dis 61:11, 1980.

424. Scherer PW: Mucus transport by cough. Chest 80(6 Suppl):830, 1981.

425. Cory RAS, Valentine EJ: Varying patterns of the lobar branches of the pulmonary artery. Thorax 14:267, 1959.

426. Elliot FM, Reid L: Some new facts about the pulmonary artery and its branching pattern. Clin Radiol 16:193, 1965.

427. Horsfield K: Morphometry of the small pulmonary arteries in man. Circ Res 42:593, 1978.

428. Singhal S, Henderson R, Horsfield K, et al: Morphometry of the human pulmonary arterial tree. Circ Res 33:190, 1973.

429. Heath D, Wood EH, DuShane JW, et al: The structure of the pulmonary trunk at different ages and in cases of pulmonary hypertension and pulmonary stenosis. J Pathol Bacteriol 77:443, 1959.

430. Reid L: Personal communication, 1984.

431. MacKay EH, Banks J, Sykes B, et al: Structural basis for the changing physical properties of human pulmonary vessels with age. Thorax 33:335, 1978.

432. Plank L, James J, Wagenvoort CA: Caliber and elastin content of the pulmonary trunk. Arch Pathol Lab Med 104:238, 1980.

433. Takahashi T, Wagenvoort N, Wagenvoort CA: The density of muscularized pulmonary arteries in normal lungs. Arch Pathol Lab Med 107:19, 1983.

434. Pump KK: The circulation in the peripheral parts of the human lung. Dis Chest 49:119, 1966.

435. Wagenvoort CA, Wagenvoort N: Pathology of pulmonary hypertension. New York, John Wiley & Sons, 1977.

436. Brinkman GL: Ultrastructure of atherosclerosis in the human pulmonary artery. Am Rev Respir Dis 105:351, 1972.

437. Moore GW, Smith RRL, Hutchins GM: Pulmonary artery atherosclerosis. Correlation with systemic atherosclerosis and hypertensive pulmonary vascular disease. Arch Pathol Lab Med 106:378, 1982.

438. Brenner O: Pathology of the vessels of the pulmonary circulation. Part I. Arch Intern Med 56:211, 1935.

439. Balk AG, Dingemans KP, Wagenvoort CA: The ultrastructure of the various forms of pulmonary arterial intimal fibrosis. Virchows Arch [A] Pathol Anat Histol 382:139, 1979.

440. Weibel ER: On pericytes, particularly their existence on lung capillaries. Microvasc Res 8:218, 1974.

441. Meyrick B, Reid L: Ultrastructural findings in lung biopsy material from children with congenital heart defects. Am J Pathol 101:527, 1980.

442. Meyrick B, Reid L: The effect of continued hypoxia on rat pulmonary arterial circulation. An ultrastructural study. Lab Invest 38:188, 1978.

443. Horsfield K, Gordon WI: Morphometry of pulmonary veins in man. Lung 159:211, 1981.

444. Hogg JC, Staub NC, Bergofsky EH, et al: Workshop on the pulmonary endothelial cell. Conference Report. Am Rev Respir Dis 119:165, 1979.

445. Heath D, Smith P: The pulmonary endothelial cell. Thorax 34:200, 1979.

446. Ryan JW, Ryan US: Pulmonary endothelial cells. Fed Proc 36:2683, 1977.

447. Nohl HC: An investigation into the lymphatic and vascular spread of carcinoma of the bronchus. Thorax 11:172, 1956.

448. Smith U, Ryan JW, Michie DD, et al: Endothelial projections as revealed by scanning electron microscopy. Science 173:925, 1971.

449. Ryan US, Ryan JW, Whitaker C, et al: Localization of angiotensin converting enzyme (kininase II). II. Immunocytochemistry and immunofluorescence. Tissue Cell 8:125, 1976.

450. Smith U, Ryan JW: Substructural features of pulmonary endothelial caveolae. Tissue Cell 4:49, 1972.

451. Strum JM, Junod AF: Radioautographic demonstration of 5-hydroxytryptamine-3 H uptake by pulmonary endothelial cells. J Cell Biol 54:456, 1972.

452. Pietra GG, Sampson P, Lanken PN, et al: Transcapillary movement of cationized ferritin in the isolated perfused rat lung. Lab Invest 49:54, 1983.

453. Schneeberger EE: Structural basis for some permeability properties of the air-blood barrier. Fed Proc 37:2471, 1978.

454. Schneeberger-Keeley EE, Karnovsky MJ: The ultrastructural basis of alveolar-capillary membrane permeability to peroxidase used as a tracer. J Cell Biol 37:781, 1968.

455. Yoneda K: Regional differences in the intercellular junctions of the alveolar-capillary membrane in the human lung. Am Rev Respir Dis 126:893, 1982.

456. Assimacopoulos A, Guggenheim R, Kapanci Y: Changes in alveolar capillary configuration at different levels of lung inflation in the rat. An ultrastructural and morphometric study. Lab Invest 34:10, 1976.

457. Rosenquist TH, Bernick S, Sobin SS, et al: The structure of the pulmonary interalveolar microvascular sheet. Microvasc Res 5:199, 1973.

458. Glazier JB, Hughes JMB, Maloney JE, et al: Measurements of capillary dimensions and blood volume in rapidly frozen lungs. J Appl Physiol 26:65, 1969.

459. Jefferson KE: The normal pulmonary angiogram and some changes seen in chronic nonspecific lung disease. I. The pulmonary vessels in the normal pulmonary angiogram. Proc Roy Soc Med 58:677, 1965.

460. Chang CH (Joseph): The normal roentgenographic measurement of the right descending pulmonary artery in 1,085 cases. Am J Roentgenol 87:929, 1962.

461. Simon G: Principles of Chest X-Ray Diagnosis. 3rd ed. London, Butterworth, 1971.

462. Liu Y-Q: Personal communication, 1981.

463. Coussement AM, Gooding CA: Objective radiographic assessment of pulmonary vascularity in children. Radiology 109:649, 1973.

464. Wójtowicz J: Some tomographic criteria for an evaluation of the pulmonary circulation. Acta Radiol (Diagn) 2:215, 1964.

465. Burko H, Carwell G, Newman E: Size, location, and gravitational changes of normal upper lobe pulmonary veins. Am J Roentgenol 111:687, 1971.

466. Genereux GP: Conventional tomographic hilar anatomy emphasizing the pulmonary veins. Am J Roentgenol 141:1241, 1983.

467. Heitzman ER: The Mediastinum. Radiologic Correlations with Anatomy and Pathology. St. Louis, CV Mosby, 1977, pp 216–334.

468. Heitzman ER: Radiologic diagnosis of mediastinal lymph node enlargement. J Can Assoc Radiol 29:151, 1978.

469. Davies DV, Coupland RE (eds): Gray's Anatomy. 34th ed. London, Longmans, Green, 1967, pp 774, 881.

470. Brash JC (ed): Cunningham's Textbook of Anatomy. 9th ed. London, Oxford University Press, 1951, p 1243.

471. Yamashita H: Roentgenologic Anatomy of the Lung. Tokyo, Igaku-Shoin, 1978, pp 10–25, 70–107.

472. Shevland JE, Chiu LC, Shapiro RL, et al: The role of conventional tomography and computed tomography in assessing the resectability of primary lung cancer. A preliminary report. CT 2:1, 1978.

473. Favez G, Willa C, Heinzer F: Posterior oblique tomography at an angle of 55° in chest roentgenology. Am J Roentgenol 120:907, 1974.

474. Felson B: Chest Roentgenology. Philadelphia, WB Saunders, 1973, p 185.

475. Schinz HR, Baensch WE, Frommhold W, et al: In Schinz HR, Baensch WE (eds): Roentgen Diagnosis. 2d ed. New York, Grune & Stratton, 1975, p 21.

476. Friedman PJ: Practical radiology of the hila and mediastinum. Postgrad Radiol 1:269, 1981.

477. Vix VA, Klatte EC: The lateral chest radiograph in the diagnosis of hilar and mediastinal masses. Radiology 96:307, 1970.

478. Proto AV, Speckman JM: The left lateral radiograph of the chest. 1. Med Radiogr Photogr 55:30, 1979.

479. Proto AV, Speckman JM: The left lateral radiograph of the chest. 2. Med Radiogr Photogr 56:38, 1980.

480. Fraser RG, Fraser RS, Renner JW, et al: The roentgenologic diagnosis of chronic bronchitis: A reassessment with emphasis on parahilar bronchi seen end-on. Radiology 120:1, 1976.

481. Schnur MJ, Winkler B, Austin JHM: Widening of the posterior wall of the bronchus intermedius: A sign on lateral chest radiographs of congestive heart failure, lymph node enlargement, and neoplastic infiltration. Radiology 139:551, 1981.

482. Webb WR, Gamsu G: Computed tomography of the left retrobronchial stripe. J Comput Assist Tomog 7:65, 1983.

483. Janower ML: Fifty-five-degree posterior oblique tomography of the pulmonary hilum. J Can Assoc Radiol 29:158, 1978.

484. McLeod RA, Brown LR, Miller WE, et al: Evaluation of the pulmonary hila by tomography. Radiol Clin North Am 14:51, 1976.

485. Brown LR, DeRemee RA: Fifty-five-degree oblique hilar tomography. Mayo Clin Proc 51:89, 1976.

486. Osborne DR, Korobkin M, Ravin CE, et al: Comparison of plain radiography, conventional tomography and computed tomography in detecting intrathoracic lymph node metastases from lung carcinoma. Radiology 142:157, 1982.

487. Naidich DP, Khouri NF, Scott WW, et al: Computed tomography of the pulmonary hila: Normal anatomy. J Comput Assist Tomogr 5:459, 1981.

488. Webb WR, Glazier G, Gamsu G: Computed tomography of the normal pulmonary hilum. J Comput Assist Tomogr 5:476, 1981.

489. Naidich DP, Khouri NF, Scott WW, et al: Computed tomography of the pulmonary hila: Abnormal anatomy. J Comput Assist Tomogr 5:468, 1981.

490. Webb WR, Glazier G, Gamsu G: Computed tomography of the abnormal pulmonary hilum. J Comput Assist Tomogr 5:485, 1981.

491. Itoh H, Murata K, Todo G, et al: Anatomy of pulmonary lung tissue in the hilum. Jpn J Clin Radiol 29:1459, 1984.

492. Partain CL, Price RR, Patton JA, et al: Nuclear magnetic resonance imaging. RadioGraphics 4:5, 1984.

493. Harms SE, Morgan TJ, Yamanashi WS, et al: Principles of nuclear magnetic resonance imaging. RadioGraphics 4(Sp Ed):26, 1984.

494. Pavlicek W, Modic M, Weinstein M: Pulse sequence and significance. RadioGraphics 4(Sp Ed):49, 1984.

495. Pykett IL: NMR imaging in medicine. Sci Am 246:78, 1982.

496. Young SW: Nuclear Magnetic Resonance Imaging: Basic Principles. New York, Raven Press, 1984.

497. Axel L: Blood flow effects in magnetic resonance imaging. Am J Roentgenol 143:1157, 1984.

498. Bradley WG Jr, Waluch V, Lai K-S, et al: The appearance of rapidly flowing blood on magnetic resonance imaging. Am J Roentgenol 143:1167, 1984.

499. Farmer DW, Moore E, Amparo E, et al: Calcific fibrosing mediastinitis: Demonstration of pulmonary vascular obstruction by magnetic resonance imaging. Am J Roentgenol 143:1189, 1984.

500. Amparo EG, Higgins CB, Hoddick W, et al: Magnetic resonance imaging of aortic disease: Preliminary results. Am J Roentgenol 143:1203, 1984.

501. Moore EH, Webb WR, Verrier ED, et al: MRI of chronic posttraumatic false aneurysms of the thoracic aorta. Am J Roentgenol 143:1195, 1984.

502. Cohen AM, Creviston S, LiPuma JP, et al: NMR evaluation of hilar and mediastinal lymphadenopathy. Radiology 148:739, 1983.

503. Gamsu G, Webb WR, Sheldon P, et al: Nuclear magnetic resonance imaging of the thorax. Radiology 147:473, 1983.

504. Axel L, Kressel HY, Thickman D, et al: NMR imaging of the chest at 0.12 T: Initial clinical experience with a resistive magnet. Am J Roentgenol 141:1157, 1983.

505. O'Donovan PB, Ross JS, Sivak ED, et al: Magnetic resonance imaging of the thorax: The advantages of coronal and sagittal planes. Am J Roentgenol 143:1183, 1984.

506. Webb WR, Jensen BG, Gamsu G, et al: Coronal magnetic resonance imaging of the chest: Normal and abnormal. Radiology 153:729, 1984.

507. Webb WR, Gamsu G, Stark DD, et al: Evaluation of magnetic resonance sequences in imaging mediastinal tumors. Am J Roentgenol 143:723, 1984.

508. Glazer HS, Levitt RG, Lee JKT, et al: Differentiation of radiation fibrosis from recurrent pulmonary neoplasm by magnetic resonance imaging. Am J Roentgenol 143:729, 1984.

509. Dooms GC, Hricak H, Crooks LE, et al: Magnetic resonance imaging of the lymph nodes: Comparison with CT. Radiology 153:719, 1984.

510. Yu PN: Pulmonary Blood Volume in Health and Disease. Philadelphia, Lea & Febiger, 1969.

511. Roughton FJW, Forster RE: Relative importance of diffusion and chemical reaction rates in determining rate of exchange of gases in the human lung, with special reference to true diffusing capacity of pulmonary membrane and volume of blood in the lung capillaries. J Appl Physiol 11:290, 1957.

512. Bates DV, Varvis CJ, Donevan RE, et al: Variations in the pulmonary capillary blood volume and membrane diffusion component in health and disease. J Clin Invest 39:1401, 1960.

513. Newman F, Smalley BF, Thomson ML: Effect of exercise, body and lung size on CO diffusion in athletes and nonathletes. J Appl Physiol 17:649, 1962.

514. Johnson RL Jr, Taylor HF, Lawson WH Jr, with the technical assistance of Prengler: Maximal diffusing capacity of the lung for carbon monoxide. J Clin Invest 44:349, 1965.

515. Weibel ER: Morphometrische Analyse von Zahl, Volumen and Oberfläche der Alveolen und Kapillären der menschlichen Lunge. Z Zellforsch Mikrosk Anat 57:648, 1962.

516. Cander L, Forster RE: Determination of pulmonary parenchymal tissue volume and pulmonary capillary blood flow in man. J Appl Physiol 14:541, 1959.

517. Caro CG: Physics of blood flow in the lung. Br Med Bull 19:66, 1963.

518. Maeda H, Itoh H, Ishii Y, et al: Pulmonary blood flow distribution measured by radionuclide-computed tomography. J Appl Physiol 54:225, 1983.

519. Nemery B, Wijns W, Piret L, et al: Pulmonary vascular tone is a determinant of basal lung perfusion in normal seated subjects. J Appl Physiol 54:262, 1983.

520. Permutt S, Howell JBL, Proctor DF, et al: Effect of lung inflation on static pressure-volume characteristics of pulmonary vessels. J Appl Physiol 16:64, 1961.

521. Howell JBL, Permutt S, Proctor DF, et al: Effect of inflation of the lung on different parts of the pulmonary vascular bed. J Appl Physiol 16:71, 1961.

522. Thomas LJ, Griffo ZJ, Roos A: Effect of negative-pressure inflation of the lung on pulmonary vascular resistance. J Appl Physiol 16:451, 1961.

523. Whittenberger JL, McGregor M, Berglund E, et al: Influence of state of inflation of the lung on pulmonary vascular resistance. J Appl Physiol 15:878, 1960.

524. Hakim TS, Michel RP, Chang HK: Effect of lung inflation on pulmonary vascular resistance by arterial and venous occlusion. J Appl Physiol 53:1110, 1982.

525. Culver BH, Butler J: Mechanical influences on the pulmonary microcirculation. Annu Rev Physiol 42:187, 1980.

526. Isawa T, Teshima T, Hirano T, et al: Regulation of regional perfusion distribution in the lungs: Effect of regional oxygen concentration. Am Rev Respir Dis 118:55, 1978.

527. Fishman AP: Vasomotor regulation of the pulmonary circulation. Annu Rev Physiol 42:211, 1980.

528. Marshall C, Marshall B: Site and sensitivity for stimulation of hypoxic pulmonary vasoconstriction. J Appl Physiol 55:711, 1983.

529. Hakim TS, Michel RP, Minami H, et al: Site of pulmonary hypoxic vasoconstriction studied with arterial and venous occlusion. J Appl Physiol 54:1298, 1983.

530. Linehan JH, Dawson CA: A three-compartment model of the pulmonary vasculature: Effects of vasoconstriction. J Appl Physiol 55:923, 1983.

531. Sylvester JT, Mitzner W, Ngeow Y, et al: Hypoxic constriction of alveolar and extra-alveolar vessels in isolated pig lungs. J Appl Physiol 54:1660, 1983.

532. Volkel N, Kaukel E, Trautmann J: Accumulation of histamine and cyclic nucleotides in lung tissue during chronic hypobaric hypoxia. Lung 155:277, 1978.

533. Bergofsky EH, Lehr DE, Fishman AP: The effect of changes in hydrogen ion concentration on the pulmonary circulation. J Clin Invest 41:1492, 1962.

534. Silove ED, Inoue T, Grover RF: Comparison of hypoxia, PH and sympathomimetic drugs on bovine pulmonary vasculature. J Appl Physiol 24:355, 1968.

535. Downing SE, Lee JC: Nervous control of the pulmonary circulation. Annu Rev Physiol 42:199, 1980.

536. Bergofsky EH: Humoral control of the pulmonary circulation. Annu Rev Physiol 42:221, 1980.

537. Georg J, Lassen NA, Millemgaard K, et al: Diffusion in the gas phase of the lungs in normal and emphysematous subjects. Clin Sci 29:525, 1965.

538. von Hyek H: Cellular structure and mucus activity in the bronchial tree and alveoli. In deReuck AVS, O'Connor M (eds): Ciba Foundation Symposium on Pulmonary Structure and Function. London, J. & A. Churchill, 1962, p 100.

539. Jameson AG: Diffusion of gases from alveolus to precapillary arteries. Science 139:826, 1963.

540. Bates DV, Macklem PT, Christie RV: Respiratory Function in Diseases; An Introduction to the Integrated Study of the Lung. 2nd ed. Philadelphia, WB Saunders, 1971.

541. Finley TN, Swenson EW, Comroe JH Jr: The cause of arterial hypoxemia at rest in patients with "alveolar-capillary block syndrome." J Clin Invest 41:618, 1962.

542. Read J, Williams RS: Pulmonary ventilation/blood flow relationships in interstitial disease of the lungs. Am J Med 27:545, 1959.

543. Forster RE, Craw MR, Constantine HP, et al: Gas exchange processes in the pulmonary capillaries. In de Reuck AVS, O'Connor M (eds): Ciba Foundation Symposium on Pulmonary Structure and Function. London, J. & A. Churchill, 1962, pp 215–231.

544. Crapo JD, Crapo RO: Comparison of total lung diffusion capacity and the membrane component of diffusion capacity as determined by physiologic and morphometric techniques. Resp Physiol 51:183, 1983.

545. Riley RL, Cournand A: "Ideal" alveolar air and the analysis of ventilation-perfusion relationships in the lungs. J Appl Physiol 1:825, 1949.

546. Badeer HS: Gravitational effects on the distribution of pulmonary blood flow: Hemodynamic misconceptions. Respiration 43:408, 1982.

547. Milic-Emili J, Henderson JAM, Dolovich MB, et al: Regional distribution of inspired gas in the lung. J Appl Physiol 21:749, 1966.

548. Milic-Emili J: Interregional distribution of inspired gas. Prog Resp Res 16:33, 1981.

549. Milic-Emili J, Mead J, Turner JM: Topography of esophageal pressure as a function of posture in man. J Appl Physiol 19:212, 1964.

550. Glazier JB, Hughes JMB, Maloney JE, et al: Vertical gradient of alveolar size in lungs of dogs frozen intact. J Appl Physiol 23:694, 1967.

551. Ball WC Jr, Stewart PB, Newsham LGS, et al: Regional pulmonary function studied with xenon133. J Clin Invest 41:519, 1962.

552. West JB, Dollery CT: Distribution of blood flow and ventilation-perfusion ratio in the lung, measured with radioactive CO_2. J Appl Physiol 15:405, 1960.

553. Glazier JB, DeNardo GL: Pulmonary function studied with the xenon133 scanning technique. Normal values and a postural study. Am Rev Respir Dis 94:188, 1966.

554. Bentivoglio LG, Beerel F, Stewart PB, et al: Studies of regional ventilation and perfusion in pulmonary emphysema using xenon133. Am Rev Respir Dis 88:315, 1963.

555. West JB, Dollery CT, Hugh-Jones P: The use of radioactive carbon dioxide to measure regional blood flow in the lungs of patients with pulmonary disease. J Clin Invest 40:1, 1961.

556. Kaneko K, Milic-Emili J, Dolovich MB, et al: Regional distribution of ventilation and perfusion as a function of body position. J Appl Physiol 21:767, 1966.

557. Engel LA, Grassino A, Anthonisen NR: Demonstration of airway closure in man. J Appl Physiol 38:1117, 1975.

558. Prefaut C, Engel LA: Vertical distribution of perfusion and inspired gas in supine man. J Appl Physiol 43:209, 1981.

559. Bake B, Wood L, Murphy B, et al: Effect of inspiratory flow rate on regional distribution of inspired gas. J Appl Physiol 37:8, 1974.

560. Fixley MS, Roussos CS, Murphy B, et al: Flow dependence of gas distribution and the pattern of inspiratory muscle contraction. J Appl Physiol 45:733, 1978.

561. Bake B, Bjure J, Widimsky J: The effects of sitting and graded exercise on the distribution of pulmonary blood flow in healthy subjects studied with the 133xenon technique. Scand J Clin Lab Invest 22:99, 1968.

562. Bryan AC, Bentivoglio LG, Beerel F, et al: Factors affecting regional distribution of ventilation and perfusion in the lung. J Appl Physiol 19:395, 1964.

563. Gledhill N, Froese AB, Buick FJ, et al: VA/Q inhomogeneity and $AaDo_2$ in man during exercise: Effect of SF_6 breathing. J Appl Physiol 45:512, 1978.

564. Ewan PW, Jones HA, Nosil J, et al: Uneven perfusion and ventilation within lung regions studies with nitrogen-13. Resp Physiol 34:45, 1978.

565. Fenn WO, Rahn H, Otis AB: A theoretical study of the composition of alveolar air at altitude. Am J Physiol 146:637, 1946.

566. Raymond W: The alveolar air equation abbreviated. Chest 74:675, 1978.

567. Minh VD, Patakas DA, Davies PL, et al: A single-breath method of alveolar O_2 determination. Respiration 37:66, 1979.

568. Turek Z, Kreuzer F: Effects of shifts of the O_2 dissociation curve upon alveolar-arterial O_2 gradients in computer models of the lung with ventilation-perfusion mismatching. Resp Physiol 45:133, 1981.

569. West JB: Ventilation-perfusion inequality and overall gas exchange in computer models of the lung. Resp Physiol 7:88, 1969.

570. Staub NC: Alveolar-arterial oxygen tension gradient due to diffusion. J Appl Physiol 18:673, 1963.

571. Dantzker DR, Wagner PD, West JB: Instability of lung units with low VA/Q ratios during O_2 breathing. J Appl Physiol 38:886, 1975.

572. Harf A, Pratt T, Hughes JMB: Regional distribution of VA/Q in man at rest and with exercise measured with krypton-81m. J Appl Physiol 44:115, 1978.

573. Wagner PD, Saltzman HA, West JB: Measurement of continuous distribution of ventilation-perfusion ratios: Theory. J Appl Physiol 36:588, 1974.

574. Davenport HW: The ABC of Acid-Base Chemistry; The Elements of Physiological Blood-Gas Chemistry for Medical Students and Physicians. 5th ed. Chicago, University of Chicago Press, 1969.

575. Frisell WB: Acid-Base Chemistry in Medicine. New York, Macmillan, 1968.

576. Masaro EJ, Siegel PD: Acid-Base Regulation: Its Physiology and Patho-Physiology. Philadelphia, WB Saunders, 1971.

577. Hills AG: Acid-Base Balance; Chemistry, Physiology, Patho-physiology. Baltimore, Williams & Wilkins, 1973.

578. Siggaard-Andersen O: The Acid-Base Status of the Blood. 4th ed. Baltimore, Williams & Wilkins, 1974.

579. Winters RW, Engel K, Dell RB: Acid-Base Physiology in Medicine. A Self-Instruction Program. Cleveland, The London Company, 1967.

580. Ruch TC, Patton HD (eds): Physiology and Biophysics. II. Circulation, Respiration and Fluid Balance. Philadelphia, WB Saunders, 1974.

581. Siegel PD: The physiologic approach to acid-base balance. Med Clin North Am 57:863, 1974.

582. Oliva PB: Lactic acidosis. Am J Med 48:209, 1970.

583. Gennari FJ, Goldstein MB, Schwartz WB: The nature of the renal adaptation to chronic hypocapnia. J Clin Invest 51:1722, 1972.

584. Northfield TC, Kirby BJ, Tattersfield AE: Acid-base balance in acute gastrointestinal bleeding. Br Med J 2:242, 1971.

585. Fulop M, Horowitz M, Aberman A, et al: Lactic acidosis in pulmonary edema due to left ventricular failure. Ann Intern Med 79:180, 1973.

586. Aberman A, Fulop M: The metabolic and respiratory acidosis of acute pulmonary edema. Ann Intern Med 76:173, 1972.
587. Pierce NF, Fedson DS, Brigham KL, et al: The ventilatory response to acute base deficit in humans. Time course during development and correction of metabolic acidosis. Ann Intern Med 72:633, 1970.
588. Pitts RF: Physiology of the Kidney and Body Fluids: An Introductory Text. 2nd ed. Chicago, Year Book Medical Publishers, 1968.
589. Kurtzman NA, White MG, Rogers PW: Pathophysiology of metabolic alkalosis. Arch Intern Med 131:702, 1973.
590. Goldring RM, Cannon PJ, Heinemann HO, et al: Respiratory adjustment to chronic metabolic alkalosis in man. J Clin Invest 47:188, 1968.
591. Lifschitz MD, Brasch R, Cuomo AJ, et al: Marked hypercapnia secondary to severe metabolic alkalosis. Ann Intern Med 77:405, 1972.
592. Goldring RM, Turino GM, Heinemann HO: Respiratory-renal adjustments in chronic hypercapnia in man. Extracellular bicarbonate concentration and the regulation of ventilation. Am J Med 51:772, 1971.
593. Schwartz WB, Brackett NC Jr, Cohen JJ: The response of extracellular hydrogen ion concentration to graded degrees of chronic hypercapnia: The physiologic limits of the defense of pH. J Clin Invest 44:291, 1965.
594. Brackett NC Jr, Cohen JJ, Schwartz WB: Carbon dioxide titration curve of normal man. Effect of increasing degrees of acute hypercapnia on acid-base equilibrium. N Engl J Med 272:6, 1965.
595. Arbus GS, Hebert LA, Levesque PR, et al: Characterization and clinical application of the "significance band" for acute respiratory alkalosis. N Engl J Med 280:117, 1969.
596. Brackett NC Jr, Wingo CF, Muren O, et al: Acid-base response to chronic hypercapnia in man. N Engl J Med 280:124, 1969.
597. Arbus GS: An in vivo acid-base nomogram for clinical use. Can Med Assoc J 109:291, 1973.
598. Flenley DC: Another non-logarithmic acid-base diagram? Lancet 1:961, 1971.
599. Austin WH: Acid-base balance. A review of current approaches and techniques. Am Heart J 69:691, 1965.
600. Botenga ASJ: Selective Bronchial and Intercostal Arteriography. Leiden, HE Stenfert Kroese, NV, 1970.
601. Cudkowicz L: Bronchial arterial circulation in man. Normal anatomy and responses to disease. In Moser KM (ed): Pulmonary Vascular Diseases. New York, Marcel Dekker, 1979, p 111.
602. Liebow AA, Hales MR, Lindskog GE: Enlargement of the bronchial arteries, and their anastomoses with the pulmonary arteries in bronchiectasis. Am J Pathol 25:211, 1949.
603. Turner-Warwick M: Systemic arterial patterns in the lung and clubbing of the fingers. Thorax 18:238, 1963.
604. Glaen C: Tractationes Frobenianae (liber 6, capritulum 3). Basel, 1562.
605. Ruysch F: Epistola Anatomica. Amsterdam, 1732.
606. Reisseisen FD, Von Sommering ST: Ueber den Bau der Lungen. Berlin, 1808.
607. Cudkowicz L: Leonardo da Vinci and the bronchial circulation. Br J Tuberc 47:23, 1953.
608. Cauldwell EW, Siekert RG, Linenger RE, et al: The bronchial arteries: An anatomic study of 150 cadavers. Surg Gynecol Obstet 86:395, 1948.
609. Tobin CE: The bronchial arteries and their connection with other vessels in the human lung. Surg Gynecol Obstet 95:741, 1952.
610. Verloop MC: The arterial bronchiales and their anastomoses with the arterial pulmonalis in the human lung: A microanatomical study. Acta Anat (Basel) 5:171, 1948.
611. Cudkowicz L, Armstrong JB: Observations on the normal anatomy of the bronchial arteries. Thorax 6:343, 1951.
612. Pump KK: The bronchial arteries and their anastomoses in the human lung. Dis Chest 43:245, 1963.
613. Newton TH, Preger L: Selective bronchial arteriography. Radiology 84:1043, 1965.
614. Liebow AA: Patterns of origin and distribution of the major bronchial arteries in man. Am J Anat 117:19, 1965.
615. Marchand P, Gilroy JC, Wilson VH: An anatomical study of the bronchial vascular system and its variations in disease. Thorax 5:207, 1950.
616. Moberg A: Anastomoses between extracardiac vessels and coronary arteries. I. Via bronchial arteries. II. Via internal mammary arteries. Acta Radiol [Diagn] (Stockh) 6:177, 263, 1967.
617. Johnsson K-A: Collateral circulation between bronchial and coronary arteries. Acta Radiol [Diagn] (Stockh) 8:393, 1969.
618. Av, do DM: The Lung Circulation. Vol 1. New York, Pergamon Press, 1965, Chapter 4.
619. Berry JL, Daly I de B: The relation between the pulmonary and bronchial vascular systems. Proc R Soc Lond [Biol] 109:319, 1931.
620. Baile EM, Nelems JM, Schulzer M, et al: Measurements of regional bronchial arterial blood flow and bronchovascular resistance in dogs. J Appl Physiol 53:1044, 1982.
621. Baile EM, Ling H, Heyworth JR, et al: Bronchopulmonary anastomotic and non-coronary collateral blood flow in humans during cardiopulmonary bypass. Chest 87(6):749, 1985.
622. Salisbury PF, Weil P, State D: Factors influencing collateral blood flow to the dog's lung. Circ Res 5:303, 1957.
623. Modell HI, Beck K, Butler J: Functional aspects of canine bronchopulmonary vascular communications. J Appl Physiol 50:1045, 1981.
624. Baile EM, Albert RK, Kirk W, et al: Positive end-expiratory pressure decreases bronchial blood flow in the dog. J Appl Physiol 56:1289, 1984.
625. Baile EM, Pare PD: Response of the bronchial circulation to acute hypoxemia and hypocardia in the dog. J Appl Physiol 55:1474, 1983.
626. Brunner HD, Schmidt CF: Blood flow in the bronchial artery of the anesthetized dog. Am J Physiol 148:648, 1947.
627. Martinez L, de Letona J, Castro de la Mata R, et al: Local and reflex effects of bronchial arterial injection of drugs. J Pharmacol Exp Ther 133:295, 1961.
628. Lung MAKY, Wang JCC, Cheng KK: Bronchial circulation: An autoperfusion method for assessing the vasomotor activity and the study of alpha and beta adrenoceptors in the bonchial artery. Life Sci 19:577, 1976.
629. McFadden ET Jr: Respiratory heat and water exchange: Physiological and clinical implications. J Appl Physiol 54:331, 1983.
630. McLaughlin RF, Tyler WS, Canada RO: Subgross pulmonary anatomy in various mammals and man. JAMA 175:694, 1961.
631. Pietra GG, Szidon JP, Leventhal MN, et al: Histamine and interstitial pulmonary edema in the dog. Circ Res 29:323, 1971.
632. Baile EM, Dahlby RW, Wiggs BJR, et al: Role of tracheal and bronchial circulation in respiratory heat exchange. J Appl Physiol 58:217, 1985.
633. Baile EM, Osborne S, Wiggs BJR, et al: Mechanism for increased airway blood flow during warm dry air hyperventilation. Fed Proc 44:1754, 1985.
634. Viola AR, Abbate EH: Respiratory function and effective collateral flow 8 years after ligation of the left pulmonary artery. Am Rev Respir Dis 108:1216, 1973.
635. Fritts HW Jr, Harris P, Chidsey CA III, et al: Estimation of flow through bronchopulmonary vascular anastomoses with use of T-1824 dye. Circulation 23:390, 1961.
636. Robertson HT, Jindal S, Lakshminarayan S, et al: Gas exchange properties of the bronchial circulation in a dog lobe. Am Rev Respir Dis 129:A229, 1984.
637. Virchow R: Gesammelte Abhandlungen zur wissenschaftlichen Medicin. Frankfurt am Main, 1856, p 285.
638. Malik AB, Tracy SE: Bronchovascular adjustments after pulmonary embolism. J Appl Physiol 49:476, 1980.
639. Block ER, Stalcup SA: Metabolic functions of the lung—of what clinical relevance. Chest 81:215, 1982.
640. Rannels DE, Low RB, Youdale T, et al: Use of radioisotopes in quantitative studies of lung metabolism. Fed Proc 41:2833, 1982.
641. Freiman DG, Suyemoto J, Wessler S: Frequency of pulmonary thromboembolism in man. N Engl J Med 272:1278, 1965.
642. Attwood HD, Park WW: Embolism to the lungs by trophoblast. J Obstet Gynaecol Br Comm 68:611, 1961.
643. Sharnoff JG, Scardino V: Pulmonary megakaryocytes in human fetuses and premature and full-term infants. Arch Pathol 69:27/139, 1960.
644. Sharnoff JG, Kim ES: Evaluation of pulmonary megakaryocytes. Arch Pathol 66:176, 1958.
645. Aabo K, Hansen KB: Megakaryocytes in pulmonary blood vessels. I: Incidence at autopsy; clinicopathological relations especially to disseminated intravascular coagulation. Acta Pathol Microbiol Scand 86:285, 1978.
646. Wells S, Sissons M, Hasleton PS: Quantitation of pulmonary megakaryocytes and fibrin thrombi in patients dying from burns. Histopathology 8:517, 1984.
647. Hansen KB, Aabo K, Myhre-Jensen O: Response of pulmonary (circulating) megakaryocytes to experimentally induced consumption coagulopathy in rabbits. Acta Path Microbiol Scand Sect A, 87:165, 1979.
648. Kaufman RM, Airo R, Pollack S, et al: Circulating megakaryocytes and platelet release in the lung. Blood 26:720, 1965.
649. Pedersen NT: Occurrence of megakaryocytes in various vessels and their retention in the pulmonary capillaries in man. Scand J Haematol 21:369, 1978.
650. Kallinikos-Maniatis A: Megakaryocytes and platelets in central venous and arterial blood. Acta Haematol 42:330, 1969.
651. Martin JF, Slater DN, Trowbridge EA: Abnormal intrapulmonary platelet production: A possible cause of vascular and lung disease. Lancet 2:793, 1983.
652. DeCoteau WE: The role of secretory IgA in defense of the distal lung. Ann NY Acad Sci 221:214, 1974.
653. Said SI: The lung as a metabolic organ. N Engl J Med 279:1330, 1968.

654. Orr TSC: Mast cells and allergic asthma. Br J Dis Chest 67:87, 1973.
655. Uvnäs B: Mechanism of histamine release in mast cells. Ann NY Acad Sci 103:278, 1963.
656. Massaro D, Weiss H, Simon MR: Protein synthesis and secretion by lung. Am Rev Respir Dis 101:198, 1970.
657. Yeager H Jr, Massaro G, Massaro D: Glycoprotein synthesis by the trachea. Am Rev Respir Dis 103:188, 1971.
658. Fisher AB, Pietra GG: Comparison of serotonin uptake from the alveolar and capillary spaces of isolated rat lung. Am Rev Respir Dis 123:74, 1981.
659. Fanburg BL: Prostaglandins and the lung. Am Rev Respir Dis 108:482, 1973.
660. Edmonds JF, Berry E, Wyllie JH: Release of prostaglandins caused by distension of the lungs. Br J Surg 56:622, 1969.
661. Adkinson NJ Jr, Newball HH, Findlay S, et al: Anaphylactic release of prostaglandins from human lung in vitro. Am Rev Respir Dis 121:911, 1980.
662. Hollinger MA, Giri SN, Patwell S, et al: Effect of acute lung injury on angiotensin converting enzyme in serum, lung lavage and effusate. Am Rev Respir Dis 121:373, 1980.
663. Block ER, Schoen FJ: Effect of alpha-naphthylthiourea on uptake of 5-hydroxytryptamine from the pulmonary circulation. Am Rev Respir Dis 123:69, 1981.
664. Dobuler KJ, Catravas JD, Gillis CN: Early detection of oxygen-induced lung injury in conscious rabbits—reduced in vivo activity of angiotensin converting enzyme and removal of 5-hydroxytryptamine. Am Rev Respir Dis 126:534, 1982.
665. Geddes DM, Nesbitt K, Traill T, et al: First pass uptake of 14C propranolol by the lung. Thorax 34:810, 1979.
666. Pang JA, Geddes DM: The biochemical properties of the pulmonary circulation (review). Lung 159:231, 1981.
667. Siddik ZH, Trush MA, Gram TE: Pulmonary accumulation of drugs in vitamin A deficiency. Lung 157:209, 1980.
668. Hislop A, Reid L: Development of the acinus in the human lung. Thorax 29:90, 1974.
669. Have-Opbroek AAWT: The development of the lung in mammals: An analysis of concepts and findings. Am J Anat 162:201, 1981.
670. Langston C, Kida K, Reed M, et al: Human lung growth in late gestation and in the neonate. Am Rev Respir Dis 129:607, 1984.
671. Hodson WA: Development of the lung. In Hodson WA (ed): Development of the Lung. New York, Marcel Dekker, 1977.
672. Thurlbeck WM: Postnatal growth and development of the lung. Am Rev Respir Dis 111:803, 1975.
673. Bucher U, Reid L: Development of the intrasegmental bronchial tree: The pattern of branching and development of cartilage at various stages of intra-uterine life. Thorax 16:207, 1961.
674. Sinclair-Smith CC, Emery JL, Gadsdon D, et al: Cartilage in children's lungs: A quantitative assessment using the right middle lobe. Thorax 31:40, 1976.
675. Tos M: Development of the mucous glands in the human main bronchus. Anat Anz 123:376, 1968.
676. Boyden EA, Tompsett DH: The changing patterns in the developing lungs of infants. Acta Anat 61:164, 1965.
677. Thurlbeck WM: Postnatal human lung growth. Thorax 37:564, 1982.
678. Davies G, Reid L: Growth of the alveoli and pulmonary arteries in childhood. Thorax 25:669, 1970.
679. Hogg JC, Williams J, Richardson JB, et al: Age as a factor in the distribution of lower-airway conductance and in the pathologic anatomy of obstructive lung disease. N Engl J Med 282:1283, 1970.
680. Wailoo MP, Emery JL: Normal growth and development of the trachea. Thorax 37:584, 1982.
681. Hislop A, Reid LM: Formation of the pulmonary vasculature. In Hodson WA (ed): Development of the Lung. New York, Marcel Dekker, 1977, p 37.
682. Hislop A, Reid L: Pulmonary arterial development during childhood: Branching pattern and structure. Thorax 28:129, 1973.
683. Hislop A, Reid L: Fetal and childhood development of the intrapulmonary veins in man: Branching pattern and structure. Thorax 28:313, 1973.
684. Smith BT, Fletcher WA: Pulmonary epithelial-mesenchymal interactions: Beyond organogenesis. Hum Pathol 10:248, 1979.
685. Adamson IYR, King GM: Sex differences in development of fetal rat lung. II. Quantitative morphology of epithelial-mesenchymal interactions. Lab Invest 50:461, 1984.
686. Smith BT: Lung maturation in the fetal rat: Acceleration by injection of fibroblast-pneumocyte factor. Science 204:1094, 1979.
687. Vaccaro C, Brody JS: Ultrastructure of developing alveoli. 1. The role of the interstitial fibroblast. Anat Rec 192:467, 1978.
688. Maksvytis HJ, Vaccaro C, Brody JS: Isolation and characterization of the lipid-containing interstitial cell from the developing rat lung. Lab Invest 45:248, 1981.
689. Emery JL: The postnatal development of the human lung and its implications for lung pathology. Respiration 27(Suppl):41, 1970.
690. Kida K, Thurlbeck WM: The effects of β-aminopropionitrile on the growing rat lung. Am J Pathol 101:693, 1980.
691. Das RM: The effect of β-aminopropionitrile on lung development in the rat. Am J Pathol 101:711, 1980.
692. Wigglesworth JS, Winston RML, Bartlett K: Influence of the central nervous system on fetal lung development. Arch Dis Child 52:965, 1977.
693. Fewell JE, Lee CC, Kitterman JA: Effects of phrenic nerve section on the respiratory system of fetal lambs. J Appl Physiol 51:293, 1981.
694. Liggins GC, Vilos GA, Campos GA, et al: The effect of spinal cord transection on lung development in fetal sheep. J Dev Physiol 3:267, 1981.
695. Torday JS, Nielsen HC, Fencl MDM, et al: Sex differences in fetal lung maturation. Am Rev Respir Dis 123:205, 1981.
696. Castleman WL: Alterations in pulmonary ultrastructure and morphometric parameters induced by para-influenza (sendai) virus in rats during postnatal growth. Am J Pathol 114:322, 1984.
697. Das RM: The effects of intermittent starvation on lung development in suckling rats. Am J Pathol 117:326, 1984.
698. Weibel ER: Functional morphology of the growing lung. In Pathophysiology: 1. Pre- and neonatal anatomy in relation to some pathology in children. Respiration 27(Suppl):27, 1970.
699. Dawes GS: Breathing before birth in animals and man. An essay in developmental medicine. N Engl J Med 290:557, 1974.
700. Sant'Ambrogio G: Information arising from the tracheobronchial tree of mammals. Physiol Rev 62:531, 1982.
701. Richardson J, Beland J: Nonadrenergic inhibitory nervous system in human airways. J Appl Physiol 41:764, 1976.
702. Richardson JB, Ferguson CC: Morphology of the airway. In Nadel JA (ed): Physiology and Pharmacology of the Airways. New York, Marcel Dekker, 1980, p 1.
703. Fisher AWF: The intrinsic innervation of the trachea. J Anat 98:117, 1964.
704. Larsell O, Dow RS: The innervation of the human lung. Am J Anat 52:125, 1933.
705. Gaylor JB: The intrinsic nervous mechanism of the human lung. Brain 57:143, 1934.
706. Spencer H, Leof D: The innervation of the human lung. J Anat 98:599, 1964.
707. Fillenz M, Widdicombe JG: Receptors of the lungs and airways. In Neil E (ed): Enteroceptors. New York, Springer-Verlag, 1972, p 81.
708. Fox B, Bull TB, Guz A: Innervation of alveolar walls in the human lung: An electron microscopic study. J Anat 131:6832, 1980.
709. Hung K-S, Hertweck MS, Hardy JD, et al: Electron microscopic observations of nerve endings in the alveolar walls of mouse lungs. Am Rev Respir Dis 108:328, 1973.
710. Taylor DR, Muir AL, Fleetham JA: Effect of rapid saline infusion on breathing pattern in normal man. Clin Invest Med 7:86, 1984.
711. Russell JA: Nonadrenergic inhibitory innervation of canine airways. J Appl Physiol 48:16, 1980.
712. Richardson JB: State of the Art—nerve supply to the lungs. Am Rev Respir Dis 119:785, 1979.
713. Richardson JB: Recent progress in pulmonary innervation. Am Rev Respir Dis 128:65, 1983.
714. Nadel JA, Barnes PJ: Autonomic regulation of the airways. Annu Rev Med 35:451, 1984.
715. Barnes PJ: Localization and function of airway autonomic receptors. Eur J Respir Dis 65:187, 1984.
716. Richardson JB: Nonadrenergic inhibitory innervation of the lung. Lung 195:315, 1981.
717. Chesrown SE, Venugopalan CS, Gold WM, et al: In vivo demonstration of nonadrenergic inhibitory innervation of the guinea pig trachea. J Clin Invest 65:314, 1980.
718. Irvin CG, Martin RR, Macklem PT: Nonpurinergic nature and efficacy of nonadrenergic bronchodilatation. J Appl Physiol 52:562, 1982.
719. Souhrada JF, Kivity S: The effect of some factors on the inhibitory nervous systems of airway smooth muscle. Respir Physiol 48:297, 1982.
720. Said SI: Vasoactive peptides in the lung, with special reference to vasoactive intestinal peptide. Exp Lung Res 3:343, 1982.
721. Sheppard MN, Polak JM, Allen JM: Neuropeptide tyrosine (NPY): A newly discovered peptide is present in the mammalian respiratory tract. Thorax 39:326, 1984.
722. Diamond L, Richardson JB: Inhibitory innervation to airway smooth muscle. Exp Lung Res 3:379, 1982.
723. Taylor SM, Pare PD, Schelenberg RR: Cholinergic and non-adrenergic mechanisms in human and guinea pig airways. J Appl Physiol 56:958, 1984.
724. Osorio J, Russak M: Reflex changes in the pulmonary and systemic pressures elicited by stimulation of baroreceptors in the pulmonary artery. Circ Res 10:664, 1962.
725. Krahl VE: The glomus pulmonale: A preliminary report. Bull School Med Univ Maryland 45:36, 1960.
726. Edwards C, Heath D: Microanatomy of glomic tissue of the pulmonary trunk. Thorax 24:209, 1969.
727. Korn D, Bensch K, Liebow AA, et al: Multiple minute pulmonary tumors resembling chemodectomas. Am J Pathol 37:641, 1960.

728. Kuhn C III, Askin FB: The fine structure of so-called minute pulmonary chemodectomas. Hum Pathol 6:681, 1975.

729. De Gasperis C, Miani A: Observations sur l'ultrastructure du mésothélium pleural de l'homme. Bull Assoc Anat 145:188, 1970.

730. Kawai T, Suzuki M, Kageyama K: Reactive mesothelial cell and mesothelioma of the pleura. Virchows Arch [Pathol Anat] 393:251, 1981.

731. Jaurand M-C, Kaplan H, Thiollet J, et al: Phagocytosis of chrysotile fibers by pleural mesothelial cells in culture. Am J Pathol 94:529, 1979.

732. Ryan GB, Grobety J, Majno G: Mesothelial injury and recovery. Am J Pathol 71:93, 1973.

733. Policard A, Galy P: Considérations histophysiologiques sur la plèvre pulmonaire chez l'homme. Bull Hist Appl Techn Micros 18:67, 1941.

734. Miller WS: The vascular supply of the pleura pulmonalis. Am J Anat 7:389, 1907.

735. Agostoni E: Mechanics of the pleural space. Physiol Rev 52:57, 1972.

736. Lennon EA, Simon G: The height of the diaphragm in the chest radiograph of normal adults. Br J Radiol 38:937, 1965.

737. Felson B: The lobes and interlobar pleura: Fundamental roentgen considerations. Am J Med Sci 230:572, 1955.

738. Raasch BN, Carsky EW, Lane EJ, et al: Radiographic anatomy of the interlobar fissures: A study of 100 specimens. Am J Roentgenol 138:1043, 1982.

739. Felson B: Chest Roentgenology. Philadelphia, WB Saunders, 1973.

740. Ritter H, Eyband M: Der diagnostische Wert eines lageveränderten Ober-Mittellappenspaltes im Lungensagittalbild. (The diagnostic significance, in the sagittal chest film, of a shift in the upper and middle lobe fissures). Fortschr Roentgenstrahl 86:431, 1957.

741. Marks BW, Kuhns LR: Identification of the pleural fissures with computed tomography. Radiology 134:139, 1982.

742. Fisher MS: Letters to the editor: Adam's lobe. Radiology 154:547, 1985.

743. Speckman JM, Gamsu G, Webb WR: Alterations in CT mediastinal anatomy produced by an azygos lobe. Am J Radiol 137:47, 1981.

744. Boyden EA: The distribution of bronchi in gross anomalies of the right upper lobe, particularly lobes subdivided by the azygos vein and those containing pre-eparterial bronchi. Radiology 58:797, 1952.

745. Schaffner VD: Chest. In Shanks SC, Kereley P (eds): A Textbook of X-Ray Diagnosis. Vol II, 2nd ed. Philadelphia, WB Saunders, 1950–52, p 241.

746. Rigler LG, Ericksen LG: The inferior accessory lobe of the lung. Am J Roentgenol 29:384, 1933.

747. Godwin JD, Tarver RD: Accessory fissures of the lung. Am J Roentgenol 144:39, 1985.

748. Boyden EA: Cleft left upper lobes and the split anterior bronchus. Surgery 26:167, 1949.

749. Davis LA: The vertical fissure line. Am J Roentgenol 84:451, 1960.

750. Webber MM, O'Loughlin BJ: Variations of the pleural vertical fissure line. Radiology 82:461, 1964.

751. Friedman E: Further observations on the vertical fissure line. Am J Roentgenol 97:171, 1966.

752. Black LF: The pleural space and pleural fluid. Mayo Clin Proc 47:493, 1972.

753. Yamada S: Uber die seröse Flüssigkeit in der Pleurahöhle der gesunden Menschen. Z Ges Exp Med 90:342, 1933.

754. Müller R, Löfstedt S: The reaction of the pleura in primary tuberculosis of the lungs. Acta Med Scand 122:105, 1945.

755. Rohrer F: Physiologie der Atembewegung. In Bethe A, von Bergmann G, Embden G, et al (eds): Handbuch der Normalen und Pathologischen Physiologie. Vol II. Berlin, Springer, 1925, pp 70–127.

756. Miserocchi G, Agostoni E: Contents of the pleural space. J Appl Physiol 30:208, 1971.

757. Agostoni E., D'Angelo E, Roncoroni G: The thickness of the pleural liquid. Resp Physiol 5:1, 1968.

758. Agostoni E, Mead J: Statics of the respiratory system. In Fenn WO, Rahn H (eds): Handbook of Physiology. Section 3: Respiration. Vol I. Washington, DC, American Physiological Society, 1964, pp 387–409.

759. Agostoni E, Taglietti A, Setnikar I: Absorption force of the capillaries of the visceral pleura in determination of the intrapleural pressure. Am J Physiol 191:277, 1957.

760. Stewart PB: The rate of formation and lymphatic removal of fluid in pleural effusions. J Clin Invest 42:258, 1963.

761. Stewart PB: Personal communication, 1967.

762. Courtice FC, Simmonds WJ: Absorption from the lungs. J Physiol 109:103, 1949.

763. Burgen ASV, Stewart PB: A method for measuring the turnover of fluid in the pleural and other serous cavities. J Lab Clin Med 52:118, 1958.

764. Courtice FC, Simmonds WJ: Physiological significance of lymph drainage of the serous cavities and lungs. Physiol Rev 34:419, 1954.

765. Lauweryns JM: The blood and lymphatic microcirculation of the lung. In Sommers SC (ed): Pulmonary Pathology Decennial; 1966–1975. New York, Appleton-Century-Crofts, 1975, p 1.

766. Hendin AS, Greenspan RH: Ventilatory pumping of human pulmonary lymphatic vessels. Radiology 108:553, 1973.

767. Lauweryns JM, Baert JH: Alveolar clearance and the role of the pulmonary lymphatics. State of the art. Am Rev Respir Dis 115:625, 1977.

768. Lauweryns JM: The juxta-alveolar lymphatics in the human adult lung. Histologic studies in 15 cases of drowning. Am Rev Dis 102:877, 1970.

769. Warren MF, Drinker CK: The flow of lymph from the lungs of the dog. Am J Physiol 136:207, 1942.

770. Yoffey JM, Courtice FC: Lymphatics, Lympha and the Lymphomyeloid Complex. New York, Academic Press, 1970, p 294.

771. Drinker CK: Extravascular protein and the lymphatic system. Ann NY Acad Sci 46:807, 1946.

772. Fleischner FG: The butterfly pattern of acute pulmonary edema. Am J Cardiol 20:39, 1967.

773. Hendin AS: Postmortem demonstration of inspiratory constriction of deep lymphatic vessels of the human lung. Radiol 9:1, 1974.

774. Trapnell DH: Recognition and incidence of intrapulmonary lymph nodes. Thorax 19:44, 1964.

775. Greenberg HB: Benign subpleural lymph node appearing as a pulmonary "coin" lesion. Radiology 77:97, 1961.

776. Rosenberger A, Abrams HL: Radiology of the thoracic duct. Am J Roentgenol 11:807, 1971.

777. Fuchs WA, Galeazzi RL: The radiographic anatomy of the thoracic duct (in German). Radiologe 10:180, 1970.

778. Abramson DI: Blood Vessels and Lymphatics. New York, Academic Press, 1962, p 703.

779. Leeds SE, Uhley HN, Sampson JJ, et al: A new method for measurement of lymph flow from the right duct in the dog. Am J Surg 98:211, 1959.

780. Uhley HN, Leeds SE, Sampson, JJ, et al: Some observations on the role of the lymphatics in experimental acute pulmonary edema. Circ Res 9:688, 1961.

781. Uhley HN, Leeds SE, Sampson JJ, et al: Role of pulmonary lymphatics in chronic pulmonary edema. Circ Res 11:966, 1962.

782. Leeds SE, Uhley HN, Sampson JJ, et al: Significance of changes in the pulmonary lymph flow in acute and chronic experimental pulmonary edema. Am J Surg 144:254, 1967.

783. Leeds SE, Reich S, Uhley HN, et al: The pulmonary lymph flow after irradiation of the lungs of dogs. Chest 59:203, 1971.

784. Beck E, Beattie EJ Jr. The lymph nodes in the mediastinum. J Int Coll Surg 29:247, 1958.

785. Heitzman ER: Royal College Lecture: Radiologic diagnosis of mediastinal lymph node enlargement. J Can Assoc Radiol 29:151, 1978.

788. Yamashita H: Anatomy of hilar lymph nodes. In Roentgenologic Anatomy of the Lung. New York, Igaku-Shoin, 1978.

789. Glazer GM, Gross BH, Quint LE, et al: Normal mediastinal lymph nodes: Number and size according to American Thoracic Society mapping. Am J Roentgenol 144:261, 1985.

790. Leigh TF, Weens HS: The Mediastinum. Springfield, IL, Charles C Thomas, 1959, pp 16–27.

791. Osborne DR, Korobkin M, Ravin CE, et al: Comparison of plain radiography, conventional tomography, and computed tomography in detecting intrathoracic lymph node metastases from lung carcinoma. Radiology 142:157, 1982.

792. Moak GD, Cockerill EM, Farber MO, et al: Computed tomography vs. standard radiology in the evaluation of mediastinal adenopathy. Chest 82:69, 1982.

793. Mintzer RA, Malave SR, Neiman HL, et al: Computed vs. conventional tomography in evaluation of primary and secondary pulmonary neoplasms. Radiology 132:653, 1979.

794. Hirleman MT, Yie-Chiu VS, Chium LC, et al: The resectability of primary lung carcinoma: A diagnostic staging review. CT 4:146, 1980.

795. Khan A, Khan FA, Garvey J, et al: Oblique hilar tomography and mediastinoscopy; A correlative prospective study in 100 patients with bronchogenic carcinoma. Chest 86:424, 1984.

796. McLoud TC, Wittenburg J, Ferruci JT: Computed tomography of the thorax and standard radiographic evaluation of the chest: Comparative study. Radiology 132:539, 1979.

797. Faling LJ, Pagatch RD, Jung-Leggy Y, et al: Computed tomographic scanning of the mediastinum in the staging of bronchogenic carcinoma. Am Rev Respir Dis 124:690, 1981.

798. Janower ML: Fifty-five-degree posterior oblique tomography of the pulmonary hilum. J Can Assoc Radiol 29:158, 1978.

799. Khan A, Gersten KC, Garvey J, et al: Oblique hilar tomography, computed tomography, and mediastinoscopy for prethoracotomy staging of bronchogenic carcinoma. Radiology 156:295, 1985.

800. Glazer GM, Francis IR, Shirazi KK, et al: Evaluation of the pulmonary hilum: Comparison of conventional radiography, 55° posterior oblique tomography, and dynamic computed tomography. J Comput Assist Tomogr 7:983, 1983.

801. Rea HH, Shevland JE, House AJS: Accuracy of computed tomographic scanning in assessment of the mediastinum in bronchial carcinoma. J Thorac Cardiovasc Surg 81:825, 1981.

802. Baron RL, deVitt RG, Sagel SS, et al.: Computed tomography in the preoperative evaluation of bronchogenic carcinoma. Radiology 145:727, 1982.

803. Ekholm S, Albrechtsson U, Kugelberg J, et al: Computed tomography in pre-operative staging of bronchogenic carcinoma. J Comput Assist Tomogr 4:763, 1977.

804. Glazer GM, Gross BH, Quint LE, et al: Normal mediastinal lymph nodes: Number and size according to American Thoracic Society mapping. Am J Roentgenol 144:261, 1985.

805. Schnyder PA, Gamsu G: CT of the pretracheal retrocaval space. Am J Roentgenol 136:303, 1981.

806. Shevland JE, Chium LC, Schapiro RL, et al: The role of conventional tomography and computed tomography in assessing the resectability of primary lung cancer: A preliminary report. CT 2:1, 1978.

807. Underwood GH Jr, Hooper RG, Axelbaum SP, et al: Computed tomographic scanning of the thorax in the staging of bronchogenic carcinoma. N Engl J Med 300:777, 1979.

808. Genereux GP, Howie JL: Normal mediastinal lymph node size and number: CT and anatomic study. Am J Roentgenol 142:1095, 1984.

809. Baron RL, Lee JKT, Sagel SS, et al: Computed tomography of the normal thymus. Radiology 142:121, 1982.

810. Sone S, Higashihara T, Morimoto S, et al: CT anatomy of hilar lymphadenopathy. Am J Roentgenol 140:887, 1983.

811. American Joint Committee: Manual for Staging of Cancer 1978. Chicago, Whitting, 1978.

812. Glazer GM, Orringer MB, Gross BH, et al: The mediastinum in non–small cell lung cancer: CT-surgical correlation. Am J Roentgenol 152:1101, 1984.

813. Heelan RT, Martini N, Westcott JW, et al: Carcinomatous involvement of the hilum and mediastinum: Computed tomographic and magnetic resonance evaluation. Radiology 156:111, 1985.

814. Webb WR, Jensen BG, Sollitto R, et al.: Bronchogenic carcinoma: Staging with MR compared with staging with CT and surgery. Radiology 156:117, 1985.

815. Bowden DH, Adamson IYR: Endothelial regeneration as a marker of the differential vascular responses in oxygen-induced pulmonary edema. Lab Invest 30:350, 1974.

816. Stocker JT, Malczak HT: A study of pulmonary ligament arteries: Relationship to intralobar pulmonary sequestration. Chest 86:611, 1984.

817. Islam MS: Mechanisms of controlling residual volume and emptying rate of the lung in young and elderly health subjects. Respiratory 40:1, 1980.

818. Wang N-S: Anatomy and physiology of the pleural space. Symposium on Pleural Disease. Clin Chest Med 6:3, 1985.

819. Mariassy AT, Wheeldon EB: The pleura: A combined light microscopic, scanning, and transmission electron microscopic study in the sheep. I. Normal pleura. Exp Lung Res 4:293, 1983.

820. Wang N-S: The regional difference of pleural mesothelial cells in rabbits. Am Rev Respir Dis 110:623, 1974.

821. Andrews PM, Porter KR: The ultrastructural morphology and possible functional significance of mesothelial microvilli. Anat Rec 177:409, 1973.

822. Rennard SI, Jaurand M-C, Bignan J, et al: Role of pleural mesothelial cells in the production of the submesothelial connective tissue matrix of lung. Am Rev Respir Dis 130:267, 1984.

823. Whitaker D, Papadimitriou JM, Walters MN-I: The mesothelium: Its fibrinolytic properties. J Pathol 136:291, 1982.

824. Whitaker D, Papadimitriou JM: Mesothelial healing: Morphological and kinetic investigations. J Pathol 145:159, 1985.

825. Wheeldon EB, Mariassy AT, McSporran KD: The pleura: A combined light microscopic and scanning and transmission electron microscopic study in the sheep. II. Response to injury. Exp Lung Res 5:125, 1983.

826. Yamashita H: Roentgenologic Anatomy of the Lung. New York, Igaku-Shoin, 1978, pp 46–58.

827. Proto AV, Ball JB: Computed tomography of the major and minor fissures. Am J Roentgenol 140:439, 1983.

828. Proto A, Speckman JM: The left lateral radiograph of the chest. Med Radiogr Photogr 55, No 1, 1979.

829. Proto AV, Ball JB: The superolateral major fissures. Am J Roentgenol 140:431, 1983.

830. Marks BW, Kuhns LR: Identification of the pleural fissures with computed tomography. Radiology 143:139, 1982.

831. Goodman LR, Golkow RS, Steiner RM, et al: The right mid-lung window: A potential source of error in computed tomography of the lung. Radiology 143:135, 1982.

832. Rabinowitz JG, Cohen BA, Mendleson DS: The pulmonary ligament. Radiol Clin North Am 22:659, 1984.

833. Rost RC, Proto AV: Inferior pulmonary ligament: Computed tomographic appearance. Radiology 14:479, 1983.

834. Cooper C, Moss AA, Buy J, et al: CT of the pulmonary ligament. Am J Roentgenol 141:231, 1983.

835. Godwin JD, Bock P, Osborne DR: CT of the pulmonary ligament. Am J Roentgenol 141:231, 1983.

836. Hyde, I: Traumatic para-mediastinal air cysts. Br J Radiol 44:380, 1971.

837. Fagan CJ, Swischuk LE: Traumatic lung and para-mediastinal pneumatoceles. Radiology 120:11, 1976.

838. Ravin CE, Smith GW, Lester PD, et al: Post-traumatic pneumatocele in the inferior pulmonary ligament. Radiology 121:39, 1976.

839. Friedman PJ: Adult pulmonary ligament pneumatocele: A loculated pneumothorax. Radiology 155:575, 1985.

840. Godwin JD, Merten DF, Baker ME: Paramediastinal pneumatocele: Alternative explanations to gas in the pulmonary ligament. Am J Roentgenol 145:525, 1985.

841. Tombropoulos EG: Lipid synthesis by lung subcellular particles. Arch Intern Med 127:408, 1971.

842. McCort JJ, Robbins LL: Roentgen diagnosis of intrathoracic lymph-node metastases in carcinoma of the lung. Radiology 57:339, 1951.

843. Rouvière H: Anatomy of the Human Lymphatic System (translated by MJ Tobias). Ann Arbor, MI, Edwards, 1938.

844. Klingenberg I: Histopathologic findings in the prescalene tissue from 1,000 post-mortem cases. Acta Chir Scand 127:57, 1964.

845. Baird JA: The pathways of lymphatic spread of carcinoma of the lung. Br J Surg 52:868, 1965.

846. Leszczyński SZ, Pawlicka L (in collaboration): Purulent and Fibrous Mediastinitis. Radiological Diagnosis. Warsaw, PZWL (Polish Medical Publishers), 1972.

847. Davies DV, Coupland RE (eds): The respiratory system. In Gray's Anatomy; Descriptive and Applied. London, Longmans, Green, and Company, 1958.

848. Zylak CJ, Pallie W, Jackson R: Correlative anatomy and computed tomography: A module on the mediastinum. RadioGraphics 2:555, 1982.

849. Naidich DP, Zerhouni EA, Siegelman SS: Computed Tomography of the Thorax. New York, Raven Press, 1984.

850. Proto AV, Simmons JD, Zylak CJ: The anterior junction anatomy. CRC Crit Rev Diagn Imaging 19:111, 1983.

851. Proto AV, Simmons JD, Zylak CJ: The posterior junction anatomy. CRC Crit Rev Diagn Imaging 20:121, 1983.

852. Felson B: The mediastinum. Sem Roentgenol 4:31, 1969.

853. Oliphant M, Wiot JF, Whalen JP: The cervicothoracic continuum. Radiology 120:257, 1976.

854. Baron RL, Lee, JKT, Sagel SS, et al: Computed tomography of the normal thymus. Radiology 142:121, 1982.

855. Day DL, Gedgaudas E: The thymus. Radiol Clin North Am 22:519, 1984.

856. Kattan KR, Felson B, Holder LE, et al: Superior mediastinal shift in right lower lobe collapse. The "upper triangle sign." Radiology 116:305, 1975.

857. Proto AV, Speckman JM: The Left Lateral Radiograph of the Chest. Med Radiogr Photogr, 55, No. 2, 1980.

858. Jemelin C, Candardjis G: Retrosternal soft tissue: Quantitative evaluation and clinical interest. Radiology 109:7, 1973.

859. Whalen JP, Oliphant M, Evans JA: Anterior extrapleural line: Superior extension. Radiology 115:525, 1975.

860. Branscom JJ, Austin JHM: Aberrant right subclavian artery: Findings seen on plain chest roentgenograms. Am J Roentgenol 119:539, 1973.

861. Ball JB Jr, Proto AV: The variable appearance of the left superior intercostal vein. Radiology 144:445, 1982.

862. Friedman AC, Chambers E, Sprayregen S: The normal and abnormal left superior intercostal vein. Am J Roentgenol 131:599, 1978.

863. McDonald CJ, Castellino RA, Blank N: The aortic nipple: The left superior intercostal vein. Radiology 96:533, 1970.

864. Lane EJ, Heitzman ER, Dinn WM: The radiology of the superior intercostal veins. Radiology 120:263, 1976.

865. Blank N, Castellino RA: Patterns of pleural reflections of the left superior mediastinum: Normal anatomy and distortions produced by adenopathy. Radiology 102:585, 1972.

866. Heitzman ER, Lane EJ, Hammack DB, et al: Radiological evaluation of the aortic-pulmonic window. Radiology 116:513, 1975.

867. Ramirez-Rivera J, Schwartz B, Dowell AR, et al: Biochemical composition of human pulmonary washings. Arch Intern Med 127:395, 1971.

868. Schinz HR, Baensch W, Friedl E: Lehrbuch der Röntgendiagnostik. 1st ed. Leipzig, Thieme, 1928.

869. Lachman E: A comparison of the posterior boundaries of the lungs and pleura as demonstrated on the cadaver and on the roentgenogram of the living. Anat Rec 83:521, 1942.

870. Brailsford JF: The radiographic posteromedial border of the lung, or the linear thoracic shadow. Radiology 41:34, 1943.

871. Dalton CJ, Schwartz SS: Evaluation of the paraspinal line in roentgen examination of the thorax. Radiology 66:195, 1956.

872. Garland LH: The posteromedial pleural line. Radiology 41:29, 1943.

873. Gupta SK, Mohan V: The thoracic paraspinal line: Further significance. Clin Radiol 30:329, 1979.

874. Heitzman ER: The Mediastinum. Radiologic Correlations with Anatomy and Pathology. St. Louis, CV Mosby, 1977, pp 33–66, 198–206.

875. Genereux GP: The posterior pleural reflections. Am J Roentgenol 141:141, 1983.

876. Lane EJ, Carsky EW: Epicardial fat: Lateral plain film analysis in normals and in pericardial effusion. Radiology 91:1, 1968.

877. Trackler RT, Brinker RA: Widening of the left paravertebral pleural line on supine chest roentgenogram in free pleural effusions. Am J Roentgenol 96:1027, 1966.

878. Lane EJ, Proto AV, Phillips TW: Mach bands and density perception. Radiology 121:9, 1976.

879. Grant JCB: In Brash JC (ed): Respiratory System. Cunningham's Text-book of Anatomy. New York, Oxford University Press, 1951, p 1331.

880. Savoca CJ, Austin JHM, Goldberg HI: The right paratracheal stripe. Radiology 122:295, 1977.

881. Bachman AL, Teixidor HS: The posterior tracheal band: Reflector of local superior mediastinal abnormality. Br J Radiol 48:352, 1975.

882. Yrjana J: The posterior tracheal band and recurrent esophageal carcinoma. Radiology 136:615, 1980.

883. Kormano M, Yrjana J: The posterior tracheal band: Correlation between computed tomography and chest radiography. Radiology 136:689, 1980.

884. Putman CE, Curtis AM, Westfried M, et al: Thickening of the posterior tracheal stripe: A sign of squamous cell carcinoma of the esophagus. Radiology 121:533, 1976.

885. Palayew MJ: The tracheo-esophageal stripe and the posterior tracheal band. Radiology 132:11, 1979.

886. Figley M: Mediastinal minutiae. Semin Roentgenol 4:22, 1969.

887. Proto AV, Lane EJ: Air in the esophagus: A frequent radiographic finding. Am J Roentgenol 129:433, 1977.

888. Cimmino CV: The esophageal-pleural stripe on chest teleroentgenograms. Radiology 67:754, 1956.

889. Cimmino CV: Further notes on the esophageal-pleural stripe. Radiology 77:974, 1961.

890. Ormond RS, Jaconette JR, Templeton AW: The pleural esophageal reflection: An aid in the evaluation of esophageal disease. Radiology 80:738, 1963.

891. Austin JHM, Thorsen MK: Normal azygos arch: Retrotracheal visualization on frontal chest tomograms. Am J Radiol 137:1205, 1981.

892. Keats TE, Lipscomb GE, Betts CS III: Mensuration of the arch of the azygos vein and its application to the study of cardiopulmonary disease. Radiology 90:990, 1968.

893. Felson B: Letter from the editor. Semin Roentgenol 2:323, 1967.

894. Doyle FH, Read AE, Evans KT: The mediastinum in portal hypertension. Clin Radiol 12:114, 1961.

895. Milne ENC, Pistolesi M, Miniati M, et al: The vascular pedicle of the heart and the vena azygos. Part I: The normal subject. Radiology 152:1, 1984.

896. Pistolesi M, Milne ENC, Miniati M, et al: The vascular pedicle of the heart and the vena azygos. Part II: Acquired heart disease. Radiology 152:9, 1984.

897. Milne E, Imray TJ, Pistolesi M, et al: The vascular pedicle and the vena azygos. Part III: In trauma—the "vanishing" azygos. Radiology 153:25, 1984.

898. Heitzman ER, Scrivani JV, Martino J, et al: The azygos vein and its pleural reflections. I. Normal roentgen anatomy. Radiology 101:249, 1971.

899. Heitzman ER, Scrivani JV, Martino J, et al: The azygos vein and its pleural reflections. II. Applications in the radiological diagnosis of mediastinal abnormality. Radiology 101:259, 1971.

900. Onitsuka H, Kuhns LR: Dextroconvexity of the mediastinum in the azygoesophageal recess. Radiology 135:126, 1980.

901. Gammill SL, Krebs C, Meyers P, et al: Cardiac measurements in systole and diastole. Radiology 94:115, 1970.

902. Castellino RA, Blank N: Adenopathy of the cardiophrenic angle (diaphragmatic) lymph nodes. Am J Roentgenol 114:509, 1972.

903. Berger AJ, Mitchell RA, Severinghaus JW: Regulation of respiration (first of three parts). N Engl J Med 297:92, 1977.

904. Berger AJ, Mitchell RA, Severinghaus JW: Regulation of respiration (second of three parts). N Engl J Med 297:138, 1977.

905. Berger AJ, Mitchell RA, Severinghaus JW: Regulation of respiration (third of three parts). N Engl J Med 297:194, 1977.

906. Derenne JP, Macklem PT, Roussos CL: The respiratory muscles: Mechanics, control and pathophysiology. Am Rev Respir Dis 118:1119, 1978.

907. Hornbein TF, Lenfant C (eds): Regulation of breathing, Parts One and Two. Lung Biology in Health and Disease. New York, Marcel Dekker, 1981.

908. In Williams MH (ed): Disturbance of Respiratory Control. Clinical Chest Med I. Philadelphia, WB Saunders, 1980.

909. Pavlin EG, Hornbein TF: Basics of respiratory disease. American Thoracic Society 7:26, 1979.

910. McDonald DM: Peripheral chemoreceptors: Structure, function, relationship of the carotid body. In Hornbein TF, Lenfant C (eds): Regulation of Breathing, Part One. Lung Biology in Health and Disease. New York, Marcel Dekker, 1981, p 321.

911. Biscoe TJ, Willshaw P: Stimulus-response relationships of the peripheral arterial chemoreceptors. In Hornbein TF, Lenfant C (eds): Regulation of Breathing, Part One. Lung Biology in Health and Disease. New York, Marcel Dekker, 1981.

912. Lugliani R, Whipp BJ, Seard C, et al: Effect of bilateral carotid body resection on ventilatory control at rest and during exercise in man. N Engl J Med 285:1105, 1971.

913. Phillipson EA, Sullivan CE: Arousal: The forgotten response to respiratory stimuli (editorial). Am Rev Respir Dis 118:807, 1978.

914. Bledsoe SW, Hornbein TF: Central chemosensors and the regulation of their chemical environment. In Hornbein TF, Lenfant C (eds): Regulation of Breathing. Part One. Lung Biology in Health and Disease. New York, Marcel Dekker, 1981, p 347.

915. Widdicombe JG: Nervous receptors in the respiratory tract and lungs. In Hornbein TF, Lenfant C (eds): Regulation of Breathing, Part One. Lung Biology in Health and Disease. New York, Marcel Dekker, 1981, p 429.

916. McBride B, Whitelaw WA: A physiological stimulus to upper airway receptors in humans. J Appl Physiol 51:1189, 1981.

917. Burgess KR, Whitelaw WA: Reducing ventilatory response to carbon dioxide by breathing cold air. Am Rev Respir Dis 129:687, 1984.

918. Sant'Ambrogio G, Mathew OP, Fisher JT, et al: Laryngeal receptors responding to transmural pressure, airflow and local muscle activity. Resp Physiol 54:317, 1983.

919. Mathew OP: Upper airway negative-pressure effects on respiratory activity of upper airway muscles. J Appl Physiol 56:500, 1984.

920. Duron B: Intercostal and diaphragmatic muscle endings and afferents. In Hornbein TF, Lenfant C: Regulation of Breathing, Part One. Lung Biology in Health and Disease, New York, Marcel Dekker, 1981, p 473.

921. Ford GT, Whitelaw WA, Rosenal TW, et al: Diaphragm function after upper abdominal surgery in humans. Am Rev Respir Dis 127:431, 1983.

922. Road JD, Burgess KR, Ford GT: Diaphragm function after upper versus lower abdominal surgery in dogs. Physiologist 25:331, 1982.

923. Mitchell RA: Neural regulation of respiration. Clin Chest Med 1:3, 1980.

924. Mitchell RA, Berger AJ: Neural regulation of respiration. In Hornbein TF, Lenfant C: Regulation of Breathing, Part One. Lung Biology in Health and Disease. New York, Marcel Dekker, 1981, p 541.

925. Martin J, Aubier M, Engel LA: Effects of inspiratory loading on respiratory muscle activity during expiration. Am Rev Respir Dis 125:352, 1982.

926. von Euler C: On the central pattern generator for the basic breathing rhythmicity. J Appl Physiol 55:1647, 1983.

927. Phillipson EA, McClean PA, Sullivan CE, et al: Interaction of metabolic and behavioural respiratory control during hypercapnia and speech. Am Rev Respir Dis 117:903, 1978.

928. Fitzgerald RS: The respiratory control system. Chest 85:585, 1984.

929. Phillipson EA, Duffin J, Cooper JD: Critical dependence of respiratory rhythmicity on metabolic CO_2 load. J Appl Physiol 50:45, 1981.

930. Milic-Emili J: Recent advances in clinical assessment of control of breathing. Lung 160:1, 1982.

931. Jammes Y, Auran Y, Gouvernet J, et al: The ventilatory pattern of conscious man according to age and morphology. Bull Eur Physiopathol Resp 15:527, 1979.

932. Tobin MJ, Jenouri G, Sackner MA: Effect of naloxone on change in breathing pattern with smoking. Chest 82:530, 1982.

933. Tobin MJ, Chadha TS, Jenouri G, et al: Breathing patterns. 2. Diseased subjects. Chest 84:286, 1983.

934. Tobin MJ, Chadha TS, Jenouri G, et al: Breathing patterns. 1. Normal Subjects. Chest 84:202, 1983.

935. Askanazi J, Milic-Emili J, Broell JR, et al: Influence of exercise and CO_2 on breathing pattern of normal man. J Appl Physiol 47:192, 1979.

936. Collins DD, Scoggin CH, Zwillich CW, et al: Hereditary aspects of decreased hypoxic response. J Clin Invest 62:105, 1978.

937. Kawakami Y, Yamamoto H, Yoshikawa T, et al: Respiratory chemosensitivity in smokers—studies on monozygotic twins. Am Rev Respir Dis 126:986, 1982.

938. Kawakami Y, Yoshikawa T, Shida A, et al: Control of breathing in young twins. J Appl Physiol 52:537, 1982.

939. Kawakami Y, Yamamoto H, Yoshikawa T, et al: Chemical and behavioural control of breathing in adult twins. Am Rev Respir Dis 129:703, 1984.

940. Michiels TM, Light RW, Mahutte CK: Naloxone reverses ethanol-

induced depression of hypercapnic drive. Am Rev Respir Dis 128:823, 1983.

941. Stanley NN, Galloway JM, Gordon B, et al: Increased respiratory chemosensitivity induced by infusing almitrine intravenously in healthy man. Thorax 38:200, 1983.

942. Laksminarayan S, Sahn SA, Weil JV: Effect of aminophylline on ventilatory responses in normal man. Am Rev Respir Dis 117:33, 1978.

943. Baier H, Somani P: Ventilatory drive in normal man during semi-starvation. Chest 85:222, 1984.

944. Folgering H, Braakhekke J: Ventilatory response to hypercapnia in normal subjects after propranolol, metoprolol and oxprenolol. Respiration 39:139, 1980.

945. Bosisio E, Sergi M, Sega R, et al: Respiratory response to carbon dioxide after propranolol in normal subjects. Respiration 37:197, 1979.

946. Hutchinson PF, Harrison RN: Effect of acute and chronic beta-blockade on carbon dioxide sensitivity in normal man. Thorax 35:869, 1980.

947. Knill RL, Gelb AW: Ventilatory responses to hypoxia and hypercapnia during halothane sedation and anesthesia in man. Anesthesiology 49:244, 1978.

948. Leitch AG: The hypoxic drive to breathing in man. Lancet 1:428, 1981.

949. Fleetham JA, Arnup ME, Anthonisen NR: Familial aspects of ventilatory control in patients with chronic obstructive pulmonary disease. Am Rev Respir Dis 129:3, 1984.

950. Byrne-Quinn E, Weil JV, Sodal IE, et al: Ventilatory control in the athlete. J Appl Physiol 30:91, 1971.

951. Schoene RB: Control of ventilation in climbers to extreme altitude. J Appl Physiol 53:886, 1982.

952. Bradley BL, Mestas J, Forman J, et al: The effect on respiratory drive of a prolonged physical conditioning program. Am Rev Respir Dis 122:741, 1980.

953. Douglas NJ, White DP, Weill JV, et al: Effect of breathing route on ventilation and ventilatory drive. Resp Physiol 51:209, 1983.

954. Sheldon MI, Green JF: Evidence for pulmonary CO_2 chemosensitivity effects on ventilation. J Appl Physiol 52:1192, 1982.

955. Whipp J: Ventilatory control during exercise in humans. Annu Rev Physiol 45:393, 1983.

956. Whipp BJ: The control of exercise hyperpnea. In Hornbein TF, Lenfant C (eds): Regulation of Breathing, Part Two. Lung Biology in Health and Disease. New York, Marcel Dekker, 1981, p 1069.

957. Hesse B, Kanstrup I-L, Christensen NJ, et al: Reduced norepinephrine response to dynamic exercise in human subjects during O_2 breathing. J Appl Physiol 51:176, 1981.

958. Flenley DC, Brash H, Clancy L: Ventilatory response to steady-state exercise in hypoxia in humans. J Appl Physiol 46:438, 1979.

959. Cherniack NS, Altose MD: Respiratory responses in ventilatory loading. In Hornbein TF, Lenfant C (eds): Regulation of Breathing, Part Two. Lung Biology in Health and Disease. New York, Marcel Dekker, 1981, p 905.

960. Kelsen SG, Prestel TF, Cherniack NS, et al: Comparison of the respiratory responses to external resistive loading and bronchoconstriction. J Clin Invest 67:1761, 1981.

961. Burki NK, Davenport PW, Safdar F, et al: The effects of airway anesthesia on magnitude estimation of added inspiratory resistive and elastic loads. Am Rev Respir Dis 127:2, 1983.

962. Campbell EJM, Guz A: Breathlessness. In Hornbein TF, Lenfant C (eds): Regulation of Breathing, Part Two. Lung Biology in Health and Disease. New York, Marcel Dekker, 1981, p 1181.

963. Stubbing DG, Killian KJ, Campbell EJM: The quantification of respiratory sensations by normal subjects. Resp Physiol 55:251, 1981.

964. Killian KJ, Campbell EJM: Dyspnea and exercise. Annu Rev Physiol 45:465, 1983.

965. Killian KJ, Mahutte CK, Howell JBL, et al: Effect of timing, flow, lung volume, and threshold pressures on resistive load detection. J Appl Physiol 49:958, 1980.

966. Killian KJ, Campbell EJM, Howell JBL: The effect of increased ventilation on resistive load discrimination. Am Rev Respir Dis 120:1233, 1979.

967. Zechman FW, Wiley RL, Davenport PW: Ability of healthy men to discriminate between added inspiratory resistive and elastic loads. Resp Physiol 45:111, 1981.

968. Stubbing DG, Killian KJ, Campbell EJM: Weber's law and resistive load detection. Am Rev Respir Dis 127:5, 1983.

969. Mahutte CK, Campbell EJM, Killian KJ: Theory of resistive load detection. Resp Physiol 51:131, 1983.

970. Remmers JE: Control of breathing during sleep. In Hornbein TF, Lenfant C (eds): Regulation of Breathing, Part Two. Lung Biology in Health and Disease. New York, Marcel, Dekker, 1981, p 1197.

971. Weiner D, Mitra M, Salamone J: Effect of chemical stimuli on nerves supplying upper airway muscles. J Appl Physiol 52:530, 1982.

972. Bartlett D Jr, Knuth SL, Knuth KV: Effects of pulmonary stretch

973. Brouilette RT, Thach BT: A neuromuscular mechanism maintaining extrathoracic airway patency. J Appl Physiol 46:772, 1979.

974. Korl RC, Knuth SL, Bartlett D: Selective reduction of genioglossal muscle activity by alcohol in normal human subjects. Am Rev Respir Dis 129:247, 1984.

975. Phillipson EA: State of the art—control of breathing during sleep. Am Rev Respir Dis 118:909, 1978.

976. Remmers JE, Anch AM, deGroot WJ: Respiratory disturbances during sleep. Clin Chest Med 1:57, 1980.

977. Cherniack NS: Respiratory dysrhythmias during sleep. N Engl J Med 305:325, 1981.

978. Douglas NJ, White DP, Pickett CK, et al: Respiration during sleep in normal man. Thorax 37:840, 1982.

979. Gothe B, Altose MD, Goldman MD, et al: Effect of quiet sleep on resting and CO_2 stimulated breathing in humans. J Appl Physiol 50:724, 1981.

980. Douglas NG, White DP, Weil JV, et al: Hypercapnic ventilatory response in sleeping adults. Am Rev Respir Dis 126:758, 1982.

981. Douglas J, White P, Weil V, et al: Hypoxic ventilatory response decreases during sleep in normal men. Am Rev Respir Dis 125:286, 1982.

982. Berthon-Jones M, Sullivan CE: Ventilatory and arousal responses to hypoxia in sleeping humans. Am Rev Respir Dis 125:632, 1982.

983. White DP, Douglas NJ, Pickett CK, et al: Sleep deprivation and the control of ventilation. Am Rev Respir Dis 128:948, 1983.

984. Strohl KP: Upper airway muscles of respiration. Am Rev Respir Dis 124:211, 1981.

985. Derenne J-P, Macklem PT, Roussos CL: The respiratory muscles: Mechanics, control and pathophysiology. I. Am Rev Respir Dis 118:119, 373, 581, 1978.

986. Luce JM, Culver BH: Respiratory muscle function in health and disease. Chest 81:82, 1982.

987. Mathew OP, Abu-Osba YK, Thach BT: Influence of upper airway pressure changes on genioglossus muscle respiratory activity. J Appl Physiol 52:438, 1982.

988. Mathew OP, Abu-Osba YK, Thach BT: Genioglossus muscle responses to upper airway pressure changes: Afferent pathways. J Appl Physiol 52:445, 1982.

989. Onal E, Lopata M, O'Connor TD: Diaphragmatic and genioglossal electromyogram responses to CO_2 rebreathing in humans. J Appl Physiol 50:1052, 1981.

990. Hwang J, Bartlett D Jr, St. John WM: Characterization of respiratory-modulated activities of hypoglossal motoneurons. J Appl Physiol 55:793, 1983.

991. Gottfried SB, Strohl KP, Van De Graff W, et al: Effects of phrenic stimulation on upper airway resistance in anesthetized dogs. J Appl Physiol 55:419, 1983.

992. Hyland RH, Hutcheon MA, Perl A, et al: Upper airway occlusion induced by diaphragmatic pacing for primary alveolar hypoventilation: Implications for the pathogenesis of obstructive sleep apnea. Am Rev Respir Dis 124:180, 1981.

993. Gal TJ, Goldberg SK: Diaphragmatic function in healthy subjects during partial curarization. J Appl Physiol 48:921, 1980.

994. Edwards RHT: The diaphragm as a muscle. Mechanisms underlying fatigue. Am Rev Respir Dis 119:Part 2(Suppl)81, 1979.

995. De Troyer A: Mechanical role of the abdominal muscles in relation to posture. Resp Physiol 53:341, 1983.

996. Sharp JT: Respiratory muscles: A review of old and newer concepts. Lung 157:185, 1980.

997. De Troyer A, Sampson M, Sigrist S, et al: The diaphragm: Two muscles. Science 213:237, 1981.

998. Gauthier GF, Padykula HA: Cytological studies of fiber types in skeletal muscle—a comparative study of the mammalian diaphragm. J Cell Biol 28:333, 1966.

999. Burke RE, Levine DN, Tsairis P, et al: Physiological types and histochemical profiles in motor units of the cat gastrocnemius. J Physiol 234:723, 1973.

1000. Belman MJ, Sieck GS: The ventilatory muscles—fatigue, endurance and training. Chest 82:761, 1982.

1001. Rochester D: Is diaphragmatic contractility important (editorial)? N Engl J Med 30:305, 1981.

1002. Faulkner JA, Maxwell LC, Ruff GL, et al: The diaphragm as a muscle. Contractile properties. Am Rev Respir Dis 119(Suppl):89, 1979.

1003. Keens TG, Bryan AC, Levison H, et al: Developmental pattern of muscle fiber types in human ventilatory muscles. J Appl Physiol 44:909, 1978.

1004. Lieberman DA, Maxwell LC, Faulkner JA: Adaptation of guinea pig diaphragm muscle to aging and endurance training. Am J Physiol 222:556, 1972.

1005. Faulkner JA, Maxwell LC, Lieberman DA: Histochemical characteristics of muscle fibers from trained and detrained guinea pigs. Am J Physiol 222:836, 1972.

1006. Leak LV: Gross and ultrastructural morphologic features of the diaphragm. Am Rev Respir Dis 119(Suppl):3, 1979.

1007. Wang N-S: The preformed stomas connecting the pleural cavity and the lymphatics in the parietal pleura. Am Rev Respir Dis 111:12, 1975.

1008. Thurlbeck WM: Diaphragm and body weight in emphysema. Thorax 33:483, 1978.

1009. Butler C: Diaphragmatic changes in emphysema. Am Rev Respir Dis 114:155, 1976.

1010. Warwick R, Williams PL (eds): Gray's Anatomy. 35th British ed. Philadelphia, WB Saunders, 1973, p 667.

1011. Comtois A, Gorczyca W, Grassino A: Microscopic anatomy of the arterial diaphragmatic circulation. Clin Invest Med 7:81, 1984.

1012. Rochester DF, Briscoe AM: Metabolism of the working diaphragm. Am Rev Respir Dis 119:101, 1979.

1013. DeTroyer A, DeBeyl DZ, Thirion M: Function of the respiratory muscles in acute hemiplegia. Am Rev Respir Dis 123:631, 1981.

1014. Derenne J-PH, Macklem PT, Roussos CH: State of the art. The respiratory muscles: Mechanics, control and pathophysiology. Part II. Am Rev Respir Dis 118:373, 1978.

1015. Altose MD, DiMarco AF, Gottfried SB, et al: The sensation of respiratory muscle force. Am Rev Respir Dis 126:807, 1982.

1016. Guz A: Sensory aspects of the diaphragm. Am Rev Respir Dis 119(Suppl):65, 1979.

1017. Campbell EJM: The effect of muscular paralysis induced by curarization on breath holding in normal subjects. Am Rev Respir Dis 119(Suppl):67, 1979.

1018. Young DA, Simon G: Certain movements measured on inspiration-expiration chest radiographs correlated with pulmonary function studies. Clin Radiol 23:37, 1972.

1019. Wittenborg MH, Aviad I: Organ influence on the normal posture of the diaphragm: A radiological study of inversions and heterotaxies. Br J Radiol 36:280, 1963.

1020. Simon G, Bonnell J, Kazantzis G, et al: Some radiological observations on the range of movement of the diaphragm. Clin Radiol 20:231, 1969.

1021. Alexander C: Diaphragm movements and the diagnosis of diaphragmatic paralysis. Clin Radiol 17:79, 1966.

1022. Schmidt S: Anatomic and physiologic aspects of respiratory kymography. Acta Radiol (Diagn) 8:409, 1969.

1023. Edwards RHT: Human muscle physiology and metabolism. Br Med Bull 36:159, 1980.

1024. Human muscle fatigue (editorial). Lancet 2:729, 1981.

1025. Luce JM, Culver BH: Respiratory muscle function in health and disease. Chest 81:82, 1982.

1026. Loh L, Goldman M, Newsom-Davis J: The assessment of diaphragm function. Medicine 56:165, 1977.

1027. Newman SL, Road JD, Grassino A: Diaphragmatic contraction in postural changes. Fed Proc 42:1010, 1983.

1028. Braun NMT, Aora NS, Rochester DF: Force-length relationship of the normal human diaphragm. J Appl Physiol 53:405, 1982.

1029. Roussos C, Macklem PT: The respiratory muscles. N Engl J Med 307:786, 1982.

1030. Rousson CS, Macklem PT: Diaphragmatic fatigue in man. J Appl Physiol 43:189, 1977.

1031. Moxham J, Morris AJR, Spiro SG, et al: Contractile properties and fatigue of the diaphragm in man. Thorax 36:164, 1981.

1032. Rochester DF, Briscoe AM: Metabolism of the working diaphragm. Am Rev Respir Dis 119(Suppl):101, 1979.

1033. Roussos CH: The failing ventilatory pump (review). Lung 160:59, 1982.

1034. Macklem PT: Respiratory muscles: The vital pump. Chest 78:753, 1980.

1035. Roussos C, Macklem PT: The respiratory muscles. N Engl J Med 307:786, 1982.

1036. Gandevia SC, McKenzie DK, Neering IR: Endurance properties of respiratory and limb muscles. Resp Physiol 53:47, 1983.

1037. Derenne J-PH, Macklem PT, Roussos CH: State of the art. The respiratory muscles: Mechanics, control and pathophysiology. Part III. Am Rev Respir Dis 118:581, 1978.

1038. Arora NS, Rochester DF: Effect of body weight and muscularity on human diaphragm muscle mass, thickness, and area. J Appl Physiol 52:64, 1982.

1039. Hughes RL, Katz H, Sahgal V, et al: Fiber size and energy metabolites in five separate muscles from patients with chronic obstructive lung disease. Respiration 44:321, 1983.

1040. Field S, Kelly SM, Macklem PT: The oxygen cost of breathing in patients with cardiorespiratory disease. Am Rev Respir Dis 126:9, 1982.

1041. Jardim J, Farkas G, Prefaut C, et al: The failing inspiratory muscles under normoxic and hypoxic conditions. Am Rev Respir Dis 124:274, 1981.

1042. Vellody VPS, Nassery M, Balasaraswathi K, et al: Compliances of human rib cage and diaphragm-abdomen pathways in relaxed versus paralyzed states. Am Rev Respir Dis 118:479, 1978.

1043. Gilbert R, Auchincloss JH, Peppi D: Relationship of rib cage and abdomen motion to diaphragm function during quiet breathing. Chest 80:607, 1981.

1044. Cohen CA, Zagelbaum G, Gross D, et al: Clinical manifestations of inspiratory muscle fatigue. Am J Med 73:308, 1982.

1045. Roussos C, Fixley M, Gross D, et al: Fatigue of inspiratory muscles and their synergic behaviour. J Appl Physiol 46:896, 1979.

1046. Williams TJ, Ahmad D, Morgan WKC: A clinical and roentgenographic correlation of diaphragmatic movement. Arch Intern Med 141:878, 1981.

1047. Black LF, Hyatt RE: Maximal respiratory pressures; Normal values and relationship to age and sex. Am Rev Respir Dis 99:696, 1969.

1048. Konno K, Mead J: Measurement of the separate volume changes of rib cage and abdomen during breathing. J Appl Physiol 22:407, 1967.

1049. Macklem PT: Respiratory muscles—the vital pump. Chest 78:753, 1980.

1050. Lopata M, Zubillaga G, Evanich MJ, et al: Diaphragmatic EMG response to isocapnic hypoxic and hyperoxic hypercapnia in humans. J Lab Clin Med 91:698, 1978.

1051. Gross D, Grassino A, Ross W, et al: Electromyogram pattern of diaphragmatic fatigue. J Appl Physiol 46:1, 1979.

1052. Moxam J, Edwards R, Aubier M, et al: Changes in EMG power spectrum (high-to-low ratio) with force fatigue in humans. J Appl Physiol 53:1094, 1982.

1053. Onal E, Lopatal M, Ginzburg AS, et al: Diaphragmatic EMG and transdiaphragmatic pressure measurements with a single catheter. Am Rev Respir Dis 124:563, 1981.

1054. Macklem PT: Normal and abnormal function of the diaphragm. Thorax 36:161, 1981.

1055. DeTroyer A, Estenne M: Limitations of measurement of transdiaphragmatic pressure in detecting diaphragmatic weakness. Thorax 36:169, 1981.

1056. Gibson GJ, Clark E, Pride NB: Static transdiaphragmatic pressures in normal subjects and in patients with chronic hyperinflation. Am Rev Respir Dis 124:685, 1981.

1057. Nickerson BH, Keens TG: Measuring ventilatory muscle endurance in humans as sustainable inspiratory pressure. J Appl Physiol 52:768, 1982.

1058. Aubier M, Farkas G, De Troyer A, et al: Detection of diaphragmatic fatigue in man by phrenic stimulation. J Appl Physiol 50:538, 1981.

1059. Field S, Kelly SM, Macklem PT: The oxygen cost of breathing in patients with cardiorespiratory disease. Am Rev Respir Dis 126:9, 1982.

1060. Aubier M, DeTroyer A, Sampson M, et al: Aminophylline improves diaphragmatic contractility. N Engl J Med 305:249, 1981.

1061. Sigrist S, Thomas D, Howell S, et al: The effect of aminophylline on inspiratory muscle contractility. Am Rev Respir Dis 126:46, 1982.

1062. Howell S, Roussos C: Isoproterenol and aminophylline improve contractility of fatigued canine diaphragm. Am Rev Respir Dis 129:118, 1984.

1063. Pardy RL, Rivington RN, Despas PJ, et al: The effects of inspiratory muscle training on exercise performance in chronic air flow limitation. Am Rev Respir Dis 123:426, 1981.

1064. Goldenberg DB, Brogdon BG: Congenital anomalies of the pectoral girdle demonstrated by chest radiography. J Can Assoc Radiol 18:472, 1967.

1065. Scheff S, Laforet EG: The internal thoracic muscle and the lateral chest roentgenogram. Radiology 86:27, 1966.

1066. Shopfner CE, Jansen C, O'Kell RT: Roentgen significance of the transverse thoracic muscle. Am J Roentgenol 103:140, 1968.

1067. Whalen JP, Meyers MA, Oliphant M, et al: The retrosternal line: A new sign of an anterior mediastinal mass. Am J Roentgenol 117:861, 1973.

1068. King JB: Calcification of the costal cartilages. Br J Radiol 12:2, 1939.

1069. Sanders CF: Sexing by costal cartilage calcification. Br J Radiol 39:233, 1966.

1070. Christensen EE, Dietz GW: The supraclavicular fossa. Radiology 118:37, 1976.

1071. Ominsky S, Berinson HS: The suprasternal fossa. Radiology 122:311, 1977.

1072. Navani S, Shah JR, Levy PS: Determination of sex by costal cartilage calcification. Am J Roentgenol 108:771, 1970.

1073. Vastine JH II, Vastine MF, Arango O: Genetic influence on osseous development with particular reference to the deposition of calcium in the costal cartilages. Am J Roentgenol 59:213, 1948.

1074. Zawadowski W: Über die Schattenbildunger an der Lungen-Weichteilgrenze. Fortschr Roentgenstr 53:306, 1936.

1075. Gluck MC, Twigg HL, Ball MF, et al: Shadows bordering the lung on radiographs of normal and obese persons. Thorax 27:232, 1972.

1076. Vix VA: Extrapleural costal fat. Radiology 112:563, 1974.

1077. Foley WJ, Whitehouse WM: Supernumerary thoracic ribs. Radiology 93:1333, 1969.

1078. Köhler A: Borderlands of the Normal and Early Pathologic in Skeletal Roentgenology. 10th ed. New York, Grune & Stratton, 1956.

1079. Parsons FG: On the proportions and characteristics of the modern English clavicle. J Anat 51:71, 1917.

1080. Shauffer IA, Collins WV: The deep clavicular rhomboid fossa. Clinical significance and incidence in 10,000 routine chest photofluorograms. JAMA 195:778, 1966.

1081. Cockshott WP: The coracoclavicular joint. Radiology 131:313, 1979.

1082. Cigtay OS, Mascatello VJ: Scapular defects: A normal variation. Am J Radiol 132:239, 1979.

1083. Shoop JD: Transthoracic rib. Radiology 93:1335, 1969.

1084. Kermond AJ: Supernumerary intrathoracic rib—an easily recognized rare anomaly. Australas Radiol 15:131, 1971.

1085. Freed C: Intrathoracic rib: A case report. S Afr Med J 46:1165, 1972.

1086. Sullivan D, Cornwell WS: Pelvic rib: Report of a case. Radiology 110:355, 1974.

1087. Goodman LR, Teplick SK, Kay H: Computed tomography of the normal sternum. Am J Roentgenol 141:219, 1983.

1088. Goldman HI, Becklake MR: Respiratory function tests: Normal values at median altitudes and the prediction of normal results. Am Rev Tuberc 79:457, 1959.

1089. Rosenblum LJ, Mauceri RA, Wellenstein DE, et al: Density patterns in the normal lung as determined by computed tomography. Radiology 137:409, 1980.

1090. Flatley FJ, Constantine H, McCredie RM, et al: Pulmonary diffusing capacity and pulmonary capillary blood volume in normal subjects and in cardiac patients. Am Heart J 64:159, 1962.

1091. Bucci G, Cook CD: Studies on respiratory physiology in children. VI. Lung diffusing capacity, diffusing capacity of the pulmonary membrane and pulmonary capillary blood volume in congenital heart disease. J Clin Invest 40:1431, 1961.

1092. Jonsson B, Linderholm H, Pinardi G: Atrial septal defect: A study of physical working capacity and hemodynamics during exercise. Acta Med Scand 159:275, 1957.

1093. Westermark N: On the roentgen diagnosis of lung embolism. Acta Radiol 19:357, 1938.

1094. Joseph AEA, Lacey GJ, Bryant THE, et al: The hypertransradiant hemithorax. The importance of lateral decentering, and the explanation for its appearance due to rotation. Clin Radiol 29:125, 1978.

1095. Lavender JP, Doppman J: The hilum in pulmonary venous hypertension. Br J Radiol 35:303, 1962.

1096. Daley R, Goodwin JF, Steiner RF (eds): Clinical Disorders of the Pulmonary Circulation. London, J. & A. Churchill, 1960.

1097. Spiro RG: Glycoproteins: Their biochemistry, biology and role in human disease, part 1. N Engl J Med 281:991, 1969.

1098. Redding RA, Douglas WHJ, Stein M: Thyroid hormone influence upon lung surfactant metabolism. Science 175:994, 1972.

1099. Dollery CT, West JB, Wilcken DEL, et al: A comparison of the pulmonary blood flow between left and right lungs in normal subjects and patients with congenital heart disease. Circulation 24:617, 1961.

1100. Friedman WF, Braunwald E, Morrow AG: Alterations in regional pulmonary blood flow in patients with congenital heart disease studied by radioisotope scanning. Circulation 37:747, 1968.

1101. Chen JTT, Robinson AE, Goodrich JK, et al: Uneven distribution of pulmonary blood flow between left and right lungs in isolated valvular pulmonary stenosis. Am J Roentgenol 107:343, 1969.

1102. Riley RL: Effect of lung inflation upon the pulmonary vascular bed. In de Reuck AVS, O'Connor M (eds): Ciba Foundation Symposium on Pulmonary Structure and Function. London, J. & A. Churchill, 1962, pp 261–272.

1103. Rigler LG: Functional roentgen diagnosis: Anatomical image—physiological interpretation. Am J Roentgenol 82:1, 1959.

1104. Whitley JE, Martin JF: The Valsalva maneuver in roentgenologic diagnosis. Am J Roentgenol 91:297, 1964.

1105. Westermark N: On the influence of the intra-alveolar pressure on the normal and pathological structure of the lungs. Acta Radiol 25:874, 1944.

1106. Amundsen P: Planigraphy in Möller and Valsalva experiments. Acta Radiol 40:387, 1953.

1107. Garland LH: Studies on the accuracy of diagnostic procedures. Am J Roentgenol 82:25, 1959.

1108. Garland LH: On the scientific evaluation of diagnostic procedures. Radiology 52:309, 1949.

1109. Garland LH, Cochrane AL: Results of international test in chest roentgenogram interpretation. JAMA 149:631, 1952.

1110. Felson B, Morgan WKC, Bristol LJ, et al: Observations on the results of multiple readings of chest films on coal miners' pneumoconiosis. Radiology 109:19, 1973.

1111. Tuddenham WJ: Problems of perception in chest roentgenology: Facts and fallacies. Radiol Clin North Am 1:277, 1963.

1112. Tuddenham WJ: Visual search, image organization, and reader error in roentgen diagnosis: Studies of the psychophysiology of roentgen image perception. (Memorial Fund Lecture). Radiology 78:694, 1962.

1113. Tuddenbaum WJ, Calvert WP: Visual search patterns in roentgen diagnosis. Radiology 76:255, 1961.

1114. Tuddenham WJ: The visual physiology of roentgen diagnosis. A. Basic concepts. Am J Roentgenol 78:116, 1957.

1115. Riebel FA: Use of the eyes in x-ray diagnosis. Radiology 70:252, 1958.

1116. Kundel HL, Nodine CF: Interpreting chest radiographs without visual search. Radiology 116:527, 1975.

1117. Kundel HL, LaFollette PS Jr: Visual search patterns and experience with radiological images. Radiology 103:523, 1972.

1118. Kundel HL, Wright DJ: The influence of prior knowledge of visual search strategies during the viewing of chest radiographs. Radiology 93:315, 1969.

1119. Kundel HL: Visual sampling and estimates of the location of information on chest films. Invest Radiol 9:87, 1974.

1120. Carmody DP, Nodine CF, Kundel HL: Global and segmented search for lung nodules of different edge gradients. Invest Radiol 15:224, 1980.

1121. Newell RR, Garneau R: The threshold visibility of pulmonary shadows. Radiology 56:409, 1951.

1122. Kelsey CA, Moseley RD Jr, Mettler FA Jr, et al: Original investigations. Observer performance as a function of viewing distance. Invest Radiol 16:435, 1981.

1123. Shea FJ, Ziskin MC: Visual system transfer function and optimal viewing distance for radiologists. Invest Radiol 7:147, 1972.

1124. Berkson J, Good CA, Carr DT, et al: Identification of "positives" in roentgenographic readings. Am Rev Respir Dis 81:660, 1960.

1125. Spratt JS Jr, Ter-Pogossian M, Long RTL: The detection and growth of intrathoracic neoplasms: The lower limits of radiographic distinction of the antemortem size, the duration, and the pattern of growth as determined by direct mensuration of tumor diameters from random thoracic roentgenograms. Arch Surg 86:283, 1963.

1126. Goldmeier E: Limits of visibility of bronchogenic carcinoma. Am Rev Respir Dis 91:232, 1965.

1127. Resnik JEJ: Is a roentgenogram of fine structures a summation image or a real picture? Acta Radiol 32:391, 1949.

1128. Greening RR, Pendergrass EP: Postmortem roentgenography with particular emphasis upon the lung. Radiology 62:720, 1954.

1129. Beilin DS, Fink JP, Leslie LW: Correlation of postmortem pathological observations with chest roentgenograms. Radiology 57:361, 1951.

1130. de Geer G, Webb WR, Gamsu G: Normal thymus: Assessment with MR and CT. Radiology 158:313, 1986.

1131. Francis IR, Glazer GM, Bookstein FL, et al: The thymus: Reexamination of age-related changes in size and shape. Am J Roentgenol 145:249, 1985.

1132. Griscom NT, Wohl ME: Dimensions of the growing trachea related to age and gender. Am J Roentgenol 146:233, 1986.

1133. Rhodes CG, Wollmer P, Fazio F, et al: Quantitative measurement of regional extravascular lung density using positron emission and transmission tomography. Comput Assist Tomogr 5:783, 1981.

1134. Hedlund LW, Vock P, Effmann EL: Evaluating lung density by computed tomography. Semin Respir Med 5:76, 1983.

1135. Hedlund LW, Vock P, Effmann EL: Computed tomography of the lung: Densitometric studies. Radiol Clin North Am 21:775, 1983.

1136. Rosenblum LJ, Mauceri RA, Wellenstein DE, et al: Density patterns in the normal lung as determined by computed tomography. Radiology 137:409, 1980.

1137. Genereux GP: Computed tomography and the lung: Review of anatomic and densitometric features with their clinical application. Assoc Radiol 36:88, 1985.

1138. Wegener OH, Koeppe P, Oeser H: Measurement of lung density by computed tomography. Comput Assist Tomogr 2:263, 1978.

1139. Goddard PR, Nicholson EM, Laszlo G, et al: Computed tomography in pulmonary emphysema. Clin Radiol 33:379, 1982.

1140. Genereux GP: CT of acute and chronic distal air-space (alveolar) disease. Semin Roentgenol 19:211, 1984.

1141. Simon G: Personal communication, 1965.

1142. Piiper J, Haab P, Rahn H: Unequal distribution of pulmonary diffusing capacity in the anesthetized dog. J Appl Physiol 16:499, 1961.

1143. Bhalla DK, Crocker TT: Tracheal permeability in rats exposed to ozone. Am Rev Respir Dis 134:572, 1986.

1144. Richardson J, Bouchard T, Ferguson CC: Uptake and transport of exogenous proteins by respiratory epithelium. Lab Invest 35:307, 1976.

1145. Gonzalez S, von Bassewitz DB, Grundmann E, et al: Rudimentary cilia in hyperplastic, metaplastic, and neoplastic cells of the lung and pleura. Pathol Res Pract 180:511, 1985.

1146. Smallman LA, Gregory J: Ultrastructural abnormalities of cilia in the human respiratory tract. Hum Pathol 17:848, 1986.

1147. Balis JU, Paterson JF, Paciga JE, et al: Distribution and subcellular localization of surfactant-associated glycoproteins in human lung. Lab Invest 52:657, 1985.

1148. Gosney JR, Sissons MCJ, O'Malley JA: Quantitative study of endocrine cells immunoreactive for calcitonin in the normal adult human lung. Thorax 40:866, 1985.

1149. Torikata C, Mukai M, Kawakita H, et al: Neurofilaments of Kultschitsky cells in human lung. Acta Pathol Jap 36:93, 1986.

1150. Starcher BC: Elastin and the lung. Review article. Thorax 41:577, 1986.

1151. Spicer SS, Schulte BA, Chakrin LW: Ultrastructural and histochemical observations of respiratory epithelium and gland. Exp Lung Res 4:137, 1983.

1152. Pierce JA, Ebert RV: Fibrous network of the lung and its change with age. Thorax 20:469, 1965.

1153. Hansen JE, Ampaya EP: Human air space shapes, sizes, areas, and volumes. J Appl Physiol 38:990, 1975.

1154. Bowden DH, Adamson IYR: Role of monocytes and interstitial cells in the generation of alveolar macrophages: I. Kinetic studies of normal mice. Lab Invest 42:511, 1980.

1155. Lehnert BE, Valdez YE, Stewart CC: Translocation of particles to the tracheobronchial lymph nodes after lung deposition: Kinetics and particle-cell relationships. Exp Lung Res 10:245, 1986.

1156. Shimura S, Boatman ES, Martin CJ: Effects of aging on the alveolar pores of Kohn and on the cytoplasmic components of alveolar type II cells in monkey lungs. J Pathol 148:1, 1986.

1157. du Bois RM: The alveolar macrophage. Editorial. Thorax 40:321, 1985.

1158. Shellito J, Kaltreider HB: Heterogeneity of immunologic function among subfractions of normal rat alveolar macrophages. Am Rev Respir Dis 131:678, 1985.

1159. Nugent KM, Glazier J, Monick MM, et al: Stimulated human alveolar macrophages secrete interferon. Am Rev Respir Dis 131:714, 1985.

1160. Murara K, Itoh H, Todo G, et al: Bronchial venous plexus and its communication with pulmonary circulation. Invest Radiol 21:24, 1986.

1161. Muller NL, Webb WR: Radiographic imaging of the pulmonary hila. Invest Radiol 20:661, 1985.

1162. Bhattacharya J, Staub NC: Direct measurement of microvascular pressures in the isolated perfused dog lung. Science 210:327, 1980.

1163. Hakim TS, Michel RP, Chang HK: Partitioning vascular resistance in dogs by arterial and venous occlusion. J Appl Physiol Respir Environ 52:710, 1982.

1164. Graham R, Skoog C, Oppenheimer L, et al: Critical closure in the canine pulmonary vasculature. Circ Res 50:566, 1982.

1165. West JB, Dollery CT, Naimark A: Distribution of blood flow in isolated lung: Relation to vascular and alveolar pressures. J Appl Physiol 19:713, 1964.

1166. West JB: Regional differences in the lung. Chest 74:426, 1978.

1167. Stahlman MT, Gray ME: Ontogeny of neuroendocrine cells in human fetal lung. Lab Invest 51:449, 1984.

1168. Laitinen A: Ultrastructural organization of intraepithelial nerves in the human airway tract. Thorax 40:488, 1985.

1169. Laitinen A, Partanen M, Hervonen A, et al: Electron microscopic study on the innervation of the human lower respiratory tract: Evidence of adrenergic nerves. Eur J Respir Dis 67:209, 1985.

1170. Barnes PJ: The third nervous system in the lung: Physiology and clinical perspective. Thorax 39:561, 1984.

1171. Bray BA, Keller S, Mandl I, et al: Collagenous membrane from the surface of human visceral pleura. Lung 163:361, 1985.

1172. Bolen JW, Hammar SP, McNutt MA: Reactive and neoplastic serosal tissue. Am J Surg Pathol 10:34, 1986.

1173. Gale ME, Greif WL: Intrafissural fat: CT correlation with chest radiography. Radiology 160:333, 1986.

1174. Postmus PE, Kerstjens JM, Breed A, et al: A family with lobus venae azygos. Chest 90:298, 1986.

1175. Austin JHM: The left minor fissure. Radiology 161:433, 1986.

1176. Glazer HS, Aronberg DJ, Sagel SS, et al: CT demonstration of calcified mediastinal lymph nodes: A guide to the new ATS classification. AJR 147:17, 1986.

1177. Woodring JH, Daniel TL: Medical analysis emphasizing plain radiographs and computed tomograms. Med Radiogr Photogr 62:1, 1986.

1178. Chasen MH, McCarthy MJ, Gilliland JD, et al: Concepts in computed tomography of the thorax. RadioGraphics 6:793, 1986.

1179. Kittredge RD: The right posterolateral tracheal band. J Comp Assist Tomogr 3:348, 1979.

1180. Fleischner FG, Udis SW: Dilatation of the azygos vein: A roentgen sign of venous engorgement. Am J Roentgenol 67:569, 1952.

1181. Alter AJ, Kargas GA, Kargas SA, et al: The influence of ambient and viewbox light upon visual detection of low-contrast targets in a radiograph. Invest Radiol 17:402, 1982.

1182. Begin R, Renzetti AD: Alveolar-arterial oxygen pressure gradient: I. Comparison between an assumed and actual respiratory quotient in stable chronic pulmonary disease; II. Relationship to aging and closing volume in normal subjects. Respir Care 22:491, 1977.

1183. Kendall MW, Eissman E: Scanning electron microscopic examination of human pulmonary capillaries using a latex replication method. Anat Rec 196:275, 1980.

1184. Georges R, Sauman G, Loiseau A: The relationship of age to pulmonary membrane conductance and capillary blood volume. Am Rev Respir Dis 117:1069, 1978.

1185. Hutchins GM, Haupt HM, Moore GW: A proposed mechanism for the early development of the human tracheobronchial tree. Anat Rec 201:635, 1981.

1186. Boffa P, Stovin P, Shneerson J: Lung developmental abnormalities in severe scoliosis. Short reports. Thorax 39:681, 1984.

1187. Kradin RL, Spirn PW, Mark EJ: Intrapulmonary lymph nodes—Clinical, radiologic, and pathologic findings. Chest 87:662, 1985.

1188. Jolles PR, Shin MS, Jones WP: Aortopulmonary window lesions: Detection with chest radiography. Radiology 159:647, 1986.

1189. Sullivan TY, Yu P-L: Airway anesthesia effects on hypercapnic breathing pattern in humans. J Appl Physiol Respir Environ 55:368, 1983.

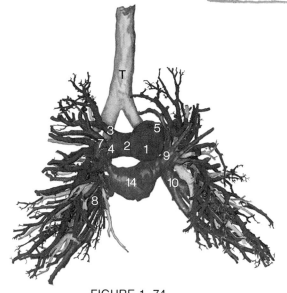

FIGURE 1–74

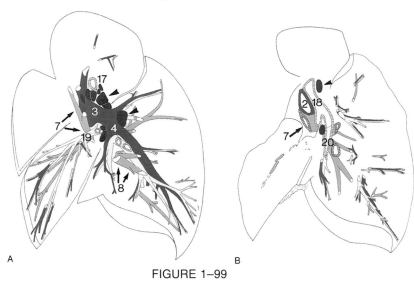

A

B

FIGURE 1–99

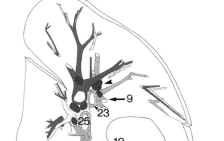

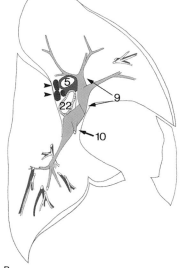

A

B

FIGURE 1–100

2
CHAPTER
Methods of Roentgenologic and Pathologic Investigation

315

ROENTGENOLOGIC EXAMINATION

In this book the approach to the diagnosis of chest disease involves two basic steps in a logical sequence of events: first, *identification* of a pathologic process roentgenologically; and second, through *correlation* of these preliminary roentgenographic findings *with the clinical picture,* arrival at a diagnosis that takes into account the results of special roentgenographic procedures, laboratory tests, pulmonary function tests, scintillation scanning, and other procedures such as bronchoscopy and pathologic examination of cytology and biopsy specimens. In this chapter the roentgenographic and pathologic methods we employ are described. Emphasis is placed on the techniques that have proved most valuable in our experience. Procedures that others have employed to advantage but we have found unrewarding are described briefly, together with our reasons for regarding them as unprofitable.

The cornerstone of roentgen diagnosis is the plain roentgenogram. This statement cannot be overemphasized. All other roentgen procedures, such as fluoroscopy, conventional and computed tomography, and special contrast studies, are strictly ancillary. With a few exceptions, to which we refer later on, establishing the *presence* of a disease process by plain roentgenography of the chest should constitute the first step; if this first examination does not show clearly the nature and extent of the lesion, additional studies can be carried out to *complement* the plain roentgenogram.

CONVENTIONAL ROENTGENOGRAPHY

Routine Projections

Roentgenologists vary in their appreciation of which projections of the thorax constitute the most satisfactory basic or "routine" views for preliminary evaluation. The great majority, including us, prefer posteroanterior and lateral projections. Although stereoscopic films in posteroanterior projection may be almost as informative to the experienced viewer, they fail to depict with sufficient clarity certain anatomic structures that are clearly seen on lateral roentgenograms.[6] Consequently, we do not recommend posteroanterior stereoscopy except possibly as a screening procedure for patients in whom chest disease is not suspected. As basic projections of the thorax, posteroanterior and lateral roentgenograms provide the essential requirement of a three-dimensional view of the chest. No pathologist is satisfied with examining a gross specimen from only one aspect. He or she must not only turn it over and view all aspects but also must incise it and view its inner structure. Therefore the roentgenologist—who is actually a gross morphologist—should not be satisfied to examine as complex a structure as the thorax in one direction only, except as a screening procedure in asymptomatic subjects. Roentgenography of the chest as a screening procedure (as used in mass surveys) is carried out on such a colossal scale that it has become economically unsound to take more than a single posteroanterior view. One cannot be overly critical of this practice, since the subjects are ostensibly asymptomatic. At the other end of the scale are those roentgenologists who are not satisfied with only two views of the thorax and whose routine includes a third projection, such as an overpenetrated view in posteroanterior projection. There is little doubt that such a routine allows a more thorough assessment of the thoracic contents than is possible with only two views, but it is unlikely that the diagnostic yield justifies the additional time and expense.

From an analysis of over 10,000 chest roentgenographic examinations of a hospital-based population, Sagel and his colleagues[7] concluded that routine screening examinations, obtained solely because of hospital admission regulations or scheduled surgery, are not warranted in patients under 20 years of age and that the lateral projection can be safely eliminated from routine screening examinations in patients 20 to 39 years of age but should be included whenever chest disease is suspected and in screening examinations of patients 40 or more years of age. Similar conclusions were drawn in two more recent reviews, one dealing with routine preoperative examinations[8] and the other with routine admission chest roentgenograms.[9] In the former study of 905 surgical admissions, the investigators carried out clinical screening for the presence of factors that would make patients more likely to have abnormal preoperative chest roentgenograms: of the 368 who had no risk factors, only one had an abnormal chest roentgenogram; by contrast, of the 504 patients who had identifiable risk factors, 114 (22 per cent) were found to have serious abnormalities on their preoperative chest roentgenograms. In the second study, by Hubbell and his colleagues,[9] dealing with a Veterans Administration population known to have a high prevalence of cardiopulmonary disease, roentgenographic abnormalities were identified in 106 (36 per cent) of 294 patients; in only 20 of these were the findings new or unexpected, and treatment was changed because of roentgenographic results in only 12 (4 per cent) of the patients. Of even greater importance was the observation that in only one of these patients might appropriate treatment have been omitted if a chest roentgenogram had not been obtained. From this study, the investigators concluded that the impact of routine admission chest roentgenograms on patient care is very small, even in a population with a high prevalence of cardiopulmonary disease.

In an analysis of the charts and routine preoperative chest roentgenograms of 350 children admitted for elective pediatric surgery,[10] it was found that for the most part such roentgenograms revealed no useful information and that they were not indicated in the absence of clinical suspicion of pulmonary or cardiovascular disease. Similar conclusions were drawn in a retrospective study of routine prenatal chest roentgenograms of 12,109 pregnant women delivered consecutively at the Mayo Clinic;[11] of the 48 patients who showed appreciable roentgenographic abnormalities, *all* had a positive history or abnormal physical findings that would have suggested the presence of disease and the requirement for chest roentgenography. Another study with a somewhat different slant was carried out by a Harvard group;[12] this study assessed the contribution of chest radiography to diagnosis in 1102 consecutive patients with chest complaints at the emergency ward and ambulatory screening clinic of a large hospital. The workers found that 96 per cent of the patients less than 40 years of age had no acute roentgenographic abnormalities, a normal physical examination of the chest, and no hemoptysis; if roentgenograms in the below-40-year age group had been limited to patients with an abnormal physical examination or hemoptysis, 58 per cent of the patients in that group would have been spared the examination, and only 2.3 per cent of the acute roentgenographic abnormalities in the entire population of patients under age 40 years would have gone undetected. It is of some interest that these researchers found that in patients over 40 years of age, chest symptoms were a sufficient indication for chest roentgenography, a conclusion also reached by Sagel and his colleagues.[7]

In a recent statement promulgated by the American College of Radiology,[13] the following referral criteria for routine screening chest x-ray examinations were recommended: that all routine prenatal chest x-ray examinations be discontinued; that routine chest roentgenograms not be required solely because of hospital admission; that routine periodic examinations unrelated to job exposure be discontinued; and that mandated chest x-ray examinations as a condition of initial or continuing employment have not been shown to be of sufficient productivity to justify their continued use for tuberculosis detection.

Now that the high costs of medical care are being critically examined, the physician should give due consideration to the observations and conclusions reached in the foregoing studies. A risk-benefit analysis of routine chest x-ray examinations has recently been reviewed by Robin and Burke.[667]

ROENTGENOGRAPHIC TECHNIQUE

The basic principles of roentgenographic technique are:

(1) Positioning must be such that the x-ray beam is properly centered, the patient's body is not rotated, and the scapulae are rotated sufficiently anteriorly so as to be projected free of the lungs.

(2) Respiration must be fully suspended, preferably at total lung capacity (TLC). In this regard, the studies of Crapo and his associates[14] are important: these investigators showed that in erect chest roentgenography, normal subjects routinely inhale to approximately 95 per cent of TLC *without coaxing*; thus, such roentgenograms can be of value in estimating lung volume and, by comparison with subsequent roentgenograms, in appreciating increase or decrease in volume as a result of disease.

(3) Exposure factors should be such that the resultant roentgenogram permits faint visualization of the thoracic spine *and* the intervertebral discs so that lung markings behind the heart are clearly visible; exposure should be as short as possible, consistent with the production of adequate contrast.

(4) In heavy subjects, appropriate grids must be employed to reduce scatter radiation to a minimum.

Unfortunately, all too frequently technical factors are such that optimal roentgenographic density is achieved over the lungs generally but without adequate penetration of the mediastinum or the left side of the heart (Fig. 2–1), a tendency that seriously limits roentgen interpretation. As has been stressed by Tuddenham,[31] moderate overexposure can be easily compensated for by bright illumination; underexposure, on the other hand, cannot be compensated for by any viewing technique and, since it prevents visualization of vital areas of the thorax, should not be tolerated in any circumstances. With perseverance, it is always possible to develop roentgenographic techniques that obviate problems of underexposure.

Of the more than 67,000 roentgenograms obtained in the "black lung" program to the end of 1972, 2098 (approximately 3 per cent) were rejected by expert readers.[15] These roentgenograms were rejected for various technical reasons, including poor processing, roentgenographic overexposure or

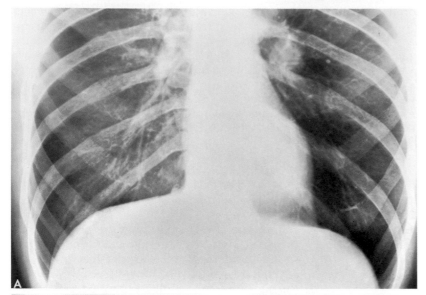

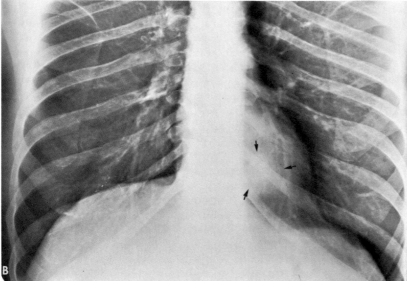

Figure 2–1. The Hazard of Roentgenographic Underexposure. *A,* A roentgenogram of the lower half of the thorax in posteroanterior projection reveals no obvious abnormalities. The mediastinum and left side of the heart are underpenetrated. *B,* A more heavily penetrated view (in slight lordotic projection) demonstrates a somewhat poorly defined nodular mass situated in the lung behind the left heart (*arrows*). Even in retrospect, this lesion is not visible in *A.*

underexposure, and in some cases bad geometry. Trout and his colleagues[15] concluded that problems of quality did not lie so much with equipment or processing as with the willingness to accept a poor product. In the vast majority of circumstances the responsibility belongs to the radiologist, and it is clear that only continual surveillance of all aspects of roentgenographic exposure and processing will guarantee the excellence—not merely the acceptability—of roentgenographic quality to which all radiologists should aspire. Trout and Kelley[660] designed a phantom model for evaluating chest roentgenographic techniques and equipment. This inexpensive, relatively uncomplicated apparatus, composed of generally available materials, is recommended to those who wish to maintain a high standard of roentgenography.

At this juncture, an appropriate question might be "What radiographic technique provides the optimal chest roentgenogram?" To answer that question, at least in part, we review some of the deliberations of a symposium entitled The Optimization of Chest Radiography held in Madison, Wisconsin, in 1979, at which many experts in the field discussed the multiple factors involved in obtaining and interpreting the optimal chest roentgenogram.[661] Although this conference was held some years ago, we believe that the conclusions reached are valid today. As one might imagine, opinions on certain matters were divided, sometimes widely. For example, although it was generally agreed that the large x-ray absorption differences in various areas of the chest make it most difficult to obtain a chest roentgenogram with ideal exposure and diagnostic quality in all areas, there was some dissension as to what constitutes the ideal kilovoltage. One group of observers[18] stated that a high kVp technique reduces the dominance of bone and provides a better match to film latitude, resulting in better visibility of vasculature, nodular lesions, air-tissue interfaces, and diffuse low-contrast soft tissue features. Steiner and his group,[19] in a comparative study of 350 and 120 kVp techniques, found that neither was superior in all categories but that each played a complementary role in image perception in the thorax. Further, Tuddenham[20] suggested that the perception of diagnostically critical shadows in a chest roentgenogram is more often limited by subjective factors than by the technical characteristics of the recording. He argued that the characteristics of the various structures in the chest are so dissimilar that "ideal" imaging of all structures in a single recording is simply not possible. He concluded that the radiologist must either adopt a technique that selectively optimizes the recording of the type of structure of greatest diagnostic interest in a particular clinical situation, recognizing that the recording of other structures may be inferior, or must accept a compromise recording in which all structures are reasonably well but none ideally imaged.

The technique that we have employed with consistent success for over 15 years is based upon the output obtainable from a 1000 ma, 3-phase, 12-pulse generator with a maximum rating of 150 kVp. The kVp is fixed at 145, the ma is variable from 400 to 600, and exposure is controlled by phototiming. A time range of 10 to 60 msec establishes the exposure range of 5 to 30 mas for most examinations. A constant focal film distance of 10 ft is employed, with a fixed 6 inch air gap. This air gap technique, described originally by Watson[16] and modified by Jackson,[17] interposes a space of 6 inches between the patient and the x-ray film; since the air gap reduces radiation scatter by distance dispersion, no grid is required. To achieve adequate exposure of the mediastinum while maintaining a proper level of exposure of the lung, we use a tunnel-wedge filter.[21] Wedge filtration was advocated by Lynch[22] for equalizing the densities of the thinner apical regions of the chest with those of basal regions; in addition to reducing exposure to the apices, it provides increased exposure over the width of the mediastinum. The wedge filter is constructed of various thicknesses of 0.003 inch copper foil to a maximum thickness of approximately 0.3 mm; in addition to the advantages of such filtration just described, it has been shown[24] that a copper filter of 0.32 mm thickness reduces the entrance exposure to the patient by 30 to 40 per cent—a decided advantage in these days of worry over radiation hazard. The filter is mounted over the tube aperture of a rectangular brass cone 61 cm long. This cone, permanently mounted on the x-ray tube, collimates the x-ray beam to a precise 14 × 17 inch area at a distance of 10 ft, precluding excessive field coverage. The film changer system has a multifilm magazine that feeds each film into an evacuated screen-film compression device, thereby producing excellent screen contact during exposure. Completion of the exposure activates photoidentification of the film; this is fed automatically into a 90 sec processor,

which permits dry film viewing approximately 2 min after exposure. Of some interest is a recent study[528] in which the effectiveness of a wedge filter in improving the detection of nodules and infiltrates (sic) was assessed: it was found that the filter technique was not significantly different from the conventional (nonfilter) technique in the depiction of infiltrates (sic) but was slightly worse for the identification of nodules.

The high kilovoltage technique[22, 23] has several advantages over that in the standard (60 to 80) kVp range. Since the coeffcents of x-ray absorption of bone and soft tissue approximate each other in the higher kV ranges, roentgenographic visibility of the bony thorax is reduced with only slight change in the overall visibility of lung structures. Further, the mediastinum is better penetrated, permitting visibility of lung behind the heart and of the many mediastinal lines whose identification is so important to the overall assessment of both mediastinum and lungs. This technique can produce chest roentgenograms superior in all respects to those obtained with other techniques; in addition to the better penetration of the mediastinum, these films yield a clearer visibility of the pulmonary vasculature than can be obtained with more standard techniques. In a study designed to compare the detection of pulmonary nodules on chest roentgenograms exposed at 70 kVp and 120 kVp, Kelsey and his colleagues[25] found a clear improvement in observer performance with the higher kilovoltage, presumably as a result of the wider latitude provided by this technique. The only possible drawback of the high kV technique is the diminished visibility of calcium, resulting from the lower coefficient of x-ray absorption, but this has not proved troublesome in practice.

In a comparative study of air gap and grid techniques in chest roentgenography, Trout and his colleagues[26] found that the former can provide contrasts equal to those obtained with grids, and that of the various combinations of distances possible, a focal film distance of 10 ft and an air gap of 6 inches provide a good compromise. Patient exposure with an air gap technique was comparable to a no grid, no air gap technique and was less than that obtained with a grid.

Magnification roentgenography is achieved by altering the position of the object so that the object-film distance is increased and the target-object distance decreased. A ratio of 1:1 magnifies the object to twice normal size. Disregarding other important factors that affect image sharpness (such as intensifying screens), the smaller the focal spot of the anode the sharper the definition. It is stressed that with the usual target-film distances used in clinical roentgenography, anatomic structures approximately the same size as or smaller than the focal spot of the x-ray tube cannot be reproduced with sharp definition[28] (at the time of writing, the smallest practical focal spot size is 0.3 mm). This limita-

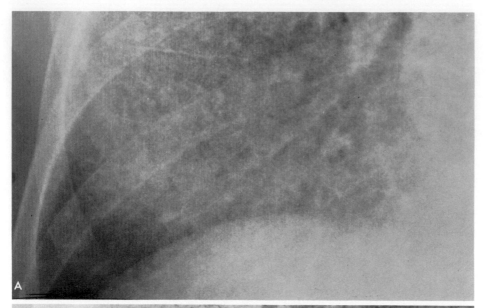

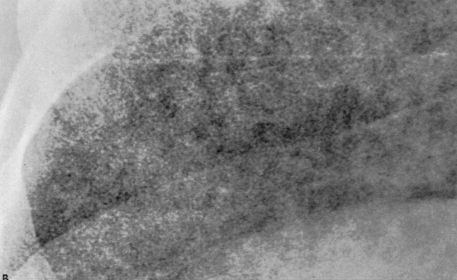

Figure 2–2. Value of Roentgenographic Magnification. *A*, A section of the lower portion of the right lung of a posteroanterior roentgenogram (photographically magnified) of a patient with pulmonary alveolar microlithiasis. The tiny calcispherytes can be visualized but tend to be confluent and thus indistinct. *B*, The same area of a roentgenogram made at 2:1 roentgenographic magnification using a 0.3 mm focus tube. Significant improvement in visibility of the individual calcispherytes has been obtained.

tion is based on the geometric unsharpness created by penumbra and obviously is increased as the object-film distance becomes greater. Magnification is helpful only in resolving high contrast shadows so closely approximated as to be distinguished with difficulty on standard roentgenograms (Fig. 2–2);[31] such a situation pertains, for example, when the myriad of tiny vessels in the lung periphery are opacified during angiography.[32] With rather limited experience to date, we have found magnification roentgenography of the chest confusing rather than clarifying, although Lefcoe[27] has sung its praises in the evaluation of diffuse pulmonary disease. Of a somewhat different nature is the electronic magnification capability of digital radiography, which decidedly improves definition and visibility of low-contrast pulmonary shadows, particularly with edge enhancement (*see* page 325).

The *lordotic projection* can be made in anteroposterior projection or in a modified posteroanterior projection as recommended by Simon.[30] A modification of the anteroposterior view suggested by Jacobson and Sargent[29] seems to possess some merit: instead of assuming the rather uncomfortable lordotic pose, the patient stands erect and the x-ray tube is angled 15 degrees cephalad. The chief advantage of this modification is its reproducibility. The lordotic projection frequently is advocated to improve visibility of the lung apices, superior mediastinum, and thoracic inlet; for locating a lesion by parallax; and for identifying the minor fissure in suspected cases of atelectasis of the right middle lobe.[33, 34] We are not particularly impressed by the value of this projection. Much time and money are wasted by performing examinations in lordotic projection when a direct approach by conventional or computed tomography would yield more information.

Inspiratory-Expiratory Roentgenography

Roentgenograms exposed in full inspiration (total lung capacity) and maximal expiration (residual volume) may supply useful imformation in two specific situations.

1. The main indication for such studies is the investigation of air trapping, either general or local. When air trapping is widespread, as in spasmodic asthma or emphysema, diaphragmatic excursion is reduced symmetrically and lung density changes little; in order to demonstrate these features convincingly, however, expiration must be forced and preferably timed. When air trapping is local, as results from bronchial obstruction or from lobar emphysema, the expiratory roentgenogram reveals restricted ipsilateral diaphragmatic elevation, a shift of the mediastinum toward the contralateral hemithorax, and relative absence of density change in involved bronchopulmonary segments (Fig. 2–3).

2. When pneumothorax is suspected, and the visceral-pleural line is not visible on the standard inspiratory roentgenogram or the findings are equivocal, a film taken in full expiration may show the line more clearly (Fig. 2–4). This is because at full expiration (a) the volume of air in the pleural space is relatively greater in relation to the volume of lung, providing better separation of the pleural surfaces, and (b) the relationship of the pleural line to overlying ribs changes. Furthermore, in cases of established pneumothorax (discussed in detail in Chapter 4; *see* page 683), comparison of the volume of the ipsilateral lung on roentgenograms exposed at TLC and RV may provide information about the size of the pleural defect. If the lung's volume is greatly decreased by expiration, it can be assumed that most of its air content was expired via the tracheobronchial tree and that the visceral-pleural defect is closed or very small; if lung volume is little changed, it can be assumed that the pleural defect is open.

Valsalva and Mueller Maneuvers

As discussed in Chapter 1, these maneuvers may aid in determining the vascular or solid nature of intrathoracic masses. Since for accurate comparison lung volumes must be roughly the same on the two roentgenograms, use of a spirometer is advisable to control the degree of lung inflation; the end of quiet inspiration probably is the most satisfactory position from which to institute both maneuvers. Pressures can be measured on a simple water manometer, plus 40 to 50 cm water for the Valsalva and minus 40 to 50 cm water for the Mueller. Pressures should be sustained for approximately 10 sec before exposure. Either the erect or recumbent position can be employed, depending upon the information sought.

Roentgenography in the Lateral Decubitus Position

In this technique, the patient lies on one side and the x-ray beam is oriented horizontally. Since

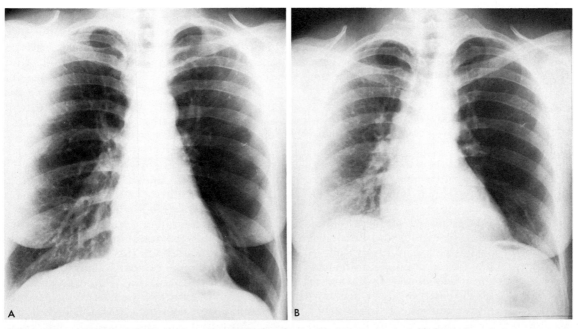

Figure 2–3. Value of Inspiratory-Expiratory Roentgenography in the Assessment of Air Trapping. *A*, A roentgenogram in full inspiration (TLC) of a 31-year-old woman with unilateral obliterative bronchiolitis (Swyer-James syndrome). *B*, In full expiration (RV), the presence of left-sided air trapping is evidenced by a shift of the mediastinum to the right, reduction in left hemidiaphragmatic excursion, and a marked discrepancy in overall density of the two lungs. (From Paré JAP, Fraser R: Synopsis of Diseases of the Chest. Philadelphia, WB Saunders, 1983, p 103.)

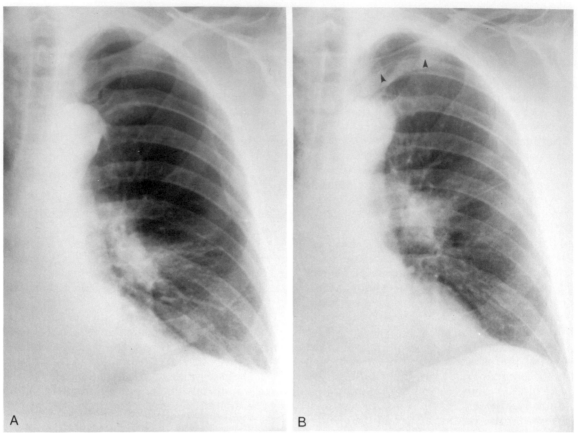

Figure 2–4. The Value of Expiration (RV) in the Demonstration of a Small Pneumothorax. Detail of left lung from a posteroanterior chest roentgenogram: *A* was obtained at total lung capacity and *B*, at residual volume. A small left apical pneumothorax is revealed. The visceral pleural line cannot be identified with conviction in *A* but can be seen clearly on the expiratory film (*arrowheads*).

in the majority of instances the dependent hemithorax is the side being specifically examined, it is desirable to elevate the thorax on a nonabsorbing support such as a foam cushion or mattress. The technique is invaluable for the identification of small pleural effusions. Less than 100 ml of fluid may be identified on well-exposed roentgenograms in this position, whereas those taken with the patient erect seldom reveal pleural effusions of less than 300 ml.[35] Roentgenography in lateral decubitus position is useful also to demonstrate a change in position of an air-fluid level in a cavity or to ascertain whether a structure that forms part of a cavity represents a freely moving intracavitary loose body (*e.g.,* a fungus ball or mycetoma) (*see* Figure 4–90, page 591).

A modification of the standard lateral decubitus projection was introduced by Müller and Löfstedt[36] to identify more precisely small amounts of fluid in the pleural space. They placed a pillow under the patient's hip so that the trunk sloped downward at an angle of about 20 degrees; the lower arm was extended above the head and the trunk rotated dorsally so that the scapula paralleled the horizontal table (to prevent the scapula from obscuring the lower thoracic margin) (Fig. 2–5). Roentgenography was carried out at full expiration, when the

reduced volume of the thoracic cavity raised the fluid level to its maximum. (Although the rationale is undoubtedly correct, we believe that a film taken at moderate inspiration would provide better contrast between the relatively deflated lung and adjacent pleural fluid.) With this method, Müller and Löfstedt[36] identified fluid collections as small as 3 to 5 ml, and Hessén,[37] in his superb treatise on the roentgen examination of pleural fluid, confirmed the superiority of this technique in identifying small pleural effusions.

Still another variation on the standard lateral decubitus position for the identification of pleural fluid consists of an oblique semisupine position described by Möller.[38] With this technique, the patient assumes a position roughly 45 degrees erect and 45 degrees oblique, thus providing clear viewing of the posterolateral gutters inferiorly and permitting evaluation of the presence or absence of pleural effusion on both sides simultaneously. Möller contends that the technique facilitates demonstration of encapsulated as well as free fluid. We have had no experience with this technique.

An additional indication for roentgenography in the lateral decubitus position has been described. Expiratory films are very useful—in fact, frequently essential—for demonstrating the air trapping char-

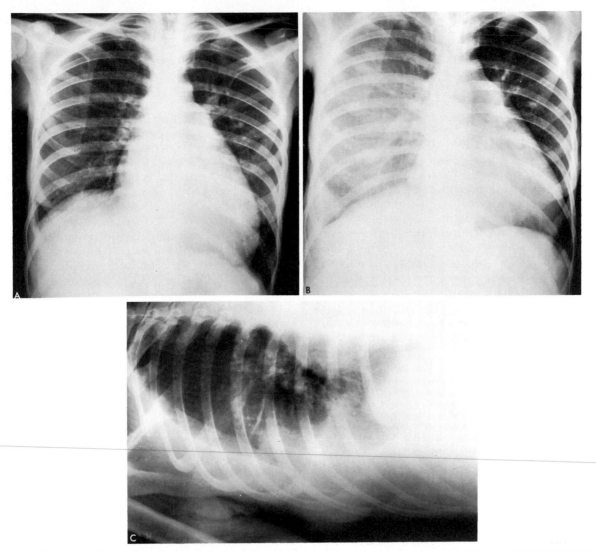

Figure 2–5. Value of Lateral Decubitus Roentgenography in the Assessment of Pleural Effusion. A posteroanterior roentgenogram in the erect position (*A*) reveals what appears to be marked elevation of the right hemidiaphragm, although slight thickening of the axillary pleura in the region of the costophrenic sulcus suggests the possibility of infrapulmonary effusion. Roentgenography in the supine position (*B*) reveals a marked increase in the opacity of the right hemithorax, owing to the presence of fluid in the posterior pleural space; the right hemidiaphragm is now viewed in proper perspective, whereas in *A* it was obscured by subpulmonic effusion. A lateral decubitus roentgenogram (*C*) shows the fluid to much better advantage along the costal margin and reveals how much fluid can be accommodated in the subpulmonic space.

(From Paré JAP, Fraser R: Synopsis of Diseases of the Chest. Philadelphia, WB Saunders, 1983, p 104.)

acteristic of endobronchial foreign bodies, usually in infants and young children. Because of the frequent lack of communication with the patient and resultant difficulty in obtaining good-quality expiratory roentgenograms, Capitanio and Kirkpatrick[39] have adopted lateral decubitus roentgenography as a satisfactory alternative. They point out that when a child is placed on his or her side the dependent hemithorax is splinted, restricting movement of the thoracic cage on that side. As a consequence, in normal children inflation of the dependent lung tends to be less than that of the upper lung; however, when air trapping is present in the dependent lung, the affected lobe or segment tends to remain hyperlucent.

Roentgenography in the Oblique Position

Oblique studies are sometimes useful in locating a disease process (e.g., pleural plaques in asbestosis), with or without prior fluoroscopy, but in most situations we prefer to employ more searching techniques, such as conventional or computed tomography.

BEDSIDE ROENTGENOGRAPHY

The number of requests for roentgenographic examination of the chest with mobile apparatus at a patient's bedside (traditionally and almost universally called "portable," with semantic inaccuracy) has increased enormously in recent years, owing partly to a remarkable growth of intensive care units and partly to the introduction of complex cardiovascular surgical procedures that require close postoperative surveillance. For example, in one of our institutions (Medical Center, University of Alabama at Birmingham), fully 55 per cent of all roentgenographic examinations of the chest are obtained at the bedside, and discussions with colleagues at several other tertiary care institutions suggest that this high figure is not too uncommon. By and large, such roentgenograms are almost invariably technically inferior to those obtained in the standard manner in a radiology department. This inferior quality derives from multiple factors, some of which are uncontrollable (e.g., the patient's supine position, a short focus-film distance, and the restricted ability of many such patients to suspend respiration or to achieve full inspiration to total lung capacity). Other factors, including the technical ones employed in the exposure, are subject to control. Frequently, these roentgenograms are over- or underexposed, sometimes to a degree that limits or even precludes recognition of the subtle changes that are so important in the postoperative period. These difficulties often result in the radiologist either accepting an inferior product or arranging a repeat examination, with associated patient discomfort, increased radiation exposure, and increased costs. To obviate these problems, we and others[40] strongly recommend the use of a high kVp technique or, as an alternative, a technique employing a double-screen/double-film combination in a single cassette.[41] Currently under investigation and clinical study is the digitization and processing of x-ray exposures on either x-ray film or a specially designed cassette or plate, with the resulting digital image being subject to contrast manipulation on cathode ray tube (CRT) monitors; it is anticipated that this technique will achieve considerable success (see further discussion in the section on digital radiography, page 325).

Circumstances often demand that the patient be supine, usually postoperatively or in cases of severe illness. Because of the shorter focus-film distance usually required and the anteroposterior direction of the x-ray beam, magnification of the heart and superior mediastinum often amounts to 15 to 20 per cent, compared with 5 per cent in conventional posteroanterior teleroentgenography. Care must be taken not to misinterpret the magnification as organic enlargement. Roentgenography in supine patients is liable to result in diagnostic error in relation to the pulmonary vascular shadows also. As discussed in Chapter 1, pulmonary blood volume is approximately 30 per cent greater in supine than in erect subjects, and, therefore, the pulmonary vascular shadows usually appear larger. In the upper lungs, this dilatation is enhanced by removal of the effects of gravity and consequent

increased flow to upper lung zones. This must not be misinterpreted as evidence of pulmonary venous hypertension.

All too frequently the degree of elevation of the patient on bedside roentgenograms is not recorded, a deficiency that can hamper interpretation, particularly with respect to upper zone vessel size; a University of Vermont group[42] has described a simple device to measure patient position, and we have employed this to advantage for some years.

The diagnostic efficacy of bedside chest radiography has been the subject of two recent studies, one by Henschke and her associates[43] and the other by Janower and his colleagues.[44] Henschke and associates analyzed 1132 consecutive bedside roentgenograms obtained on 140 patients admitted to surgical and medical intensive care units over a 2 month period: their findings included malpositioning of endotracheal or tracheostomy tubes (in 12 per cent of patients in whom tubes were present), malpositioning of central venous catheters (in 9 per cent of patients in whom catheters were present), and such interval changes as pneumothorax, atelectasis, and pulmonary edema (present in 44 per cent of roentgenograms subsequent to the initial study). Overall, new findings or changes affecting the patient's management were present in 65 per cent of the roentgenograms. Janower and his coworkers[44] discovered positive roentgenographic findings in 45.4 per cent of the bedside examinations they analyzed; although they concluded that such examinations were indicated in 94 per cent of their cases, in only 56 per cent should the examination have been requested as an emergency procedure. In a letter to the editor in which he commented on these two papers, Hall[45] questioned the appropriateness of the "daily routine" bedside chest roentgenogram even on ICU patients receiving mechanical ventilation; he takes the position that the "cookbook" (sic) practice of obtaining chest roentgenograms only at arbitrary time intervals is open to criticism and is somewhat analogous to the equally common practice of obtaining chest roentgenograms solely on the condition of hospital admission, anticipated surgery, or prospective employment.

ROENTGENOLOGIC PROCEDURES FOR THE EVALUATION OF INTRATHORACIC DYNAMICS

Fluoroscopy

The fluoroscopic screen registers a constant image of the object being examined and thus allows appreciation of the dynamic activity of roentgenographically visible intrathoracic structures. *With few exceptions, fluoroscopy should be restricted to this purpose.* The work by Greenspan and his colleagues[46] on timed expiratory roentgenography in the detection of air trapping lends support to our contention that fluoroscopy is seldom superior to roentgenography even in the assessment of such rapid events as diaphragmatic elevation and mediastinal swing. Assessing local and general air trapping, these researchers used a 1 sec forced expiratory roentgenogram (FEV_1) in addition to films exposed at TLC and RV. In over 200 subjects studied, local air trapping was identified in 16, 12 of whom had a normal spirographic trace. In nine patients, trapping could be detected only on the FEV_1 roentgenogram, both TLC and RV films being within normal limits. Admittedly, FEV_1 roentgenography is more difficult and time-consuming, but it provides a permanent record of pathophysiologic events and, unlike fluoroscopy, permits objective assessment.

Identification of abnormalities of esophageal position or contour can be important in roentgenologic diagnosis. As has been emphasized by Fleischner[47] and by Middlemass,[48] deformity caused by enlarged mediastinal lymph nodes may constitute a cardinal sign in the diagnosis of bronchogenic cancer or in the assessment of operability once the diagnosis has been established. Disturbed esophageal dynamics, as in achalasia or scleroderma, may be the chief indication of the origin of the patchy consolidation seen in aspiration pneumonitis or the diffuse reticular pattern of interstitial fibrosis. Fluoroscopy should always precede roentgenography in the investigation of esophageal disease: not only is it the only method for revealing abnormalities of dynamics (e.g., aperistalsis), but it also allows appreciation of minimal but persistent irregularities of contour that might appear insignificant on roentgenograms of the barium-filled esophagus. When attention is directed toward a specific area, spot films can be obtained for permanent record. Since deformity may be small and local, as when caused by a single enlarged lymph node, fluoroscopic inspection should always be carried out in several projections.

Roentgen Densitometry

This technique (synonyms: fluorodensimetry, fluoroscopic densography, statidensigraphy, and cinedensigraphy) has received considerable attention in recent years as a roentgenologic method for studying pulmonary ventilation and perfusion.[49–66] It involves measurement of the flux of x-rays or gamma rays penetrating selected lung zones during the respiratory cycle. Photomultiplier tubes pick up the radiation and transform it into an electric signal, which is amplified and fed into a recorder. Thus, it provides a continuous record of variations in density during quiet respiration, forced expiration, and cough, providing a comparison of the ventilatory capacity of various portions of the lung. Vascular pulsation can be recorded when the breath is held, and ventilation and pulsation can be related to simultaneous spirometric and electrocardiographic tracings. This technique has great possibilities and

apparently can provide much the same information as the radioactive xenon method of estimating regional ventilation and perfusion. Further reference to its use is made in the section dealing with roentgenologic methods of assessing lung function.

DIGITAL RADIOGRAPHY

Since its inception, the discipline of diagnostic radiology has depended on photographic film as the primary vehicle for recording and interpreting the radiologic image, and this dependence has served us well. However, a change in this traditional approach is taking place in the form of digital techniques: for example, digitization is already an integral part of the imaging process in diagnostic ultrasound, nuclear medicine, CT, MRI, and digital subtraction angiography (DSA). Only conventional radiography of the chest and other body parts has lagged behind, but current developments in industry suggest that we are now on the threshold of closing the loop on digital imaging, particularly of the thorax.

Research in the production of digital roentgenographic images of the thorax is progessing along four different fronts.

(1) One involves the digitization of the television signal in image-intensified fluorography, a technique that has been employed with limited success in the production of chest images: the approach yields good temporal resolution but degrades the spatial and contrast resolution and provides a limited dynamic range; in addition, it is subject to a variety of distortions and requires a very large intensifying screen sufficient to cover the average chest. This technique is also the basis of DSA, an imaging modality that is discussed in a subsequent section (see page 339).

(2) The second method that has achieved some success is the digitization and processing of x-ray exposures on a specially designed cassette or plate (Fig. 2–6). This system employs a storage phosphor incorporated into a cassette or high sensitivity detection plate. During exposure, the receptor stores the x-ray energy and is then scanned by a laser beam, which results in the creation of visible or infrared radiation the intensity of which corresponds to the x-ray energy. The resultant luminescence is then converted to digital signals and processed. Subsequently, the digital signals are converted back to analog and reproduced on single-emulsion film by laser camera. The system's image-processing capability provides automated control of image contrast and density and can be extended to effect edge enhancement.

(3) An alternative method is digital processing of radiographic film,[67] in which a radiograph is digitized using a high-intensity laser scanner:

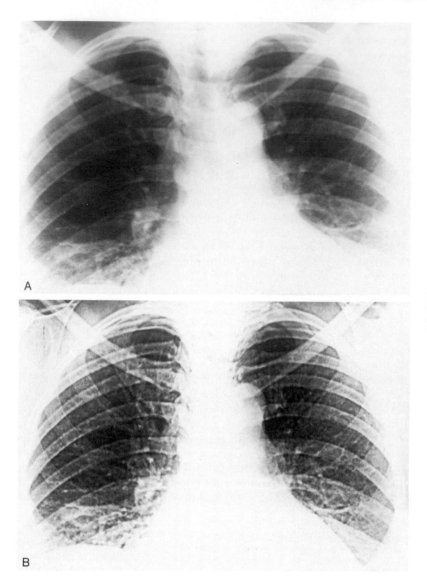

Figure 2–6. Digital Radiography: Storage Phosphor Technique. A conventional roentgenogram is reproduced in *A*, and a digital image in *B*. Appreciation of lung markings is clearly enhanced in *B*. (Courtesy of Dr. Chris Merritt, Ochsner Clinic, New Orleans, LA.)

the recorded image data are then subjected to a wide variety of processing options, with display of processed images on CRT monitors. Images are of a quality comparable to those illustrated in Figure 2–6. Through the use of a specially designed, energy-selective cassette, this technique also permits dual-energy imaging from two films effectively exposed to different x-ray energy spectra.

The second and third of these techniques provide excellent spatial resolution but suffer from a lack of scatter suppression. However, because of the facility for image manipulation, they have been shown to be excellent techniques for bedside radiography; they seldom require repeat studies, and since bedside radiography is becoming almost as frequent as conventional examinations in the x-ray department, this quality in itself should prove a boon. The second and third techniques are now being employed in some centers to provide full departmental digitization.[68]

(4) The fourth approach to digital radiography involves the use of detectors for direct conversion from an analog to a digital electronic signal of x-rays transmitted through a patient. This technique, termed scan projection radiography, is under development by a number of manufacturers who are working in two different but related directions: one employs a pencil beam of x-rays that scans a patient transversely from top to bottom and is capable of producing an image of the chest with an extremely low radiation dose to the patient. The second technique employs a fan beam of x-rays that scans across the patient and is intercepted by a vertical row of scintillation detectors. We have had most experience in the latter method, and it is the one that we would like to describe in some detail, particularly with respect to its potential for dual-energy subtraction.

Since early 1982, a prototype digital unit dedicated to chest radiography (designed and constructed by Picker International) has been on clinical trial in the Department of Radiology of the Medical Center of the University of Alabama in Birmingham.[69, 70] Briefly, the unit employs a vertical x-ray fan beam that scans transversely across the patient (Fig. 2–7). The beam is defined by a 0.5 mm foreslit collimator positioned between the x-ray tube and the patient, and a 1.0 mm aftslit collimator positioned between the patient and detector array. After traversing the patient and aftslit collimator, the x-ray beam strikes a vertically oriented detector array that consists of 1024 photodiodes coupled to a gadolinium oxysulfide screen. The diodes measure 0.5 mm and are contiguous, resulting in a total array length of 512 mm (1024 pixels) or 20 inches. An equal number of horizontal values is obtained by sampling the pixels over a transverse scan of 20 inches. The photodiode signals are digitized with 12 bit precision by analog-to-digital converters and subsequently compressed to 8 bits. The x-ray tube, collimator slits, and detector array are mechanically

linked together and scan across the patient in 4.5 seconds. The viewing console consists of four 525-line CRT monitors, one for communication with the computer and three for displaying images—one in PA projection, one in lateral projection, and the third providing a two-times magnification zoom image of any selected region of either projection. Images appear on the monitors within 4 seconds of radiographic exposure and can be viewed in either the negative or positive phase. Density and brightness levels can be varied by window and level settings much the same as on CT apparatus. Film copies of the CRT images in either the negative or positive phase can be made with a laser multiformat camera. In contrast to conventional screen/film systems, scatter is virtually nonexistent. The 26 mR entrance skin exposure is comparable to the United States' national average in 1982.

Over a period of a year, approximately 800 patients underwent conventional chest radiography on a dedicated high kV chest unit, followed within

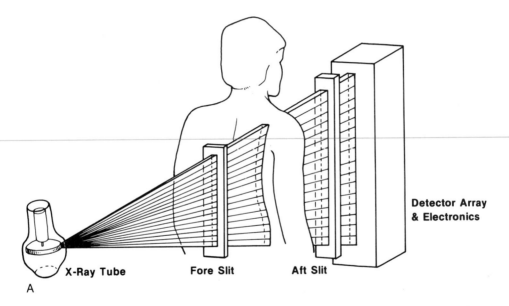

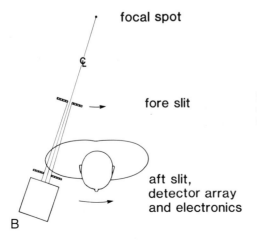

Figure 2–7. Technique of Scanned Digital Radiographic Unit. *A,* Viewed from the side. *B,* Viewed from the top. *See* text for description.

minutes by identical projections on the digital unit across the hall. From these, 50 were selected whose conventional radiographs displayed a variety of appearances, including no abnormality and a wide range of pathologic states (Fig. 2–8). These images were randomized and submitted to seven Board-certified radiologists in order to determine the efficiency of the digital system to depict normal anatomic structures and pathologic states with a degree of accuracy at least equivalent to that of conventional radiographs. The results follow.[71]

(1) The visibility of seven anatomic structures in the mediastinum was consistently better on the digital images than on conventional roentgenograms. In each case, the difference was statistically significant. The improvement was clearly attributable to the facility of digital image manipulation through the window/level capability and the resultant increase in exposure latitude and low contrast detectability.

(2) With minor exceptions, pathologic states were equally well seen in the two systems and in no case was the difference in detectability of abnormalities greater than would be anticipated from interobserver variability.

One of the more exciting developments in digital radiography lies in the technique of dual-energy subtraction. Quantitative radiology—a study by which quantitative data can be obtained for more explicit characterization of normal and pathologic tissues—has been a practical method of investigation for many years, particularly in the field of nuclear medicine and to a lesser extent ultrasound. Similarly, measurements of quantifiable parameters with MRI look very promising although they are still in a rather embryonic stage of development. We now know that the potential exists for digital radiography to provide useful information in tissue characterization, particularly in the identification of calcification. As will be discussed shortly, CT has already made major inroads into the assessment of the calcium content of solitary pulmonary nodules,[72-74] and it is becoming apparent that digital fan-beam radiography of the chest can accomplish the same thing more quickly and less expensively.

The concept of utilizing two photon energies to obtain information on tissue characteristics was first suggested in the early 1950s and has been employed in a variety of techniques ever since. In x-ray imaging, the approach that has generally been employed to obtain the different x-ray photon energy information has been to switch the x-ray tube voltage;[73] typically, x-rays produced at 85 and 135 kV are employed, with additional filtration added to the high kV beam; this technique has been applied to both CT and scan projection radiography but possesses a number of inherent problems and limitations that can be obviated by employing a constant high kV and a dual-energy sensitive x-ray detector.

The latter technique is the one used in the second generation Picker digital radiographic apparatus:[75] a moderately low atomic number phosphor coupled to a photodiode is followed by a high atomic number phosphor/photodiode combination to form a receptor sandwich. The low atomic number section preferentially absorbs the low energy x-ray photons and transmits the majority of high energy photons, a large percentage of which are stopped in the second, higher atomic number section. The resultant image can be separated electronically into two images, one of which depicts structures of high calcium content such as bone, and the other of which reproduces only the soft tissue. The benefits to be derived are obvious, particularly with regard to the identification of calcium within solitary pulmonary nodules and the resultant differentiation of benign and malignant lesions.

Over a three month period in 1985 at the University of Alabama at Birmingham, the potential value of this technique was established beyond reasonable question.[76] Forty-one patients with solitary (occasionally multiple) pulmonary nodules were examined with this technique, employing second-generation fan-beam equipment; all images were subjected to dual-energy subtraction, and the amount of calcium within the nodule or mass was estimated visually on CRT monitors (*see* Figure 4–96, page 597). Twenty-eight nodules or masses were noncalcified, and 13 were calcified. Of the former, 20 were

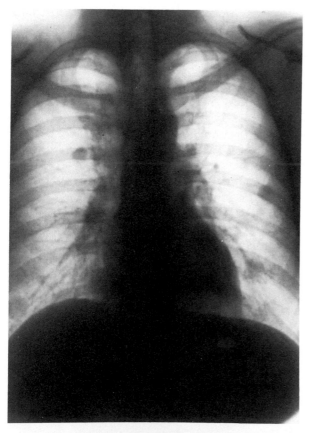

Figure 2–8. Digital Radiography: Image from Prototype Scanned Projection Unit. The image is reproduced in the positive (reverse) phase because of superior rendition of lung detail. Patient has metastatic teratocarcinoma of the testis.

pathologically proved, 16 being malignant and 4 benign (2 granulomas, 2 bronchiectasis); in 3 of the remaining 8, a presumptive diagnosis is reasonably certain (1 granuloma, 2 metastases) while in 5 the diagnosis has not been made. In 8 of the 13 calcified lesions, the diagnosis can reasonably be regarded as confirmed as granulomas; the remaining 5 are being followed with that presumptive diagnosis. It is emphasized that these assessments of the presence or absence of calcium were made by visual inspection of CRT monitors. Algorithms incorporated into the computer software permit precise measurement of the amount of calcium per gram of tissue,[668] and we anticipate that application of these techniques will provide more positive information than is obtainable by simple visual inspection.

CONVENTIONAL TOMOGRAPHY

Techniques

Tomography (synonyms: body section roentgenography, planigraphy, laminagraphy, stratigraphy, and sectional roentgenography) allows selective visibility of a particular layer of tissue to the exclusion of structures lying superficial or deep to it. Regardless of the type of motion employed, the technique involves reciprocal movement of the x-ray tube and film at proportional velocity. The reciprocal motion causes blurring of all structures not continuously "in focus" during excursions of the tube and film, so that the image of only a thin "slice" is recorded in detail on the roentgenogram. The level of tomographic "cut" is controlled by the ratio of the tube-object distance to the object-film distance, so that this level can be altered by varying the ratio. The thickness of the "cut" is governed by the length of tube-film travel—the shorter the excursion, the thicker the layer recorded (zonography). Various reciprocal movements of tube and film have been developed, including rectilinear, circular, elliptic, and hypocycloidal.

Although rectilinear tomography is probably the simplest to perform and most widely available, Littleton and his colleagues[77] have concluded from a recent tomographic study of a fresh frozen human cadaver that a rectilinear tomogram is not a true sectional image and that it does not truthfully represent the planar anatomy of the intended layer; by contrast, pluridirectional tomograms, particularly trispiral, accurately depict the anatomic section in fine detail. These researchers strongly recommend the use of pluridirectional techniques in chest tomography. However, in a more recent study in which full lung linear and pluridirectional tomography were compared in the detection of pulmonary nodules, Bein and associates[78] found no superiority of the latter method, ostensibly because small nodules could remain undetected on slices at 1-cm intervals with the extremely thin (1 mm) focal plane characteristic of the pluridirectional technique.

Indications

With the increasing availability and improved technical quality of CT, we are becoming convinced that this technique should replace conventional tomography in virtually all situations in which morphologic clarification is required. However, for those physicians for whom CT is not available, there are two main indications for standard tomography of the thorax.

1. The need for precise knowledge of the morphologic characteristics of lesions visible on plain roentgenograms, the nature of which is obscured by superimposed images lying superficial and deep to them. Perhaps the best example of this indication is the detection of unsuspected pulmonary cavitation (Fig. 2–9). In a study of 271 tomograms of 172 patients with pulmonary tuberculosis,[79] in 10.7 per cent tomography revealed cavitation unsuspected on conventional roentgenograms: conversely, in 18.8 per cent tomography failed to show cavities suspected on plain roentgenograms. Other examples of this indication include identification of calcium in pulmonary nodules and the separation of potentially confusing hilar shadows.

2. Clearer visibility of shadows that on plain roentgenograms are indistinct because of image summation. The prime example of this indication is study of the bronchi and the pulmonary vasculature. Visibility of the trachea and proximal large bronchi is very clear tomographically. Posterior oblique tomography at an angle of 55 degrees has been recommended for displaying a clearer outline of the anatomic components of the hila.[80]

For some years, the place of full lung tomography in the investigation of metastatic disease has been disputed, but certain general principles now appear to be fairly well accepted. It is well known that if a primary malignant lesion has been eradicated, removal of a single metastasis from the lungs may be curative; therefore, when a single metastatic lesion is identified in a lung on standard roentgenograms, therapeutic and prognostic implications demand thorough tomographic search of both lungs for other metastatic foci. In patients in whom no metastases are identified on plain roentgenograms, the situation is not quite so simple. There is now no doubt that in some patients metastatic lesions will be discovered on full lung tomograms that are not seen on plain roentgenograms: of 410 patients with a variety of malignant neoplasms studied retrospectively by Sindelar and his colleagues,[81] 54 had confirmed metastatic disease; of these, metastases were identified by full lung tomography in 51 patients (94.4 per cent) but in only 36 patients (66.7 per cent) on standard chest roentgenograms. Thus, in this series 15 of the patients with normal chest roentgenograms had metastatic lesions demonstrated on tomograms. This suggests that full lung tomography is indicated in all patients with primary malignant neoplasms arising outside the thorax in whom surgical resection (rather than cytotoxic ther-

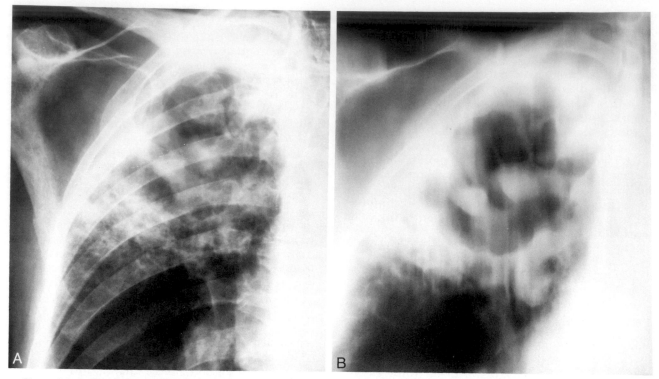

Figured 2–9. The Value of Conventional Tomography in the Demonstration of Pulmonary Cavitation. *A,* A detail view from a conventional posteroanterior chest roentgenogram reveals inhomogeneous consolidation in the subapical region of the right upper lobe. The possibility of a cavity in the consolidation was questioned by the referring radiologist. *B,* An anteroposterior tomogram through the consolidation shows an irregular, thick-walled cavity. The patient is an elderly man who had cough and hemoptysis; *M. tuberculosis* was identified in abundance in the patient's sputum.

apy) is the treatment of choice. However, we suspect that cost-benefit analysis of *all* patients with extrathoracic cancer would show that tomography is of real value only in those with neoplasms that show propensity for spread to the lungs, notably malignant melanoma and primaries arising in the urogenital and skeletal systems. This attitude is lent some support by a recent study by Curtis and her colleagues[82] of 144 patients with proven breast carcinoma and a negative chest roentgenogram in which it was shown convincingly that full lung tomography is not warranted as a screening procedure in these patients, chiefly because of the low propensity for carcinoma of the breast to metastasize to the lungs. Incidentally, if full lung tomography is to be performed for the detection of metastatic pulmonary nodules, a recent study comparing full lung tomograms obtained at 1 and 2 cm intervals showed that the detection rate was significantly improved with 1 cm sections.[78]

Still open to question is the issue of whole lung tomography versus computed tomography (CT) in the investigation of metastatic disease. One of the most thorough studies that has been performed in this regard is that of Muhm and his colleagues,[83] in which 91 patients with known malignancy were studied by both whole lung tomography and computed tomography of the lungs. In 32 (35 per cent) of the 91 patients, more pulmonary nodules were detected by CT than by whole lung tomography. In 5 of the 32 patients, whole lung tomography showed

no pulmonary nodules but CT showed one or more; in 13 patients, one nodule was seen on whole lung tomography but two or more were detected by CT; in an additional 13 patients, bilateral pulmonary nodules were detected by CT after whole lung tomography had demonstrated nodules in only one lung. Of considerable interest was the observation that in 4 of the 91 patients in this series fewer nodules were detected by CT than by whole lung tomography. It seems to us that the final answer is not yet in place on this controversy. The interested reader is directed to two excellent critical reviews of articles dealing with the subject of whole lung tomography and CT in the investigation of pulmonary nodules in metastatic disease.[84]

In summary, there is now little doubt that in patients with primary malignancies that show a propensity for metastasizing to lungs, and for whom surgical rather than cytotoxic therapy is planned, tomography should be carried out before attacking the primary lesion. Evidence that has accumulated to date suggests that the preferred technique in this regard is computed rather than conventional tomography.

COMPUTED TOMOGRAPHY (CT)

Techniques

Since the introduction of this revolutionary British invention into North America in 1973, clinical evaluation of the technique has burgeoned and has demonstrated beyond question its enormous value in the investigation and diagnosis of disease. Although initially its use in the diagnosis of intracranial disease was undoubtedly of greatest value, the development of the body scanner has enabled us to look into the thorax and abdomen and see things heretofore beyond the scope of diagnostic techniques. CT of the thorax serves as a noninvasive technique capable of demonstrating soft tissue structures and of detecting small differences in their densities.

A computed tomographic scan consists of a group of images of the body in a series of transverse slices. It replaces the standard transmission roentgenographic image with a system that measures the quantity of x-ray photons that are absorbed by the different elements within the body. Briefly, the technique involves the rotation of a single beam of x-rays 360 degrees around the body in 1 degree steps, taking measurements of the transmitted radiation at each interval during rotation. The x-ray beam is collimated to a width ranging from 5 to 12 mm so that each scan represents a slice of body of that thickness. Obviously, multiple slices are required to cover the whole thorax.

As in most roentgenographic procedures, the variable forming the CT image is the difference in x-ray attenuation properties of various tissues; for example, the attenuation coefficient of fat is less than that of muscle, which is less than that of bone, thus permitting their distinction. In CT, a series of profiles of x-ray attenuations is obtained at different angles to the object examined. By the use of a computer-applied algorithm, these profiles yield cross-sectional images of the x-ray attenuation coefficients. These images depict anatomic structures and pathologic alterations invisible by conventional radiologic techniques. As pointed out by Ter-Pogossian,[85] the success of CT stems from three factors: (1) utilization of a narrow beam of x-rays and highly collimated detectors to provide a signal that is nearly free of scattered radiation; (2) the properties of CT detectors to be significantly more free of noise than conventional screen-film combinations; and (3) reconstruction of a cross-sectional image unencumbered by superimposed activity. Anatomic structures often can be identified by CT although the difference in their attenuation coefficients is negligible, provided these structures are separated by interfaces of different attenuation properties; for instance, in the abdomen the liver and pancreas can be distinguished from each other and from other structures because of the presence of fat-containing interfaces of low attenuation. In addition, the attenuation coefficient of one tissue compared with another can be established in relative terms by determining their "CT numbers." This simple procedure can be greatly aided by the intravenous injection of a contrast medium, which brings about a rise in CT numbers in proportion to the blood content of the tissue being measured; for example, contrast enhancement will usually permit distinction of a mediastinal cyst from an aortic aneurysm or a highly vascular solid neoplasm.

A spate of articles appears each year describing new indications for CT of the thorax, and it is difficult or impossible to keep up with the flood, particularly in a textbook to be published some years in the future. However, we have selected a few articles that have been published in recent years that have attempted to place the subject in reasonable perspective, and these are recommended for further reading.[86–91] Throughout the remainder of this book, indications for CT examination in specific disease entities are discussed in the appropriate sections.

The Society for Computed Body Tomography published a series of indications for body CT;[92] the following, with some modification, represent the recommendations of that organization. Although these undoubtedly will be modified as experience grows, they constitute a reasonable summary of current indications. These indications can conveniently be divided into abnormalities affecting the mediastinum, lungs, pleura, and chest wall.

MEDIASTINUM

Evaluation of Problems Identified on Standard Chest Roentgenograms. The differentiation of the cystic or solid nature of mediastinal masses, the localization of such masses relative to other mediastinal structures and to some extent the determination of their composition (*e.g.*, adipose tissue); the assessment of whether mediastinal widening is pathologic or is simply an anatomic variation or caused by physiologic fat deposition; the distinction of a solid mass from a vascular anomaly or aneurysm (generally by contrast enhancement); the differentiation of a dilated pulmonary artery from a solid mass in a hilum (*e.g.*, enlarged lymph nodes) when conventional tomography fails or is not capable of making this distinction (however, see further on); the differentiation of lymph node enlargement, vascular abnormality, or anatomic variant in the presence of deformity of the paraspinal line; and finally, determination of the presence and extent of mediastinal spread in patients with pulmonary carcinoma.

Search for Occult Thymic Lesions. The detection of thymoma or hyperplasia in selected patients with myasthenia gravis when standard chest roentgenograms are negative or suspicious.

LUNGS

Search for Pulmonary Lesions. The detection of occult pulmonary metastases when extensive surgery is planned for a known primary neoplasm with a high propensity for lung metastases or when a solitary lung metastasis is identified on a chest roentgenogram; the detection of a primary neoplasm in a patient with positive sputum cytology and negative chest roentgenography and fiberoptic bronchoscopy.

Search for Diffuse or Central Calcification. The search for calcium in a pulmonary nodule when conventional tomography is indeterminate. In this regard, the exciting results obtained by Siegelman and his colleagues in the differentiation of benign and malignant solitary pulmonary nodules are worthy of note.[93] By assessing CT numbers from thin sections of 91 apparently noncalcified pulmonary nodules in 88 patients, these investigators showed that benign lesions had relatively high CT numbers, presumably because of diffuse calcification, and that malignant lesions had comparatively lower numbers.

PLEURA

Detection of Pleural Effusion. When its presence may be obscured by a pulmonary opacity and when simpler roentgenographic techniques or ultrasound fail to clarify; assessment of the postpneumonectomy fibrothorax for recurrent disease.

Determination of the Extent of Pleural Involvement. In the investigation of selected patients with pulmonary carcinoma.

CHEST WALL

Determination of the Extent of Neoplastic Disease. Assessment of bone, muscle, and subcutaneous tissue involvement and the detection of intrusion into the thoracic cavity or spinal canal.

Additional indications might include assisting in the percutaneous biopsy of lesions such as mediastinal masses when fluoroscopic guidance is inadequate; the localization of loculated collections of fluid within the pleural space when standard roentgenographic, fluoroscopic, or ultrasonic techniques prove inadequate; and (possibly) the early detection of pulmonary emphysema and determination of its severity.[94]

In a prospective study, Mintzer and his colleagues[95] compared the value of conventional chest tomography and CT in the evaluation of 100 patients with proved chest malignancies. Generally, the mediastinum was better assessed by CT, particularly in identifying neoplastic invasion. By contrast, conventional tomograms were found to be more useful in evaluating the hila. In the study as a whole, either full lung tomography or CT (or both) directly affected therapy in 18 patients. In a more recent study in which plain roentgenography, conventional tomography, and computed tomography were compared in the detection of intrathoracic lymph node metastases from lung carcinoma,[96] it was shown that all modalities demonstrated about the same accuracy; however, in patients with hilar or mediastinal lymph node enlargement (or both),

CT was more sensitive but not more specific than the other two, and conventional tomography was no more accurate than CT for hilar evaluation.

MAGNETIC RESONANCE IMAGING (MRI)

When certain atomic nuclei are placed in a magnetic field and stimulated by radio waves of a particular frequency, they will re-emit some of the absorbed energy in the form of radio signals. This phenomenon, known as nuclear magnetic resonance, has been used since shortly after World War II by organic chemists, biochemists, and physicists to identify and analyze spectroscopically intricate molecules in liquids or solids. During the early 1970s, several investigators began exploring the possibility that the technique could also produce images of sufficient resolution for medical purposes, and with the advances that have been made during the past two years there is no doubt that MR imaging will have a major impact on the practice of medicine in the future. The physical principles involved in the production of an MR image are highly complex and have been detailed in a number of review articles.[97–103]

PHYSICAL PRINCIPLES

With the exception of the hydrogen nucleus, which consists of a single proton, atomic nuclei contain both protons and neutrons. The constituent nucleons (the generic term for a proton or neutron) each possess an intrinsic angular moment or "spin"; however, since pairs of protons or neutrons align in such a way that their spins cancel out, a *net* spin will exist for a nucleus only when it contains an odd (unpaired) proton or an odd neutron or both. This intrinsic spin has an associated magnetic moment so that each nucleus may be considered to act as a small bar magnet. When these nuclei are exposed to a magnetic field, they experience a torque, their axis of spin rotating about the field direction as the nuclei attempt to line up parallel to the magnetic field. Any nucleus possesses a characteristic resonant or "precessional" frequency that is determined by the magnetic field strength and a constant (the gyromagnetic ratio which takes into account the magnetic properties of the nuclear species in question); the pulse of radio frequency (RF) radiation must be of precisely the same frequency as the precessional frequency of the nucleus (also known as the Larmor frequency). The coordinates of the magnetic field and the net magnetization vectors are usually described using a three-dimensional coordinate system in which the z axis is parallel to the magnetic lines of force and the x and y axes are perpendicular both to each other and to the z axis (Fig. 2–10).

To induce the magnetic resonance phenomenon, a short RF pulse is applied via a coil surround-

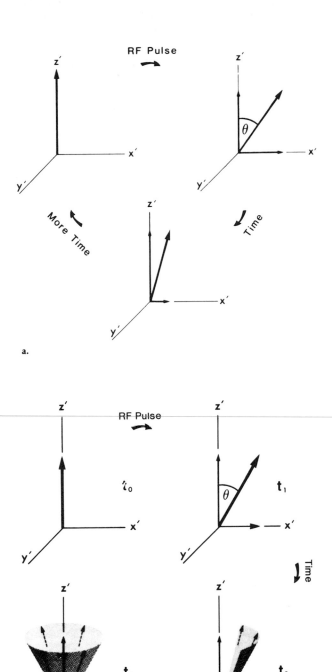

a.

b.

c.

Figure 2–10. Relaxation Behavior of the Macroscopic Magnetic Moment in the Rotating Reference Frame, and Decay of the Nuclear Signal. The coordinate axes rotating at the Larmor frequency are denoted x', y', and z'.

A, Before the RF pulse, the magnetic moment is aligned with the z' axis. Immediately following a $\theta°$ pulse, the vector makes an angle θ with the z' axis. The component in the x' direction generates the nuclear signal. The vector then relaxes back to its equilibrium position, and the z' component of magnetization increases exponentially with a time constant T_1. T_1 relaxation is one mechanism responsible for reduction of the x' component and hence also for diminution of the amplitude of the nuclear signal.

B, Immediately following the RF pulse, the vector is displaced from the z' axis. T_2 relaxation then occurs simultaneously with spin-lattice (T_1) relaxation. Internuclear magnetic interactions and field inhomogeneities slightly alter the local magnetic fields experienced by the various nuclei, and some begin to precess at different rates. The components of magnetization in the x',y' plane therefore fan out, the RF signal becomes out of phase, and the signal starts to decay with a time constant T_2. Eventually, the components of magnetization in the x',y' plane will be randomly distributed. There will be no net signal emitted, even though complete spin-lattice relaxation may not yet have occurred.

C, The exponential fall of the free induction decay (FID) signal arises from dephasing of the transverse (x',y' plane) components of magnetization. At time t_1 immediately following application of the RF pulse, the nuclei all precess in phase and the nuclear signal strength is greatest. At time t_2, some dephasing of the magnetization has occurred and the signal is diminished. At time t_3, the components of magnetization are distributed randomly in the x',y' plane, and the FID amplitude approaches zero.

(From Pykett IL, Newhouse JH, Buonanno FS, et al: Radiology *143*:157, 1982.)

ing the sample, the RF radiation being equivalent to the application of a second, smaller magnetic field (Fig. 2–10). The radio frequency signal changes the state of the protons in the magnetic field from one of equilibrium to one of excitation. This excited state is inherently unstable and will naturally decay toward the equilibrium state over a period of time. As the nuclei "relax" to their original alignment in the magnetic field, they radiate to their surroundings the absorbed energy at their characteristic or Larmor frequency. The re-emitted energy provides a signal that can be detected by a receiver coil wrapped around the sample; if there are a sufficient number of these signals and if they can be spatially resolved, an image of the distribution of the emitting nuclei can be formed.

The signal strength during emission diminishes exponentially with a characteristic "relaxation time" that is determined in part by the general environment of the nuclei. The greater the facility to pass energy to neighboring nuclei, the more rapidly the irradiated nuclei can return to their original energy state; hence, a shorter relaxation time. There are two relaxation times, T_1 and T_2.

T_1: Once nuclei have been energized by an RF pulse, T_1 is the time constant corresponding to the exponential restoration of the magnetization *parallel* to the external field (Fig. 2–11); to put it another way, T_1 represents the time required for the component of the net magnetization vector in the z direction to return to its initial value after it has been perturbed by the RF pulse (Figs. 2–10 and 2–11). T_1 is also known as the spin-lattice or longitudinal relaxation time. In a pure liquid, the return to equilibrium is exponential, and after three T_1s have elapsed, 95 per cent of the original magnetization will have been restored.

T_2: T_2 is the time constant corresponding to the exponential decay of the magnetization *perpendicular* to the external field and is also known as the spin-spin relaxation time. After an RF pulse has tipped the nuclear magnetization vector toward the transverse plane, the components of this vector all precess together or "in phase" and therefore appear to be stationary in the rotating reference frame. However, the precession does not remain in phase. Subtle local alterations of the magnetic field strength cause some nuclei to precess at different rates from others; the RF waves from individual nuclei dephase and cancel each other out, and the sum of nuclear magnetization vectors in the transverse plane decays to zero. The time constant for this dephasing or decay is called T_2. The T_2 or spin-spin relaxation time provides additional data about the local environment in which the hydrogen nuclei reside. During the measuring pulse, the precessing protons are brought into phase with the frequency of the radio signal (Fig. 2–11). When the signal is turned off, all the dipoles are rotating together in phase; however, with the passage of time some of the dipoles will precess more rapidly than others,

becoming progressively more out of phase relative to one another. When they have become sufficiently out of phase, all the dipoles are canceled by an equal and opposite dipole interaction, causing the signal to cease. The time that it takes the signal to stop is called T_2.

For water and simple liquids, T_1 and T_2 are equal and about 5 sec, whereas for solids, T_2 is distinctly shorter than T_1. The factors that determine T_1 and T_2 are numerous; for example, the two relaxation times are most sensitive to the degree of molecular motion. In solids and at low temperatures, there is little molecular motion, and T_1 may be many seconds whereas T_2 is only microseconds. However, in liquids and at higher temperatures, T_1 and T_2 are almost equal. T_2 can never be longer than T_1 and is often substantially shorter. Thus, if the ratio of T_2 to T_1 approaches unity, the sample may be assumed to be relatively liquid-like; if the ratio is very small, the sample may be assumed to be relatively solid.

Currently MR images with a 256×256 array of data points are being acquired in times of 4 to 8 minutes. Although there are grounds for believing that future MR images with higher spatial resolution and more favorable signal-to-noise ratios will be produced, they will continue to be time dependent and in all likelihood will be slower in acquisition than is CT. Since the data used to produce an MR image are averaged, motion results in decreased spatial resolution rather than complete image distortion as in CT, although there is little doubt that gating, both cardiac and respiratory, will markedly diminish reconstruction artifacts because of motion.

MR Pulse Sequences

The radiofrequency pulse duration determines the extent to which the net magnetization rotates with respect to its original alignment. For example, a 90° pulse rotates the net magnetization 90°; similarly, a 180° pulse rotates the net magnetization 180°. An appropriate sequence of radiofrequency pulses may be used to emphasize either the T_1 or T_2 portion of the MR signal or to improve the efficiency of data accumulation.[104] The more common pulse sequences include saturation recovery, inversion recovery, and spin-echo.

Saturation Recovery. This sequence utilizes two 90° pulses separated by a time interval, T. This time interval is set to be longer than T_2 but shorter than T_1; thus, the second pulse arrives before T_1 relaxation is complete. The signal obtained depends upon the extent of relaxation that has occurred during time interval T.[104]

Inversion Recovery. If a 180° pulse is applied to a sample in equilibrium with a magnetic field, the net magnetization rotates so that it points in the opposite direction to the field. The magnetization will at once begin to revert to its original state at a rate determined by T_1. After some particular time,

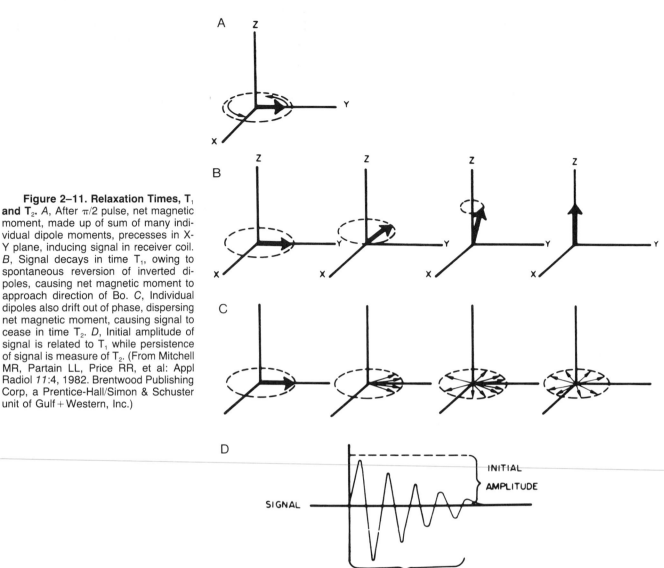

Figure 2–11. Relaxation Times, T$_1$ and T$_2$. *A*, After $\pi/2$ pulse, net magnetic moment, made up of sum of many individual dipole moments, precesses in X-Y plane, inducing signal in receiver coil. *B*, Signal decays in time T$_1$, owing to spontaneous reversion of inverted dipoles, causing net magnetic moment to approach direction of Bo. *C*, Individual dipoles also drift out of phase, dispersing net magnetic moment, causing signal to cease in time T$_2$. *D*, Initial amplitude of signal is related to T$_1$ while persistence of signal is measure of T$_2$. (From Mitchell MR, Partain LL, Price RR, et al: Appl Radiol *11*:4, 1982. Brentwood Publishing Corp, a Prentice-Hall/Simon & Schuster unit of Gulf + Western, Inc.)

the residual net magnetization, whether it is still opposed to or aligned with field, can be measured by rotating it by 90°, so that it produces a coherent induced signal in a measuring coil. The amplitude of this signal will depend on the time interval between the 180° and 90° pulses and on T$_1$, so that the latter can be estimated by measuring the signal obtained at two or more different time intervals.

Spin-Echo (SE). In this sequence, a 90° pulse rotates the net magnetization into the xy plane. The nuclear magnets, which are initially phase coherent, will begin to spin out of phase; after a time period, T, a 180° pulse is applied following which the magnetization partially refocuses to form an echo signal after a time (Fig. 2–12).[104] According to Gore and associates,[97] the effect is like that on a group of runners, who, because they move at different speeds, spread out as they get farther from the start line; if they are suddenly told that they are running in the wrong direction, they will all turn around and, since the farthest away are the fastest, will all

arrive back at the start line together.[105] Spin-echo may be used to determine T$_2$ without contamination from inhomogeneity effects of the magnetic field.[102]

In addition to these sequences is the MR parameter, free induction decay (FID) or spin density, the number of nuclear signals per unit volume or the concentration of nuclei of interest in the area to be studied. Assuming an adequate spin-density, an MR image is dependent largely upon relaxation times and selected pulse sequences.

IMAGING NUCLEI

The most commonly studied nucleus is the proton contained in the hydrogen atoms of water and fat because of its strong signal and its abundance in human tissue. The development of other imaging nuclei has been the goal of several groups, but the difficulties imposed by their relative scarcity and weak signal strength have proved formidable. For example, since the ratio of ^{31}P to protons in

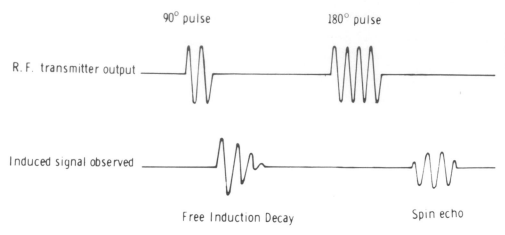

Figure 2–12. A Spin-Echo 90-τ-180-τ Pulse Sequence for Measuring T_2. The 90° pulse produces a signal proportional to the initial magnetization induced by the static field. The signal decays partly because of spin-spin interactions but also because the static field is not perfectly homogeneous. The 180° pulse applied after time τ reflects the spins about a fixed axis normal to the field direction so that they refocus to give an echo signal at time 2τ. The echo amplitude, M(2τ), is given by

$$M(2\tau) = M(o)e - \frac{2\tau}{T_2}$$

independent of field imperfections. (From Gore JC, Emery EW, Orr JS, et al: Invest Radiol *16*:269, 1981.)

human organs and tissues is 10^{-3} to 10^{-5} and since ^{31}P MR signals are weak, images comparable to those produced by proton MR at present are exceedingly difficult or impossible to obtain. Other potential nuclei include ^{13}C, ^{15}N, [17]O, ^{19}F, [23]Na, [33]S, [35]Cl, and [39]K.[106] Contrast agents for proton imaging such as gadolinium (Gd-DTPA) may also prove of value with time.[107]

POTENTIAL CLINICAL USES

Certain supporters of MRI have promoted the concept that although disease has traditionally been regarded in pathologic/anatomic terms, MR techniques may allow investigation in chemical/physiologic terms. Since chemical and physiologic alterations may precede changes in anatomy or pathology, MR becomes an especially attractive diagnostic method. For example, malignant tissue generally has a longer relaxation time than normal tissue although there is much overlap in the value of relaxation times. The following is a rough cross-section of the recent literature dealing with various thoracic diseases; each of these will be discussed in more detail in pertinent chapters of the book.

Hilar Masses and Lymph Nodes. In a retrospective study of 144 patients,[108] MR and CT gave similar results with abnormal lymph nodes measuring more than 13 or 15 mm in diameter, but MR displayed these nodes better because of its excellent soft tissue contrast resolution. In 12 patients with unilateral or bilateral hilar masses, Webb and his colleagues[109] were able to differentiate the mass from hilar vasculature more easily with MR than with contrast-enhanced CT; in 5 of these patients, hilar lymph nodes approximately 1 cm in diameter were easily seen using MR but were difficult or impossible to appreciate prospectively on CT.

Mediastinal Masses. In eight patients with benign mediastinal masses who underwent both CT and MR imaging, Gamsu and his colleagues[110]

found that the intensity difference between mass and surrounding mediastinal fat was greater on MR than on CT; however, although the masses were clearly identified with both modalities, delineation of a mass from surrounding mediastinal structures was better on CT. A number of articles have emphasized the advantage of coronal and sagittal images of the thorax in the evaluation of mediastinal disease:[111–113, 669] in two of three patients with thoracic masses reported in one of these series,[111] sagittal or coronal MR provided significant anatomic information that was either less evident or invisible on transaxial MR or CT images or reformations. In a more recent MR study of 75 patients with mediastinal masses, von Schulthess and his colleagues[4] found that MR depicted all masses and demonstrated compromise of vessels and cardiac chambers as a result of the inherent contrast between the masses and cardiovascular structures; in fact, vascular compromise was better assessed with MR than with CT. They concluded that while the anatomic information is comparable to that produced by CT, MR provides some insight into the composition of the mass.

Pulmonary Embolism. In an experimental study in dogs, Gamsu and his coworkers[114] found that MR imaging possesses considerable potential for the demonstration of relatively small pulmonary emboli and recommended clinical trials in patients. Two reports[115, 116] have documented the detection of pulmonary emboli by MRI in individual patients.

Pulmonary Edema. In a study by Skalina and his associates[117] of the effect of permeability pulmonary edema on proton MR relaxation times, a linear relationship was found between the relaxation times and the amount of extravascular lung water. They pointed out that any diffuse alveolar process, including edema, may increase proton density. In a more recent MR study of permeability and hydrostatic edema in animals, Schmidt and his associates[5] showed that hydrostatic pulmonary edema demonstrated similar T_1 but markedly shorter T_2 relaxation times than permeability edema, and that MRI can be used to estimate the severity of both types of edema.

Radiation Fibrosis. In one patient, MRI accurately differentiated recurrent pulmonary neoplasm from contiguous radiation fibrosis by dint of the presence of two components—a high intensity part (the recurrent cancer) and a contiguous low intensity part (the radiation fibrosis).[118]

Fibrosing Mediastinitis. In two patients with pulmonary vascular occlusion caused by fibrosing mediastinitis, MRI and CT findings were similar; however, because of the high contrast between flowing blood and vessel wall afforded by a spin-echo sequence, obstruction of mediastinal vessels was demonstrated by MRI without the use of contrast media.[119]

Aortic Disease. In four patients with aortic dissection, MRI permitted identification of intimal flaps and determination of the origin of aortic branches from either of two lumens.[120] MRI has also been found to be useful in the initial diagnosis and postoperative follow-up of a patient with a posttraumatic false aortic aneurysm.[121]

Thoracic Disease in Children. MRI has been reported to be particularly valuable in delineating mediastinal and parenchymal masses from adjacent vascular structures without the need for contrast media enhancement.[122] In addition, the absence of an irradiation hazard is of obvious importance in this age group.

COMPARISON OF MR AND CT IMAGING

MRI possesses a number of general advantages over CT that are of considerable importance: for example, in contrast to the radiation hazard in CT imaging, there is no known significant biologic risk to the use of magnetic and RF probes in the human body at current imaging levels. Also, MR imaging requires no moving parts; therefore, the permutations in MRI are the result of bioelectronic manipulation, eliminating the mechanical problems that occur with CT. This allows tomographic reconstruction of planes in the coronal, sagittal, transverse, or oblique directions without movement of the patient.

A few comparison studies of the diagnostic efficacy of the two modalities have been reported, and many more can be anticipated. The efficacy of MRI of the mediastinum and hila was investigated by Cohen and his colleagues,[123] who performed MR scans in 22 patients selected on the basis of an abnormal CT: in all cases the high contrast resolution of MRI in the mediastinum allowed clear definition of 19 malignant and 4 benign processes, and in 6 patients MRI demonstrated a greater extent of disease than did CT. It was concluded that MRI is as useful as CT, or more so, in the evaluation of malignant disease of the hila and mediastinum. In another comparison study,[124] it was concluded that with current technology without respiratory or car-

diac gating, MRI offers little improvement over contrast-enhanced CT in the diagnosis of benign and malignant processes involving the pleura, chest wall, mediastinum, hila, and pulmonary parenchyma: of 18 patients examined with both modalities, 15 of the MR scans were considered to be as diagnostic as CT in demonstrating abnormalities. However, in two cases CT was superior to MR, and in one case without adequate vascular opacification on CT, MR was superior in differentiating a mass from the pulmonary artery.

Undoubtedly the most comprehensive study to date was performed at the Mayo Clinic and reported in February, 1985, by Baker and his colleagues.[125] These researchers analyzed the results of MRI in the first 1000 consecutive patients studied by this technique, emphasizing the value of this procedure in comparison with CT and other imaging modalities. The unit employed a 0.15-tesla resistive magnet. Within the chest, because spatial resolution was noticeably better with CT than with MRI and because small pulmonary tumors and mediastinal masses were generally obscured by motion (there was no capability for gating, either cardiac or respiratory), CT was preferred by most observers. However, the superior density discrimination and the additional data collected from the sagittal and coronal images of MRI were deemed to be of considerable diagnostic value in many cases. Distinguishing hilar nodes or masses from pulmonary vessels was more easily accomplished with MRI than with CT without contrast enhancement. More specifically, MRI was found to be superior to CT in detecting certain lesions in pediatric patients, equal to CT in detecting many chest lesions, and inferior to CT in detecting thymoma, parathyroid adenoma, and small pulmonary nodules.

In three more recent articles dealing with the efficacy of MR and CT in the staging of pulmonary carcinoma[1, 2] and in the imaging of mediastinal and hilar masses,[3] it was generally agreed that CT and MR provide comparable information regarding the presence and size of mediastinal lymph nodes and the curative resectability or nonresectability of bronchogenic carcinoma. However, in each of these studies it was seen that small, contiguous lymph nodes shown individually by CT can appear as a single, enlarged mass by MR as a result of partial-volume averaging, and that although MR better discriminates mediastinal nodes from vascular structures, apparently enlarged nodes may not contain neoplasm. Levitt and his colleagues[3] concluded that because of the requirement for patient selection and the identified pitfalls of MRI, CT remains, for the present, the imaging procedure of choice in the staging of patients with pulmonary carcinoma.

BRONCHOGRAPHY

Physicians in general and radiologists in particular are becoming increasingly concerned about the efficacy of certain roentgenologic procedures in clarifying the nature of an illness. This concern derives partly from a desire to reduce the burgeoning costs of medical care (by restricting diagnostic procedures to their most productive minimum) and partly from a growing awareness that the discovery rate of some procedures is low in relation to patient benefit. In our opinion,[126] bronchography is one of these procedures. Avery joins in this opinion by suggesting that bronchography may be an "outmoded procedure."[127]

Perhaps more than any other roentgenologic procedure, bronchography has been the subject of controversy as to its value in the diagnosis of pulmonary disease. Supporters of the procedure (who, we suspect, are in the minority) speak enthusiastically of its ability to distinguish infectious from neoplastic pulmonary lesions by revealing characteristic deformity of the airways.[128] Although bronchography probably can provide this differentiation in some situations, the question remains: if efficacious treatment depends on identification of the offending microorganisms or neoplastic cells, why employ bronchography to make a *general* distinction between the two processes in the first place? With few exceptions, to which reference is made further on, the *diagnosis* of pulmonary disease depends on microbiologic or morphologic examination, and the many recently developed procedures to obtain adequate material for study permit precise diagnosis in most cases without recourse to bronchography. Biopsies of most lesions affecting the major airways can be performed bronchoscopically, and prior roentgenographic location of the lesion is usually as accurate by tomography as by bronchography—and with considerably less hazard. With few exceptions, biopsies of lesions in the lung periphery beyond the reach of the bronchoscope can be done by transthoracic needle or bronchial brush—or the diagnosis may have been confirmed already by cytologic examination of sputum or bronchial washings.

Despite its ease of performance, bronchography should never be carried out without due consideration of its potential hazards. Apart from the very real danger of allergic reaction to either the topical anesthesia or the bronchographic medium itself or both (ranging from bronchospasm through iodism to frank anaphylaxis and death), bronchography gives rise to a temporary impairment of ventilation and diffusion that should not be disregarded, especially in patients with respiratory insufficiency.[129, 130] Furthermore, the injection of 10 to 15 ml of foreign material into a lung must give rise to a foreign body reaction, to however small a degree.[131–138] Another potential hazard of bronchography, particularly but not exclusively in infants and children, is the pulmonary collapse that results from airway obstruction, chiefly due to occlusion of distal airways.[139] Robinson and his colleagues detected segmental pulmonary collapse in 75 of 165 pediatric bronchograms (45 per cent).[140] Pulmonary collapse appeared to correlate with the

more readily diffusible gas mixtures used in general anesthesia, particularly halothane, with a contribution by aqueous contrast agents. There was no apparent correlation with the amount of contrast material used, duration of the study, or premedication. In subsequent experiments by the same researchers,[140] in which bronchography was performed on anesthetized dogs, segmental collapse occurred in 10 of 11 dogs given 100 per cent oxygen during bronchography but in none of 9 ventilated with room air; the mean reduction in arterial oxygen tension was 58 per cent in the former group but only 30 per cent in the latter. In view of the high incidence of pulmonary collapse with general anesthesia for bronchography in children, Wilson and colleagues[141] advocate topical anesthesia in such circumstances: no serious complications occurred in 575 infants and children thus studied. Although probably the gaseous mixture used for ventilation was the major cause of collapse in the Robinson study, obstruction by the bronchographic medium undoubtedly played a role. It would seem logical, therefore, to use a contrast medium such as powdered tantalum that tends to coat the bronchial mucosa rather than plug its lumen. This advantage was confirmed by Gamsu and his coworkers,[142] who reported absence of pulmonary collapse following a total of 15 bronchograms with powdered tantalum in 13 patients ranging in age from 13 days to 16 years.

Indications

As with most special diagnostic procedures, the indications for bronchography vary widely in different institutions. Our own experience has led us to adopt a conservative approach, not only because more direct diagnostic procedures are more informative and less hazardous, but also because with some conditions (e.g., hemoptysis in association with normal chest roentgenogram) bronchography has a low discovery rate.

In our view, there is only one indication for bronchography—the investigation of the presence and extent of bronchiectasis, and then only when the clinical state of the patient is such that surgical resection of local disease could be performed with benefit. Although the plain roentgenogram reveals bronchiectasis in approximately 93 per cent of patients with the disease,[143] only bronchography shows its severity and distribution. Whenever bronchiectasis is suspected or proved and surgery is contemplated, all 19 bronchopulmonary segments must be identified bronchographically to exclude abnormality in areas in which no changes are apparent on the plain roentgenogram. One cautionary note: simple dilatation of segmental bronchi without destruction—reversible bronchiectasis—is a frequent concomitant of acute pneumonia and, although temporary, may persist as long as 3 to 4 months. During this period, bronchography may reveal bronchial deformity indistinguishable from irreversible cylindrical bronchiectasis; despite clinical suspicion of chronic disease, therefore, definitive investigation should be postponed for at least 4 months after acute pneumonia.

It is emphasized that in a patient with hemoptysis and a normal chest roentgenogram, bronchography rarely reveals abnormality and seldom is indicated, an opinion with which Forrest and his associates are in complete agreement.[144] We believe that the most logical next step in the investigation of these patients should be CT; should this prove unrevealing and if the hemoptysis is potentially exsanguinating, pulmonary or bronchial arteriography (or both) can be resorted to. A similar but more vexing problem develops when sputum cytology findings are repeatedly positive for malignant cells but the plain roentgenographic and bronchoscopic appearances are normal. In such cases, we find bronchography just as unrevealing as in cases of hemoptysis from an unidentified site; as with hemoptysis, we feel that the most logical next step in the investigation of these patients is a CT scan. If the scan is normal, watchful waiting is recommended, with plain roentgenograms taken at 3 month intervals or less until either a lesion is demonstrated or the length of the follow-up has excluded a reasonable possibility of neoplasm (false-positive cytologic findings).

The bronchographic techniques most widely used include supraglottic injection, the transglottic catheter method (the catheter is inserted through the glottis via the nose or mouth), and the percutaneous cricothyroid technique (administration directly through a needle,[145] or by a modified Seldinger technique[135, 146, 147]). We prefer the transglottic technique, in which a soft rubber urethral catheter is inserted through the larynx via a naris and into a selected site in the bronchial tree.

ANGIOGRAPHY

This includes all procedures in which contrast media are injected into the vascular structures of the thorax for investigating thoracic disease. These methods include pulmonary angiography, angiocardiography, aortography, bronchial arteriography, superior vena cava angiography, and azygography. Only the general indications for their use are considered here; detailed discussion in relation to specific diseases is presented in relevant chapters.

Our attitude toward thoracic angiography is clearly more conservative than that of many others. In several situations in which others successfully employ angiography, such as assessing the operability of lung cancer, we rely more heavily on traditional methods of roentgenologic investigation, including CT scanning. It is inevitable that the contents of this book reflect this attitude. However, to disregard the experience of others would be negligent; therefore, wherever these procedures are mentioned, our discussion of angiographic techniques and findings is based largely on the observations of others.

Pulmonary Angiography

TECHNIQUE

Depending upon individual circumstances, pulmonary angiography can be performed by various routes: (a) by venous injection into one arm or both arms simultaneously, through a needle or, preferably, a catheter; (b) via a catheter into the superior vena cava, right atrium, right ventricle, or main pulmonary artery; or (c) by selective injection into the right or left pulmonary artery or one of its branches. In pulmonary angiography, as in all other special angiographic procedures, individual requirements for each examination must be determined in relation to the specific circumstances. For example, when there is a pulmonary neoplasm arising in the paramediastinal zone and the integrity of the superior vena cava is in doubt, substantially more information can be gained if pulmonary angiography is performed via an arm vein rather than by intracardiac or pulmonary artery injection.

Generally speaking, however, direct injection into the main pulmonary artery or one of its branches invariably produces clearer opacification of the pulmonary vascular tree than does venous or intracardiac injection; the superior visibility usually outweighs any disadvantage inherent in the catheterization procedure. An additional benefit of selective injection has been described by Cicero and del Castillo.[148] These investigators performed 146 examinations on 137 patients, each of whom was subjected to two procedures—filling of the entire pulmonary arterial tree by injection into the right side of the heart, and segmental angiography by placement of the catheter in the artery of the segment being studied—and reported superior results with the second method. This finding relates to the fact that a diseased segment of the arterial tree causes blood to be shunted away from that segment, so that a flood injection tends to opacify comparatively normal branches remote from the disease. Similarly, wedge angiography[149] and magnification techniques[150, 151] provide improved visibility of small peripheral arterial and venous branches.[152] Visibility of the mediastinal portion of the pulmonary arteries can be improved by caudal angulation of the x-ray tube perpendicular to the long axis of the main pulmonary artery;[153] the method is said to minimize superimposition of major vessels.

Digital subtraction angiography (DSA) is an imaging modality whose clinical application at the time of writing has been somewhat controversial; the technique has had considerable success in angiography of the cervical and the abdominal vessels[163–165] but has received mixed reviews as a method of examining the pulmonary vasculature, chiefly in the investigation of possible pulmonary embolism.[166–170]

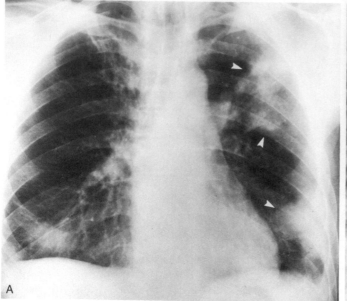

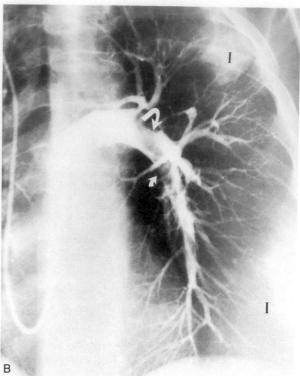

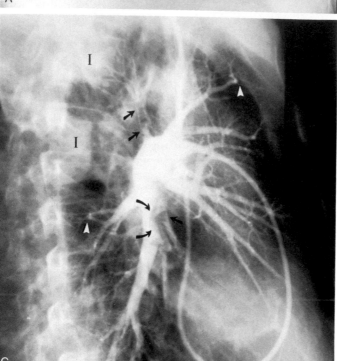

Figure 2–13. The Value of Pulmonary Angiography in the Demonstration of Thromboembolism. *A,* A conventional posteroanterior chest roentgenogram discloses multiple areas of consolidation (*arrowheads*) that relate closely to a pleural surface. A selective left pulmonary angiogram in oblique (*B*) and lateral (*C*) projection (arterial phase) demonstrates multiple intraluminal filling defects (*arrows*) and amputated peripheral arteries (*arrowheads*). Note that the vascular abnormalities subtend the infarcts identified on the conventional study (*I* in *B* and *C*). Similar findings were present in the right pulmonary artery (not shown). Features are diagnostic of pulmonary thromboembolism and infarction. The patient is a 26-year-old man who had acute dyspnea and pleuritic chest pain 48 hours following an extended intercontinental airplane flight.

In a study of 14 patients suspected of having pulmonary embolism,[171] useful clinical information was obtained in 13; in 9 critically ill patients, the procedure was performed through pulmonary artery catheters already in place for monitoring pressures. Problems have arisen from two main sources: the limited area of coverage provided by currently available image intensifiers and the misregistration of the subtraction images caused by respiratory motion. Electrocardiographic gating has been shown to improve image sharpness[168] but may not be effective in patients with marked tachycardia. Despite these problems, preliminary studies in both animals[168, 169] and humans[166, 170] have produced promising results, and it is possible that future improvements in equipment design will result in DSA becoming a safe and reliable technique for the diagnosis of pulmonary embolism.

INDICATIONS

(a) Detection of congenital abnormalities of the pulmonary vascular tree, including agenesis or hypoplasia of a pulmonary artery, coarctation of one or more pulmonary arteries (peripheral pulmonic stenosis), idiopathic dilatation of a pulmonary artery, arteriovenous malformation of the lung, anomalous pulmonary venous drainage, and pulmonary venous varix.

(b) Investigation of acquired disease of the

pulmonary arterial and venous circulation: primary pulmonary arterial hypertension, secondary pulmonary arterial and venous hypertension, and conditions of obscure origin leading to pulmonary venous obstruction (e.g., mediastinitis).

(c) Rarely, the investigation of active pulmonary hemorrhage.[154]

(d) Investigation of thromboembolic disease of the lungs (Fig. 2–13). The important role that pulmonary angiography can play in the investigation of thromboembolic disease is no longer in dispute; in selected cases it may be of great diagnostic importance.[155–162]

No significant side effects of pulmonary angiography have been observed. In an experimental study in dogs, Julien and Gamsu[172] demonstrated transient bronchoconstriction that reached a maximum of 15 sec after injection and disappeared by 1 min; interruption of vagal conduction prevented changes in airway diameter, indicating that the bronchoconstriction was mediated via a vagal reflex arc. The only caveat in the performance of pulmonary angiography is in patients with primary pulmonary arterial hypertension, in which the risk of morbidity or mortality is increased.

Aortography

TECHNIQUE

The preferred technique is direct catheterization of the thoracic aorta percutaneously,[173] with either flooding of the aorta or selective catheterization of a particular vessel. An alternative method is digital subtraction aortography following injection into an arm vein or superior vena cava; this technique provides satisfactory opacification in selected cases when direct catheterization of the aorta is contraindicated.

INDICATIONS

(a) Aortography is imperative in patients in whom mediastinal widening is observed following severe deceleration injuries.[175] When the widening is recognized, emergency aortography is indicated (1) to distinguish purely venous hematoma from major arterial injury, and (2) to show the number and sites of arterial lesions. In some cases, CT may precede or replace aortography.

(b) Precise identification of aortic anomalies, such as patent ductus arteriosus or aortic coarctation.

(c) Identification of anomalous vessels, such as an artery supplying a sequestered lobe.[180, 181]

Bronchial and Intercostal Arteriography

TECHNIQUE

Optimal opacification can be achieved only by selective catheterization, usually via a percutaneous

transfemoral approach;[174, 176–178] the tip of the catheter is wedged into a bronchial artery at the level of the fifth or sixth thoracic vertebra. With this technique, Miyazawa and associates[179] satisfactorily opacified the bronchial arteries in 67 (66 per cent) of 101 patients. Botenga's treatise[174] is recommended for detailed study.

When the bronchial arteries are markedly hypertrophied and tortuous, they can be opacified in some cases by an aortic flood technique.

INDICATIONS

It is questionable whether bronchial arteriography can aid in the diagnosis or management of pulmonary disease, although as a research procedure it has provided much information about the pathophysiology and pathology of several pulmonary abnormalities associated with increased bronchial collateral circulation (chronic suppurative disease and chronic pulmonary oligemia).[176, 182–186] The procedure is of limited value for investigating peripheral pulmonary lesions, since both primary and metastatic neoplasms may receive their blood supply from the bronchial arteries,[176] and even some benign neoplasms show a "tumor blush."[187]

Bronchial arteriography has been recommended for investigating severe hemoptysis, particularly when a possible source of bleeding is not apparent from the plain roentgenogram. In patients with cataclysmic, life-threatening hemoptysis in whom resectional surgery is contraindicated for one reason or another, the technique of therapeutic embolization of bronchial arteries has been gaining increasing attention.[189–192] A number of substances can be employed for occlusion, including Gianturco coils, Ivanlon, Gelfoam, or inflatable balloons. A similar technique has been employed for controlling severe hemorrhage from pulmonary arteries, such as from a Rasmussen aneurysm[189] and from multiple pulmonary artery fistulas.[193]

North and associates have emphasized the importance of combined bronchial and intercostal arteriography in studies of pulmonary collateral blood flow.[188] They showed that selective catheterization of bronchial and intercostal arteries may demonstrate either or both supplying systemic blood to the lung in pathologic conditions; pleural disease is necessary for participation of the intercostal artery. When such patients present cataclysmic hemoptysis, it is important to recognize that the nonbronchial systemic vessels often can be the source of bleeding, particularly in patients with chronic infection and pleural involvement; in such cases it can be exceedingly difficult to decide what vessel or vessels to embolize.[192]

Superior Vena Cava Angiography

TECHNIQUE

This procedure can be carried out by unilateral or simultaneous bilateral arm vein injection or via a catheter inserted into the superior vena cava or one of its large tributary veins.

To investigate obstruction of the superior vena cava (the superior vena cava syndrome).

ROENTGENOLOGIC METHODS IN THE ASSESSMENT OF LUNG FUNCTION

It is inevitable that over the years roentgenographic techniques have been devised to estimate parameters of lung function.[194, 195] Some, notably the determination of lung volume, are very accurate compared with physiologic methods of measurement; the majority, however, either lack sufficient precision or necessitate the use of highly complex apparatus not generally available. Whereas the refined techniques of pulmonary function testing described in Chapter 3 serve as the sheet anchor of physiologic investigation in most cases, certain roentgenologic procedures are useful as rough screening methods or when physiologic techniques are not available.

Determination of Lung Volumes

Many roentgenographic methods have been devised for determining lung volume;[196] unfortunately, most of these are inaccurate except as a rough gauge. This lack of accuracy is due largely to the awkward shape of the thorax and to the difficulty in estimating the volumetric contributions of the diaphragmatic domes, heart, pulmonary blood volume, and tissue volume. However, in 1960 an ingenious method was described by Barnhard and his associates[197] in which the lungs were pictured as a stack of five horizontal elliptical cylindroids. The volume of each of these five segments was measured and their total was the capacity of the thorax. The volumes of the heart, the right and left hemidiaphragms, the intrathoracic extracardiac blood, and the lung tissue were totaled and subtracted from the thoracic capacity to yield the total volume of gas in the lungs. Measurements thus obtained approximated those obtained by conventional means in healthy subjects and in patients with congestive heart failure, but were significantly greater in patients with emphysema when compared with figures obtained by gas dilution measurement of TLC. A more recent study,[198] however, showed comparable TLC values obtained with the Barnhard technique and plethysmographically in patients with various chest diseases. Similarly, Loyd and associates,[199] who modified Barnhard's technique in the light of new physiologic data on pulmonary tissue and blood volume, compared results obtained with their roentgenographic method with plethysmographically determined TLC. Results were comparable in normal subjects and in patients with pulmonary fibrosis, sarcoidosis, emphysema, or

pulmonary neoplasm, but in emphysema, as might be anticipated, values obtained with the roentgenographic method were more accurate than those with gas dilution techniques. When TLC was known, RV was readily obtained by subtracting the spirometrically obtained vital capacity (VC). An experienced observer could make the measurements in less than 30 min and the technique was highly reproducible.

In 1971 Harris and his colleagues[200] described a comparably accurate method for estimating TLC from chest roentgenograms that is faster and much simpler than the Barnhard or Loyd technique. The outlines of the lungs on posteroanterior and lateral roentgenograms are traced, their areas measured with a planimeter, and a regression equation applied to these measurements. More recently, Jaffe[201] devised a technique by which TLC can be determined from chest roentgenograms in less than 40 sec: a tracking device or *cursor* held by the operator traces the outline of the lungs on an opaque fiberglass *platen*, and the coordinates of any point on the board are electrically determined. The operation is controlled by a programmable computer, and the output is displayed on an X–Y plotter. This method employs Simpson's rule—which, Jaffe states, obviates any major correction equation—through the use of very narrow horizontal slices. In comparing results thus obtained with water displacement measurements of various phantoms, he reported volume estimates that differed from true volume by −8 to +16 per cent. He did not report comparison of results with his technique with plethysmographically determined TLC in patients. Recently, TLC has been measured satisfactorily without operator intervention by a computer analysis of posteroanterior and lateral roentgenograms.[662] Even more promising is the technique recently described by Herman and his coworkers,[663] which employs computerized graphic-to-digital conversion of tracings directly from posteroanterior and lateral roentgenograms. The procedure can be performed in less than 60 sec, and in a test on 53 subjects showed good correlation with physiologic measurements (r = 0.85).

On the strength of the fact that CT reveals a true cross-sectional area of a segment of the chest, Friedman and his colleagues[202] found that measurement of this area of the lung at several adjacent levels permits calculation of a geometrically defined volume: the best correlation between linear dimensions and true volume was obtained with equations that used lung width and AP diameter of each scan, maximum AP lung diameter, and relative scan level from apex to base. The method compared favorably with previous regression or geometric approximation methods for estimating total lung volume.

Studies of Ventilation

Fluoroscopy and *roentgenography* may be useful as rough screening measures in the investigation of pulmonary ventilation. Estimates of diaphragmatic and costal excursion during quiet and forced respiration may indicate restricted ventilation, either bilaterally symmetric, as in diffuse bronchospasm or emphysema, or asymmetric, as may occur in association with bronchial obstruction by neoplasm or foreign body. The technique of FEV_1 roentgenography described by Greenspan and his colleagues[46] seems preferable to standard untimed expiratory roentgenography for assessing local or general air trapping. In their study of over 200 persons, including 60 normal subjects, these workers found 9 patients in whom air trapping could be detected only on the FEV_1 roentgenogram, standard inspiratory and expiratory roentgenograms being normal; in 12 of 16 patients with local air trapping, the spirographic trace was normal, the roentgenogram providing the only evidence for disease. This technique is at present rather cumbersome and time-consuming, and we are not convinced that it provides information not obtainable from a roentgenogram exposed following a forced vital capacity breath. However, both methods may detect disease not apparent on standard inspiratory roentgenograms and unsuspected clinically or from standard tests of pulmonary function.

Studies of Perfusion

Since the volume of extravascular interstitial tissue presumably is constant, the roentgenographic density of lung parenchyma is dependent upon the ratio of the amount of blood in peripheral vessels to the amount of gas in air spaces. At any one time, therefore, at a given degree of lung inflation, lung density should reflect the absolute amount of blood within the vascular tree, including capillaries. Oligemia or pleonemia, if of sufficient degree, can be appreciated on standard roentgenograms of the chest through assessment of decrease or increase, respectively, in the size of pulmonary vascular markings. Similarly, local oligemia can often be recognized by a reduction in background haze compared with zones of normal or increased perfusion, particularly when full lung tomography is employed. However, when oligemia is general (as in emphysema), alteration in pulmonary capillary volume is seldom appreciable by subjective evaluation of background lung density but can be revealed by roentgen densitometry. In two independent studies[57, 59] in which densitometric recordings of the periphery of the lung were compared with simultaneous electrocardiograms, the densitometric record permitted identification of the various phases of the pulmonary pulse and proved to be a true record of pulmonary pulsation and perfusion. Similarly, Laws and Steiner[58] found good correlation between densitometric records and pulmonary artery pressures obtained simultaneously during cardiac catheterization. They consider that density variations must be related to changes in the volume of blood in the lungs.

The most widely used method of assessing regional pulmonary ventilation and perfusion is lung scintiscanning. Techniques most commonly used are described in the following section.

LUNG SCINTISCANNING

Although the number of indications for lung scanning has increased over the years, the major clinical application is in two relatively narrow fields of interest—thromboembolic disease and ventilation-perfusion studies of lung function.

It is beyond the scope of this book to describe in detail the imaging techniques, radiopharmaceuticals, and methods of interpretation of lung scans. They are only summarized here, and the interested reader is directed to excellent monographs on the use and interpretation of the lung scan.[203–205] Articles dealing with specific aspects are cited in this and other relevant sections.

Instrumentation

Generally speaking, the use of radioactive isotopes in lung studies involves the recording on sensitive devices of the gamma radiation produced by radionuclides injected intravenously into the bloodstream or inhaled into the air spaces. The imaging devices are basically of two types—the rectilinear scanner, which covers the field of interest in "strips," and the scintillation or gamma camera, which records in a single exposure the flux of gamma radiation from the lungs (Fig. 2–14). The latter is much more versatile, permitting viewing of a large area at one time; in addition, the gamma camera permits isotopic angiography and angiocardiography.

A more recent addition to the armamentarium that is said to possess advantages over conventional planar imaging in the diagnosis of pulmonary embolism[206] is the whole-body emission tomographic scanner that images the lungs in a manner analogous to that of the CT scanner.

Quantification of pulmonary scans has received increasing emphasis, particularly for measuring regional pulmonary ventilation and perfusion.[204, 207–210] A gamma camera-computer system is used: the camera interfaces an analog-to-digital converter, a memory system, and a magnetic tape recorder for data storage, and the data displayed are density changes as a percentage variation from the mean density change[207] or three-dimensional images of pulmonary ventilation and perfusion.[208]

Loken and his colleagues[211] successfully employ two scintillation cameras to view both anterior and posterior lung areas. Scintiphotograms are obtained from both cameras throughout the course of both perfusion and ventilation portions of the study, and computer processing of data permits quantitative information to be obtained on perfusion, ventilation, and clearance of ^{133}Xe from selected regions of both anterior and posterior lung zones.

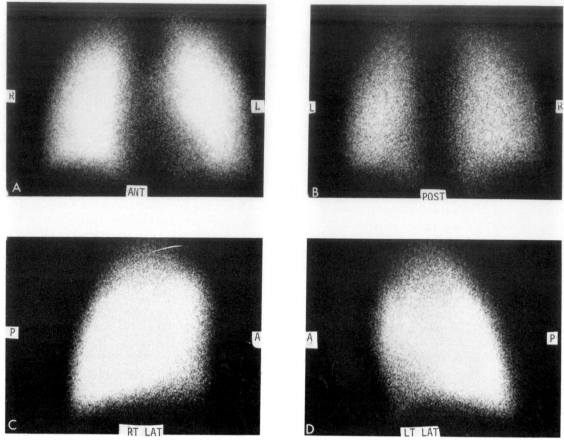

Figure 2–14. Normal Perfusion Lung Scan. Anterior (A), posterior (B), right lateral (C), and left lateral (D) views recorded with a gamma camera following intravenous injection of ⁹⁹ᵐTc MAA.

Although the standard scintillation camera is the more popular instrument for quantifying lung function with ¹³³Xe, there is an almost equal trend toward the use of special purpose multidetector systems. Multiple discrete scintillation detectors cover both front and back of the chest, resolving each lung into approximately eight regions for assessment of ventilation and perfusion.

For transmission scanning, a flat-field, high-activity radioactive source is placed behind the patient, and the transmitted radioactivity is scanned with a gamma camera or rectilinear scanner. This records relative absorption and attenuation of gamma rays through the body, and thus is analogous to photon transmission in standard roentgenography. This technique has limited application in the chest, being used chiefly in the diagnosis of pericardial effusion.

Radiopharmaceuticals

These substances may be particulate or gaseous. The former has the advantage of allowing more time for scanning. For this, an intravenous injection is given of a standard quantity of tagged MAA (macroaggregates of human serum albumin) containing radioactive particles largely in the range of 10 to 50 μ in diameter. Being larger than the capillaries, they lodge in the first capillary bed encountered. Since the particles remain lodged for a considerable time before they disintegrate, they can be scanned with either the relatively slow, widely available rectilinear scanner or the gamma camera. Imaging with gaseous radionuclides—¹³³Xe, for example—requires performance of the scan over a relatively brief period, necessitating use of the scintillation camera.

For studies of the pulmonary circulation with particulates, the commonest vehicle for the radionuclide is MAA, which is prepared by heating human serum albumin to 100°C. The resultant particle sizes range from 10 to 100 μ in diameter, depending largely upon a constant pH of 5.4 to 5.5.[212–215] The albumin (or other particle) may be labeled with ¹³¹I, ⁹⁹ᵐTc, or ¹¹³ᵐIn.[212, 216, 221, 222] Other radiopharmaceuticals recommended include ⁹⁹ᵐTc-sulfur colloid MAA[217] and radioactive albumin microspheres, the latter mainly because of their uniform size.[218–220] The properties of commonly used radiopharmaceuticals in lung scanning are summarized in Table 2–1.

Table 2–1. Properties of Commonly Used Lung Scanning Agents

RADIO-NUCLIDE	PHYSICAL T½	PRINCIPAL GAMMA KEV	BETA	PARTICLE	BIOLOGIC LUNG T½	SCANNING DOSE ROUTE	RADIATION TO LUNGS
[131]I	8 days	364	Yes	Macroaggregated albumin	8 hr	300 µCi IV	1.2–1.8 rad
[113m]In	100 min	390	No	Ferric hydroxide	4–12 hr	2 mCi IV	1.5 rad
[99m]Tc	6 hr	140	No	Macroaggregated albumin		2 mCi IV	0.8 rad
[99m]Tc	6 hr	140	No	Ferric hydroxide	6–20 hr	2 mCi IV	1.2 rad
[99m]Tc	6 hr	140	No	Albumin microsphere	4.5 hr	2 mCi IV	0.8 rad
[113m]In	100 min	390	No	Albumin microsphere		2 mCi IV	1.5 rad
[133]Xe	5.27 days	81 31	Yes	Aqueous solution	0.5 min	10 mCi IV	28–50 mrad

(From Mishkin FS, Brashear RE: Use and Interpretation of the Lung Scan. Springfield, IL, Charles C Thomas, 1971.)

Since the procedure is based on trapping particles within the small vessels of the lung, particle size is critical. The majority of those less than 10 µ in diameter pass through the lung "sieve" into the reticuloendothelial system, largely in the liver and spleen,[214, 215, 223] whereas particles exceeding 100 µ in diameter may obstruct larger vessels, with resultant deleterious effects. A particle size of 10 to 50 µ in diameter has been found optimal. It has been recommended[225] that a minimum of 60,000 albumin microspheres be administered to avoid false-positive scans resulting from an insufficient number of particles when using currently available instrumentation; the optimum number of particles is about 100,000. Disappearance time from the lungs is nearly exponential, biologic half-life ranging from 4 to 20 hours[204] (Table 2–1). Radioactivity of ^{131}I disappears from the lung in 24 hours. With rare exceptions,[224] extensive clinical experience[212–215] has revealed no significant toxicity or morbidity associated with the injection of human serum albumin; radiation dosage rates are well within tolerable limits.

The gaseous radiopharmaceutical most widely used for studying the pulmonary circulation is [133]Xe. The [133]Xe (10 mCi dissolved in saline) is injected intravenously; while the patient holds his or her breath, a gamma camera picture records perfusion. Since the xenon passes almost instantly into the alveoli, during subsequent respiration the distribution of xenon throughout all areas of ventilated lung, including those poorly perfused, can be recorded. Xenon is cleared from the lungs in 3 to 4 min in normally ventilated regions but is delayed in poorly ventilated regions (that is, those with air trapping).

Techniques for assessing pulmonary ventilation involve the inhalation of a radioactive gas (such as ^{133}Xe or [81m]Kr) or a nebulized aerosol of a radioactive material (such as albumin labeled with ^{131}I or ^{99m}Tc) (Fig. 2–15). For the latter, the particles must be sufficiently small—less than 1 µ in diameter—to reach the alveoli. A single-breath radio-aerosol-inhalation technique has been described that purports to maximize peripheral lung deposition.[670]

Indications

Of the several indications for lung scanning summarized by Deland and Wagner,[205] the following five seem to be the most clinically useful.

(a) Detection of pulmonary thromboemboli.

(b) Monitoring the natural history or treatment of thromboembolism.

(c) Quantitative evaluation of the distribution of infectious, obstructive, and other pulmonary diseases.

(d) Preoperative evaluation of patients with emphysema, neoplasms, and bronchiectasis.

(e) Early detection of carcinoma of the lung (e.g., in patients with positive cytologic findings and a normal chest roentgenogram).

Several other indications for lung scan have been reported: identification of lung neoplasms and their differentiation from nonmalignant lesions, with [197]HgCl or ^{67}Ga;[226, 227] detection of pulmonary bacterial infections with labeled thyroid hormones and pertechnetate;[228] identification of *Aspergillus niger* infection with [85]Sr;[229] quantification of extravascular lung water;[230, 231, 234] detection of endobronchial foreign bodies in infants and children;[232] location of deep venous thrombi with ^{131}I-labeled fibrinogen;[233] and the identification of the sites of hemoptysis with ^{99m}Tc sulfur colloid and ^{99m}Tc-labeled red blood cells.[235]

Of these several additional indications, perhaps the most important are those relating to the use of [67]gallium citrate. In a review of the use of ^{67}Ga in pulmonary disorders, Siemsen and colleagues[236] pointed out that this isotope possesses limited value in the differential diagnosis of pulmonary diseases because of its nonspecific affinity for both neoplastic and inflammatory processes. However, based on personal observations of over 1100 patients with a variety of pulmonary diseases, they concluded that the judicious use of ^{67}Ga in selected patients can be of value in a number of clinical situations, specifically in the preoperative evaluation of hilar and mediastinal involvement in pulmonary neoplasms, in the differential diagnosis of pulmonary infarction and bacterial pneumonia, in the assessment of activity in patients with sarcoidosis (including evaluation

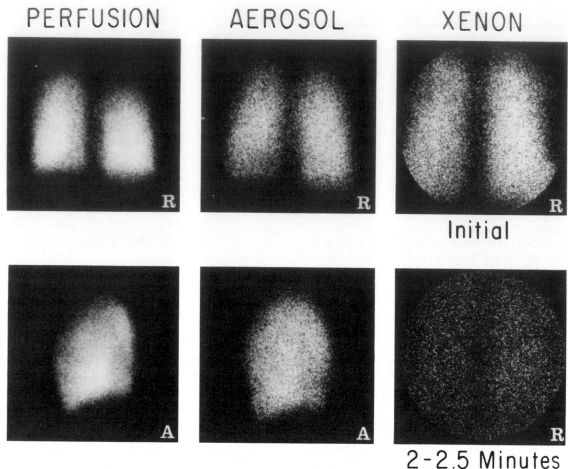

Figure 2–15. Normal Perfusion Airway Patency, and Ventilation Lung Scans. The two perfusion lung images on the left (posterior and lateral) were obtained following injection of ^{99m}Tc MAA, the airway patency images in the middle following inhalation of ^{99m}Tc sulfur colloid, and the inhalation images on the right following injection of ^{133}Xe. In all three procedures, the radiopharmaceutical was delivered and the images recorded in the erect position with a gamma camera. Note that the upper lung zones are better ventilated than perfused. The initial xenon image was made during breath-holding; washout is nearly complete in 2.0 to 2.5 minutes. (Courtesy of the late Dr. George Taplin, University of California, Los Angeles.)

of the effects of corticosteroid therapy), in the early detection of neoplastic and infectious diseases before roentgenographic abnormality becomes apparent (particularly in diffuse carcinomatosis and *Pneumocystis carinii* pneumonia), and in the interstitial pulmonary disease caused by bleomycin therapy.[237] Because of its affinity for active inflammatory tissue, ^{67}Ga can be of value in estimating the degree of activity in patients with cryptogenic fibrosing alveolitis and in following the response to therapy, a feature emphasized by Line and his colleagues.[238] It has also been reported to be useful in following the response to therapy in patients with lymphoma.[239] In a recent review of 111 patients who had had lung resection for carcinoma, Hatfield and coworkers[671] concluded that routine postoperative whole-body gallium scanning can facilitate early detection of recurrence in some cases. In summarizing their experience in over 1100 cases, Siemsen and his colleagues[236] concluded, "It remains to be seen whether gallium imaging statistically provides essential additional information in these indications when compared to cheaper conventional techniques."

Large amounts of ^{85}Sr may be deposited in lungs undergoing diffuse active calcification, presumably by heterionic exchange. Chaudhuri and associates,[240] describing a patient with multiple myeloma whose serum level of calcium was increased (the chest roentgenogram was normal), stated that most of the ^{87m}Sr administered for bone scan was taken up by the lungs. They postulated that the strontium combined with the excess phosphate to form macroaggregates and that these were trapped in the pulmonary capillaries.

The major indication for lung scanning is the investigation of thromboembolic diseases.[241, 242] Briefly, studies with tagged MAA are of diagnostic value only when the scan image is compared with the chest roentgenogram. Many physiologic and pathologic conditions (such as the patient's posture during tracer injection, obesity, cardiomegaly, and cardiac decompensation) alter lung images and must be taken into account for correct interpretation.[243] Since any disease characterized by consolidation or atelectasis or both can diminish pulmonary artery perfusion, and since the airless lung can absorb radiation, reduced or absent radioactivity on

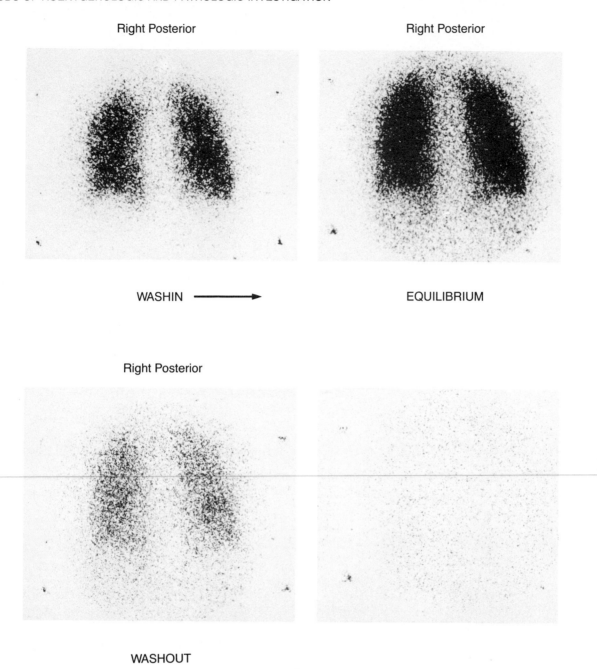

Illustration continued on following page

Figure 2–16. The Value of Ventilation/Perfusion Lung Scans in the Diagnosis of Thromboembolism. *A*, A [133]xenon posterior inhalation lung scan discloses normal ventilation parameters during the washin, equilibrium, and washout phases.

scanning does not necessarily indicate embolism. When the clinical picture suggests embolism, however, and the chest roentgenogram shows no opacity, scintillation studies may be diagnostic. This is especially true when the perfusion scan shows one or more defects and the ventilation scan is normal (just as a normal lung scan virtually excludes a major pulmonary embolus) (Fig. 2–16). Since pulmonary embolism may be medically or surgically curable, the diagnosis must be made by whatever tools are at the physician's disposal. In many cases the diagnosis can be established by isotopic studies,

but *the majority of pulmonary emboli can be identified only by integrating information gained from all methods of investigation.*[244]

A recent study[245] of healthy adults in whom some type of perfusion defect was detected in 10 (16 per cent) of 61 subjects casts some doubt on the specificity of positive perfusion lung scans in patients with suspected pulmonary thromboembolism. The defect was subtle in six, but was major enough in the other four to be indistinguishable from defects that might be anticipated from a major pulmonary embolism. In the study of Krumholz and

Anterior

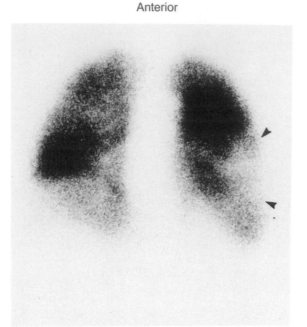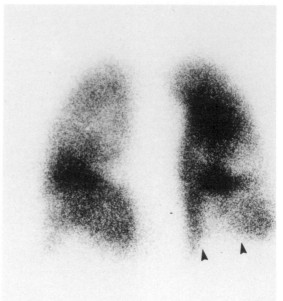

Right Posterior Oblique

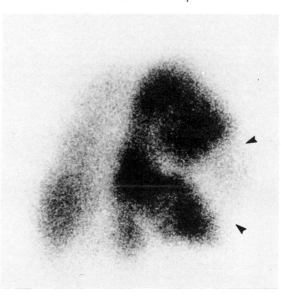

B

Figure 2–16 *Continued. B*, Corresponding ⁹⁹ᵐtechnetium MAA perfusion lung scans in anterior, posterior, and right and left posterior oblique projections identify multiple segmental filling defects throughout both lungs (*arrowheads*). These findings, in concert with the ventilation study, are virtually diagnostic (high probability) of pulmonary thromboembolism. The patient is a 65-year-old man who presented acute dyspnea.

coworkers[246] of 71 patients with chronic obstructive pulmonary disease (COPD), in which subjects showed abnormal lung volumes, flow rates, and diffusing capacity on pulmonary function testing in almost every case but many had no abnormalities on the chest roentgenogram, the degree of function test impairment correlated well with the degree of

pulmonary underperfusion revealed on the ¹³¹I lung scans. The researchers emphasized that it is not sufficient to relate lung photoscans to chest roentgenograms alone, and that in patients with COPD the assessment of scans must take into account function derangements shown by pulmonary function studies.

In view of these observations,[245, 246] it may be that an abnormal lung scan associated with a normal chest roentgenogram should be taken as evidence of an embolic episode only if serial scans reveal disappearance of the perfusion defect. Certainly more studies of this type are required to delineate the appearance of a "normal" scan.

DIAGNOSTIC ULTRASOUND

This technique has limited but potentially important applications within the thorax. The limitations are imposed by the physical composition of the intrathoracic structures in that neither air nor bone transmits sound, instead absorbing or reflect-

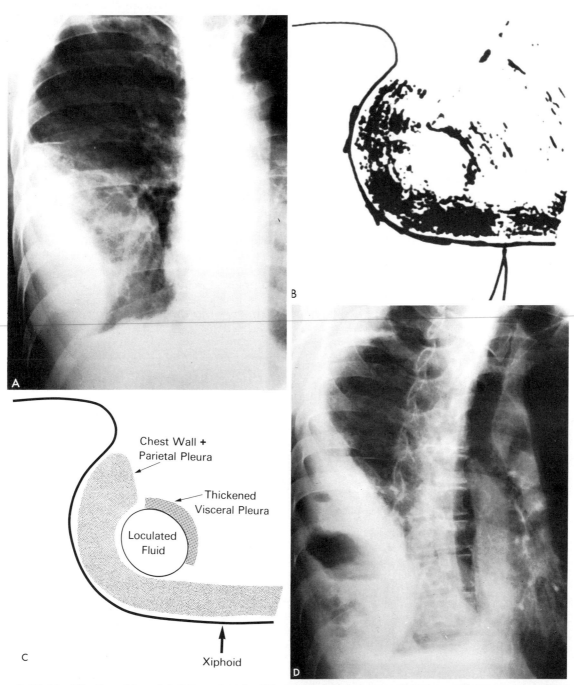

Figure 2–17. Identification of Loculated Empyema by Ultrasonography. An anteroposterior roentgenogram (*A*) reveals a large, homogeneous opacity in the right lower hemithorax laterally whose configuration strongly suggests fluid loculation. An ultrasonic B-scan of the lower chest (*B*) shows a roughly elliptical, sharply demarcated sonolucent space posterolaterally, possessing the typical characteristics of a fluid-filled space. A drawing (*C*) indicates important landmarks. Thoracentesis was carried out, pus withdrawn, and air introduced; an oblique roentgenogram (*D*) reveals the space corresponding to the sonolucent zone in the ultrasound recording. (Courtesy of Dr. Reggie Greene, Massachusetts General Hospital, Boston.)

(From Paré JAP, Fraser R: Synopsis of Diseases of the Chest. Philadelphia, WB Saunders, 1983, p 115.)

ing incoming sonic energy and preventing the collection of information about acoustic interfaces behind ribs or lung tissue. But there are "windows" in the thorax through which ultrasonography can garner information useful in the investigation of thoracic disease. Undoubtedly the most important of these are the intercostal spaces, through which ultrasonic beams can be directed toward the heart and pericardium. In this field of echocardiography ultrasonography has made its greatest impact in the assessment of thoracic disease, particularly in establishing the nature of valvular deformity, the volume of cardiac chambers, and the thickness of their walls. It is also valuable for detecting pericardial effusion, assessing its size, and differentiating it from cardiomegaly.

In selected cases, ultrasonic examination may provide useful information concerning three other areas: the subcostal pleura (via the intercostal spaces), the right hemidiaphragm and contiguous pleura and subphrenic space (via the liver), and mediastinal masses in close proximity to the thoracic cage.

The most useful application of ultrasonography in the evaluation of diseases of the lungs and pleura is in the assessment of local pleural thickening, usually caused by loculated empyema.[247–251] Differentiation of liquid from solid pleural collections, which may be exceedingly difficult with standard roentgenographic techniques, can often be achieved easily with ultrasonography (Fig. 2–17), particularly

with high resolution real-time sonographic sector scanning. Furthermore, it provides an assessment of the amount of fluid loculated in a pleural pocket, indicates the anatomic point for thoracentesis, and simplifies fluid aspiration by permitting insertion of a needle directly through a special transducer. This procedure can be carried out at the patient's bedside with mobile ultrasonic apparatus, thus obviating the need for special roentgenographic projections. Marks and his associates[252] have emphasized the superiority of real-time ultrasonography over articulated-arm B-scanners in the assessment of pleura-based fluid collections: they found that a change in a pleural opacity's shape with respiration, or the presence of septations within the collection with demonstrated motion, constitutes a reliable indicator that fluid can be aspirated.

The criteria for a fluid-containing structure are that it (1) is free of echoes, (2) has a sharp posterior wall, and (3) demonstrates increased transmission of sound deep to the collection of fluid.[253] Employment of high resolution real-time sector scanning can facilitate assessment of fluid collections as demonstrated by Hirsch and his associates[254] in their evaluation of 50 patients with roentgenographic evidence of pleural or pleura-based opacities: of those cases selected for thoracentesis, fluid sufficient for diagnosis was obtained in 90 per cent; further, complex septated pleural loculations were found to contain an exudative effusion in 74 per cent of the patients while anechoic areas yielded exudative and

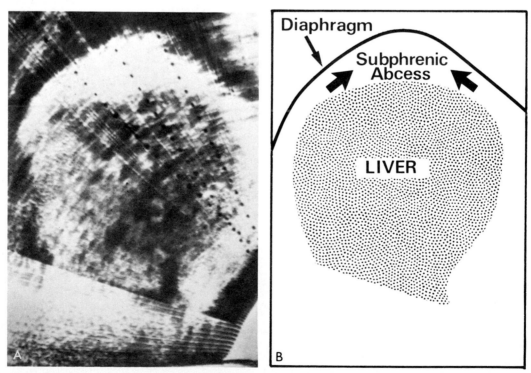

Figure 2–18. Identification of Subphrenic Abscess by Ultrasonography. *A*, B-scan of the right upper abdomen with a gray scale technique, the probe scanning upward from just below the lowest costal cartilage anteriorly. A sonolucent space representing fluid separates the right hemidiaphragm from the liver. Note the typical inhomogeneous pattern of the liver. *B*, A drawing illustrates important landmarks. (Courtesy of the Montreal General Hospital.)

transudative effusions with almost equal frequency. Even an anechoic area does not always represent a fluid collection, as emphasized by Shin and Gray:[255] in a case report, they describe a large, elliptic echo-free area deep to the chest wall that closely simulated a large pleural collection but which proved at autopsy to be caused by massive replacement of lung parenchyma by Hodgkin's tissue. It appears that this paradox is the result of the homogeneity of tissue replacing the lung parenchyma; it should not be a problem in distinguishing pleural fluid from such pulmonary abnormalities as atelectasis or pneumonia.

Pleural fluid in the subpulmonic area of the right lung and collections of fluid in the subphrenic space (subphrenic abscess) can be similarly assessed (Fig. 2–18). Connell and his colleagues[256] have pointed out a potential pitfall in the diagnosis of subpulmonic pleural effusions: such a collection can easily be missed if the ultrasonic examination is carried out with the patient supine; such examinations should always be performed with the patient erect. Also, since the liver is trans-sonic, the right hemidiaphragm is accessible, permitting evaluation of its mobility and determination of fluid collections above and below it.[257]

The acoustic properties of mediastinal masses in close proximity to the thoracic cage can be determined,[258] although CT is undoubtedly the procedure of choice in such evaluation. Ultrasonic studies are limited at present to the differentiation of solid from liquid masses (e.g., thymoma from pericardial cyst in the anterior mediastinum). Goldberg correctly diagnosed cystic, solid, or complex patterns in 28 of 30 mediastinal masses (92 per cent accuracy), using A-mode and M-mode ultrasonic displays.[259] The development of more sophisticated scanners with gray scale almost certainly will expand the capabilities of ultrasonography in this area. In fact, one report describes the demonstration of a subcarinal bronchogenic cyst in each of two children by real-time ultrasonography using the parasternal approach.[260]

MASS CHEST ROENTGENOGRAPHY AS A SCREENING PROCEDURE

Over the past two decades the medical use of ionizing radiation has increased enormously. In the United States, for example, the estimated number of roentgenographic examinations of the thorax increased by 23 per cent from 53×10^6 in 1964 to 65×10^6 in 1970.[261] Similarly, in the 10 year period from 1956 to 1965, the average number of all roentgenologic examinations in hospitals increased by 3.5 per cent *per annum* in England and 6.5 per cent *per annum* in France.[262] In Japan, in the same period the number of medical x-ray films used increased by approximately 10 per cent annually[263]—and photofluorographic examinations

as part of mass chest surveys increased from approximately 8 million in 1950 to 40 million in 1970.[264]

This vastly increasing use of ionizing radiation in the diagnosis of chest disease, particularly in mass chest roentgenography, has caused many to ponder the efficacy of such programs, especially in relation to the potentially harmful effect of such huge quantities of radiation on populations as a whole. A most useful, succinct policy statement stemming from these deliberations was prepared by the Bureau of Radiological Health of the (then) United States Department of Health, Education, and Welfare, in collaboration with the American Colleges of Radiology and Chest Physicians.[265] The pertinent recommendations embodied in this statement are presented later on, but first we should review the discovery rate of mass chest roentgenography over the past few years. We are indebted to the aforementioned HEW report for much of the following information.

Mass chest roentgenography—usually defined as a survey of the general population with mobile or portable x-ray units—has been the basic technique for detecting tuberculosis in the United States for more than 30 years. The rationale for its use has been that most unknown, active cases of tuberculosis could be discovered early so that treatment could be instituted before irreparable lung damage occurred. In recent years, studies of the efficacy of these programs have shown this premise to be false, largely because of the rapid decline in the incidence of pulmonary tuberculosis during the past decade. In fact, in many areas of the country the disease is now almost nonexistent. In 1958, 6534 new active cases of tuberculosis were reported; by 1971, this number had been almost halved. Results of local screening programs illustrate their present low yield. The 109,000 mobile chest x-ray examinations performed in Cleveland in 1969 revealed only 18 (0.016 per cent) new cases of active pulmonary tuberculosis.[266] (Of even greater significance is the fact that these 18 cases constituted only 5 per cent of the 335 new active cases reported in Cleveland during that year, suggesting that most are discovered when patients seek medical advice for symptoms of illness.) The discovery rate was similar in Denver, Colorado, during 1965–1970: screening of 276,658 persons revealed only 54 (0.019 per cent) active cases of tuberculosis.[267]

The results are similar for the discovery rate of chest diseases other than tuberculosis. For example, a 1971 Report of the Inter-Society Commission for Heart Disease Resources[268] stated that the yield is low when compared with the cost in radiation exposure, money, and time of trained medical personnel; relatively few patients with previously unknown heart disease amenable to treatment are identified in this way. Similarly, a 1972 report from the Philadelphia Pulmonary Neoplasm Research Project[269] concluded that semiannual screening contributes little toward solving the lung cancer problem: of 6136 male volunteers who had semiannual chest roentgenograms for the detection of bronchogenic carcinoma, 121 (2 per cent) developed cancer, but only 10 (8 per cent) of these survived 5 years.

In addition to these low discovery rates, the potential injurious effects of ionizing radiation must be taken into account. Such effects cannot be predicted with certainty, but estimates of the potentially harmful effects of mass screening surveys have been attempted. Kitabatake and his colleagues,[264] who admit that their conclusions are based on certain assumptions, predict that the 40 million photofluorographic studies carried out in Japan during 1968 will result in leukemia in 46 patients and incurable pulmonary cancer in 7 during the subsequent 25 years; in addition, they estimate that 150 genetic deaths will occur until the tenth generation. Despite the foregoing, it has been estimated that the risk of one chest x-ray taken in a good hospital (risk being defined as an increased chance of death of one part in a million) is equivalent to smoking 1.4 cigarettes, living 2 days in New York or Boston, or drinking Miami drinking water for a year![672]

In view of these considerations, we reproduce here verbatim the recommendations contained in the policy statement referred to earlier, which has been endorsed by the American Lung Association and the Centers for Disease Control. We enthusiastically endorse these recommendations.

1. Community chest x-ray surveys among the general population are not productive as a screening procedure for the detection of tuberculosis and should not be done. In a high tuberculosis incidence area where fixed x-ray facilities are limited or not available, it may be necessary to screen selected groups of the population by x-ray in conjunction with the tuberculin skin test. In such circumstances, full follow-up treatment facilities must be available as an essential component of the community tuberculosis control program. Tuberculin skin tests should be performed for those under age 21 in lieu of chest x-ray examinations, even if periodic physical examinations are required for food handlers or school employees. Those jurisdictions requiring chest x-ray examinations should re-evaluate this procedure. The primary screening of grade and high school children for tuberculosis should not be by x-ray examination. The chest x-ray examination would thus be restricted to the positive reactors to the tuberculin test in the younger age groups. In low prevalence groups, consideration should also be given to the tuberculin skin test as the initial screening examination for case finding. X-ray examination should be restricted to the positive reactors.

2. Community chest x-ray surveys among the general population for detection of other pulmonary disease or heart disease have not proved sufficiently rewarding and should not be done.

3. When radiologic screening of selected groups of the general population may be productive, the full size film is preferred. The use of the photofluorographic unit as a screening device is justified only under the following conditions:

a. A definitive interpretation must be made by qualified physicians, such as certified radiologists or other physicians with demonstrated competence in the interpretation of chest radiographs.

b. The radiographs and the reports should be made available upon request to the private physician and public health and hospital agencies for a period of at least 5 years.

c. The equipment used must meet the requirements of the NCRP Report No. 33, or appropriate State and Federal regulations.

4. While community chest x-ray surveys among the general population are not recommended, x-ray facilities for individuals should be available. These may be located in a public health department, private office, or health center.

PATHOLOGIC EXAMINATION

In many pulmonary diseases, diagnosis is not possible despite the combined use of roentgenographic, clinical, and special laboratory and function studies. In these cases, it is necessary to obtain cells or tissue for pathologic examination, on the basis of which a definitive diagnosis is possible in many instances. The techniques employed to obtain this material as well as a brief summary of the principles involved in its examination are discussed in this section.

CYTOLOGY

Cytology is concerned primarily with the morphologic features of individual or small clusters of cells. Although it is most useful in the diagnosis of malignancy, occasionally it can also detect noncellular material or cellular changes suggestive of specific benign disease. Further details of technique, application, and interpretation are described in several comprehensive texts and review articles.[270–275, 673]

Cytology of Tracheobronchial Secretions

Cells and other material suitable for cytologic examination are most often obtained from the lungs by the spontaneous or induced expectoration of sputum, by bronchial washing or brushing performed during endoscopy, and by bronchoalveolar lavage (BAL). It has also been suggested that in some anesthetized patients, analysis of secretions suctioned from the endotracheal tube might be useful as a screening procedure for carcinoma.[674]

BAL is performed by wedging a fiberoptic bronchoscope in a peripheral bronchus and instilling and withdrawing quantities of sterile saline. Cells are counted and a differential determined from the recovered material. Although still primarily a research procedure, BAL is also being actively promoted as a method of diagnosing, staging, and determining therapy in patients with diseases such as sarcoidosis, eosinophilic granuloma, and eosinophilic pneumonia.[276–279]

Sputum is best collected by having the patient rinse his or her mouth with water and then expectorate a deep cough specimen into a wide-mouthed collecting jar; the optimal time is considered to be early morning just after rinsing. Inadequate samples are fairly common, accounting for as many as 29 per cent of specimens in some series;[280, 281] the commonest causes are insufficient material or lack of sputum altogether (indicated by the absence of alveolar macrophages).[281] Careful explanation to the patient of the necessity for a deep cough should help reduce this incidence of inadequate specimens. When sputum production is truly minimal and specimens are repeatedly inadequate, it may be helpful to induce deep expectoration by having the patient inhale aerosolized heated solutions of saline, propylene glycol, or sulfur dioxide.[282–288] It is also important to obtain postbronchoscopic specimens for analysis; the procedure itself leads to repeated deep coughing that often proves fruitful in producing diagnostic specimens.

Once collected, sputum may be processed in several ways.

(1) In one widely used method, the freshly expectorated sample is brought to the laboratory where it is examined for tissue fragments or for areas of discolored, blood-tinged mucus. Specimens from these areas as well as from randomly chosen mucus are then smeared evenly over glass slides and immediately fixed in 95 per cent ethyl alcohol or by cytospray without air drying. Since the number of unsatisfactory and negative specimens decreases as the number of smears increases,[289] at least three slides should be prepared. The slides are then stained, usually by the Papanicolaou method, and examined by the cytotechnician or cytopathologist.

Although widely used, this direct smear technique has two disadvantages: first, the lack of fixative in the collecting jar makes it difficult to obtain either multiple specimens over an extended period of time or a single specimen at a site remote from the laboratory; second, and more important, since only a small portion of the expectorated mucus is usually sampled, the potential for missing malignant cells is considerable. A variety of prefixation and concentration techniques have been proposed to overcome these objections. One method has been to dissolve the mucus to yield a less viscous fluid that can either be passed through a Millipore filter[290, 291] or centrifuged to provide a cell-rich residue that can be smeared on a slide.[292] Many mucolytic substances have been employed, including urea, hydrogen peroxide, detergents, enzymes (including hyaluronidase, papain, ficin, pancreatin, trypsin, and chymotrypsin[290, 293]), acetylcysteine,[294] and several commercial agents.[291, 292]

(2) In a second method, proposed by Saccomanno and associates in 1963,[295] sputum is expectorated into a jar containing 50 per cent ethyl or isopropyl alcohol (which itself contains 2 per cent polyethylene glycol); the alcohol acts as a fixative that permits the collection of sputum specimens over several days. In the laboratory, the sputum-alcohol mixture is placed in a household-type food blender and blended at highest speed for a short period of time, effectively emulsifying the mucus and resulting in a fluid that can be centrifuged. When the supernatent is discarded, the residual concentrated cellular material is smeared on glass slides, dried, and stained. This procedure results in a substantial increase in the number of cells, both benign and malignant, available for examination. Saccomanno found that this technique increased the number of satisfactory smears (containing at least a few alveolar macrophages) from about 70 per cent in the direct smear method to 92 per cent in the blender method. In a study investigating the number of positive smears derived from sputum to which a known number of malignant cells had been experimentally added, Ellis and Kernosky[296] found malignant cells in 14 of 39 slides prepared by the direct smear method in samples containing approximately 49 malignant cells per ml of sputum; this discovery rate dropped to only 2 of 40 slides when the concentration was decreased to 24 cells per ml. By contrast, in specimens prepared by the Saccomanno method, all 42 slides prepared from sputum containing 6 cells per ml were positive. The researchers concluded that there was a 24-fold increased efficiency of detection by the Saccomanno method.

(3) The sample may be formalin-fixed and embedded in paraffin, yielding blocks from which multiple sections can be cut and stained in the same manner as tissue fragments obtained by biopsy.[297] However, since the discovery rate of neoplastic cells is low and details of cellular morphology are often suboptimal,[271] this technique is not commonly used.

The problems involved with sputum processing are not encountered in samples obtained by endoscopic bronchial washings or brushings since the amount of mucus is usually minimal. Specimens obtained by bronchial brushing can be smeared directly onto glass slides and rapidly fixed in the endoscopy room; it has also been suggested that the cell-rich fluid obtained by agitating the brush in saline should be filtered in an attempt to increase the yield of diagnostic cells.[298] Bronchial washings should be passed through a membrane filter and, if sufficient in amount, centrifuged; the cellular residue can then be smeared or prepared into a cell block for histologic examination.

The principal purpose of cytologic examination of sputum and specimens obtained by bronchial washings and brushings is the detection of malignancy. It has been repeatedly shown that such examination is worthwhile: in large series of patients with confirmed lung cancer, positive diagnoses range from 50[299] to 90 per cent.[282, 300–305] Although the yield from sputum specimens has been reported to be at least equal to that from bronchial washings,[300, 306] the latter will be available for cytologic examination in most cases since fiberoptic bronchoscopy is almost always indicated in patients with suspected pulmonary carcinoma. In most cases, malignant cells derived by one technique will also be identified in specimens from the other two; in a small but important minority, however, the use of the three modes of investigation is complementary. For example, in one study of 57 patients subsequently proved to have carcinoma, brush specimens were positive in 52 (91 per cent) and washings in 50 (88 per cent); the combined positive yield was 96 per cent.[307]

False-positive results (the reporting of malignant cells in the absence of true neoplasm) in specimens of sputum and in bronchial washings and brushings are uncommon, being reported in only 1 to 3 per cent of cases in most series.[302, 306, 308] Reasons include inexperience of the cytologist, evaluation of poorly preserved or inadequately prepared specimens, and misinterpretation of reactive epithelial atypia as neoplastic. The last-named is most common in the presence of pneumonia[309] or pulmonary infarction[310, 311] or in association with cytotoxic drugs.[312] Although malignant cells may be found in the absence of clinical signs and symptoms or roentgenographic abnormality (e.g., in carcinoma *in situ*), this situation should always be viewed with suspicion: the slides should be reviewed in consultation with the reporting cytopathologist, and, if the material is still felt to indicate malignancy, the possibility of specimen mix-up should be considered and confirmatory samples obtained.

In addition to the inexperience of the cytopathologist and inadequate collection and preparation of specimens, several other reasons for false-negative results exist. It has been repeatedly shown that the yield of malignant cells increases with the number of specimens examined,[281, 299, 303, 313, 314] regardless of whether the specimens are sputum, washings, brushings, or a combination of these. The increase in yield can be substantial: for example, in one study of 449 cases of proved lung carcinoma, positive diagnosis obtained by sputum cytology increased from 40.3 per cent on the first sample to 79.9 per cent on the fifth.[281] Positive cytologic diagnoses are made more often with central than with peripheral neoplasms and with large than with small tumors.[281, 300, 313, 315] For example, in one series, the true positive rate for tumors less than 2 cm in diameter was only 15 per cent whereas for those greater than 2 cm the rate was 82 per cent.[281] Although histopathologic type has been shown to correlate with positive diagnosis, squamous cell carcinoma having a higher incidence than adenocarcinoma or large cell carcinoma,[281, 314, 315] this is probably explained by the much more frequent central location and intrabronchial growth of the squamous cell variety. Some investigators have found that lesions in the upper lobes are associated with a smaller yield than those in the lower lobes.[314, 315] Metastatic neoplasms are less commonly detected than are primary lung carcinomas, possibly because

they tend to invade pulmonary parenchyma rather than the proximal airways; nevertheless, discovery rates of 30 to 54 per cent have been reported.[288, 316, 675]

In benign disease, examination of sputum and bronchial washings and brushings is usually unrewarding. The most useful application is in the detection and characterization of infectious or parasitic organisms [including Gram or acid-fast staining of bacteria which is usually performed in the microbiology laboratory and is discussed later (*see* page 412)]. Virus-induced cytopathologic changes may be suggestive of a specific organism[317] and may provide supportive evidence of the etiology of a pneumonia before results of serologic or cultural investigations are available. Many fungi and parasites are identifiable when stained by the Papanicolaou technique, and examination of tracheobronchial secretions occasionally leads to specific diagnosis. In some instances, identification of specific organisms is fairly common: for example, Vercelli-Retta and colleagues reported finding structures diagnostic of *Echinococcus granulosus* in 8 (33 per cent) of 24 cases of hydatid disease;[318] similarly, the definitive diagnosis of *Pneumocystis carinii* pneumonia can be made in many cases by identifying silver-positive organisms in specimens obtained from bronchial washings and brushings or from induced sputum in patients with acquired immunodeficiency syndrome (AIDS).[676]

Cytologic examinations in noninfectious, nonneoplastic diseases are even less likely to be productive although there are a few exceptions: for example, in the appropriate clinical setting, the presence of macrophages containing lipid supports a diagnosis of lipoid pneumonia or fat emoblism.[319, 677] Similarly, the finding of hemosiderin-laden macrophages indicates previous intrapulmonary hemorrhage and is consistent with the diagnosis of either Goodpasture's syndrome or idiopathic pulmonary hemorrhage. The identification of elastin fibers in potassium hydroxide preparations of sputum has been said to be supportive evidence for the presence of necrotizing pneumonia.[320]

Cytology of Pleural Fluid

For cytologic examination, pleural fluid should be collected in a clean jar and transported to the laboratory as soon as possible. If rapid transportation is not feasible, cellular morphology will usually be reasonably well preserved without fixative for up to 24 hours at refrigerator temperature.[270] If sufficient fluid is available, one portion can be passed through a membrane filter and another centrifuged to yield a cell-rich residue from which smears or, if possible, a cell block can be made. As with transthoracic needle aspiration (TTNA), the latter procedure frequently yields small tissue fragments on which histochemical and immunohistochemical investigations can be performed. Bloody effusions can be difficult to evaluate, not only because of problems in making smears but because of the large number of red cells that obscure cellular morphology; a variety of techniques have been proposed to obviate these problems, including density-gradient centrifugation, sedimentation, filtration, and microhematocrit procedures.[321, 322] Cells within pleural fluid can be examined by both scanning and transmission electron microscopy and by immunohistochemical techniques, ancillary procedures that may be of diagnostic importance. Details of these techniques and their indications are discussed in subsequent sections (*see* pages 374 and 375).

As with cytologic examination of pulmonary secretions, the primary feature of diagnostic importance in pleural fluid is the exclusion or confirmation of malignancy. In addition, the number and nature of inflammatory and other cells within the effusion may provide valuable clues concerning etiology. Finally, in a number of uncommon conditions noncellular material or unusual cellular alterations may suggest a diagnosis.

ERYTHROCYTES

Light and associates found red blood cell (RBC) counts greater than 10,000 per mm^3 common to all types of effusion and therefore of no discriminatory value.[323] Counts exceeding 100,000 per mm^3 were most often associated with malignant neoplasm, pulmonary infarction, or trauma. A grossly bloody effusion suggests the possibility of a "bloody tap," in which case the RBC count is high only in the first part of the aspirate. A grossly bloody effusion or one containing 100,000 RBC per mm^3 is much more likely to be of neoplastic than of tuberculous origin.

NEUTROPHILS

A large number of neutrophils in pleural fluid usually indicate the presence of bacterial pneumonia but this can also occur in association with pancreatitis and pulmonary infarction and occasionally with malignant neoplasms and tuberculosis.[323] Although polymorphonuclear leukocytosis predominates in the early stages of tuberculous effusion, it is rapidly superseded by lymphocytosis;[324] thus, an effusion that has been present for longer than a few days that contains more than 50 per cent neutrophils is almost certainly not caused by tuberculosis.

LYMPHOCYTES

In contrast to the "50 per cent rule" for neutrophils and tuberculosis, an effusion containing 50 per cent or more lymphocytes is almost certainly either tuberculous or neoplastic:[323, 325] of 102 patients studied in one series,[323] 31 with an exudative effusion showed a predominant cellular response of small lymphocytes and 30 of these were proved

to be caused by either tuberculosis or cancer. Although lymphocyte predominance may be seen in either disease, most effusions caused by neoplasm contain an admixture of other cell types, resulting in a polymorphous cellular population; by contrast, the lymphocyte-rich effusion of tuberculosis typically contains a paucity of mesothelial or other mononuclear or polymorphonuclear inflammatory cells;[270, 323] in fact, the cellular uniformity may be so marked as to suggest the possibility of well-differentiated lymphocytic lymphoma.[326]

EOSINOPHILS

Eosinophilic pleural effusion may or may not be associated with blood eosinophilia and occurs in a variety of conditions. One of the more common associations is pleural trauma: in a series of 127 effusions with greater than 20 per cent eosinophils, Spriggs and Boddington found a history of recent operation, trauma, spontaneous pneumothorax, or thransthoracic aspiration in 81 (63 per cent).[270] The development of an eosinophilic effusion has also been documented following the induction of artificial pneumothorax in the therapy of tuberculosis.[327] The pathogenesis of eosinophilia in these situations is not clear. The presence of air within the pleural space has been proposed as the common denominator,[328, 329] but the experimental production of eosinophilia by the intraperitoneal injection of blood[330] suggests that other factors may also be operational.

Several other associated clinical conditions have been implicated but are less common;[329, 331–333] in fact, quite frequently there is no clinical correlation at all.[329, 331] Pulmonary infections, including histoplasmosis, coccidioidomycosis, and actinomycosis are occasional causes of eosinophilic effusion,[323, 332, 334] as are parasitic infestations such as amebiasis, ascariasis, and ruptured hydatid cyst. An especially high incidence has been noted in patients with paragonamiasis, presumably related to the transpleural migration of this organism. Effusions that accompany immunologic abnormalities such as rheumatoid disease[270, 332] and drug-induced hypersensitivity[331, 335] are only occasionally associated with increased eosinophils. A high proportion of "benign asbestos effusions" have been found to show eosinophilia,[329] and pulmonary infarction is also said to be a relatively frequent cause.[270]

Perhaps the most important point to take away from this discussion of etiologies is that tuberculous and neoplastic effusions only occasionally contain substantial numbers of eosinophils.[270, 323, 332, 336]

MALIGNANT CELLS

The incidence of positive cytologic examination of pleural effusions of malignant origin ranges from 33 to 87 per cent;[323] most series report an accuracy of about 50 per cent.[323, 337–339] Definitive diagnosis may be difficult, chiefly as a result of the cytologically atypical changes that can occur in reactive mesothelial cells. As with the cytologic investigation of bronchial secretions, repeated examinations are likely to increase the yield of positive diagnoses.[323] Combining cytogenetic analysis with cytologic examination is said to increase the true positive yield to over 80 per cent;[339] flow cytometric DNA analysis[678] and electron microscopy[340, 341] may also be of benefit in selected cases (*see* page 374). Immunocytochemical analysis is an especially promising area of investigation, several studies having reported success in determining specific cell type as well as in distinguishing reactive mesothelial cells from malignant cells on the basis of their antigenic characteristics (*see* page 375).[342–344] Tissue culture of aspirated cells has also been shown to be diagnostic,[345] but results are not substantially better than those using conventional cytologic techniques.

A review of the literature in 1981 showed an overall false-positive rate of only 0.44 per cent for several combined series, although false-negative rates are considerably higher.[346] In patients with cancer in whom no malignant cells are identified in the effusion, it is possible that the effusion is secondary to either pneumonia distal to an obstructing bronchogenic carcinoma or to lymphatic obstruction. This explanation was supported in one study by the finding that 5.5 per cent of patients with proved lung carcinoma and cytologically negative pleural effusion survived for 3 to 14 years.[347] As discussed in the section on pleural biopsy, direct biopsy with a Cope or Abrams needle is a more efficient diagnostic procedure than is exfoliative cytology.

MISCELLANEOUS CYTOLOGIC FINDINGS

Benign disease may be diagnosed or suggested from the examination of material or altered cells within a pleural effusion, but this is very uncommon. Examples include endometriosis,[348] parasitic and infectious diseases like echinococcosis[349] and aspergillosis,[350] rheumatoid disease,[353] ruptured mediastinal teratoma,[679] and systemic lupus erythematosus.[351, 352]

Needle Aspiration

Unlike other procedures such as transthoracic needle biopsy and mediastinoscopy, which produce true tissue fragments, needle aspiration results in a specimen that consists predominantly of individual or small clusters of cells. In recent years, it has become evident that it is a technique with high reliability and minimal discomfort and complication to the patient; it has thus become one of the principal methods in the diagnosis of lung cancer. Aspirates can be taken across the chest wall (transthoracic needle aspiration), the bronchial wall (transbronchial needle aspiration), or directly during mediastinoscopy or thoracotomy (intraoperative needle aspiration).

TRANSTHORACIC NEEDLE ASPIRATION

Transthoracic needle aspiration (TTNA; also known as fine or skinny needle aspiration) was first described by Leyden in the late 19th century, at which time it was designed to obtain microorganisms responsible for acute pneumonia.[354] Shortly thereafter[355] and during the next few decades,[356, 357] reports appeared of its use in the diagnosis of lung cancer. A half century later, a cutting needle for biopsying the lung was introduced;[358] along with several technical modifications, this allowed the removal of an actual core of tissue and resulted in rapid replacement of the fine needle aspiration technique. With the recognition in recent years of a considerable morbidity and mortality associated with the cutting method without the advantage of a greater diagnostic yield, most physicians have rediscovered TTNA, and the cutting needle has now become virtually extinct. This preference has undoubtedly been influenced by the growing expertise of the cytologist and of the operators performing the procedure. This subject has been reviewed in detail by Sterrett and his colleagues.[274]

TTNA consists of the suction of fluid and cells into a syringe through a long, narrow-gauge needle inserted percutaneously into parenchymal lesions. Most clinicians now use needles of 19 to 22 gauge (equivalent to an external diameter of 0.7 to 1.1 mm),[359–368] although some advocate the use of an ultrathin needle of 24 to 25 gauge, asserting fewer complications and an exceptionally good yield.[363] A minority remain proponents of a larger-bore needle (18 gauge or less), which they consider provides the advantages of both an aspiration and a cutting needle, i.e., less risk and more tissue. However, recent reports from these investigators[369, 370] indicate that the morbidity and mortality consequent on the use of this larger-bore "aspiration" needle may be equivalent to that of the Vim-Silverman and other cutting needles that have been largely discarded.

The prone position is recommended during the procedure to reduce the possibility of air embolism, and the patient should be instructed to breath-hold during needle insertion. Fluoroscopic television monitoring is usually employed to ensure accurate positioning of the needle within the lesion.[364, 366, 371–373, 375] CT scanning has also been used as an aid to localization prior to aspiration;[366, 376] if necrosis is suspected within the lesion, contrast enhancement may be performed to position the needle accurately in viable tissue.[377] When the needle is judged to be inserted properly, it is rotated and withdrawn while applying vigorous suction.[368] Some investigators stress the importance of making from three to six separate aspirations[368, 378] and of repeating the procedure should the results initially prove negative.[371, 375, 379] The considerable disparity in results in different series may relate partly to the operator's degree of perseverance. Sinner has stated that lesions smaller than 1 cm in diameter may require more than one needle insertion to obtain sufficient representative material for evaluation (in his study the diameter ranged from 4 to 20 mm).[379] This also has been the experience of others,[380, 381] including Nordenström, who advised us in personal communication that he will puncture a lesion several times if malignant cells are not recovered from one aspiration. Thus, it is possible that the dilemma of false-negative reports can be overcome at least partly by repeated biopsies, an observation attested to by the almost unbelievable results achieved by Nordenström. Regardless of the number of passes made, roentgenograms of the chest should be obtained immediately after the procedure and possibly several hours later to detect complicating pneumothorax.

Aspirated material may be evacuated directly onto glass slides, smeared, and immediately fixed by cytospray technique or in 95 per cent alcohol. The needle should be rinsed with saline and the resulting material either passed through a membrane filter or centrifuged to yield a cell-rich residue that can be smeared or fixed and processed into a cell block. This procedure has been shown to increase the number of positive cases substantially.[298] The preparation of a cell block is particularly desirable, since it frequently provides tissue fragments for histologic examination and for histochemical and immunohistochemical analysis. In many cases, the determination of a specific type of malignancy is greatly facilitated by these procedures. If indicated, a portion of the aspirated sample can be processed for electron microscopic examination.[382, 383, 680] Although slides may be stained in the laboratory by standard Papanicolaou or other techniques, some researchers[384–386] have proposed immediate staining of smears at the time of the aspiration (in a manner analogous to performing frozen sections on tissue). This enables rapid assessment of the adequacy of the specimen so that repeat aspirations may be performed immediately in an attempt to increase yield.

The two main indications for fine needle aspiration cytology are diagnosis of pulmonary or mediastinal malignancy and determination of the etiology of serious pneumonia when noninvasive diagnostic methods have failed. Since even in the hands of operators with the greatest experience there is a definite although small false-negative yield, the procedure is not indicated if there is intention to proceed with resection of a lesion regardless of the results of the test. Although some authorities believe that a diagnosis of small cell cancer precludes surgery, even in operable patients, this opinion is not held by all. We feel that biopsy of a peripheral lesion strongly suspected of being a cancer merely to establish diagnosis or cell type preoperatively is not warranted. An exception to this "rule" may apply in geographic regions in which TTNA yields a relatively high proportion of specific benign diagnoses such as in areas where coccidioidomycosis or histoplasmosis is endemic. In patients with suspected cancer, there are thus three clear-cut indications for TTNA: (1) the establishment of a cytologic diagnosis in a patient judged to be unresectable on clinical or roentgenologic grounds; (2) the determination of cell type in a lesion suspected of representing either a metastasis[387] or a second primary pulmonary carcinoma;[388] and (3) the establishment of a diagnosis in a patient who is a poor surgical risk and in whom a positive biopsy would permit acceptance of the risk.

Contraindications to the procedure include a suspicion that the lesion may be an echinococcal cyst, the presence of severe pulmonary arterial hypertension, a patient with a bleeding disorder or on anticoagulant therapy, the inability of the patient to tolerate a complicating pneumothorax, or a patient with an uncontrollable cough.[360] Serious complications of TTNA are rare: in their review of the literature, Sterrett and colleagues[274] documented 12 deaths, most of which were caused by hemorrhage; air embolism[389–391] and massive pneumothorax[274] are also occasional causes. A small pneumothorax is a much more common complication, possessing an overall incidence of approximately 30 per cent; however, less than a third of these patients require aspiration of the pleural space, through either a malleable sigmoid needle or an intercostal drainage tube.[372, 375, 392–395] It is interesting that in one series assessing the usefulness of needle biopsy in chest lesions in different locations, the incidence of pneumothorax was lower in central than in peripheral lesions; the complication rate did not differ between large and small lesions.[396]

Significant bleeding into the lung or pleural space is rare when the needle employed is 1 mm or less in cross section;[397–399] employing an ultrathin needle of 24 or 25 gauge, Zavala and Schoell[363] performed TTNA on 50 patients and obtained an incidence of pneumothorax and hemorrhage of 8 and 4 per cent respectively; these low figures compare with an incidence of 30 and 10 per cent respectively in 2062 patients culled from the literature who were biopsied with 16 to 20 gauge needles. As a result of having produced cardiac tamponade (requiring pericardiocentesis) in two patients, one group of experienced investigators[400] has advised against biopsying lesions too close to the mediastinum. There have been occasional reports of tumor implantation along the needle tract.[392, 401–403, 681] The procedure itself usually results in little discomfort for the patient; it is interesting that pain upon puncture of the lesion, although rare in most tumors, is relatively common in neurogenic tumors of the mediastinum.[404]

The accuracy of cytologic diagnosis in TTNA has been assessed in two investigations of intra- and inter-observer reproducibility.[405, 406] In one,[405] a review of 100 cases showed concordance in the diagnosis of malignancy of 90 per cent between two observers and 94 per cent by the same observers at different times. Agreement as to the cell type of malignant tumors was 80 per cent between observers and 85 per cent by the same cytologist. In the second study,[406] also of 100 cases, interobserver agreement in the diagnosis of malignancy was 85 per cent; intraobserver reproducibility was 100 per cent for the cytologist experienced with TTNA and 90 per cent for a relatively inexperienced observer, implying the benefit to accurate diagnosis of repeated exposure.

As with other cytologic techniques, the most important use of TTNA is in the establishment of a diagnosis of malignancy, the diagnostic yield being highest in peripheral pulmonary lesions over 1 cm in diameter[407] and in superior sulcus neoplasms;[408] although yield is lower in central lesions, diagnostic accuracy is still appreciable. In one study in which the diagnostic yield of TTNA was compared with sputum cytology, the former was superior irrespective of the location of the tumor.[409] A review of the recent literature reveals an average overall accuracy of approximately 85 per cent (15 per cent false-negatives) for TTNA of the lung in series with subsequent histologic proof of malignancy or adequate clinical follow-up.[361–364, 370, 372, 375, 394, 395, 398, 410–412] Only a few investigators[362, 375, 395] have been able to achieve the sensitivity of over 90 per cent previously reported by Nordenström[371] and by Sinner.[379] False-positives rarely exceed 5 per cent and in most series range from 0.5 to 2 per cent.[274] The most common condition leading to a false-positive diagnosis is tuberculosis.[274]

Metastatic neoplasm may be differentiated from primary lung carcinoma in a substantial number of cases. In many instances, comparison of tissue fragments within a cell block with slides of a known extrathoracic primary will provide the diagnosis. In addition, cytologic features of some neoplasms (such as renal cell carcinoma or colonic adenocarcinoma[413]) are occasionally sufficiently characteristic to suggest a source without examination of actual tissue fragments. Electron microscopic and immunohistochemical examinations occasionally can prove useful in determining the cell type, either of primary lung carcinoma or of a metastasis.[368, 414–418]

Although the principal application of TTNA is in the determination of malignancy and its cell type, a specific diagnosis of a benign condition is occasionally possible. Since small tissue fragments are often included in the aspirate, especially when larger-bore needles are used, virtually any pulmonary disease that has characteristic histopathologic changes may be identified.[274] The most important of these are infections. Obviously, culture of aspirated material is the most important aspect of tissue analysis in these cases, and material for this purpose should always be submitted to the microbiology laboratory when there is a suspicion that a lesion might be of infectious etiology. However, as in the examination of tracheobronchial secretions, cytologic examination occasionally can provide the initial or only etiologic diagnosis of the pneumonia. *Pneumocystis carinii*, *Actinomyces* and *Legionella* species, and a variety of fungi[673] and parasites[682] may be identified, either by routine or special stains or by immunofluorescent techniques. In the appropriate clinical and roentgenologic setting, the presence of bacteria within an acute inflammatory exudate may suggest a diagnosis of abscess. Fragments identifiable as granulomas can be detected on smears and filters prepared from TTNA; the presence of finely granular or calcified necrotic material, corresponding to areas of caseous necrosis, is also suggestive of a granulomatous process.[683] The most common underlying lesion in these cases is tuberculosis; morphologic findings in aspirates from them have been described in detail by Dahlgren and Ekstrom.[684]

Many benign neoplastic and non-neoplastic lesions can also be definitely diagnosed by TTNA, including hamartomas,[419] nodular amyloidosis,[420] thymomas, posterior mediastinal neurogenic tumors, and lipomas.[274] The diagnosis of other non-neoplastic conditions may also be suggested by the cellular background of the smear: for example, the presence of fragments of vegetable material implies the probability of aspiration pneumonia,[685] and the finding of numerous blood cells and hemosiderin-laden macrophages suggests the diagnosis of pulmonary infarction[686] or other processes associated with pulmonary hemorrhage.

TRANSBRONCHIAL NEEDLE ASPIRATION

Although needle aspiration of mediastinal lesions may be carried out percutaneously (TTNA),[374, 393, 421–428] a transbronchial approach is becoming increasingly popular.[359, 365, 366, 393, 399, 429] Transbronchial needle aspiration (TBNA) may be accomplished through either a rigid or a flexible fiberoptic bronchoscope. When the latter instrument is employed, lesions that are more peripherally situated in the bronchial tree can be aspirated, particularly when these are not visible through the bronchoscope.[359, 374, 426] The technique is most useful in the upper lobes. It has been used both in establishing a primary diagnosis[359, 374, 426] and in the staging of known lung carcinoma[425] and should be regarded as a procedure that is complementary to washings and brushings. The yield of positive diagnosis is somewhat less than that for peripheral lung masses and is particularly low in mediastinal lymphomas.

INTRAOPERATIVE NEEDLE ASPIRATION

Fine needle aspiration is used by some surgeons to make a definitive diagnosis of malignancy during thoracotomy or mediastinoscopy in patients in whom the diagnosis of lung cancer was not confirmed preoperatively. The diagnostic accuracy ranges from 95 to 100 per cent, and smears prepared at the operating table can be stained and interpreted within 10 minutes.[430–432]

Aspiration from Intravascular Catheters

Examination of cells and tissue fragments in blood aspirated from a "wedged" Swan-Ganz catheter has been advocated as a means of diagnosing fat and amniotic fluid embolism and lymphangitic carcinoma.[687] Although reports of its use in these situations are few, the technique may prove to be valuable in certain situations.

BIOPSY

In a number of cases of malignancy and in the majority of cases of benign disease, cytologic investigations alone do not provide a definitive diagnosis. In these circumstances, tissue biopsy is usually necessary and can be accomplished by a number of techniques, each of which has its own type and rate of complication as well as diagnostic yield. The physician must decide which method is the most appropriate for any particular patient and clinical situation. It is unrealistic to make hard-and-fast rules as to what type of lesion requires a biopsy and which procedure should be used. Each case must be considered individually, taking into account all the variables involved in the decision.

The following pages outline the principles involved in making this decision. Before discussing specific techniques, however, it is appropriate to emphasize several features that are common to all.

(1) Despite the fact that reported instances of mortality are rare and that morbidity is seldom serious although fairly common, every method of obtaining tissue can result in complications. High-risk patients are those with pulmonary hypertension, bleeding diathesis, bullae, and limited respiratory reserve. Even in these circumstances, however, biopsy may be indicated on the chance that it will provide information indicating specific therapy. Although biopsy "activists"—proponents of the policy of getting a tissue diagnosis "no matter what"—support their position by citing the very low reported mortality rate and the easily controlled complications, we suspect that some deaths and serious complications go unreported.

(2) When considering the merits of a particular technique, it is necessary to take into account the experience of its proponents, who will generally obtain results superior to those of less experienced investigators. In fact, the various techniques have been infrequently compared by the same observer. Burt and associates[433] carried out a prospective comparative study of TTNA, cutting needle biopsy, transbronchial biopsy (TBB), and open lung biopsy (OLB) on 20 consecutive patients with pulmonary

disease, usually diffuse but either acute or chronic; each patient had all four types of biopsy. The diagnostic yield was as follows: aspiration, 29 per cent; cutting, 53 per cent; TBB, 59 per cent; and OLB, 94 per cent. In an extensive review of the literature in which the results of biopsies in chronic diffuse lung disease were compared,[434] the combined results of a number of investigators gave total yields of 63 per cent for cutting, 72 per cent for drill, 72 per cent for TBB, and 94 per cent for OLB.

(3) Although biopsy is usually performed to obtain material for histologic study, in many cases it is essential that some tissue be sent to the laboratory for bacteriologic and mycologic analysis or preferably inoculated on culture media in the operating room; this is especially true for specimens obtained by OLB.

(4) It is important to remember that a biopsy samples only a small portion of a particular disease process. Thus, because of possible variation in distribution and severity, especially in diffuse pulmonary disease, the findings in one biopsy specimen cannot be absolutely extrapolated to all regions.

(5) Finally, it must be stressed that correlation of clinical, roentgenologic, and pathologic findings is likely to provide a far more precise diagnosis than that of which each alone is capable, and close cooperation between each specialist should be avidly encouraged.

For the most part, patients requiring biopsy for definitive diagnosis have one of two distinct types of roentgenographic presentation: local or general pulmonary disease. "General" disease implies widespread involvement of all or most of both lungs whereas "local" disease includes all other disease processes: the latter may be unifocal (such as a solitary pulmonary nodule or cavity) or multifocal (such as multiple pulmonary nodules or cavities). From the point of view of both the indications for biopsy and the technique to be employed, the manner in which these two patterns are approached is quite different.

In patients with a solitary pulmonary nodule, several factors influence the decision to perform a biopsy. For example, it would be reasonable to assume that a small, uncalcified, peripheral nodule discovered on a screening chest roentgenogram of an asymptomatic person under 30 years of age was granulomatous, particularly if the patient lived in an endemic zone of histoplasmosis. Watchful waiting and repeat roentgenograms every 3 to 6 months for 2 years are probably sufficient to establish the benign nature of the lesion. By contrast, in the absence of distinguishing roentgenographic features, especially in older patients at risk of cancer by virtue of a smoking history, biopsy may be warranted to determine whether the lesion is malignant.

In patients who have widespread or general pulmonary disease, the differential diagnosis includes a multitude of diseases, and the roentgeno-graphic appearances are seldom sufficiently characteristic for specific diagnosis. Although most patients with diffuse roentgenographic abnormality have chronic disease, often of insidious onset, in some the clinical presentation is acute and fulminating. Many of the latter group are compromised hosts, in which case an invasive diagnostic procedure clearly is justified to identify the responsible microorganism so that appropriate antibiotic therapy can be instituted promptly. In patients with chronic disease, the indications for lung biopsy are less clear-cut. When disease has produced symptoms and is obviously progressive, biopsy is mandatory unless the patient is too old or too ill to warrant the slight risk; like others,[435] we have seen several such patients for whom biopsy results led to the diagnosis of a treatable condition. A more detailed discussion of roentgenographic patterns of disease in relation to biopsy techniques can be found on page 365.

Bronchial Abnormalities, Including Tumors

The bronchial approach for obtaining histologic or cytologic material for diagnosis is being used with increasing frequency, not only because of its high yield but also because of the low incidence of complications. Tissue can be obtained directly from lesions visible through the bronchoscope or from bronchoscopically invisible lesions in the lung periphery. Malignant cells or microorganisms can be obtained by brushing bronchoscopically visible lesions or those which are only roentgenographically visible and whose location for biopsy is established fluoroscopically. Cytologic studies also can be performed on aspirated washings from such areas. The method and complications of bronchoscopy are considered in detail on page 406. Here, we will discuss the indications and results of its use for obtaining tissue and cells.

The principal value of proximal airway bronchoscopic biopsy is in the diagnosis of malignancy and the establishment of cell type. A diagnosis of sarcoidosis also can often be confirmed by this technique. Less commonly, other lesions such as benign endobronchial neoplasms and endobronchial tuberculosis also can be detected. Endoscopically visible lesions in the proximal bronchial tree can be brushed, washed, aspirated with a needle, or biopsied with forceps. The first three of these procedures have already been discussed in the section on cytology; with respect to total yield, they are complementary to tissue biopsy.[307]

The great visual range of the flexible fiberoptic bronchoscope (FFB) represents a distinct advantage of this instrument over the rigid bronchoscope, especially in the upper lobes. One group of investigators estimated that two thirds of 700 primary pulmonary carcinomas were visible with the FFB compared with only one third with the rigid scope.[436] In a combined retrospective study of the experience at Guys and Brompton Hospitals in London, England, of 68 lesions from which positive biopsies had been obtained by FFB, 23 were judged to be out of range of the rigid scope.[437] Overall diagnostic yield from tumors that are bronchoscopically visible ranges from 90 to over 95 per cent with the FFB compared with about 85 per cent with the rigid instrument.[438–440] Popovich and associates[440] reported a diagnostic yield of 92 per cent in central tumors when a single forceps biopsy was performed combined with cytology from brushings; this figure increased to 96 per cent when up to four forceps biopsies were carried out. Fortunately, the diagnosis of small cell carcinoma from tissue specimens is very dependable (and only slightly less so by cytology); this is particularly important since it is generally accepted that central varieties of this neoplasm should be treated primarily by radiation or chemotherapy (or both) rather than by surgical resection.[439, 441]

Lung

Transbronchial Biopsy (TBB)

Transbronchial biopsy (TBB) has been proved to be of value in the diagnosis of sarcoidosis, lymphangitic carcinomatosis, and diffuse opportunistic infections, but of relatively low yield in interstitial pneumonitis and fibrosis and in bacterial pneumonia.[442–444] In opportunistic infections, its success can be attributed more to the ancillary technique of FFB (see page 409) than to tissue biopsy itself. In chronic interstitial disease, a biopsy is best obtained with the forceps inserted into a small peripheral bronchus;[445, 446] however, the recommendation made by Andersen and Fontana and associates[445, 446] that the forceps should be closed in expiration does not appear to be warranted since a study in dogs has revealed no difference in material obtained in inspiration and expiration.[447]

The yield obtained from TBB of peripheral pulmonary nodules is dependent in large measure on the thoroughness and ingenuity of the investigator and increases with the number of biopsies taken.[440] Cells can be obtained by needle aspiration (TBNA), brushing, washing, and a variety of cutting instruments,[448–451] techniques that are complementary.[307] Biplane fluoroscopy[440, 448–454] is essential for localizing the lesion, and it is not surprising that those who do not use this facility have a very poor yield.[455] With prior mapping of the location of lesions by selective bronchography, and using a double-hinged curette through a FFB under fluoroscopic guidance, Ono and coworkers obtained a positive cytologic diagnosis in 45 of 46 peripheral carcinomas less than 2 cm in diameter.[451] When fluoroscopy is used without bronchography, the diagnostic yield in malignant lesions ranges from 70 to 90 per cent.[440, 449, 452, 454, 456–459, 461] The yield with benign lesions is considerably lower.[454, 460]

TRANSTHORACIC NEEDLE BIOPSY (TTNB)

Although microscopic fragments of lung or tumor tissue are sometimes obtained with TTNA (especially with larger-bore needles), a true core of tissue can be procured only with a cutting needle. Three techniques have been used: punch biopsy, trephine drill biopsy, and suction-excision biopsy. Although some investigators espouse the virtues of TTNB,[688] it appears that all three procedures are gradually being replaced by TTNA, not only because it possesses a significantly lower complication rate but because the diagnostic yield of the four procedures is comparable.

Punch Biopsy. The needle originally designed for punch biopsy, the Vim-Silverman, consists of an inner, split, cutting needle that is driven into the lung, and an outer needle that is inserted over and compresses the cutting blades. Both needles are rotated 180° and then removed, with a thin sliver of tissue trapped between the blades.[358] A number of modifications have been introduced over the years:[462] the type and gauge of needle employed varies widely from institution to institution, ranging from the 17 gauge aspiration and core-cutting Lee needle[463] through a slotted 20 gauge thin-walled needle[464] to the 23 gauge flexible, stainless steel Chiba needle.[465] Although a number of reports indicate better results with thin-walled aortographic or 18 gauge lumbar puncture needles,[397, 398, 466] we have been impressed by the lack of any major difference in the incidence of positive results or complications with the gauge of needle employed.

Although satisfactory lung specimens have been obtained in approximately 80 per cent of cases with various types of cutting needles, a precise tissue diagnosis can be expected in only 65 per cent and in half this number if the diagnosis of nonspecific pulmonary fibrosis is excluded.[461, 467, 468] The diagnostic accuracy is considerably higher if the procedure is confined to peripheral masses,[369, 469, 470] although even in these cases the yield is no better than that reported by a number of workers employing TTNA.[361–364, 370, 375, 394, 395, 397, 398, 411, 412, 472]

Cutting needles result in pneumothorax in 20 to 25 per cent of patients and in hemoptysis in 10 to 15 per cent;[369, 468–471] this incidence is approximately the same as that encountered with TTNA using a 16 to 20 gauge needle but is considerably higher than that reported for an ultrathin needle of 24 to 25 gauge.[363] In addition, hemorrhage is usually more severe and life-threatening, and the mortality rate is undoubtedly higher.[369, 411, 468–471, 473–477]

Trephine Biopsy. This technique employs a high-speed drill with an outside diameter ranging from 2.1 to 3.0 mm; it can be performed more rapidly and with less pain than the conventional form of cutting needle biopsy. The yield is equivalent to that of punch biopsy, and the complication rate may be somewhat lower;[434] however, several deaths have been reported.[478–480]

Suction-excision Biopsy. To our knowledge, there have been only two reports in the literature of the use of this instrument.[481, 482] Negative pressure applied with a syringe draws lung tissue into the side portal of a biopsy needle inserted through the pleural cavity. By its very nature, suction-excision biopsy of the lung should be used only for diffuse disease involving the subpleural parenchyma; limited data suggest that the yield leaves something to be desired.[481, 482]

THORACOSCOPIC BIOPSY

Thoracoscopy (pleuroscopy) is a procedure in which the pleura is directly examined visually. In the days when artificial pneumothorax was the accepted treatment for tuberculosis, the technique was universally employed to sever adhesions between the visceral and parietal pleura. In recent years, there has been a revival of the technique for diagnosing pulmonary and pleural disease, predominantly in Europe[483–486] but also in North America.[487–491]

After the induction of pneumothorax, an endoscope (thoracoscope, fiberoptic bronchoscope, or mediastinoscope) is inserted through an incision in an intercostal space and the pleura examined; biopsy of the pleura or underlying lung can be performed through the same or a second opening in the thoracic cage. Anesthesia can be local,[447] regional,[491] or general.[485] The procedure appears to be well tolerated by both children and adults[492, 493, 664] and even by patients who demonstrate some degree of hypoxemia prior to initiation of the procedure.[494] Biopsy specimens of lung parenchyma measure 2 to 5 mm, being considerably larger than those obtained by TBB. As with other biopsy procedures, it is desirable to obtain multiple specimens. A coagulative device connected to the biopsy forceps can be used to seal ruptured bullae or blebs in cases of spontaneous pneumothorax.

In the few reported series of patients with diffuse interstitial disease, the diagnostic yield of thoracoscopic biopsy ranges from 90 to 100 per cent.[485, 486] Complications include hemorrhage (which is usually mild) and pneumothorax (which may be persistent).[485, 486] The technique has been used successfully in immunocompromised hosts.[486, 491] Despite the encouraging reports to date, it is obvious that further experience is required before this procedure can be accepted as an alternative diagnostic approach to open lung biopsy.

OPEN LUNG BIOPSY (OLB)

Open lung biopsy (OLB) is recommended particularly for cases of chronic diffuse lung disease, but it is also useful in some cases of acute and presumably infectious disease when other, less risky, procedures have been unproductive. The chest is opened through a standard thoracotomy incision or through a limited incision large enough to allow removal of a fragment of tissue measuring 2 to 3 cm in diameter. Gaensler and Carrington[495] prefer a modified Chamberlain approach, entering the thorax in the second interspace for easy access to all pulmonary lobes and the mediastinum; a general anesthetic is recommended in case the incision must be extended.[435] When a small incision is used, pulmonary parenchyma is ballooned out by exerting positive pressure on the lung, a clamp is applied, and the tissue is removed. Originally described by Andrews and Klassen,[496] this technique is particularly applicable when the disease is so diffuse that any portion of the lung is likely to reveal the pathology. When disease is more confined, a full thoracotomy incision is recommended; the operator can then examine the lung and choose the best site for biopsy. The larger incision is not associated with higher morbidity or mortality but usually necessitates a longer hospital stay.

Selection of the appropriate site for biopsy is clearly of paramount importance. Areas of discrete disease should be removed *en bloc* if small enough to be included in the specimen; if more extensive disease is present, the biopsy should include an area of transition between abnormal and apparently normal lung. Samples from more than one site should be taken if surgically feasible. Intraoperative frozen sections may be examined to help ensure the adequacy of the tissue sample. The tips of the lingula and middle lobe are not uncommon sites of chronic vascular changes and fibrosis[689] and should be avoided; similarly, it is unwise to biopsy very abnormal areas since these often show end-stage disease of unrecognizable origin.[495] Computed tomography has recently been used to identify a precise area for biopsy at minithoracotomy;[497] the CT scan is performed in the operative position and the optimal area to biopsy is indicated by a radiopaque marker placed on the skin.

In general, the biopsy specimens should be submitted to a pathologist as soon as possible after excision. Portions may then be selected for electron microscopic or immunofluorescent examination, and frozen sections can be performed to provide a preliminary diagnosis or to assess adequacy of biopsy material. The remaining tissue can then be fixed and used for permanent histologic sections. Techniques have been described for inflating biopsy specimens to help eliminate difficulties in interpretation associated with alveolar collapse.[498, 499]

When performed by an experienced surgeon, OLB has a mortality rate roughly equivalent to that of needle biopsy, especially if seriously ill patients are excluded.[435, 665] In a review of 502 patients subjected to OLB for the diagnosis of chronic interstitial lung disease, Gaensler and Carrington reported a mortality rate of 0.3 per cent and a complication rate of 2.5 per cent.[495] However, from a review of 2290 cases in the literature, Gaensler and associates calculated mortality and complication rates of 1.8 and 7.0 per cent respectively, figures that are probably more realistic estimates of the true incidence.[434] Gaensler and Carrington also reported a diagnostic yield of 92.2 per cent, a remarkable success rate which is perhaps open to some question when it is recognized that the final diagnosis in 3.4 per cent was "honeycombing," in 2.2 per cent, bronchiolitis obliterans, and in 5.6 per cent, "nonspecific."

OLB appears to be gaining in popularity as the most dependable diagnostic procedure in immunocompromised patients with roentgenographic evidence of acute pulmonary disease whose etiology has not been established by noninvasive methods. Although it is associated with a high incidence of complications, the mortality rate is surprisingly low and the yield of a definitive diagnosis high.[500, 501]

Pleura

NEEDLE BIOPSY

The most common method of obtaining fragments of pleural tissue for histologic examination is transthoracic needle biopsy (TTNB), a procedure that can be performed at the same time as thoracentesis (described on page 410).[502] The two needles most commonly used are the Cope and Abrams (a recent modification of the Abrams needle is the addition during manufacture of a three-way tap).[503] Success with these instruments depends largely upon the skill of the operator, the selection of patients, and the number of biopsies taken. The last of these is very important: in one series of 55 patients with pleural effusion, 33 were found to be malignant or granulomatous; up to 10 biopsies were obtained on individual patients from one site only, and in 32 of the 33 patients the pathologic abnormality was present in only some of the specimens.[504]

The chief value of TTNB of the pleura is in the diagnosis of cancer and tuberculosis. Since granulomatous disease other than tuberculosis seldom involves the pleura, the finding of necrotizing or non-necrotizing granulomas is usually accepted as an indication of tuberculous infection, even when microorganisms are not identified. Rarely, histologic findings in patients with rheumatoid disease permit the assumption that the pleural effusion is a manifestation of this condition.[505] Only rarely has pleural granulomatous inflammation consistent with sarcoidosis been associated with an effusion.[506, 507] Although the diagnosis of tuberculous pleurisy with effusion is usually made pathologically by identification of granulomatous inflammation rather than by discovery of acid-fast organisms,[513, 514] cultures of pleural fluid are occasionally positive despite negative biopsy results.[511] Culture of pleural tissue fragments has also been reported to be positive in a high proportion of cases.[507]

The diagnostic yield in patients with neoplastic involvement of the pleura ranges from 40 to 75 per cent (average, 62 per cent).[504, 508–512, 515] Sensitivity in the diagnosis of tuberculosis is somewhat higher, ranging from 70 to 88 per cent (average, 79 per cent).[504, 508–512, 516] Combined use of biopsy and cell blocks from pleural fluid has been reported to have a yield as high as 87 per cent in the diagnosis of cancer.[517]

In patients in whom the nature of a pleural effusion has not been established, needle biopsy of the pleura should be carried out whenever thoracentesis is performed, and always before starting treatment for tuberculous effusion. Like other workers,[518, 519] we remove fluid for cytology, culture, and biochemical studies and then take several pieces of tissue by needle biopsy; if this yields no diagnostic material, we recommend direct pleural biopsy through a limited thoracotomy incision or by thoracoscopy.

Although complications are rare and usually mild, we have encountered two instances of rather severe hemorrhage into the chest wall and pleural cavity. Mediastinal and subcutaneous emphysema have been reported,[504, 511] and there have been at least three instances of pulmonary neoplasm developing along needle tracks;[512, 520, 521] the incidence of implantation and growth of mesothelioma cells following needle biopsy is much higher.

THORACOSCOPIC BIOPSY

There is good evidence that thoracoscopic biopsy is the diagnostic method of choice in the investigation of patients with persistent pleural effusion in whom a diagnosis has not been established by cytology and needle biopsy. It appears to be a less traumatic procedure than open pleural biopsy, and its yield of positive diagnoses is remarkably good. In one series of 150 patients with malignant effusion, the diagnosis was established in 131 (87 per cent) whereas the combined yield of needle biopsy and pleural fluid cytology was only 41 per cent.[484] In another study of 11 patients in whom a diagnosis was not established by thoracentesis or closed pleural biopsy, a positive diagnosis of cancer was made in 9 by thoracoscopic biopsy.[487] The technique has also been employed to obtain tissue for hormone receptor determination in patients with pleural effusion caused by metastatic breast carcinoma.[690]

OPEN BIOPSY

Some physicians prefer to obtain a biopsy specimen of the pleura directly, contending that tissue specimens are superior and that the procedure is no more difficult to perform than needle biopsy.[666] We do not agree with this: because of the added risk of the general anesthetic that we consider to be essential for direct pleural biopsy, even with a limited thoracotomy incision,[522] we restrict open pleural biopsy to patients with pleural effusion in whom needle biopsy or thoracoscopic biopsy has not yielded a specific diagnosis.

A major decision that must be made in patients with pleural effusion of undetermined etiology is whether to administer treatment for tuberculosis. Although some investigators[523, 524] feel that a negative needle biopsy excludes a tuberculous etiology, the experience of others is against sole reliance on the percutaneous method: for example, Scerbo and coworkers[511] obtained no granulomatous tissue by needle biopsy in 3 of 14 patients proved to have tuberculous pleurisy with effusion.

Despite the use of immunohistochemistry and electron microscopy, malignant mesothelioma and metastatic carcinoma can be difficult to diagnose from the small tissue fragments obtained by TTNB and thoracoscopic biopsy.[525] When malignancy is suspected from evidence provided by clinical, roentgenologic, or histologic findings, open biopsy is indicated to obtain adequate tissue samples. It may be advantageous before thoracotomy to induce pneumothorax followed by chest roentgenography, to outline the tumor as an aid to the surgeon in selecting the best area to biopsy.

Mediastinum

Three procedures can be used to obtain tissue from the mediastinum: mediastinoscopy,[526] open biopsy,[527] and biopsy through a catheter.[530–532] The main indications for these techniques are the staging and (less often) the diagnosis of pulmonary carcinoma. Primary mediastinal neoplasms also can be diagnosed by these means, as can certain benign conditions such as sarcoidosis. Involvement of mediastinal lymph nodes in patients with pulmonary carcinoma is associated with a very poor prognosis: despite the contention of some authorities that mediastinal lymph nodes are regional and therefore potentially resectable,[529] it is the opinion of most observers that involvement of these nodes portends a negligible chance of 5 year survival.[533, 534] As pointed out by Pearson,[535] these differences of opinion may derive from the fact that, at least in part, prognosis depends on how far up the mediastinum lymph node involvement has extended; for example, patients with metastases in lymph nodes contiguous with involved bronchopulmonary nodes may survive for 5 years. Pearson reviewed three papers dealing with patients in whom positive mediastinal nodes were identified at mediastinoscopy and who subsequently were subjected to resection without adjuvant therapy: there were no 5 year survivors. Other workers have also reported a zero postoperative survival rate of patients with positive mediastinal nodes.[536, 537] By contrast, Pearson cites his own experience with 42 patients with squamous cell carcinoma and positive mediastinoscopy who received preoperative radiation followed by resection: 9.5 per cent survived 5 years, a result that may reflect the site of mediastinal node involvement, or the therapy, or a combination of both.[535]

Mediastinal lymph node biopsy also can be useful in the diagnosis of nonmalignant disease affecting hilar or mediastinal nodes, particularly sarcoidosis. A review of eight studies reporting the incidence of positive results of node biopsy in patients with clinical diagnosis of sarcoidosis showed that the yield of diagnostic material from mediastinoscopy ranged from 84 to 100 per cent.[538]

OPEN BIOPSY

This procedure permits direct inspection of mediastinal lymph nodes through the usual thoracotomy incision or limited mediastinotomy.[527, 539, 540] It has the advantage of permitting more extensive exploration of the mediastinum and more accurate assessment of neoplastic extension to the hila.

Because of the barrier produced by the arch of the aorta on the left, mediastinoscopy results in a lower positive yield in neoplasms of the left lung than of the right. For example, in one study of 162 patients with pulmonary carcinoma unassociated with roentgenographic evidence of mediastinal lymph node enlargement, cervical mediastinoscopy yielded 16 per cent with lymph node invasion—19.7 per cent on the right and only 10.6 per cent on the left.[541] By contrast, of 45 similar patients with left-sided tumors who underwent left anterior mediastinotomy, 28.9 per cent were found to be positive.[541] Because of this, a left anterior mediastinotomy is advocated for exploration of the mediastinum in cases of left-sided tumors. In primary carcinomas arising in the lower lobes, mediastinal biopsy by either mediastinoscopy or mediastinotomy seldom results in a positive yield; in one series of 39 patients in which mediastinal nodes showed neoplastic involvement, the primary was situated in a lower lobe in only one.[541]

CATHETER BIOPSY

Catheter biopsy of the mediastinum, a technique developed by Nordenström, who experienced considerable success without serious complications, can be done via a transjugular, paraxiphoid, or paravertebral approach.[530–532] In lesions of the posterior mediastinum, he used carbon dioxide to separate fascial planes.[532] We have been unable to find evidence from the literature that others have attempted to emulate him.

MEDIASTINOSCOPIC BIOPSY

As originally described by Carlens,[526] mediastinoscopy is carried out through an incision in the suprasternal notch; the soft areolar tissues are dissected along the trachea, and biopsy material is removed under direct vision through an instrument similar to that used for pediatric esophagoscopy. The space explored comprises the upper half of the mediastinum, including tissues around the intrathoracic portion of the trachea, the tracheal bifurcation, and the proximal part of the major bron-

chi. Complications are uncommon and usually not serious; one review of the literature estimated their incidence at 3 to 4 per cent.[537] The most serious is hemorrhage, usually venous;[537, 542, 543] in one review of 740 cases,[543] serious hemorrhage occurred in eight patients, requiring thoracotomy for control in two. A laryngeal nerve, usually the left recurrent, is occasionally injured: in a study of 47 patients by indirect laryngoscopy, both pre- and postoperatively, Widström[544] found that four (6 per cent) developed this complication. Pneumothorax and wound infections are very uncommon.[537, 542, 543] That the incidence of complications can be reduced with experience was amply demonstrated by Sarin and Nohl-Oser,[545] who encountered two severe hemorrhages in their first 50 mediastinoscopies and no morbidity whatever in the next 350.

If mediastinoscopy fails to reveal lymph node metastases, resectability of lung tissue at thoracotomy is almost assured, being reported in 67 (93 per cent) of 72 patients in one series[542] and in 140 (96 per cent) of 147 in another.[545] On the other hand, mediastinoscopy is of considerable value in reducing the number of thoracotomies at which disease is found to be unresectable: for example, Gunstensen and Wade[546] decreased unnecessary thoracotomies from 28 to 15 per cent, Marchand[547] from 25 to 8 per cent, and Doctor[548] by an estimated 30 per cent. Over a 13 year period, Ashraf and associates[549] were able to exclude 236 (27 per cent) of 874 patients from thoracotomy on the strength of findings at mediastinoscopy; follow-up of 210 of the 236 showed that only 4 (1.7 per cent) were alive after 5 years whereas 24.5 per cent of the 638 patients who were subjected to resection were 5 year survivors.

Biopsy of mediastinal lymph nodes in patients with proved pulmonary carcinoma has an overall positive yield of approximately 30 per cent.[549, 551, 552] The incidence of positive results varies with the cell type; for example, in Sarin's and Nohl-Oser's series of 296 patients,[545] mediastinal nodes were involved in 149 (50 per cent)—in 54 (37.5 per cent) of 144 cases of squamous cell carcinoma, in 15 (50 per cent) of 29 cases of adenocarcinoma, and in 65 (75 per cent) of 90 cases of small cell carcinoma (the cell type was not clearly established in 15). Based on their experience over a three year period, Smith and coworkers[550] concluded that mediastinoscopy should be performed prior to thoracotomy in all patients with a central carcinoma and in those with a peripheral carcinoma measuring 4 or more cm in diameter; those with peripheral lesions less than 4 cm in diameter could be taken directly to thoracotomy. Employing these criteria for mediastinoscopy, these workers found mediastinal metastases in 82 of 203 patients (40 per cent)—in 13 (20 per cent) of 64 squamous cell carcinomas, 24 (33 per cent) of 73 adenocarcinomas, 25 (60 per cent) of 41 large cell carcinomas, and 20 (80 per cent) of 25 small cell carcinomas. Only 44 of the 82 patients with positive mediastinoscopy showed mediastinal involvement on conventional chest roentgenograms. With the general availability of fourth generation CT apparatus nowadays, this examination is playing an increasing role in the staging of lung cancer; its impact on the requirement for mediastinoscopy and the advantages and disadvantages of the two procedures are discussed at some length in Chapter 8.

Scalene Lymph Nodes

Scalene lymph node biopsy, first described by Daniels in 1949,[553] consists of the removal of tissue lying on the scalene group of muscles in the supraclavicular fossa, including the medial fat pad. Its main applications have been in the determination of spread beyond the thorax in cases of proved or suspected pulmonary carcinoma and in the diagnosis of sarcoidosis. Mediastinoscopy with node biopsy has largely replaced the latter application, chiefly because it provides a greater yield of pathologic material and does not increase risk.

Following Rouvière's assertion[554] that lymph from the right lung and the lower half of the left lung drains to the right supraclavicular lymph nodes, it was customary for surgeons to biopsy the right scalene areas whenever disease involved these lung regions. However, Rouvière's conclusions were based on studies of fetuses and infants, and it has now been shown that they do not apply to adults.[529, 555, 556] Baird[556] found that lymphatic spread of carcinoma is usually ipsilateral, and that when contralateral it is just as often from right to left as from left to right. However, Brantigan and associates[529] found a considerable incidence of contralateral spread and concluded that both scalene areas should be biopsied in all cases of proved or suspected carcinoma of the lung.

Scalene lymph nodes that are palpable almost always contain pathologic tissue:[529, 557] in a review of the literature, Brantigan and colleagues[529] found that palpable nodes were involved by neoplasm pathologically in 475 (83 per cent) of 576 cases of pulmonary carcinoma. As expected, the positive yield is not nearly as high when scalene nodes are not palpable: in the review of Brantigan and colleagues, biopsy of nonpalable nodes was positive in only 452 (20 per cent) of 2254 patients with pulmonary carcinoma; approximately the same incidence (23.8 per cent) of positive biopsy findings of nonpalpable nodes was found in their own series of 341 cases of histologically proved carcinoma of the lung.[529] In a more recent study of 101 consecutive patients with pulmonary carcinoma who were otherwise considered appropriate candidates for pulmonary resection, Schatzlein and coworkers[558] found only 9 to have positive pathologic results on biopsy of nonpalpable scalene nodes; in this series, no patient with a peripheral primary lesion, regardless of size or cell type, had metastases to scalene nodes. These investigators also found that bilateral biopsy of the scalene area was no more likely to yield positive results than ipsilateral biopsy alone.

The yield of positive results of scalene lymph node biopsy increases in proportion to the number of patients with sarcoidosis included in the series; even when such nodes are not palpable, they contain granulomas in 70 to 80 per cent of patients with proved sarcoidosis.[559–562]

Scalene node biopsy is a relatively minor procedure *in experienced hands* but should not be relegated to inexperienced members of the house staff. Major complications include local large vessel injury, lymphatic fistulas, Horner's syndrome, and infection extending into the mediastinum. A review of 186 scalene lymph node biopsies at the Massachusetts General Hospital showed a 6 per cent incidence of serious complications, fatal in two cases;[563] another study[564] reported a lymphatic fistula in one patient and a fatal complicating pneumothorax in two.

In summary, since mediastinoscopic lymph node biopsy results in a higher diagnostic yield, biopsy of scalene areas should be restricted to patients with palpable nodes.

SUMMARY AND RECOMMENDATIONS

Out of the vast experience accumulated over the past three or four decades, we will attempt to summarize the indications for the use of specific techniques to obtain material for pathologic examination. Although we have taken the extensive experience of other investigators into due consideration, our recommendations largely reflect the approaches we have adopted on the basis of personal experience. It is emphasized at the outset that no specific rules apply to every situation; each patient must be considered individually and the merits of all the variables must be weighed before making a decision. Despite this, the following general recommendations should apply in *all* situations in which thought is being given to obtain material for pathologic examination.

1. The procedure with the least risk and discomfort to the patient should have the highest priority. Thus, an invasive procedure is not indicated if a diagnosis can be established by simpler, noninvasive techniques such as sputum culture or cytology. Similarly, TTNA of a peripheral nodule is preferred to thoracotomy and open biopsy when definitive surgical treatment is not possible.

2. Biopsy is not indicated if the possibility of malignancy has been excluded by certain clinical findings or roentgenographic signs. For example, calcification within a solitary pulmonary nodule or confirmation of lack of change in the size of a solitary nodule over time both imply a benign process; special procedures to establish the presence of calcification (conventional or computed tomogra-

phy, or dual-energy digital radiography) should be performed before any invasive procedure is attempted; similarly, a concerted search for previous roentgenograms should be made.

3. The patient's general condition must be such that it does not by itself contraindicate the procedure; for example, TTNA of a small peripheral nodule for purposes of diagnosis alone might be justified in a patient with severe COPD in whom a thoracotomy and surgical resection would not be feasible, but the patient should have enough breathing reserve to withstand a possible complicating pneumothorax.

4. It is important to recognize that the confidence that is placed in any particular technique is proportional to the ability to exclude false results. Apart from inherent deficiencies in the method itself, this ability is largely determined by the expertise of the persons performing the procedure and interpreting the results and will clearly vary among different institutions and individuals. The value of a particular method should thus be questioned when it is associated with an appreciable number of false-negative or false-positive results.

5. The patient's age is very important in some situations; for example, a solitary peripheral nodule in a 25-year-old woman and a 50-year-old man require different approaches.

6. Features in the patient's history may be of major importance in influencing the decision whether or not to biopsy. For example, a history of exposure to carcinogens such as cigarette smoke, asbestos, or radioactive materials should increase the suspicion of a malignant process; similarly, a definitive history of exposure to a patient with tuberculosis would increase the likelihood of this disease.

7. The presence or absence of symptoms of disease elsewhere in the body is an essential factor; for example, entirely different approaches are needed in the investigation of multiple pulmonary nodules in a patient with polyarthritis, in one with a large renal mass, and in one with nasal ulceration and hematuria.

8. Finally, time is an important consideration in all cases. We have seen patients whose roentgenograms revealed a lesion of unknown etiology for which biopsy was being considered for definitive diagnosis; however, the lesion had either diminished in size or had disappeared altogether on roentgenograms obtained a few days later. In many instances, therefore, it is advisable to delay an invasive procedure for at least a week, particularly when a lesion is likely to be infectious in origin.

In six basic roentgenographic patterns of pulmonary disease the indications for and techniques of biopsy are different. In the recommendations that follow, these patterns are discussed in relation to variables of major importance to each, leading to a decision as to whether to recommend an invasive procedure and which procedure is most appropriate for each lesion.

SOLITARY PERIPHERAL PULMONARY NODULE 2 CM OR LESS IN DIAMETER
(Fig. 2–19)

Such a lesion in a patient under 30 years of age is almost certainly benign; biopsy is not warranted even if previous roentgenograms are unavailable for comparison or an earlier film did not show a similar shadow. In such cases, however, roentgenograms should be obtained every 3 months for at least a year to confirm the benign nature of the lesion. Calcium within the lesion (not eccentrically situated) establishes its benign nature beyond reasonable doubt and indicates no further need for follow-up. Eccentric calcification should raise the possibility of so-called scar carcinoma, and such a lesion should either be investigated promptly or watched closely.

In patients over 30 years of age, particularly those aged 40 to 60 years, a solitary, noncalcified lesion must be regarded as cancer until proved otherwise. If previous roentgenograms are not available for comparison or if such roentgenograms fail to reveal a lesion or show a smaller lesion than is now apparent, the patient should be investigated initially by examination of multiple sputum specimens and by bronchoscopy with washings and brushings. If these are negative and if there is no evidence of metastatic disease in the mediastinum or elsewhere, in most cases we recommend proceeding directly to thoracotomy. Although in these circumstances some would advocate TTNA to obtain preoperative diagnosis, for a variety of reasons we feel that in the majority of cases this procedure is not justified. If intraoperative frozen sections of mediastinal lymph nodes are negative, excisional biopsy with frozen sections of the nodule should be performed; if this proves malignancy, definitive surgical excision can then be undertaken.

If a patient with a solitary pulmonary nodule refuses surgery or if surgery is contraindicated by severe impairment of lung function or evidence of metastatic disease, there is reasonable justification for an invasive procedure such as TTNA or TBNA. The rationale in each of these circumstances is twofold—to exclude rare benign conditions that can simulate malignancy and to help establish prognosis. Another situation in which TTNA might be the procedure of choice is the patient with an extrapulmonary primary malignancy without known metastases who develops a solitary pulmonary nodule. In these circumstances, it may be justified to consider the pulmonary nodule as a second primary; however, the increased likelihood of it representing a metastasis makes thoracotomy less appealing as an initial diagnostic procedure. Depending to some extent on the type of extrapulmonary neoplasm (e.g., melanoma, colorectal carcinoma, prostatic carcinoma), in some cases TTNA combined with immunocytochemical and electron microscopic examinations can provide a definite answer as to the primary or metastatic nature of the nodule.

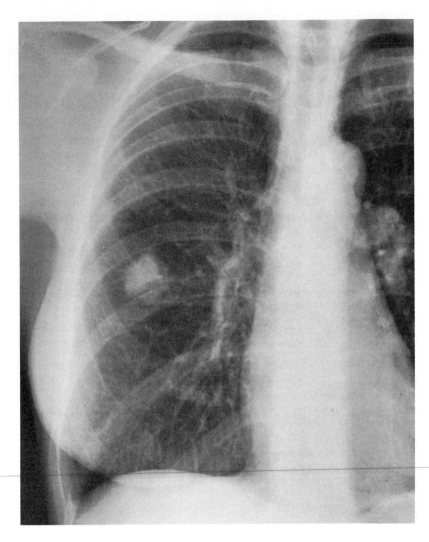

Figure 2–19. Solitary Pulmonary Nodule 2 cm in Diameter. This nodule is of uniform density and contains no demonstrable calcium. A roentgenogram from several years previously revealed no lesion. Surgical resection was carried out without biopsy study of the nature of the lesion. Anaplastic carcinoma. The patient is 51-year-old woman.

SOLITARY PERIPHERAL PULMONARY NODULE LARGER THAN 2 CM IN DIAMETER
(Fig. 2–20)

Since larger nodules are more likely to be malignant, the age-related conservative approach just described for some patients is not warranted, and management should proceed as described for a nodule in the 40- to 60-year-old age group. If cavitation is present in a lesion of this size, the etiology may be infectious even in the absence of fever, constitutional symptoms, or leukocytosis; since such lesions are usually caused by anaerobic organisms, a therapeutic trial of penicillin may be indicated if the clinical history is compatible with such a diagnosis.

SEGMENTAL CONSOLIDATION OF LUNG PARENCHYMA, USUALLY ASSOCIATED WITH LOSS OF VOLUME
(Fig. 2–21)

In most patients with this pattern, an endobronchial lesion is causing atelectasis or obstructive pneumonitis, and bronchoscopy with brushings,

washings, and biopsy usually establishes the diagnosis. Despite the potential hazard of biopsy-related hemorrhage from vascular lesions, it is desirable to establish a diagnosis before thoracotomy in order to detect cases of small cell carcinoma or the occasional benign neoplasm.

MULTIPLE PULMONARY NODULES WITH OR WITHOUT CAVITATION
(Fig. 2–22)

In many patients with this roentgenographic pattern, the diagnosis is apparent without recourse to cytologic or histologic examination of tissue; the majority of patients have either an established primary neoplasm elsewhere or multiple infectious granulomas. Positive skin tests to specific antigens or a history of residence or travel in an endemic zone may be helpful in establishing the latter diagnosis. If these investigations are unproductive, we believe that a direct approach by TTNA is the procedure of choice; open lung or cutting needle biopsy should be reserved for patients in whom less traumatic procedures have yielded negative results. In patients with an established primary malignancy,

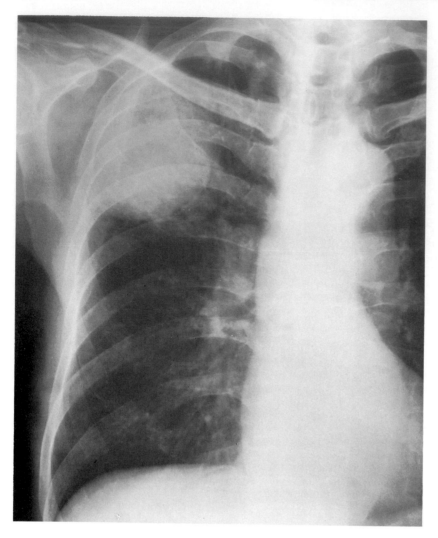

Figure 2–20. Large Peripheral Mass. A large, ill-defined mass of uniform density is present in the right upper lobe, its lateral border contiguous to the visceral pleura. The diagnosis of adenocarcinoma was established by biopsy with cutting forceps via a fiberoptic bronchoscope.

biopsy confirmation of the metastatic nature of multiple pulmonary nodules is usually unnecessary. In patients in whom the primary site is unknown, roentgenographic investigation of multiple organ systems in search of a primary neoplasm is so often unrewarding that we feel that it is seldom indicated. When metastases and multiple granulomas have been excluded, the remaining diagnostic possibilities are rather limited and include Wegener's granulomatosis, rheumatoid necrobiotic nodules, and multiple pyemic abscesses. In most of these cases, careful attention to signs and symptoms of extrathoracic disease and to laboratory findings should enable one to make a confident diagnosis.

ACUTE DIFFUSE PULMONARY DISEASE
(Fig. 2–23)

The great majority of patients with this pattern are immunocompromised hosts. Respiratory symptoms are often absent when an abnormality is first discovered on a chest roentgenogram, but in some cases cough and dyspnea develop and rapidly worsen, creating a situation that requires immediate

decisions regarding management. Such patients are likely to be receiving immunosuppressive drugs, corticosteroids, chemotherapeutic agents, or antibiotics, and a drastic reduction in dosage or complete withdrawal of medications frequently results in clinical and roentgenologic improvement; an early decision to take this action before the onset of severe dyspnea and hypoxemia will permit assessment of roentgenologic response before it becomes necessary to commit the patient to an invasive diagnostic procedure. If resolution does occur, it can be assumed that either there has been an improvement in host defenses with consequent control of infection or the disease was the result of a drug reaction. If clearing does not occur, the etiology of the diffuse pulmonary disease is probably an opportunistic microorganism. Since it is unusual for such opportunists to be identified with certainty in either sputum or tracheal aspirates, in most instances an immediate invasive procedure is indicated for diagnosis, and we recommend that bronchoscopy with TBB and ancillary procedures such as BAL should be performed first. If these prove negative, thoracoscopic or open lung biopsy can be performed as a final resort.

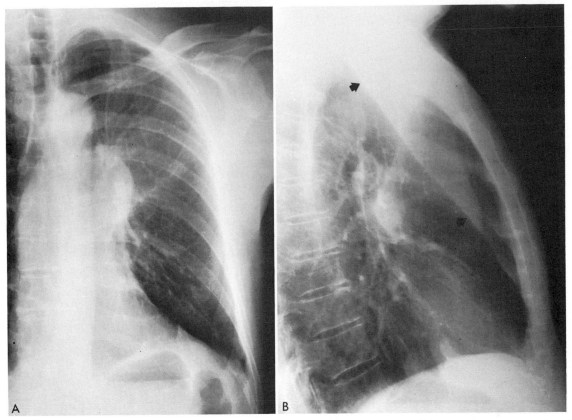

Figure 2–21. Obstructive Pneumonitis, Left Upper Lobe. Posteroanterior (*A*) and lateral (*B*) roentgenograms reveal moderate loss of volume of the left upper lobe (*arrows* in *B* point to anteriorly displaced major fissure). The collapsed lobe is uniformly opaque and shows no air bronchogram. Bronchoscopic biopsy revealed squamous cell carcinoma. The patient is a 63-year-old man.

CHRONIC DIFFUSE PULMONARY DISEASE
(Fig. 2–24)

The roentgenographic pattern of disease usually indicates predominant involvement of either the interstitium or airspaces, more often the former, and onset is usually insidious. Many of these patients are asymptomatic, and it is debatable whether an invasive diagnostic procedure is justified despite the low risk. For example, the patient with a diffuse reticular pattern, hilar lymph node enlargement, and anergy almost certainly has sarcoidosis and requires no further investigation. However, there are many patients in whom diffuse progressive disease has produced symptoms and in whom the roentgenographic pattern and clinical picture provide no clues to the diagnosis. In this situation, unless the patient is too old or too ill to warrant the slight risk, biopsy is mandatory to establish the diagnosis of a potentially treatable condition. Open lung biopsy is the procedure of choice, although the results of thoracoscopic biopsy suggest that this technique might be of value in some circumstances.

Occasionally, patients become so disabled by dyspnea that we hesitate to recommend open biopsy; in such circumstances, we think it wise to restrict invasive procedures to those least likely to provoke complications since therapy other than with corticosteroids is unlikely to be indicated regardless of the biopsy result. As the first step, we recommend a transbronchial approach for biopsy of the peripheral parenchyma with a cutting instrument; should this prove unrewarding, open lung biopsy can then be performed if absolutely necessary. In our opinion, the low yield of needle biopsy contraindicates this procedure.

EXAMINATION OF EXCISED LOBES AND WHOLE LUNGS

Pulmonary lobes that have been surgically excised or whole lungs that have been removed either surgically or at autopsy can be examined by a variety of techniques. To some extent, the method of examination depends on the suspected nature of the underlying disease: for example, injection of the pulmonary artery with contrast medium might be the procedure of choice in a case of suspected arteriovenous fistula, and incineration of lung tissue and analysis of the residue may be desirable in the presence of pneumoconiosis. However, these special techniques are impractical and unnecessary as a routine, and in the great majority of cases the most appropriate method of investigation is inflation and fixation of the lung with liquid formalin followed by serial slicing. The easiest and most widely utilized

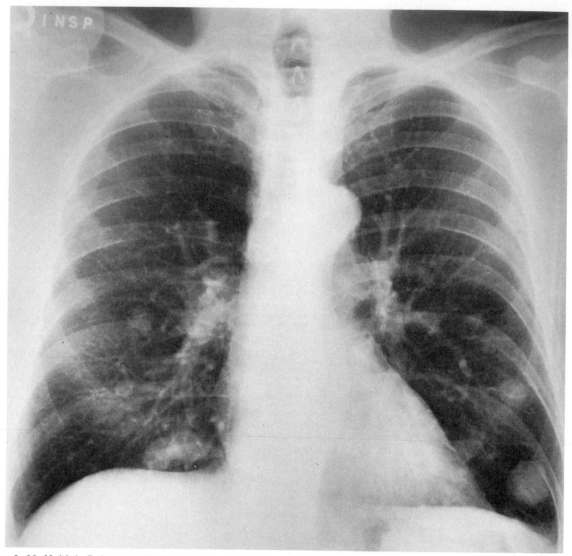

Figure 2–22. Multiple Pulmonary Nodules Without Cavitation. This 62-year-old man had had a malignant melanoma excised from his neck 3 years previously. At the time of this roentgenogram, he was asymptomatic.

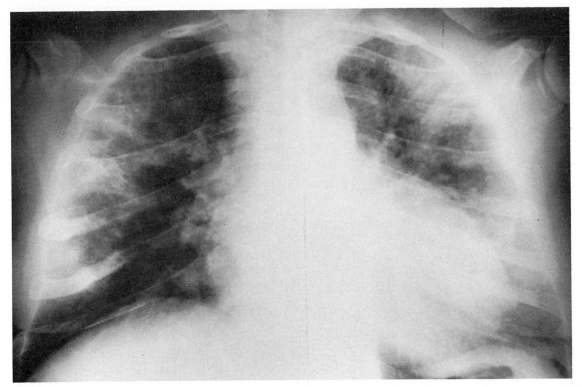

Figure 2–23. Acute Diffuse Lung Disease. This 32-year-old renal transplant patient who was on immunosuppressive therapy presented low-grade fever, increasing dyspnea, and cough. Sputum and transtracheal aspirates failed to reveal an etiologic agent, but bronchial brushing showed *Pneumocystis carinii* organisms.

method of fixation is to distend the lung to apparent full inflation with formalin introduced into the bronchi under positive pressure. This is conveniently performed from a container elevated above the lung, the most suitable maximal pressure head ranging from 25 to 50 cm of formalin; a smaller pressure head can be obtained by raising the lung in relation to the fluid level in the reservoir. A full head of pressure may be required to inflate the lungs of patients who died in status asthmaticus, with lower pressures for lungs of older patients and those suspected of having emphysema. Although variations on this basic technique have been proposed,[565] the additional information derived from them is not sufficient to warrant their routine use.

After inflation, the most proximal airways are clamped and the lung or lobe left for a period of time in a large vat of formalin. Although the tissue may be firm enough to be adequately cut after only 2 to 3 hours, specimens are best left overnight and examined the following morning. After examination of the pleural surface, they should be cut with a sharp knife or commercial meat slicer in even sections 1 to 1.5 cm thick; sectioning may occur in any plane, but we find the sagittal direction most convenient. The cut slices can be rinsed in running water to remove formalin and then laid out on a cutting board for detailed examination. In addition to systematic inspection of parenchyma, airways, vessels, and lymph nodes, palpation of grossly unremarkable areas should be performed to identify the occasional abnormality that is not apparent visually.

Examination of a slice under the dissecting microscope may reveal abnormalities in greater detail than can be achieved with either the naked eye or light microscope; this is particularly useful in the assessment of emphysema, especially when the tissue is impregnated with barium and floated under water (as originally described by Heard).[566] In some cases, the technique developed by Gough and Wentworth[567] of mounting whole lung sections on paper may be useful for recording observations and preserving specimens and is especially helpful in the assessment of the extent and severity of emphysema. A rapid method of preparing these sections has been described;[568] a modified technique has also been described by Ferencz and Greco[569] for the study of normal and diseased pulmonary arteries.

Although slicing after expansion to apparent full inflation and fixation is the easiest and most valuable method for examining lungs or lobes, the technique can be criticized on several points. (1) It is not known how much artifact may result from overinflation. After its removal from the body, the lung's expansion is no longer limited by the chest wall, so that *in vitro* inflation to maximal capacity theoretically can produce volumes larger than existed *in vivo*. However, it has been established that lung volumes at apparent full inflation are similar to predicted TLC values,[570] implying that lung size is limited to some extent by the pleura. Thus, the

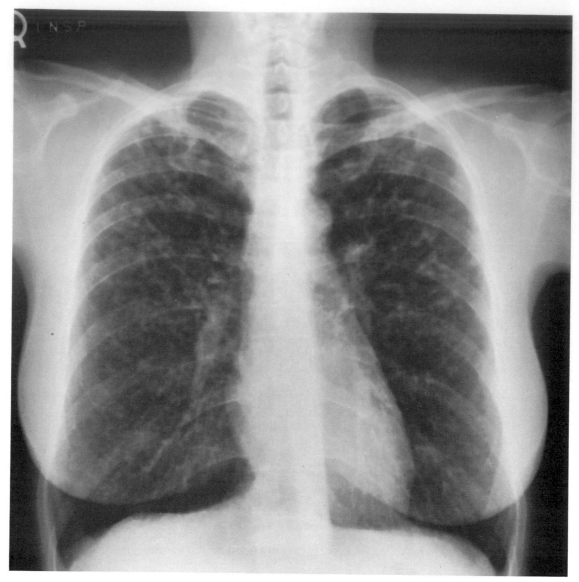

Figure 2–24. Chronic Diffuse Lung Disease. This 46-year-old woman presented with a 6-month history of increasing shortness of breath on exertion and mild, nonproductive cough. A rather coarse reticulonodular pattern is present, with moderate upper zone predominance. Open lung biopsy revealed eosinophilic granuloma.

potential deleterious effects of overinflation do not appear to pose a significant problem. (2) When a lung is distended and left without a constant head of pressure, it diminishes 20 to 30 per cent in volume, even when the bronchus is clamped. The greater part of this decrease in volume occurs in the first few hours after inflation, and it is largely complete within 12 hours. Much of it is the result of leakage through pleural tears, but it also occurs in air-tight lungs in which it presumably results from tissue shrinkage and from solution and diffusion of gas and fixative. Although not a significant factor for routine diagnosis, this volume loss can be minimized if necessary by the use of constant pressure during fixation; an apparatus for accomplishing this has been described by Heard and his colleagues.[571] (3) Obviously, culture is not possible once the lung has been fixed, and it is inevitable that in a number of cases routine examination of lungs by inflation and fixation will lead to the lack of specific identification of an infectious organism. Thus, in surgically excised specimens in which a preoperative diagnosis has not been made, it is mandatory that appropriate swabs or portions of abnormal tissue or both be taken for culture before fixation. The same applies to lungs removed postmortem from patients with suspected pneumonia, especially when the host is immunocompromised or may have an unusual pulmonary disease. In most cases, the pleural incision used to obtain the appropriate tissue can be sutured or clamped and the lung subsequently inflated to a degree adequate for proper examination. (4) It is somewhat more difficult to dissect pulmonary arteries and bronchi in sliced specimens than in intact lung. Nevertheless, in cases in which this is necessary, these structures can be dissected in continuity by careful comparison of each slice with its neighbor. (5) Pulmonary edema may be difficult to recognize in fixed inflated specimens as a result of the flooding of airspaces by formalin; when this diagnosis is suspected, a small portion of lung can be excised and fixed intact and the incision clamped. (6) Postmortem roentgenograms for radiologic-pathologic correlation are not possible.

Despite these potential disadvantages, we believe that the identification and topography of lesions can be much better appreciated in distended, fixed lung slices than in the distorted, limp tissue of uninflated, unfixed lung. In addition, appreciation of the nature and extent of disease microscopically is vastly superior in the former situation. Thus, we feel that the advantages of this technique far outweigh the disadvantages and recommend that simple distention by liquid formalin be the routine procedure for the examination of all lungs, whether of necropsy or surgical origin.

Several additional techniques have been advocated to obtain specimens suitable for special investigations such as morphometric analysis and radiologic-pathologic correlation. Some researchers have advocated inflation and fixation by formaldehyde gas rather than fluid.[572-575] This results in specimens that are said to be ideal for demonstration purposes and for the study of three-dimensional morphology;[572] in addition, excellent radiologic-pathologic correlation can be achieved.[573, 574] However, depending to some extent on the temperature of the formaldehyde vapor as well as the severity of parenchymal disease, the tissue may be inadequately fixed and the histology poor.[575] Inflation by formalin steam does not dehydrate the lungs as rapidly as gas alone, and preservation for histologic studies is said to be much better.[575, 576] Some workers have also suggested using a combination of liquid inflation-fixation and air-drying.[577, 578] In this technique, a mixture of formalin, polyethylene glycol, and alcohol is insufflated into the bronchi. After fixation (about 48 hours), the lung is dried by blowing air through the bronchus at a constant pressure of about 20 mm mercury.[578] These techniques result in adequately preserved specimens from which excellent gross and histologic correlation with radiologic patterns can be appreciated.[579-582]

Radiologic-pathologic correlation has also been attempted by postmortem radiography. The appearance of the chest roentgenogram using this technique is similar to one taken antemortem during quiet breathing or at expiration.[691] It is desirable to employ special halters to suspend the body in a vertical position.

SPECIAL PATHOLOGIC TECHNIQUES

Examination of the Pulmonary Vasculature and Airways

Several substances have been used for pulmonary *angiography*. The most satisfactory of these is the Schlesinger mass,[583] the basic ingredient of which is gelatin that is kept liquid at room temperature by potassium iodide and that solidifies upon the addition of formalin. Barium sulfate or other radiopaque material can be added to obtain roentgenographic visibility, and dyes can be used to define different components of the vasculature. A technique to obtain postmortem roentgenographic visibility of the bronchial arteries has been described by Cudkowicz and Armstrong.[584] *Bronchography* can be performed using either the Schlesinger mass or fine-particle barium or lead insufflated into the bronchial tree. *Corrosion casts* of the pulmonary vasculature or bronchial tree have been made with several materials, including wax, celluloid,[585] vinyl resin,[586] unsaturated polyester resins,[585] and, most recently, silicone rubber.[587] After the selected material has hardened, the surrounding lung is digested in acid, leaving permanent casts of the injected structure. A method of preparing a hollow cast of the bronchial tree has also been described.[588]

Postmortem Lung Cultures

Although postmortem lung cultures should always be taken in the appropriate circumstances, their results must be assessed with caution. The major problems in their interpretation are the high incidence of positive cultures in the absence of clinical or pathologic evidence of true infection[589-591] and the poor correlation in some studies between antemortem and postmortem cultures.[590] The reasons for the high percentage of positive cultures obtained in the absence of apparent infection include (1) inadequacy of sterile technique during the procurement of the culture; (2) the presence of commensal organisms in chronically diseased lung such as chronic bronchitis or cystic fibrosis; and (3) terminal aspiration of oropharyngeal secretions into distal airways. It has also been suggested that some organisms can be present normally in otherwise unremarkable pulmonary tissue.[592]

The most meaningful culture results may be obtained with the following procedures:[593]

(1) Cultures should be taken under sterile conditions immediately after the thorax has been entered and before the large vessels and gastrointestinal tract have been incised.

(2) The pleural surface of a palpably or visibly abnormal area of lung should be seared with a hot spatula or soldering iron. The pleura should then be incised with a scalpel within the seared area and the underlying parenchyma either swabbed or cut into a small tissue fragment with sterile instruments.

(3) The lung parenchyma adjacent to the cultured area should be sectioned and fixed for histologic examination.

Confidence in the clinicopathologic significance of a positive culture requires the presence of at least some of the following: (a) the absence of organisms normally considered skin or oropharyngeal commensals such as *Staphylococcus epidermidis* or *Streptococcus viridans*; (b) the presence of a pure culture of one organism in more than one site, either in lung and blood or in two different foci in the same or both lungs; (c) the presence of histologic evidence of infection in the tissue adjacent to that yielding the positive culture (inflammation, with or without the presence of organisms with Gram or other stains); and (d) a heavy growth of organisms. To the extent that these findings are absent, the relevance of a positive culture must be questioned.

It has been suggested that qualitative determination of bacterial growth may be important in determining which postmortem cultures are significant. In a postmortem study of 50 lungs, Knapp and Kent[594] found histologic evidence of pneumonia or bronchitis in 18 cases; in these 18, culture from the adjacent lung parenchyma grew greater than 10^5 organisms per ml of tissue in all but one instance. By contrast, although 21 of 50 cases without histologic infection had positive cultures, in only 3 were the counts greater than 10^5 per ml. A technique of culture from prints derived from fresh[692] or microtome sections of frozen lung tissue has also been said to yield reliable results.[595]

Electron Microscopy

It is usually unnecessary to examine pulmonary tissue or cells by electron microscopy for diagnostic purposes, the application of this technique in lung disease being primarily in research. Nevertheless, in some instances its use is helpful and occasionally indispensable in establishing a precise diagnosis. Some of these applications have been reviewed by Wang.[596]

TRANSMISSION ELECTRON MICROSCOPY

In transmission electron microscopy (TEM), an electron beam is focused on an ultrathin section of tissue and an image produced by collecting the transmitted electrons on a screen or photographic plate. Because of the necessity for a small tissue specimen (usually in the order of 0.25×0.25 mm in the final prepared state), one of the major limitations of the technique is related to sampling, diagnostic conclusions being considered reliable only when the tissue examined is representative of the disease process. Careful handling and fixation of tissue is essential since autolysis rapidly results in ultrastructural changes that can obscure proper interpretation, especially in diseased lungs.[597] A convenient and adequate fixative is a cold buffered mixture of 4 per cent formaldehyde and 1 per cent glutaraldehyde, although a buffered solution of either alone may be adequate for initial fixation. Tissue fragments should be small (1 mm) to allow for adequate fixative penetration. Specimens obtained at bronchoscopy or TTNA can be placed directly in fixative by the endoscopist or aspirator, although open lung biopsy specimens should be referred immediately to a pathologist who can appropriately sample and mince the tissue. Fluid aspirated from the pleural space can be centrifuged and the resulting cellular pallet fixed and processed for TEM; preservation of ultrastructural detail in this instance has been reported to be adequate even after delay in fixation.[340]

Although generally not as adequate for interpretation as biopsy material, tissue obtained at autopsy also can be used, and several techniques have been advocated to obviate postmortem autolysis. Trump and his colleagues[598] performed "immediate autopsies" within 3 to 5 minutes of death, a procedure that is cumbersome and probably impractical in most situations although it results in adequate tissue preservation. Bachofen and his coworkers[597] injected glutaraldehyde into the lung percutaneously within 30 minutes of death, mixing it with a dye to localize the injected region upon evisceration; although useful for examining normal lungs or diffuse lung disease, this technique is less helpful for focal abnormalities in which precise localization of the areas to inject may be difficult. Tracheobronchial tissue obtained up to 5 hours postmortem and placed in Krebs-Henseleit solution perfused with oxygen and carbon dioxide may be remarkably well preserved.[599] Samples for TEM can also be retrieved from paraffin-embedded tissue or from cut and stained sections on glass slides. Although in these circumstances cellular details are usually obscured, structures such as neurosecretory granules or viral particles may be sufficiently well preserved to help establish a diagnosis.[600]

Only a brief review of some of the diagnostic applications of TEM will be given here. Although the identity of the etiologic agent in pneumonia is determined most reliably by culture and less often by light microscopy, ultrastructural examination occasionally will establish the presence of an organism and may indicate specific type; this is particularly true of viral infections in which variation in size and morphology enables precise characterization of some species. Preservation of viral particles is usually reasonably good, and tissue or cells obtained from blocks or even slides years after fixation have been found to harbor recognizable virions.[600, 601] TEM is essential for the diagnosis and characterization of the immotile cilia syndrome,[602] since currently the basic abnormality cannot be accurately determined by other means.

Although usually not essential, electron microscopic findings are sufficiently characteristic to help confirm the diagnosis of a variety of metabolic abnormalities, including amyloidosis, alveolar proteinosis, and some storage diseases.[603] Intracytoplasmic "X-bodies" are characteristic of the Langerhans cells of eosinophilic granuloma, and their identification may help confirm the diagnosis; although this is usually not necessary in specimens obtained by OLB, analysis of cells obtained by TBB or BAL may obviate the need for such an invasive procedure.[604, 605] TEM examination of the lungs, unlike that of the kidneys, is usually unrewarding in immunologic disease of presumed immune complex origin; only rarely have basement membrane–dense deposits consistent with such complexes been identified.[606]

Of more widespread use is the application of TEM to the diagnosis of pulmonary neoplasms. This occasionally can be the definitive diagnostic technique in such uncommon neoplasms as carcinoid tumor, tracheobronchial gland carcinomas,[607, 608] benign clear cell tumor,[609, 610] and others.[611, 612] The finding of neurosecretory granules may aid in the diagnosis of small cell carcinoma, especially when only small amounts of tissue are available from transbronchial biopsy or TTNA. A clear-cut histogenetic diagnosis of pulmonary sarcoma is often aided by ultrastructural findings, and most neoplasms with a sarcomatous appearance should be examined in this fashion (in conjunction with immunohistochemical techniques) before a specific diagnosis is applied. In pleural effusions,[340, 613, 614] TEM is useful in differentiating mesothelioma from metastatic carcinoma. It can also be helpful occasionally in distinguishing primary from metastatic lung carcinoma[341] and lymphoma from carcinoma, the latter particularly in lymph nodes biopsied at mediastinoscopy.

There is debate as to whether the classification of non–small cell pulmonary carcinoma by TEM is either useful or appropriate.[615–617] There is no doubt that ultrastructural examination of these neoplasms can show evidence of differentiation that is not detectable by light microscopic examination;[617–620] this is particularly true of poorly differentiated carcinoma, which is sometimes shown to have both glandular and squamous features ultrastructurally when neither characteristic is identifiable by light microscopy. Although these observations are important in understanding the nature of the disease, as yet there is little if any evidence to justify the routine use of TEM in the classification of pulmonary carcinoma from the viewpoint of either prognosis or therapy.

SCANNING ELECTRON MICROSCOPY

The technique and application of scanning electron microscopy (SEM) have been reviewed in detail[621–624, 693] and will be only briefly described here. Basically, an electron beam sweeps over and interacts with the surface of the specimen, resulting in several forms of secondary radiation. Depending on the nature of the radiation and the means utilized to image it, important characteristics of a specimen can be revealed.[621, 625] SEM is not encumbered by the two major problems encountered with tissue used for TEM. Tissue preservation is not as essential since fine ultrastructural detail is not observed, so that formalin-fixed, paraffin-embedded material is adequate. In addition, substantially larger tissue sections can be examined, making the problem of sampling considerably less important. Techniques have been described for examining cells obtained from bronchial secretions and pleural fluid by both light microscopy and SEM.[626–628]

SEM images that are familiar to most physicians are produced when secondary electrons are collected and amplified, resulting in an exquisitely detailed three-dimensional representation of the surface morphology of an object (see Fig. 1–7, page 7). Although undoubtedly beautiful and of value in understanding the pathogenesis and morphology of pulmonary disease, such images are usually not helpful in establishing a diagnosis. However, some investigators have suggested that they can be of value in differentiating benign, atypical, and malignant cells in pleural effusions.[626, 629–631]

Of far greater importance in diagnosis are other forms of emitted radiation. Back-scattered electrons are emitted in numbers proportional to the atomic number of the material from which they emanate. Since most foreign substances have an atomic number greater than that of carbon, they cause a brighter image than does surrounding tissue, and the technique is thus useful in identifying such substances in very small amounts (up to 50 nm in diameter).[621, 693] In addition, x-rays emitted from an object can be examined by wave-length or energy dispersion spectrometry to provide a precise analysis of the elemental composition of the portion of the sample examined. The primary use of SEM is thus in the study of the pneumoconioses, in which particulate material can be identified and its composition precisely analyzed. Since the different images can be correlated, the technique can provide accurate information about the location of specific particulates within cells or tissues.

Immunochemistry

The development of techniques for the immunochemical demonstration of tissue antigens has been one of the major advances in diagnostic pathology in recent years. The extent of their application, especially in relation to monoclonal antibodies, is only beginning to be appreciated at the time of this writing, and no doubt an abundance of information will be forthcoming on this subject in the near future.

Immunofluorescence tests are performed by applying an antibody conjugated with fluorescein dye to a tissue section.[632] After washing, the tissue is examined with a fluorescent microscope, enabling appreciation of the fluorescent antibody-antigen complex. In the lung, the technique has had its widest application in the study of immunologic abnormalities, especially Goodpasture's syndrome and hypothesized immune complex disease. Its use in the former condition has been the most rewarding,[633] and in patients in whom this diagnosis is suspected tissue should always be taken and examined by immunofluorescence. The technique has also been used for identifying infectious organisms such as *Legionella* species[634] and subtypes of *S. pneumoniae*.[635] The potential for other uses is limited predominantly by the ingenuity of pulmonary researchers and by the development of specific antibodies:[632] for example, Pertschuk and colleagues have reported a high sensitivity and specificity of anti-angiotensin–converting enzyme antibody for the granulomas of sarcoidosis.[636] Other applications are likely to be developed in the near future.

Immunofluorescence tests have three major problems: (1) the necessity in most cases for using frozen tissue (ideally snap frozen at $-70°C$ or less at the time of excision); (2) the difficulty in some instances of localizing the foci of positive immuno-fluorescence histologically; and (3) the natural fading of fluorescence in many cases, resulting in the lack of a permanent tissue record. To overcome these difficulties, a variety of *immunoenzymatic* techniques have been developed:[637] these can be used on formalin-fixed paraffin-embedded tissue, and the application of an appropriate counterstain results in histologic details that are of sufficient clarity to locate regions of positive reactivity precisely. Methods have also been developed for use on cells exfoliated from the airways or aspirated from pleural fluid or parenchymal tumors.[344, 638, 694]

Basically, immunoenzymatic techniques involve the conjugation of a diagnostic antibody with an enzyme (most frequently peroxidase), the application of this combination to a tissue section, and the addition of a substrate (such as diaminobenzidine in the case of peroxidase) that reacts with the enzyme to produce a visible compound. Although these techniques have been used in the study of immunologic lung disease[639] and for the identification of microorganisms,[640] their major application has been in the diagnosis of pulmonary and mediastinal neoplasms.[695] A variety of antibodies have been developed in an attempt to characterize subtypes of pulmonary carcinoma more precisely[418, 641–643] and to distinguish neoplasms such as mesothelioma from metastatic adenocarcinoma[644–646] or mediastinal lymphoma from thymoma.[647] Other applications include distinguishing metastatic from primary pulmonary neoplasms[416] and reactive from malignant mesothelial cells,[342, 343, 646] the identification of bronchioloalveolar cell carcinoma,[417] and the precise characterization of pulmonary sarcomas. As with immunofluorescent tests, the potential benefit of immunoenzymatic techniques in diagnostic pathology is substantial, and the full scope of their use awaits further development.

Analysis of Tissue Contents

In some cases of pneumoconiosis, it may be useful to identify the type of retained dusts within excised lung tissue. Techniques for this purpose include high temperature ashing, micro-incineration, plasma ashing and etching, and wet-chemical or enzyme digestion. These have been discussed and referenced in detail by Vallyathan and colleagues.[624] Although still in an investigative stage, it has been suggested that the analysis of tumor content of hyaluronic acid may be helpful in the diagnosis of mesothelioma[648–650] and that the determination of tissue enzymes may help establish prognosis in patients with pulmonary carcinoma.[528]

Lung Morphometry

Morphometry is concerned with the estimation of quantity or of measurements such as diameter, volume, and thickness by counting points and line segments superimposed on a two-dimensional image.[654] In the lung, the latter is usually a standard H&E-stained tissue section or a TEM photomicrograph. Although its application in the study of normal lung was pioneered by Weibel in 1963[651] and it has been used extensively for this purpose since then, the use of morphometry as a diagnostic procedure in pulmonary disease has been minimal. Its greatest application has been in developmental anomalies, in which it is of value in characterizing such conditions as pulmonary hypoplasia[655, 656] and neonatal lobar emphysema.[652, 653] It is also possible that computer-generated diagnoses based on morphometric analysis will be available in the future in certain specific situations.[696]

Cytogenetics

The principal use of cytogenetic investigation in the diagnosis of chest disease is in relation to malignant pleural effusions;[339, 657–659, 697] when combined with routine cytologic examination, diagnostic accuracy has been reported to be as high as 83 per cent.[659] There is evidence that the technique might be especially useful in effusions caused by leukemia or lymphoma.[659]

REFERENCES

1. Webb WR, Jensen BG, Sollitto R, et al: Bronchogenic carcinoma: Staging with MR compared with staging with CT and surgery. Radiology 156:117, 1985.
2. Heelan RT, Martini N, Westcott JW, et al: Carcinomatous involvement of the hilum and mediastinum: Computed tomographic and magnetic resonance evaluation. Radiology 156:111, 1985.
3. Levitt RG, Glazer HS, Roper CL, et al: Magnetic resonance imaging of mediastinal and hilar masses: Comparison with CT. Am J Roentgenol 145:9, 1985.
4. von Schulthess GK, McMurdo K, Tscholakoff D, et al: Mediastinal masses: MR imaging. Radiology 158:289, 1986.
5. Schmidt HC, Tsay DG, Higgins CB: Pulmonary edema: An MR study of permeability and hydrostatic types in animals. Radiology 158:297, 1986.
6. Vix VA, Klatte EC: The lateral chest radiograph in the diagnosis of hilar and mediastinal masses. Radiology 96:307, 1970.
7. Sagel SS, Evens RG, Forrest JV, et al: Efficacy of routine screening and lateral chest radiographs in a hospital-based population. N Engl J Med 291:1001, 1974.
8. Rucker L, Frye EB, Staten MA: Usefulness of screening chest roentgenograms in preoperative patients. JAMA 250:3209, 1983.
9. Hubbell FA, Greenfield S, Tyler JL, et al: Special Article. The impact of routine admission chest x-ray films on patient care. N Engl J Med 312:209, 1985.
10. Farnsworth PB, Steiner E, Klein RM, et al: The value of routine preoperative chest roentgenograms in infants and children. JAMA 244:582, 1980.
11. Bonebrake CR, Noller KL, Loehnen CP, et al: Routine chest roentgenography in pregnancy. JAMA 240:2747, 1978.
12. Benacerraf BR, McLoud TC, Rea JT, et al: An assessment of the contribution of chest radiography in outpatients with acute chest complaints: A prospective study. Radiology 138:293, 1981.
13. Harris JH (Report from Chairman of the Board): Referral criteria for routine screening chest x-ray examinations. Am Coll Radiol Bull 38:17, 1982.
14. Crapo RO, Montague T, Armstrong J: Inspiratory lung volume achieved on routine chest films. Invest Radiol 14:137, 1979.
15. Trout ED, Jacobson G, Moore RT, et al: Analysis of the rejection rate of chest radiographs obtained during the coal mine "black lung" program. Radiology 109:25, 1973.
16. Watson W: Gridless radiography at high voltage with air gap technique. X-Ray Focus 2:12, 1958.
17. Jackson FI: The air-gap technique, and an improvement by anteroposterior positioning for chest roentgenography. Am J Roentgenol 92:688, 1964.
18. Charbonnier F, Barbour J: The physical basis for high voltage chest radiography. Am J Roentgenol 134:200, 1980.
19. Steiner RM, Tuddenham W, McArdle G, et al: High kilovoltage chest radiography: A comparison of 350 and 120 kVp techniques. Am J Roentgenol 134:200, 1980.
20. Tuddenham WJ: Rationale for high kVp chest radiography. Am J Roentgenol 134:200, 1980.
21. Wilkinson GA, Fraser RG: Roentgenography of the chest. Appl Radiol 4:41, 1975.
22. Lynch PA: A different approach to chest roentgenography: Triad technique (high kilovoltage, grid, wedge filter). Am Roentgenol 93:965, 1965.
23. Tuddenham WJ, Gibbons JF, Hale J, et al: Supervoltage and multiple simultaneous roentgenography—new technics for roentgen examination of the chest. Radiology 63:184, 1954.
24. Rossi RP, Harnisch G, Hendee WR: Reduction of radiation exposure in radiography of the chest. Radiology 144:909, 1982.
25. Kelsey CA, Moseley RD, Mettler FA, et al: Comparison of nodule detection with 70-kVp and 120-kVp chest radiographs. Radiology 143:609, 1982.
26. Trout ED, Kelley JP, Larson VL: A comparison of an air gap and a grid in roentgenography of the chest. Am J Roentgenol 124:404, 1975.
27. Lefcoe MS: Direct magnification radiography of the chest in diffuse pulmonary disease. J Can Assoc Radiol 27:3, 1976.
28. Corry P: Personal communication, 1967.
29. Jacobson G, Sargent EN: Apical roentgenographic views of the chest. Am J Roentgenol 104:822, 1968.
30. Simon G: Principles of Chest X-Ray Diagnosis. 3rd. ed. London, Butterworth, 1971.
31. Tuddenham WJ: Problems of perception in chest roentgenography: Facts and fallacies. Radiol Clin North Am 1:277, 1963.
32. Sandor T, Adams DF, Herman PG, et al: The potential of magnification angiography. Am J Roentgenol 120:916, 1974.
33. Zinn B, Monroe J: The lordotic position in fluoroscopy and roentgenography of the chest. Am J Roentgenol 75:682, 1956.
34. Rundle FF, DeLambert RM, Epps RG: Cervicothoracic tumors: A technical aid to their roentgenologic localization. Am J Roentgenol 81:316, 1959.
35. Rigler LG: Roentgen diagnosis of small pleural effusion: A new roentgenographic position. JAMA 96:104, 1931.
36. Müller R, Löfstedt S: The reaction of the pleura in primary tuberculosis of the lungs. Acta Med Scand 122:105, 1945.
37. Hessén I: Roentgen examination of pleural fluid: A study of the localization of free effusion, the potentialities of diagnosing minimal quantities of fluid and its existence under physiological conditions. Acta Radiol (Suppl) 86, 1951.
38. Möller A: Pleural effusion. Use of the semi-supine position for radiographic detection. Radiology 150:245, 1984.
39. Capitanio MA, Kirkpatrick JA: The lateral decubitus film: An aid in determining air-trapping in children. Radiology 103:460, 1972.
40. Tabrisky J, Herman MW, Torrance DJ, et al: Mobile 240 kVp phototimed chest radiography. Am J Roentgenol 135:295, 1980.
41. Wilkinson GA, Fraser RG: Use of double screen-film combination in bedside chest roentgenography. Radiology 117:222, 1975.
42. Gallant TE, Dietrich PA, Shinozaki T, et al: Technical notes. Simple device to measure patient position on portable chest radiographs. Am J Roentgenol 131:169, 1978.
43. Henschke CI, Pasternack GS, Schroeder S, et al: Bedside chest radiography: Diagnostic efficacy. Radiology 149:23, 1983.
44. Janower ML, Jennas-Nocera Z, Mukai J: Utility and efficacy of portable chest radiographs. Am J Roentgenol 142:265, 1984.
45. Hall FM: Indications for bedside radiographs. Letter to editor. Am J Roentgenol 143:684, 1984.
46. Greenspan RH, Sagel S, McMahon J, et al: Timed expiratory chest films in the detection of air-trapping (abstract). Invest Radiol 8:264, 1973.
47. Fleischner FG: The esophagus and mediastinal lymphadenopathy in bronchial carcinoma. Radiology 58:48, 1952.
48. Middlemass IBD: Deformity of the oesophagus in bronchogenic carcinoma. J Fac Radiol 5:121, 1953.
49. Marchal M: De l'enregistrement des pulsations invisibles du poumon à l'état normal et à l'état pathologique. (Recording of invisible pulsations of the lung in normal and pathological states.) Acad Sci (Paris) 222:1314, 1946.
50. Kourilsky R, Marchal M: Étude cinédensigraphique de la circulation artérielle du poumon dans différentes affections pathologiques du poumon, des bronches et du médiastin. (Cinestudy of pulmonary arterial circulation in various pathological conditions of the lungs, bronchi and mediastinum.) J Fr Med Chir Thorac 7:113, 1953.
51. Marchal M, Marchal MT: Perfectionnements en stat-densigraphie. (Progress in statidensigraphy.) Acad Sci (Paris) 238:2560, 1954.
52. Steiner RE, Laws JW, Gilbert J, et al: Radiological lung-function studies. Lancet 2:1051, 1960.
53. Marchal M, Marchal MT, Kourilsky R: Enregistrement photo-elétrique de la ventilation des poumons separés dans les stenoses bronchiques par la stati-densigraphie. (Photoelectric recording of the ventilation of each lung in bronchial stenoses by statidensigraphy.) Bronches 11:102, 1961.
54. Kourilsky R, Marchal M, Marchal MT: A new method of functional x-ray exploration of the lungs: Photoelectric stati-densigraphy. Dis Chest 42:345, 1962.
55. Karwowski J: L'exploration de la ventilation pulmonaire par la nouvelle méthode électronique de stati-densigraphie; Corrélation avec la bronchospirométrie. (The exploration of pulmonary ventilation by the new electronic method of statidensigraphy. Correlation with bronchospirometry.) J Fr Med Chir Thorac 17:101, 1963.
56. Oderr C: Air trapping, pulmonary insufficiency and fluorodensimetry. Am J Roentgenol 92:501, 1964.
57. Kourilsky R, Marchal M, Marchal MT: Recording respiratory function by x-rays: Basic principles. Thorax 20:428, 1965.

2

58. Laws JW, Steiner RE: X:ray densitometry in the study of pulmonary ventilation and the pulmonary circulation. Br J Radiol 38:512, 1965.

59. Standertskjöld-Nordenstam CG: The pulmonary circulation during pneumonia. A cinedensigraphic study. Acta Radiol (Suppl) 239:1, 1965.

60. Oderr C: Radiologic assessment of pulmonary insufficiency and cough effectiveness. Dis Chest 49:46, 1966.

61. Sutherland GR, Leask E, Samuel E: Pulmonary vascular and ventilatory changes in bronchial carcinoma studies by fluorodensitometry. Clin Radiol 19:269, 1968.

62. Zelefsky MM, Schulz RJ: Evaluation of regional pulmonary ventilation by gamma ray densigraphy. Radiology 91:1208, 1968.

63. Cattrell VG, Franklin DH, Kirkpatrick AE: Gamma densitometry in the study of ventilation and the pulmonary circulation. Clin Radiol 21:396, 1970.

64. Hutchison DCS, Cattrell VG, Kirkpatrick AE, et al: The measurement of regional pulmonary density, ventilation and perfusion by gamma-ray densitometry. Br J Radiol 44:955, 1971.

65. Reiss KH, Schuster W: Quantitative measurements of lung function in children by means of Compton backscatter. Radiology 102:613, 1972.

66. Silverman NR: Clinical video-densitometry; Pulmonary ventilation analysis. Radiology 103:263, 1972.

67. Sommer FG, Smathers RL, Wheat RL, et al: Digital processing of film radiographs. Am J Roentgenol 144:191, 1985.

68. Margulis A: Personal communication, December, 1984.

69. Tesic MM, Mattson RA, Barnes GT, et al: Digital radiography of the chest: Design features and considerations for a prototype unit. Radiology 148:259, 1983.

70. Barnes GT, Sones RA, Tesic MM: Digital chest radiography: Performance evaluation of a prototype unit. Radiology 154:801, 1985.

71. Fraser RG, Breatnach ES, Barnes GT: Digital radiography of the chest: Clinical experience with a prototype unit. Radiology 148:1, 1983.

72. Siegelman SS, Zerhouni EA, Leo FP, et al: CT of the solitary pulmonary nodule. Am J Roentgenol 135:1, 1980.

73. Cann CE, Gamsu G, Birnberg FA, et al: Quantification of calcium in solitary pulmonary nodules using single- and dual-energy CT. Radiology 145:493, 1982.

74. Zerhouni EA, Spivey JF, Morgan RH, et al: Factors influencing quantitative CT measurements of solitary pulmonary nodules. J Comput Assist Tomogr 6:1075, 1982.

75. Barnes GT, Sones R, Tesic MM, et al: Detector for dual energy digital radiography. Radiology 154:801, 1985.

76. Fraser RG, Barnes GT, Hickey N, et al: Potential value of digital radiography: Preliminary observations on the use of dual-energy subtraction in the evaluation of pulmonary nodules. Chest (Suppl) 89:249S, 1986.

77. Littleton JT, Durizch ML, Callahan WP: Linear vs. pluridirectional tomography of the chest: Correlative radiographic anatomic study. Am J Roentgenol 134:241, 1980.

78. Bein ME, Greenberg M, Liu P-Y, et al: Pulmonary nodules: Detection in 1 and 2 cm full lung linear tomography. Am J Roentgenol 135:513, 1980.

79. Favis EA: Planigraphy (body section radiography) in detecting tuberculous pulmonary cavitation. Dis Chest 27:668, 1955.

80. Janower ML: Fifty-five-degree posterior oblique tomography of the pulmonary hilum. J Can Assoc Radiol 29:158, 1978.

81. Sindelar WF, Bagley DH, Felix EL, et al: Lung tomography in cancer patients. Full-lung tomograms in screening for pulmonary metastases. JAMA 240:2060, 1978.

82. Curtis AM, Ravin CE, Collier PE, et al: Detection of metastatic disease from carcinoma of the breast: Limited value of full lung tomography. Am J Roentgenol 134:253, 1980.

83. Muhm JR, Brown LR, Crowe JK, et al: Comparison of whole lung tomography and computed tomography for detecting pulmonary nodules. Am J Roentgenol 131:981, 1978.

84. Goldberg HI: Critical reviews: Detection of pulmonary nodules by computed tomography. Invest Radiol 12:474, 1977.

85. Ter-Pogossian MM: The challenge of computed tomography. Am J Roentgenol 127:1, 1976.

86. McLoud TC, Wittenberg J, Ferrucci JT Jr: Computed tomography of the thorax and standard radiographic evaluation of the chest: A comparative study. J Comp Assist Tomogr 3:170, 1979.

87. Robbins AH, Pugatch RD, Gerzof SG, et al: Further observations on the medical efficacy of computed tomography of the chest and abdomen. Radiology 137:719, 1980.

88. Heitzman ER: Fleischner Lecture. Computed tomography of the thorax: Current perspectives. Am J Roentgenol 136:2, 1981.

89. Raval B, Lamki N, Carey LS: Computed tomography in chest diseases. CT 5:91, 1981.

90. Sones PJ Jr, Torres WE, Colvin RS, et al: Effectiveness of CT in evaluating intrathoracic masses. Am J Roentgenol 139:469, 1982.

91. Baron RL, Levitt RG, Sagel SS, et al: Body computed tomography.

92. Society for Computed Body Tomography: Special report. New indications for computed body tomography. Am J Roentgenol 133:115, 1979.

93. Siegelman SS, Zerhouni EA, Leo FP, et al: CT of the solitary pulmonary nodule. Am J Roentgenol 135:1, 1980.

94. Rosenblum LJ, Mauceri RA, Wellenstein DE, et al: Computed tomography of the lung. Radiology 129:521, 1978.

95. Mintzer RA, Malave SR, Neiman HL, et al: Computed vs. conventional tomography in evaluation of primary and secondary pulmonary neoplasms. Radiology 132:653, 1979.

96. Osborne DR, Korobkin M, Ravin CE, et al: Comparison of plain radiography, conventional tomography, and computed tomography in detecting intrathoracic lymph node metastases from lung carcinoma. Radiology 142:157, 1982.

97. Gore JC, Emery EW, Orr JS, et al: Medical nuclear magnetic resonance imaging: I. Physical principles. Invest Radiol 16:269, 1981.

98. The new wave in medicine: Nuclear magnetic resonance. JAMA 247:151, 1982.

99. Brownell GL, Budinger TF, Lauterbur PC, et al: Positron tomography and nuclear magnetic resonance imaging. Science 215:619, 1982.

100. James AE, Partain CL, Holland GN, et al: Review. Nuclear magnetic resonance imaging: The current state. Am J Roentgenol 138:201, 1981.

101. Crooks L, Arakawa M, Hoenninger J, et al: Work in Progress. Nuclear magnetic resonance whole-body imager operating at 3.5 KGauss. Radiology 143:169, 1982.

102. Pykett IL, Newhouse JH, Buonanno FS, et al: Nuclear magnetic resonance. Principles of nuclear magnetic resonance imaging. Radiology 143:157, 1982.

103. Mitchell MR, Partain CL, Price RR, et al: NMR: State of the art in medical imaging. Reflections from National Cancer Institute/Bowman Gray/Vanderbilt International Symposium. Appl Radiol July/Aug 1982, p 19.

104. Harms SE, Morgan TJ, Yamanashi WS, et al: Principles of nuclear magnetic resonance imaging. RadioGraphics 4(Sp. Issue):26, 1984.

105. Pavlicek W, Modic M, Weinstein M: Pulse sequence and significance. RadioGraphics 4(Sp. Issue):49, 1984.

106. Partain CL, Price RR, Patton JA, et al: Nuclear magnetic resonance imaging. RadioGraphics 4(Sp. Issue):5, 1984.

107. Wolf GL, Baum S: Nuclear magnetic resonance contrast agents for proton imaging. RadioGraphics 4(Sp. Issue):66, 1984.

108. Dooms GC, Hricak H, Crooks LE, et al: Magnetic resonance imaging of the lymph nodes: Comparison with CT. Radiology 153:719, 1984.

109. Webb WR, Gamsu G, Stark DD, et al: Magnetic resonance imaging of the normal and abnormal pulmonary hila. Radiology 152:89, 1984.

110. Gamsu G, Stark DD, Webb WR, et al: Magnetic resonance imaging of benign mediastinal masses. Radiology 151:709, 1984.

111. Webb WR, Gamsu G, Crooks LE: Multisection sagittal and coronal magnetic resonance imaging of the mediastinum and hila. Radiology 150:475, 1984.

112. Webb WR, Jensen BG, Gamsu G, et al: Coronal magnetic resonance imaging of the chest: Normal and abnormal. Radiology 153:729, 1984.

113. O'Donovan PB, Ross JS, Sivak ED, et al: Magnetic resonance imaging of the thorax: The advantages of coronal and sagittal planes. Am J Roentgenol 143:1183, 1984.

114. Gamsu G, Hirji M, Moore EH, et al: Experimental pulmonary emboli detected using magnetic resonance. Radiology 153:467, 1984.

115. Thickman D, Kressel HY, Axel L: Demonstration of pulmonary embolism by magnetic resonance imaging. Am J Roentgenol 142:921, 1984.

116. Moore EH, Gamsu G, Webb WR, et al: Pulmonary embolus: Detection and follow-up using magnetic resonance. Radiology 153:471, 1984.

117. Skalina S, Kundel HL, Wolf G, et al: The effect of pulmonary edema on proton nuclear magnetic resonance relaxation times. Invest Radiol 19:7, 1984.

118. Glazer HS, Levitt RG, Lee JKT, et al: Differentiation of radiation fibrosis from recurrent pulmonary neoplasm by magnetic resonance imaging. Am J Roentgenol 143:729, 1984.

119. Farmer DW, Moore E, Amparo E, et al: Calcific fibrosing mediastinitis: Demonstration of pulmonary vascular obstruction by magnetic resonance imaging. Am J Roentgenol 143:1189, 1984.

120. Amparo EG, Higgins CB, Hoddick W, et al: Magnetic resonance imaging of aortic disease: Preliminary results. Am J Roentgenol 143:1203, 1984.

121. Moore EH, Webb WR, Verrier ED, et al: MRI of chronic posttraumatic false aneurysms of the thoracic aorta. Am J Roentgenol 143:1195, 1984.

Computed tomography in the preoperative evaluation of bronchogenic carcinoma. Radiology 145:727, 1982.

122. Brasch RC, Gooding CA, Lallemand DP, et al: Magnetic resonance imaging of the thorax in childhood (Work in Progress). Radiology 150:463, 1984.
123. Cohen AM, Creviston S, LiPuma JP, et al: Nuclear magnetic resonance imaging of the mediastinum and hili: Early impressions of its efficacy. Am J Roentgenol 141:1163, 1983.
124. Ross JS, O'Donovan PB, Novoa R, et al: Magnetic resonance of the chest: Initial experience with imaging and in vivo T₁ and T₂ calculations. Radiology 152:95, 1984.
125. Baker HL Jr, Berquist TH, Kispert DB, et al: Magnetic resonance imaging in a routine clinical setting. Mayo Clin Proc 60:75, 1985.
126. Fraser RG: Editorial: Bronchography 1972. J Can Assoc Radiol 23:236, 1972.
127. Avery ME: Bronchography: Outmoded procedure? Pediatrics 46:333, 1970.
128. Molnar W, Riebel FA: Bronchography: An aid in the diagnosis of peripheral pulmonary carcinoma. Radiol Clin North Am 1:303, 1963.
129. Christoforidis AJ, Nelson SW, Tomashefski JF: Effects of bronchography on pulmonary function. Am Rev Respir Dis 85:127, 1962.
130. Suprenant E, Wilson A, Bennett L, et al: Changes in regional pulmonary function following bronchography. Radiology 91:736, 1968.
131. Björk L, Lodin H: Pulmonary changes following bronchography with Dionosil oily (animal experiments). Acta Radiol 47:177, 1957.
132. Luridiana N: Distribution and injurious effects of bronchographic contrast media in the lungs; Roentgen-histological studies of 100 specimens from pulmonary resection. G Ital Tuberc 12:188, 1958.
133. Holden WS, Cowdell RH: Late results in bronchography using Dionosil oily. Acta Radiol 49:105, 1958.
134. Widdicombe JG: Respiratory reflexes from the trachea and bronchi of the cat. J Physiol (Lond) 123:55, 1954.
135. Wilson JKV: Cricothyroid bronchography with a polyethylene catheter: Description of a new technique. Am J Roentgenol 81:305, 1959.
136. Dunbar JS, Skinner GB, Wortzman G, et al: An investigation of effects of opaque media on the lungs with comparison of barium sulfate, lipiodol and Dionosil. Am J Roentgenol 82:902, 1959.
137. Light JP, Oster WF: Clinical and pathological reactions to the bronchographic agent Dionosil aqueous. Am J Roentgenol 98:468, 1966.
138. Smith TR, Frater, R, Spataro J: Delayed granuloma following bronchography. Chest 64:122, 1973.
139. Robinson AE: Dimensional response of large airways during bronchography in the paediatric patient. Invest Radiol 8:121, 1973.
140. Robinson AE, Hall KD, Yokoyama KN, et al: Pediatric bronchography: The problem of segmental pulmonary loss of volume. 1. A retrospective study of 165 pediatric bronchograms. Invest Radiol 6:89, 1971.
141. Wilson JF, Peters GN, Fleshman K: A technique for bronchography in children. An experience with 575 patients using topical anesthesia. Am Rev Respir Dis 105:564, 1972.
142. Gamsu G, Platzker A, Gregory G, et al: Powdered tantalum as a contrast agent for tracheobronchography in the pediatric patient. Radiology 107:151, 1973.
143. Gudbjerg CE: Bronchiectasis; radiological diagnosis and prognosis after operative treatment. Acta Radiol (Suppl) 143, 1957.
144. Forrest JV, Sagel SS, Omell GH: Bronchography in patients with hemoptysis. Am J Roentgenol 126:597, 1976.
145. Beck E, Hobbs AA Jr: A technique for bronchography. Am J Roentgenol 79:269, 1958.
146. Steckel RJ, Grillo HC: Catheterization of the trachea and bronchi by a modified Seldinger technic: A new approach to bronchography. Radiology 83:1035, 1964.
147. Sargent EN, Turner AF: Percutaneous transcricothyroid membrane selective bronchography: A simple, safe technique for selective catheterization and visualization of segmental and subsegmental bronchi. Am J Roentgenol 104:792, 1968.
148. Cicero R, del Castillo H: Lobar and segmental angiopneumography in pulmonary disease. Acta Radiol 45:42, 1956.
149. Jacobson G: Peripheral pulmonary (wedge) arteriography—a standardized technique for the single film arteriogram. Clin Radiol 14:326, 1963.
150. Takaro T, Scott SM: Angiography using direct roentgenographic magnification in man. Am J Roentgenol 91:448, 1964.
151. Greenspan RH, Simon AL, Ricketts HJ, et al: In vivo magnification angiography. Invest Radiol 2:419, 1967.
152. Tsuiki K, Miyazawa K, Ishikawa K, et al: Correlation of magnifying pulmonary wedge angiogram and pulmonary hemodynamics. Am Rev Respir Dis 104:899, 1971.
153. Kattan KR: Angled view in pulmonary angiography: A new roentgen approach. Radiology 94:79, 1970.
154. Wagner RB, Baeza DR, Stewart JE: Active pulmonary hemorrhage localized by selective pulmonary angiography. Chest 67:121, 1975.
155. Cooley RN: Pulmonary thromboembolism—the case for the pulmonary angiogram (editorial). Am J Roentgenol 92:693, 1964.
156. Montes M, Alder RH, Brennan JC: Bronchiolar apocrine tumor. Am Rev Respir Dis 93:946, 1966.
157. Stoney WS, Adams JE: The diagnosis of acute pulmonary embolism by arteriography. Am Rev Respir Dis 83:26, 1961.
158. Williams JR, Wilcox WC: Pulmonary embolism: Roentgenographic and angiographic considerations. Am J Roentgenol 89:333, 1963.
159. Dexter L, Smith GT: Quantitative studies of pulmonary embolism. Am J Med Sci 247:641, 1964.
160. Allison PR, Dunnill MS, Marshall R: Pulmonary embolism. Thorax 15:273, 1960.
161. Ferris EJ, Stanzler RM, Rourke JA, et al: Pulmonary angiography in pulmonary embolic disease. Am J Roentgenol 100:355, 1967.
162. Sautter RD, Fletcher FW, Emanuel DA, et al: Pulmonary arteriography in the operating room. Chest 57:423, 1970.
163. Chilcote WA, Modic MT, Pavlicek WA, et al: Digital subtraction angiography of the carotid arteries: A comparative study in 100 patients. Radiology 139:287, 1981.
164. Buonocore E, Meaney TF, Borkowski GP, et al: Digital subtraction angiography of the abdominal aorta and renal arteries. Radiology 139:281, 1981.
165. Meaney TF, Weinstein MA, Buonocore E, et al: Digital subtraction angiography of the human cardiovascular system. Am J Roentgenol 135:1153, 1980.
166. Ludwig JW, Verhoeven LAJ, Kersbergen JJ, et al: Digital subtraction and angiography of the pulmonary arteries for the diagnosis of pulmonary embolism. Radiology 147:639, 1983.
167. Slutsky RA, Higgins CB: Analysis of the pulmonary circulation using digital intravenous angiography. Radiology 146:219, 1983.
168. Hirji M, Gamsu G, Webb WR, et al: EKG-gated digital subtraction angiography in the detection of pulmonary emboli. Radiology 152:19, 1984.
169. Chiles C, Guthaner DF, Djang WT: Detection of pulmonary emboli in dogs using digital subtraction angiography. Invest Radiol 18:507, 1983.
170. Ferris EJ, Holder JC, Lim WN, et al: Angiography of pulmonary emboli: Digital studies and balloon-occlusion cineangiography. Am J Roentgenol 142:369, 1984.
171. Goodman PC, Brant-Zawadzki M: Digital subtraction. Pulmonary angiography. Am J Roentgenol 139:305, 1982.
172. Julien PJ, Gamsu G: The effect of pulmonary angiography on bronchomotor tone. Invest Radiol 9:297, 1974.
173. Seldinger SI: Catheter replacement of the needle in percutaneous arteriography: A new technique. Acta Radiol 39:368, 1953.
174. Botenga ASJ: Selective Bronchial and Intercostal Arteriography. Leiden, HE Stenfert Kroese, NV, 1970.
175. Davies ER, Roylance J: Aortography in the investigation of traumatic mediastinal haematoma. Clin Radiol 21:297, 1970.
176. Viamonte M Jr: Angiographic evaluation of lung neoplasms. Radiol Clin North Am 3:529, 1965.
177. Nordenström B: Selective catheterization and angiography of bronchial and mediastinal arteries in man. Acta Radiol 6:13, 1967.
178. Darke CS, Lewtas NA: Selective bronchial arteriography in the demonstration of abnormal systemic circulation in the lung. Clin Radiol 19:357, 1968.
179. Miyazawa K, Katori R, Ishikawa K, et al: Selective bronchial arteriography and bronchial blood flow: Correlative study. Chest 57:416, 1970.
180. Sutton D, Samuel RH: Thoracic aortography in intralobar lung sequestration. Clin Radiol 14:317, 1963.
181. Turk LN III, Lindskog GE: The importance of angiographic diagnosis in intralobar pulmonary sequestration. J Thorac Cardiovasc Surg 41:299, 1961.
182. Turner-Warwick M: Systemic arterial patterns in the lung and clubbing of the fingers. Thorax 18:238, 1963.
183. Liebow AA: Recent observations on pulmonary collateral circulation. Med Thorac 19:609, 1962.
184. Greenspan RH, Capps JH: Pulmonary angiography: Its use in diagnosis and as a guide to therapy in lesions of the chest. Radiol Clin North Am 1:315, 1963.
185. Liebow AA, Hales MR, Harrison W, et al: The genesis and functional implications of collateral circulation of the lungs. Yale J Biol Med 22:637, 1950.
186. Heimburg P: Bronchial collateral circulation in experimental stenosis of the pulmonary artery. Thorax 19:306, 1964.
187. Kahn PC, Paul RE, Rheinlander HF: Selective bronchial arteriography and intra-arterial chemotherapy in carcinoma of the lung. J Thorac Cardiovasc Surg 50:640, 1965.
188. North LB, Boushy SF, Houk VN: Bronchial and intercostal arteriography in non-neoplastic pulmonary disease. Am J Roentgenol 107:328, 1969.
189. Remy J, Smith M, Lemaitre L, et al: Treatment of massive hemoptysis by occlusion of a Rasmussen aneurysm. Am J Roentgenol 135:605, 1980.

190. Remy J, Arnaud A, Fardou H, et al: Treatment of hemoptysis by embolization of bronchial arteries. Radiology 122:33, 1977.

191. MacErlean DP, Gray BJ, FitzGerald MX: Bronchial artery embolization in the control of massive haemoptysis. Br J Radiol 52:558, 1979.

192. Vujic I, Pyle R, Hungerford GD, et al: Angiography and therapeutic blockade in the control of hemoptysis. The importance of nonbronchial systemic arteries. Radiology 143:19, 1982.

193. Castaneda-Zuniga W, Epstein M, Zollikofer C, et al: Embolization of multiple pulmonary artery fistulas. Radiology 134:309, 1980.

194. Barden RP, Comroe JH Jr: Roentgenologic evaluation of pulmonary function: A correlation with physiologic studies of ventilation. Am J Roentgenol 75:668, 1956.

195. Barder RP: Glimpses through the pulmonary window. Interpretation of the radiologic evidence in disorders of the lungs. Hickey Lecture, 1966. Am J Roentgenol 98:269, 1966.

196. Gildenhorn HL, Hallett WY: An evaluation of radiological methods for the determination of lung volumes. Radiology 84:754, 1965.

197. Barnhard HG, Pierce JA, Joyce JW, et al: Roentgenographic determination of total lung capacity. A new method evaluated in health, emphysema and congestive heart failure. Am J Med 28:51, 1960.

198. O'Shea J, Lapp NL, Russakoff AD, et al: Determination of lung volumes from chest films. Thorax 25:544, 1970.

199. Loyd HM, String ST, DuBois AB: Radiographic and plethysmographic determination of total lung capacity. Radiology 86:7, 1966.

200. Harris TR, Pratt PC, Kilburn KH: Total lung capacity measured by roentgenograms. Am J Med 50:756, 1971.

201. Jaffe CC: A new technique for rapid determination of quantitative data from radiographs. Radiology 103:451, 1972.

202. Friedman PJ, Brimm JE, Botkin MC, et al: Measuring lung volumes from chest films using equations derived from computed tomography. Invest Radiol 19:263, 1984.

203. Freeman LM, Blaufox MD (eds): Seminars in Nuclear Medicine. Vol I. New York, Grune & Stratton, 1971, pp 121-262. (Ten articles on use and interpretation of the lung scan.)

204. Mishkin FS, Brashear RE: Use and Interpretation of the Lung Scan. Springfield, IL, Charles C Thomas, 1971.

205. Deland FH, Wagner HN Jr: Atlas of Nuclear Medicine. Vol II: Lung and Heart. Philadelphia, WB Saunders, 1970.

206. Khan O, Ell PJ, Jarritt PH, et al: Radionuclide section scanning of the lungs in pulmonary embolism. Br J Radiol 54:586, 1981.

207. Potchen EJ, Evens RG, Hill R, et al: Regional pulmonary function in man: Quantitative transmission radiography as an adjunct to lung scintiscanning. Am J Roentgenol 108:724, 1970.

208. Goodrich JK, Jones RH, Coulam CM, et al: Xenon[133] measurement of regional ventilation. Radiology 103:611, 1972.

209. Loken MK, Medina JR, Lillehei JP, et al: Regional pulmonary function evaluation using xenon[133], a scintillation camera, and computer. Radiology 93:1261, 1969.

210. L'Heureux P, Loken M, Ponto R, et al: Regional evaluation of pulmonary function in chronic obstructive pulmonary disease: A technique using xenon[133], a scintillation camera, and computer analysis of data. Radiology 100:107, 1971.

211. Loken MK, Ponto RA, Kronenberg RS, et al: Dual camera studies of pulmonary function with computer processing of data. Am J Roentgenol 121:761, 1974.

212. Taplin GV, Johnson DE, Dore EK, et al: Suspensions of radioalbumin aggregates for photoscanning the liver, spleen, lung and other organs. J Nucl Med 5:259, 1964.

213. Rosenthall L: Lung scanning with radioiodinated macroaggregates of human serum albumin. J Can Assoc Radiol 16:30, 1955.

214. Wagner HN Jr, Sabiston DC Jr, McAfee JG, et al: Diagnosis of massive pulmonary embolism in man by radioisotope scanning. In Quinn JL III (ed): Scintillation Scanning in Clinical Medicine (based on a Symposium sponsored by the Department of Radiology of the Bowman Gray School of Medicine). Philadelphia, WB Saunders, 1964, pp 125-141.

215. Quinn JL III, Whitley JE: Lung scintiscanning. In Quinn JL III (ed): Scintillation Scanning in Clinical Medicine (based on a Symposium sponsored by the Department of Radiology of the Bowman Gray School of Medicine). Philadelphia, WB Saunders, 1964, pp 142-157.

216. Loken MK, Telander GT, Salmon RJ: Technetium[99m] compounds for visualization of body organs. JAMA 194:152, 1965.

217. Thomas J, Wiener SN: ^{99m}Tc-sulfur colloid macroaggregated albumin for lung imaging. Radiopharmaceutical properties in animals. Radiology 107:591, 1973.

218. Rhodes BA, Zolle I, Buchanan JW, et al: Radioactive albumin microspheres for studies of the pulmonary circulation. Radiology 92:1453, 1969.

219. Burdine JA, Sonnemaker RE, Ryder LA, et al: Perfusion studies with technetium[99m] human albumin microspheres (HAM). Radiology 95:101, 1970.

220. Rhodes BA, Stern HS, Buchanan JA, et al: Lung scanning with ^{99m}Tc-microspheres. Radiology 99:613, 1971.

221. Stern HS, Goodwin DA, Wagner HN Jr, et al: In[133m]—a short-lived isotope for lung scanning. Nucleonics 24:57, 1966.

222. Ferrari M, Paez A, Soto CL, et al: Basic physiopathological patterns of perfusion and inhalation pulmonary scintigraphy. Thorax 24:695, 1969.

223. Rosenthal L: Personal communication, 1968.

224. Dworkin HJ, Smith JR, Bull FE: A reaction following administration of macroaggregated albumin (MAA) for lung scan. Am J Roentgenol 98:427, 1966.

225. Heck LL, Duley JW Jr: Statistical considerations in lung imaging with ^{99m}Tc albumin particles. Radiology 113:675, 1974.

226. Rosenthall L, Greyson ND, Eidenger SL: Positive identification of lung neoplasm with [197]HgCl₂. J Can Assoc Radiol 21:181, 1970.

227. Ito Y, Okuyama S, Awano T, et al: Diagnostic evaluation of ^{67}Ga scanning of lung cancer and other diseases. Radiology 101:355, 1971.

228. Adelberg HM, Siemsen JK, Jung RC, et al: Scintigraphic detection of pulmonary bacterial infections with labelled thyroid hormones and pertechnetate. Radiology 99:141, 1971.

229. Ray GR, DeNardo GL, King GH: Localization of strontium[85] in soft tissue infected by Aspergillus niger. Radiology 101:119, 1971.

230. Potchen EJ: Photons and physiology: New Horizons for Radiologists Lecture. Radiology 103:1, 1972.

231. Jones T, Clark JC, Buckingham PD, et al: The use of oxygen[15] labelled water for the measurement of pulmonary extravascular water (abstract). Br J Radiol 45:630, 1972.

232. Rudavsky AZ, Leonidas JC, Abramson AL: Lung scanning for the detection of endobronchial foreign bodies in infants and children: Clinical and experimental studies. Radiology 108:629, 1973.

233. Dugan MA, Kozar JJ 3rd, Charkes MD, et al: The use of iodinated fibrinogen for localization of deep venous thrombi by scintiscanning. Radiology 106:445, 1973.

234. Critchley M, Prichard H, Grime JS, et al: Radionuclide assessment of extravascular lung water in minimal pulmonary oedema. Clin Radiol 32:607, 1981.

235. Winzelberg GG, Wholey MH, Jarmolowski CA, et al: Patients with hemoptysis examined by Tc-99m sulfur colloid and Tc-99m-labeled red blood cells: A preliminary appraisal. Radiology 153:523, 1984.

236. Siemsen JK, Grebe SF, Waxman AD: The use of gallium-67 in pulmonary disorders. Semin Nucl Med 8:235, 1978.

237. Richman SD, Levenson SM, Bunn PA, et al: [67]Ga accumulation in pulmonary lesions associated with bleomycin toxicity. Cancer 36:1966, 1975.

238. Line BR, Fulmer JD, Reynolds HY, et al: Gallium-67 citrate scanning in the staging of idiopathic pulmonary fibrosis: Correlation with physiologic and morphologic features and bronchoalveolar lavage. Am Rev Respir Dis 118:355, 1978.

239. Turner DA, Forham EW, Ali A, et al: Gallium-67 imaging in the management of Hodgkin's disease and other malignant lymphomas. Semin Nucl Med 8:205, 1978.

240. Chaudhuri TK, Muilenburg ML, Christie JH: Abnormal deposition of radiostrontium in lungs. Chest 61:190, 1972.

241. Krahl VE: The lung as a target organ in thromboembolism. In Sasahara AA, Stein M (eds): Pulmonary Embolic Disease. New York, Grune & Stratton, 1965, pp 13–22.

242. Wagner HN Jr: Current status of lung scanning (editorial). Radiology 91:1235, 1968.

243. Poe ND, Swanson LA, Taplin GV: Physiological factors affecting lung scan interpretations. Radiology 89:66, 1967.

244. MacLean LD, Shibata HR, McLean APH, et al: Pulmonary embolism: The value of bedside scanning, angiography and pulmonary embolectomy. Can Med Assoc J 97:991, 1967.

245. Tetalman MR, Hoffer PB, Heck LL, et al: Perfusion lung scan in normal volunteers. Radiology 106:593, 1973.

246. Krumholz RA, Burnham GM, DeLong JF: Lung scan utilization in the diagnosis of pulmonary disease. Chest 62:4, 1972.

247. Joyner CR Jr, Herman RJ, Reid JM: Reflected ultrasound in the detection and localization of pleural effusion. JAMA 200:399, 1967.

248. Viikeri M, Jaaskelainen J, Tahti E: Ultrasonic examination of pleural thickenings and calcifications in occupational asbestosis. Dis Chest 54:17, 1968.

249. Viikeri M: Ultrasound examination of pleural plaques; Experimental, pathologic and clinical studies. Acta Radiol (Suppl) 301:7, 1970.

250. Sandweiss DA, Hanson JC, Gosink BB, et al: Ultrasound in diagnosis, localization, and treatment of loculated pleural empyema. Ann Intern Med 82:50, 1975.

251. Doust BD, Baum JK, Maklad NF, et al: Ultrasonic evaluation of pleural opacities. Radiology 114:135, 1975.

252. Marks WM, Filly RA, Callen PW: Real-time evaluation of pleural lesions: New observations regarding the probability of obtaining free fluid. Radiology 142:163, 1982.

253. Rosenberg ER: Ultrasound in the assessment of pleural densities. Chest 84:283, 1983.

254. Hirsch JH, Hogers JV, Mack LA: Real-time sonography of pleural opacities. Am J Roentgenol 136:297, 1981.

255. Shin MS, Gray PW Jr: Pitfalls in ultrasonic detection of pleural fluid. J Clin Ultrasound 6:421, 1978.
256. Connell DG, Crothers G, Cooperberg PL: The subpulmonic pleural effusion: Sonographic aspects. J Can Assoc Radiol 33:101, 1982.
257. Lewandowski BJ, Winsberg F: Sonographic demonstration of the right paramediastinal pleural space. Radiology 145:127, 1982.
258. Tanaka M, Oka S, Ebina T, et al: The diagnostic application of ultrasound to disease in mediastinal organs. III. The ultrasonocardiotomography in living human subjects. Sci Rep Res Inst Tohoku Univ (Med) 14:1, 1967.
259. Goldberg BB: Mediastinal ultrasonography. J Clin Ultrasound 1:114, 1973.
260. Ries T, Currarino G, Nikaidoh H, et al: Real-time ultrasonography of subcarinal bronchogenic cysts in two children. Radiology 145:121, 1982.
261. US Department of Health, Education, and Welfare: Public Health Service, Food and Drug Administration: Population Exposure to X-Rays, United States, 1970. Washington DC, DHEW Publication (FDA) 73–8047, 1973.
262. International Commission on Radiological Protection: Protection of the Patient in X-Ray Diagnosis. Publication 16. New York, Pergamon Press, 1970.
263. Hashizume T, Kato Y, Maruyama T, et al: Population mean marrow dose and leukaemia: Significant dose from diagnostic medical x-ray examinations in Japan, 1969. Health Phys 23:845, 1972.
264. Kitabatake T, Yokoyama M, Sakka M, et al: Estimation of benefit and radiation risk from mass chest radiography. Radiology 109:37, 1973.
265. US Department of Health, Education and Welfare, in collaboration with the American College of Radiology and the American College of Chest Physicians: The Chest X-Ray as a Screening Procedure for Cardiopulmonary Disease. A Policy Statement. Washington, DC, Publication No. (FDA) 73-8036, 1973.
266. Lewis WW: Mobile x-ray units: A critical look. Natl Tuberc Resp Dis Assoc Bull Oct, 1971.
267. Sbarbaro JA: Mobile x-ray units: Too much effort, too few results. Natl Tuberc Resp Dis Bull Oct, 1971.
268. Abrams HL, Adelstein SJ, Elliott LP, et al: Report of Inter-Society Commission for Heart Disease Resources. Circulation 43:A-135, 1971.
269. Boucot KR, Weiss W: Is curable lung cancer detected by semiannual screening? JAMA 224:1361, 1973.
270. Spriggs AI, Boddington MM: The Cytology of Effusions. New York, Grune & Stratton, 1968, pp 1–39.
271. Johnston WW, Frable WJ: Diagnostic Respiratory Cytopathology. New York, Masson Publishing, 1979.
272. Dahlgren S, Nordenström B: Transthoracic Needle Biopsy. Stockholm, Almquist and Wiksell, 1966.
273. Kato H, Konaka C, Ono J, et al: Cytology of the Lung; Techniques and Interpretation. New York, Igaku-Shoin, 1983.
274. Sterrett G, Whitaker D, Glancy J: Fine-needle aspiration of lung, mediastinum and chest wall. A clinicopathologic exercise. In Sommers SC, Rosen PP: Pathology Annual 17 (Part 2), 1982, p 197.
275. Bonfiglio TA: Cytopathologic interpretation of transthoracic fine-needle biopsies. In Johnston WS (ed): Masson Monographs in Diagnostic Cytopathology. New York, Masson Publishing, 1983.
276. Crystal RG, Gadek JE, Ferrans VJ, et al: Interstitial lung disease: Current concepts of pathogenesis, staging and therapy. Am J Med 70:542, 1981.
277. Hunninghake GW, Kawanami O, Ferrans VJ, et al: Characterization of the inflammatory and immune effector cells in the lung parenchyma of patients with interstitial lung disease. Am Rev Respir Dis 123:407, 1981.
278. Greening AP: Bronchoalveolar lavage. Br Med J 284:1896, 1982.
279. Garvey J, Guarneri J, Khan F, et al: Clinical evaluation of bronchopulmonary lavage using the flexible fiberoptic bronchoscope. Ann Thorac Surg 30:427, 1980.
280. Ahlbom G, Winslov J: Outpatient sputum cytology in the diagnosis of lung cancer. Scand J Resp Dis 58:227, 1977.
281. Ng ABP, Horak GC: Factors significant in the diagnostic accuracy of lung cytology in bronchial washing and sputum samples. II. Sputum samples. Acta Cytol 27:397, 1983.
282. Umiker WO: Diagnosis of bronchogenic carcinoma: An evaluation of pulmonary cytology, bronchoscopy and scalene lymph node biopsy. Dis Chest 37:82, 1960.
283. Olsen CR, Froeb HF, Palmer LA: Sputum cytology after inhalation of heated propylene glycol: A clinical correlation. JAMA 178:668, 1961.
284. Kim BM, Froeb HF, Palmer L, et al: Clinical experience with cytologic examination of sputum obtained by heated aerosols. Am Rev Respir Dis 87:836, 1963.
285. Leilop L, Garret M, Lyons HA: Evaluation of technique and results for obtaining sputum for lung carcinoma screening: A study by blind technique. Am Rev Respir Dis 83:803, 1961.
286. Umiker WO, Korst DR, Cole RP, et al: Collection of sputum for cytologic examination: Spontaneous vs. artificially produced sputum. N Engl J Med 262:565, 1960.
287. Umiker WO: A new vista in pulmonary cytology: Aerosol induction of sputum. Dis Chest 39:512, 1961.
288. Fontana RS, Carr DT, Woolner LB, et al: An evaluation of methods of inducing sputum production in patients with suspected cancer of the lung. Proc Mayo Clin 37:113, 1962.
289. Russell WO, Neidhardt HW, Mountain CF, et al: Cytodiagnosis of lung cancer. A report of a four-year laboratory, clinical, and statistical study with a review of the literature on lung cancer and pulmonary cytology. Acta Cytol 7:1, 1963.
290. Chang JP, Anken M, Russell WO: Liquefaction and membrane filtration of sputum for the diagnosis of cancer. Am J Clin Pathol 37:584, 1962.
291. McCarty SA: Solving the cytopreparation problem of mucoid specimens with a mucoliquefying agent (Mucolexx) and nucleopore filters. Acta Cytol 16:221, 1972.
292. Liu W: Concentration and fractionation of cytologic elements in sputum. Acta Cytol 10:368, 1966.
293. Pharr SL, Farber SM: Cellular concentration of sputum and bronchial aspirations by tryptic digestion. Acta Cytol 6:447, 1962.
294. Bonime RG: Improved procedure for the preparation of pulmonary cytology smears. Acta Cytol 16:543, 1972.
295. Saccomanno G, Saunders RP, Ellis H, et al: Concentration of carcinoma or atypical cells in sputum. Acta Cytol 7:305, 1963.
296. Ellis HD, Kernosky JJ: Efficiency of concentrating malignant cells in sputum. Acta Cytol 7:372, 1963.
297. Abramson W, Dzenis V, Hicks S: Cytologic study of sputa and exudates using paraffin tubes. Acta Cytol 8:306, 1964.
298. Smith MJ, Kini SR, Watson E: Fine needle aspiration and endoscopic brush cytology. Comparison of direct smears and rinsings. Acta Cytol 24:456, 1980.
299. Johnston WW, Bossen EH: Ten years of respiratory cytopathology at Duke University Medical Center. 1. The cytopathologic diagnosis of lung cancer during the years 1970 to 1974, noting the significance of specimen number and type. Acta Cytol 24:103, 1980.
300. Rosa UW, Prolla JC, da Silva Gastal E: Cytology in diagnosis of cancer affecting the lung. Results in 1,000 consecutive patients. Chest 63:203, 1973.
301. Allan WB, Whittlesey P: The results of the experimental use of sulfur dioxide in the production of material for cell studies in lung cancer. Ann Intern Med 52:326, 1980.
302. Hinson KFW, Kuper SWA: The diagnosis of lung cancer by examination of sputum. Thorax 18:350, 1963.
303. Oswald NC, Hinson KFW, Canti G, et al: The diagnosis of primary lung cancer with special reference to sputum cytology. Thorax 26:623, 1971.
304. Hartveit F: Time and place of sputum cytology in the diagnosis of lung cancer. Thorax 36:299, 1981.
305. Ng ABP, Horak GC: Factors significant in the diagnostic accuracy of lung cytology in bronchial washing and sputum samples. 1. Bronchial washings. Acta Cytol 27:391, 1983.
306. Lerner MA, Rosbash H, Frank HA, et al: Radiologic localization and management of cytologically discovered bronchial carcinoma. N Engl J Med 264:480, 1961.
307. Muers MF, Boddington MM, Cole M, et al: Cytological sampling at fiberoptic bronchoscopy: Comparison of catheter aspirates and brush biopsies. Thorax 37:457, 1982.
308. Laurie W: Sputum cytology in the diagnosis of bronchial carcinoma. Med J Aust 1:205, 1966.
309. Johnston WW: Ten years of respiratory cytopathology at Duke University Medical Center. III. The significance of inconclusive cytopathologic diagnoses during the years 1970 to 1974. Acta Cytol 26:759, 1982.
310. Bewtra C, Dewan N, O'Donahue WJ Jr: Exfoliative sputum cytology in pulmonary embolism. Acta Cytol 27:489, 1983.
311. Scoggins WG, Smith RH, Frable WJ, et al: False-positive cytological diagnosis of lung carcinoma in patients with pulmonary infarcts. Ann Thorax Surg 24:474, 1977.
312. Koss LG, Melamed MR, Mayer K: The effect of busulfan on human epithelia. Am J Clin Pathol 44:385, 1965.
313. Ng ABP, Horak GC: Factors significant in the diagnostic accuracy of lung cytology in bronchial washing and sputum samples. 1. Bronchial washings. Acta Cytol 27:391, 1983.
314. Umiker WO: False-negative reports in the cytologic diagnosis of cancer of the lung. Am J Clin Pathol 28:37, 1957.
315. Clee MD, Sinclair DJM: Assessment of factors influencing the result of sputum cytology in bronchial carcinoma. Thorax 36:143, 1981.
316. Rosenberg BF, Spjut HJ, Gedney MM: Exfoliative cytology in metastatic cancer of the lung. N Engl J Med 261:226, 1959.
317. Naib ZM, Stewart JA, Dowdle WR, et al: Cytological features of viral respiratory tract infections. Acta Cytol 12:162, 1968.
318. Vercelli-Retta J, Mañana G, Reissenweber NJ: The cytologic diagnosis of hydatid disease. Acta Cytol 26:159, 1982.

2

319. Losner S, Volk BW, Slade WR, et al: Diagnosis of lipoid pneumonia by examination of sputum. Am J Clin Pathol 20:539, 1950.

320. Shlaes DM, Lederman M, Chmielewski R, et al: Elastin fibers in the sputum of patients with necrotizing pneumonia. Chest 83:885, 1983.

321. Yam LT, Janckila AJ: A simple method of preparing smears from bloody effusions for cytodiagnosis. Acta Cytol 27:114, 1983.

322. Nagasawa T, Nagasawa S: Enrichment of malignant cells from pleural effusions by Percoll density gradients. Acta Cytol 27:119, 1983.

323. Light RW, Erozan YS, Ball WC Jr: Cells in pleural fluid. Their value in differential diagnosis. Arch Intern Med 132:854, 1973.

324. Antony VB, Repine JE, Harada RN, et al: Inflammatory responses in experimental tuberculosis pleurisy. Acta Cytol 27:355, 1983.

325. Mestitz P, Pollard AC: The diagnosis of tuberculous pleural effusion. Br J Dis Chest 53:86, 1959.

326. Spieler P: The cytologic diagnosis of tuberculosis in pleural effusions. Acta Cytol 23:374, 1979.

327. Schwartz S, Broadbent M: Eosinophiles and other components of pleural effusions. Trans Clin Climatol Assoc 55:96, 1939.

328. Spriggs AI: Pleural eosinophilia due to pneumothorax (letter). Acta Cytol 23:425, 1979.

329. Adleman M, Albelda SM, Gottlieb J, et al: Diagnostic utility of pleural fluid eosinophilia. Am J Med 77:915, 1984.

330. Chapman JS, Reynolds RC: Eosinophilic response to intraperitoneal blood. J Lab Clin Med 51:516, 1958.

331. Veress JF, Koss LG, Schreiber K: Eosinophilic pleural effusions. Acta Cytol 23:40, 1979.

332. Campbell GD, Webb WR: Eosinophilic pleural effusion: A review with the presentation of seven new cases. Am Rev Respir Dis 90:194, 1964.

333. Béthoux L, Merle M, Nony J: Les pleurésies à éosinophiles. (Étude de 11 observations.) Eosinophilic pleurisy. (A report of 11 cases.) Rev Tuberc (Paris) 25:354, 1961.

334. Curran WS, Williams AW: Eosinophilic pleural effusion: A clue in differential diagnosis. Arch Intern Med 111:809, 1963.

335. Petusevsky ML, Faling J, Rocklin RE, et al: Pleuropericardial reaction to treatment with dantrolene. JAMA 242:2772, 1979.

336. Järvinen KAJ, Kahanpää A: Prognosis in cases with eosinophilic pleural effusion: 17 cases followed for five to twelve years. Acta Med Scand 164:245, 1959.

337. Naylor B, Schmidt RW: The case for exfoliative cytology of serous effusions. Lancet 1:711, 1964.

338. Chrétien J: Needle biopsy of the pleura: A simple procedure often more efficient than the classical methods. Abbottempo 1:25, 1963.

339. Dewald GW, Hicks GA, Dines DE, et al: Cytogenetic diagnosis of malignant pleural effusions: Culture methods to supplement direct preparations in diagnosis. Mayo Clin Proc 57:488, 1982.

340. Gondos B, McIntosh KM, Renston RH, et al: Application of electron microscopy in the definitive diagnosis of effusions. Acta Cytol 22:297, 1978.

341. Posalaky Z, McGinley D, Posalaky IP: Electron microscopic identification of the colorectal origins of tumor cells in pleural fluid. Acta Cytol 25:45, 1981.

342. To A, Coleman DV, Dearnaley DP, et al: Use of antisera to epithelial membrane antigen for the cytodiagnosis of malignancy in serous effusions. J Clin Pathol 34:1326, 1981.

343. Woods JC, Harris H, Spriggs AI, et al: A new marker for human cancer cells. 3. Immunocytochemical detection of malignant cells in serous fluids with Ca1 antibody. Lancet 2:512, 1982.

344. Walts AE, Said JW: Specific tumor markers in diagnostic cytology. Immunoperoxidase studies of carcinoembryonic antigen, lysozyme, and other tissue antigens in effusions, washes, and aspirates. Acta Cytol 27:408, 1983.

345. Monif GRG, Stewart BN, Block AJ: Living cytology. A new diagnostic technique for malignant pleural effusions. Chest 69:626, 1976.

346. Kutty CPK, Remeniuk E, Varkey B: Malignant-appearing cells in pleural effusion due to pancreatitis. Case report and literature review. Acta Cytol 24:412, 1980.

347. Decker DA, Dines DE, Payne WS, et al: The significance of a cytologically negative pleural effusion in bronchogenic carcinoma. Chest 74:640, 1978.

348. Zaatari GS, Gupta PK, Bhagavan BS, et al: Cytopathology of pleural endometriosis. Acta Cytol 26:227, 1982.

349. Jacobson ES: A case of secondary echinococcosis diagnosed by cytologic examination of pleural fluid and needle biopsy of pleura. Acta Cytol 17:76, 1973.

350. Reyes CV, Kathuria S, MacGlashan A: Diagnostic value of calcium oxalate crystals in respiratory and pleural fluid cytology. A case report. Acta Cytol 23:65, 1979.

351. Kelley S, McGarry P, Hutson Y: Atypical cells in pleural fluid characteristic of systemic lupus erythematosus. Acta Cytol 15:357, 1971.

352. Osamura RY, Shioya S, Handa K, et al: Lupus erythematosus cells in pleural fluid; Cytologic diagnosis in two patients. Acta Cytol 21:215, 1977.

353. Nosanchuk JS, Naylor B: A unique cytologic picture in pleural fluid from patients with rheumatoid arthritis. Am J Clin Pathol 50:330, 1968.

354. Leyden EV von: Ueber infectiose Pneumonie. Dtsch Med Wochenschr 9:52, 1883.

355. Ménétrier P: Cancer primitif du poumon. Bull Soc Anat (Paris) 61:643, 1886.

356. Horder TJ: Lung puncture: A new application of clinical pathology. Lancet 2:1345, 1909.

357. Dudgeon LS, Patrick CV: A new method for the rapid microscopical diagnosis of tumors: With an account of 200 cases so examined. Br J Surg 15:250, 1927.

358. Silverman I: A new biopsy needle. Am J Surg 40:671, 1938.

359. Rosenberger A, Adler O: Fine needle aspiration biopsy in the diagnosis of mediastinal lesions. Am J Roentgenol 131:239, 1978.

360. Flower CDR, Verney GI: Percutaneous needle biopsy of thoracic lesions: An evaluation of 300 biopsies. Clin Radiol 30:215, 1979.

361. Dull WL: Needle aspiration biopsy in suspected pulmonary carcinoma. Respiration 39:291, 1980.

362. Tao LC, Pearson FG, Delarue NC, et al: Percutaneous fine-needle aspiration biopsy: 1. Its value to clinical practice. Cancer 45:1480, 1980.

363. Zavala DC, Schoell JE: Ultra-thin needle aspiration of the lung in infectious and malignant disease. Am Rev Respir Dis 123:125, 1981.

364. Todd TRJ, Weisbrod G, Tao LC, et al: Aspiration needle biopsy of thoracic lesions. Ann Thorac Surg 32:154, 1981.

365. van Sonnenberg E, Lin AS, Deutsch AL, et al: Percutaneous biopsy of difficult mediastinal, hilar, and pulmonary lesions by computed tomographic guidance and a modified coaxial technique. Radiology 148:300, 1983.

366. Adler OB, Rosenberger A, Peleg H: Fine-needle aspiration biopsy of mediastinal masses: Evaluation of 136 experiences. Am J Roentgenol 140:893, 1983.

367. Sterrett G, Whitaker D, Shilkin KB, et al: The fine-needle aspiration cytology of mediastinal lesions. Cancer 51:127, 1983.

368. Berkman WA, Chowdhury L, Brown NL, et al: Value of electron microscopy in cytologic diagnosis of fine-needle biopsy. Am J Roentgenol 140:1253, 1983.

369. Ballard GL, Boyd WR: A specially designed cutting aspiration needle for lung biopsy. Am J Roentgenol 130:899, 1978.

370. Lalli AF, McCormack LJ, Zelch M, et al: Aspiration biopsies of chest lesions. Radiology 127:35, 1978.

371. Nordenström B: Transthoracic needle biopsy. N Engl J Med 276:1081, 1967.

372. Dahlgren S, Nordenström B: Transthoracic Needle Biopsy. Stockholm, Almqvist and Wiksells, 1966.

373. Berquist TH, Bailey PB, Cortese DA, et al: Transthoracic needle biopsy: Accuracy and complications in relation to location and type of lesion. Mayo Clin Proc 55:475, 1980.

374. Shure D, Fedullo PF: Transbronchial needle aspiration of peripheral masses. Am Rev Respir Dis 128:1090, 1983.

375. Poe RH, Tobin RE: Sensitivity and specificity of needle biopsy in lung malignancy. Am Rev Respir Dis 122:725, 1980.

376. Reuter K, Raptopoulos V, Reale F, et al: Diagnosis of peritoneal mesothelioma: Computed tomography, sonography, and fine-needle aspiration biopsy. Am J Roentgenol 140:1189, 1983.

377. Pinstein ML, Scott RL, Salazar J: Avoidance of negative percutaneous lung biopsy using contrast-enhanced CT. Am J Roentgenol 140:265, 1983.

378. Jereb M, Us-Krasovec M: Thin needle biopsy of chest lesions: Timesaving potential. Chest 78:288, 1980.

379. Sinner WN: Transthoracic needle biopsy of small peripheral malignant lung lesions. Invest Radiol 8:305, 1973.

380. Flower CDR, Verney GI: Percutaneous needle biopsy of thoracic lesions—an evaluation of 300 biopsies. Clin Radiol 30:215, 1979.

381. Gobien RP, Valicenti JF, Paris BS, et al: Thin-needle aspiration biopsy: Methods of increasing the accuracy of a negative prediction. Radiology 145:603, 1982.

382. Akhtar M, Aii MA, Owen E, et al: Technical methods. A simple method for processing fine-needle aspiration biopsy specimens for electron microscopy. J Clin Pathol 33:1214, 1980.

383. Collins VP, Ivarsson B: Tumor classification by electron microscopy of fine needle aspiration biopsy material. Acta Pathol Microbiol Scand 89:103, 1981.

384. Yam LT, Levine H: Rapid cytologic diagnosis of percutaneous needle aspirates of peripheral pulmonary lesions. Am J Clin Pathol 59:648, 1973.

385. Pak HY, Yokota S, Teplitz RL, et al: Rapid staining techniques employed in fine needle aspirations of the lung. Acta Cytol 25:178, 1981.

386. Pak HY, Yokota SB, Teplitz RL: Rapid staining techniques employed in fine needle aspiration (letter). Acta Cytol 27:81, 1983.

387. Lillington GA: The utility of needle aspiration biopsy of the lung. Mayo Clin Proc 55:516, 1980.

388. Sinner WN: Fine-needle biopsy of double or multiple primary carcinomas of the lung. ROFO 139:420, 1983.

389. Lauby VW, Burnett WE, Rosemond GP, et al: Value and risk of biopsy of pulmonary lesions by needle aspiration: Twenty-one years' experience. J Thorac Cardiovasc Surg 49:159, 1965.

390. Westcott JL: Air embolism complicating percutaneous needle biopsy of the lung. Chest 63:108, 1973.

391. Woolf CR: Applications of aspiration lung biopsy with a review of the literature. Dis Chest 25:286, 1954.

392. Gibney RTN, Man GCW, King EG, et al: Aspiration biopsy in the diagnosis of pulmonary disease. Chest 80:300, 1981.

393. Jereb M, Us-Krasovec M: Transthoracic needle biopsy of mediastinal and hilar lesions. Cancer 40:1354, 1977.

394. Sagel SS, Ferguson TB, Forrest JV, et al: Percutaneous transthoracic aspiration needle biopsy. Ann Thorac Surg 26:399, 1978.

395. Allison DJ, Hemingway AP: Percutaneous needle biopsy of the lung. Br Med J 282:875, 1981.

396. Jereb M: The usefulness of needle biopsy in chest lesions of different sizes and locations. Radiology 134:13, 1980.

397. Fontana RS, Miller WE, Beabout JW, et al: Transthoracic needle aspiration of discrete pulmonary lesions: Experience in 100 cases. Med Clin North Am 54:961, 1970.

398. Zelch JV, Lalli AF, McCormack LJ, et al: Aspiration biopsy in diagnosis of pulmonary nodule. Chest 63:149, 1973.

399. Sanders DE, Thompson DW, Pudden BJE: Percutaneous aspiration lung biopsy. Can Med Assoc J 104:139, 1971.

400. Kucharczyk W, Weisbrod GL, Cooper JD, et al: Cardiac tamponade as a complication of thin needle aspiration lung biopsy. Chest 82:120, 1982.

401. Dumont A, Durieu H, Declerq F, et al: À propos des dangers de la ponction-biopsie transpariétale des tumeurs du poumon. J Fr Med Chir Thorac 5:453, 1951.

402. Allbritten FF Jr, Nealon T, Gibbon JH, et al: The diagnosis of lung cancer. Surg Clin North Am 32:1657, 1952.

403. Ochsner A, DeBakey M, Dixon JL: Primary cancer of the lung. JAMA 135:321, 1947.

404. Dahlgren SE, Ovenfors C-O: Aspiration biopsy diagnosis of neurogenous mediastinal tumours. Acta Radiol Diagn 10:289, 1970.

405. Taft PD, Szyfelbein WM, Greene R: A study of variability in cytologic diagnoses based on pulmonary aspiration specimens. Am J Clin Pathol 73:36, 1980.

406. Francis D, Hojgaard K: Transthoracic aspiration biopsy. A study on diagnostic reproducibility. Acta Pathol Microbiol Scand 85:889, 1977.

407. Clark RA, Grech R, Robinson A, et al: Limitations of fibre-optic bronchoscopy under fluoroscopy in the investigation of peripheral lung lesions. Br J Radiol 51:432, 1978.

408. Walls WJ, Thornbury JR, Naylor B: Pulmonary needle aspiration biopsy in the diagnosis of Pancoast tumors. Radiology 111:99, 1974.

409. Dahlgren SE, Lind B: Comparison between diagnostic results obtained by transthoracic needle biopsy and by sputum cytology. Acta Cytol 16:53, 1972.

410. Philips J, Goodman B, Kelly V: Percutaneous thoracic aspiration needle biopsies. Pathology 14:211, 1981.

411. Zavala DC: The diagnosis of pulmonary disease by nonthoracotomy techniques. Chest 64:100, 1973.

412. Sargent EN, Turner AF, Gordonson J, et al: Percutaneous pulmonary needle biopsy: Report of 350 patients. Am J Roentgenol 122:758, 1974.

413. Michel RP, Lushpihan A, Ahmed MN: Pathologic findings of transthoracic needle aspiration in the diagnosis of localized pulmonary lesions. Cancer 51:1663, 1983.

414. Akhtar M, Ali MA, Owne EW: Application of electron microscopy in the interpretation of fine-needle aspiration biopsies. Cancer 48:2458, 1981.

415. Collins VP, Ivarson B: Tumor classification by electron microscopy of fine needle aspiration biopsy material. Acta Pathol Microbiol Scand [A] 89:103, 1981.

416. Craig ID, Shum DT, Desrosiers P, et al: Choriocarcinoma metastatic to the lung. A cytologic study with identification of human choriogonadotropin with an immunoperoxidase technique. Acta Cytol 27:647, 1983.

417. Singh G, Katyal SL, Torikata C: Carcinoma of type II pneumocytes. Immunodiagnosis of a subtype of "bronchioloalveolar carcinomas." Am J Pathol 102:195, 1981.

418. Said JW, Nash G, Sassoon AF, et al: Involucrin in lung tumors. A specific marker for squamous differentiation. Lab Invest 49:563, 1983.

419. Dahlgren S: Needle biopsy of intrapulmonary hamartoma. Scand J Resp Dis 47:187, 1966.

420. Tomashefski JF Jr, Cramer SF, Abramowsky C, et al: Needle biopsy diagnosis of solitary amyloid nodule of the lung. Acta Cytol 24:224, 1980.

421. Schieppati EE: Mediastinal lymph node puncture through the tracheal carina. Surg Gynecol Obstet 107:243, 1958.

422. Simeček C: Cytological investigation of intrathoracic lymph nodes in carcinoma of the lung. Thorax 21:369, 1966.

423. Bridgman AH, Duffield GD, Takaro T: An appraisal of newer diagnostic methods for intrathoracic lesions. Dis Chest 53:321, 1968.

424. Lundgren R, Bergman F, Angstrom T: Comparison of transbronchial fine needle aspiration biopsy, aspiration of bronchial secretion, bronchial washing, brush biopsy and forceps biopsy in the diagnosis of lung cancer. Eur J Respir Dis 64:378, 1983.

425. Wang KP, Terry P, Marsh B: Bronchoscopic needle aspiration biopsy of paratracheal tumors. Am Rev Respir Dis 118:17, 1978.

426. Buirski G, Calverley PMA, Douglas NJ, et al: Bronchial needle aspiration in the diagnosis of bronchial carcinoma. Thorax 36:508, 1981.

427. Lemer J, Malberger E, Konig-nativ R: Transbronchial fine needle aspiration. Thorax 37:270, 1982.

428. Wang KP, Marsh BR, Summer WR, et al: Transbronchial needle aspiration for diagnosis of lung cancer. Chest 80:48, 1981.

429. Dahlgren SE, Ovenfors C-O: Aspiration biopsy diagnosis of neurogenous mediastinal tumours. Acta Radiol (Diagn) 10:289, 1970.

430. McCarthy WJ, Christ ML, Fry WA: Intraoperative fine needle aspiration biopsy of thoracic lesions. Ann Thorac Surg 30:24, 1980.

431. DeCaro LF, Pak HY, Yokota S, et al: Intraoperative cytodiagnosis of lung tumors by needle aspiration. J Thorac Cardiovasc Surg 85:404, 1983.

432. Pantzar P, Meurala H, Koivuniemi A, et al: Preoperative fine needle aspiration biopsy of lung tumors. Scand J Thorac Cardiovasc Surg 17:51, 1983.

433. Burt ME, Flye MW, Webber BL, et al: Prospective evaluation of aspiration needle, cutting needle, transbronchial and open lung biopsy in patients with pulmonary infiltrates. Ann Thorac Surg 32:146, 1981.

434. Wall CP, Gaensler EA, Carrington CB, et al: Comparison of transbronchial and open biopsies in chronic infiltrative lung diseases. Am Rev Respir Dis 123:280, 1981.

435. Gaensler EA, Moister VB, Hamm J: Open-lung biopsy in diffuse pulmonary disease. N Engl J Med 270:1319, 1964.

436. Taylor FH, Evangelist FA, Barham BF: The flexible fiberoptic bronchoscope: Diagnostic tool or medical toy? Ann Thorac Surg 29:546, 1980.

437. Webb J, Clarke SW: A comparison of biopsy results using rigid and fiberoptic bronchoscopes. Br J Dis Chest 74:81, 1980.

438. Dreisin RB, Albert RK, Talley PA, et al: Flexible fiberoptic bronchoscopy in the teaching hospital: Yield and complications. Chest 74:144, 1978.

439. Rudd RM, Gellert AR, Boldy DAR, et al: Bronchoscopic and percutaneous aspiration biopsy in the diagnosis of bronchial carcinoma cell type. Thorax 37:462, 1982.

440. Popovich J Jr, Kvale PA, Eichenhorn MS, et al: Diagnostic accuracy of multiple biopsies from flexible fiberoptic bronchoscopy—a comparison of central versus peripheral carcinoma. Am Rev Respir Dis 125:521, 1982.

441. Zisholtz BM, Eisenberg H: Lung cancer cell type as a determinant of bronchoscopy yield. Chest 84:428, 1983.

442. Haponik EF, Summer WR, Terry PB, et al: Clinical decision making with transbronchial lung biopsies: The value of nonspecific histologic examination. Am Rev Respir Dis 125:524, 1982.

443. Puksa S, Hutcheon MA, Hyland RH: Usefulness of transbronchial biopsy in immunosuppressed patients with pulmonary infiltrates. Thorax 38:146, 1983.

444. Zellweger J-P, Leuenberger PJ: Cytologic and histologic examination of transbronchial lung biopsy. Eur J Respir Dis 63:94, 1982.

445. Andersen HA, Fontana RS: Transbronchoscopic lung biopsy for diffuse pulmonary diseases: Technique and results in 450 cases. Chest 62:125, 1972.

446. Andersen HA, Fontana RS, Harrison EG Jr: Transbronchoscopic lung biopsy in diffuse pulmonary disease. Dis Chest 48:187, 1965.

447. Shure D, Abraham JL, Konopka R: How should transbronchial biopsies be performed and processed? Am Rev Respir Dis 126:342, 1982.

448. Nordenström B, Carlens E: Bronchial biopsy in connection with bronchography. Acta Radiol (Diagn) 3:37, 1965.

449. Willson JKV, Eskridge M, Scott EL: Transbronchial biopsy of benign and malignant peripheral lung lesions: Description of three new instruments. Radiology 100:541, 1971.

450. Esguerra A, Wetmore J, Rickert RR: Transbronchial lung biopsy. Laboratory evaluation of a biopsy instrument capable of obtaining specimens suitable for histologic studies. Am Rev Resp Dis 102:808, 1970.

451. Ono R, Loke J, Ikeda S: Bronchofiberoscopy with curette biopsy and bronchography in the evaluation of peripheral lung lesions. Chest 79:162, 1981.

452. Willson JKV, Eskridge M: Bronchial brush biopsy with a controllable brush. Am J Roentgenol 109:471, 1970.

453. Fennessy JJ, Lu C-T, Variakojis D, et al: Transcatheter biopsy in the diagnosis of diseases of the respiratory tract. Radiology 110:555, 1974.

454. Radke JR, Conway WA, Eyler WR, et al: Diagnostic accuracy in

peripheral lung lesions: Factors predicting success with flexible fiberoptic bronchoscopy. Chest 76:176, 1979.

455. Clark RA, Gray PB, Townshend RH, et al: Transbronchial lung biopsy: A review of 85 cases. Thorax 32:546, 1977.

456. Beerman H, Kirshbaum BA: Some associated pulmonary and cutaneous diseases: A review of recent literature. Am J Med Sci 242:494, 1961.

457. Fry WA, Manalo-Estrella P: Bronchial brushing. Surg Gynecol Obstet 130:67, 1970.

458. Fennessy JJ: Bronchial brushing. Ann Otol Rhinol Laryngol 79:924, 1970.

459. Penido JRF, Lance JS, Cotton BH, et al: Endobronchial brush biopsy in the diagnosis of pulmonary lesions. Arch Surg 105:44, 1972.

460. Wallace JM, Deutsch AL: Flexible fiberoptic bronchoscopy and percutaneous needle lung aspiration for evaluating the solitary pulmonary nodule. Chest 81:665, 1982.

461. Zavala DC, Rossi NP, Rodman NF, et al: A new mobile catheter for obtaining bronchial brush biopsies. Diagnostic results in 50 patients with suspicious pulmonary lesions and negative bronchoscopies. Am Rev Respir Dis 106:541, 1972.

462. Kremp RE, Klatte EC, Collins RD: Technical considerations of percutaneous pulmonary biopsy. Radiology 100:285, 1971.

463. Vine HS, Kasdon EJ, Simon M: Technical developments and instrumentation. Percutaneous lung biopsy using the Lee needle and a track-obliterating technique. Radiology 144:921, 1982.

464. Westcott JL: Direct percutaneous needle aspiration of localized pulmonary lesions: Results in 422 patients. Radiology 137:31, 1980.

465. Chin WS, Yee IS: Percutaneous aspiration biopsy of malignant lung lesions using the Chiba needle. An initial experience. Clin Radiol 29:617, 1978.

466. Kline TS, Neal HS: Needle biopsy. A pilot study. JAMA 224:1143, 1973.

467. Youmans CR Jr, Middleton JM, Derrick JR, et al: Percutaneous needle biopsy of the lung for diffuse parenchymal disease. Dis Chest 54:105, 1968.

468. Vitums VC: Percutaneous needle biopsy of the lung with a new disposable needle. Chest 62:717, 1972.

469. Mehnert JH, Brown MJ: Percutaneous needle core biopsy of peripheral pulmonary masses. Am J Surg 136:151, 1978.

470. McEvoy RD, Begley MD, Antic R: Percutaneous biopsy of intrapulmonary mass lesions: Experience with a disposable cutting needle. Cancer 51:2321, 1983.

471. Zavala DC, Bedell GN: Percutaneous lung biopsy with a cutting needle. An analysis of 40 cases and comparison with other biopsy techniques. Am Rev Respir Dis 106:186, 1972.

472. Black LF, Hyatt RE: Maximal respiratory pressures: Normal values and relationship to age and sex. Am Rev Respir Dis 99:696, 1969.

473. Bandt PD, Blank N, Castellino RA: Needle diagnosis of pneumonitis. Value in high-risk patients. JAMA 220:1578, 1972.

474. Adamson JS Jr, Bates JH: Percutaneous needle biopsy of the lung. Arch Intern Med 119:164, 1967.

475. Smith WG: Needle biopsy of lung. Lancet 2:318, 1964.

476. Meyer JE, Ferrucci JT Jr, Janower ML: Fatal complications of percutaneous lung biopsy. Review of the literature and report of a case. Radiology 96:47, 1970.

477. Lung biopsy in the acutely ill—when and how? Clinical conference in pulmonary disease. Chest 62:484, 1972.

478. Steel SJ, Winstanley DP: Trephine biopsy of the lung and pleura. Thorax 24:576, 1969.

479. Wilson JR, Jones RL, Mielke B, et al: Trephine lung biopsy. Can Med Assoc J 108:704, 1973.

480. Castillo G, Ahmad M, Vanordstrand HS, et al: Trephine drill biopsy of the lung. Cleveland Clinic experience. JAMA 228:189, 1974.

481. Martiny O, Berson SD, Solomon A, et al: An evaluation of needle punch biopsy specimens in the diagnosis of diffuse lung disease. Am Rev Respir Dis 107:209, 1973.

482. Newhouse MT: Suction excision biopsy for diffuse pulmonary disease. Chest 63:707, 1973.

483. Brandt H-J, Loddenkemper R, Mai J: Atlas der Diagnostischen Thorakoskopie: Indikationen, Technik. Stuttgart, Georg Thieme Verlag,

484. Boutin C, Viallat JR, Cargnino P, et al: Thoracoscopy in malignant pleural effusions. Am Rev Respir Dis 124:588, 1981.

485. Boutin C, Viallat JR, Cargnino P, et al: Thoracoscopic lung biopsy: Experimental and clinical preliminary study. Chest 82:44, 1982.

486. Dijkman JH, van der Meer JWM, Bakker W, et al: Transpleural lung biopsy by the thoracoscopic route in patients with diffuse interstitial pulmonary disease. Chest 82:76, 1982.

487. Miller JI, Hatcher CR Jr: Thoracoscopy: A useful tool in the diagnosis of thoracic disease. Ann Thorac Surg 26:68, 1978.

488. Williams T, Thomas P: The diagnosis of pleural effusions by fiberoptic bronchoscopy and pleuroscopy. Chest 80:566, 1981.

489. Weissberg D, Kaufman M: Diagnostic and therapeutic pleuroscopy: Experience with 127 patients. Chest 78:732, 1980.

490. Weissberg D, Kaufman M, Zurkowski Z: Pleuroscopy in patients with pleural effusion and pleural masses. Ann Thorac Surg 29:205, 1980.

491. Rodgers BM, Ryckman FC, Moazam F, et al: Thoracoscopy for intrathoracic tumors. Ann Thorac Surg 31:414, 1981.

492. Heine F: Die Probeexcision aus Veränderungen in Thoraxraum und Lunge unter thorakoskopischer Sicht. Beitr Klin Tuberk 116:615, 1957.

493. Lloyd MS: Thoracoscopy and biopsy in the diagnosis of pleurisy with effusion. Q Bull Sea View Hosp 14:128, 1953.

494. Faurschou P, Madsen F, Viskum K: Thoracoscopy: Influence of the procedure on some respiratory and cardiac values. Thorax 38:341, 1983.

495. Gaensler EA, Carrington CB: Open biopsy for chronic diffuse infiltrative lung disease: Clinical, roentgenographic and physiological correlations in 502 patients. Ann Thorac Surg 30:411, 1980.

496. Andrews NC, Klassen KP: Eight years experience with pulmonary biopsy. JAMA 164:1061, 1957.

497. Daly BDT, Pugatch RD, Faling LJ, et al: Computed-tomographic-guided minithoracotomy. A preliminary report of a new approach to open lung biopsy. Radiology 146:543, 1983.

498. Churg A: An inflation procedure for open lung biopsies. Am J Surg Pathol 7:69, 1983.

499. Brody AR, Craighead JE: Preparation of human lung biopsy specimens by perfusion-fixation. Am Rev Respir Dis 112:645, 1975.

500. Rossiter SJ, Miller DC, Churg AM, et al: Open lung biopsy in the immunosuppressed patient. Is it really beneficial? J Thorac Cardiovasc Surg 77:338, 1979.

501. Hasse J, Perruchoud A, Dalquen P, et al: Open lung biopsy in diffuse pulmonary disease. Lung 159:23, 1981.

502. DeFrancis N, Klosk E, Albano E: Needle biopsy of the parietal pleura: A preliminary report. N Engl J Med 252:948, 1955.

503. Anderson JP: A modification of the Abrams's pleural biopsy punch. Br J Dis Chest 75:408, 1981.

504. Mungall IPF, Cowen PN, Cooke NT, et al: Multiple pleural biopsy with the Abrams needle. Thorax 35:600, 1980.

505. Tserkézoglou A, Metakidis S, Papastamatiou-Tsimara H, et al: Solitary rheumatoid nodule of the pleura and rheumatoid pleural effusion. Thorax 33:769, 1978.

506. Gardiner IT, Uff JS: Acute pleurisy in sarcoidosis. Thorax 33:124, 1978.

507. Nelson DG, Loudon RG: Sarcoidosis with pleural involvement. Am Rev Respir Dis 108:647, 1973.

508. Levine H, Cugell DW: Blunt-end needle biopsy of pleura and rib. Arch Intern Med 109:516, 1962.

509. Niden AH, Burrows B, Kasik JE, et al: Percutaneous pleural biopsy with a curetting needle. Special reference to biopsy without effusion. Am Rev Respir Dis 84:37, 1961.

510. Cope C, Bernhardt H: Hook-needle biopsy of pleura, pericardium, peritoneum and synovium. Am J Med 35:189, 1963.

511. Scerbo J, Keltz H, Stone DJ: A prospective study of closed pleural biopsies. JAMA 218:377, 1971.

512. Mestitz P, Purves MJ, Pollard AC: Pleural biopsy in the diagnosis of pleural effusion: A report of 200 cases. Lancet 2:1349, 1958.

513. Weiss W: Needle biopsy of the parietal pleura in tuberculosis. Am Rev Respir Dis 78:17, 1958.

514. Reese O Jr, McLean RL, Raaen TD: Acid-fast bacilli in pleural biopsy specimens. Arch Intern Med 108:438, 1961.

515. Deluccia VC, Reyes EC: Percutaneous needle biopsy of parietal pleura: Analysis of 50 cases. NY State J Med 77:2058, 1977.

516. Cope C: New pleural biopsy needle; Preliminary study. JAMA 167:1107, 1958.

517. Sison BS, Weiss Z: Needle biopsy of the parietal pleura in patients with pleural effusions. Br Med J 2:298, 1962.

518. Donohoe RF, Katz S, Matthews MJ: Pleural biopsy as an aid in the etiologic diagnosis of pleural effusion: Review of the literature and report of 132 biopsies. Ann Intern Med 48:344, 1958.

519. Shaw RK, Hallett WY: Biopsy of the parietal pleura. Am J Med Sci 241:593, 1961.

520. Schachter EN, Basta W: Subcutaneous metastasis of an adenocarcinoma following a percutaneous pleural biopsy. Am Rev Respir Dis 107:283, 1973.

521. Jones FL Jr: Subcutaneous implantation of cancer: A rare complication of pleural biopsy. Chest 57:189, 1970.

522. Carr DT, Soule EH, Ellis FH Jr: Management of pleural effusions. Med Clin North Am 48:961, 1964.

523. Arrington CW, Hawkins JA, Richert JH, et al: Management of undiagnosed pleural effusions in positive tuberculin reactors. Am Rev Respir Dis 93:587, 1966.

524. Richert JH, Wier JA, Salyer JM, et al: The reliability of tissue diagnosis of pleurisy: A preliminary report. Ann Intern Med 52:320, 1960.

525. Herbert A, Gallagher PJ: Pleural biopsy in the diagnosis of malignant mesothelioma. Thorax 37:816, 1982.

526. Carlens E: Mediastinoscopy: A method for inspection and tissue biopsy in the superior mediastinum. Dis Chest 36:343, 1959.

527. Chandler SB, Stemmer EA, Calvin JW, et al: Mediastinal biopsy for indeterminate chest lesions. Thorax 21:533, 1966.

528. Kelsey CA, Lane RG, Moseley RD, et al: Chest radiographs obtained with shaped filters: Evaluation by observer performance tests. Radiology 159:653, 1986.

529. Brantigan JW, Brantigan CO, Brantigan OC: Biopsy of nonpalpable scalene lymph nodes in carcinoma of the lung. Am Rev Respir Dis 107:962, 1973.

530. Nordenström B: Transjugular approach to the mediastinum for mediastinal needle biopsy: A preliminary report. Invest Radiol 2:134, 1967.

531. Nordenström B: Paraxiphoid approach to the mediastinum for mediastinography and mediastinal needle biopsy: A preliminary report. Invest Radiol 2:141, 1967.

532. Nordenström B: Paravertebral approach to the posterior mediastinum for mediastinography and needle biopsy. Acta Radiol (Diagn) 12:298, 1972.

533. Palva T, Viikari S, Inberg M: Pulmonary carcinoma: Mediastinoscopic criteria for curative resections. Dis Chest 56:156, 1969.

534. Paulson DL, Urschel HC Jr: Selectivity in the surgical treatment of bronchogenic carcinoma. J Thorac Cardiovasc Surg 62:554, 1971.

535. Pearson FG: Use of mediastinoscopy in selection of patients for lung cancer operations. Ann Thorac Surg 30:205, 1980.

536. Gibbons JRP: The value of mediastinoscopy in assessing operability in carcinoma of the lung. Br J Dis Chest 66:162, 1972.

537. Hájek M, Homan van der Heide JN: Early detection of mediastinal spread of pulmonary carcinoma by mediastinoscopy. Thorax 25:720, 1970.

538. Ross JK, Mikhail JR, Drury RAB, et al: Mediastinoscopy. Thorax 25:312, 1970.

539. McNeill TM, Chamberlain JM: Diagnostic anterior mediastinotomy. Ann Thorac Surg 2:532, 1966.

540. Evans DS, Hall JH, Harrison GK: Anterior mediastinotomy. Thorax 28:444, 1973.

541. Deneffe G, Lacquet LM, Gyselen A: Cervical mediastinoscopy and anterior mediastinotomy in patients with lung cancer and radiologically normal mediastinum. Eur J Respir Dis 64:613, 1983.

542. Van Der Schaar PJ, Van Zanten ME: Experience with mediastinoscopy. Thorax 20:211, 1965.

543. Editorial: Mediastinoscopy. Lancet 1:1219, 1972.

544. Widström A: Palsy of the recurrent nerve following mediastinoscopy. Chest 67:365, 1975.

545. Sarin CL, Nohl-Oser HC: Mediastinoscopy: A clinical evaluation of 400 consecutive cases. Thorax 24:585, 1969.

546. Gunstensen J, Wade JD: Mediastinoscopy. An analysis of 320 consecutive cases. Br J Surg 59:209, 1972.

547. Marchand P: Mediastinoscopy. S Afr Med J 46:285, 1972.

548. Doctor AH: Mediastinoscopy: A critical evaluation of 220 cases. Ann Surg 174:965, 1971.

549. Ashraf MH, Milson PL, Walesby RK: Selection by mediastinoscopy and long-term survival in bronchial carcinoma. Ann Thorac Surg 30:208, 1980.

550. Smith SR, Hooper RG, Beechler CR, et al: Indications for mediastinal lymph node evaluation. Chest 81:599, 1982.

551. Bergh NP, Rydberg B, Scherstén T: Mediastinal exploration by the technique of Carlens. Dis Chest 46:399, 1964.

552. Maassen W, Kirsch M, Thümmler M: Indikationen und vorläufige Ergebnisse bei 300 Mediastinoskopien. (The results of 300 mediastinoscopies.) Prax Pneumol 18:65, 1964.

553. Daniels AC: A method of biopsy useful in diagnosing certain intrathoracic diseases. Dis Chest 16:360, 1949.

554. Rouvière H: Anatomy of the Human Lymphatic System (trans by Tobias MJ). Ann Arbor, MI, Edwards, 1938.

555. Klingenberg I: Histopathologic findings in the prescalene tissue from 1,000 post-mortem cases. Acta Chir Scand 127:57, 1964.

556. Baird JA: The pathways of lymphatic spread of carcinoma of the lung. Br J Surg 52:868, 1965.

557. Lal S, Poole GW: Scalene-node biopsies. Lancet 2:112, 1963.

558. Schatzlein MH, McAuliffe S, Orringer MB, et al: Scalene node biopsy in pulmonary carcinoma: When is it indicated? Ann Thorac Surg 31:322, 1981.

559. Aikens RL: Scalene node biopsy. Can Med Assoc J 81:891, 1959.

560. Tarnowski CE: One hundred consecutive lymph gland biopsies by Daniels' method in cases of obscure pulmonary disease. Acta Tuberc Scand 41:192, 1962.

561. Lillington GA, Jamplis RW: Scalene node biopsy. Ann Intern Med 59:101, 1963.

562. Shields TW, Lees WM, Fox RT: The diagnostic value of biopsy of nonpalpable scalene lymph nodes in chest diseases. Ann Surg 148:184, 1958.

563. Skinner DB: Scalene-lymph-node biopsy: Reappraisal of risks and indications. N Engl J Med 268:1324, 1963.

564. Thomas HS, Bloomer WE, Orloff MJ: Scalene lymph node biopsy. Dis Chest 53:316, 1968.

565. Hartung W: Gefrier-Grossschnitte von ganzen Organen, speziell der Lunge. (Frozen large sections of total organs, especially the lungs.) Zentralbl Allg Pathol 100:408, 1960.

566. Heard BE: A pathological study of emphysema of the lungs with chronic bronchitis. Thorax 13:136, 1958.

567. Gough J, Wentworth JE: The use of thin sections of entire organs in morbid anatomical studies. J Roy Micr Soc 69:231, 1949.

568. Whimster WF: Rapid giant paper sections of lungs. Thorax 24:737, 1969.

569. Ferencz C, Greco J: A method for the three-dimensional study of pulmonary arteries. Chest 57:428, 1970.

570. Thurlbeck WM: The geographic pathology of pulmonary emphysema and chronic bronchitis. I. Review. Arch Environ Health 14:16, 1967.

571. Heard BE, Esterly JR, Wootliff JS: A modified apparatus for fixing lungs to study the pathology of emphysema. Am Rev Respir Dis 95:311, 1967.

572. Blumenthal BJ, Boren HG: Lung structure in three dimensions after inflation and fume fixation. Am Rev Respir Dis 79:764, 1959.

573. Wright BM, Slavin G, Kreel L, et al: Postmortem inflation and fixation of human lungs. A technique for pathological and radiological correlations. Thorax 29:189, 1974.

574. Mittermayer C, Wybitul K, Rau WS, et al: Standardized fixation of human lung for radiology and morphometry; Description of a "two chamber" system with formaldehyde vapor inflation. Pathol Res Pract 162:115, 1978.

575. Silverton RE: Gross fixation methods used in the study of pulmonary emphysema. Thorax 20:289, 1965.

576. Weibel ER, Vidone RA: Fixation of the lung by formalin steam in the controlled state of air inflation. Am Rev Respir Dis 84:856, 1961.

577. Markarian B: A simple method of inflation-fixation and air drying of lungs. Am J Clin Pathol 63:20, 1975.

578. Sutinen S, Pääkkö P, Lahti R: Post-mortem inflation, radiography and fixation of human lungs. A method for radiological and pathological correlations and morphometric studies. Scand J Resp Dis 60:29, 1979.

579. Pääkkö P, Sutinen S, Lahti R: Pattern recognition in radiographs of excised air-inflated human lungs. I. Circulatory disorders in non-emphysematous lungs. Eur J Respir Dis 62:21, 1981.

580. Pääkkö P, Sutinen S, Lahti R: Pattern recognition in radiographs of excised air-inflated human lungs. II. Acute inflammation in non-emphysematous lungs. Eur J Respir Dis 62:33, 1981.

581. Pääkkö P: Pattern recognition in radiographs of excised air-inflated human lungs. III. Chronic interstitial and granulomatous inflammation, scars, and lymphangitis carcinomatosa in non-emphysematous lungs. Eur J Respir Dis 62:289, 1981.

582. Sutinen S, Pääkkö P, Lohela P, et al: Pattern recognition in radiographs of excised air-inflated human lungs. IV. Emphysema alone and with other common lesions. Eur J Respir Dis 62:297, 1981.

583. Schlesinger MJ: New radiopaque mass for vascular injection. Lab Invest 6:1, 1957.

584. Cudkowicz L, Armstrong JB: Observations on the normal anatomy of the bronchial arteries. Thorax 6:343, 1951.

585. Tompsett DH: Anatomical Techniques. London, E. & S. Livingstone, 1970.

586. Liebow AA, Hales MR, Lindskog GE, et al: Plastic demonstrations of pulmonary pathology. J Bull Int Assoc Med Museums 27:116, 1947.

587. Phalen RF, Oldham MJ: Airway structures. Tracheobronchial airway structure as revealed by casting techniques. Am Rev Respir Dis 128:S1, 1983.

588. Timbrell V, Bovan NE, Davies AS, et al: Hollow casts of lungs for experimental purposes. Nature 225:97, 1970.

589. Dolan CT, Brown AL Jr, Ritts RE Jr: Microbiological examination of postmortem tissues. Arch Pathol 92:206, 1971.

590. Koneman EW, Davis MA: Postmortem bacteriology. III. Clinical significance of microorganisms recovered at autopsy. Am J Clin Pathol 61:28, 1974.

591. Koneman EW, Minckler TM, Shires DG, et al: Postmortem bacteriology: II. Selection of cases for culture. Am J Clin Pathol 55:17, 1971.

592. Minckler TM, Newell GR, O'Toole WF, et al: Microbiology experience in collection of human tissue. Am J Clin Pathol 45:85, 1960.

593. de Jongh DS, Loftis JW, Green GS, et al: Postmortem bacteriology. A practical method for routine use. Am J Clin Pathol 49:424, 1968.

594. Knapp BE, Kent TH: Postmortem lung cultures. Arch Pathol 85:200, 1968.

595. Zanen-Lim OG, Zanen HC: Postmortem bacteriology of the lung by printculture of frozen tissue. A technique for in situ culture of microorganisms in whole frozen organs. J Clin Pathol 33:474, 1980.

596. Wang N-S: Applications of electron microscopy to diagnostic pulmonary pathology. Hum Pathol 14:888, 1983.

2

597. Bachofen M, Weibel ER, Roos B: Postmortem fixation of human lungs for electron microscopy. Am Rev Respir Dis *111*:247, 1975.

598. Trump BF, Valigorsky JM, Jones RT, et al: The application of electron microscopy and cellular biochemistry to the autopsy. Observations on cellular changes in human shock. Hum Pathol *6*:499, 1975.

599. Ferguson CC, Richardson JB: A simple technique for the utilization of postmortem tracheal and bronchial tissues for ultrastructural studies. Hum Pathol *9*:463, 1978.

600. Pinkerton H, Carroll S: Fatal adenovirus pneumonia in infants. Correlation of histologic and electron microscopic observations. Am J Pathol *65*:543, 1971.

601. Smith J, Coleman DV: Electron microscopy of cells showing viral cytopathic effects in Papanicolaou smears. Acta Cytol *27*:605, 1983.

602. Editorial: "Immotile-cilia" syndrome and ciliary abnormalities induced by infection and injury. Am Rev Respir Dis *124*:107, 1981.

603. Skikne MI, Prinsloo I, Webster I: Electron microscopy of lung in Niemann-Pick disease. J Pathol *106*:119, 1972.

604. Basset F, Soler P, Jaurand MC, et al: Ultrastructural examination of bronchoalveolar lavage for diagnosis of pulmonary histiocytosis X: Preliminary report on four cases. Thorax *32*:303, 1977.

605. Kullberg FC, Funahashi A, Siegesmund KA: Pulmonary eosinophilic granuloma: Electron microscopic detection of X-bodies on lung lavage cells and transbronchoscopic lung biopsy in one patient. Ann Intern Med *96*:188, 1982.

606. Kuhn C: Systemic lupus erythematosus in a patient with ultrastructural lesions of the pulmonary capillaries previously reported in the *Review* as due to idiopathic pulmonary hemosiderosis. Am Rev Respir Dis *106*:931, 1972.

607. Heard BE, Dewar A, Firmin RK, et al: One very rare and one new tracheal tumour found by electron microscopy: Glomus tumour and acinic cell tumour resembling carcinoid tumours by light microscopy. Thorax *37*:97, 1982.

608. Heilman E, Feiner H: The role of electron microscopy in the diagnosis of unusual peripheral lung tumours. Hum Pathol *9*:589, 1978.

609. Hoch WS, Patchefsky AS, Takeda M, et al: Benign clear cell tumor of the lung. An ultrastructural study. Cancer *33*:1328, 1974.

610. Becker NH, Soifer I: Benign clear cell tumor ("sugar tumor") of the lung. Cancer *27*:712, 1971.

611. Chumas JC, Lorelle CA: Pulmonary meningioma. A light- and electron-microscopic study. Am J Surg Pathol *6*:795, 1982.

612. Katzenstein A-LA, Maurer JJ: Benign histiocytic tumor of lung. A light- and electron-microscopic study. Am J Surg Pathol *3*:61, 1979.

613. Warhol MJ, Hickey WF, Corson JM: Malignant mesothelioma. Ultrastructural distinction from adenocarcinoma. Am J Surg Pathol *6*:307, 1982.

614. Domagala W, Woyke S: Transmission and scanning electron microscopic studies of cells in effusions. Acta Cytol *19*:214, 1975.

615. Sobin LH: The histologic classification of lung tumors: The need for a double standard. Hum Pathol *14*:1020, 1983.

616. Nash G: The diagnosis of lung cancer in the 80s: Will routine light microscopy suffice? Hum Pathol *14*:1021, 1983.

617. Leong AS-Y: The relevance of ultrastructural examination in the classification of primary lung tumors. Pathology *14*:37, 1982.

618. Churg A: The fine structure of large cell undifferentiated carcinoma of the lung. Evidence for its relation to squamous cell carcinomas and adenocarcinomas. Hum Pathol *9*:143, 1978.

619. Auerbach O, Frasca JM, Parks VR, et al: A comparison of World Health Organization (WHO) classification of lung tumors by light and electron microscopy. Cancer *50*:2079, 1982.

620. Gould VE, Chejfec G: Ultrastructural and biochemical analysis of "undifferentiated" pulmonary carcinomas. Hum Pathol *9*:377, 1978.

621. Abraham JL: Recent advances in pneumoconiosis: The pathologist's role in etiologic diagnosis. Chapter 6. *In* Thurlbeck WM, Abell MR (eds): The Lung: Structure, Function, and Disease. Baltimore, Williams and Wilkins, 1978.

622. Lapenas DJ, Davis GS, Gale PN, et al: Mineral dusts as etiologic agents in pulmonary fibrosis: The diagnostic role of analytical scanning electron microscopy. Am J Clin Pathol *78*:701, 1982.

623. Ghadially FN: Invited review. The technique and scope of electron-probe x-ray analysis in pathology. Pathology *11*:95, 1979.

624. Vallyathan NV, Green FHY, Craighead JE: Recent advances in the study of mineral pneumoconiosis. *In* Sommers SC, Rosen PP (eds): Pathology Annual, Part 2. Vol 15. New York, Appleton-Century-Crofts, 1980.

625. Hayes TL, Pease RFW, McDonald LW: Applications of the scanning electron microscope to biologic investigations. Lab Invest *15*:1320, 1966.

626. Domagala W, Kahan AV, Koss LG: A simple method of preparation and identification of cells for scanning electron microscopy. Acta Cytol *23*:140, 1979.

627. Mikel UV, Johnson FB: A simple method for the study of the same cells by light and scanning electron microscopy. Acta Cytol *24*:252, 1980.

628. Becker SN, Wong JY, Marchiondo AA, et al: Scanning electron microscopy of alcohol-fixed cytopathology specimens. Acta Cytol *25*:578, 1980.

629. Takenaga A, Matsuda M, Horai T, et al: Scanning electron microscopy in the study of lung cancer. New technique of comparative studies on the same lung cancer cells by light microscopy and scanning electron microscopy. Acta Cytol *21*:90, 1977.

630. Kaneshima S, Kiyasu Y, Kudo H, et al: An application of scanning electron microscopy to cytodiagnosis of pleural and peritoneal fluids. Comparative observation of the same cells by light microscopy and scanning electron microscopy. Acta Cytol *22*:490, 1978.

631. Gondos B, Lai CE, King EB: Distinction between atypical mesothelial cells and malignant cells by scanning electron microscopy. Acta Cytol *23*:321, 1979.

632. Pertschuk LP, Kim DS, Brigati DJ: Nonrenal practical applications of immunofluorescence in diagnostic pathology. *In* Sommers SC, Rosen PP (eds): Pathology Annual. Part 1, Vol 14. New York, Appleton-Century-Crofts, 1979.

633. Beechler CR, Enquist RW, Hunt KK, et al: Immunofluorescence of transbronchial biopsies in Goodpasture's syndrome. Am Rev Respir Dis *121*:869, 1980.

634. Lowry BS, Vega FG Jr, Hedlund KW: Localization of *Legionella pneumophila* in tissue using FITC-conjugated specific antibody and a background stain. Am J Clin Pathol *77*:601, 1982.

635. Wicher K, Kalinka C, Mlodozeniec P, et al: Fluorescent antibody technic used for identification and typing of *Streptococcus pneumoniae*. Am J Clin Pathol *77*:72, 1982.

636. Pertschuk LP, Silverstein E, Friedland J: Immunohistologic diagnosis of sarcoidosis; Detection of angiotensin-converting enzyme in sarcoid granulomas. Am J Clin Pathol *75*:350, 1981.

637. Falini B, Taylor OR: New developments in immunoperoxidase techniques and their application. Arch Pathol Lab Med *107*:105, 1983.

638. To A, Dearnaley DP, Ormerod MG, et al: Indirect immunoalkaline phosphatase staining of cytologic smears of serous effusions for tumor marker studies. Acta Cytol *27*:109, 1983.

639. Fox B, Shousha S, James KR, et al: Immunohistological study of human lungs by immunoperoxidase technique. J Clin Pathol *35*:144, 1982.

640. Suffin SC, Kaufmann AF, Whitaker B, et al: *Legionella pneumophila*. Identification in tissue sections by a new immunoenzymatic procedure. Arch Pathol Lab Med *104*:283, 1980.

641. Lehto VP, Stenman S, Miettinen M, et al: Expression of a neural type of intermediate filament as a distinguishing feature between oat cell carcinoma and other lung cancers. Am J Pathol *110*:113, 1983.

642. Said JW, Nash G, Banks-Schlegel S, et al: Keratin in human lung tumors. Patterns of localization of different-molecular-weight keratin proteins. Am J Pathol *113*:27, 1983.

643. Springall DR, Lackie P, Levene MM, et al: Immunostaining of neuron-specific enolase is a valuable aid to the cytological diagnosis of neuroendocrine tumours of the lung. J Pathol *143*:259, 1984.

644. Corson JM, Pinkus GS: Mesothelioma: Profile of keratin proteins and carcinoembryonic antigen. An immunoperoxidase study of 20 cases and comparison with pulmonary adenocarcinomas. Am J Pathol *108*:80, 1982.

645. Wang N-S, Huang S-N, Gold P: Absence of carcinoembryonic antigen–like material in mesothelioma. An immunohistochemical differentiation from other lung cancers. Cancer *44*:937, 1979.

646. Kahn HJ, Hanna W, Yeger H, et al: Immunohistochemical localization of prekeratin filaments in benign and malignant cells in effusions. Comparison with intermediate filament distribution by electron microscopy. Am J Pathol *109*:206, 1982.

647. Battifora H, Sun T-T, Bahu RM, et al: The use of antikeratin antiserum as a diagnostic tool: Thymoma versus lymphoma. Hum Pathol *11*:635, 1980.

648. Waxler B, Eisenstein R, Battifora H: Electrophoresis of tissue glycosaminoglycans as an aid in the diagnosis of mesotheliomas. Cancer *44*:221, 1979.

649. Arai H, Kang K-Y, Sato H, et al: Significance of the quantification and demonstration of hyaluronic acid in tissue specimens for the diagnosis of pleural mesothelioma. Am Rev Respir Dis *120*:529, 1979.

650. Chiu B, Churg A, Tengblad A, et al: Analysis of hyaluronic acid in the diagnosis of malignant mesothelioma. Cancer *54*:2195, 1984.

651. Weibel ER: Morphometry of the human lung. New York, Academic Press, 1963.

652. Hislop A, Reid L: New pathological findings in emphysema of childhood: 2. Overinflation of a normal lobe. Thorax *26*:190, 1971.

653. Henderson R, Hislop A, Reid L: New pathological findings in emphysema of childhood: 3. Unilateral congenital emphysema with hypoplasia—and compensatory emphysema of contralateral lung. Thorax *26*:195, 1971.

654. Loud AV, Anversa P: Biology of disease. Morphometric analysis of biologic processes. Lab Invest *50*:250, 1984.

655. Cooney TP, Thurlbeck WM: Pulmonary hypoplasia in Down's syndrome. N Engl J Med 307:1170, 1982.
656. Williams AJ, Vawter G, Reid LM: Lung structure in asphyxiating thoracic dystrophy. Arch Pathol Lab Med 108:658, 1984.
657. Hansson A, Korsgaard R: Cytogenetical diagnosis of malignant pleural effusions. Scand J Respir Dis 55:301, 1974.
658. Hansteen I-L., Hillestad I., Thomassen OK: Chromosome analysis and cell cytology in effusions. A comparative study. Scand J Respir Dis 58:51, 1977.
659. DeWald G, Dines DE, Weiland LH, et al: Usefulness of chromosome examination in the diagnosis of malignant pleural effusions. N Engl J Med 295:1494, 1976.
660. Trout ED, Kelley JP: A phantom for the evaluation of techniques and equipment used for roentgenography of the chest. Am J Roentgenol 117:771, 1973.
661. Symposium: The Optimization of Chest Radiography. Madison, WI, University of Wisconsin, 1979.
662. Paul JL, Levine MD, Fraser RG, et al: The measurement of total lung capacity based on a computer analysis of anterior and lateral radiographic chest images. IEEE Trans Biomed Eng 21:444, 1974.
663. Herman PG, Sandor T, Mann BE, et al: Rapid computerized lung volume determination from chest roentgenograms. Am J Roentgenol 124:477, 1975.
664. Janik JS, Nagaraj HS, Groff DB: Thoracoscopic evaluation of intrathoracic lesions in children. J Thorac Cardiovasc Surg 83:408, 1982.
665. Theodos PA: Lung biopsy in the diagnosis of the pneumoconioses. Dis Chest 53:271, 1968.
666. Hill HE, Hensler NM, Breckler IA: Pleural biopsy in diagnosis of effusion: Results in fifty cases of pleural disease observed consecutively. Am Rev Respir Dis 78:8, 1958.
667. Robin ED, Burke CM: Routine chest x-ray examinations. Chest 90:258, 1986.
668. Hickey NM, Niklason LT, Sabbagh E, et al: Dual-energy digital radiographic quantification of calcium in simulated pulmonary nodules. AJR 148:19, 1987.
669. Poon PY, Bronskill MJ, Henkelman RM, et al: Magnetic resonance imaging of the mediastinum. J Can Assoc Radiol 37:173, 1986.
670. Elam DA, Poe ND: A single-breath radioaerosol-inhalation technique. Radiology 145:542, 1982.
671. Hatfield MK, MacMahon H, Ryan JW, et al: Postoperative recurrence of lung cancer: Detection by whole-body gallium scintigraphy. AJR 117:911, 1986.
672. Wilson R: Analyzing the daily risks of life. Technology Review, Feb 1979, pp 41–46.
673. Johnston WW: Cytologic diagnosis of lung cancer: Principles and problems. Pathol Res Pract 181:1, 1986.
674. Chalon J, Tang CK, Klein GS, et al: Routine cytodiagnosis of pulmonary malignancies. Arch Pathol Lab Med 105:11, 1981.
675. Kern WH, Schweizer CW: Sputum cytology of metastatic carcinoma of the lung. Acta Cytol 20:514, 1976.
676. Pitchenik AE, Ganjei P, Torres A, et al: Sputum examination for the diagnosis of Pneumocystis carinii pneumonia in the acquired immunodeficiency syndrome. Am Rev Respir Dis 133:226, 1986.
677. Corwin RW, Irwin RS: The lipid-laden alveolar macrophage as a marker of aspiration in parenchymal lung disease. Am Rev Respir Dis 132:576, 1985.
678. Hostmark J, Vigander T, Skaarland E: Characterization of pleural effusions by flow-cytometric DNA analysis. Eur J Respir Dis 66:315, 1985.
679. Cobb CJ, Synn J, Cobb SR, et al: Cytologic findings in an effusion caused by rupture of a benign cystic teratoma of the mediastinum into a serous cavity. Acta Cytol 29:1015, 1985.
680. Akhtar M, Bakry M, Nash E: An improved technic for processing aspiration biopsy for electron microscopy. Am J Clin Pathol 85:57, 1986.
681. Muller NL, Bergin CJ, Miller RR, et al: Seeding of malignant cells into the needle track after lung and pleural biopsy. J Can Assoc Radiol 37:192, 1986.
682. Hawkins AG, Hsiu J-G, Smith RM, et al: Pulmonary dirofilariasis diagnosed by fine needle aspiration biopsy: A case report. Acta Cytol 29:19, 1985.
683. Silverman JF, Johnsrude IS: Fine needle aspiration cytology of granulomatous cryptococcosis of the lung. Acta Cytol 29:157, 1985.
684. Dahlgren SE, Ekstrom P: Aspiration cytology in the diagnosis of pulmonary tuberculosis. Scand J Respir Dis 53:196, 1972.
685. Covell JL, Feldman PS: Fine needle aspiration diagnosis of aspiration pneumonia (phytopneumonitis). Acta Cytol 28:77, 1984.
686. Silverman JF, Weaver MD, Shaw R, et al: Fine needle aspiration cytology of pulmonary infarct. Acta Cytol 29:162, 1985.
687. Masson RG, Ruggieri J: Pulmonary microvascular cytology: A new diagnostic application of the pulmonary artery catheter. Chest 88:908, 1985.
688. Strobel SL, Keyhani-Rofagha S, O'Toole RV, et al: Nonaspiration-needle smear preparations of pulmonary lesions: A comparison of cytology and histology. Acta Cytol 29:1047, 1985.
689. Newman SL, Michel RP, Wang N-S: Lingular lung biopsy: Is it representative? Am Rev Respir Dis 132:1084, 1985.
690. Levine MN, Young JEM, Ryan ED, et al: Pleural effusion in breast cancer: Thoracoscopy for hormone receptor determination. Cancer 57:324, 1986.
691. Hampton AO, Castleman B: Correlation of postmortem chest teleroentgenograms with autopsy findings. With special reference to pulmonary embolism and infarction. Am J Roentgenol 43:305, 1940.
692. Fung JC, Sun T, Kilius I, et al: Printcultures for postmortem microbiology. Ann Clin Lab Sci 13:83, 1983.
693. McMahon JT: Analytical electron microscopy in pneumoconiosis. Cleveland Clin Q 52:503, 1985.
694. Dalquen P, Bittel D, Gudat F, et al: Combined immunoreaction and Papanicolaou's stain on cytological smears. Path Res Pract 181:50, 1986.
695. Tubbs RR: Pulmonary immunohistology. Cleveland Clin Q 52:473, 1985.
696. Stratton-Hans L, Stratton-Hans H: Methods in laboratory investigation: Applications of computerized interactive morphometry in pathology. II. A model for computer generated diagnosis. Lab Invest 54:708, 1986.
697. Bousfield LR, Greenberg ML, Pacey F: Cytogenetic diagnosis of cancer from body fluids. Acta Cytol 29:768, 1985.
698. Greengard O, Head JF, Goldberg SL, et al: Enzyme pathology and the histologic categorization of human lung tumors: The continuum of quantitative biochemical indices of neoplasticity. Cancer 49:460, 1982.

2

3

Methods in Clinical, Laboratory, and Functional Investigation

CLINICAL HISTORY

The fundamental importance of precise history-taking in arriving at the correct diagnosis becomes evident in subsequent chapters, in which the multifarious clinical conditions that can give rise to similar roentgenographic patterns are considered. With any abnormality seen roentgenographically, a logical diagnosis may be made on the information elicited by careful history-taking, findings during meticulous physical examination, and intelligently directed laboratory or pulmonary function tests. In pulmonary disease the key to solution of abnormal roentgenographic shadows most often lies in thorough awareness of the patient's complaints. In some cases, despite symptoms indicating advanced and disabling disease, the chest roentgenogram may be normal, a finding which, in itself, limits the diagnostic possibilities and excludes diseases invariably associated with an abnormal roentgenogram. The differential diagnosis of respiratory disorders with normal roentgenograms is discussed in the appropriate chapter in Volume IV.

Good history-taking is an art. It requires that the patient be at ease, confident in the doctor's ability, and prepared to divulge all pertinent details that will enable the physician to identify the cause of the malady. Of particular importance is the avoidance of an atmosphere of haste, although often the physician must patiently return a digressing patient to a discussion of pertinent information. After the initial description of complaints by the patient, the physician should elicit further details. For example, arriving at the significance of dyspnea requires more information as to its onset: was it sudden or gradual? Concerning its severity: does it occur when the patient is walking slowly in the street, or only when he or she runs upstairs? Does it require exertion to develop or occur even at rest? At what time of day is it particularly obvious? Is it made worse by lying flat? The patient's answers to these questions and to others intended to clarify other major symptoms frequently give the physician a good idea of the diagnosis by the time the history has been taken. Then any pertinent information concerning past illnesses and personal habits should be elicited. Of prime importance in lung disease is such information as to the patient's tobacco consumption, in what form and what quantity. Areas of residence and travel should be ascertained; even a brief exposure elsewhere can result in an infection or infestation that otherwise might be overlooked. Similarly, a complete and chronologic occupational history may indicate that the patient's complaints are due to exposure to a specific substance known to be an occupational hazard, or may identify a nonspecific dust or fume to which chronic cough and expectoration may be attributable. Finally, since lung disease frequently is only one manifestation of a more general process, or is secondary to a disease involving other organs, an account of the function of other body systems is essential.

The symptoms of respiratory disease are cough and expectoration, shortness of breath, chest pain, and hemoptysis. These will be considered individually and in greater detail, after which further consideration will be given to the pertinence of personal, occupational, and residential history and to disease of other organ systems commonly associated with respiratory disorders.

SYMPTOMS OF RESPIRATORY DISEASE

Cough and Expectoration

Cough is a defensive mechanism designed to rid the conducting passages of mucus and foreign material. The afferent pathways of the cough reflex are in the trigeminal, glossopharyngeal, superior laryngeal, and vagus nerves. The nerve endings in the upper respiratory tract are sensitive to contact with foreign material and to volume change in their vicinity (mechanoreceptors) and respond to sulfur dioxide and, presumably, other noxious chemical agents (chemoreceptors) in the smaller bronchi.[1, 2] Lauweryns and associates[3, 4] described neuroepithelial bodies in the tracheobronchial tree that extend distally as far as the small bronchioles and alveoli, both of which appear in electron microscopic studies to be supplied by nerves; however, the function of these bodies is thought to be purely secretory or chemoreceptive,[4] and it is generally accepted that the acinar units do not contain nerve endings for the initiation of coughing. The cough reflex is stimulated when material originating from disease in the alveoli arrives in the larger airways. The efferent pathways of the cough reflex arc lie in the recurrent laryngeal nerve, which causes closure of the glottis, and in the phrenic and spinal nerves, which effect contraction of the diaphragm and other respiratory muscles against a closed glottis. The most sensitive areas of the conducting system are in the larynx and epicarina and at the bifurcation of the major bronchi.

Cough unassociated with wheezing or dyspnea may be caused by asthma, even when routine pulmonary function tests are normal.[5] These patients can be recognized by the demonstration of hyperreactivity of their bronchi to inhalational challenge tests with histamine, methacholine, or carbachol, and by amelioration of the cough following administration of bronchodilators.[6, 7]

Cough can be precipitated by irritation of nerve endings in airway passages by foreign material or by extraluminal distortion or compression of airways that can occur within the mediastinum or lung parenchyma from interstitial edema or fibrosis. In addition, cough can result from stimulation of the parietal pleura, pericardium, stomach, or external auditory meatus.[8]

The character of a cough rarely indicates the disease process responsible. However, patients frequently describe a cough that originates from a need to "clear the throat" and that both physician and patient visualize as coming from the upper respiratory tract. These patients usually have a chronic postnasal drip, and the cough is often described as "hacking"—a short, dry, frequently repeated cough, different from the deep, "loose" cough of patients with disease of more peripheral regions, in the bronchi or lung parenchyma. Patients with tracheal lesions sometimes have a "brassy" cough, whereas a "bovine" sound has been described in association with laryngeal paralysis.

A cough may be dry or productive. An acute dry cough often develops in the early stages of virus infections involving both upper and lower respiratory tracts. A dry cough may occur in association with bronchogenic carcinoma, although the majority of these patients smoke many cigarettes and therefore have bronchitis and produce some mucoid expectoration. A dry, very irritating cough, often occurring in spasms, may be an early symptom of left-sided heart failure. A short, dry cough may be a nervous habit; this is usually recognized as such by the patient or his or her family and medical advice rarely is sought for this complaint. Psychogenic cough in children may be croupy and explosive and can be recognized by the fact that it never occurs during sleep and is not affected by antitussive drugs. Nevertheless it is wise to carry out a bronchial reactivity inhalational challenge test on such patients to exclude the possibility of asthma.[9]

Most dry coughs, if sufficiently prolonged, eventually become productive. The expectorated material is clear and mucoid when the stimulus to cough and to hypersecretion by bronchial mucous glands is viral in origin or due to foreign substances such as smoke or atmospheric pollution, but otherwise it becomes colored and purulent, with secondary bacterial infection.

The time of occurrence of the cough may be useful in determining its origin. Most people with a chronic cough complain that it is worse when they lie down at night; this is particularly true of those who have bronchiectasis or a postnasal drip from chronic sinusitis. The patient with chronic bronchitis or bronchiectasis also expectorates on arising in the morning. Spasms of coughing due to bronchial asthma or left-sided heart failure frequently occur at night and may awaken the patient. A cough in association with or shortly after ingestion of food may indicate aspiration into the tracheobronchial tree.

The character and quantity of expectorated material may suggest the diagnosis. The patient with chronic bronchitis expectorates daily in small quantities, usually mucoid material, but with "colds" this may become yellow or green and sometimes slightly blood-streaked. Saccular bronchiectasis gives rise to copious, purulent, and often blood-streaked expectoration every day. The gelatinous, "rusty" expectoration formerly associated with pneumococcal pneumonia rarely has been seen

since the advent of antibiotics, and bacterial pneumonia is now more commonly associated with thick yellow or greenish sputum. A foul or fetid odor indicates infection from fusospirochetal or anaerobic organisms, usually in cases of lung abscess. Bronchial tree casts, consisting of inspissated mucus, are seen in cases of bronchitis, spasmodic asthma, or mucoid impaction, the last often in association with hypersensitivity aspergillosis (see Chapter 6). Rarely, the mucoid material expectorated greatly exceeds the amount generally seen in productive bronchitis. In some instances this so-called bronchorrhea is a presenting symptom of bronchiolo-alveolar carcinoma,[10] and then the very quantity of material establishes the diagnosis. In many cases, however, the etiology is obscure,[11] and it may be difficult to differentiate sputum from saliva; in such circumstances analysis of the material for neuraminic acid will aid differentiation, the content of it being greater in the latter.[11]

Although a cough itself may not indicate the underlying disease process, its combination with other symptoms may be highly suggestive. If it occurs suddenly during an acute febrile episode and is associated with hoarseness, viral laryngotracheobronchitis is very likely the cause. When it is accompanied by stridor, some intrinsic or extrinsic obstruction to the upper respiratory passages is present. An associated generalized wheeze usually indicates acute bronchospasm, although rarely an endotracheal or mediastinal lesion in the region of the carina may be responsible. A persistent local wheeze during expiration often indicates an intrinsic bronchogenic lesion, such as carcinoma. A cough that develops and persists after resection for bronchogenic carcinoma does not necessarily indicate a recurrence of the neoplasm but may be secondary to exposed sutures within the bronchial stump.[12]

An alarming although rare symptom following a spasm of coughing is syncope; patients usually are of stocky build and smoke and drink heavily. Although commonly attributed to cerebral ischemia from decreased cardiac output secondary to the abrupt rise in intrathoracic pressure, syncope can occur before a decline in peripheral blood pressure and after a single cough;[13] in such situations, the electroencephalographic pattern may suggest cerebral concussion, the likely mechanism being a rapid rise in cerebrospinal fluid pressure.[665] Cough syncope has been reported to occur as a complication of whooping cough in both children[651] and adults[14] and in association with neoplastic or cerebrovascular disease.[15]

The onset of cough often is so insidious that the patient is unaware of the symptom; this is particularly common among heavy smokers, who at first may deny this symptom and then make light of it, fearful that the doctor may suggest their giving up the habit. The association of cigarette smoking and bronchitis is discussed at greater length in the sections on chronic bronchitis and emphysema (see

Chapter 11), but it may be well to emphasize here that any change in the character of a cough may indicate pulmonary malignancy, just as a change in bowel habit may be indicative of carcinoma of the lower bowel.

Hoarseness

In neonates, this symptom is usually caused by laryngomalacia or laryngeal paralysis. In children, an acute onset of hoarseness is attributable to an acute infective swelling of the larynx or to aspiration of a corrosive agent or foreign body. The infectious causes include croup (acute laryngotracheitis), usually caused by parainfluenza infection, laryngotracheobronchitis following measles, parainfluenza or respiratory syncytial virus infection, and acute epiglottitis, caused most commonly by *Haemophilus influenzae*, type B.

In adults, laryngeal disease generally does not cause upper airway obstruction. Hoarseness is the major symptom, occurring whenever a normal smooth vocal cord fails to come into firm apposition with its fellow. Sudden onset indicates infection, trauma, allergic edema, or inhalation of noxious fumes.[16] Acute laryngitis is caused by one of a variety of different viruses; patients who talk a lot, either from habit or in their occupation, may regain their normal voice only with difficulty. If the symptom persists for more than 3 weeks, the vocal cords should be examined for evidence of an intrinsic "singer's nodule," contact ulcer, granuloma, leukoplakia, or cancer.[16] The most common pulmonary cause of persistent hoarseness is unilateral abductor paralysis that results from recurrent laryngeal nerve involvement, usually from extension of a bronchogenic carcinoma into the aortopulmonary window.

Shortness of Breath

The symptom of dyspnea or awareness of breathing is caused by inappropriateness between respiratory motor neuron output and the resulting ventilation. Decreased ventilation at a given level of neural drive may relate to increased impedance of the respiratory system (increased resistance or decreased compliance) or to respiratory muscle weakness or fatigue. A more complete discussion of the mechanisms leading to dyspnea can be found in Chapter 1, page 260.

This symptom probably includes several sensations. In normal subjects made hyperpneic, the sensation experienced differed from one subject to another but remained the same in a particular individual, whether produced by breathing 7 per cent carbon dioxide, exercise, or the intravenous infusion of vanillic acid diethylamide.[17] The anxious patient "unable to take a deep breath," the patient with emphysema having difficulty in tying his or her shoelaces, and the athlete who has just run 100 yards in under 9.5 seconds are almost certainly

experiencing different types of discomfort; nevertheless, all will agree that they are short of breath. Thus, in determining the diagnosis, the physician must obtain not only a thorough description of the sensation perceived but also an account of the circumstances that tend to precipitate this sensation and its association with other symptoms.[652]

A detailed description is most useful in differentiating organic causes of shortness of breath from functional or psychoneurotic dyspnea. The latter variety, which is related to tension or anxiety, is the commonest cause of shortness of breath; it is said to occur in 10 per cent of patients of specialists in internal medicine.[18] It often is associated with various other symptoms but can occur independently. Usually it is described as an inability to take a deep breath or to get air "down to the bottom of the lungs," and patients often spontaneously demonstrate by taking a deep breath. If not, it is helpful to ask them to breathe as they do when short of breath. They will respond by taking a deep breath, and, as history-taking continues, may unconsciously repeat the sighing respirations from time to time. In dyspnea of organic cause, on the other hand, the sensation is more difficult to describe; the patients may say they are "short-winded" or "puff" and on request will demonstrate hyperpnea, breathing more deeply and perhaps more rapidly than normal.

The circumstances in which this sensation occurs should be elucidated. Patients who are short of breath at rest and not during exercise almost invariably have functional dyspnea; they may say that shortness of breath occurs when they are at home after a busy day, or while they are "sitting around doing nothing." An exception to this rule is the patient with spasmodic asthma, who may be able to indulge in strenuous exercise without shortness of breath in the intervals between periodic attacks of extreme dyspnea. On direct questioning the patient with functional dyspnea may give a history of chronic tension or of episodes of acute nervous tension precipitating this complaint, but just as frequently such an association is denied.

During pregnancy, dyspnea is physiologic[19, 20] and should cause concern only if it develops abruptly in preeclampsia, when it may be caused by pulmonary edema, or during the third trimester, when pulmonary embolism must be ruled out. Approximately 15 per cent of pregnant women complain of shortness of breath during the first trimester, 50 per cent before 19 weeks, and 76 per cent by 31 weeks of gestation; however, this symptom rarely increases in severity during the final weeks before delivery.[19] It is very likely that the complaint of dyspnea by a pregnant woman results from a combination of the hyperventilation produced by increased circulating progesterone and the elevated diaphragm.

Inability to lie flat because of a feeling of suffocation or waking during the night with shortness of breath strongly suggests organic disease. Since attacks of asthma often occur during the night, this symptom does not necessarily indicate left ventricular failure, but it should arouse suspicion and a careful physical examination should be directed toward exclusion of this possibility. Although the desire for three or four pillows under one's head while in bed commonly relates to mitral stenosis or left ventricular failure, many patients with chronic bronchitis and emphysema are more comfortable in this position, particularly when the disease is advanced or when coughing and expectoration are severe.

Shortness of breath only during exertion is strong evidence for organic disease and renders functional dyspnea unlikely. The degree of exertion necessary to provoke it and whether this sensation occurs invariably in the same circumstances should be ascertained. Most patients with established emphysema perceive little difference in the amount of exertion that produces shortness of breath from day to day; significant daily variation, invariably due to changes in the degree of spasm or bronchial secretions, is a diagnostic indication of asthma or an asthmatic form of chronic bronchitis. All varieties of chronic obstructive lung disease may deteriorate suddenly, with increasing dyspnea, in an atmosphere of smog. Some patients do not complain of undue dyspnea during exertion but state that it develops afterward, while they are at rest. Often this indicates some form of left-sided heart failure, but it may be due to a variant of chronic bronchitis or asthma in which bronchospasm or increase in bronchial secretions is precipitated by exercise.

In contrast to the patients with chronic bronchitis and emphysema, who gradually and almost imperceptibly experience more severe shortness of breath with lesser degrees of exertion, the person who has been in good health and in whom this symptom develops suddenly usually has pneumothorax. More rarely, it may represent the initial episode of bronchospasm due to allergic asthma or the first indication of mitral stenosis or acute myocardial infarction. Acute dyspnea may occur also with pneumonia or diffuse bronchiolitis, but in these conditions there are usually premonitory symptoms of fever and cough, with or without infection of the upper respiratory tract, which readily differentiates them. The sudden onset of dyspnea, often with obvious hyperpnea and tachycardia, in an ill or a postoperative patient may denote pulmonary embolism.

Of equal importance to the event that precipitates it is the relationship of dyspnea to other symptoms. In bronchitis or emphysema, dyspnea that develops during exertion is almost invariably preceded by a long history of cough and expectoration; dyspnea is perceived and gradually increases in severity, occurring with less and less exertion. In angina pectoris, shortness of breath may be so closely linked to "tightness" in the chest that patients with coronary insufficiency may have difficulty in determining which symptom limits their activity and even may be unable to differentiate one sensation from the other. In such patients this combination of symptoms is usually associated with exertion and characteristically requires immediate and complete cessation of activity—in contrast to dyspnea during exertion in patients with emphysema, which may allow continuance at a slower pace. Patients with heart disease who cannot increase their cardiac output to meet the tissues' demand for extra oxygen during exercise may experience not only shortness of breath but also weakness.[21] Dyspnea of functional or psychoneurotic origin may be associated with a great variety of symptoms. The dyspnea may be confused with weakness and fatigue, and many of these patients describe these sensations as if they were identical. Some symptoms may relate to resultant hyperventilation, and others probably are directly due to tension or anxiety. A sensation of "pins and needles" in the fingertips may be complained of, especially in situations that are likely to induce anxiety such as a visit to a crowded supermarket.[22] Normal subjects rendered hypocapneic and alkalotic through hyperventilation experienced a feeling of unreality and lightheadedness, as well as some alteration in awareness.[23] They also noted tingling and numbness of the hands, feet and circumoral area, sensations presumably due to hypocapnia, but were not bothered by precordial discomfort or sweating, symptoms often described by chronically anxious patients who complain of shortness of breath and are considered to have hyperventilation syndrome. Shortness of breath due to bronchospasm may be difficult to diagnose when patients are seen in the interval between episodes, with no signs of the disease; a diagnosis of bronchial asthma is suggested by a history of coughing, and particularly wheezing, during or after episodes of dyspnea, since these symptoms are not associated with functional disorders. Asthmatics frequently experience increased cough and dyspnea at night or in the early hours of the morning.

Chest Pain

The great majority of incidences of chest pain that require evaluation are acute in nature; however, chronic chest pain can occasionally present as a difficult and sometimes unsolvable diagnostic problem. Pain within the thorax falls into three main etiologic categories: pleural irritation, affections of the mediastinum, and abnormalities of the thoracic wall. The many and varied causes of acute chest pain have recently been the subject of an extensive review.[24]

Pleural Pain

Although disease involving the thoracic cage and its contents can give rise to multifarious pains, disease of the lung itself may progress to an advanced stage and result in death without producing even minor chest pain; this is because the lung tissue and visceral pleura lack a sensory apparatus to detect pain. The parietal pleura, on the other hand, is richly supplied with sensory nerves deriving from the intercostal nerves and the nerves to the diaphragm. The nerve endings are stimulated by inflammation and stretching of the membrane, and not, as was thought in the past, by the friction of visceral pleura against parietal pleura. Pleural pain may vary in degree, from lancinating discomfort during slight inspiratory effort to a less severe but still sharp pain that may "catch" the patient at the end of a maximal inspiration. Pleural pain often disappears or is reduced to a dull ache during expiration or breath-holding. Pressure over the intercostal muscles in the area of pain may not elicit discomfort, and when it does, the pain is mild compared to the subjective sensation. This is in contrast to chest wall pain, which is associated with a palpable zone of extreme tenderness, often localized to a very small area of muscle. Except when it involves the diaphragm, the diseased area of pleura, which often is secondary to a pulmonary parenchymal lesion, typically underlies the area in which pain is perceived. The central part of the diaphragm is innervated by the phrenic nerve, and the sensory afferent fibers enter the cervical cord mainly in the third and fourth cervical posterior nerve roots; hence, irritation of the central portion of the diaphragmatic pleura is referred to the neck and the upper part of the shoulder. The outer parts of the diaphragmatic pleura are supplied by lower intercostal nerves, which enter the thoracic cord in the seventh to twelfth dorsal posterior nerve roots; irritation of this portion of the pleura causes referred pain in the lower thorax. Pleural pain usually signifies inflammatory or malignant disease but also may accompany pneumothorax. The mechanism by which the parietal pleura is irritated in pneumothorax is not known; the pain may be made worse by deep inspiration, may have an aching quality, or may be felt simply as a tightness in the chest.

MEDIASTINAL PAIN

In contrast to pleural pain, which is fairly characteristic and originates in the parietal pleura, pain from the mediastinal area may vary in quality and be caused by various diseases. The trachea, esophagus, pericardium, aorta, thymus gland, and many lymph nodes are situated in the mediastinum, and disease involving any of these may cause pain in that region. It should be borne in mind that inflammation or neoplastic infiltration of the mediastinal compartment itself may cause discomfort locally. The quality, intensity, and radiation of the pain and the precipitating factors are important in determining the origin of the sensation. It may be felt in the retrosternal or precordial area and may radiate to the neck or arms or through to the back.

The most common retrosternal pain is that due to myocardial ischemia; this is described as "squeezing," "pressing," or "choking" and may extend to the neck or down the left arm or both arms; onset is abrupt and the pain may be associated with circulatory collapse. The severe pain due to myocardial infarction may be closely simulated in other entities; these include massive pulmonary embolism, in which the mechanism of the pain is not completely understood but is thought to result from acute pulmonary hypertension. A "squeezing" or "pressing" pain identical to that of angina pectoris may be experienced by patients with severe chronic pulmonary hypertension due to mitral stenosis or multiple small pulmonary emboli. Acute pericarditis may cause pain confusingly similar to that produced by myocardial disease; the pain often has a precordial distribution and may be made worse by breathing or swallowing and be relieved by bending forward.[25] Dissecting aneurysm of the aorta also may give rise to similar pain and should be suspected when pain is severe from the outset, instead of gradually increasing, and when it radiates to the back and down the abdomen into the lower limbs. A local aneurysm of the aorta may cause "boring" retrosternal or back pain when it erodes sternum, ribs, or vertebrae. Esophageal disease may give rise to "burning" pain and usually is clearly associated with the ingestion of food. Those who have regurgitation of acid gastric juice complain that the pain is worse when they recline and may be relieved when they stand. A common retrosternal sensation, which presumably originates in sensory nerve endings of the tracheal mucosa, is the painful rawness under the sternum experienced by patients with infection of the upper respiratory tract and dry, hacking cough.

In some instances, the etiology of acute chest pain that resembles angina pectoris and that is severe enough to warrant admission to an intensive care unit is not established. Of 89 such patients who were considered to have no evidence of myocardial infarction or ischemia on their original admission, 2 were subsequently readmitted with myocardial infarction;[26] after 1 year of follow-up, 75 per cent of the remainder were in their original employment compared with only 36 per cent of a group of patients considered to have heart disease.

CHEST WALL PAIN

Pain originating in or referred to the chest wall, not due to parietal pleural irritation, is common. When this pain appears to originate in intercostal muscle fibers there may be a history of trauma which produced strain or even tearing, but more often there is no obvious precipitating cause and the condition is labeled as myositis or fibrositis. In our experience, local pain and tenderness in chest muscle is frequently associated with acute infection of the tracheobronchial tree, accompanied by residual dry cough, often paroxysmal. In such cases tenderness may be elicited by pressure over the painful area, usually in the anterolateral lower intercostal muscles. This pain can be differentiated from true "pleural pain" by its limited or lack of increase during deep inspiration, its aggravation by coughing or trunk movement, and its persistence between paroxysms of coughing. Muscle pain not associated with the dry cough of an acute respiratory infection or with direct trauma to the intercostal muscles requires careful investigation to exclude other conditions that may cause referral of pain.

Another chest wall pain is that due to pressure or inflammation irritating the posterior nerve root. Called radicular pain, this follows the specific intercostal nerve distribution and radiates around the chest from behind or, in some cases, is localized to one area. Usually it is described as dull and aching and is made worse by movement, particularly coughing. It may be due to a protruded intervertebral disk, rheumatoid spondylitis, malignant disease involving the vertebrae, or inflammatory or malignant disease within the spinal canal. A variety of intercostal nerve root pain whose origin may be difficult to identify in the early stages, before the appearance of the typical rash, is that due to herpes zoster. The pain is usually described as "burning," most often over a wide area unilaterally along the pathway of one or more intercostal nerves.

Pain confined to vertebral and paravertebral areas may originate in inflammatory or neoplastic disease of the vertebrae, and percussion over the vertebral spines may elicit local tenderness due to disease in the underlying vertebral body. An unusual form of pain, usually in bone, is that experienced by patients with Hodgkin's disease or other neoplasms; this lasts for an hour or more after the ingestion of even small amounts of alcohol.[27]

Pain in the chest wall may be due to disease of the ribs. In addition to those of known traumatic origin, rib fractures may result from prolonged episodes of severe coughing. The costochondral junctions of the ribs may be the site of perichondritis, often associated with tenderness and swelling (Tietze's syndrome); usually the pain is persistent and described as "gnawing" or "aching." The ribs may be involved in a metastatic process or multiple myeloma and rarely by a primary tumor such as a fibrosarcoma; the pain usually is appreciated before the mass develops, at first poorly localized but later as a dull, boring ache over the area of invasion.

A benign transitory pain of undetermined origin has been described by the name "precordial catch."[28] Probably this syndrome of anterior chest pain is familiar to most practicing physicians because of personal experience of the sensation.[29] It is a severe, sharp pain, occurring at rest or during mild activity over the left side of the chest, usually at the cardiac apex, and lasting from 30 sec to 5 min.[25] It comes on suddenly during inspiration, and the invariable reaction is a brief suspension of respiration; then breathing is maintained at a shallow level while the pain disappears gradually. Its onset often is associated with poor posture, improvement in which sometimes relieves the pain. The mechanism is unknown, the condition is very common, and its importance lies solely in its differentiation from other chest pain of more serious consequence.

Hemoptysis

This is often a presenting complaint in an otherwise asymptomatic patient, who is understandably alarmed and who regards this finding as indicative of serious disease. The physician should do likewise and should never reassure and then dismiss the patient, since every patient who complains of an initial episode of hemoptysis should have at least a chest roentgenogram; many require extensive investigation.

The source of bleeding may be from the upper respiratory tract. The patient may have a nosebleed, with some blood trickling into the pharynx and causing coughing and expectoration. The pharynx itself may bleed because of its involvement in an ulcerative process. Bleeding from these sites usually can be distinguished clinically from hemoptysis originating in the lower respiratory tract. When there is doubt as to the source of bleeding, the patient should be assumed to have lung disease and should be examined accordingly. Patients with a history of acute or chronic bronchitis sometimes expectorate blood-streaked sputum, but it must not be forgotten that even a trace of blood in the sputum may be the first indication of bronchogenic carcinoma. Bleeding is a common complaint of patients with carcinoid tumor. In bronchiectasis, bloody expectoration may be the only symptom; usually it is abundant and originates in granulation tissue. Less frequent causes of bleeding from the bronchial tree are the erosion of broncholiths through the wall of the bronchus and dilatation of bronchial veins in association with mitral stenosis. Rarely, a dramatic, exsanguinating hemoptysis results from rupture of an aortic aneurysm into a bronchus.

Bleeding from the lung itself may be due to a local lesion, such as pulmonary infarction, pneumonia, lung abscesses and cysts, and various granulomata, including tuberculosis, mycotic infections, and Wegener's granuloma. Although systemic disorders with a bleeding tendency are rarely if ever manifested by isolated bleeding from the lower respiratory tract, they may give rise to severe hemoptysis accompanied by bleeding into other viscera and the skin, or the bleeding may be massive and confined to the lungs without associated expectoration of blood.[30] The possibility of pulmonary or bronchial lesions as a source of bleeding should be investigated when patients on anticoagulant therapy cough up blood. A few patients who complain of blood "welling up" in the throat have hematemesis from esophageal varices, a possibility that should not be overlooked, particularly when bleeding is brisk and the blood is dark.

Although the amount of hemoptysis is of little value in establishing the diagnosis, the character of the bloody sputum may suggest the underlying disease process. As already mentioned, simple streaking of mucoid material can occur in bronchitis, but may denote a more serious condition such as tuberculosis or bronchogenic carcinoma. When the sputum is frankly bloody and does not contain mucoid or purulent material it is more likely due to pulmonary infarction than to pneumonia, particularly if it persists unchanged for several days. Bloody material mixed with pus should suggest pneumonia or lung abscess in acute illness and bronchiectasis in chronic disease. When the blood is diluted, giving it a pink and sometimes frothy appearance, pulmonary edema from left heart failure should be suspected.

Any attempt to determine the major causes of hemoptysis from a review of the literature is unlikely to lead to any valid statistical conclusion. There appears to be a general lack of agreement as to the definition of the term; for example, many recorders would not include simple blood streaking under this designation. If patients with chronic bronchitis with blood-streaked sputum are included, bronchitis and bronchiectasis are the commonest causes when a specific diagnosis can be made;[31-33] this applies in Western countries, in which the diagnosis is established in approximately 50 per cent of patients with hemoptysis—obviously, the major causes depend to a great extent on the degree of control of pulmonary tuberculosis and, in certain areas, of the lung fluke *Paragonimus westermani*. In Western Europe and North America, bronchogenic carcinoma is said to be responsible for hemoptysis in 5 to 10 per cent of cases.[31-33] Bronchiectasis associated with inactive tuberculosis of the upper lobes has been reported to be a commoner cause than active tuberculosis,[32] and this has been our experience.

Factitious or simulated hemoptysis is rare but should not be overlooked as a possible explanation for sudden and dramatic episodes of apparent bleeding. A "profile" has been described for potential perpetrators of this form of Munchausen syndrome; a neurotic and aggressive young woman with a history of multiple previous hospital admissions and procedures, and with medical knowledge obtained through family contacts or as a result of paramedical employment.[34, 35]

When the physician is informed that a patient has coughed up blood, two main decisions are required: (1) If the hemoptysis is small in amount, how much investigation is necessary? and (2) if the hemoptysis is massive, how should it be managed?

In any circumstance, minor hemoptysis is an indication for a chest roentgenogram and acid-fast cultures. If the patient is a nonsmoker and no findings on the chest roentgenogram suggest a neoplasm, bronchoscopy is not required. If hemoptysis recurs at regular intervals despite antibiotic therapy for presumed endobronchial infection, direct vision of the airways is indicated. In an attempt to form guidelines for bronchoscopic intervention, Weaver and associates[36] concluded that in three groups of patients it was not required: (1) those with a strong clinical history of a non-neoplastic disease process that can explain the bleeding (e.g., bronchiectasis); (2) those with a demonstrated site of extrapulmonary bleeding; and (3) those whose clinical status is so poor that no action would be taken regardless of the bronchoscopic findings.

A somewhat more controversial recommendation made by the same group of investigators was to forego bronchoscopy in patients under 40 years of age whose chest roentgenogram was normal and whose hemoptysis did not last for more than 1 week. In reaction to this last recommendation, two editorials[37, 38] emphasized the point that a normal chest roentgenogram does not exclude central bronchogenic carcinoma, a fact that is borne out by our own experience and by that of others.[39–41] However, no published data indicate the incidence of pulmonary carcinoma in patients less than 40 years of age who have hemoptysis lasting less than 1 week and a normal chest roentgenogram (we suspect that the figure is very low). In contrast to the rigid bronchoscopy advisable in patients who are actively and copiously bleeding, those with mild hemoptysis and those who have stopped bleeding should undergo flexible fiberoptic bronchoscopy. Using FFB during active but relatively minor bleeding, one group of investigators localized the segment from which the blood was coming in 93 per cent of 71 patients.[42] In another study of 129 patients,[43] the clinical efficacy of early and delayed FFB was compared; although the bleeding site was identified considerably more often in the former group, it was concluded that the difference was neither diagnostically nor therapeutically decisive. It has been shown that the prognosis for patients with hemoptysis and normal chest roentgenograms and FFB is very good; in the majority of cases the hemoptysis ceases within 6 months with no serious cause detected.[653, 654]

An area of great confusion and controversy in pulmonary medicine concerns "massive" or "major" hemoptysis. The amount of bleeding required for classification into this category is by no means agreed upon, and the management is equally controversial despite dogmatic opinions from various investigators. Occasionally, patients die from asphyxiation or exsanguination as a result of massive intrabronchial and intrapulmonary hemorrhage; although we appear to have the means at our disposal to prevent such catastrophes, unfortunately it is difficult to identify the likely victims. One body of opinion holds that patients who are admitted to hospitals with copious hemoptysis are in danger of dying unless drastic measures such as pulmonary resection or bronchial artery embolization are carried out as quickly as possible, but there is no certainty of this. On the other hand, patients with minor degrees of hemoptysis are not necessarily immune from sudden massive hemorrhage. In one review,[44] the unpredictability of massive hemoptysis was emphasized: of 123 cases, 8 deaths occurred from sudden catastrophic hemorrhage in seemingly stable patients awaiting endoscopy or surgery. Nevertheless, we agree with what appears to be a general consensus in the literature that patients with copious bleeding on admission are at greater risk from asphyxiation or exsanguination than are those with mild hemorrhage. From a review of their 10 year experience in the surgical management of patients with massive hemoptysis, Garzon and Gourin found that those who survived surgery had expectorated about half the amount of blood preoperatively as had those who died.[45]

But what is massive hemoptysis? If we are to accept the proposition that the expectoration of a specific quantity of blood leaves a patient in jeopardy, we must come to some reasonable conclusion as to how much that is. Crocco and associates[46] found a mortality rate of 37 per cent among patients who lost 600 ml of blood within a period of 48 hours, figures that are perhaps the most quoted in the literature.[47] Others define massive hemoptysis as the expectoration of 600 ml within 24 hours,[44, 45, 48] more than 500 ml in a single expectoration, or more than 1000 ml in smaller increments over a period of several days.[49] One group of workers differentiates between massive and exsanguinating hemoptysis, the latter being the loss of 1000 ml at a rate of 150 ml or more per hour.[50]

The underlying diseases responsible for copious hemoptysis appear to be the same in several large series reported in the literature. Those most frequently cited are bronchiectasis, tuberculosis (either active or inactive), mycetoma, lung abscess, pulmonary carcinoma, broncholith, and A-V aneurysm.[44, 45, 47, 51–54, 655] Iatrogenic causes are infrequent, the most common being in association with the use of the Swan-Ganz catheter.[55–57]

A review of the surgical literature suggests that all doubts about how to manage the patient with "massive" hemoptysis have been eliminated. For stable patients with adequate breathing reserve, surgical resection is recommended after the site of bleeding has been identified by rigid bronchoscopy.[46, 47, 58] For patients whose physical status is less than optimum but who nevertheless are capable of undergoing subsequent resectional surgery, temporary measures are recommended, including lavage with cold saline,[44, 48] Fogarty catheterization of the appropriate bronchus, and bronchial artery embolization.[45, 49–51, 59–65] Careful scrutiny of these studies suggests that surgical authorities have a tendency to relegate to the "control" or medically managed group those patients who exsanguinate suddenly prior to management decision and those who are considered inoperable. Unfortunately, few control

studies exist; as has been pointed out, "in evaluating the merits of surgical versus medical treatment of hemoptysis, it is important to compare only patients who are operable and in whom there was a choice between surgical and medical treatment."[66] It has been our experience that the majority of patients with serious hemoptysis can be managed conservatively, an opinion that is suported by a number of reported surveys.[53, 66–68] In a review of their experience with 728 patients with cystic fibrosis, Stern and coworkers identified 38 (5 per cent) with massive hemoptysis (defined as more than 300 ml in 24 hours), all of whom stopped bleeding without surgical intervention; antibiotics and blood transfusions were administered when indicated.[68]

In conclusion, it is perhaps appropriate to propose certain guidelines for the management of patients with copious hemoptysis, even in a book concerned primarily with diagnosis. Three main groups can be recognized.

1. Patients who are actively bleeding and who have expectorated an amount of blood estimated to be more than 1000 ml should have bronchoscopy immediately, preferably with a rigid scope. The bleeding site should be identified and the appropriate bronchus occluded with a Fogarty catheter or washed with cold saline. If the chest roentgenogram has revealed a cavity containing a mycetoma or one whose appearance is compatible with a Rasmussen's aneurysm (tuberculosis cavity), surgical resection should be performed following blood replacement.

2. With lesser amounts of hemoptysis (estimated at between 500 and 1000 ml), it is probably preferable to carry out bronchoscopy and to occlude the bronchus leading to the site of bleeding; this should be followed by a period of watchful waiting, with immediate availability of cross-matched blood.

3. When the quantity of blood expectorated is judged to be less than 500 ml, conservative management with subsequent bronchoscopy is indicated; however, if bleeding continues in appreciable amounts over a 4 day period, and assuming that the site is known, consideration should be given to surgical resection.

It is our opinion that the efficacy of bronchial artery embolization has now been proved conclusively.

Miscellaneous Symptoms

Fever should suggest pneumonia, particularly when the chest roentgenogram reveals an air space or segmental opacity; if the fever is accompanied by a teeth-chattering chill, the pneumonia is likely pneumococcal in origin. Fever can also occur with malignancies, especially lymphomas and related diseases, and pulmonary infarction. As with hemoptysis, fever may be factitious, in which circumstance it tends to occur as one of the causes of fever of unknown origin in paramedical employees with psychiatric problems.[69]

Confusion, irrationality, and even *coma* can occur as a result of underlying pulmonary disease, particularly in the elderly; these signs are usually associated with hypoxemia or hypercapnia and often with impairment of cerebral circulation. When they develop abruptly, a number of precipitating disease processes should be considered, including pneumonia, thrombotic or fat embolism, and hypercalcemia secondary to squamous cell carcinoma. In such a clinical setting, it is important to rule out infectious or metastatic lesions of the meninges or cerebrum.

Halitosis is multifactorial in origin[70] and is most commonly caused by some disorder of the oral cavity; however, it can be a major clue to the presence of an anaerobic infection in the oropharynx or in the lung itself.

PAST ILLNESSES AND PERSONAL HISTORY

Establishing the correct diagnosis may depend upon a knowledge of the patient's medical history or personal habits: the respiratory symptoms or abnormal chest roentgenogram simply may represent previous active lung disease that has left its imprint on the pulmonary parenchyma, or a lung lesion may be a belated metastasis from a primary malignancy elsewhere that was removed many years earlier. A patient's memory should be jogged for recall of dates and places of previous chest roentgenograms, and these should be obtained for comparison with the present one. Patients should be questioned about medication: many acute and chronic bacterial and mycotic infections occur in patients on long-term antibiotic and corticosteroid therapy, and lipoid pneumonia may follow the use of nose drops or laxatives containing mineral oil. Respiratory failure may be wholly or partly attributable to recent sedation. A patient's cigarette consumption may be of significance in suspected cases of bronchogenic carcinoma or bronchitis and emphysema. As with corticosteroid therapy, poor diet and heavy alcohol intake may play a major part in lowering resistance to infection; this statement is supported by clinical evidence, and experimental work[71] indicates that all three of these factors, as well as hypoxia, appear to inhibit clearing of bacteria from the normally sterile lower respiratory tract. The personal history is not complete without inquiry about contact with animals, domestic and wild. This pertains not only to the patient with allergies, whose bronchospasm may be due to a household pet, but also, for example, to the patient with an acute pneumonic lesion who may have contracted ornithosis from a sick bird in his or her home, tularemia from skinning a wild rabbit, or Q fever from inhalation of dust contaminated by sheep or cattle.

Family History

In pulmonary disease, this aspect is most important in relation to a potential source of infection. Tuberculosis remains the most serious of the pulmonary diseases that spread in the home, but many acute viral and mycoplasma infections may be disseminated throughout a household, and a recent occurrence may be significant in the investigation of patients with acute pneumonitis.

Some pulmonary diseases have a familial incidence, presumably on a genetic basis. They include cystic fibrosis, some forms of pulmonary emphysema,[72–74] a hereditary form of fibrosing alveolitis (familial fibrocystic pulmonary dysplasia), hereditary telangiectasia, ciliary dyskinesia (immotile ciliary syndrome), pulmonary myomatosis, and alveolar microlithiasis. Most of these diseases are rare and may be recognized only when a familial incidence is revealed. They are considered in greater detail in other chapters.

Occupational and Residential History

A complete occupational history from the time of first employment is essential when the chest roentgenogram reveals diffuse pulmonary disease. Although silicosis remains the commonest pneumoconiosis, an ever-growing list of pulmonary diseases due to occupational exposure must be kept in mind. In addition to the pneumoconioses that cause diffuse granulomatous and fibrotic parenchymal disease, exposure to various chemical fumes, such as high concentrations of sulfur dioxide, may result in severe bronchial damage, and the fumes and dust present in many occupations may elicit severe, although in some cases reversible, bronchitis and bronchospasm. Farmers appear to be particularly liable to occupational lung disease; exposure to moldy hay may cause severe bronchospasm and result in diffuse pulmonary granulomata, a disease known as "farmer's lung." Droppings from wild[75, 76] and domestic birds provide a favorable nitrogenous substrate for the growth of fungi, particularly *Histoplasma capsulatum*, to which workers on poultry farms may be heavily exposed. High concentrations of the nitrogen dioxide in fresh silage may cause severe bronchiolitis, pulmonary edema, and bronchiolitis fibrosa obliterans; this condition is known as "silo-filler's disease." Residence in an area of heavy atmospheric pollution may lead to the development of disease. Pollution, mainly from industry, not only can have a nonspecific irritating effect on patients with asthma and chronic obstructive pulmonary disease but also can sensitize the airways and induce a bronchospastic state. Industrial air may contain inorganic compounds, such as asbestos and beryllium, which are known to cause granuloma and fibrosis and even mesothelioma in patients who live in the vicinity of mines and industrial plants where these substances are used.

A history of residence in, and even travel

through, an area where coccidioidomycosis or histoplasmosis is endemic may be pertinent, and parasitic diseases should be suspected in emigrants from areas in which they are endemic. Patients who have resided recently in India and who have bronchospasm, severe leukocytosis, and eosinophilia very likely have tropical eosinophilia, caused by a filarial parasite. A pulmonary mass in a young farmer from Greece or Italy may well be a hydatid cyst. Chronic cor pulmonale in an Egyptian suggests the possibility of schistosomiasis. The patient from central China who has chronic hemoptysis may have paragonimiasis and not tuberculosis.

Systemic Inquiry

Since lung involvement may be only one manifestation of a general disease process, inquiry concerning all body systems may prove revealing. In some instances, the mere fact that certain other organs or tissues are involved may suggest the diagnosis; for instance, the patient with diffuse lung disease who has Raynaud's phenomenon and difficulty in swallowing almost certainly has scleroderma, and multiple lung cavities in association with severe nasal trouble and hematuria undoubtedly represent Wegener's disease. Systemic inquiry may reveal symptoms indicating a primary site for multiple discrete nodules in the lung which had been suspected of being metastatic deposits. Bronchogenic small cell carcinoma may be associated with abnormality in almost any organ or tissue, and symptoms of the extrapulmonary manifestations of this unusual neoplasm can be elicited by systemic inquiry. Similarly, a diagnosis of chronic pulmonary insufficiency and respiratory failure may be made after eliciting a history of headache, confusion, tremor, twitching, or somnolence,[77, 78] and can be confirmed by determination of the PCO_2 of the arterial blood.

PHYSICAL EXAMINATION

The diagnosis of chest disease requires competence in examination of the chest. The physician who does not become proficient in this art and who makes judgments regarding underlying pathology purely on the basis of roentgenologic findings inevitably is guilty of diagnostic errors and sloppy management. The roentgenogram has not replaced the physician's eyes, ears, and hands; rather, it is an additional, valuable diagnostic method, complementary to the technique of physical examination, providing information the latter cannot give.

The present-day student is fortunate in having roentgenography and pulmonary function tests as indispensable aids in perfecting his technique in physical examination. Only when students have become skilled in this method can they judge how thorough the examination of any specific patient should be. Circumstances will arise in which they will have to depend upon their senses to make decisions concerning therapy that may fundamentally affect the patient's life; this may occur in the home, where roentgenography is unavailable, or even in the hospital when the patient is too sick to be moved or circumstances dictate an immediate decision such as the removal of air in the case of tension pneumothorax.

Physical signs are judged to be abnormal on the basis of deviation from norms determined through the examination of many patients with healthy lungs, and the quality of the changes indicates the underlying pathologic process. Roentgenology also attempts to define pathology by a deviation from accepted normal standards, through interpretation of patterns of decreased or increased density. The chest roentgenogram may be interpreted as being normal when there is serious and advanced pulmonary disease detectable only by physical examination; conversely, roentgenography may reveal severe abnormality when physical findings are normal.

METHOD OF EXAMINATION AND SIGNIFICANT CHEST SIGNS

The front of the thorax is best examined when the patient is supine, and the back in the sitting or standing position; patients who are too weak to sit upright unaided should be supported by someone standing at the foot of the bed and holding their hands. When this is impossible because of extreme weakness or serious illness, the patient should lie on the right side and then roll over on the left side, the uppermost hemithorax being examined in turn. It is important to keep in mind always that examination of the chest is a comparative exercise. Each region of one side is compared with the same area on the other side; this rule applies equally for inspection, palpation, percussion, and auscultation.

Inspection

Inspection of the patient is well under way by the time the physical examination has begun. Throughout history-taking the physician has had ample opportunity to note the character of a cough, the presence or absence of hyperpnea, sighing respirations, or grimaces of pain accompanying cough or respiration. In the examining room the thoracic cage is inspected for evidence of deformity and the skin for its color and evidence of collateral venous circulation. Chest movement is observed and the rate of respiration is noted. The respiratory rate can be a valuable early indicator of respiratory dysfunction. Its usefulness as a screening method for detecting lower respiratory infection has recently been demonstrated in the postoperative period[79] and in geriatric patients.[80] Estimating the depth of respiration is a notoriously difficult clinical judgment, particularly in patients who have predominantly diaphragmatic breathing. A local lag during inspiration may not be obvious during quiet breathing, and for this reason the patient should be asked to take a deep breath and the movements of the chest cage on the two sides should be compared.

Of even greater importance than establishing asynchrony between the two hemithoraces is the assessment of respiratory muscle function. In Chapter 1, we have already described abdominal motion and its pertinence to diaphragmatic contraction (see page 269). In physical examination of the respiratory system, the most important aspect of inspection is undoubtedly observation of the patient in the supine position to determine the relative contribution of diaphragmatic and intercostal muscle function. Indrawing of the abdominal wall on inspiration, or cyclic preponderance of abdominal and thoracic movement, suggests paralysis or fatigue of the diaphragm and constitutes a clear indication of the cause of dyspnea or of impending ventilatory failure. Some patients with severe COPD may manifest two patterns of breathing: slow deep breathing (being more obvious while the patient is awake) alternating with rapid shallow breathing (typically occurring during sleep).[81]

A lag during inspiration or an area of diminished movement seen or felt and involving all or part of a hemithorax may be the only physical sign indicating disease of the lung or pleura. It indicates loss of elasticity of the underlying tissues, or compensatory spasm of intercostal and disphragmatic musculature in the vicinity to avoid pain on movement. This sign is present in acute disease such as atelectasis, pneumonia, or pleurisy; or it may indicate a long-standing chronic or inactive fibrotic process of the lung or pleura, and then often is associated with scoliosis of the dorsal spine, with the concavity to the diseased side. When the loss of volume is considerable, whether due to an acute or chronic lesion, there may be a shift of the mediastinum; this is detectable as displacement of the apical cardiac impulse and the trachea toward the involved side. With fibrosis, and particularly with atelectasis, the lower intercostal spaces may be abnormally sucked in during inspiration.

Palpation

A suspected lag detected on inspection of the chest may be confirmed when a hand is placed on each hemithorax while the patient breathes deeply. The relative contribution of the respiratory muscles can also be assessed by palpation of the abdominal, intercostal, and accessory muscles during inspiration. The apical cardiac impulse and the trachea should be palpated, a shift from normal position indicating loss of volume or a relative increase in volume of one hemithorax in comparison with the other. The left parasternal region should be palpated to determine whether a heave is present, denoting right ventricular hypertrophy. The intercostal spaces and ribs should be palpated for tumor masses and to elicit any tenderness to pressure. The axillae and the cervical region should be explored carefully to detect enlarged lymph nodes.

Percussion

The chest wall is then percussed, once again comparing identical areas on the two sides. Since the degree of resonance is influenced by the thickness of the chest wall and the volume of lung underlying the percussion finger, "normal" percussion differs not only from patient to patient but also from area to area in the same patient. The percussion note in disease and in health may vary from tympanitic (over the stomach gas bubble) to flat (over the liver), sounds readily detectable by even the inexperienced; between these extremes are degrees of hyperresonance and dullness whose significance can be evaluated only with experience. The percussion note is produced by vibration of the percussed finger and sympathetic vibrations of the chest wall and underlying tissues and organs. The quality of the note is composed of its loudness, pitch, and timbre. The amplitude of vibrations (loudness) is much less over solid organs, such as the heart and liver, than over healthy lung, which, because of its elasticity, vibrates more. The loudness also depends upon the force of the stroke and the thickness of the chest wall. An accumulation of fluid between the percussed finger and underlying lung reduces intensity or loudness. Resonance elicited by percussion over healthy aerated lung is distinguishable from the dull note obtained over a solid organ by the rapidity of vibrations (pitch) and by overtones superimposed on the basic note (timbre); the resonant note has a lower pitch and more overtones. The difference between the normal, resonant note and the tympanitic note—as is heard on percussion over gas in the stomach—is due largely to difference in timbre.

In the presence of lung disease the percussion note varies from the impaired resonance heard over an area of pneumonia that is partially consolidated, to the dullness over a completely consolidated or collapsed segment or lobe, and to the extreme dullness or flatness that indicates a large accumulation of pleural fluid. At the other end of the scale, the note is hyperresonant in cases of emphysema and pneumothorax and sometimes is tympanitic over large superficial cavities or pneumothorax. An unusual form, known as "skodaic resonance," is heard sometimes over a partly compressed upper lung region when the lower portion is collapsed by pleural effusion; the note has a "boxy" quality and the mechanism of its production is unknown.

Guarino[82] has described the technique "auscultatory percussion of the chest" that he asserts permits identification of parenchymal lesions of less than 2 cm in diameter. This is done by auscultating the chest posteriorly while gently percussing the manubrium, comparing one side with the other. Limited experience with this technique has not convinced us of its dependability or of its necessity in view of the ready availability and accuracy of chest roentgenography.

Before turning from percussion to a consideration of auscultatory findings, it should be stressed that the lung tissue assessed by the percussing finger is only the superficial 5 cm. No matter how much force is used in this method of examination, the central portion of the lung remains "silent." Also, the differences in note are perceived not only by the ears but also by touch; over solid tissue the examining fingers appreciate a difference in vibration as well as a sensation of resistance that can be distinguished from the elasticity felt over air-containing areas.

Auscultation

Auscultation of the lungs is best performed with a stethoscope with small internal volume and small end piece–skin contact.[83] The quality and intensity of the breath sounds, as well as the presence or absence of adventitious noises, are ascertained by listening while the patient breathes quietly and then deeply, with the bell or diaphragm held firmly against the chest. The quality of breath sounds varies from region to region, even in normal subjects, depending upon the proximity of larger bronchi to the chest wall. In the axillae or at the lung bases a vesicular sound is heard during inspiration and often early in expiration that has been likened to the rustle of wind in the trees. The sound of air flow has a somewhat different quality over the trachea and upper retrosternal area; the pitch is higher, and expiration is clearly audible and lasts longer than the inspiratory phase. Between the scapulae and anteriorly under the clavicles, particularly on the right side, the breath sounds assume characteristics of both vesicular and bronchial air flow and are described as bronchovesicular.

The intensity of "air entry" of breath sounds should be appraised. Again, this depends upon the thickness of the chest wall and the region of the lung examined, as well as upon the depth of respiration. Recent renewed interest in the technique of phonopneumography has confirmed some clinical assumptions concerning the intensity of breath sounds.[84–90] This technique employs magnetic tape to record breath sounds; the phase of respiration and air flow velocity are correlated by a pneumotachygraph signal. Using phonopneumography to analyze breath sounds in normal subjects with controlled lung volume and air flow, LeBlanc and his colleagues[84] could detect gravity-related unevenness of regional pulmonary ventilation, as has been demonstrated with radioactive xenon.[91, 92] When a subject sitting erect inspires from residual volume, air first enters the uppermost part of the lungs, so that in apical zones the maximal intensity of breath sounds occurs at low lung volumes and is synchronous with maximal air flow. By contrast, over the lung bases the intensity is maximal somewhat later

in the inspiratory cycle, at approximately 30 to 50 per cent of vital capacity, again associated with maximal air flow. Thus, the study of LeBlanc and coworkers validates use of the term "air entry" to describe regional pulmonary ventilation, since it relates air entry to the intensity of breath sounds. In patients with emphysema, others[93, 94] have compared the intensity of breath sounds heard through a stethoscope with regional ventilation of the lungs estimated by radioactive xenon. They found a good correlation between weak and absent breath sounds and poor ventilation.

The mechanism of production of breath sounds is not thoroughly understood. Forgacs and colleagues,[95] who measured the intensity of breath sounds at the mouth while eliminating such adventitious sounds as wheezing and stridor, found that the sound of breathing is generated by turbulent flow in the upper respiratory tract; when turbulent flow was reduced by the inspiration of helium, breath sounds were eradicated. These investigators also showed that reduction in bronchial caliber, as in asthma, increases turbulence by increasing flow velocity, thus augmenting the intensity of the inspiratory sound. Auscultation over the glottis normally reveals a high-pitched noise during inspiration, followed by a pause and then by a higher-pitched, louder, longer expiration. This sound, which is heard very well over the trachea, is modified slightly in the bronchial tubes, in which expiration becomes even more high-pitched. However, at the periphery of the lung the character of the sound is radically changed: inspiration is louder than expiration, which is short and may not even be heard.[85] There is no pause between inspiration and expiration, and the sound has a soft, rustling quality known as "vesicular breathing." This alteration in the noise caused by turbulence in the larger airways is believed to be caused by both a dampening effect of the spongy lung tissue and the entry of air from thousands of narrow terminal bronchioles into acinar units.[84] Coope likened the additive effect of all these tiny murmurs to "the murmuring of innumerable bees" when a single bee at a distance may not be heard.[96]

The exact mechanism of production of breath sounds is still controversial. Kraman[97] has recorded the peripheral vesicular sound in normal volunteers during quiet breathing; the volunteers then produced a laryngeal sound that was not picked up at the periphery. He concluded that the vesicular inspiratory sound is produced by turbulence in airways larger than 2 mm but probably excluding the main stem bronchi and trachea; by contrast, the expiratory sound partly originates from the main stem bronchi and trachea but not the glottis.

Many factors may contribute to reduction or complete abolition of vesicular breathing. It may be difficult to hear breath sounds during shallow breathing due to weakness or neuromuscular disease. Diminished air entry, due to complete obstruction of a lobar or segmental bronchus or reduction in compliance resulting from edema or fibrosis of interstitial tissue, respectively, may eliminate or diminish the vesicular murmur. Complete destruction of acinar units, as in chronic obstructive emphysema, may result in very faint air entry. The transmission of breath sounds may be interrupted by an excess of subcutaneous fat or may be completely suppressed by fluid or air in the pleural cavity.

The quality of breath sounds changes from vesicular to bronchovesicular or bronchial when underlying parenchyma partly or completely loses its air content; this occurs in pneumonia and in "nonobstructive" atelectasis. Consolidated or airless lung tissue is an excellent conductor of high-pitched, prolonged expiratory sounds that emanate from adjacent bronchi. Occasionally, when the lung is consolidated, a cavity serves as a resonating chamber; breaths have a hollow, reverberating, low-pitched quality known as "cavernous." Another modification of the noise of bronchial air flow is "amphoric" breathing, when there is a tense pneumothorax over a collapsed lung, usually with an open bronchopleural fistula; this sound is high-pitched and metallic.

The voice sounds may provide clues to pathologic changes. Normally, soft, confused, barely audible sound is heard over lung distant from large bronchi. In the presence of consolidation or nonobstructive atelectasis, voice sounds become more distinct and produce a noise known as "bronchophony"; in many cases of consolidation the words are distinctly audible over the involved area when the patient whispers "ninety-nine"; this "whispering pectoriloquy" is a useful confirmatory sign of pneumonic consolidation. In some cases, when large accumulations of fluid compress the lower portion of the lung the voice sounds have a nasal quality over the upper lung (analogous to skodaic resonance on percussion).

Unfortunately, the terminology of adventitious sounds is not standard, and it almost appears that every doctor has his or her own classification. The student is further confused by the imaginative physician who introduces subjective and fanciful terms of no benefit in teaching the art of physical examination. "Rale" is derived from "death rattle," a coarse, discontinuous, bubbling sound that emanates from the trachea and large bronchi of dying patients who are too weak to cough. Laennec[98] considered the words "rale" and "rhonchus" synonymous; the lack of distinction has resulted in considerable confusion, since the Latin word "rhonchus" translates in English to "wheeze," a descriptive term more appropriate to describe the continuous noise caused by partial obstruction of bronchial tubes. Subsequent writers attempted to resolve this confusion by subdividing the adventitious sounds of air passing in and out of the bronchi and alveoli into rhonchi (continuous noises) and crepitations (discontinuous noises).[99] This has not met with general acceptance, and most physicians reserve the term crepitations for the very fine, discontinuous noises believed to represent the separation of sticky, moist surfaces as air enters the acinar unit or the actual penetration of air into alveolar spaces containing edema or exudate. Particularly confusing is the term "dry rales," which may be used synonymously with rhonchi (continuous noises), in contradistinction to "moist rales" (discontinuous noises). We use a terminology that is descriptive and simple and probably is the most widely accepted by present-day physicians (Table 3–1).

Adventitious sounds are divided into those having their origin in the bronchopulmonary tree and those indicating disease of the pleura. *Rales* (synonym: crackles[99, 100]) are discontinuous noises, which may be fine (usually at the end of inspiration, as air enters the acinar unit), medium (often during both inspiration and expiration, as air flows by an excess of fluid in the smaller bronchi), and coarse (the low-pitched, bubbling sounds that result from the accumulation of secretions in larger bronchi and the trachea). Rales are present more often during inspiration, when air flow is faster. They may be elicited during a rapid, deep breath, or—particularly when they are fine—during a deep breath after maximal expiration ended by a cough (posttussive rales). Fine rales are sometimes detected at the lung bases at the end of a deep inspiration, even in normal subjects; such individuals are likely to be

Table 3–1. A Classification of Adventitious Lung Sounds Widely Used

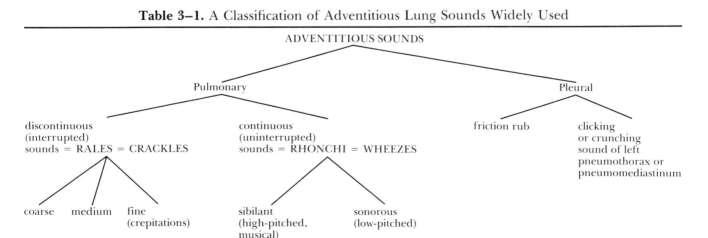

obese. In healthy volunteers, these crackles can be heard and recorded anteriorly at the lung bases near the end of a slow inspiration from residual volume;[101–103] they are believed to represent the inflation of atelectatic acini[101] or the opening of collapsed basilar bronchioles.[103] Fine rales, however, are usually persistent and multiple and often occur in showers; they indicate pulmonary edema or the alveolar exudate of pneumonia. They may be modified in the proximity of a cavity or pneumothorax; these act as resonating chambers and alter the timbre. In cases of diffuse interstitial disease associated with general loss of lung volume, they have a high-pitched superficial quality; they do not disappear on coughing and may represent the passage of air into innumerable atelectatic units, the resulting sound being intensified by adjacent airless pulmonary parenchyma. Reproducing breath sounds and adventitious sounds visually, Weiss and Carlson[87] clearly showed different patterns of crepitations in cases of pulmonary fibrosis and pulmonary edema. The patterns were finer and more regularly distributed throughout inspiration in pulmonary fibrosis. Mori and coworkers[104] separate the waveform of crackles into two segments—a starting segment, in which the sound is determined by the pressure ratio at the site of the airway opening, and a decay segment, which they speculate is modified by the resonant frequency and the quality factor of the lung as a resonator. Medium and coarse rales are heard as edema fluid or exudate moves up the bronchial tree and may be audible in patients with bronchopneumonia, bronchiectasis, or chronic granulomatous diseases such as tuberculosis or the mycoses.

Other adventitious sounds that originate in the bronchopulmonary tree are the high-pitched (sibilant) and low-pitched (sonorous) continuous noises that should be called *rhonchi*. These indicate partial obstruction in the bronchial lumen by thick mucus, edema, spasm, or a local lesion of the bronchial wall. They are louder during expiration when the bronchial passages are narrower but may be heard in both phases. A wheeze is the sound of a rhonchus heard at a distance without the aid of a stethoscope or which the patient himself can detect. Local wheezing appreciated as such by the patient or a local rhonchus audible with the stethoscope that does not disappear with coughing may indicate organic obstruction by neoplasm. The term "wheezing respirations" is used sometimes to denote the persistent inspiratory and expiratory rhonchi, usually of the musical, sibilant variety, heard all over the chest during bronchospasm. That wheezing in patients with chronic airflow obstruction indicates bronchospasm has been shown in a comparative bronchodilator study of those with and without wheezing:[105] only the former showed a positive response. In patients with asthma there is an association between the proportion of the respiratory cycle occupied by wheeze, the intensity and pitch of the wheeze, and the severity of airway obstruction.[656, 657] Rhonchi not appreciated during quiet breathing may become audible when the rate of air flow is increased during fast, deep breathing or when the bronchial tubes are narrowed during maximal expiration. A particular form of rhonchus or wheeze is known as a stridor. It is an especially loud musical sound of constant pitch[106] and is caused by obstruction in the larynx or trachea; it may be heard during either inspiration or expiration or throughout the entire respiratory cycle.

The other group of adventitious sounds represents manifestations of pleural disease, in which inflammation of the pleura roughens these membranes and covers them with sticky, fibrinous exudate. During both inspiration and expiration, and particularly in areas in which excursion of the thoracic cage is greatest, a rubbing, rasping, or leathery sound may be heard as the visceral lining moves against the parietal lining. The noise usually is associated with pain. Its disappearance during breath-holding, but not during coughing, renders it unlike rhonchi due to partial bronchial obstruction by mucus, which can closely resemble pleural friction rub. This sound indicates primary pleural disease due to trauma, neoplasm, or inflammation or secondary to an underlying pulmonary neoplasm, infarction, or pneumonia; it disappears when fluid forms and separates the two membranes.

Several sounds relate to the presence of air, with or without fluid, in the pleural cavity. Most of these, such as the Hippocratic succussion splash and the bell sound described by Fagge[107] (the latter produced by tapping one coin against another placed on the chest wall), are of historic rather than diagnostic interest. Hamman[108] described a crunching or clicking sound over the lower retrosternal area, synchronous with the heart beat, which he thought was pathognomonic of air in the mediastinum. Scading and Wood[109] commented that this sound is often audible through a stethoscope and is noticed by the patient only when he or she is lying on the left side, and they found it more commonly associated with a small left pneumothorax, an opinion now held by most. In a series of 24 patients in whom this sound was heard, 22 had left-sided pneumothorax and only 2 had pneumomediastinum.[110] This sign is of diagnostic importance in that it may indicate small, roentgenologically undectable collections of air in the mediastinum. It was heard in some patients with left-sided pneumothorax whose standard posteroanterior chest roentgenogram in full inspiration was reported as normal but whose expiration film showed air in the pleural cavity.[110]

A sign has been described in seven patients that should prove useful in differentiating alveolar air leak from a bronchopleural fistula:[106] with a tube in the pleural cavity, the patient is asked to perform a Valsalva maneuver and the operator detects a squeak on auscultation over the affected hemithorax; this "leak squeak" disappears if the tube is clamped. In contrast to a lesser gradient across an alveolar air leak, this sign is thought to represent turbulence across a bronchopleural fistula caused by a high transbronchial pressure gradient.

A continuous murmur heard on auscultation over the lung in locations inconsistent with a cardiac or aortic origin may indicate pulmonary arteriovenous fistula or severe bronchiectasis. A search for the former may be initiated by the discovery on a chest roentgenogram of a solitary nodule whose characteristics suggest arteriovenous communication, with or without clinically evident mucocutaneous lesions suggesting multiple hereditary telangiectasia (Weber-Osler-Rendu disease).[111, 112] More frequently, a continuous murmur is a chance finding in severe bronchiectasis, particularly of the upper lobes;[113] in these circumstances the murmur originates from bronchial artery–pulmonary artery anastomoses, the pressure gradient causing an audible murmur and palpable thrill. The anastomoses may be of such magnitude that flow in the main pulmonary artery is reversed.[113]

Clinical examination of the heart is essential in every suspected case of pulmonary disease, since certain abnormalities may provide important clues to the etiology. For example, disease affecting either the parenchyma or the pulmonary vasculature may cause pulmonary arterial hypertension; this is evidenced by right ventricular heave, accentuated second pulmonic sound, or pulmonic or tricuspid regurgitant murmurs. In a minority of cases of diffuse pulmonary edema secondary to mitral stenosis or acute left ventricular decompensation, convincing roentgenographic evidence of cardiac enlargement is absent; in such cases, a mitral valve murmur, severe arterial hypertension, or clinical signs of left ventricular strain suggest the cause of the edema. Pulsus paradoxus, an abnormality usually associated with cardiac tamponade, may be observed in patients with obstructive pulmonary disease, particularly severe asthma. Normally the systolic arterial pressure falls 5 mm Hg or less during inspiration. Pulsus paradoxus consists of an exaggerated inspiratory fall in systemic blood pressure, usually when venous return to the right side of the heart during inspiration is impaired (as in shock), right ventricular failure, cardiac tamponade, and massive pulmonary embolism. Paradoxical pulse also may be found when the intrathoracic pressure swing is excessive, as may occur with obstruction of either upper or lower airways or even in some normal young subjects. *Reversed* pulsus paradoxus—a *rise* in arterial systolic and diastolic pressures during inspiration—has been described[114] in patients with congenital subaortic stenosis and in those receiving intermittent inspiratory positive pressure breathing for left ventricular failure; the rise in blood pressure during inspiration apparently results from the increased stroke output of the left ventricle.

EXTRATHORACIC MANIFESTATIONS OF PULMONARY DISEASE

Complete physical examination is essential in every case of lung disease. The diagnosis may be suggested by discovery of a mass or an enlarged abdominal organ. The skin and the endocrine and central nervous systems are most commonly involved. Many pulmonary lesions have cutaneous manifestations; this subject was reviewed by Beerman and Kirshbaum[115] and is discussed in relation to differential diagnosis in other chapters. Endocrinopathies and many other extrapulmonary manifestations have been linked to bronchogenic carcinoma. The neurologic symptoms of respiratory failure have been referred to; the signs are of equal importance[116] and are discussed in Chapter 11 in reference to advanced emphysema. Peripheral neuropathies in association with bronchogenic carcinoma are discussed more fully in the section relating to this disease. Studies of electromyograms and nerve biopsies suggest that the muscular wasting that occurs in some cases of chronic obstructive lung disease may be due to abnormal metabolism of Schwann cells.[117] The section that follows is concerned primarily with clubbing and cyanosis, one or both of which are found in many and must be sought in all cases of pulmonary or pleural disease.

Clubbing and Hypertrophic Osteoarthropathy (HOA)

These are not synonymous: clubbing frequently occurs in the absence of full-blown osteoarthropathy, and the latter occasionally occurs without clubbing. Confusion of simple clubbing with hypertrophic pulmonary osteoarthropathy (HPO) is probably responsible for the great variation in reported incidence of these two conditions in patients with bronchogenic carcinoma, ranging from 2 to 48 per cent. Thyroid acropachy, a rare disorder that occurs in association with various diseases of the thyroid gland, should probably be regarded as a distinct entity; it consists of clubbing of the fingers and toes and periosteal new bone formation that involves the hands and feet predominantly rather than the long bones.[118]

There are four generally accepted criteria for clubbing: (1) increased bulk of the terminal tuft; (2) change in the angle between the nail and the proximal skin to greater than 180 degrees; (3) sponginess of the nailbed when pressure is applied to the nail; and (4) increased nail curvature. When all these changes are present, or when at least one is of severe degree, clubbing is readily recognizable. Unfortunately, however, its detection at an early stage is highly subjective and frequently controversial and its recognition subject to considerable interobserver variation. Methods of objectively assessing the presence and degree of clubbing have been devised and are of particular use in epidemiologic studies.[119, 120]

In cyanotic congenital heart disease, cryptogenic fibrosing alveolitis, and subacute bacterial endocarditis, clubbing is common but hypertrophic osteoarthropathy (HOA) is rare.[118] Clubbing is occasionally unilateral in patients wtih vascular abnormalities of a limb or with brachial plexus pressure; it has also been reported on the affected side in patients with severe hemiplegia and in the toes (with or without involvement of the left hand) in those with patent ductus arteriosus with reversal of blood flow.[118] In patients with acquired symmetric clubbing of the fingers and toes, blood flow to the digits is increased.[121, 122] Although the precise pathogenesis of this phenomenon is not known, it is probable that the opening of arteriovenous anastamoses (Sucquet-Hoyer canals) in the fingers allows for the increased blood flow, and it has been suggested that some vasodilator substance that is normally inactivated escapes into the systemic circulation in the presence of pulmonary disease, making this shunting possible.[118] Numerous vasodilators, including ferritin, bradykinin, adenine nucleotides, 5-hydroxytryptamine, and the prostaglandins, would fit this role, but there is no good evidence to incriminate any one of them. Ferritin appears to have been excluded as a suspect through the use of an immunoradiometric assay that measures the concentration of this substance in the blood.[123] Patients with cystic fibrosis and clubbing have been shown to have more severe pulmonary disease and higher concentrations of both prostaglandin E and prostaglandin $F_{2\alpha}$ than do those in whom clubbing is not present.[124]

The clinical diagnosis of HOA requires the presence of deep-seated pain or joint symptoms, including arthralgia with swelling and stiffness affecting mainly the fingers, wrists, ankles, and knees. Roentgenograms usually show subperiosteal new bone formation in the long bones of the lower extremities, and some consider this finding essential to diagnosis.[225] There is no relationship between the severity of clubbing and HOA. Except in the rare idiopathic form of osteoarthropathy, which roentgenographically may appear identical to pulmonary osteoarthropathy, clubbing or osteoarthropathy is virtually pathognomonic of visceral disease, the primary organ of involvement having either vagal or glossopharyngeal innervation.[118, 126] HOA can be associated with disease of the larynx, diaphragm, esophagus, stomach, bowel, and heart[126, 127] and is a rare accompaniment of pregnancy[127, 128] and of purgative abuse[129]; thus, not all cases of osteoarthropathy are pulmonary in origin and it is important semantically to distinguish HOA from HPO. Malignant chest neoplasms account for 90 per cent of typical HPO, the majority being primary[130] but a few metastatic;[131, 132] the commonest metastatic neoplasm is soft tissue sarcoma associated with a pleurabased mass.[133] Lymphomas of the lung or medias-

tinum may be causative,[134, 135] but interstitial lung diseases[658] and adult cystic fibrosis are rarely so.[659] Osteoarthropathy is usually detected before or at the time of diagnosis of the underlying disease but occasionally can become manifest years later.[136] Clubbing is still reported from developing countries in patients with far-advanced tuberculosis,[137] but HOA does not occur in this disease: of 309 patients admitted consecutively to a tuberculosis sanatorium, none of the 3 patients with HPO had pulmonary tuberculosis (2 had cancer and 1, a pyogenic abscess).[138]

The pathogenesis of HOA is not fully understood, but it is generally agreed that the earliest morphologic change in the limbs is an overgrowth of highly vascular connective tissue, followed by subperiosteal new bone formation. As in simple clubbing, blood flow to the extremities is increased; in HOA, however, most of this augmented flow appears to be shunted through arteriovenous communications in the areas of osteoarthropathy.[139] In the great majority of cases, the increase in blood flow to the extremities appears to be secondary to a reflex mechanism, the vagus nerve serving as the afferent pathway; the efferent pathway is unknown but is considered to be hormonal (neuropeptide) rather than neuronal.[118] The stimulus to this reflex arc presumably comes indirectly from abnormal intrathoracic "masses" or ischemic tissue distal to them.[140] Sometimes a vagal reflex mechanism cannot be invoked to explain the development of this disorder. Blood flow to the fingers is not invariably increased by vagotomy, even when intrathoracic disease is present.[141] HOA localized to the toes has been described in three separate case reports in patients with Dacron grafts and intestinal fistulas of the aorta,[142–144] suggesting that in some way the Dacron must stimulate adjacent vascular endothelium to produce a vasoactive compound. In one of these patients,[142] ligation of the prosthesis and creation of an aortofemoral bypass led to a disappearance of the lower limb clubbing and HOA. The inability to affect limb blood flow in the recipient in cross-circulation experiments in dogs[145] and the absence of arterial hypoxemia in many cases of bilateral upper and lower limb HOA do not support the hypothesis of hormonal or hypoxemic stimuli in the majority of cases of this disorder. However, increased estrogen production has been reported in some cases of HOA of variable etiology,[146] and there is evidence that increased levels of circulating estrogens may at least exacerbate symptoms, as in the rare cases of HOA that develop in pregnant women in whom symptoms promptly abate after delivery.[128]

Some cases of HOA are primary or idiopathic and are not associated with demonstrable disease elsewhere in the body. This unusual condition, known as pachydermoperiostosis, is recognized as having an autosomal form of inheritance with marked variability in expressivity, males being more severely affected than females.[147] It has its onset around puberty and is associated with a distinctive thickening and furrowing of the skin of the forehead, face, and scalp (cutis verticis gyrata), severe facial acne, clubbing, and periosteal new bone formation.[147, 148] Pachydermoperiostosis should not be confused with primary or hereditary digital clubbing, which is present at birth and is usually not accompanied by the symptoms or roentgenologic findings of HOA. Although to the best of our knowledge there have been no studies directed at elucidating the early pathogenesis of pachydermoperiostosis, physiologic and roentgenologic investigation of this condition in its established state has clearly shown a decrease in circulation to the extremities, [147, 149] presumably accounting for the excessive resorption of the distal phalanges of the hands and feet (acrolysis).[148]

It must be borne in mind that most patients with acquired clubbing do not recognize the change in their terminal phalanges when it is first brought to their attention; this failure to recognize such a subtle, insidious change resulting from a potentially treatable disease emphasizes the importance of not accepting without question patients' statements that their fingers have looked the same all their lives; further investigation is essential before the primary or familial nature of the abnormality can be established.

HOA usually resolves with removal of the "causal" tumor. It has also been shown to respond to chemotherapy without objective response in the primary lesion,[150] to respond to radiotherapy of a metastatic lesion without treatment of the primary lung tumor,[151] and to undergo spontaneous resolution.[152]

Cyanosis

Many patients with lung disease have blue or bluish-gray skin and mucous membranes; this is most obvious in the nailbeds or buccal mucosa and usually reflects severe hypoxemia of arterial blood due to ventilation-perfusion inequality. Cyanosis is best appreciated in adequate daylight and is virtually unrecognizable under a fluorescent lamp.[153] It is estimated that 5 grams of hemoglobin per dl of blood have to be reduced before cyanosis is visible, and, therefore, this sign is never present in patients with severe anemia.[154] It may be due to inadequate saturation of arterial blood leaving the left side of the heart, excessive slowing in the peripheral capillaries, or both.

The central or hypoxemic variety associated with lung disease is commonest in patients with chronic obstructive emphysema and then indicates that many acinar units have low alveolar ventilation-perfusion ratios ($\dot{V}A/\dot{Q}$); in other words, a large part of underventilated lung is still being perfused with venous blood. Another rarer variety of central hypoxemia that may lead to cyanosis in lung disease is that due to pulmonary arteriovenous fistula. In this condition a true shunt takes place—a complete bypass of the acinar unit—in which venous blood passes into the arterial circulation without an opportunity to collect oxygen in the lungs. Right-to-left cardiac shunts may become evident in pulmonary diseases when for one reason or another pulmonary vascular resistance increases, allowing for blood flow to occur from right to left atrium through a patent foramen ovale; we have seen this in pulmonary thromboembolic disease, and it has been reported to occur following pneumonectomy in a patient with chronic obstructive pulmonary disease.[155] In other lung diseases, such as severe acute alveolar pneumonia with circulatory collapse, both central and peripheral factors undoubtedly play a part: the venous blood in pulmonary capillaries encounters airless acini, and the same blood stagnates in systemic capillaries and allows excessive removal of oxygen by the tissues. Probably both factors are responsible for the cyanosis so common in patients who have diffuse pulmonary infiltration with clubbing; even when they have only mild arterial oxygen unsaturation the nailbeds are definitely dusky blue. Cardiac conditions with a right-to-left shunt may engender a central form of cyanosis, but are differentiated from pulmonary conditions by the clinical findings and the results of pulmonary function tests. Arterial oxygen unsaturation due to shunting also occurs in association with cirrhosis of the liver, but then is rarely severe enough to incur cyanosis.

Peripheral cyanosis either is paroxysmal and precipitated by cold, as in Raynaud's disease, or general and prolonged, in the latter case often with systemic hypotension and indications of circulatory collapse. The former type occurs in scleroderma, which not uncommonly involves the lung; the latter is commoner in primary heart disease, such as myocardial infarction, than in lung conditions but may occur in association with cor pulmonale and hypoxemia and then indicates a very poor prognosis.

When cyanosis is central in origin the nailbeds usually are deep blue or blue-gray and the skin is warm, whereas peripheral cyanosis is usually associated with cold, clammy skin and dusky, livid nailbeds. Frequently it is not possible on appearance alone to differentiate with certainty between central and peripheral cyanosis, and other clinical findings may not indicate the cause. However, the degree of oxygen saturation of arterial blood will give the answer.

When the pathogenesis of cyanosis appears obscure, methemoglobinemia or sulfhemoglobinemia should be considered. Rarely, methemoglobinemia is primary and congenital. More commonly, the coffee-colored pigment results from the administration of drugs, including nitrates, chlorates, quinones, aniline dyes, sulfonamide derivatives, acetanilid, and phenacetin. Sulfhemoglobinemia and methemoglobinemia may occur simultaneously, usually from ingestion of the same drugs, and then the cyanosis is lead colored. When either of these conditions is present, the venous blood is brownish even after being shaken in air for 15 minutes. The diagnosis can be confirmed by spectroscopic analysis to identify the absorption bands.

THE DEPENDABILITY OF PHYSICAL FINDINGS

Although physical examination of the chest may reveal information that cannot be obtained from roentgenography, it is inexcusable to rely upon physical findings alone and ignore the roentgenographic method of diagnosis when these facilities are available. This error in judgment usually occurs when the patient is treated at home for symptoms and signs suggestive of the early stages of pneumonia. When this condition improves with therapy the physician may neglect to arrange a follow-up roentgenogram and may realize the mistake only when the patient again complains of symptoms referable to the lungs and roentgenography shows a central bronchogenic carcinoma that undoubtedly was responsible for the previous obstructive pneumonitis. Similarly, hospital patients with pneumonia should be followed closely until the chest roentgenogram has cleared completely.

The dependability of physical findings also should be considered from the viewpoint of error. It is disturbing to note the disagreement in detecting abnormal physical signs.[156, 157] Smylie and associates[156] concluded that it was difficult to visualize how observer error could be reduced, since it appeared to reflect neither experience nor the method of clinical teaching. In recent years the significance of some signs of pulmonary disease has been assessed using physiologic methods, and the results of such studies have already been discussed under physical examination of the chest (see page 398). Such validation of empirically accepted clinical findings strengthens the importance of the physical examination. It has been noted that the degree of airflow obstruction can be assessed by the length of a forced expiration after full inspiration, measured with a stethoscope or a stopwatch.[158] In our opinion, an even better test for assessing obstructive disease is to have the patient breathe in and out as rapidly as possible for 10 to 15 sec while one listens with the stethoscope. This is the clinical counterpart of maximal breathing capacity (MBC), which, with a little experience, can be closely predicted on the basis of this simple procedure. Regional lung ventilation, as assessed by radioactive gas techniques (see Pulmonary Function Tests), can be correlated with clinical findings and provide a useful, objective index of the intensity of breath sounds. We are impressed by the correlation between local intensity of breath sounds detected by the stethoscope and

the vascular pattern seen on the roentgenogram in patients with emphysema. In many cases the breath sounds and the pulmonary vasculature to that area of lung are similarly decreased, indicating either coincidental destruction of pulmonary parenchyma and vessels or a compensatory mechanism by which pulmonary blood supply is diverted from poorly ventilated to better ventilated units. A comprehensive objective assessment of contemporary clinical methods of examining the chest might serve to revitalize the art of physical diagnosis.

Differences of opinion among observers are not confined to chest signs and are apparent in the recognition of such extrapulmonary signs as cyanosis and clubbing. In Comroe and Botelho's study,[159] observers could not detect cyanosis until the arterial oxygen saturation had fallen to 80 per cent, and one quarter failed to appreciate this sign when saturation was 70 to 75 per cent. Thus, even when cyanosis is not clinically detected, analysis of the arterial blood PO_2 or oxygen saturation may reveal hypoxemia of severe degree.

Although advanced clubbing is unlikely to lead to any difference of opinion among observers, early clubbing is frequently the subject of controversy.[160] In one study,[161] discrepancies in its detection were equally divided among experienced examiners and medical students.

SPECIAL DIAGNOSTIC PROCEDURES

ENDOSCOPIC EXAMINATION

Laryngoscopy

The larynx can be examined indirectly, by use of a mirror, or directly; the latter may be combined with bronchoscopy.

Laryngoscopy should be performed in any patient who complains of a persistent, dry, hacking or brassy cough, particularly when this is associated with hoarseness. The vocal cords should be well seen, not only to exclude a local lesion but also to detect paralysis which would account for the hoarseness. In the latter instance, roentgenography may reveal a mediastinal lesion involving a recurrent laryngeal nerve. When the larynx appears healthy and the vocal cords move freely, bronchoscopy is indicated to rule out an endotracheal or endobronchial origin for the patient's symptoms.

Bronchoscopy

The development of the flexible fiberoptic bronchoscope (FFB) has popularized this form of examination, making it relatively easy for both patient and physician. In most major hospitals this procedure is now generally performed by internists and surgeons specializing in lung disease. Although the indications for endoscopic examination of the lower airways have multiplied, the commonest application of the FFB continues to be in the diagnosis of pulmonary carcinoma; since it is the surgeon who requires a clear picture of the extent of the lesion and its position in the bronchial tree in order to assess resectability and to determine how much lung should be removed, he or she is the logical person to perform bronchoscopy in patients with suspected cancer. An experienced bronchoscopist may recognize fixation of the mediastinum or loss of the normal "sharpness" of the carina, indicating compression of bronchi by involved lymph nodes.

Satisfactory bronchoscopy requires the patient's confidence in the bronchoscopist; explanation of the procedure and reassurance of the patient take only a few minutes and may greatly facilitate examination. Differences of opinion exist as to the need for prebronchoscopic sedation, the type of anesthesia, the indications, if any, for rigid as against flexible fiberoptic bronchoscopy, and the method of insertion of the instrument. There appears to be general agreement among bronchoscopists that atropine sulfate is indicated prior to bronchoscopy; this drug not only reduces bronchial secretions but prevents bradycardia and reflex bronchoconstriction produced by stimulation of vagal nerve endings.[162] In one study,[163] atropine given by the intramuscular route was felt to be superior to inhalation in inhibiting the vasovagal response. Some form of sedation is commonly advocated and almost certainly is to be recommended for children to be examined under local anesthesia; however, it is questionable whether it is needed in adults.[164] Local anesthesia is preferred, certainly in adults;[165, 166] it allows for cooperation of the patient during the procedure, which is mandatory if an adequate specimen is to be obtained by bronchial lavage. The local anesthetic is applied first with a nebulizer and subsequently by spraying the vocal cords and trachea under direct view. Since an essential feature of most bronchoscopies is bronchial lavage to obtain secretions from the bronchial tree, it should be borne in mind that some local anesthetics have antibacterial action; for example, tetracaine (Pontocaine) severely inhibits cultural growth of *Mycobacterium tuberculosis*,[167, 168] and lidocaine (Xylocaine) is said to inhibit the growth of fungi and nontuberculous bacteria.

When general rather than local anesthesia is indicated, the patient should be closely monitored in the postbronchoscopic period for hypoventilation occasioned by the anesthetic or by neuromuscular blocking agents.[169]

Bronchoscopy can be performed with either a rigid or a fiberoptic bronchoscope. Since the development of the FFB by Ikeda in 1970[170] and its introduction to America by Smiddy and colleagues,[171] this instrument has superseded the rigid bronchoscope for most purposes.[165, 166] Two recognized disadvantages of the FFB are the small size of biopsy specimens and inadequate suction capability if active and copious bleeding is present.[172] The rigid bronchoscope is preferred by many in the investigation of massive hemoptysis (*see* page 394) and by some for endoscopic examination of children, particularly for the removal of foreign bodies and as a means of inserting the FFB.[166]

The FFB can be introduced through the nose or through a rigid metal bronchoscope or endotracheal tube. Sackner and Landa[173] favor a soft latex nasopharyngeal airway; others[166, 174] recommend an endotracheal tube; and a minority use a rigid bronchoscope through which they insert the FFB. Some preferences in the method of insertion are undoubtedly dictated by ethnic differences in the sizes of the nasal passages.[165, 166]

Ideally, fluoroscopic and resuscitative facilities should be available in a special room set aside for endoscopic procedures. However, the FFB has a role to play in emergency situations at the bedside as well,[173, 175–178] notably in the ICU.[179] Hypoxic patients should be given supplemental oxygen during the procedure; a special adapter is available to prevent air leak for those patients who are being artificially ventilated.[180–183]

A major indication for bronchoscopy is roentgenographic evidence of bronchial obstruction, usually consisting of loss of volume of a lung, a lobe, or a segment. Bronchoscopy is indicated in all instances of suspected central bronchogenic carcinoma; it has been estimated that the FFB permits observation of 10 to 15 per cent more of these neoplasms than does the rigid scope (*see* page 360). In some patients, the pediatric FFB can reveal distal lesions in adults.[660] Another frequent indication for bronchoscopy is hemoptysis, the complete management of which has been considered previously (*see* page 394). Washings and bronchoscopic biopsy specimens may be obtained in difficult undiagnosed cases of pulmonary infection using special catheters constructed to avoid oropharyngeal contamination. Other indications for FFB include the following: (1) to ascertain whether tracheal intubation can be safely prolonged beyond the third day;[182] (2) to perform sensitive bronchography via a catheter;[184] (3) to remove foreign bodies or secretions causing obstruction postoperatively or in bronchial asthma (the rigid scope may be useful for these purposes);[178, 180] and (4) for draining peripheral abscesses and extracting mucoid impactions.[185] FFB has also been used in research endeavors: the performance of bronchoalveolar lavage in studies of the pathogenesis of interstitial lung diseases, the insertion of small Teflon discs into the trachea and the recording of their movements in the investigation of tracheal mucous velocity (*see* page 69), and the assessment of lobar and segmental function of the lungs in humans.[186]

The risk inherent in the bronchoscopic examination itself appears slight; most complications occur following biopsy procedures. However, the hemodynamic effects are substantial and are probably related largely to a reflex sympathetic discharge caused by mechanical irritation of the larynx and bronchi.[187] In their study of ten patients, Lundgren and associates recorded mean increases in systemic arterial pressure of 30 per cent, in heart rate of 43 per cent, in cardiac index of 28 per cent, and in pulmonary artery occlusion pressure of 86 per cent.[187] PaO_2 fell an average of 7 mm Hg during bronchial suctioning and in the postbronchoscopic period. Cardiac arrhythmias are common and correlate with the passage of the bronchoscope through the vocal cords and with the hypoxemia consequent on suctioning.[188–192] Administration of lidocaine[191] or oxprenolol[189] can reduce the number of disturbances in cardiac rhythm. In their report of 24,521 bronchoscopies, Credle and associates found the incidence of complications with local anesthetic to be much higher with tetracaine (Pontocaine) than with lidocaine (Xylocaine);[193] in this series, the commonest complication of the procedure itself was laryngospasm, which the researchers thought could have been avoided if sufficient local anesthetic had been used. Major reported complications of FFB include pneumonia (five instances),[194–198] pneumothorax, and hemorrhage (the last two almost always associated with transbronchial biopsy).[165, 195, 199] In two large series of 908[195] and 4595[199] patients, the overall mortality consequent on bronchoscopy was reported to be 0.1 per cent, whereas in two others of 24,521[193] and 1223[165] patients, deaths occurred in 0.01 per cent and 0.00 per cent respectively.

It has recently been shown that in patients in whom bronchoscopy is contraindicated or is refused, CT can be a reliable alternative in the investigation of bronchial disease:[661] of 64 cases in which lesions were detected bronchoscopically, CT was positive in 59; CT correctly excluded disease in 35 (92 per cent) of 38 cases that were subsequently verified to be normal by fiberoptic bronchoscopy.

Esophagoscopy

Pulmonary disease may occur in association with esophageal lesions, and diagnosis may be facilitated by direct endoscopic examination of the esophagus. The procedure should be preceded by fluoroscopy and roentgenography.

Aspiration pneumonia may be secondary to diverticula, achalasia, or stenosis, or a result of peptic ulceration or neoplasm of the esophagus. When the origin of expectorated blood is not known, direct view of the lower esophagus may be indicated to detect bleeding varices. Diffuse pulmonary lesions can occur in association with dysphagia in patients with scleroderma, in which case esophagoscopy, fluoroscopy, and cinefluorography may be required to confirm the diagnosis.

BACTERIOLOGY IN PULMONARY DISEASE

Collection of Material

SPUTUM

A most important aid to the definitive diagnosis of lung disease lies in the proper collection of sputum and the diagnostic methods used in its examination. Unfortunately, the chest physician and the microbiologist appear to live in different worlds in most hospitals and their talents are seldom combined to full advantage. Frequently a specimen of "sputum" arrives in the bacteriology laboratory as a faint, rapidly drying stain at the bottom of the sputum box. Almost every clinical situation in chest disease requires that the bacteriology laboratory receive a fresh specimen of sputum, preferably from well down in the lungs and at least from the posterior pharynx. The physician whose patient has acute pneumonia accomplishes two purposes by watching the patient cough and spit into the sputum box: gross examination of the material may indicate an important clue to diagnosis, and he can ensure that some dependable person (in many cases, preferably himself) immediately conveys the expectorated material to the bacteriology laboratory. If the physician delivers the sample, the clinical problem can be discussed with the bacteriologist, who then can determine the bacteriologic diagnostic method most appropriate to the clinical picture. In the case of outpatients, the expectorated material should be collected in a screw-capped glass jar that has been thoroughly cleaned and placed in boiling water for at least 3 min. The patient should be instructed to cough up material from deep in the lungs upon arising in the morning and to arrange for its immediate transport to the hospital where it should be inoculated on culture medium at once. Proper in-hospital collection of material for culture perhaps requires even more physician supervision. This statement applies particularly to diagnostic specimens obtained in the operating room, where excised tissue is often promptly deposited in formalin, thus eliminating any possibility of detecting a potential infectious etiology.

Fresh specimens are required in bacterial, mycotic, and viral diseases. The only indications for collecting expectorated material over a prolonged period are to determine its quantity and quality and to obtain material for acid-fast culture, which is positive most often when sputum is collected for 24 to 72 hours. However, since acid-fast bacilli are often detectable on film smears of freshly expectorated material, longer collection may not be necessary in many cases of cavitary disease or lobar consolidation suspected to be due to tuberculosis.

Unfortunately, many patients who are admitted to the hospital with pneumonia have been given antibiotics before admission, with the result that significant pathogens fail to grow on culture. When this occurs, it is wise to repeat the culture, bearing in mind that immediate inoculation of a fresh specimen is essential. When a patient fails to respond to antibiotic therapy appropriate to the pathogen originally detected, further cultures should be made, since another pathogenic agent, perhaps acquired in the hospital, may be responsible for the lack of clinical improvement.

Induction of sputum is a much neglected procedure. Inhalation of an aerosolized solution of propylene glycol, sulfur dioxide, or distilled water may stimulate a productive cough resulting in diagnostic specimens; this method is particularly useful in patients with tuberculosis who lack spontaneous expectoration, in which situation it has proved complementary to gastric lavage.[200–202]

Swabs of the upper respiratory tract may also yield tubercle bacilli in patients with suspected tuberculosis who do not expectorate. Swabs of the pharynx or nasopharynx, which frequently are taken from patients with suspected viral disease, should be placed immediately in a liquid solution containing salt and either gelatin or bovine albumin, with or without antibiotics.[203] This material should be delivered immediately to the laboratory for inoculation; when preparation is delayed for a few hours the specimen should be kept at $-40°C$ or, if for longer, at $-70°C$.

TRACHEAL ASPIRATION AND LAVAGE

Since potential pathogens may inhabit the oropharynx and upper respiratory tract without causing disease, it is evident that positive cultures of a pathogenic bacterium do not necessarily signify that a pneumonic process is due to the cultured organism. In one study, 27 of 61 cultures from patients without pneumonia contained reportable pathogens, most being gram-negative bacteria but a minority being *S. pneumoniae*.[204] When the growth is heavy or pure, more reliance can be placed on this finding, but decisions concerning therapy and management must be based on clinical features as well. Some workers attempt to solve this problem by washing sputum repeatedly before culturing and by quantitative culture.[205, 206] If a potential pathogen is present in excess of 10^6 organisms per milliliter of secretions, it is considered significant.[204] The combination of sputum washing and quantitative culture appears to be a valid method of increasing diagnostic accuracy in patients with pneumonia, but the time consumed in carrying out these two procedures makes such methods impractical for most laboratories on a routine basis.[207, 208] The assumption that the mere presence of polymorphonuclear phagocytes and bacteria on a Gram stain indicates at least 10^5 organisms per milliliter and hence provides immediate quantitative bacteriology to permit the clinican to make therapeutic decisions[209] is almost certainly unfounded, despite some clinical evidence for the usefulness of this finding.[210, 211]

Because of these limitations, a technique for bypassing the upper respiratory passages and for obtaining material directly from the trachea became widely used.[212–215] This procedure, described by Pecora in 1963[216] and known as transtracheal aspiration (TTA), is performed by introducing a 14-gauge needle through the cricothyroid membrane and anterior tracheal wall, followed by the insertion of a polyethylene catheter through the needle; suction is applied to the catheter to obtain material for smear and culture. False-negative results are uncommon,[208, 212] estimated by one observer at 1 per cent.[217] By contrast, false-positive cultures are frequent and have been attributed to underlying bronchitis associated with colonization of the lower respiratory tract. In one study, 22 of 26 patients with bronchitis or bronchiectasis had positive cultures of material obtained by TTA, usually in heavy growth;[218] in another study of 335 patients with postive TTA cultures, 89 were not considered to have bacterial pneumonia, comprising a false-positive yield of 27 per cent.[217] In a young military population, Gram stain of TTA offered no advantages over sputum Gram stain in the initial management of acute pneumonia.[662] Further, in a study of 31 clinically uninfected patients with carcinoma, organisms were obtained by TTA in all.[219] False-negative results are considered to occur as a result of acute air space pneumonia in which the responsible organism is confined to the area of involvement; with this in mind, Peltier and associates[220] modified the TTA procedure by inserting a fluoroscopically guided wire to the lesion, followed by brushing and washing. Despite this added feature, they still reported false-negative results in a group of 20 immunosuppressed patients. Because of such findings but, more importantly, because of the inherent risk of severe complications such as hemorrhage, cardiac arrythmias due to hypoxia, subcutaneous and mediastinal emphysema, and occasional reported fatalities,[221–224] this procedure has lost some of its popularity. In its place there has been a tendency to turn to transbronchial biopsy, washings, and brushings; to TTNA; or to open lung biopsy as safer and more productive methods of establishing the etiology of difficult pneumonias.

TRANSBRONCHIAL BIOPSY (TBB)

Obtaining specimens for smear and culture through the bronchoscope is subject to the same likelihood of contamination by oropharyngeal organisms as in sputum expectoration. If smear or culture growth shows a pathogenic microorganism not ordinarily present as a commensal in the oropharynx, such as *M. tuberculosis*, *B. dermatitidis*, *H. capsulatum*, or *P. carinii*, the result can be accepted as a true positive.[225–230] In an attempt to overcome the inevitable contamination of the intranasally or orally inserted flexible fiberoptic bronchoscope, Wimberley and associates[231] placed a sterile sampling brush within a telescoping double catheter occluded by a distal polyethylene glycol plug.* When the desired site of sampling was reached, the plug was extruded and the inner catheter and brush advanced 3 to 4 cm before obtaining the specimen. These researchers and others[232] have stressed the importance of using an aerosolized local anesthetic rather than one that runs down the bronchoscope and thus serves as a potential vehicle for contamination. Using the same plugged telescoping catheter (PTC), other investigators[232–234, 663, 664] have shown a good yield of presumed pathogens with few false-positives. However, more recent reports of PTC use[235, 236] have not been so encouraging, a positive bacterial yield being obtained by one group in 21 of 25 normal subjects, with or without prior rhinovirus inoculation.[235] In order to distinguish pathogens from non-pathogens,[237] the original proponents of this technique now advise performing quantitative aerobic and anaerobic cultures in addition to the PTC aspiration. Teague and associates[210] advocate the use of a sheathed, non-plugged sterile brush passed under fluoroscopic control and combined with a quantitative culture technique, but others[231, 232] have failed to confirm the efficiency of this technique.

In the diagnosis of pulmonary infections, bronchoscopy is usually confined to brushing and washing, but some workers include a tissue biopsy.[229, 238] Complications of TBB are rare and seldom serious, particularly if the procedure is confined to brushing; serious hemorrhage may occur with actual tissue biopsy, even in compromised hosts who have received platelet transfusion prior to the biopsy.[229, 238] In compromised hosts suspected of having *Pneumocystis carinii* pneumonia, bronchoalveolar lavage (BAL) is almost always diagnostic.[239]

TRANSTHORACIC NEEDLE ASPIRATION (TTNA)

Although TTNA plays its greatest role in the diagnosis of peripheral nodules or masses (*see* page 356), its value in determining the etiology of severe air space pneumonia, undiagnosed by all other means, is becoming more apparent.[240, 241] In one series of 108 immunocompromised patients in whom biplane fluoroscopy was employed for needle placement, 1 or more etiologic organisms were identified in 79 presumed infectious episodes.[242] In most instances, complications are rare and minor[243, 244] and usually can be avoided by the use of ultrathin needles.[240] In very ill patients with underlying disease, severe bleeding, air embolism, and even death may occur, and in these cases an open lung biopsy is perhaps advisable.[245]

OPEN LUNG BIOPSY (OLB)

In patients with suspected pneumonia, this procedure should be largely restricted to immunocom-

*Medi-Tech Model BFW/1.0/70/90; Cooper Scientific Corp., Watertown, MA.

promised hosts with overwhelming disease.[246–248] In this clinical setting, the yield can be expected to be approximately 80 per cent:[247, 248] specific treatable infections can sometimes be recognized that have not been diagnosed by TBB.[238, 246] The complication rate is probably no higher than with TTNA or TBB in patients with equally severe illness.

EXAMINATION OF STOOL

As can be appreciated from Table 3–2, microscopic examination of slides (with coverslip) of fecal material is indicated in many parasitic diseases of the lungs; also, viruses can often be isolated in stools. Centrifugation filtration methods can be used to concentrate parasites or eggs.[249]

BLOOD

A culture should be made at the height of fever, using an aseptic technique, in every case of acute fulminating pneumonia. In cases of lung disease thought to be viral, the blood should be drawn early in the disease; part of the aliquot should be used for culture and part for identifying antibodies to pathogens (*see* later discussion).

PLEURAL EFFUSION

The presence of pleural effusion is determined by the roentgenographic appearance and physical signs. The area of maximal accumulation is judged from posteroanterior and lateral roentgenograms; it is confirmed by percussion of the chest wall or, when available, by reflected ultrasound.[250–253] In most cases thoracentesis is performed through the interspace at the site of maximal dullness, usually posteriorly or posterolaterally. If the amount of pleural fluid is small or if the fluid is loculated, ultrasonography is the method of choice to guide thoracentesis.[254] However, in many cases of pleural effusion apparent roentgenographically, the history or physical examination or both may arouse suspicion of an underlying parenchymal lesion. In such cases as much fluid as possible should be removed to give a clearer view of underlying lung parenchyma that may be hidden by the opacification of a large accumulation of effusion. In these circumstances the needle should be inserted low in the thoracic cage.

The patient sits on the bed, either with the head of the bed raised at a right angle or with his legs over the side of the bed and his feet on a chair, with his arms resting on a pillow on a bedside stand. The hand on the side of the proposed thoracentesis should be placed on the opposite shoulder, to widen the intercostal space. This procedure should not cause severe pain; one should reassure the patient beforehand and make sure he is comfortably positioned. The skin should be sterilized over an area of at least three interspaces and the patient should be draped. In our experience, the key to a successful thoracentesis and a comfortable patient is the use of plenty of local anesthetic—at least 5 ml of 1 per cent or

Table 3–2. Identification of Parasitic Pulmonary Infestations

ORGANISM	MICROSCOPIC AND CULTURAL CHARACTERISTICS	SEROLOGIC TESTS	SKIN TESTS	WBC*
Ancylostoma duodenale, Necator americanus	Ova or mature worms in stools	Nil	Yes	leuk to mod eos
Ascaris lumbricoides	Adult worms or typical mamillated outer shell ova in stools	Nil	Nil	mild to mod eos
Cysticercus cellulosae	Ova or mature worms in stools; biopsy of subcutaneous nodules	Complement-fixation and indirect hemagglutination of limited value	Yes	norm to mild eos
Echinococcus granulosus	Scolices found in sputum	Complement-fixation, indirect hemagglutination, and bentonite flocculation	Yes	norm to mod slight eos
Entamoeba histolytica	Amebae in sputum or stool; cysts in stool	Indirect hemagglutination, indirect immunofluorescence, CIE, agglutination and precipitation	Nil	mod + – eos
Filaria sp. (tropical eosinophilia)	Lung biopsy or microfilaria larvae in nocturnal blood rarely	Complement-fixation of limited value	Yes	con eos + +
Paragonimus sp.	Typical operculated eggs in sputum or stool	Complement-fixation	Yes	norm no eos
Pneumocystis carinii	1 to 3 micron, irregular organism may be found in sputum or in lung biopsy	Direct and indirect immunofluorescence	Nil	mild to con neut
Schistosoma mansoni, S. japonicum, S. haematobium	Typical ova of each variety in stool, urine, and rarely in sputum; lung biopsy	Specific complement-fixation and precipitation; flocculation and fluorescent antibody of limited value	Yes	mod eos
Strongyloides stercoralis	Larvae in stools and rarely in sputum	Filarial complement-fixation	Nil	mild to con eos
Toxocara sp. (visceral larva migrans)	Larvae seen in eosinophilic granuloma in liver biopsy	Indirect hemagglutination of limited value	Nil	con eos + +
Toxoplasma gondii	Inoculation of mice with suspected material and demonstration of intracellular crescent-shaped protozoan	Sabin-Feldman dye, fluorescent antibody, and complement-fixation	Yes	norm with some lymph
Trichinella spiralis	Larvae seen in muscle biopsy specimens 10 days postinfection	Precipitation, complement-fixation, flocculation, and indirect immunofluorescence	Yes	mild to con eos

*LEUKOCYTE (WBC) COUNT:
<5000 = leukopenia (leuk)
5000–10,000 = normal
10,000–12,000 = mild
10,000–15,000 = moderate (mod)
>15,000 = considerable (con)

CIE = countercurrent immunoelectrophoresis
eos = eosinophilia
lymph = lymphocytosis
neut = neutrophilia

2 per cent lidocaine hydrochloride (Xylocaine) or a similar anesthetic and, for the patient with a very thick chest wall, as much as 10 ml. When the skin is frozen the needle is introduced gradually through the chest wall, allowing some anesthetic to infiltrate intercostal muscle. The patient usually complains of a twinge of pain when the parietal pleura is touched. Anesthetic should be liberally injected in this area, with the needle withdrawn and reinserted at different angles until a satisfactorily large area of parietal pleura in that interspace is anesthe-tized. The No. 25 needle used for anesthetizing the skin surface is replaced by a No. 22 needle for infiltrating the muscle down to the parietal pleura and to penetrate the pleura and remove fluid. Usually 20 ml of fluid are sufficient when thoracentesis is carried out solely for diagnostic purposes. A 5 to 10 ml syringe is used during induction of anesthesia and is replaced by a 20 ml syringe for collection of fluid. If large amounts of fluid are to be withdrawn, the needle is best replaced by an intravenous catheter.[255]

It is our opinion that in the majority of cases, initial thoracentesis should be combined with biopsy of the parietal pleura. When the diagnosis has been positively established (e.g., the effusion is considered to be secondary to pneumonia or is grossly a transudate in a patient with cardiac, liver, or renal failure), pleural biopsy is not required.

We prefer the Abrams needle for pleural biopsy. When the anesthetic has been infiltrated and the No. 22 needle is in the effusion, a clamp is applied on the needle, flush with the skin; 20 ml of pleural fluid are drawn into the syringe, and the syringe and needle are withdrawn. A clamp is applied on the Abrams biopsy needle the same distance from the sharp trocar tip as from the point of the No. 22 needle to its clamp. A small incision is made with a scalpel through anesthetized skin and the needle, with its inner (cutting) cylinder in the closed position and with a three-way stopcock and 50 ml syringe attached to the needle adapter, is introduced through the anesthetized muscle and pleura until the clamp reaches the thoracic wall. Then the inner cutting cylinder is rotated, allowing fluid to pass through the side opening in the needle and into the syringe. Often the fluid is slightly blood-tinged from trauma of the trocar, which is why specimens for diagnostic purposes should be taken before the pleural biopsy needle is introduced. When most of the fluid has been removed the biopsy needle is withdrawn slowly, with some pressure on the needle toward the side containing the biopsy notch; the notch is placed laterally to avoid intercostal vessels, and when the parietal pleura slips into the notch the needle's withdrawal is suddenly interrupted. When this happens the cutting cylinder is rotated and the biopsy needle containing the specimen is withdrawn. It is wise to take several specimens, even when the first appears satisfactory, for bacteriologic culture as well as pathologic examination. Inability to obtain fluid may indicate empyema, the material being too thick to pass through a No. 22 needle. When the clinical circumstances suggest this, a No. 16 should be inserted after production of a satisfactory degree and extent of anesthesia. Empyema can be diagnosed on gross examination of aspirated fluid. In cases of loculated effusion the exploring needle should be withdrawn and reinserted at different angles. It is in these circumstances that adequate infiltration of anesthetic in the parietal pleura is so important. When no fluid is withdrawn at the first attempt despite strong evidence of its presence, thoracentesis should be repeated in higher or lower interspaces, after further anesthesia.

Complications from thoracentesis are rare; however, when accompanied by biopsy they are more common and may be serious. Bleeding can be copious and presumably occurs from trauma to an intercostal artery; in theory, hemorrhage can be avoided by biopsying in the plane of the intercostal space, either laterally or medially, and by carefully avoiding the area immediately under the rib where the intercostal artery is situated. When only a small amount of pleural fluid is present, the needle may penetrate the lung, an occurrence that is usually readily recognizable by the aspiration of blood and air; this complication is not uncommon and, although it may induce a pneumothorax, it seldom causes serious bleeding. It can be avoided by contin-

uous pull on the barrel of the syringe as it is slowly introduced through the parietal pleura; this enables the operator to find even a thin film of pleural fluid between the membranes. The amount of fluid withdrawn depends upon the circumstances; the chief indication for complete removal is to obtain a clearer view of the underlying lung or because the fluid is making the patient dyspneic. It is unwise to remove fluid too rapidly from patients who are in heart failure or who have severe anemia, since acute pulmonary edema is likely to develop: only a limited amount should be removed at any one time, and use of a vacuum bottle is contraindicated.

Smears and Cultures

All patients who are acutely ill with pneumonia when admitted to the hospital should be encouraged to cough and spit into a sputum box as soon as possible; if they are unable to expectorate because of the severity of their illness, TTNA, TBB, or OLB should be undertaken; which of these diagnostic methods is to be employed depends on the suspected etiology of the pneumonia and the expertise of the examiner. The fresh sputum or aspirate should be smeared on a slide, Gram-stained, and inoculated on a culture medium. The choice of antibiotic should be made on the basis of the Gram stain, before obtaining culture and sensitivity results from the bacteriology laboratory. Patients with the relevant clinical picture whose smears show organisms predominantly gram-negative or with the morphologic appearance of staphylococci should be diagnosed as having these forms of pneumonia, and the appropriate antibiotics should be given. This does not mean that one can diagnose the etiologic agent of pneumonia by the smear alone; subsequent culture may reveal a pathogen different from that suspected from the preliminary smear. However, since patients with severe acute pneumonia may die before the results of culture are forthcoming, this smear represents the most dependable method of making a tentative diagnosis and instituting appropriate therapy. Although most healthy individuals have a sterile tracheobronchial tree, all have upper respiratory tracts that contain nonpathogenic cocci and bacilli that are readily apparent on routine smear; in cases of fulminating pneumonia, therefore, it is essential that specimens be obtained from the lower respiratory tract.

Furthermore, even positive sputum cultures of a pathogenic bacterium do not necessarily signify that a pneumonic process is due to the cultured organism. When the growth is heavy or pure, more reliance can be placed on this finding, but decisions concerning therapy and management must be based on clinical features as well. It has been suggested that the results of culture are more reliable if expectorated sputum is repeatedly washed beforehand.[205] Another technique advocated by some investigators is "quantitative" culture of sputum,[206] in which the sputum is liquefied with acetylcysteine in a sterile glass tube containing sterile glass beads; the contents are mixed and serially diluted, then streaked on various culture media.[205, 206] When patients are critically ill and the clinical situation and smear do not indicate the likely diagnosis, most workers find washing of sputum and quantitative culture too time-consuming and prefer to use TTNA, TBB, or OLB.

Hemolytic coagulase-positive *Staphylococcus aureus* is usually not pathogenic for a healthy adult but may well cause pneumonia if the patient has had influenza recently or is suffering from a debilitating disease, particularly if the organism was acquired in the hospital and is penicillin-resistant. Most patients admitted to the hospital with bronchopulmonary infection have had some antibiotic therapy before admission, and the finding of only nonpathogenic, gram-negative organisms may be due simply to antibiotic suppression of more sensitive bacteria; also, the causal pathogen may be a virus, the identity of which may (or may not) be disclosed by subsequent serologic studies. Clinical clues, such as the gross appearance of sputum,[256] increased numbers of polymorphonuclear leukocytes in the peripheral blood, and roentgenographic evidence of air-space pneumonia may indicate that the pneumococcus cultured is in fact the cause of the disease. If there is satisfactory clinical response, changing the antibiotic or adding another as successive cultures grow different potential pathogens represents an irresponsible and often dangerous approach to the care of patients with pneumonia.

Mycobacterium tuberculosis and other mycobacteria may be apparent in sputum smears stained by the Ziehl-Neelsen method. A presumptive diagnosis of tuberculosis can be made on this evidence but definitive diagnosis can be made only when culture reports are received. Homogenization of the sputum with 2 per cent sodium hydroxide and acetylcysteine before inoculation on culture media is advocated.[257, 258] At least two media should be used for culture of these organisms, since some strains grow better on one type than on another. The organism is identifiable by the colony appearance and rate of growth. Diagnosis can be made quickly by use of fluorescence microscopy.[259] The fluorescent dye localizes in acid-fast bacilli and renders them visible on the dark background.

Table 3–3 summarizes the bacteriologic features of the many bacterial and viral diseases that may affect the lungs.

Positive cultures for various saprophytic fungi are often obtained after the administration of antibiotics, and evaluation of their pathogenicity requires careful appraisal of the clinical picture. In otherwise healthy persons, little significance attaches to the finding of species of *Candida*, including *Candida albicans*, even in heavy growth; this organism can be considered pathogenic only when it is grown on culture and is seen histologically in lung biopsy.[260, 261] Other potentially pathogenic fungi, such as *Geotrichum*, *Mucor*, and *Aspergillus*, are commonly saprophytic, and the clinical findings lead to a suspicion of pathogenicity only when there is evidence of impaired host defense.[262]

Isolation of the organism, whether it be bacterium, virus, rickettsia, or fungus, is the only conclusive means of diagnosing infectious disease, but the culture of some pathogens is fraught with danger and may lead to laboratory-acquired disease. The etiologic agents of tularemia[263] and Q fever[264] fall into this category, and great care should be taken in handling material in cases of suspected or known disease of this type. It may even be wise to settle for a presumptive diagnosis based on the results of serologic and skin tests. Fungus disease also has been reported to originate in the laboratory due to *Coccidioides immitis*[265] and *Histoplasma capsulatum*.[266]

Animal Inoculation

Although the use of animals for the isolation of bacteria largely has been abandoned because of improvements in culture techniques, guinea pig inoculation is still used in tuberculosis and may prove complementary to other diagnostic tests. The pathogens of Q fever and psittacosis can be isolated by intraperitoneal inoculation of guinea pigs or mice, but extreme care must be exercised to avoid laboratory-acquired infection. Goodwin and associates[267] stated that the early stage of chronic pulmonary histoplasmosis, before the development of cavitation, is not readily diagnosed by the usual methods; in the majority of their 28 cases a positive culture was obtained only after passage through mice. The use of animal inoculation in various infectious diseases is summarized in Tables 3–3 and 3–4.

SEROLOGIC AND SKIN TESTS

These methods are particularly useful in the diagnosis of pulmonary viral or mycotic infections. They portray the antigen-antibody reactions that take place in the skin and the test tube, usually as a result of the development of antibodies in the patient; therefore, in the more acute viral diseases the findings may not indicate the etiologic agent until the convalescent state of the disease is reached. These tests are widely used in diagnosing a number of chronic pulmonary disorders and epidemiologically to establish the prevalence of diseases of infectious origin in specific geographic areas.[268] Since the patient has usually recovered by the time the antibody titer rises, indicating the diagnosis, these tests are seldom of direct diagnostic value in individual cases, but they are useful in identifying the etiologic agents of various diseases in population groups.[269–276]

Table 3–3. Identification of Bacterial, Rickettsial, and Viral Pulmonary Infections

ORGANISM	MICROSCOPIC AND CULTURAL CHARACTERISTICS	SEROLOGIC TESTS	SKIN TESTS	WBC*
Streptococcus pneumoniae	Tentative identification on smear; blood culture on blood agar; mouse inoculation	Specific antiserum to identify serogroup; CIE to detect antigen	Nil	con neut
Streptococcus pyogenes	Tentative on smear; Lancefield group A on culture; beta hemolysis on blood agar	Antibodies to antistreptolysin O	Nil	con neut
Staphylococcus aureus, S. epidermidis	Tentative on smear; colonies hemolyze blood agar; organism is coagulase positive (*aureus*), coagulase negative (*epidermidis*)	Nil	Nil	con neut
Bacillus anthracis	Tentative on smear; culture on peptone agar	Indirect fluorescent antibody, agar gel–diffusion of limited value	Nil	norm to con neut
Listeria monocytogenes	Motile organism showing hemolysis on blood agar; conjunctival inoculation in rabbit or guinea pig	Agglutination	Nil	mod with lymph
Pseudomonas aeruginosa, P. cepacia	Tentative on smear; heavy growth on artificial medium required for pathogenicity	Nil	Nil	leuk to mod
Pseudomonas pseudomallei	Aerobic or anaerobic standard culture media; motile pleomorphic with one or two flagella at one pole	Hemagglutination and complement-fixation	Nil	norm to mod
Pseudomonas mallei	Species differentiated antigenically; culture on enriched agar; guinea pig inoculation	Agglutination, complement-fixation	Yes	leuk to norm
Klebsiella aerogenes	Tentative on smear; mucoid, gelatinous colonies on agar; biochemical tests and type-specific antibody	Specific antiserum to identify type	Nil	leuk to mod
Escherichia coli	Tentative on smear and with heavy growth on artificial medium; diagnosis with positive blood culture	Nil	Nil	norm to mod
Proteus sp.	Tentative on smear and with heavy growth on artificial medium; diagnosis with positive blood culture	Nil	Nil	norm to con
Salmonella sp.	Tentative on smear; *S. typhi* or *S. choleraesuis*, usually; differentiation on basis of biochemical tests and agglutination	Agglutination to identify specific serotypes	Nil	leuk to mod
Acinetobacter	Large white or mucoid colony on agar; inability to reduce nitrates	Nil	Nil	mild to mod
Legionella sp.	Growth of gram-negative bacteria on charcoal yeast extract	Direct and indrect immunofluorescence. ELISA and radioimmunoassay for antigen	Nil	mod to con
Haemophilus influenzae	Encapsulated organism with capsular swelling in appropriate biologic fluid; nasopharyngeal swab culture on blood agar in children	Specific antiserum to identify type; CIE for antigen	Nil	norm to mod
Bordetella pertussis	Smear nasopharyngeal swab on Bordet-Gengou agar	Fluorescent antibody, complement-fixation, and agglutination	Nil	mod to con lymph
Francisella tularensis	Tentative on smear; body fluids cultured on blood agar directly or after passage through mouse or guinea pig	Agglutination	Yes	norm to mod

*LEUKOCYTE (WBC) COUNT:
<5000 = leukopenia (leuk)
5000–10,000 = normal
10,000–12,000 = mild
10,000–15,000 = moderate (mod)
<15,000 = considerable (con)

CIE = countercurrent immunoelectrophoresis
ELISA = enzyme-linked immunosorbent assay
eos = eosinophilia
lymph = lymphocytosis
neut = neutrophilia

Table continued on opposite page

Table 3–3. Identification of Bacterial, Rickettsial, and Viral Pulmonary Infections *Continued*

ORGANISM	MICROSCOPIC AND CULTURAL CHARACTERISTICS	SEROLOGIC TESTS	SKIN TESTS	WBC*
Yersinia pestis	Tentative on smear; body fluids cultured on blood agar directly or after passage through mouse or guinea pig	Fluorescent antibody, agglutination, and complement-fixation	Nil	mod to con
Brucella sp.	10% CO_2 needed for *B. abortus* culture on tryptose phosphate; differentiate species on basis of biochemical and serologic tests	Agglutination and complement-fixation	Yes	leuk to norm
Neisseria meningitidis	Growth on enriched culture media at 37° C in atmosphere of CO_2	Specific antiserum to identify serogroup	Nil	mod
Bacterium of cat scratch fever	Gram-negative silver-stained bacterium in lymph nodes	Direct immunofluorescence	Yes	norm
Bacteroides sp.	Anaerobic culture required of transtracheal or needle-aspirated material; frequently combined with anaerobic streptococci and fusospirochetes	Nil	Nil	norm to mod
Mycobacterium sp.	Tentative identification on smear; colony appearance identifies strain; animal inoculation	Agar–double diffusion and hemagglutination of limited value	Yes	norm to mild with mono-cytosis
Mycoplasma pneumoniae	Growth of pleuropneumonia-like organisms on enriched agar or beef broth; cultivation in simian cell tissue culture and chorioallantoic membrane	Cold agglutination, complement-fixation, fluorescent antibody, and CIE for antigen	Nil	norm to mild to con
Influenza virus	Human and simian cell tissue culture; inoculation of chick embryo	Complement-fixation, hemagglutination and neutralization, fluorescent antibody	Nil	mild to con with neut
Parainfluenza virus	Human and simian cell tissue culture	Neutralization, complement-fixation, and hemabsorption with guinea pig erythrocytes	Nil	norm to mod
Respiratory syncytial virus	Human, simian, and bovine cell tissue culture from nasal or pharyngeal secretions	Neutralization, complement-fixation, and hemagglu-tination-inhibition	Nil	norm
Rubeola virus	Human and simian cell tissue culture; inoculation of chick embryos; giant cells in urine or throat washings	Hemagglutination-inhibition, neutralization, and complement-fixation	Nil	norm to mod
Coxsackie virus	Culture in human amnion or rhesus monkey kidney	Neutralization	Nil	leuk to mod
ECHO viruses	Human and simian cell tissue culture	Neutralization, complement-fixation	Nil	norm to mod
Adenoviruses	Human and simian cell tissue culture	Complement-fixation, neutralization	Nil	norm to mild
Herpes zoster (varicella)	Human cell tissue culture; intranuclear inclusion bodies in sputum cells in pneumonia	Complement-fixation, neutralization, fluorescent antibody. Cross-react with herpes simplex	Nil	norm to con
Cytomegalovirus	Human cell tissue culture	Complement-fixation, immunofluorescent antibody	Nil	norm
Epstein-Barr virus (infectious mononucleosis)	May be cultured from saliva or blood—of little value in diagnosis	Heterophil antibody agglutination, EBV antibodies by immunofluorescence, complement-fixation or immunodiffusion	Nil	leuk to con lymph
Chlamydia trachomatis, C. psittaci	Inoculation of mice or chick embryos with sputum or blood	Complement-fixation	Nil	leuk to mod
Coxiella burnettii (Q fever)	Culture of body fluids in chick embryos, guinea pigs; direct fluorescence in tissue	Complement-fixation	Nil	norm to mod

Table 3–4. Identification of Mycotic Pulmonary Infections

ORGANISM	MICROSCOPIC AND CULTURAL CHARACTERISTICS	SEROLOGIC TESTS	SKIN TESTS	WBC*
Histoplasma capsulatum	On glucose agar at 30° C mycelial growth with tuberculate spores; on cysteine blood agar at 37° C or in tissues stained with silver nitrate 2 by 4 μ yeast cells occur; mice inoculation useful	Complement-fixation with mycelial and yeast antigens, latex agglutination, agar gel–double diffusion, and indirect fluorescent antibody	Yes	norm to mild leuk in disseminated cases
Coccidioides immitis	On glucose agar at 30° C mycelial growth with arthrospores; in human body fluids or tissues or after inoculation into mice or guinea pigs 20 to 80 μ spherules seen	Agar gel–double diffusion latex agglutination, tubular precipitation, and complement-fixation	Yes	norm to mod eos with *E. nodosum*
Blastomyces dermatitidis	On glucose agar grows slowly as mycelia with conidia; on blood agar grows as single budding, doubly refractile, walled yeast organisms	Agar gel–double diffusion and indirect fluorescent antibody for yeast form only and of limited value	Nil	norm to mod rarely con
Cryptococcus neoformans	On glucose agar and on blood agar at 37° C, 4 to 20 μ yeast cells; these spherical organisms with a thick capsule may be identified in body fluids with India ink stain	Indirect fluorescence and complement-fixation for antibody; agglutination for both antibody and antigens	Nil	norm to mod
Actinomyces sp.	On enriched agar under anaerobic conditions delicate gram-positive hyphae; in tissues or body fluids mycelial clumps (sulfur granules) may be identified	Indirect fluorescent antibody to differentiate species	Nil	norm to mod
Nocardia sp.	On glucose agar and on blood agar under aerobic conditions delicate branching filamentous hyphae; organism gram-positive and some strains acid-fast	Nil	Yes (much cross-reaction)	mod neut or leuk or lymph
Aspergillus sp.	On glucose agar broad septate hyphae with characteristic conidiophores expanding into large vesicle form	Precipitation, CIE and ELISA tests for antigen of uncertain value	Yes	norm to mod sometimes eos
Candida sp.	On corn-meal agar thick-walled chlamydospores; in body fluids and tissues, 2 to 4 μ, thin-walled, oval budding yeasts seen	Agglutination, immuno-diffusion, and ELISA test for antigen	Nil	norm to mod
Phycomycetes (mucormycosis)	On glucose agar wide, nonseptate hyphae bearing large (100 μ) globular sporangia form	Nil	Nil	—
Geotrichum sp.	On glucose agar oval or spherical arthrospores separated from hyphae; in sputum may be large rectangular arthrospores with rounded ends	Nil	Nil	eos in bronchial form
Sporothrix schenckii	On glucose agar at 30° C delicate hyphae supporting conidiophores; on enriched media at 37° C cigar-shaped gram-positive found	Agglutination, complement-fixation, agar gel–diffusion, and indirect fluorescent antibody	Nil	norm to mod
Paracoccidioides brasiliensis	On glucose agar mycelial growth with branching hyphae and conidia; in tissues or on culture at 37° C multiple budding yeast organisms seen	Tube precipitation, complement-fixation, agar gel–double diffusion, latex agglutination, and fluorescent antibody	Yes	—
Pseudallescheria boydii	On glucose agar thin hyphae with stalks bearing single conidium; large (50 to 200 μ) flask-shaped ascospores also seen	Immunodiffusion	Nil	—
Torulopsis glabrata	On glucose agar reproduces by budding but fails to produce septate hyphae	Nil	Nil	norm

*LEUKOCYTE (WBC) COUNT:
    <5000 = leukopenia (leuk)
    5000–10,000 = normal
    10,000–12,000 = mild
    10,000–15,000 = moderate (mod)
    >15,000 = considerable (con)

CIE = countercurrent immunoelectrophoresis
ELISA = enzyme-linked immunosorbent assay
eos = eosinophilia
lymph = lymphocytosis
neut = neutrophilia

Serologic Testing

This technique is most often used to determine the causative pathogens in various bacterial, viral, mycotic, and parasitic diseases (*see* Tables 3–2, 3–3, and 3–4). In the great majority of instances the test is dependent upon the development in the patient's serum of antibodies that cause agglutination, precipitation, or complement fixation, when exposed to specific antigens. Although very high titers on one occasion may strongly suggest the specific etiologic agent, rising or falling titers in serial or paired serologic tests some time apart constitute much stronger evidence. In those diseases in which the antigen is a bacterium in the sputum, the diagnostic test can be carried out, after the organism has been cultured, within a few days of onset of the illness. This applies to pneumococcal and Klebsiella pneumonia, for which specific antisera can be used to determine the type or strain of the organism.

Serologic testing is of most practical value in relation to chronic pulmonary disease, and this is well exemplified in fungal infections.[277, 278] The two major pathogenic mycoses in which serologic tests play a distinct role in diagnosis are coccidioidomycosis and histoplasmosis. Richert and Campbell[279] correlated positive results in skin and serologic tests with the findings of *Histoplasma capsulatum* in pathologic material from 123 patients: the skin test was positive in 117, while serologic testing gave a positive response in only 73 (48 per cent), with a titer of 1:32 or higher in only 16, presumably indicating inactivity of the disease in most cases at that time. The most useful serologic test in histoplasmosis is the complement-fixation (CF) test, using both histoplasmin and a saline suspension of yeast form as antigens. Using these two antigens, positive results will be obtained in approximately 95 per cent of culturally proved cases of progressive pulmonary disease.[278] The yeast form gives a positive result earlier. In disseminated infections the CF reaction is less reliable, giving positive results in 56 to 80 per cent of cases.[278] In 84 per cent of cases of culturally proved nondisseminated histoplasmosis the titer will be higher than 1:16.[280] Other serologic tests of value in detecting histoplasmosis are the latex agglutination test (positive only in detecting acute primary infections), the agar gel-double diffusion test (useful in resolving whether positive CF results are due to cross-reactions), and the fluorescent antibody test used in detecting the yeast form of *H. capsulatum* in tissues or clinical specimens.[278] Immunoelectrophoretic studies by Walter[281] in 146 patients with chronic histoplasmosis revealed that 96.5 per cent of sera contained precipitins; in only 5 cases did the serum fail to demonstrate precipitins, and these patients had disseminated histoplasmosis or had sputum that remained culturally positive for *H. capsulatum* for 5 to 7 years despite courses of amphotericin B therapy. These cases probably reflected far-advanced disease that overwhelmed the patient's immune defense mechanisms.

In coccidioidomycosis, screening is recommended with agar gel–double diffusion as well as a latex particle agglutination test, and positive reactors should be tested by complement-fixation and tubular precipitin. The CF test is used primarily to determine whether the disease is disseminated: a titer rising above 1:16 should arouse suspicion of dissemination. Precipitins may be detected within 1 to 3 weeks after the onset of primary infections; the CF test, however, is not usually positive until 4 to 6 weeks after infection, by which time the precipitin test usually has reverted to negative. Spherulin (antigen prepared from the sporangium (spherule) of *C. immitis*) is more sensitive than coccidioidin (antigen derived from the mycelial form).[282]

Less common mycotic infections caused by pathogenic (in contrast to opportunistic) fungi in which serologic testing may prove useful are sporotrichosis and paracoccidioidomycosis (South American blastomycosis). Results of serologic tests are negative in cutaneous sporotrichosis but the complement-fixation test is highly specific and usually positive in the active pulmonary form.[283] Fluorescent antibody reagents against the yeast form are useful in overcoming the difficulty of identifying these organisms.[278] In paracoccidioidomycosis, the agar gel–double diffusion method reveals precipitins early in the clinical course of the disease and can be demonstrated in the sera of virtually all patients with proved disease. Complement-fixation is similarly useful in following patients with rising titers indicating dissemination.[278]

The detection of antibodies as a reflection of host tissue invasion may be extremely useful in opportunistic fungal infections, whereas the culture of fungi from sputum or transtracheal aspirates is of limited value since these organisms are common commensals. However, they cause disease in compromised hosts, in whom significant antibody production is often not forthcoming because of defective immune response. This appears to be the case in invasive aspergillosis (in which antibodies are not detectable) in contrast to allergic aspergillosis and aspergilloma (in which high levels of precipitins are present). On the other hand, the sera of patients with systemic candidiasis may contain both agglutinating and precipitating antibodies,[284, 285] but not invariably.[286] Serologic testing may also be useful in detecting antigen in patients with suspected fungal infections, best exemplified by the latex agglutination technique in detecting cryptococcal polysaccharide antigen in CSF. Using antibody prepared in rabbits, Goodman and associates[287] demonstrated antigen in 36 of 39 patients with culturally proved meningeal cryptococcosis. More importantly, they obtained positive titers for latex agglutinating antibodies in three cases with negative cultures, India ink preparations, and CSF antibodies (measured by indirect fluorescent antibody and tube precipitin methods); two of these patients responded to amphotericin B, whereas the third died and was found to have cryptococcal granulomas in the arachnoid space. A 1973 report[278] of an American College of Chest Physicians Committee recommended an indirect fluorescence antibody technique combined with tubular agglutination and latex particle agglutination for detecting cryptococcosis.

Serologic tests may also assist in the diagnosis of several parasitic diseases; for example, invasive amebiasis can be detected by both gel diffusion precipitin and indirect hemagglutination tests. Obviously the results of such tests are more reliable in North Americans than in patients from areas in which these diseases are highly endemic, on whom they must be interpreted with caution.[288] The three most reliable serologic tests for diagnosing toxoplasmosis are the indirect fluorescent antibody, indirect hemagglutination, and Sabin-Feldman dye tests; the last-named is costly, and its use of living organisms renders it potentially hazardous.[288] Although disease endemism varies regionally, antibodies can be demonstrated in a significant percentage of asymptomatic persons; however, a rise in antibody titer is the surest way to establish the presence of toxoplasmosis, and an initial examination that reveals a titer much higher than usual in asymptomatic people should suggest active disease. Antibody titers rise rapidly during the first 6 to 8 weeks after infestation, level off for a few weeks, and then fall steadily over the next year or so; eventually they reach levels commonly found in an asymptomatic populace presumed to have had subclinical infection as evidenced by slight elevations in antibody titers.[289] Hydatid disease is almost always associated with the production of antibodies, and rupture of a cyst often results in a rise in titer.[290] Several antigens have been prepared from these cysts, and a great variety of immunologic methods has been used to detect serum antibodies. Perhaps the most reliable method is indirect hemagglutination, which has been reported to give positive results in approximately 90 per cent of cases of hepatic cysts and 30 per cent of pulmonary cysts.[291] Serologic testing is also used in trichinosis, although here its value is limited by the short clinical course of the infestation and by delay in the development of antibodies; 1 week after the onset of symptoms, the bentonite flocculation and complement-fixation tests are positive in only 20 to 30 per cent of patients, reaching a peak of 80 to 90 per cent by the fourth to fifth week.[292]

In addition to the more or less specific antibodies, nonspecific cold agglutination antibodies and antibodies to *Streptococcus MG* are found in approximately 50 per cent of patients with *Mycoplasma pneumoniae* infections and constitute strong evidence of this disease. However, cold agglutinins sometimes develop in other infectious diseases involving the lungs.

The mixing of specific serum with an antigen from the patient comprises a different form of antigen-antibody reaction which is not strictly a serologic test; this technique has thrown new light on the early immunologic diagnosis of infectious diseases.[293] Antigen and specific antibody, one of which is labeled with fluorescent dye, are mixed and processed; the histologic sections are washed thoroughly to remove unbound reagent, and antigen-antibody reactions become apparent as fluorescent areas. In most instances antiserum to the suspected organism is mixed with tracheobronchial secretions or cultures of this material. This is the direct method, which requires labeling of the specific antibody to the suspected antigen. An indirect method, which does not require fluorescent dye tagging of specific antibody, is of even greater practical value: this consists of an anti-immunoglobulin to one species of animal prepared in another species. This antiglobulin fluorescent conjugate can then be mixed with the patient's serum or overlaid on the histologic preparation; in this way a number of specific antibodies can be looked for at the same time.[294] This procedure permits diagnosis in the acute phase of various infections, including those caused by *Mycoplasma pneumoniae*,[295, 296] *H. capsulatum*,[297, 298] *Legionella* sp., respiratory syncytial virus,[299] and many other organisms (*see* Tables 3–2, 3–3, and 3–4).

Skin Tests

These tests can be divided into those used to detect hypersensitivity to allergens that produce immediate reactions and those used to diagnose bacterial, fungal, and parasitic diseases that usually give rise to delayed reactions.

IMMEDIATE REACTIVITY

Scratch or intradermal tests are used to detect atopy, seasonal and perennial rhinitis, and asthma, using common inhalants such as pollens, molds, dusts, and danders; foods and drugs are used when the patient's history indicates specific sensitivity. Application of the allergens provokes more or less specific reactions. Some have a nonspecific irritating quality. Pollen extracts are almost always specific and usually of clinical significance. This is true also for mold spore extracts and for many danders and some foods, but not for house dust, feathers, wool, kapok, and silk. Skin tests are particularly useful when they confirm a history indicating specific allergy and form the basis of a desensitization program.

SKIN TESTS FOR BACTERIA, FUNGI, AND PARASITES

Tables 3–2, 3–3, and 3–4 summarize the uses of these reactions for diagnostic purposes. Skin tests of value for diagnosing bacterial infections are those used in suspected mycobacterial disease and tularemia.

Diagnostic skin testing for mycobacterial infections in man can be of great value, particularly in identifying tuberculosis. Until recent years it was accepted that virtually all patients with tuberculosis had positive test reactions; for example, one report[300] described 99.6 per cent positive reactivity to intermediate strength tuberculin (0.0001 mg PPD or 5 TU PPD) in 468 patients with active disease. A negative tuberculin skin reaction with both intermediate and second strength PPD (or OT 1:1000 and 1:100) has been regarded as virtually conclusive evidence of the absence of tuberculosis.[301] However, recent studies have shown that the tuberculin test is by no means so dependable, not only because of errors resulting from inactive injected material or faulty technique, but because a certain percentage of patients with active disease appear to be totally anergic or specifically anergic to PPD or have not yet developed skin hypersensitivity.[302]

The material used for mycobacterial skin testing is purified protein derivatives (PPD) of various mycobacterial species. Mycobacterial PPD is obtained from filtrates of heat-killed cultures of bacilli that have grown on a synthetic medium and have then been precipitated by trichloroacetic acid or neutral ammonium sulfate.[303] An international PPD-tuberculin is designated PPD-S; all other PPDs of tuberculin are designated as such by lot number and producer. Commonly used PPDs of nontuberculous (atypical) organisms are PPD-Y (*M. kansasii*), PPD-G (scotochromogen "Gause"), PPD-B (*M. intracellulare*), and PPD-F (*M. fortuitum*).

Intermediate strength PPD (0.0001 mg; 5 TU) is usually employed for diagnostic skin testing for tuberculosis. If the clinical and roentgenographic findings strongly suggest active disease, PPD first strength (1 TU) should be used initially, since sensitive persons may have severe reactions to tuberculin. This was demonstrated by the systemic symptoms and local tissue destruction that occurred in students who received 10,000 TU (0.2 mg) in error.[304] If a patient fails to react to intermediate strength PPD, a second strength (PPD-S 250 TU) can be used, although a positive reaction at this strength is less significant.

The skin test is carried out as follows. The solution (0.1 ml) is injected intradermally through disposable 26 or 27 gauge short-beveled needles on the volar aspect of the forearm, with the needle bevel pointing upward.[305] Jet injection or multiple puncture, such as the Heaf and the Disk tine test, should not be used for diagnostic purposes but is useful for epidemiologic surveys, particularly in children.[303, 306, 307] The patch test is no longer considered reliable. Tests should be read on the second or third day after injection, the diameter of induration being measured transversely to the long axis of the forearm and recorded in millimeters. The degree of erythema is of no significance and need not be estimated, although its presence should suggest the possibility that injection was subcutaneous rather than intracutaneous.[303] Since 1969 most observers have accepted the recommendations of the American Thoracic Society[308] that a Mantoux reaction of 10 mm or larger is positive, 5 to 9 mm is doubtful, and less than 5 mm is negative.

A positive tuberculin reaction is strong evidence that a patient has or has had tuberculosis, particularly if the induration is 10 mm or more in diameter. False-positive reactions are rare; they usually occur when induration is smaller than 10 mm in diameter or when reaction to PPD-S is negative at 5 TU and positive at 250 TU. These false-positive reactions represent cross-reactions caused by infection from atypical mycobacteria. Several studies indicate that the larger the size of the tuberculin reaction the greater the risk of clinical tuberculosis in the future.[303, 304, 306, 307, 309, 310]

The major drawback to the tuberculin test lies in the considerable incidence of false-negative reactions. (For practical diagnostic purposes, a false-negative reaction is one in which the intracutaneous injection of 0.1 ml of 5 TU PPD-S results in induration less than 5 mm in diameter or, if the American Thoracic Society recommendations are accepted, less than 10 mm.) False-negative reactions may be due to (1) faulty technique of administration, (2) faulty interpretation of the reaction, (3) lack of potency of the injected material, or (4) diminished immunologic response to tuberculin.[311, 312] Accepted errors in technique include the injection of too little antigen (possibly due to leakage from the syringe) and subcutaneous rather than intradermal injection; however, recent work[313] has raised doubts that these apparent "errors" in technique can in fact occasion negative results. Errors in reading are due mainly to inexperience. In addition, there may be interobserver disagreement in reading;[312] for example, great variation has been recorded in the interpretation of repeated tuberculin reactions from year to year[307] and even from week to week on known positive reactors by the same person using the same antigen.[314] The injected material may be faulty as a result of improper dilution, degeneration, or adsorption of the PPD to glass or plastic containers; the original observation by Parish and O'Brien in 1935[315] that adsorption or adhesion of tuberculin to glass or plastic can result in major error has been confirmed by many other observers.[316–321] Magnusson and associates[322] showed that the addition of Tween 80, a detergent, stabilizes tuberculin solution and prevents its adsorption on glass and plastic. Nonstabilized tuberculin solution stored in glass containers and subsequently taken into glass or plastic syringes loses most of its potency within hours to weeks after preparation.[318–321] The larger the surface area to which the test material is exposed the more adsorption will occur, with proportional loss of potency.[321] One can only conclude from these reports that nonstabilized tuberculin solution is unreliable, and that only material that has been stabilized with Tween 80 (5 ppm) should be used to determine a patient's reactivity to tuberculin.

False-negative reactions to tuberculin may also be caused by a patient's diminished immunologic response. Patients infected with *M. tuberculosis* show negative reactions during the 3 to 9 weeks of incubation while the cell-mediated delayed hypersensitivity is developing. Various acute exanthemata, particularly measles, transiently depress the tuberculin reaction; a more permanent diminution or loss of delayed skin hypersensitivity may occur in sarcoidosis, lymphoma, chronic leukemia, amyloidosis, syphilis, hypothyroidism, and advanced carcinoma.[323] In addition, corticosteroids may render previously positive reactors negative.

In addition to the well-documented diminution or disappearance of a positive reaction related to certain acute and chronic diseases, it is generally accepted that reaction to tuberculin may wane with advancing age and may decrease or disappear with the treatment of the infection in its earliest stages.[303, 304, 306, 307, 325] "Waning" may not be the correct term to explain a loss of skin sensitivity with advancing years, since in one study it was concluded that it was not a gradual reduction but an "all or none phenomenon," the proportion of patients with anergy increasing with each decade.[324] Detection of the disease in the earliest stages of infection requires documentation of the patient's conversion from negative to positive tuberculin reaction. It is obvious that the development of delayed skin hypersensitivity is contingent upon the use of equally potent material for sequential Mantoux testing.[318] A *bona fide* tuberculin converter is one whose skin test has changed from negative to positive but whose chest roentgenogram has remained normal and whose sputum is negative on culture.[326] Documentation by serial testing is essential; it has been conclusively shown that acceptance of a patient's recollection of a previous skin test is unreliable.[327] Atuk and Hunt[328] described the effect of a year's treatment with isoniazid in the reaction to intermediate strength PPD in 20 tuberculin converters. Ten reverted to negative reactions, in five the diameter of induration decreased, and the remainder were unchanged after treatment.

In contrast to the loss of sensitivity to tuberculin that may occur with aging or with treatment of early disease, an occasional patient may show enhanced reaction associated with repeated Mantoux testing. The potential error in calling a test negative when the induration measures 5 mm or less is revealed by this phenomenon, since the booster effects of subsequent tuberculin testing may produce a positive reaction of 10 or more mm and lead to the assumption that tuberculosis has developed.[303, 329, 330] In the study by Thompson and associates,[331] boosting occurred as early as 1 week after an initial tuberculin test, rarely before that time; it occurred in all age groups although the incidence increased with age. The booster reaction is believed to reflect a remote tuberculous infection or a recent or remote sensitization by one or more of the nontuberculous mycobacteria. Its importance lies particularly in the detection of tuberculin converters in hospital infection control programs. It has been recommended[331] that a second identical skin test be given 1 week after the first, so that true conversion in serial testing can be differentiated from the booster phenomenon. Following such guidelines, a group of investigators in Alabama obtained a booster rate of 8.3 per cent;[332] by contrast, a pilot project involving testing of 416 new young employees in Rochester, New York (a nonendemic area for nontuberculous mycobacterial infection) revealed a complete absence of booster reactions.[333]

Delayed skin hypersensitivity to tuberculin is a measure of cell-mediated immunity. Other indices of cell-mediated immunity include one of particular importance in relation to the tuberculin reaction: the development *in vitro* of lymphocyte transformation (blastogenesis) using tuberculin to stimulate lymphocytes in culture.[330, 334, 335] Comparison of the lymphocyte response to tuberculin antigen from various mycobacterial species usually shows agreement with the results of skin tests.[334, 336, 337] Miller and Jones,[330] who determined the degree of delayed hypersensitivity to tuberculin PPD by sequential skin testing with first, intermediate, and second strength PPD and simultaneously challenged the subjects' lymphocytes maximally with PPD *in vitro*, found the minimal strength of tuberculin required to detect skin test sensitivity linearly related to the logarithm of the lymphocyte transformation index. The results of this study cast some doubt on the validity of assuming that induration of less than 10 mm is not specific: the occurrence of some degree of lymphocyte transformation in subjects nonreactive to the three strengths of tuberculin suggests that most skin test reactions, regardless of size, have an *in vitro* immunologic correlate. In Smith and Reichman's study[335] of *in vitro* lymphocyte transformation to PPD in patients who failed to react to intradermal PPD, six of the seven later became reactive to PPD 19 days to 3 months after *in vitro* transformation was first observed, suggesting that lymphocyte transformation may be a more sensitive and reliable method of determining tuberculous infection. These studies, as well as those of others,[307] indicate that most reactions of less than 10 mm in diameter are specific in persons who are acquiring or losing a greater degree of sensitivity to tuberculin. Kane and MacVandiviere,[338] who infected guinea pigs with various strains of mycobacteria and skin-tested them with 5 TU PPD 6 to 8 weeks after infection, stated that about 50 per cent of cases would have been missed if the criterion of a positive reaction to PPD-S was a diameter of induration of at least 10 mm.

Of prime importance in any consideration of tuberculin testing is the situation of patients whose sputum grows *M. tuberculosis* but whose tuberculin skin test is negative. Data accumulated by workers at Maybury Sanatorium in Northville, Michigan[339, 340] have thrown considerable light on this problem. Using the same batch of OT for 20 years, they found that an average of 92 per cent of patients reacted to 1/10,000 or 1/1000 OT with little variation from year to year. In their experience, most nonreactors to tuberculin were critically ill, having cavitation and evidencing recent spread of disease, with large numbers of organisms in their sputum; roentgenograms usually showed "exudation" and postmortem examination an acute exudative reaction. The cavitation, however, indicated that these persons must have been sensitive to tuberculin at one time, the loss of sensitivity leading to a reaction not necrotic or granulomatous but similar to that expected in pneumococcal pneumonia. Other investigators have shown that negative reactions to 5 TU of stable PPD (treated with Tween 80 to prevent adsorption) may occur in cases of relatively mild infection with positive sputum culture.[302, 311, 314, 320] An incidence of 10 to 17 per cent of this phenomenon has been reported in unselected series; unfortunately, serial tuberculin testing, which would reveal whether true sensitivity was developing or the patients were basically anergic, was not carried out.

Cross-reactions to mycobacterial PPD occur between antigenically related strains. A patient reacting to PPD-S, particularly in the doubtful range (5 mm), may have an atypical mycobacterial infection, in which case simultaneous testing with atypical mycobacterial antigens may be of value.[303, 341] Patients with a larger reaction to PPD-S than to atypical mycobacterial PPD are much more likely to have tuberculosis, especially if induration exceeds 10 mm in diameter. In a follow-up study of 1 million United States naval recruits who had been skin tested on enlistment,[310] by far the highest percentage of individuals in whom active disease developed had larger PPD-S than PPD-B or PPD-G reactions. However, the contrary does not hold true: many patients whose cultures are positive for atypical organisms manifest stronger reactions to PPD-S than to atypical mycobacterial PPD.[341, 342]

The skin test for tularemia is the intradermal injection of antibody that causes a reaction within 5 days of the onset of disease. This test is sensitive and specific for tularemia. Half of all patients with clinical tularemia have positive skin test reactions the day they present to the physician. It is a delayed hypersensitivity reaction read after 48 hours and can be administered easily and read at the bedside. It rarely causes a rise in antibody titer and, once positive, may remain so for as long as 4 years, even after the agglutination test has become negative.[343] Skin tests using Brucellin or Brucellergen in the diagnosis of infections due to *B. melitensis* do not reflect the degree of activity of the infection and may stimulate the formation of agglutinins. Such a test is of limited value in the rare case of pulmonary disease suspected of being due to this organism; if it is to be used, the agglutination test should be performed first. Skin tests for fungus infections aid in the diagnosis of histoplasmosis and coccidioido-

mycosis but not blastomycosis.[344] A strong argument can be made for avoiding histoplasmin intradermal skin testing in adults suspected of having active histoplasmosis. Intradermal injection of histoplasmin can increase circulating antibodies,[345, 346] although complement-fixing antibody titers seldom rise above one sixteenth.[281] If blood is drawn at the same time as or within 4 days of skin testing, a spurious rise in antibody titer will not have had time to develop. On the other hand, the first serologic tests frequently show equivocal values and repeat tests are required to ascertain activity; skin testing may thus interfere with the interpretation of serial rises in antibody titers. The yeast phase antigen is much less likely to cause a rise in serum antibodies when given intradermally.

In patients with coccidioidomycosis, sensitivity is determined by intradermal injection of antigen from lysates of the mycelial (coccidioidin) or spherule form (spherulin); both are highly specific but neither appears useful in disseminated disease. A skin test with coccidioidin has the same significance as the tuberculin reaction, becoming positive 3 to 4 weeks after infection and 12 to 20 days after the onset of clinical illness.[278] Spherulin appears to be just as specific but more sensitive than coccidioidin.[347, 348] In one study, 32 per cent more reactors were detected with spherulin.[347] However, follow-up of the patients who reacted to spherulin but not initially to coccidioidin showed the subsequent development of sensitivity to the latter, and it was concluded that latent sensitivity to this agent can be made apparent by reaction to spherulin.[347] Highly specific skin tests have been described in patients with paracoccidioidomycosis and sporotrichosis,[278] but because of the high incidence of false positive and false negative reactions, North American blastomycosis cannot be detected by skin testing.

Skin tests in patients with parasitic infestation produce varied reactions. In trichinosis, the injection of an antigen prepared from extracts of ground dry trichinae produces an immediate reaction if administered after the third week of illness. Both immediate and delayed reactions occur when the Casoni test is performed in cases of hydatid disease. Skin tests are of value in diagnosing filariasis and toxoplasmosis, although positive results may not be obtained in the latter disease until several months after onset.

BIOCHEMICAL TESTS

Sputum

Biochemical analysis of bronchopulmonary secretions has not received much attention as a diagnostic procedure. Burgi and colleagues[349] have advocated the analysis of lactic dehydrogenase (LDH) activity and semiquantification of deoxyribonucleic acid (DNA) by fluorescence microscopy as indicators of an active flare-up of infection in chronic bronchitis.

Pleural Fluid

Pleural fluid should be examined for cellular content, and aliquots should be sent to bacteriology, pathology, and biochemistry laboratories. The cytology, both malignant and benign, is considered in Chapter 2 (*see* page 354)

PROTEIN CONTENT

The terms *transudate* and *exudate* are still used in relation to pleural effusion, but the present tendency is to group effusions according to protein content rather than to specific gravity. Carr and Power,[350] who summarized 4 years of experience at the Mayo Clinic, concluded that the protein concentration almost always differentiates transudates of congestive heart failure from exudates due to cancer or tuberculosis: 84 per cent of 43 specimens of pleural fluid attributable to congestive heart failure contained less than 3.0 grams of protein per dl of fluid, whereas 92.8 per cent of 167 effusions due to cancer and all 20 tuberculous effusions had more than 3.0 grams per dl. In most cases, pleural fluid associated with hepatic cirrhosis was low in protein, whereas that due to pulmonary infarction, pneumonia, and lupus erythematosus had the higher protein concentration of an exudate.

In a prospective study of 150 pleural effusions, Light and associates[351] described a more elaborate attempt to separate transudates from exudates. Employing diagnostic criteria based on clinical presentation, they classified 47 effusions as transudates and 103 as exudates. Biochemically, there were three differentiating characteristics: (1) a fluid-to-serum protein ratio greater than 0.5; (2) pleural fluid LDH greater than 200 IU; and (3) a fluid-to-serum LDH ratio greater than 0.6. All but one of the clinically diagnosed exudates had at least one of these characteristics, whereas only one transudate had any. These investigators concluded that the simultaneous use of both protein and LDH levels in pleural fluid analysis permits better differentiation of transudates from exudates than does use of just one.

GLUCOSE CONTENT

The significance of the glucose concentration in pleural fluid is controversial. Glenert,[352] who examined 50 effusions, concluded that the glucose content does not reflect the diagnosis and is no lower in tuberculosis than in other conditions. In one study in which pleural effusions were divided to transudates and exudates on the basis of clinical evidence of etiology,[353] all but one transudate had pleural fluid glucose levels exceeding 95 mg per dl. Mean values for tuberculosis and neoplastic exudates also were within the normal range (81.7 and 109 mg, respectively), and glucose levels in four neoplastic effusions and three tuberculosis exudates were below 60 mg. Several investigators have reported very low glucose concentrations in pleural effusion secondary to tuberculosis[354] and rheumatoid arthritis,[353, 355–357] and it is probable that values below 26 mg per dl usually indicate one of these diseases. In an analysis of 76 effusions associated with rheumatoid arthritis,[358] 78 per cent had glucose levels less than 30 mg per dl. However, very low glucose content in neoplastic pleural effusions also has been reported: for example, it was less than 25 mg per dl in 8 of 88 malignant pleural effusions analyzed by Berger and Maher.[359] Low glucose values in neoplastic pleural effusions have been correlated with very large collections of fluid.[353, 359] The glucose level may be lower in empyema fluid than in the serum.[352, 360, 361] It may be useful to determine the glucose content of a further specimen of pleural fluid after giving a glucose meal, since it is said that ingested glucose increases the very low values often found in tuberculosis[362] but not those associated with rheumatoid arthritis.[363]

pH OF PLEURAL FLUID

The determination of the pH of pleural fluid is undoubtedly multifactorial. Acid can be produced in the pleural fluid or in the pleural membranes by the action of bacteria and leukocytes on glucose (with the production of CO_2 and lactate) and by direct production by tumor cells and red blood cells. Probably a more important contributor to acid-base balance is the state of the serosal membrane which, when thickened, tends to block the efflux of H^+. Pleural fluid does not have the buffering capacity of blood so that small changes in H^+ concentration are more apparent.[364] In a study of 183 patients with simultaneous blood and pleural fluid pH determination, Good and his colleagues[364] found all 36 transudates to have a pH above 7.30; 46 of 147 pleural fluid exudates had a pH of less than 7.30 in the presence of a normal blood pH. These 46 patients without acidemia and with pleural fluid acidosis had empyema, malignancy, collagen-vascular disease, hemothorax, tuberculosis, or esophageal rupture; the lowest observed pH (6.00) occurred in a patient with esophageal rupture, presumably as a result of contamination of the pleural fluid by gastric juice. The measurement of pH (H^+) may be helpful in distinguishing nonmalignant from malignant effusions,[365] particularly those caused by tuberculosis and neoplasm.[366] Light and associates found that a pH below 7.30 was highly suggestive of tuberculosis, whereas values greater than 7.40 usually indicated malignancy; however, when neoplastic effusions had been present for some time, pH values tended to fall, presumably as a result of thickening of the pleural membrane that caused an efflux block of H^+.[366] These workers also found that pH levels of pleural effusions associated with pneumonia but not grossly purulent can help in deciding the mode of therapy, particularly the need for tube drainage: complete resolution of the effusions was achieved with antibiotic therapy alone in all 19 patients with a pH greater than 7.20, whereas no improvement resulted from antibiotics and thoracentesis in the 5 patients with effusions with a pH of less than 7.20.

FAT CONTENT

Chylothorax should be suspected when the gross appearance of the effusion is cloudy or milky. The fat content exceeds 400 mg per dl, and the protein content is almost invariably greater than 3 grams per dl. In some cases effusions due to tuberculosis and rheumatoid disease contain cholesterol and may resemble chylothorax.[368]

OTHER BIOCHEMICALS IN PLEURAL EFFUSION

Pleural effusion, usually left-sided and sometimes hemorrhagic,[369–371] is present in 5 to 15 per cent of patients with acute pancreatitis.[353] Kaye[372] found elevated amylase values in 37 of 38 cases of pleural effusion associated with pancreatitis, and Light and Ball[353] found high values in all their five cases. The amylase content is greater in the pleural effusion than in blood serum in patients with esophageal perforation;[373] a study with polyacrylamide gel electrophoresis indicated that saliva is the major source of amylase in this disorder.[374]

Reduced pleural fluid complement has been reported in lupus erythematosus and rheumatoid arthritis,[375] suggesting that immune mechanisms may contribute to the development of pleuritis in these disorders. A high level of hyaluronic acid in pleural fluid suggests the diagnosis of mesothelioma.[376, 377] Some workers find pleural fluid levels of lysozyme (as well as pleural fluid-to-blood ratios of this enzyme) helpful in identifying empyema and tuberculous pleural effusion.[378]

Other diagnostic procedures that are not strictly biochemical in nature but have been advocated in pleural fluid analysis include counterimmunoelectrophoresis (CIE) (particularly useful in pneumococcal and *H. influenzae* pneumonias),[379–381] DNA analysis by automated flow cytometry to distinguish malignant from benign cells,[382] gas liquid chromatography to detect fatty acids produced by anaerobic organisms,[383] and prostaglandin-E as a marker for exudates.[384] The last two of these tests are currently more of academic interest than of practical value.

The characteristics of pleural effusions of different etiologies are summarized in Table 3–5.

Blood Serum

Since pulmonary involvement may be only part of a generalized disease, and since chronic processes in the lungs are often secondary to some other illness, many biochemistry procedures can be useful in determining the etiology of roentgenographic abnormalities. Specific tests proved to be of value are considered in the various chapters that deal with individual disease entities.

HEMATOLOGIC PROCEDURES IN PULMONARY DISEASE

Polycythemia frequently but not invariably occurs in association with chronic hypoxemia in pulmonary disease. In some patients who have endured long periods of hypoxemia and whose blood shows normal values for hematocrit and hemoglobin, the red cell mass is actually increased but is not recognized as such because of a simultaneous increase in plasma volume. In such circumstances determination of the blood volume reveals an absolute polycythemia.

Anemia is uncommon in lung disease. It may develop with a chronic infectious process or widespread malignancy, and in some cases of pulmonary hemosiderosis anemia may be noted even before the patient expectorates blood; in the last condition, anemia in a patient whose roentgenogram shows a diffuse acinar pattern may constitute an important diagnostic pointer.

The kidneys, and to a lesser extent other organs (particularly the liver and spleen), produce erythropoietin in response to hypoxia; the intraerythrocytic level of 2,3-diphosphoglycerate (DPG) increases and the oxygen dissociation curve shifts to the right. Initially, however, in acute hypoxia with respiratory alkalosis there is an opposite effect on hemoglobin-oxygen equilibrium, oxygen affinity increasing. In normal volunteers exposed to high altitude hypoxemia, Miller and associates[385] showed that this increased red cell-oxygen affinity is associated with increased urinary and serum erythropoietin. Treatment of these volunteers with acetazolamide prevented the initial respiratory alkalosis and reduced erythropoietin response; but when the hypoxia lasted more than 12 hours, 2,3-DPG levels continued to rise, counterbalancing the effect of alkalosis on oxygen affinity and leading to a prompt return of erythropoietin level to normal.

Variations in the total and differential leukocyte count may play a major role in the differential diagnosis of lung disease (see Tables 3–2, 3–3, and 3–4). A leukocytosis of over 15,000 white cells per mm^3, with a predominance of polymorphonuclear cells, is strong evidence for bacterial rather than viral pneumonia. It must be remembered, however, that fulminating bacterial pneumonia may be associated with normal or even low white cell counts. In volunteers inoculated with several viruses, Douglas and associates[386] found a leukocyte response only in those in whom symptoms developed. This response consisted of an early increase in neutrophils and decrease in lymphocytes, with reversal of these findings later in the illness. A precipitous decrease

Table 3–5. Characteristics of Pleural Effusions of Different Etiology

	TRANSUDATE	MALIGNANCY	TUBERCULOSIS	NONTUBERCULOUS PARAPNEUMONIC	RHEUMATOID DISEASE
Clinical	Signs and symptoms of congestive heart failure, cirrhosis, or nephrosis (hypoproteinemia)	Older patient; poor health prior to effusion; known primary malignancy	Younger patient, good health prior effusion; known exposure	Signs and symptoms of respiratory infection	History of arthritis ± subcutaneous rheumatoid nodules ±
Gross Appearance	Clear, straw-colored ("serous")	Serous → often sanguineous	Serous → occasionally sanguineous	Serous → sanguineous turbid (pus)	Serous → turbid or yellow-green
Microscopic Examination	0	Cytology positive, 40–87% higher with multiple samples, cell block + smears	Positive for acid-fast bacilli 30–70%; cholesterol crystals	May or may not be + for organisms	0
Cell Count + Differential	85% RBC count < 10,000 mm³; majority WBC count < 1000 mm³	40% > 100,000 RBC/mm³; WBC 1000 to 10,000, usually mononuclears predominant	In majority small lymphocytes predominant. Polymorphonuclear leukocytes may predominate initially. Rarely > 5% mesothelial cells	Polymorphonuclear predominant; 10,000/mm³ and left shift	Mononuclear cells predominant
Culture	0	0	Positive 10–70%; 10–15% sputum +/or gastric washings +	May or may not be positive	0
Protein	75% < 3 gm; pleural fluid/serum protein ratio > 0.5	90% > 3 gm; pleural fluid/serum protein ratio > 0.5	90% > 3 gm; pleural fluid/serum protein ratio > 0.5	> 3 gm; pleural fluid/serum protein ratio > 0.5	> 3 gm; pleural fluid/serum protein ratio > 0.5
Lactic Acid Dehydrogenase (LDH)	Pleural fluid/serum LDH ratio > 0.6	Pleural fluid/serum LDH ratio > 0.6	Pleural fluid/serum LDH ratio > 0.6	Pleural fluid/serum LDH ratio > 0.6; LDH level greater than 1000 IU/ml suggests complicated effusion (empyema)	Pleural fluid/serum LDH ratio > 0.6
Glucose	> 60 mg/dl	May be < 60 mg/dl; lower levels associated with poor prognosis	May be < 60 mg/dl	May be < 60 mg/dl; lower levels suggest complicated effusion (empyema)	83% < 50 mg/dl; 63% < 20 mg/dl
pH	Equal to or higher than blood pH	15% have pH < 7.20; low pH associated with poor prognosis	May be less than 7.20	May be < 7.20; lower pH suggests complicated pleural effusion (empyema)	May be < 7.20
Other	More common with right-sided heart failure	Pleural biopsy + in up to 75%	Tuberculin skin test usually positive. Adenosine deaminase levels > 30 IU/l may be specific. Pleural biopsy + for granuloma in up to 80%	Foul-smelling fluid with anaerobic organisms	Reduced complement; high rheumatoid factor (higher than serum titer); may have high cholesterol level

Table continued on opposite page

Table 3–5. Characteristics of Pleural Effusions of Different Etiology *Continued*

SYSTEMIC LUPUS ERYTHEMATOSUS	PULMONARY EMBOLISM	FUNGAL INFECTION	TRAUMATIC	CHYLOUS	CHYLIFORM
Known SLE ± young women	Predisposing factors: postoperative, immobilized, venous disease	Exposure in endemic area	History of trauma—fractured ribs	History of trauma (25%) or malignancy (50%)	Usually chronic effusions
Serous → occasionally sanguineous	Serous → often sanguineous	Serous → occasionally sanguineous	Sanguineous	Turbid whitish; turbid supernatant with centrifugation, does not clear with ethyl alcohol	Turbid whitish; turbid supernatant with centrifugation, clears with ethyl alcohol
0	0	May or may not be + for organisms	0	Fat droplets	Cholesterol crystals
Mononuclear or polymorphonuclear cells predominant	Mononuclear or polymorphonuclear cells predominant; RBC < 10,000 in 30%, RBC > 100,000 in 20%	Mononuclear or polymorphonuclear cells predominant	RBC predominant	Mononuclear cells predominant	Variable
0	0	May or may not be positive	0	0	0
> 3 gm; pleural fluid/serum protein ratio > 0.5	> 3 gm; pleural fluid/serum protein ratio > 0.5	> 3 gm; pleural fluid/serum protein ratio > 0.5	> 3 gm; pleural fluid/serum protein ratio > 0.5	> 3 gm; pleural fluid/serum protein ratio > 0.5	> 3 gm; pleural fluid/serum protein ratio > 0.5
Pleural fluid/serum LDH ratio > 0.6	Pleural fluid/serum LDH ratio > 0.6	Pleural fluid/serum LDH ratio > 0.6	Pleural fluid/serum LDH ratio > 0.6	Pleural fluid/serum LDH ratio > 0.6	Pleural fluid/serum LDH ratio > 0.6
> 60 mg/dl	> 60 mg/dl	> 60 mg/dl	> 60 mg/dl	> 60 mg/dl	May be < 60 mg/dl depending on etiology
> 7.20	> 7.20	?	May be < 7.20 with hemothorax	> 7.20	May be < 7.20 depending on etiology
Reduced complement detectable; antinuclear antibody and LE cells	Source of emboli may or may not be apparent, but venogram or impedance plethysmography usually positive	Skin and serologic tests may be helpful. Sulfur granules with actinomycosis	—	Pleural fluid triglyceride usually > 110 mg/dl	—

in total leukocyte count in peripheral blood has been found to correlate with the subsequent development of adult respiratory distress syndrome in patients at risk for this disorder. When the differential count shows eosinophilia, the diagnostic possibilities are limited: bronchial asthma, drug reactions, parasitic infestations, collagen diseases, and sometimes rarer causes, such as Hodgkin's disease, sarcoidosis, and mycotic infections.

The culture of bone marrow aspirate sometimes aids in the diagnosis of chronic infections, and the detection of malignant cells in the bone marrow may establish the nature of roentgenographically apparent pulmonary lesions.

Some researchers have found the *in vitro* reduction of nitroblue tetrazolium by neutrophils a useful indicator of bacterial infection;[387, 388] others, however, have found this test considerably less valuable than the leukocyte and differential count and other hematologic indices of infection.[389] In some hands results obtained in healthy subjects and in patients with diseases other than pyogenic infection, both microbial and nonmicrobial, have shown considerable overlap.[390, 391]

ELECTROCARDIOGRAPHY

An electrocardiogram is of fundamental importance in differentiating myocardial infarction from acute massive pulmonary embolism. It is also useful in indicating lung disease as a cause of heart failure in patients who might otherwise be considered to be suffering from coronary artery insufficiency or myocardial disease. The electrocardiographic abnormalities of diffuse lung disease[392] must be familiar to the physician specializing in this field and are reviewed in relation to cor pulmonale and pulmonary hypertension (*see* Chapter 10).

PULMONARY FUNCTION TESTS

Pulmonary function tests can play a useful role in detecting respiratory disease, in leading to a definitive diagnosis when correlated with clinical and roentgenologic findings, and in managing various pulmonary disorders through sequential objective assessment of the degree of dysfunction. Methods used for assessing pulmonary function range from simple, standardized techniques that can be performed rapidly and accurately on large groups of subjects to detailed methods for measuring disturbed respiratory physiology that are time-consuming and require sophisticated instrumentation. At one end of this spectrum, spirometry or measurement of peak expiratory flow can be performed by untrained personnel in the office, at the bedside, or in the emergency room; at the other end, the assessment of diaphragmatic muscle function may require insertion of gastric and esophageal cathe-

ters, the measurement of respiratory muscle electromyograms, and even phrenic nerve stimulation. These procedures require sophisticated recording devices and considerable technical skill. The more detailed methods that elucidate respiratory pathophysiologic abnormalities are less readily available and often represent some of the "fringe" benefits in pulmonary research centers.

The choice of which tests should be performed in a given setting depends on the purpose of the study. Indications for respiratory function tests can be broadly categorized as (1) resolving whether symptoms and signs such as dyspnea, cough, cyanosis, and polycythemia are of respiratory origin; (2) managing and following the progression of disease or response to therapy in patients with recognized pulmonary disorders; (3) assessing the risk for the development of pulmonary dysfunction and complications resulting from therapeutic interventions such as operative procedures and drugs; (4) quantifying the degree of disability in environmental or occupational lung disease; and (5) carrying out epidemiologic surveys of population groups suspected of having acquired pulmonary disease as a result of exposure to dusts or fumes.

The assessment of pulmonary function can be conveniently divided into three levels of increasing sophistication. The *first level* includes the measurement of vital capacity and maximal expiratory flow rates and an assessment of the gas-exchanging ability of the lungs by measurement of arterial blood gas tensions. Spirometry measures the forced expiratory volume in one second (FEV_1), the forced vital capacity (FVC), the ratio of FEV_1/FVC, and the peak expiratory flow (PEF). Spirometry and PEF can be readily measured with recently developed simple, inexpensive, and portable devices. Their use has been advocated as an integral part of the physical examination of adult patients and has been suggested as a means of "preventive medicine."[393] Spirometry can now be consideed as integral a part of the clinical assessment of a patient with suspected lung disease as is measurement of blood pressure in patients with cardiovascular disease. Arterial blood gas tensions can also be considered as a first line test in the assessment of respiratory dysfunction, and properly performed and interpreted tests yield valuable information regarding pulmonary and metabolic status.

The *second level* of investigation of altered lung function includes the subdivisions of lung volume and an estimate of the diffusing capacity of the lung. Measurements of functional residual capacity (FRC), total lung capacity (TLC), and residual volume (RV) using the helium dilution technique can be performed with a number of recently developed units, as can steady state or single breath diffusing capacity; coupled with spirometry and blood gas determination, these serve as the basic "screening tests" of lung function in most major hospitals.[394]

Following these tests, if doubt still exists about the nature and severity of a pulmonary disorder, a variety of *third level* procedures may be employed. More detailed description of altered lung mechanics can be obtained with measurements of airway and pulmonary resistance and the pressure-volume relationship of the lung. Respiratory control can be assessed with the ventilatory responses to O_2 and CO_2 and measurements of inspiratory and expiratory muscle strength. Quantitative and qualitative descriptions of the distribution of ventilation and perfusion can be made with radioactive gases and aerosols. The clinical usefulness of measuring nonspecific bronchial reactivity has been amply demonstrated and serves both as a means of diagnosing "reactive airway disease" and quantifying its severity and progression.

Since dyspnea on exertion is a major complaint of patients with respiratory disease, it is appropriate to study the physiology of such patients while they are exercising; circuits are now commercially available that allow measurement of workload, ventilation, O_2 uptake, CO_2 production, and the cardiovascular response to exercise. Such measurements of exercise performance also serve as an excellent objective measurement of disability.

Whatever the level, lung function tests must be interpreted and correlated with clinical and roentgenologic data to be valid. Without this added information, the interpretation of pulmonary function tests shows wide variability among individual readers.[395]

SMALL AIRWAY TESTS

Since the study of Hogg and his colleagues,[396] which showed that the major site of increased resistance in chronic obstructive pulmonary disease (COPD) is the small airways, and that of Macklem and Mead,[397] which indicated that small airways normally represent a small fraction of total airway resistance, there has been considerable research interest in the development of screening tests to detect early abnormalities of small airway function. The basic hypothesis behind these efforts is that mild small airway abnormalities undetected by conventional measurements may be the harbinger of eventual symptomatic air flow limitation.[398] The single breath nitrogen washout curve, the density dependence of maximal expiratory flow measured using a helium-oxygen mixture, and measurements of air flow at low lung volumes have all been evaluated as potential tests to detect preclinical small airway pathology. Epidemiologic studies have shown that these tests are abnormal in an appreciable number of asymptomatic smokers,[399, 400] and at the last writing of this book it was the hope that these abnormalities might allow detection of early lung dysfunction and the institution of appropriate measures to prevent progression to advanced disease.[401] Although controversy still exists regarding the value of such screening,[393, 402] it appears that the

tests may not offer advantages over simple spirometry in detecting the progression of air flow obstruction.[403, 404] One reason that small airway tests have been less discriminating than was originally hoped in identifying smokers at risk of developing progressive disease is the marked inter- and intrasubject variability in test results.[405–407] It has not been convincingly shown that the rate of decrease in forced expiratory flow in smokers correlates with abnormalities of small airway function. In summary, at present the status of "small airway tests" does not warrant their institution as routine screening procedures for the identification of patients at risk of developing COPD.

PREDICTED NORMAL VALUES OF PULMONARY FUNCTION

Interpretation of the results of pulmonary function tests is based on the degree of deviation from predicted normal values calculated from regression equations that take into account known attributes that contribute to variations of lung function. These include age, sex, height, weight, and race. A wide range of scatter among "normals" is related to genetic and environmental factors, the contribution of which has been investigated by comparing measurements of lung function in monozygotic and dizogotic twins.[408, 409] These studies suggest that both heredity and the pre- and postnatal environment influence baseline lung function, and that the response to injurious agents like cigarette smoke may in part be genetically determined.

The decision whether a measurement of lung function in an individual is abnormal is often difficult; it depends not only on the variability in a normal population of the parameter measured but also on the variability of the test itself. Although it is often advocated that lung function tests should be considered abnormal only when the value deviates by 20 or more per cent from the mean normal value, this approach is simplistic and can be misleading.[410] The definition of a normal range for a test should be constructed by calculating 95 per cent confidence limits (2 × standard error of the estimate). The commonly used +20 per cent approach assumes that the variation increases as the value increases, thus overestimating the actual variation between subjects with large lung volumes or flow rates and underestimating the variation in subjects with small volumes or flow rates.[411, 412] Ninety-five per cent confidence intervals are now available for many parameters of lung function and with computer-derived report forms can provide individualized normal ranges. The interindividual variation of lung function differs greatly between tests: for example, in a normal population the FEV_1/FVC ratio has a narrow 95 per cent confidence limit whereas the forced expiratory flow ($FEF_{25–75}$) and highly effort-dependent measurements such as maximal inspiratory and expiratory pressure have much larger limits.

Prediction equations for lung function are often inaccurate at the extremes of age—for older individuals because smaller samples of normal subjects have been examined, and for younger individuals as a result of the complex changes in lung function that occur at the interface of maturation and aging. Although most lung function variables reach their optimal value in early adult life and then decline, the age-related decline does not begin at the same age for all parameters, making the calculation of predicted normal values by backward or forward extrapolation inaccurate in young adults.[413]

The influence of weight can also be a confounding variable when included in prediction equations: in young, growing individuals, increased body weight is associated with large volumes and flows as a result of increasing respiratory muscle strength, but in later life it may be associated with decreasing lung function owing to "obesity effects."[414] For the same reasons the influence of weight may be different in tall versus short people.[415] Ethnic variations in static and dynamic lung function must also be taken into account, and normal standards for each measurement must be obtained on the population concerned.[414, 416–421] Many of the earlier prediction formulas were derived from populations that included a substantial number of smokers, but more recent studies have recognized the subtle alterations in lung function that occur in smokers, and in this group prediction equations and 95 per cent confidence limits are now available for most measurements of lung function. These will be referred to in the individual sections dealing with specific function tests.

Although one use of pulmonary function testing is to compare the values obtained in an individual with those of a normal population, following the progress of a patient over time or assessing response to acute or chronic therapy has the advantage of using the patient's own values as a control, thus permitting greater accuracy in detecting changes in lung function. The detection of a significant change or lack of change in any test over time or in response to an intervention is dependent upon the intrinsic variability of the test. This variability can be measured as the coefficient of variation of repeated tests, defined as a standard deviation of repeated tests divided by the mean. The coefficient of variation varies widely among lung function tests but in general is much narrower than the 95 per cent confidence limits observed in the population.[422] Coefficients of variation for many pulmonary function tests have been determined and will be referenced in the individual sections that follow.

Lung Volumes

Lung volumes and capacities can be appreciated by studying the diagram in Figure 3–1. There are four volumes: (1) *tidal volume* (TV), the amount of gas moved in and out of the lung with each respiratory cycle; (2) *residual volume* (RV), the amount remaining in the lung after maximal expiration and the only volume that cannot be measured directly by spirometry; (3) *inspiratory reserve volume* (IRV), the additional gas that can be inspired from the end of a quiet inspiration; and (4) *expiratory reserve volume* (ERV), the additional amount of gas that can be expired from the resting or end-expiratory level. There are also four capacities, each of which contains two or more volumes: (a) *total lung capacity* (TLC), the gas contained in the lung at the end of maximal inspiration; (b) *vital capacity* (VC), the amount that can be expired after a maximal inspiration or inspired after a maximal expiration; (c) *inspiratory capacity* (IC), the amount of gas that can be inspired from the end of a quiet expiration;

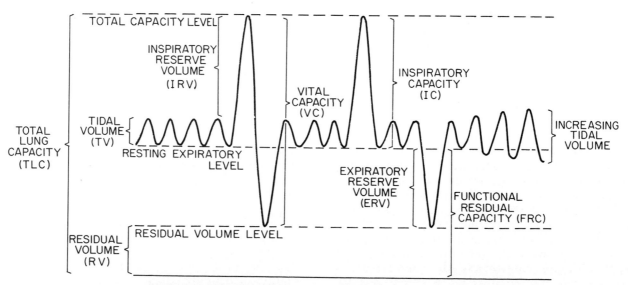

Figure 3–1. Lung Volumes and Capacities. *See* text for description.

and (d) *functional residual capacity* (FRC), the volume of gas remaining in the lung at the end of a quiet expiration.

Vital Capacity (VC)

Although this volume of gas can be measured from the end of maximal expiration to full inspiration (inspiratory vital capacity), it is usually expressed as an amount of air expelled from the lungs after a maximal inspiration (expiratory vital capacity). In fact, the most reported measurement is forced vital capacity (FVC), which is the amount of air that can be exhaled forcefully from the lung after maximal inspiration. In patients with obstructive pulmonary disease, the FVC can be significantly less than an inspired vital capacity by amounts up to 1 liter as a result of dynamic compression of airways and gas trapping on expiration and failure to detect expired volume at low flow rates.[423, 424] VC and FVC are usually measured with spirometers of various design, and predicted normal values with 95 per cent confidence limits based on age, sex, height, and in some instances weight and age are readily available.[411, 415, 425, 426] The VC varies with the position of the patient, being less in the supine than in the erect posture. The VC or FVC serves little purpose as an independent measurement of pulmonary function but can be of much value when considered in conjunction with the results of other tests; it is a simple procedure to perform and is a useful index of day-to-day changes in the clinical status of patients with neuromuscular disease, although in these patients measurements of inspiratory pressure are more sensitive in detecting improvement or deterioration. The subdivisions of VC, particularly IC and IRV, are rarely used in assessing pulmonary function. ERV may be markedly reduced in patients with obesity. TV varies greatly in normal subjects, and this measurement by itself is seldom of much value; however, multiplication of TV by the respiratory rate per minute gives the minute volume, and in some patients alveolar hypoventilation can be suggested by these two indices alone. In addition, analysis of the pattern of generation of the TV can be useful as an indicator of respiratory drive. The ratio of FEV_1/FVC is a much more useful index than the FVC alone and allows separation of patients with ventilatory abnormalities into "restrictive" or "obstructive" patterns: in patients with obstructive pulmonary disease, the FVC is relatively well maintained in relation to the FEV_1, whereas in restrictive disease the FEV_1 may be near normal and the FVC definitely decreased.

Functional Residual Capacity (FRC), Residual Volume (RV), and Total Lung Capacity (TLC)

FRC, the volume of gas in the lungs at the end of a quiet expiration, is determined chiefly by the balance between the outward recoil of the chest wall and the inward recoil of the lung, although both active inspiratory muscle activity during expiration and flow limitation during tidal breathing can increase FRC above this static value. FRC, RV, and TLC can be determined by either inert gas inhalation techniques or body plethysmography. The inert gas techniques include single and multiple breath tests, using a closed circuit and helium or an open circuit and nitrogen as the inert gases. In the open circuit technique, the patient breathes 100 per cent oxygen for 7 minutes and all expired gas is collected; FRC is calculated by multiplying the amount of gas expired during this period by the percentage of nitrogen in the expired gas. RV is then determined by subtracting ERV measured with a spirometer from the calculated FRC, and TLC is determined by adding IC to FRC. With the closed circuit method, the patient breathes from a spirometer of known volume containing helium of known concentration. At the beginning of the study, helium concentration in the lungs is zero; as the patient breathes in and out of the spirometer, the gas mixes between spirometer and lungs until the concentration of helium is the same in both. FRC is calculated from the concentration of helium before and at the end of study and the known volume of the spirometer.

$$FRC = \frac{\text{Spirometer volume} \times \text{initial He concentration}}{\text{Final He concentration}}$$

Again, RV and TLC are calculated by subtracting ERV and adding IC respectively. Both the closed circuit helium and open circuit nitrogen techniques are subject to error because they do not detect trapped gas which does not communicate with the tracheobronchial tree; they can seriously underestimate FRC, particularly in patients with obstructive lung disease, emphysematous bullae, or other intrathoracic noncommunicating accumulations of gas. In addition, they are time-consuming and repeated measurements are difficult to perform.[427] The technique has the advantage that it can be performed on anesthetized or ventilated patients.[428] The inert gas methods can be modified for use as a single breath measurement using either helium or nitrogen, but although these adaptations may be useful for screening purposes in normal subjects, they seriously underestimate FRC in patients with airway obstruction.[411, 429, 430]

The other major method of measuring FRC is based on Boyle's law and employs a body plethysmograph (body box). Boyle's law states that the product of the volume and pressure of gas is constant at constant temperature (V1 × P1 = V2 × P2). To measure FRC plethysmographically, the airway is closed at FRC and the subject pants against the closed airway, thus generating changes in mouth and pleural pressure and small increases and decreases in lung volume due to compression and decompression of thoracic gas. The relationship between changes in thoracic gas volume and mouth or pleural pressure ($\Delta V/\Delta P$) can be calibrated so that intrathoracic volume can be derived and RV and TLC obtained by having the subject perform a vital capacity maneuver immediately after measurement of FRC. The method has the theoretic advantage that all gas subjected to the swings in intrathoracic pressures is measured, whether or not it communicates with the tracheobronchial tree.

Two types of body box are commonly employed, one termed a pressure box in which the changes in thoracic volume during panting are measured by corresponding changes in pressure within the box, the other a constant pressure or volume displacement body plethysmograph in which changes in thoracic volume are measured with a highly sensitive spirometer. Although plethysmographic measurements of FRC have long been considered "the gold standard," recent evidence suggests that accuracy is affected by the pattern of panting and especially by the severity of any accompanying air flow obstruction.[431, 432] An assumption of the plethysmographic techique is that only intrathoracic and not intra-abdominal gas is subjected to swings in pressure; this has been shown to be untrue, since variable abdominal gas compression occurs when panting is accomplished by diaphragmatic or intercostal muscle action.[433, 434] The second assumption implicit in the plethysmographic method for the determination of FRC and recently shown to be erroneous is that swings in mouth pressure accurately reflect swings in alveolar pressure, which compresses and decompresses intrathoracic gas. This may be true in normal subjects, but phase and amplitude differences in alveolar and mouth pressure swings can occur as a result of a combination of intrathoracic airway narrowing and an extrathoracic compliant trachea or oral cavity; this artifact can lead to an overestimation of the true intrathoracic gas volume,[435, 436] an error that can be diminished by using intraesophageal instead of mouth pressure to measure FRC.[437-440] In patients with asthma and other obstructive pulmonary diseases, measurements of FRC and TLC provide values significantly lower with esophageal than with mouth pressure, and they are closer to measurements obtained roentgenographically or with the helium dilution technique.[441, 442] The phase and amplitude differences between mouth pressure and changes in thoracic gas volume increase with increasing airflow obstruction[437] and with increasing panting frequency.[442-445] These changes account for a significant proportion of the acute increases in TLC seen in asthmatics in whom bronchoconstriction is induced.[438, 439, 446]

The most accurate measurement of FRC and TLC in severely obstructed patients may be obtained by the plethysmographic method employing esophageal rather than mouth pressure, especially when manual support of the compliant cheeks is employed during panting at low frequency (less than 1 Hz). The measurement of thoracic gas volume by plethysmography is very reproducible, the coefficient of variation in normal subjects being approximately 4 per cent; however, this increases slightly in obstructed patients.[447] The determination of TLC based on PA and lateral chest roentgenograms has been shown to be highly accurate and can be accomplished by experienced workers in less than 5 minutes.[448, 453] Roentgenographic TLC has been shown to correlate closely with the volume of postmortem lungs fixed at 25 cm H_2O distending pressure.[454] Prediction equations for total lung capacity are available.[411, 431] RV increases with age, as does the RV/TLC ratio, but there is little change in FRC or TLC.

RESPIRATORY INDUCTIVE PLETHYSMOGRAPHY

Respiratory inductive plethysmography (RIP) is a recently described technique to measure lung volumes noninvasively.[455] The apparatus consists of coils of wire that are insulated and positioned around the rib cage and abdomen; the coils are oscillated with a high-frequency signal and emit a frequency-modulated signal that is related to the changes in enclosed volume of the rib cage and abdomen. The coils, therefore, give a signal that is proportional to the cross-sectional area enclosed within them, and with various calibration techniques the electrical output from the rib cage and abdominal coils can be summed and equated to volume change measured with a spirometer. The major advantage of RIP is that it can measure volume without the use of a mouthpiece and is thus uninfluenced by behavioral changes that may occur with such an apparatus. A number of studies have shown that the technique is reasonably accurate, although it may be affected by changes in body position.[456-460] RIP can be used for measurements of vital capacity and expiratory flow rates, although its accuracy in dynamic maneuvers is somewhat less than with the spirometer.[461, 462] Although RIP has been used to monitor ventilation during exercise, it has found its main use in studying the pattern of breathing, such as monitoring inhalation patterns during smoking and characterizing apneic periods during sleep.[452, 455]

MEASUREMENT OF FORCED EXPIRATORY VOLUME AND FLOW

The forced expiratory maneuver is the most widely used and standardized test of lung function. Expired volume can be plotted against time (Fig. 3–2) to yield a typical spirogram from which FEV_1, FVC, and FEF_{25-75} (formerly termed the maximal midexpiratory flow rate, or MMFR) can be derived. Expired volume also can be plotted against the instantaneous expiratory flow rate to yield a flow-volume curve (Fig. 3–2). Flow at specific percentages

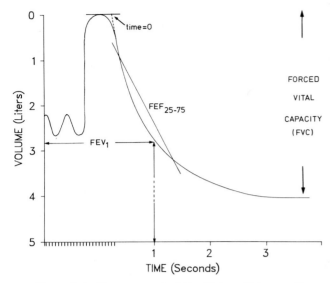

Figure 3–2. Measurement of Ventilatory Volumes. Measurements derived from a maximal forced expiration provide the most readily obtained and useful assessment of lung function. Volume in liters is plotted against time in seconds while the subject forcibly exhales from total lung capacity. The volume versus time slope is back-extrapolated to determine 0 time, and the expired volume in 1 second (FEV_1) is measured and compared with predicted values as well as to the measured forced vital capacity (FVC). The FEV_1/FVC ratio serves as a volume-independent measure of expiratory airflow obstruction. The average flow over the middle half of the forced expiratory volume (FEF_{25-75}) is obtained as the slope of the volume-time plot between 25 and 75 per cent of the FVC.

of the forced expired vital capacity, such as $VMax_{50}$ and $VMax_{25}$, can be determined from the flow-volume curve. While performance of the maximal expiratory flow maneuver is a relatively simple and standardized procedure, interpretation of the abnormalities is more complicated. The determinants of maximal expiratory flow include the elastic recoil properties of the lung, the resistance of the airways, and the compliance or collapsibility of the larger airways where flow limitation occurs.

The interest in forced expiration as a measurement of dynamic lung function stems largely from the fact that it is a relatively effort-independent measurement and is highly reproducible; three to five measurements of forced expiration are usually obtained. A number of methods have been suggested for selecting the best values for FVC, FEV_1, and FEF_{25-75}: (1) choose the forced expiration with the largest sum of FEV_1 and FVC;[463] (2) from three curves, select the largest FEV_1 and FVC even if they are not on the same curve;[412] (3) define FEV_1 and FVC as the mean of the three best of five curves;[464] and (4) construct a composite curve matched at TLC or on the descending slope of the flow-volume curve.[463] Measurement of the FEF_{25-75} is quite sensitive to changes in forced vital capacity, and it is recommended that it be calculated from the curve with the greatest sum of FEV_1 and FVC.[465] Although

the forced expiratory maneuver is effort-independent up to a point, submaximal efforts can result in paradoxically high values for FVC, FEV_1, and FEF_{25-75}, especially in patients with obstructive pulmonary disease.[466] In normal subjects, the FEV_1 and FVC have extremely narrow 95 per cent confidence limits (+5 per cent), but in obstructed patients this increases to approximately 12 per cent when measured on the same day.[422] The 95 per cent confidence limits also increase with longer time periods between measurements, presumably as a result of variability in the flow-measuring device as well as in the subject.[467]

Compared with FVC and FEV_1, there is a much higher coefficient of variation for repeated measurements of FEF_{25-75}, $VMax_{50}$, and $VMax_{25}$,[422, 468–470] a variability that increases with the degree of pulmonary dysfunction.[471] The coefficient of variation for FEF_{25-75} and $VMax_{50}$ for repeated measurements in a normal subject is 21 per cent, increasing as high as 30 per cent in obstructed patients. There is also more variation between individuals for FEF_{25-75} and $Vmax_{50}$ than for FEV_1 and FVC. The 95 per cent confidence limits for FEV_1 and FVC in a population are 21 per cent whereas in order for FEF_{25-75} and $Vmax_{50}$ to be judged abnormal, values should be more than 40 per cent below predicted.[422, 470, 472] The procedure for accurate performance of spirometry is well standardized,[469, 473] and there are excellent prediction equations based on large groups of normal nonsmokers for FEV_1, FVC, $VMax_{50}$, $VMax_{25}$, and FEF_{25-75}.[415, 426]

Bronchodilator Response

Measurements of maximal expiratory flow and volume are frequently used to quantify the reversibility of air flow obstruction in patients. To decide whether a significant improvement has occurred, it is necessary to know the reproducibility of the individual measurements:[422, 474] the 95 per cent confidence limits for acute changes in spirometric variables are 71 per cent for peak expiratory flow rate, 15 per cent for FVC, 12 per cent for FEV_1, 17 per cent for FEV_1/FVC, and 45 per cent for FEF_{25-75}.[474] A beneficial effect of bronchodilators should not be reported unless improvement beyond these limits is observed. The FEV_1 is probably the best single test for assessing bronchodilator response.[475] It is of interest that some patients with reversible bronchoconstriction respond to bronchodilators by showing a predominant increase in their flow rates (ΔFEV_1) whereas others primarily increase their expired volume (ΔFVC), and it is useful to combine the changes in these variables in assessing bronchodilator response.[476] In fact, some patients obtain considerable symptomatic relief from inhaled bronchodilators despite a decrease in the ratio of FEV_1/FVC, making this a poor estimate of bronchodilator response.[477, 478]

Density Dependence of Maximal Expiratory Flow

Maximal expiratory flow increases after patients are equilibrated with a low density gas mixture such as 80 per cent helium/20 per cent oxygen although FVC does not. In normal subjects, the flows increase over most of the vital capacity range, but at a point low in the vital capacity the flow of the two gases becomes equal (volume of isoflow—VisoV). It has been suggested that the increase in flow with the low density He/O_2 mixture and the volume of isoflow are influenced by the predominant site of airway narrowing:[479, 480] gas density has an important influence on resistance in airways where flow is turbulent but does not affect resistance where flow is laminar. Flow in the larger central airways is turbulent but gas flow in small airways is laminar because of their enormous cross-sectional area and low linear flow velocity. The theory predicts that if the major site of air flow limitation is in large airways where a turbulent flow regime exists, breathing the low density He/O_2 will substantially increase expiratory flow rates; by contrast, if the major site of flow limitation is in more peripheral airways where a laminar flow regime exists, He/O_2 will have no effect. The magnitude of the He/O_2 effect can be quantified by calculating the density dependence of maximum expiratory flow (VMax) (see equation at bottom of page). The VisoV is determined by matching the air and He/O_2 flow volume curve at TLC or RV. VMax and VisoV have been advocated as potentially sensitive tests of early small airway obstruction, but a number of clinical studies have questioned their usefulness:[481–483] part of this disenchantment stems from their marked variability and poor reproducibility,[484–487] a major problem that two separate forced expiratory maneuvers must be performed, and the vital capacity of these maneuvers frequently differs significantly. Small differences in VC can create large differences in the calculated $\Delta\dot{V}Max$ and the VisoV, and the results are very dependent upon how the two curves are matched.[488, 489] Use of a composite curve matched at TLC or RV and derived from a number of forced expiratory vital capacities on air and helium has been suggested,[488, 489] but even then the coefficients of variation are large, being greater than 22 per cent for $\Delta\dot{V}Max$ and up to 100 per cent for VisoV.[488, 490] One way to determine the reproducibility and therefore potential sensitivity of a test is to calculate the signal-to-noise ratio, which is the standard deviation of the measurement between individuals divided by the standard deviation of the measurement within an individual on repeated testing: the higher the ratio, the better the test in separating groups or measuring changes in an individual. In one study,[491] the signal-to-noise ratio for FVC was 49; for FEV_1, 26; for peak expiratory flow, 15; for VMax50, 6.5; for $\Delta\dot{V}Max50$, 0.42; for $\Delta\dot{V}Max25$, 0.29; and for VisoV, 0.7.

In addition to these problems with reproducibility and standardization, the basic assumptions underlying the use of density dependence to localize the site of air flow obstruction have been questioned.[492–494] Theoretically, all patients with established COPD in whom the major site of air flow resistance is the small airways should have decreased density dependence; however, a recent clinical study has shown density dependence to be well preserved in many patients despite advanced airflow obstruction.[495] Along with measurements of inspiratory and expiratory flow-volume curves, however, density dependence of maximal expiratory flow can be useful in the diagnosis of significant upper airway obstruction,[496] a subject considered in greater detail in Chapter 11.

Additional Tests of Forced Expiration

With the advent of practical on-line computers, flow, volume, and time signals during forced expiration can be analyzed digitally in the hope of providing additional information about the mechanisms limiting maximal expiratory flow. These include computer averaging of a number of flow-volume curves, measuring the slope ratio on the descending slope of the curve (tangent slope/chord slope at any volume), calculating the total expiratory time, and measuring the area under the maximal expiratory flow–volume curve.[497–501] In addition, partial flow-volume curves consisting of maximal expirations initiated from the end of a normal tidal breath have been suggested for some applications and have the advantage of bypassing the normal bronchodilator effect of a TLC inspiration.[502]

An interesting theoretic approach to the separation of factors limiting maximal expiratory flow is the maximal expiratory flow–elastic recoil curve.[503] As shown in Figure 3–3, the analysis of such a curve can theoretically establish the major contributor to flow limitation. Although prediction equations for normal upstream resistance have been derived, a systematic evaluation of this technique with comparison to pathologic emphysema, airway disease, and large airway abnormalities has not been performed.[503]

MAXIMAL VOLUNTARY VENTILATION (MVV)

MVV is the ventilation that can be achieved with 15 seconds of maximal effort. The test is influenced by the properties of the lung and airways

$$\Delta\dot{V}Max = \frac{\text{Maximal expiratory flow breathing } He/O_2 - \text{Maximal expiratory flow breathing air}}{\text{Maximal expiratory flow breathing air}}$$

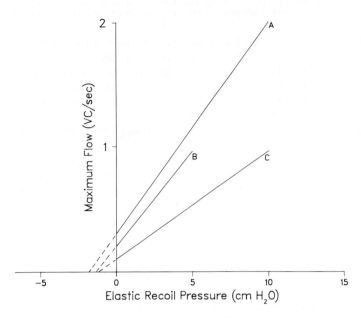

Figure 3–3. Maximal Expiratory Flow/Elastic Recoil Curve. Maximal expiratory flow can be decreased because of decreases in elastic recoil of the lung and/or increases in the resistance upstream from the flow-limiting site: upstream resistance. Theoretically, the importance of these factors can be quantified by construction of a maximal flow–elastic recoil plot. Maximal flow at different lung volumes is plotted against the measured recoil pressure at that lung volume.

Curve *A* in the figure represents a normal relationship. Peak flow reaches approximately 2 vital capacities per second, and flow diminishes as recoil decreases. The slope of the line $\Delta\dot{V}Max/\Delta P$ is upstream conductance. Curve *B* represents the relationship in a patient in whom loss of recoil is the *sole* cause of decreased flow. Maximal flow is decreased to less than half of normal due to decreased recoil pressures, but the conductance ($\Delta\dot{V}Max/\Delta P$) is normal. Curve *C* represents a patient in whom the decrease in flow is *solely* related to a narrowing of the airways and decrease in upstream conductance. The recoil pressures achieved are normal but the flow at any recoil pressure is decreased and the slope $\Delta\dot{V}Max/\Delta P_L$ is decreased.

While this is theoretically useful, we have found that the majority of patients with COPD show decreased flow from a combination of decreased recoil and decreased upstream conductance. Patients with pure emphysema, such as occurs from alpha-1-antitrypsin deficiency, show a curve like *B*.

and correlates with FEV_1, but it is also influenced by inspiratory muscle performance. The expiratory phase of such forced ventilation is determined by the mechanical properties of the airways and lung parenchyma, whereas the inspiratory portion is determined by the speed of shortening of the inspiratory muscles and is closely linked with maximal inspiratory pressures.[504–506]

PRESSURE-VOLUME CHARACTERISTICS OF THE LUNG

As discussed in Chapter 1, compliance is the relationship between the volume of air inhaled and the pressure necessary to overcome the elastic recoil of the lung. To avoid the effect of resistance and the pressure necessary to overcome it, measure-

ments of lung compliance and recoil are done during "static maneuvers." A complete pressure-volume curve of the lung is obtained by plotting lung volume in liters against the transpulmonary pressure over a range of volumes from TLC to FRC or lower. Transpulmonary pressure (P_L) is measured by a transducer that compares mouth pressure to esophageal pressure measured with a thin-walled balloon positioned in the midesophagus. Volume is measured by electrical integration of a pneumotachograph flow signal, by a spirometer, or ideally by a volume displacement body plethysmograph. The pressure-volume curve measures lung tissue elasticity, which is related to elastin and collagen fibers as well as to surface forces. Pressure-volume data are collected during quasistatic deflation from TLC or with stepwise interruption of expiratory flow from TLC (Fig. 3–4). The curves tend to be sigmoid in

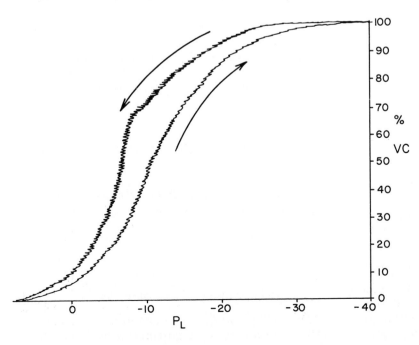

Figure 3-4. Pressure-Volume Curve. A pressure-volume tracing of a young male adult measured in both inspiration and expiration from residual volume to total lung capacity and back to residual volume. The upper curve represents the expiratory tracing. Notice the more horizontal appearance (decrease in compliance) as total lung capacity is reached.

shape,[507] but above FRC the pressure-volume data approximate an exponential function.[508–510]

A number of parameters derived from the pressure-volume curve reflect the elastic recoil properties of the lung (Fig. 3–5). The maximal elastic recoil pressure that the patient can generate at TLC (P_{LMax}) reflects the elastic recoil properties of the lung as well as the inspiratory muscle strength. Elastic recoil pressures at various percentages of TLC (P_{L90}, P_{L80}, P_{L70}, and so on) can also be employed in addition to the more standard measurement of compliance. Compliance is calculated as the volume change in liters divided by the transpulmonary pressure change over the relatively linear portion of the pressure-volume curve, near FRC. Compliance has the disadvantage of being dependent upon lung size, making comparison between individuals difficult; to circumvent this, a number of investigators have suggested fitting the pressure-volume data to an exponential equation:[508–510]

$$V = A - Be^{-KP}$$

where A is the theoretic maximal lung volume achievable at infinite transpulmonary pressure, B is the lung volume at a transpulmonary pressure of zero, and k is the shape constant that reflects the overall compliance of the lung irrespective of lung size. Prediction equations for normal values of k, P_{LMax}, and elastic recoil pressures at various percentages of TLC have been derived from study of large groups of normal, nonsmoking subjects.[511] The variability of these measurements has also been assessed in normal subjects: the elastic recoil pressure at 90 per cent of TLC (P_{L90}) and the natural logarithm of the exponential constant k have been found to be the most reproducible, possessing coefficients of variation of 9 and 6 per cent respectively.[512, 513] An increased k correlates with the severity of emphysema measured morphologically, and a decreased k has been reported in some cases of interstitial fibrosis.[509, 514] However, the curved fitting analysis was not useful in distinguishing emphysematous from nonemphysematous excised human lungs.[515] A study in which various-sized mammalian lungs were compared found that k increases with mean alveolar size; it is possible that it reflects an overall loss of elastic recoil and enlargement of air space size rather than the gross morphologic changes of emphysema.[516]

DYNAMIC COMPLIANCE

Although the compliance of the lung is normally measured during static maneuvers, dynamic compliance (C_{dyn}) can be measured during breathing as volume change divided by the changes in transpulmonary pressure at points of zero flow. In most normal subjects, C_{dyn} is very similar to static compliance over the tidal volume range and does not vary with respiratory frequencies up to 100 breaths per minute. The maintenance of the relationship between nonresistive pressure drop and volume change with increasing respiratory frequency reflects the remarkably synchronous action of acinar units throughout the lung. If there is any patchy obstruction of small airways or patchy alteration in regional lung compliance, regional time constant variations increase. With increased frequency of breathing, when the respiratory cycle time becomes shorter than the time constant of some units, C_{dyn} decreases as breathing frequency increases (frequency dependence of compliance). This decrease in compliance with increasing breathing frequencies is therefore a measure of inequalities of time constants in the lung and indirectly is a reflection of heterogeneity in small airway resistance and acinar compliance. The test has been shown to correlate with measurements of unevenness of ventilation[517] and has been advocated as a test of small airway obstruction.[518, 519] It may be one of the most specific and sensitive tests of small airway dysfunction, but it has not gained wide acceptance clinically because it requires expensive equipment, technical expertise, and the placement of an esophageal pressure catheter.[520]

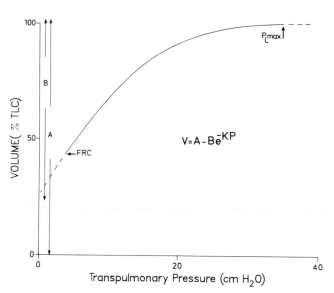

Figure 3–5. Elastic Recoil Properties of the Lung. A schematic pressure volume curve of the lung, in which lung volume as a percent of TLC (predicted or actual) is plotted against transpulmonary pressure obtained by comparing mouth and esophageal pressures. The pressure volume behavior may be described using various measurements from the P-V curve, including maximal elastic recoil (P_LMax), elastic recoil pressure at various percentages of TLC (i.e., P_{L90}, P_{L60}, and so on), and compliance—the slope of the ΔV/ΔP plot in the relatively linear range near FRC. These all have the disadvantage of describing only a portion of the curve. The whole curve can be fitted to an exponential function such as the equation described by Colebatch and associates,[508] in which V = volume, A = the theoretic maximal lung volume at infinite transpulmonary pressure, B = the volume difference between A and the 0 transpulmonary pressure intercept, P = transpulmonary pressure, and k = the exponent that describes the shape of the P-V curve. The ratio B/A defines the position of the curve whereas the exponential constant k describes the shape of the whole P-V curve.

RESISTANCE

Resistance is pressure divided by flow ($R = P/V$). In the lung, either airway resistance (R_{AW}) or pulmonary resistance (R_L) is generally measured. Airway resistance is the difference between mouth and alveolar pressure divided by flow and is obtained in a constant volume body plethysmograph. Enclosed within the body box, the subject pants through a pneumotachograph: the flow signal is plotted against alveolar pressure swings, estimated by changes in box pressure. With a closed system, box pressure varies only because alveolar gas is compressed and decompressed during panting, and variation in box pressure therefore reflects variations in alveolar pressure. Box pressure swings can be calibrated for alveolar pressure by comparing mouth and box pressure swings during obstructed breaths. Airway resistance (R_{AW}) can also be expressed as its reciprocal, conductance (G_{AW}), and since resistance varies with lung volume in a hyperbolic fashion and conductance varies with lung volume in a linear fashion, both should be corrected for the effects of lung volume. Specific airway conductance (S_{GAW}) is airway conductance per unit lung volume obtained by dividing G_{AW} by the lung volume at which it is measured; specific airway resistance (SR_{AW}) is the product of airway resistance and the thoracic gas volume at which the measurement is made.[521]

Pulmonary resistance (R) is obtained by dividing the difference between mouth and esophageal pressure (P_L) by flow. An esophageal balloon is introduced in the manner described earlier for measurement of the pressure-volume curve of the lung, and a differential pressure transducer compares mouth and pleural pressure during breathing at varying frequencies. Since the pressure difference between the mouth and the pleural space during breathing reflects not only the resistive properties of the lung but also the elastic properties, the portion of the transpulmonary pressure swing due to elastic recoil must be subtracted in order to measure the true pressure/flow relationship. This can be done electronically,[522] either by breathing at resonant frequency at which inertial and elastic forces cancel each other, or by measuring pressure changes at points of isovolume on inspiration and expiration.[523] Cardiac action can result in esophageal pressure artifacts, thus influencing the accuracy of the technique, but this can be overcome by a circuit that averages the pressure/flow relationship over a number of breaths.[524] No standardized prediction formulas or normal values are available for either airway or pulmonary resistance.

A simple noninvasive method of measuring the resistance of the respiratory system employs forced oscillations at varying frequencies during tidal breathing. Small pulses of flow are generated at the mouth by a loudspeaker, and the relationship between the output of the loudspeaker and the resultant flow can be analyzed to give values for total respiratory system resistance and reactance.[520] The respiratory system resistance can be measured over a wide range of frequencies; the frequency dependency of resistance and reactance has been suggested as a sensitive test of early small airway dysfunction.[525–527] The forced oscillation technique is easy to perform, is noninvasive, and does not require cooperation of the patient. Normal values and an estimate of reproducibility are available.[526, 528]

The measurement of airway or pulmonary resistance by whatever method represents the sum of the resistance of each generation of airways arranged in series and the airways within such generation arranged in parallel. In normal subjects, the bulk of the resistance to air flow is across the larynx and large central airways where the total cross-sectional area is least and where the flow regime is most turbulent and therefore most costly in terms of pressure loss. No noninvasive technique has been devised to measure accurately the contribution to total pulmonary resistance of various sizes and generations of airways.

THE SINGLE BREATH NITROGEN WASHOUT

The single breath nitrogen washout is the most commonly employed measure of the distribution of inspired gas. The test is carried out by having the patient inhale a vital capacity breath of pure oxygen, beginning the inhalation from residual volume and maintaining the inspiratory flow rate at less than 0.5 liter/sec. During the subsequent slow exhalation (flow 0.5 liter/sec) from TLC back to RV, the expired nitrogen concentration measured at the mouth is plotted against the expired volume on an XY recorder or oscilloscope. There are five phases to the changes in volume and nitrogen concentration during progressive exhalation (Fig. 3–6): *phase one* represents the emptying of dead space, which contains pure oxygen and no nitrogen; *phase two* represents the rapid increase in nitrogen, which occurs with the arrival of alveolar gas at the mouth; *phase three* is the slow, slight rise of nitrogen concentration that occurs during the alveolar plateau; *phase four* is the abrupt increase in nitrogen concentration that occurs in most normal subjects as residual volume is approached; and *phase five* is an irregular, abrupt decrease in nitrogen concentration, which occurs immediately before residual volume is reached.

Anatomic dead space and an inert gas dilution measurement of TLC can be calculated from the single breath nitrogen washout.[529] Closing volume is the volume above RV at which phase four begins and reflects closure of dependent airways. The addition of residual volume and closing volume gives closing capacity, which can be expressed as a percentage of TLC. The slope of the alveolar plateau (phase three) reflects the uniformity of alveolar

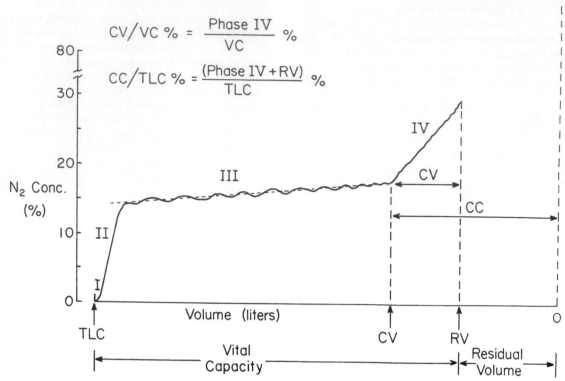

$$CV/VC\ \% = \frac{Phase\ IV}{VC}\ \%$$

$$CC/TLC\ \% = \frac{(Phase\ IV + RV)}{TLC}\ \%$$

Figure 3–6. The Single Breath Nitrogen Washout. In this test, expired nitrogen concentration (vertical axis) is plotted against expired volume starting at total lung capacity (TLC) and ending at residual volume (RV). Phase I represents dead space gas with 0 nitrogen; Phase III respresents alveolar nitrogen concentration; the slope of Phase III is increased with unevenness of distribution of ventilation. Phase IV begins at closing volume (CV) and represents the increasing contribution of gas from nitrogen-rich nondependent lung regions after basilar regions have closed. In this diagram, Phase V is not depicted.

ventilation and is calculated for the linear portion of the alveolar plateau, expressed as per cent change per liter. The upward sloping plateau normally found is related to the asynchronous emptying of lung units with different starting nitrogen concentrations; however, recent studies suggest that because of diffusive pendelluft at branch points subtending lung units of varying pathway length, an upward sloping alveolar plateau can exist despite synchronous and homogeneous volume changes throughout the lung.[530] The use of N_2 per liter as a measurement of the unevenness of alveolar ventilation was suggested by Comroe and Fowler in 1951.[531] By concentrating nitrogen within the alveolar space, continuing gas exchange during slow expiration also contributes to the upward sloping phase three and the height of phase four.[531, 532] The beginning of phase four coincides with the onset of airway closure, initially in the gravity-dependent portions of the lung. In disease, premature airway closure produces an elevated closing volume and closing capacity; the upward slope of phase three is exaggerated owing to regional differences in the distribution of the inhaled oxygen and asynchronous emptying of lung units. An increased closing capacity and slope of phase three can relate to changes in small airways or alterations in the elastic recoil of the lung secondary to elastic tissue disruption or diminished surface forces or both. The

downward sloping phase five is thought to be related to the onset of flow limitation in the uppermost regions of the lung, resulting in an increased contribution from the already flow-limited lower regions.[533]

The closing volume also can be measured by using a bolus technique that involves inhalation at RV of a small amount of xenon,[92, 534] argon,[535] or helium.[536] Since airways supplying gravity-dependent lung zones are closed at RV, the inert gas is preferentially distributed to upper lung zones, the lower zones being filled with room air or oxygen—whichever is used to complete the inspiration. During the next expiration from TLC, the inert gas is measured at the mouth and its concentration recorded against expired volume. Values for closing volume and closing capacity are similar with the bolus and single breath nitrogen washout techniques.[537] The latter can be performed on excised postmortem lungs, in which closing capacity has been shown to correlate with peripheral airway inflammation.[538] Prediction equations based on age and sex for definition of normal values and 95 per cent confidence limits are described for closing volume, closing capacity, and the slope of phase three of the single breath nitrogen washout test.[539, 540]

The distribution of inspired gas can also be measured by a multiple breath method in which the patient breathes 100 per cent O_2 for 7 minutes.[541]

When distribution of inspired air is uniform, the nitrogen content of an "alveolar" sample at the end of 7 minutes should be 2.5 or less per cent. In patients with impaired distribution, 10 to 20 minutes may elapse before the nitrogen content of poorly ventilated areas has been replaced by oxygen, so that the nitrogen content of the alveolar sample at 7 minutes may greatly exceed 2.5 per cent.

The third method for determining the distribution of inspired gas uses a helium closed-circuit apparatus; the result is expressed as the mixing efficiency.[542, 543]

THE DIFFUSING CAPACITY OF THE LUNG

As mentioned in Chapter 1, the diffusing capacity was formerly calculated for the diffusion of oxygen, but carbon monoxide has largely replaced this gas for technical reasons. The diffusing capacity for carbon monoxide (D_{LCO} or T_{LCO}) is computed as follows:

$$D_{LCO} = \frac{\text{Ml of CO taken up by capillary blood/min}}{\text{Mean alveolar } P_{CO} - \text{mean capillary } P_{CO}}$$

The amount of CO taken up by capillary blood is calculated by subtracting expired volume × CO concentration of expired gas from inspired volume × CO concentration of inspired gas. Determination of the denominator of the equation above is subject to error, especially in the presence of pulmonary disease. In normal subjects, once the dead space has been emptied, a sample of expired gas accurately reflects the mean alveolar P_{CO}, and since the normal mean capillary CO is so small that it can be ignored, the diffusing capacity can be calculated reliably. However, in diseased lungs that have relatively underventilated areas that empty late, the normal sharp division between dead space and alveolar gas is lost, and the expired gas sample might not reflect the mean alveolar P_{CO}.

Several techniques for measuring diffusing capacity with CO have been devised,[544-550] the main differences among them being the length of time that the gas is kept in the lungs and the methods of determining the mean alveolar P_{CO}. The three major methods for measuring D_{LCO} are the single breath, the rebreathing, and the steady state methods. The single breath method was originally devised by Marie Krogh[545] in an attempt to prove that oxygen was not secreted from alveolar gas into capillary blood as had been suggested by Haldane. The test was reintroduced in the early 1950s; initial technical difficulties were rectified by a number of modifications. Using standardized methodology, it is the most widely used method in North America and the United Kingdom for estimating the diffusing capacity.[469, 546, 547, 551-553] The test is accompanied by having the subject exhale to RV and then take a greater than 90 per cent vital capacity breath of a gas containing 0.3 per cent CO, 10 per cent He, 21 per cent O_2, and the balance nitrogen. After rapid inspiration of the gas, the breath is held for between 9 and 11 seconds near TLC, the first liter of expired gas is discarded, and the next liter, representative of alveolar gas it is hoped, is collected and analyzed for helium and CO. The helium dilution is used to calculate the alveolar volume (VA) as well as the initial concentration of CO in the alveolar space. The test can be repeated at brief intervals; two tests that agree within 5 per cent are required.[553] In patients with small vital capacities, a washout volume of 0.5 liter and a sample volume of 0.5 liter are recommended; alternatively, the steady state method can be used.[553]

One limitation of the single breath method is that uptake of CO from the lungs is actually occurring during the inspiratory and expiratory phase of the single breath, although the calculations assume that all CO uptake occurs during breath holding. This assumption can lead to significant error, especially with the prolonged expiration in patients with obstructive pulmonary disease. A recent modification of the technique employs a rapid response CO analyzer and three separate equations to calculate CO uptake during the inhalation, exhalation, and breath-holding periods; this gives values for D_{LCO} that are more accurate and are unaffected by prolonged expiration.[549, 554] An additional modification made feasible with the rapid response analyzer is measurement of the diffusing capacity continuously during expiration at 10 per cent lung volume decrements from 80 to 20 per cent of vital capacity. D_{LCO} is unaltered with lung volume in normal subjects but decreases at low lung volumes in patients with obstructive lung disease. This technique has the advantage that breath holding is not required, and it may be useful during exercise. Abnormalities of diffusion at low lung volumes comprise a potentially sensitive index of early disease.[550, 555]

The single breath and steady state D_{LCO} are dependent on the lung volume at which breah holding or tidal breathing occurs. For example, following pneumonectomy or with the chest wall restriction that occurs in conditions such as kyphoscoliosis, a patient may have a reduced D_{LCO} without intrinsic gas exchange abnormality in the remaining or restricted lung.[556] This had led to the suggestion that specific diffusing capacity or the diffusing capacity divided by the alveolar volume at which it was measured (D_L/VA) would be a more accurate measurement; this is abbreviated to K_{CO} in the United Kingdom.[557-559] Another method that avoids the effect of alveolar volume is measurement of the time constant of disappearance of alveolar CO during the breath-holding period.[560]

The rebreathing method involves 10 seconds of rebreathing from a small bag containing CO and helium; it is used the least in the clinical assessment of pulmonary disease. Advantages of the technique are that it can be employed in patients who are unable to breath hold, and that it is possible to perform at the bedside for the detection of alveolar hemorrhage through demonstration of an elevated D_{LCO}.[548]

The steady state techniques require inhalation of carbon monoxide gas mixtures for several breaths until alveolar P_{CO} remains constant. Knowing expired volume and mixed expired CO concentration, the uptake of carbon monoxide is easily determined, but again accurate determination of the mean alveolar P_{CO} is the source of error. A number of techniques have been employed to calculate mean alveolar P_{CO}, including end-tidal sampling, use of the Bohr equation with an assumed dead space/tidal volume ratio, and use of the Bohr equation with a measured V_D/V_T, which requires arterial puncture for measurement of arterial P_{CO_2}.[521, 561] In addition to measurement of diffusing capacity, the fractional removal of carbon monoxide (F_{CO}) can be calculated during a steady state test; this can help confirm the accuracy of the diffusing capacity value since both decrease simultaneously in most cases.[562] The fractional uptake of carbon monoxide is the amount removed divided by the amount inspired; thus

$$CO \text{ uptake per cent} = \frac{CO \text{ inspired} - CO \text{ expired}}{CO \text{ inspired}}$$

The diffusing capacity can be influenced by factors that alter the alveolar capillary membrane or pulmonary capillary blood volume. Table 3–6 summarizes the various factors that can affect the measurement of diffusing capacity (see also Fig. 1–107, page 133).[563]

Since the transfer of carbon monoxide is diffusion limited and not perfusion limited, the pulmonary blood volume (V_C) rather than pulmonary blood flow is important. The pulmonary capillary blood volume is multiplied by the kinetic constant theta (θ), which is the rate of combination of carbon monoxide and red blood cells. Theta is affected by the oxygen saturation of hemoglobin. Thus, $V_C \times \theta$ = the blood volume component of diffusing capacity. The membrane and $V_C \times \theta$ contributions to diffusing capacity can be calculated separately by measuring the diffusing capacity with different inspired P_{O_2}s. In normal subjects, the two components contribute approximately equally to the measured D_{LCO}, although morphometric techniques suggest that the $V_C \times \theta$ is the more important.[564]

The extent to which the measurement of diffusing capacity is affected by the distribution of ventilation and perfusion depends on the method used. Steady state methods are most sensitive to mismatching and are affected by the distribution of ventilation with respect to lung volume, perfusion, and diffusing capacity. The fractional uptake of carbon monoxide (F_{CO}) is least affected by the distribution of ventilation; however, it is very sensitive to the V_D/V_T and thus to respiratory frequency and tidal volume.[565] With the control of frequency, reliable prediction equations for F_{CO} have been described in normal subjects.[566]

All methods of measurement of D_{LCO} assume that the blood carboxyhemoglobin concentration and therefore the back pressure for carbon monoxide are virtually zero. However, an elevated carboxyhemoglobin concentration associated with smoking or industrial exposure can influence the measurement. Smokers can have levels of carboxyhemoglobin as high as 10 per cent, resulting in an approximate 1 per cent decrease in measured D_{LCO} for every 1 per cent increase in carboxyhemoglobin.[567] This correction does not completely return the diffusing capacity of most smokers back to normal values, however, and even asymptomatic smokers with otherwise normal pulmonary function have values for diffusing capacity that are approximately 80 per cent of predicted normal.[553] Since the diffusing capacity is dependent on pulmonary capillary blood volume or, more correctly, on the product of blood volume and hemoglobin concentration, factors that increase or decrease pulmonary blood volume or hemoglobin concentration affect the D_{LCO}. The effects of anemia and polycythemia have been investigated in a number of studies.[568–572] In one study of 50 patients free of cardiopulmonary disease whose hemoglobin values ranged from 6.7 to 16.8 grams per dl, the calculated correction factor was 7 per cent for each gram of hemoglobin.[572] From another study of 90 nonsmokers whose hematocrits ranged from 28 to 64 per cent, it was suggested that a 1.4 per cent adjustment (+ or −) be made in D_{LCO} per cent predicted for each per cent change in hematocrit above or below 44 per cent.[569]

Factors that acutely affect pulmonary capillary blood volume can also affect measured D_{LCO}: for example, the recruitment of pulmonary vascular bed during exercise results in a substantial increase in D_{LCO} within seconds.[573] D_{LCO} also increases when one breathes through an inspiratory resistance, presumably as a result of negative intrathoracic pressures and recruitment of blood volume, an effect that correlates with the D_{LCO} increase during exer-

Table 3–6. Factors Affecting Diffusing Capacity

ALVEOLAR CAPILLARY MEMBRANE
Lung volume
Surface area
"Thickness"

PULMONARY CAPILLARY BLOOD VOLUME
(Blood Volume × Hgb Concentration)
Position: increased D_{LCO} standing → sitting → lying
Mueller or Valsalva maneuvers during breath hold
Hemoglobin concentration
Hemoglobin affinity for oxygen

DISTRIBUTION OF VENTILATION RELATIVE TO PERFUSION
Affects steady state method especially
Affects F_{CO} least

BACK PRESSURE OF CARBON MONOXIDE
Cigarette smoking

cise. Asthmatic subjects frequently have an increased single breath D_{LCO}, possibly as a result of recruitment of capillary blood volume secondary to their more negative pleural pressure swings.[574] Drugs such as nitroglycerin, which can shift blood volume from the pulmonary capillary bed to the systemic capillary bed, result in a decrease in diffusing capacity.[575] The effect of increased blood volume on diffusing capacity does not distinguish increased blood volume in the vascular space of the lung from intra-alveolar blood; the diffusing capacity may be markedly increased in patients with pulmonary hemorrhage, and its measurement has been recommended for the diagnosis of this condition.[576, 577] Decreased D_{LCO} has been reported in alcoholic patients, but values may be normal when corrected for anemia and smoking.[577]

Early studies that calculated prediction equations for single breath D_{LCO} were contaminated by smokers, but more recent studies of large numbers of nonsmokers with calculated 95 per cent confidence limits are available.[558, 573, 576]

MEASUREMENT OF INEQUALITY OF VENTILATION/PERFUSION RATIOS

Methods for the assessment of disturbances of ventilation/perfusion ratios are described in detail in Chapter 1 (see page 136). The most commonly employed technique involves calculation of the alveolar-arterial gradient for oxygen using the simplified alveolar air equation. An increase in "physiologic" dead space can be measured with the Bohr equation, and venous admixture or true intrapulmonary shunt can be calculated. Bronchospirometry is now rarely used to detect differences in ventilation and perfusion in the two lungs; it involves partitioning the ventilation of the two lungs by insertion of a Carlens' catheter into the right main bronchus or by balloon occlusion of a main stem bronchus during conventional bronchoscopy.[578] Radionuclides are now more commonly used in the study of regional ventilation/perfusion inequality; the multiple inert gas technique provides the most accurate description of the distribution of ventilation/perfusion ratios in the lung, although it does not provide regional information.

CLINICAL ASSESSMENT OF RESPIRATORY CONTROL

Alveolar hypoventilation accompanied by an elevated arterial PCO_2 and the resultant fall in arterial PO_2 is the final common pathway of many pulmonary disorders. The clinical challenge is to determine why hypoventilation has occurred: is the patient hypoventilating because he or she *will not* breathe sufficiently or *cannot* breathe sufficiently?[579] Hypoventilation can have its origin in impaired central or peripheral chemoreceptor responsiveness, defective transmission of central inspiratory activity to the respiratory muscles, failure of respiratory muscle action due to muscle fatigue or weakness, or the inability of the muscular activity to generate sufficient ventilation because of increased impedance of the respiratory system. Although we normally think of alveolar hypoventilation as primarily a lung problem, it is becoming increasingly evident that metabolic, neurologic, and muscular disorders can lead to or at least contribute to hypoventilation. The list of disorders associated with depressed central ventilatory drive is ever-lengthening and includes encephalitis, cerebrovascular disease affecting the medulla, Parkinson's syndrome, myxedema, the obesity hypoventilation syndromes, narcotic addiction, bilateral spinothalamic lesions, metabolic alkalosis, bulbar poliomyelitis, carotid endarterectomy, cyanotic congenital heart disease, familial dysautonomia, and chronic exposure to high altitude.[580]

The first step in the investigation of "can't versus won't" is measurement of lung volumes and flow rates, since hypoventilation due to increased impedance does not occur unless the FEV_1 is less than about 1.2 liters. If hypoventilation is present with adequate ventilatory reserve, more detailed investigation of respiratory control is warranted.

It is difficult to quantify respiratory center output. The measurement closest to central neutral drive is the electrical neurogram of the phrenic nerve, but this is a difficult and invasive test and is rarely used. The output can also be measured by a recording of the electromyogram of the diaphragm or other inspiratory muscle, but this is already one step removed from the electrical output of the respiratory center; the EMG is also invasive and can only be applied to some of the respiratory muscles (diaphragm and intercostals). Mouth pressure measured 100 msec after obstruction of the airway[393] gives an estimate of respiratory center output unaffected by the impedance of the respiratory system, but it is influenced by the length-tension relationship and strength of the respiratory muscles. Measurements of the work of breathing or of ventilation itself are frequently used as indicators of respiratory drive but are influenced by the resistance and compliance of the lung and by neuromuscular function. A recently devised method for clinical assessment of respiratory control involves separation of the respiratory cycle into its components: tidal volume/inspiratory time (VT/Ti), a measure of mean inspiratory flow, and the ratio of inspiratory time over total respiratory cycle time, or Ti/Ttot. It has been suggested that VT/Ti is a measure of central inspiratory activity and Ti/Ttot reflects respiratory center timing.[581, 582]

Ventilatory Response Curves

The ventilatory response to carbon dioxide can be measured with a steady state or rebreathing technique.[582, 583] With the steady state method, at least two concentrations of CO_2 are employed, and relative hyperoxia is ensured during the procedure by adding a high concentration of inspired oxygen to the circuit. The difficulty with the rebreathing technique is that the arterial and brain tissue P_{CO_2} are dependent to some extent on the ventilatory response, and thus CO_2 is not a true independent variable; in addition, the technique is cumbersome to perform and requires measurement of arterial P_{CO_2} for accuracy. The most widely used method of assessing CO_2 responsiveness is the one originally devised by Read, which employs rebreathing of CO_2:[584, 585] the subject breathes from a bag containing CO_2 at approximately the level of mixed venous P_{CO_2} (7 per cent); the bag size is approximately 1 liter greater than the vital capacity and contains an enriched oxygen mixture to prevent hypoxemia during the test. The mixed venous, arterial and alveolar P_{CO_2} concentrations come into equilibrium within 30 to 60 seconds, and thereafter a linear increase in CO_2 concentration of between 3 and 6 mm Hg per min occurs owing to endogenous production of carbon dioxide. A single ventilatory response curve requires approximately 4 minutes to obtain, and reproducible tests of the ventilatory response can be obtained at intervals as short as 10 minutes.[586] The results are expressed as the slope of the ventilatory response, $\Delta V/\Delta P_{CO_2}$, and the relationship is linear with an intercept on the CO_2 axis, which reflects the starting arterial P_{CO_2} (Fig. 3–7). The range of ventilatory response to CO_2 is remarkably wide among normal healthy subjects; there is an approximate 16-fold variation of between 0.57 and 8.17 liters per min per mm Hg rise in CO_2.[583, 587] Although this can be explained in part by genetic factors (as demonstrated in studies of twins) and partly by difference in lung size, considerable residual variation exists.[588] The ventilatory response to hypercapnia is decreased if nasal rather than mouth breathing is employed, suggesting that upper airway receptors can modify the ventilatory response.[589, 590] Normal values for ventilatory responses to CO_2 have been derived.[591]

The hypoxic ventilatory response can be measured with single breath tests employing 100 per cent oxygen or 100 per cent nitrogen, or with steady state or rebreathing methods. The steady state method results in a curvilinear, hyperbolic relationship between ventilation and end-tidal or arterial P_{O_2} (Fig. 3–8). Ventilation changes little until arterial P_{O_2} reaches values of approximately 50 or 60 mm Hg, after which it increases sharply. The curvilinearity makes it difficult to fit a curve to the ventilation versus P_{O_2} relationship to obtain a meaningful quantification of the response. The most commonly used function is a hyperbolic equation in which a shape constant A is used to quantify the response.[583]

Rebuck and Campbell[592] have developed a rebreathing method to assess hypoxic ventilatory re-

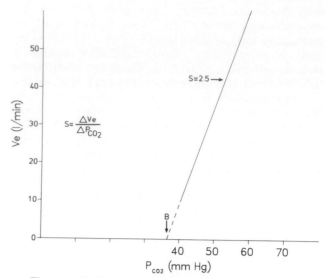

Figure 3–7. The CO_2 Ventilatory Response Curve. The ventilatory response curve to increasing levels of CO_2 serves as a measure of respiratory chemosensitivity. A linear relationship between ventilation and end-tidal CO_2 is observed with the rebreathing method and chemosensitivity is quantified as the slope of the curve

$$\frac{\Delta \dot{V}e}{\Delta P_{CO_2}}.$$

A normal curve in which the $\Delta \dot{V}e/\Delta P_{CO_2}$ is 2.5 liters per min per mm Hg is depicted. There is a wide range of normal for this slope, and the relationship can be changed by alterations in central drive, neuromuscular function, or respiratory system impedance.

sponse similar to Read's rebreathing method: with their technique, ventilation is plotted against arterial oxygen saturation measured with an ear oximeter (Fig. 3–8). The advantages are that the saturation directly reflects arterial P_{O_2} and is unaffected by any A-a O_2 gradient that may be present, unlike measurements of end-tidal P_{O_2}. The other advantage is that the relationship is linear, allowing the response to be more easily quantified; however, the fact that there is a linear relationship between saturation and ventilation does not mean that arterial saturation is the pertinent signal that stimulates the peripheral chemoreceptors. Reduction in oxygen content produced by carbon monoxide poisoning or anemia has no effect on the ventilatory response curve. The linear relationship is a fortuitous occurrence, reflecting a combination of two curvilinear relationships, one between P_{O_2} and ventilation and the other between P_{O_2} and arterial saturation.[580] The range of normal ventilatory response to hypoxemia is also extremely wide, with a mean value of 1.47 liters per min per cent fall in arterial saturation; 80 per cent of healthy normal subjects have a slope between 0.6 and 2.75.[583] It is important to maintain end-tidal P_{CO_2} constant throughout the hypoxemic ventilatory response, accomplished by adding CO_2 to the inspired circuitry. Recent studies have shown that the acute ventilatory response to

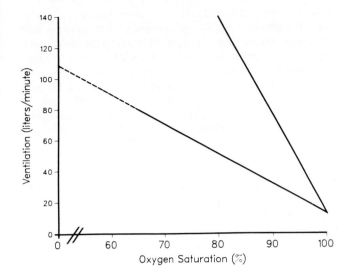

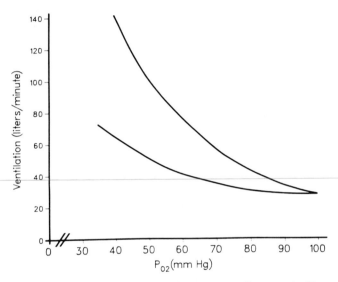

Figure 3–8. The Ventilatory Response to Hypoxemia. The ventilatory response to hypoxemia is tested by plotting ventilation versus changes in oxygen saturation (upper panel) or P_{O_2} (lower panel). A wide range of normal responses is shown by these two representative curves, which are at the upper and lower limits of normal responses. The advantage of using O_2 saturation as the independent variable is that linear relationships are produced that allow easier comparison within or between subjects. The linear relationship does not mean that the peripheral chemoreceptors sense saturation but rather is the result of combining two curvilinear relationships: that between P_{O_2} and O_2 saturation and that between P_{O_2} and ventilation.

hypoxemia, as customarily measured, overestimates the sustained hypoxemic response in normal subjects and obstructed patients.[593] A relationship exists between the ventilatory response to CO_2 and O_2 in individuals.

Additional tests to measure chemoreceptor responsiveness have been suggested, including measurement of ventilatory response during transient exposure (4 to 7 breaths) to hypoxic or hyperoxic gas mixtures and measurement of breath-holding time; however, neither of these has proved as useful

or as reproducible as the ventilatory response curves.[594, 595]

Mouth Occlusion Pressures

The ventilatory response to CO_2 and O_2 depends heavily upon the impedance of the respiratory system. Thus, a patient might have a normal neural output from a normally functioning respiratory center, but the translation of that neural output to ventilation might be impaired purely on a mechanical basis. In an attempt to get one step closer to the true output of the respiratory center, Whitelaw and colleagues[596] developed a technique to measure mouth occlusion pressure following the first 100 msec of an occluded breath. The technique is accomplished while the patient is breathing tidally at rest or during various stages of a ventilatory response curve to O_2 or CO_2. Periodically and unknown to the subject, the mouthpiece is temporarily occluded for at least 100 msec at the onset of inspiration, and the pressure generated by the inspiratory muscles at this time is termed the PO.1.[596] An occlusion this brief is undetected by the subject so that behavioral alterations in breathing pattern do not interfere with the measurement.[597] The measurement of occlusion pressure is not without its problems: recruitment of abdominal muscles during expiration can result in a decrease in FRC below the static equilibration point between lung and chest wall, so that the initial inspiratory pressure generated at the mouth will be contributed to by the sudden relaxation of the abdominal muscles and the elastic recoil of the respiratory system.[598] In obstructive lung disease, in which pleural pressure swings may be nonuniform, PO.1 measured at the mouth was significantly less than esophageal pressure at 0.1 second, presumably reflecting the same artifact that interferes with measurement of plethysmographic thoracic gas volume in these patients.[599] Despite these problems, measurement of occlusion pressure has distinct advantages over the work of breathing or ventilation as an assessment of neural drive to the inspiratory muscles since it is unaffected by the flow resistance or compliance properties of the respiratory system. PO.1 is a useful index of the neuromuscular component of the respiratory output, indicating the pressure potential available for inspiration in any given condition.[600] Using the occlusion pressure technique, studies have shown that patients with ventilatory impairment may have normal or even supranormal drive, with the decreased ventilation being attributable solely to the increased impedance of the respiratory system.[601]

Breathing Pattern Analysis

Analysis of the breathing pattern as a method of assessing the control of ventilation has been suggested by Milic-Emili.[602] Ventilation at rest or during stimulated breathing can be divided into a flow component and a timing component.

$$VE = VT/Ti \times Ti/Ttot$$

where VT/Ti is the mean inspiratory flow (tidal volume divided by inspiratory time), and $Ti/Ttot$ is the duty cycle (ratio of inspiratory time to total respiratory cycle time). Increase in ventilation can be achieved by increasing the inspiratory flow rate VT/Ti and keeping $Ti/Ttot$ constant, or by increasing $Ti/Ttot$ and keeping VT/Ti constant. The VT/Ti component is thought to reflect neural output from the respiratory center, while the $Ti/Ttot$ relationship reflects the timing element.[600] The value of separating these two components in the control of breathing in the investigation of various disease states is not yet clearly defined. It is likely, however, that continued clinical investigation will reveal specific alterations in breathing patterns in certain conditions.[594]

Electromyography and Electroneurography

Direct measurement of the electrical activity in respiratory muscles is one step closer to the respiratory center output. The EMG of the diaphragm can be recorded with surface electrodes placed on the 5th, 6th, and 7th intercostal spaces close to the costochondral junctions, or with an esophageal electrode.[600] Inspiratory intercostal muscle activity can be measured with surface electrodes in the 2nd and 3rd anterior intercostal spaces but can be contaminated with electrical activity from other muscles. Finally, electrodes can be inserted directly into inspiratory or expiratory respiratory muscles. Short of placing intracranial electrodes, direct recording of phrenic nerve electrical (ENG) activity is the closest one can come to measuring respiratory center output, but it is a procedure rarely performed in a clinical setting.[600]

TESTS OF RESPIRATORY MUSCLE PERFORMANCE

The final step in the assessment of respiratory control involves measurements of the output of the neurologic activity as reflected in respiratory muscle performance. The simplest means to test inspiratory and expiratory muscle strength is to measure maximal inspiratory and expiratory pressures (MIP and MEP) at the mouth. Simple, portable devices that can be used on a ward or in the intensive care unit have been developed for this purpose.[603] The technique involves having a subject make a maximal inspiratory and maximal expiratory effort against a closed mouthpiece in which a small leak has been constructed to avoid glottic closure and generation of pressure with the buccal and oropharyngeal muscles. The pressures generated depend on the lung volume at which the test is performed, since this influences the length-tension relationship of various respiratory muscles. Thus, maximal inspiratory pressure is generated near RV and maximal expiratory pressures near TLC when expiratory muscles are lengthened.[604] MIP and MEP are highly variable between subjects and depend upon motivation and learning; they also depend on age and to some extent on weight and height/weight. However, these variables explain little of the variance, and most of the predicted values take into account only age and sex.[603–607]

Measurement of MIP and MEP gives an overall estimate of respiratory muscle performance, but measurement of maximal transdiaphragmatic pressure (PdiMax) gives an estimate of diaphragmatic strength; this measurement is obtained by comparing pleural to gastric pressure during maximal inspiratory effort against a closed mouthpiece.[608–610] No detailed normal predicted values are available for PdiMax but have been said to be similar to PIM. Transdiaphragmatic pressure measurement has proved useful in the detection of bilateral or unilateral diaphragmatic paralysis.[608, 611] In addition to measurements of MIP and MEP that estimate strength, respiratory muscle endurance can be measured by progressively loading the inspiratory muscles with increasing resistances until maximal sustainable pressure is achieved.[612, 613]

The respiratory muscles can become fatigued in a fashion similar to that of any skeletal muscle when overloaded. The development of respiratory muscle fatigue can be detected by analysis of the electromyogram: the EMG signal is filtered into high- and low-frequency bands, and the ratio of high over low frequency decreases as fatigue develops, predating the actual failure of force generation by the muscle.[614] A simpler way to predict the development of diaphragmatic fatigue is to measure the tension-time index of the diaphragm during tidal breathing and to relate this to the maximal transdiaphragmatic pressure. The tension-time index is calculated by the average transdiaphragmatic pressure per breath as a percentage of PdiMax multiplied by the inspiratory time; when this approaches 15 per cent, fatigue is likely to ensue.[615] Obviously, the tension-time index can approach the critical value of 15 per cent as a result of a decrease in maximal transdiaphragmatic pressure secondary to respiratory muscle weakness or of an increase in the tidal Pdi swings related to increased impedance of the respiratory system.

INHALATION CHALLENGE TESTS

Since the last edition of this book was published, a veritable explosion of interest in inhalation challenge testing has occurred. Inhalation challenge tests can be broadly categorized into nonspecific and specific types. Nonspecific tests include aerosol challenge with nebulized agonists such as methacholine, histamine, and prostaglandin F_2, and protocols designed to produce cooling and drying of the airway mucosa such as by exercise and isocapnic hyperventilation. Specific challenge refers to inhalation of allergens to which the subject is known or suspected to be sensitive or to exposure to dust or environmental agents that provoke idiosyncratic lung responses in some individuals.

Nonspecific Bronchial Reactivity

During the late 1920s and early 1930s, while studying the cardiovascular effects of intravenously administered histamine, Weiss and his colleagues noted that asthmatic and emphysematous patients—but not normal subjects—manifested an exaggerated airway response characterized by wheezing and a decrease in vital capacity.[616, 617] In the mid 1940s, Curry administered acetyl-beta-methylcholine and histamine intravenously and by inhalation to normal subjects and patients with allergic rhinitis and asthma and found that both agonists produced substantially greater falls in vital capacity in the asthmatics.[618] During the mid 1950s, Tiffeneau was the first to advocate the use of nonspecific bronchial reactivity to inhaled acetylcholine as a clinical tool in the assessment and diagnosis of asthma.[619, 620] In the late 1970s, Chai,[621] Cockcroft,[622] and Juniper[623] and their associates described standardized methods to assess bronchial reactivity; since that time the systematic study of the phenomenon of nonspecific airway hyperreactivity has progressed dramatically.

METHODS

All the techniques employed to measure nonspecific bronchial reactivity (NSBR) pharmacologically involve the inhalation of an aerosol containing a known bronchoconstrictive agent. Inhalation is begun with a low concentration or dose of agonist and the "dose" is progressively increased; an index of airway narrowing is measured at each step so that a "dose-response" relationship can be constructed. A variety of techniques of delivering agonists and of measuring the response and expressing the results have been developed and are summarized in Table 3–7. The most widely used and carefully standardized technique is that described by Cockcroft and associates,[622] based on a modifi-

Table 3–7. Tests of Nonspecific Bronchial Reactivity

	AGONIST	METHOD OF ADMINISTRATION	MEASURED VARIABLE	EXPRESSION OF RESULTS
Cockcroft et al[622]	histamine or methacholine	Face mask with nose, 2 min inhalations, tidal breathing, Wright nebulizer. Output 0.13–0.16 ml/min, concentrations 0.03, 16 mg/ml in doubling steps. AMMD = 0.87 ± 1.9 μ	FEV_1 before and after diluent and after each concentration until FEV_1 has decreased 20% or greater from postdiluent value	Provocative concentration producing a 20% fall in FEV_1 (PC_{20}) calculated by interpolation
Chai et al[621]	histamine or methacholine	Devilbiss 646 nebulizer and Rosenthal French dosimeter model B-2A. 9.04 ± 0.43. 1 per nebulization. AMMD = 1.32 ± 2.5 μ, five vital capacity breaths/dose	FEV_1 after each dose till decreased 20% or greater OR specific airway conductance after each dose till 35% or greater decrease occurs	Provocative dose producing a 20% fall in FEV_1 (Pd_{20}) is calculated. Or the dose resulting in a 35% decrease in specific airway conductance (Pd_{35}-SGaw) is calculated
Lam et al[625]	methacholine	As for Cockcroft, except Bennett twin nebulizer with output 0.25 ml/min. AMMD = 3.1 μ	As for Cockcroft	As for Cockcroft, PC_{20}
Yan et al[627]	histamine	Handheld Devilbiss No. 40 glass nebulizer, bulb squeezed by technician to deliver 0.03 → 0.6 mol in doubling steps at 1 min intervals, vital capacity breaths	FEV_1 60 sec after each dose until 20% fall in FEV_1 recorded	Pd_{20} (cumulative dose calculation)
Orehek et al[626]	carbachol	Different concentrations of carbachol solution nebulized into spirometer. Varying breath number. Breath volume VT, particle size 0.1 5 m	Specific airway resistance and specific airway conductance after each dose	Sensitivity = D25 dose causing a 25% rise (cumulative). Reactivity—arithmetic relationship of dose vs. specific airway conductance (%)

cation of an earlier protocol.[624] The method employs nebulized histamine or methacholine delivered with a face mask during tidal breathing; 2 minute inhalations of increasing concentrations of histamine or methacholine are followed by measurements of FEV_1. Doubling concentrations of agonist are administered, beginning with 0.013 mg per ml and increasing to 16 mg per ml; the test is stopped when there is either a 20 per cent or greater fall in FEV_1 or when the highest concentration of agonist is reached. The level of nonspecific reactivity is calculated as the concentration of inhaled agonist that results in a 20 per cent fall in FEV_1 (PC_{20}). A minor modification of the technique has been described by Lam and associates,[625] the only differences being the use of methacholine and a Bennett twin nebulizer with a higher output.

The other technique that has been standardized and widely used to measure nonspecific bronchial reactivity has been described by Chai and associates:[621] with this technique the nebulizer is coupled to a dosimeter that delivers a known quantity of aerosol with each breath; five vital capacity breaths with increasing concentrations of agonist are inhaled and the FEV_1 or specific airway conductance measured after each dose. The dose that results in a 20 per cent decrease in FEV_1 (Pd_{20}) or a 35 per cent decrease in specific airway conductance (Pd_{35} SG_{AW}) is calculated. Orehek and colleagues[626] use carbachol, a longer-acting parasympathomimetic agent, to construct inhalation dose-response curves; they measure specific airway conductance and calculate a threshold for response ("sensitivity") as the dose producing a 25 per cent decrease in SGaw. "Reactivity" is calculated as the slope of the dose-response curve obtained by plotting the arithmetic cumulative dose of inhaled carbachol against the per cent change in specific conductance. More recently, Yan and associates[627] have described a more rapid method for measuring bronchial responsiveness that employs a handheld, bulb-operated glass nebulizer that delivers a known volume of aerosol with each squeeze of the bulb. Doubling concentrations of inhaled histamine are administered over a short time interval and a cumulative Pd_{20} calculated.

Several modifications of these basic methodologies have been suggested, including calculation of a threshold dose that causes a greater than 2 standard deviation change in FEV_1 from repeated baseline measurements; and measurement of increase in pulmonary resistance or decrease in maximal flow at 50 per cent vital capacity or on partial expiratory flow volume curves. However, none of the modifications has proved more specific or sensitive in separating normal subjects from asthmatics than has measurement of changes in FEV_1.[624, 628, 629]

The main variables determining PC_{20} in the method described by Cockcroft and associates are the output of the nebulizer, the inspiratory pattern during aerosol administration, and to a lesser ex-

tent, particle size.[630–633] To achieve reproducible and dependable results, patients must refrain from use of inhaled beta-adrenergic agonists for 8 hours prior to the study, and from short- and long-acting theophylline preparations for 24 and 48 hours respectively. Inhaled or systemic steroids have no influence on the measurement of nonspecific bronchial reactivity.[634] In stable patients, measurements of PC_{20} with histamine or methacholine show remarkable reproducibility over time; it is surprising that a close correlation exists in airway responsiveness measured with histamine, methacholine, and prostaglandin F_2.[623, 635–638] However, since histamine in high concentration tends to cause cough and flushing, since prostaglandin F_2 leads to cough and retrosternal irritation, and since carbachol is a long-acting bronchoconstricting agent, methacholine is probably the agent of choice. Measurements of NSBR have been compared using the tidal breathing method and the more complex dose metering device; the two have been found comparable and equally reproducible.[639] The more rapidly performed short test employing a handheld nebulizer has also been shown to produce results comparable to the dosimeter method, and because of ease of performance it may gain in popularity.[627] A number of population studies have been carried out to assess the sensitivity of bronchial responsiveness in distinguishing asthmatics from normal subjects.[622, 640] PC_{20} is universally lower than 8 mg per ml in asthmatic patients, whereas in subjects with normal pulmonary function and negative histories it is invariably greater than 16 mg per ml. This allows a clear separation of patients with reactive airway disease from normal subjects, although patients with chronic bronchitis, cystic fibrosis, or other chronic airway diseases may have intermediate values.

Some agreement exists among investigators concerning methods of measuring NSBR and what represents normal and abnormal reactivity, but there is continued debate about the mechanisms that cause airway responsiveness. Dose-response curves to inhaled nonspecific agonists cannot be equated to the *in vitro* smooth muscle dose-response curve in which well-characterized parameters of receptor kinetics can be described. *In vivo*, the relationship between airway smooth muscle stimulation and airway narrowing is affected by smooth muscle shortening, mucosal edema, mucous plugs, and starting airway caliber. These factors make it difficult or impossible to apply pharmacologic principles of dose-response relationships to *in vivo* dose-response curves. These misconceptions have led to an abundant literature in which the possible pathophysiologic significance of "sensitivity" and "reactivity" has been discussed.[626, 641–643] In fact, to date the distinction between sensitivity and reactivity has not been shown to be of any clinical significance.[644]

Methacholine and histamine inhalation challenges are useful in clinical practice. In doubtful cases, they can substantiate a diagnosis of asthma, especially when baseline spirometry is normal; in addition, patients whose primary complaint is cough frequently have underlying asthma that can be diagnosed by inhalation challenge testing. In patients with asthma, measurements of bronchial reactivity correlate well with the severity of symptoms and the need for medication (Fig. 3–9).[622] Bronchial reactivity can change over time: for example, intensive therapy can result in a decrease in NSBR whereas exposure to allergens or occupational sensitizers can increase it. Serial measurements of PC_{20} can be obtained to assess the efficacy of such treatment or the detrimental effect of such exposure. Measurements of bronchial responsiveness are often of clinical benefit in the pediatric asthmatic group in whom measurements of peak expiratory flow rate following inhalation of agonist can be substituted for measurements of FEV_1.[645, 646]

Specific Inhalation Challenge

Specific inhalation challenge tests are those performed on individuals who have, or are suspected of having, allergy or sensitivity to specific allergens or chemical sensitizers. The techniques of inhalation challenge with antigen and occupational agents are less well standardized than the nonspecific challenge tests with methacholine and histamine. In addition, allergy testing is time-consuming and can induce severe and prolonged responses that are potentially hazardous. Before challenging any subject with an allergen or chemical sensitizer, it is important to know the level of nonspecific airway reactivity, since the magnitude of response to the specific agent will be related to the nonspecific bronchial reactivity.[647] Inhalation of a specific antigen or chemical sensitizer can produce not only an immediate bronchoconstriction but also a delayed response that can begin anywhere from 2 to 10 hours after challenge. The delayed response may be prolonged and can result in altered nonspecific bronchial reactivity in sensitized individuals. Allergen inhalation challenge is rarely indicated in clinical practice and should be reserved for special cases being investigated in larger centers where there is expertise in the methodology. However, inhalation challenge testing with agents suspected of causing allergic alveolitis or occupational asthma may be important in establishing proof of specific sensitivity to these agents and may be required for compensation purposes.

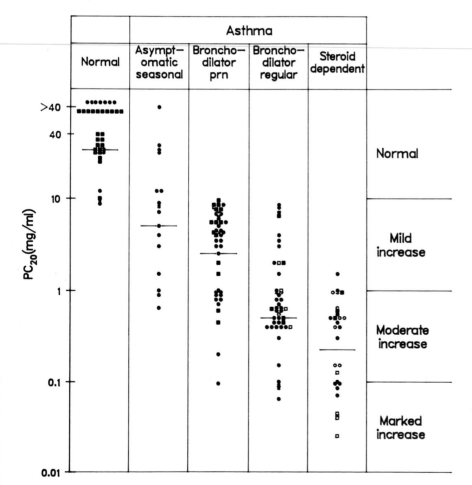

Figure 3–9. Bronchial Reactivity in Relation to Symptoms and Medication Requirement in Asthmatics. The provocative concentration of inhaled histamine resulting in a 20 per cent decrease in FEV_1 is plotted against clinical status. The data are from 35 normal subjects and 156 asthmatic patients of varying severity indicated by their medication usage. PC_{20} is on a log scale. The horizontal bars are the geometric mean for each group; the circles indicate atopic subjects; the squares indicate nonatopic subjects. The open symbols represent those in whom baseline (prehistamine) FEV_1 was less than 70 per cent predicted. There is some overlap in PC_{20} values between normal and asymptomatic allergic asthmatic patients, but the PC_{20} clearly separates normal patients from the more severely afflicted asthmatic patients. This nonspecific hyperreactivity is not related to atopic status, and, although patients with decreased starting FEV_1 tend to be more reactive (lower PC_{20}), marked airway hyperresponsiveness can occur despite normal starting expiratory flow rates. (Reprinted slightly modified from Cockcroft D, Killian D, Mellan J, et al: Clin Allergy 7:235, 1977.)

EXERCISE-INDUCED BRONCHOCONSTRICTION AND ISOCAPNIC HYPERVENTILATION

With the demonstration that the bronchoconstriction associated with exercise is caused by the breathing of cool, dry air, techniques to measure the bronchial responsiveness to such air during isocapnic hyperventilation have been developed.[648, 649] Patients are asked to hyperventilate from a source of dry air, either cold or at room temperature, and isocapnia is maintained by adding CO_2 to the inspired gas to maintain end-tidal carbon dioxide content constant. Preserving eucapnia is important because hyperventilation in the absence of exercise would produce hypocapnia, which in itself produces bronchoconstriction. Expiratory flow is measured with progressively increasing levels of hyperventilation, and the level of ventilation or the calculated respiratory heat loss producing a given fall in FEV_1 can be calculated in a fashion similar to the PC_{20}. More recently, it has been demonstrated that patients with reactive airway disease show bronchoconstriction on inhalation of ultrasonically nebulized water mist; this has been suggested as an additional nonspecific bronchial irritant in the quantification of bronchial reactivity.[650]

REFERENCES

1. Widdicombe JG: Respiratory reflexes from the trachea and bronchi of the cat. J Physiol (Lond) 123:55, 1954.
2. Widdicombe JG: Receptors in the trachea and bronchi of the cat. J Physiol (Lond) 123:71, 1954.
3. Lauweryns JM, Cokelaere M, Theunynck P, et al: Neuroepithelial bodies in mammalian respiratory mucosa. Light optical, histochemical and ultrastructural studies. Chest 65:22S, 1974.
4. Lauweryns JM, Goddeeris P: Neuroepithelial bodies in the human child and adult lung. Am Rev Resp Dis 111:469, 1975.
5. Corrao WM, Braman SS, Irwin RS: Chronic cough as the sole presenting manifestation of bronchial asthma. N Engl J Med 300:633, 1979.
6. Poe RH, Israel RH, Utell MJ, et al: Chronic cough: Bronchoscopy or pulmonary function testing? Am Rev Respir Dis 126:160, 1982.
7. Irwin RS, Corrao WM, Pratter MR: Chronic persistent cough in the adult: The spectrum and frequency of causes and successful outcome of specific therapy. Am Rev Respir Dis 123:413, 1981.
8. Editorial: Chronic cough. Lancet 2:907, 1981.
9. Shuper A, Mukamel M, Mimouni M, et al: Psychogenic cough. Arch Dis Child 58:745, 1983.
10. Storey CF, Knudtson KP, Lawrence BJ: Bronchiolar ("alveolar cell") carcinoma of the lung. J Thorac Surg 26:331, 1953.
11. Calin A: Bronchorrhoea. Br Med J 4:274, 1972.
12. Albertini RE: Cough caused by exposed endobronchial sutures. Ann Intern Med 94:205, 1981.
13. Kerr A Jr, Eich RH: Cerebral concussion as a cause of cough syncope. Arch Intern Med 108:248, 1961.
14. Jenkins P, Clarke SW: Cough syncope: A complication of adult whooping cough. Br J Dis Chest 75:311, 1981.
15. Morgan-Hughes JA: Cough seizures in patients with cerebral lesions. Br Med J 2:494, 1966.
16. Ludman H: ABC of ENT: Hoarseness and stridor. Br Med J 282:715, 1981.
17. Kontos HA, Schapiro W, Patterson JL Jr: Observations on dyspnea induced by combinations of respiratory stimuli. Am J Med 37:374, 1964.
18. Rice RL: Symptom patterns of the hyperventilation syndrome. Am J Med 8:691, 1950.
19. Milne JA, Howie AD, Pack AI: Dyspnoea during normal pregnancy. Br J Obstet Gynaecol 85:260, 1978.
20. Weinberger SE, Weiss ST, Cohen WR, et al: Pregnancy and the lung. Am Rev Respir Dis 121:559, 1980.
21. Lipscomb DJ, Edwards RHT: Computer simulation of physiological factors contributing to hyperventilation and breathlessness in cardiac patients. Br J Dis Chest 74:47, 1980.
22. Patten JP: Pins and needles. Br J Hosp Med 20:334, 1978.
23. Saltzman HA, Heyman A, Sieker HO: Correlation of clinical and physiological manifestations of sustained hyperventilation. N Engl J Med 268:1431, 1963.
24. Schneider RR, Seckler SG: Evaluation of acute chest pain. Med Clin North Am 65:53, 1981.
25. Lichstein E, Seckler SG: Evaluation of acute chest pain. Med Clin North Am 57:1481, 1973.
26. Wilcox RG, Roland JM, Hampton JR: Prognosis of patients with "chest pain ?cause." Br Med J 282:431, 1981.
27. Brewin TB: Alcohol intolerance in neoplastic disease. Br Med J 2:437, 1966.
28. Miller AJ, Texidor TA: The "precordial catch," a syndrome of anterior chest pain. Ann Intern Med 51:461, 1959.
29. Asher R: Making sense. Lancet 2:359, 1959.
30. Fireman Z, Yust I, Abramov AL: Lethal occult pulmonary hemorrhage in drug-induced thrombocytopenia. Chest 79:358, 1981.
31. Jahn O, Liener A: Contributions to the problem of pulmonary hemorrhages. Report on hospital observations from 1950–1960. Beitr. Klin Tuberk 125:399, 1962.
32. Poole G, Stradling P: Routine radiography for haemoptysis. Br Med J 1:341, 1964.
33. Johnston RN, Lockhart W, Ritchie RT, et al: Haemoptysis. Br Med J 1:592, 1960.
34. Feinsilver SJ, Raffin TA, Kornei MC, et al: Factitious hemoptysis. The case of the red towel. Arch Intern Med 143:567, 1983.
35. Roethe RA, Fuller PB, Byrd RB, et al: Munchausen syndrome with pulmonary manifestations. Chest 79:487, 1981.
36. Weaver LJ, Solliday N, Cugell DW: Selection of patients with hemoptysis for fiberoptic bronchoscopy. Chest 76:7, 1979.
37. Snider GL: When not to use the bronchoscope for hemoptysis. Chest 76:1, 1979.
38. Leading article: Haemoptysis. Br Med J 280:742, 1980.
39. Schneider L: Bronchogenic carcinoma heralded by hemoptysis and ignored because of negative chest x-ray results. NY State J Med 59:637, 1959.
40. Somner AR, Hillis BR, Douglas AC, et al: Value of bronchoscopy in clinical practice. A review of 1,109 examinations. Br Med J 1:1079, 1958.
41. Kallenbach J, Song E, Zwi S: Haemoptysis with no radiological evidence of tumour: The value of early bronchoscopy. S Afr Med J 59:556, 1981.
42. Smiddy JF, Elliot RC: The evaluation of hemoptysis with fiberoptic bronchoscopy. Chest 64:158, 1973.
43. Gong H Jr, Salvatierra C: Clinical efficacy of early and delayed fiberoptic bronchoscopy in patients with hemoptysis. Am Rev Respir Dis 124:221, 1981.
44. Conlan AA, Hurwitz SS, Krige L, et al: Massive hemoptysis. Review of 123 cases. J Thorac Cardiovasc Surg 85:120, 1983.
45. Garzon AA, Gourin A: Surgical management of massive hemoptysis: A ten-year experience. Ann Surg 187:267, 1978.
46. Crocco JA, Rooney JJ, Fankushen DS, et al: Massive hemoptysis. Arch Intern Med 121:495, 1968.
47. Sehhat S, Oreizie M, Moinedine K: Massive pulmonary hemorrhage: Surgical approach as choice of treatment. Ann Thorac Surg 25:12, 1978.
48. Conlan AA, Hurwitz SS: Management of massive haemoptysis with the rigid bronchoscope and cold saline lavage. Thorax 35:901, 1980.
49. Bredin CP, Richardson PR, King TKC, et al: Treatment of massive hemoptysis by combined occlusion of pulmonary and bronchial arteries. Rev Respir Dis 117:969, 1978.
50. Garzon AA, Cerruti MM, Golding ME: Exsanguinating hemoptysis. J Thorac Cardiovasc Surg 84:829, 1982.
51. Ferris EJ: Pulmonary hemorrhage: Vascular evaluation and interventional therapy. Chest 80:710, 1981.
52. Middleton JR, Sen P, Lange M, et al: Death-producing hemoptysis in tuberculosis. Chest 72:601, 1977.
53. Teklu B, Felleke G: Massive haemoptysis in tuberculosis. Tubercle 63:213, 1982.
54. Lin C-S, Becker WH: Broncholith as a cause of fatal haemoptysis. JAMA 239:2153, 1978.
55. Marglin SI, Castellino RA: Severe pulmonary hemorrhage following lymphography. Cancer 43:482, 1979.
56. Pape LA, Haffajee CI, Markis JE, et al: Fatal pulmonary hemorrhage after use of the flow-directed balloon-tipped catheter. Ann Intern Med 90:344, 1979.
57. Krantz EM, Viljoen JF: Haemoptysis following insertion of a Swan-Ganz catheter. Br J Anaesthesiol 51:457, 1979.
58. Baumgartner WA, Mark JBD: Recurrent major haemoptysis: Progression to pneumonectomy. Thorax 35:905, 1980.
59. Uflacker R, Kaemmerer A, Neves C, et al: Management of massive hemoptysis by bronchial artery embolization. Radiology 146:627, 1983.
60. Aspelin P, Kalen N, Svanberg: Treatment of severe haemoptysis by embolisation of the bronchial artery. A case report. Scand J Respir Dis 60:20, 1979.
61. MacErlean DP, Gray BJ, Fitzgerald MX: Bronchial artery embolization in the control of massive haemoptysis. Br J Radiol 52:558, 1979.
62. Bookstein JJ, Moser KM, Kalafer ME, et al: The role of bronchial arteriography and therapeutic embolization in hemoptysis. Chest 72:658, 1977.
63. Feloney JP, Balchum OJ: Repeated massive hemoptysis: Successful control using multiple balloon-tipped catheters for endobronchial tamponade. Chest 74:683, 1978.
64. Prioleau WH Jr, Vujic I, Parker EF, et al: Control of hemoptysis by bronchial artery embolization. Chest 78:878, 1980.
65. Magilligan DJ Jr, Ravipati S, Zayat P, et al: Massive hemoptysis: Control by transcatheter bronchial artery embolization. Ann Thorac Surg 32:392, 1981.
66. Bobrowitz ID, Ramakrishna S, Shim Y-S: Comparison of medical vs. surgical treatment of major hemoptysis. Arch Intern Med 143:1343, 1983.
67. Yang CT, Berger HW: Conservative management of life-threatening hemoptysis. Mt Sinai J Med 45:329, 1978.

3

68. Stern RC, Wood RE, Boat TF, et al: Treatment and prognosis of massive hemoptysis in cystic fibrosis. Am Rev Respir Dis *117*:825, 1978.
69. Larson EB, Featherstone HJ, Petersdorf RG: Fever of undetermined origin: Diagnosis and follow-up of 105 cases, 1970–1980. Medicine *61*:269, 1982.
70. Attia EL, Marshall KG: Halitosis. Can Med Assoc J *126*:1281, 1982.
71. Kass EH: Changing ecology of bacterial infections. Arch Environ Health *6*:19, 1963.
72. Hurst A: Familial emphysema. *In* Symposium on Emphysema and the "Chronic Bronchitis" Syndrome. Aspen, CO, 1958. Am Rev Respir Dis *80*:1959.
73. Wimpfheimer F, Schneider L: Familial emphysema. Am Rev Respir Dis *83*:697, 1961.
74. Talamo RC, Blennerhassett JB, Austen KF: Familial emphysema and alpha₁-antitrypsin deficiency. N Engl J Med *275*:1301, 1966.
75. D'Alessio DJ, Heeren RH, Hendricks SL, et al: A starling roost as the source of urban epidemic histoplasmosis in an area of low incidence. Am Rev Resp Dis *91*:725, 1965.
76. Klite PD, Young RV: Bats and histoplasmosis: A clinico-epidemiologic study of two human cases. Ann Intern Med *62*:1263, 1965.
77. Austen FK, Carmichael MW, Adams RD: Neurologic manifestations of chronic pulmonary insufficiency. N Engl J Med *257*:579, 1957.
78. Alexander JK, Amad KH, Cole VW: Observations on some clinical features of extreme obesity, with particular reference to cardiorespiratory effects. Am J Med *32*:512, 1962.
79. Gravelyn TR, Weg JG: Respiratory rate as an indicator of acute respiratory dysfunction. JAMA *244*:1123, 1980.
80. McFadden JP, Price RC, Eastwood HD, et al: Raised respiratory rate in elderly patients: A valuable physical sign. Br Med J *284*:626, 1982.
81. Castellino RA, Blank N: Etiologic diagnosis of focal pulmonary infection in immunocompromised patients by fluoroscopically guided percutaneous needle aspiration. Radiology *132*:563, 1979.
82. Guarino JR: Auscultatory percussion of the chest. Lancet *1*:1332, 1980.
83. Hampton CS, Chaloner A: Which stethoscope? Br Med J *4*:388, 1967.
84. LeBlanc P, Macklem PT, Ross WR: Breath sounds and distribution of pulmonary ventilation. Am Rev Respir Dis *102*:10, 1970.
85. Banaszak EF, Kory RC, Snider GL: Phonopneumography. Am Rev Respir Dis *107*:449, 1973.
86. Cugell DW: Use of tape recordings of respiratory sound and breathing pattern for instruction in pulmonary auscultation. Am Rev Respir Dis *104*:948, 1971.
87. Weiss EB, Carlson CJ: Recording of breath sounds. Am Rev Respir Dis *105*:835, 1972.
88. Charbonneau G, Racineux JL, Sudraud M, et al: An accurate recording system and its use in breath sounds; Spectral analysis. J Appl Physiol *55*:1120, 1983.
89. Ploysongsang Y: The lung sounds phase angle test for detection of small airway disease. Respir Physiol *53*:203, 1983.
90. Loudon RG: Auscultation of the lung. Clin Notes Respir Dis *21*:3, 1982.
91. Milic-Emili J, Henderson JAM, Dolovich MB, et al: Regional distribution of inspired gas in the lung. J Appl Physiol *21*:749, 1966.
92. Dollfuss RE, Milic-Emili J, Bates D: Regional ventilation of the lung, studied with boluses of ¹³³xenon. Respir Physiol *2*:234, 1967.
93. Nairn JR, Turner-Warwick M: Breath sounds in emphysema. Br J Dis Chest *63*:29, 1969.
94. Ploysongsang Y, Paré JAP, Macklem PT: Correlation of regional breath sounds with regional ventilation in emphysema. Am Rev Respir Dis *126*:526, 1982.
95. Forgacs P, Nathoo AR, Richardson HD: Breath sounds. Thorax *26*:288, 1971.
96. Coope R: Diseases of the Chest. 2nd ed. Edinburgh, Livingstone, 1950.
97. Kraman SS: Does laryngeal noise contribute to the vesicular lung sound? Am Rev Respir Dis *124*:292, 1981.
98. Laennec RTH: De l'Auscultation Médiate, ou Traité du Diagnostic des Maladies des Poumons et du Coeur, Fondé Principalement sur ce Nouveau Moyen d'Exploration. Paris, Brossen and Claudé, 1819.
99. Robertson AJ, Coope R: Râles, rhonchi, and Laennec. Lancet *2*:417, 1957.
100. Forgacs P: Crackles and wheezes. Lancet *2*:203, 1967.
101. Ploysongsang Y, Schonfield SA: Mechanics of production of crackles after atelectasis during low-volume breathing. Am Rev Respir Dis *126*:413, 1982.
102. Thacker RE, Kraman SS: The prevalence of auscultatory crackles in subjects without lung disease. Chest *81*:672, 1982.
103. Workum P, Holford SK, Delbano EA, et al: The prevalence and character of crackles (rales) in young women without significant lung disease. Am Rev Respir Dis *126*:921, 1982.
104. Mori M, Kinoshita K, Morinari H, et al: Waveform and spectral analysis of crackles. Thorax *35*:843, 1980.

105. Marini JJ, Pierson DJ, Hudson LD, et al: The significance of wheezing in chronic airflow obstruction. Am Rev Respir Dis *120*:1069, 1979.
106. Forgacs P: The functional basis of pulmonary sounds. Chest *73*:399, 1978.
107. Fagge CH: *In* Pye-Smith (ed): The Principles and Practice of Medicine. 2nd ed. London, Churchill, 1888.
108. Hamman L: Spontaneous mediastinal emphysema. Bull Johns Hopkins Hosp *64*:1, 1939.
109. Scadding JG, Wood P: Systolic clicks due to left-sided pneumothorax. Lancet *2*:1208, 1939.
110. Semple T, Lancaster WM: Noisy pneumothorax: Observations based on 24 cases. Br Med J *1*:1342, 1961.
111. Moyer JH, Glantz G, Brest AN: Pulmonary arteriovenous fistulas. Physiologic and clinical considerations. Am J Med *32*:417, 1962.
112. Annamalai A, Ranganathan C, Radhakrishan MA: Pulmonary arteriovenous aneurysm with a major systemic component. Indian J Radiol *13*:172, 1959.
113. Victor S, Lakshmikanthan C, Shankar G, et al: Continuous murmur as a sequel of augmented collateral circulation in suppurative lung disease: Report of three cases. Chest *62*:504, 1972.
114. Massumi RA, Mason DT, Vera Z, et al: Reversed pulsus paradoxus. N Engl J Med *289*:1272, 1973.
115. Beerman H, Kirshbaum BA: Some associated pulmonary and cutaneous diseases: A review of recent literature. Am J Med Sci *242*:494, 1961.
116. Conn O: Asterixis: Its occurrence in chronic pulmonary disease, with a commentary on its general mechanism. N Engl J Med *259*:564, 1958.
117. Appenzeller O, Parks RD, MacGee J: Peripheral neuropathy in chronic disease of the respiratory tract. Am J Med *44*:873, 1968.
118. Shneerson JM: Digital clubbing and hypertrophic osteoarthropathy: The underlying mechanisms. Br J Dis Chest *75*:113, 1981.
119. Waring WW, Wilkinson RW, Wiebe RA, et al: Quantitation of digital clubbing in children. Measurements of casts of the index finger. Am Rev Respir Dis *104*:166, 1971.
120. Sly RM, Ghazanshahi S, Buranakul B, et al: Objective assessment for digital clubbing in Caucasian, Negro, and Oriental subjects. Chest *64*:687, 1973.
121. Mendlowitz M: Measurements of blood flow and blood pressure in clubbed fingers. J Clin Invest *20*:113, 1941.
122. Racoceanu SN, Mendlowitz M, Suck AF, et al: Digital capillary blood flow in clubbing. ⁸⁵Kr studies in hereditary and acquired cases. Ann Intern Med *75*:933, 1971.
123. Shneerson JM, Jones BM: Ferritin, finger clubbing and lung diseases. Thorax *36*:688, 1981.
124. Lemen RJ, Gates AJ, Mathé AA, et al: Relationships among digital clubbing, disease severity, and serum prostaglandins $F_2\alpha$ and E concentrations in cystic fibrosis patients. Am Rev Respir Dis *117*:639, 1978.
125. Yacoub MH: Relation between the histology of bronchial carcinoma and hypertrophic pulmonary osteoarthropathy. Thorax *20*:537, 1965.
126. Doyle L: Some considerations of hypertrophic osteoarthropathy. Br J Dis Chest *74*:314, 1980.
127. Editorial: Finger clubbing and hypertrophic pulmonary osteoarthropathy. Br Med J *2*:785, 1977.
128. Borden EC, Holling HE: Hypertrophic osteoarthropathy and pregnancy. Ann Intern Med *71*:577, 1969.
129. Armstrong RD, Crisp AJ, Grahame R, et al: Hypertrophic osteoarthropathy and purgative abuse. Br Med J *282*:1836, 1981.
130. Coury C: Hippocratic fingers and hypertrophic osteoarthropathy: A study of 350 cases. Br J Dis Chest *54*:202, 1960.
131. Carlotta D, Fogel de Korc E, Bouton J: Hypertrophying osteoarthropathy and metastatic pulmonary cancer. Thorax *7*:119, 1958.
132. Golimbu C, Marchetta P, Firooznia H, et al: Hypertrophic osteoarthropathy in metastatic renal cell carcinoma. Urology *22*:669, 1983.
133. Lokich JJ: Pulmonary osteoarthropathy. Association with mesenchymal tumor metastases to the lungs. JAMA *238*:37, 1977.
134. Benfield GFA: Primary lymphosarcoma of lung associated with hypertrophic pulmonary osteoarthropathy. Thorax *34*:279, 1979.
135. Lofters WS, Walker TM: Hodgkin's disease and hypertrophic pulmonary osteoarthropathy. Complete clearing following radiotherapy. West Indian Med J *27*:227, 1978.
136. Perkins PJ: Delayed onset of secondary hypertrophic osteoarthropathy. Am J Roentgenol *130*:561, 1978.
137. Macfarlane JT, Ibrahim M, Tor-Agbidye S: The importance of finger clubbing in pulmonary tuberculosis. Tubercle *60*:45, 1979.
138. Skorneck AB, Ginsburg LB: Pulmonary hypertrophic osteoarthropathy (Periostitis): Its absence in pulmonary tuberculosis. N Engl J Med *258*:1079, 1958.
139. Rutherford RB, Rhodes BA, Wagner HN Jr: The distribution of extremity blood flow before and after vagectomy in a patient with hypertrophic pulmonary osteoarthropathy. Dis Chest *56*:19, 1969.
140. Huckstep RL, Bodkin PE: Vagotomy in hypertrophic pulmonary

osteoarthropathy associated with bronchial carcinoma. Lancet 2:343, 1958.

141. Holling HE: Pulmonary hypertrophic osteoarthropathy. Ann Intern Med 66:232, 1967.

142. King JO: Localized clubbing and hypertrophic osteoarthropathy due to infection in an aortic prosthesis. Br Med J 4:404, 1972.

143. Stein HB, Little HA: Localized hypertrophic osteoarthropathy in the presence of an abdominal prosthesis. Can Med Assoc J 118:947, 1978.

144. Gibson T, Joye J, Schumacher HR, et al: Localized hypertrophic osteoarthropathy with abdominal aortic prosthesis and infection. Ann Intern Med 81:556, 1974.

145. Holling HE, Brodey RS, Boland HC: Pulmonary hypertrophic osteoarthropathy. Lancet 2:1269, 1961.

146. Ginsburg J, Brown JB: Increased oestrogen excretion in hypertrophic pulmonary osteoarthropathy. Lancet 2:1274, 1961.

147. Rimoin DL: Pachydermoperiostosis (idiopathic clubbing and periostosis): Genetic and physiologic considerations. N Engl J Med 272:923, 1965.

148. Hedayati H, Barmada R, Skosey JL: Acrolysis in pachydermoperiostosis: Primary or idiopathic hypertrophic osteoarthropathy. Arch Intern Med 140:1087, 1980.

149. Kerber RE, Vogl A: Pachydermoperiostosis. Arch Intern Med 132:245, 1973.

150. Dalgleish AG: Hypertrophic pulmonary osteoarthropathy: Response to chemotherapy without documented tumour response. Aust NZ J Med 13:513, 1983.

151. Rao GM, Guruprakash GH, Poulose KP, et al: Improvement in hypertrophic pulmonary osteoarthropathy after radiotherapy to metastasis. Am J Roentgenol 133:944, 1979.

152. Sagar VV, Mecklenburg RL, Piccone JM: Resolution of bone scan changes in hypertrophic pulmonary osteoarthropathy in untreated carcinoma of the lung. Clin Nucl Med 3:427, 1978.

153. Kelman GR, Nunn JF: Clinical recognition of hypoxaemia under fluorescent lamps. Lancet 1:1400, 1966.

154. Lundsgaard C, Van Slyke DD: Cyanosis. Medicine 2:1, 1923.

155. Dlabal PW, Stutts BS, Jenkins DW, et al: Cyanosis following right pneumonectomy: Importance of patent foramen ovale. Chest 81:370, 1982.

156. Smylie HC, Blendis LM, Armitage P: Observer disagreement in physical signs of the respiratory system. Lancet 2:412, 1965.

157. Schneider, IC, Anderson AE Jr: Correlation of clinical signs with ventilatory function in obstructive lung disease. Ann Intern Med 62:477, 1965.

158. Rosenblatt G, Stein M: Clinical value of the forced expiratory time measured during auscultation. N Engl J Med 267:432, 1962.

159. Comroe JH, Botelho S: The unreality of cyanosis in the recognition of arterial anoxemia. Am J Med Sci 214:1, 1947.

160. Regan GM, Tagg B, Thomson ML: Subjective assessment and objective measurement of finger clubbing. Lancet 1:530, 1967.

161. Pyke DA: Finger clubbing: Validity as a physical sign. Lancet 2:352, 1954.

162. Belen J, Neuhaus A, Markowitz D, et al: Modification of the effect of fiberoptic bronchoscopy on pulmonary mechanics. Chest 79:516, 1981.

163. Zavala DC, Godsey K, Bedell GN: The response to atropine sulfate given by aerosol and intramuscular routes to patients undergoing fiberoptic bronchoscopy. Chest 79:512, 1981.

164. Pearce SJ: Fibreoptic bronchoscopy: Is sedation necessary? Br Med J 281:779, 1980.

165. Mitchell DM, Emerson CJ, Collyer J, et al: Fibreoptic bronchoscopy: Ten years on. Br Med J 281:360, 1980.

166. Oho K, Kato H, Ogawa I, et al: Present status of bronchoscopy in Japan. Br J Dis Chest 75:409, 1981.

167. Erlich H: Bacteriologic studies and effects of anesthetic solutions on bronchial secretions during bronchoscopy. Am Rev Respir Dis 84:414, 1961.

168. Conte BA, Laforet EG: The role of the topical anesthetic agent in modifying bacteriologic data obtained by bronchoscopy. N Engl J Med 267:957, 1962.

169. Godden DJ, Willey RF, Fergusson RJ, et al: Rigid bronchoscopy under intravenous general anaesthesia with oxygen Venturi ventilation. Thorax 37:532, 1982.

170. Ikeda S: Flexible bronchofibroscope. Ann Otol Rhinol Laryngol 79:916, 1970.

171. Smiddy JF, Kirby GR, Ruth WE: The flexible fiberoptic bronchoscope in pulmonary diagnosis and therapy. Transactions of the 30th VA–Armed Forces Pulmonary Disease Research Conference, Cincinnati, 1971, p 30.

172. Bates M: Fibreoptic bronchoscopy. Thorax 35:640, 1980.

173. Sackner MA, Landa JF: Bronchofiberoscopy: To intubate or not to intubate. Chest 63:302, 1973.

174. Zavala DC, Rhodes ML, Richardson RH, et al: Fiberoptic and rigid bronchoscopy: The state of the art. Chest 65:605, 1974.

175. Wanner A, Amikam B, Sackner MA: A technique for bedside bronchofiberoscopy. Chest 61:287, 1972.

176. Kovnat DM, Schaaf JT, Rath GS, et al: Bronchoscopic perspective. Chest 65:606, 1974.

177. King EG: Expanding diagnostic and therapeutic horizons—fiberoptic bronchoscopy. Chest 63:301, 1973.

178. Wanner A, Zighelboim A, Sackner MA: Nasopharyngeal airway: A facilitated access to the trachea. For nasotracheal suction, bedside bronchofiberoscopy, and selective bronchography. Ann Intern Med 75:593, 1971.

179. Barrett CR Jr: Flexible fiberoptic bronchoscopy in the critically ill patient. Methodology and indications. Chest 73(Suppl):746, 1978.

180. Barrett CR Jr, Vecchione JJ, Bell ALL Jr: Flexible fiberoptic bronchoscopy for airway management during acute respiratory failure. Am Rev Respir Dis 109:429, 1974.

181. Reichert WW, Hall WJ, Hyde RW: A simple disposable device for performing fiberoptic bronchoscopy on patients requiring continuous artificial ventilation. Am Rev Respir Dis 109:394, 1974.

182. Amikam B, Landa J, West J, et al: Bronchofiberscopic observations of the tracheobronchial tree during intubation. Am Rev Respir Dis 105:747, 1972.

183. Shinnick JP, Johnston RF, Oslick T: Bronchoscopy during mechanical ventilation using the fiberscopic. Chest 65:613, 1974.

184. Jenkins P, Dick R, Clarke SW: Selective bronchography using the fibreoptic bronchoscope. Br J Dis Chest 76:88, 1982.

185. Wanner A, Landa JF, Nieman RE Jr, et al: Bedside bronchofiberoscopy for atelectasis and lung abscess. JAMA 224:1281, 1973.

186. Williams SJ, Pierce RJ, Davies NJH, et al: Methods of studying lobar and segmental function of the lung in man. Br J Dis Chest 73:97, 1979.

187. Lundgren R, Haggmark S, Reiz S: Hemodynamic effects of flexible fiberoptic bronchoscopy performed under topical anesthesia. Chest 82:295, 1982.

188. Burman SO, Gibson TC: Bronchoscopy and cardiorespiratory reflexes. Ann Surg 157:134, 1963.

189. Stanley NN: Cardiac dysrhythmias during fibreoptic bronchoscopy: Effects of premedication with oxprenolol. Br J Dis Chest 74:418, 1980.

190. Katz AS, Michelson EL, Stawicki J, et al: Cardiac arrhythmias: Frequency during fiberoptic bronchoscopy and correlation with hypoxemia. Arch Intern Med 141:603, 1981.

191. Elguindi AS, Harrison GN, Abdulla AM, et al: Cardiac rhythm disturbances during fiberoptic bronchoscopy: A prospective study. J Thorac Cardiovasc Surg 77:557, 1979.

192. Pereira W Jr, Kovnat DM, Snider GL: A prospective cooperative study of complications following flexible fiberoptic bronchoscopy. Chest 73:813, 1978.

193. Credle WF Jr, Smiddy JF, Elliott RC: Complications of fiberoptic bronchoscopy. Am Rev Respir Dis 109:67, 1974.

194. Timms RM, Harrell JH: Bacteremia related to fiberoptic bronchoscopy. A case report. Am Rev Respir Dis 111:555, 1975.

195. Pereira W Jr, Kovnat DM, Snider GL: A prospective cooperative study of complications following flexible fiberoptic bronchoscopy. Chest 73:813, 1978.

196. Pereira W, Kovnat DM, Khan MA: Fever and pneumonia after flexible fiberoptic bronchoscopy. Am Rev Respir Dis 112:59, 1975.

197. Beyt BE Jr, King DK, Glew RH: Fatal pneumonitis and septicemia after fiberoptic bronchoscopy. Chest 72:105, 1977.

198. Hammer DL, Aranda CP, Galati V, et al: Massive intrabronchial aspiration of contents of pulmonary abscess after fiberoptic bronchoscopy. Chest 74:306, 1978.

199. Lukomsky GI, Ovchinnikov AA, Bilal A: Complications of bronchoscopy: Comparison of rigid bronchoscopy under general anesthesia and flexible fiberoptic bronchoscopy under topical anesthesia. Chest 79:316, 1981.

200. Elliott RC, Reichel J: The efficacy of sputum specimens obtained by nebulization versus gastric aspirates in the bacteriologic diagnosis of pulmonary tuberculosis. Am Rev Respir Dis 88:223, 1963.

201. Lillehei JP: Sputum induction with heated aerosol inhalations for the diagnosis of tuberculosis. Am Rev Respir Dis 84:276, 1961.

202. Carr DT, Karlson AG, Stilwell GG: A comparison of cultures of induced sputum and gastric washings in the diagnosis of tuberculosis. Mayo Clin Proc 42:23, 1967.

203. Horstmann DM, Hsiung GD: Principles of diagnostic virology. In Horsfall FL, Tamm I (eds): Viral and Rickettsial Infections of Man. 4th ed. Philadelphia, Lippincott, 1965, p 405.

204. Guckian JC, Christensen WD: Quantitative culture and gram stain of sputum in pneumonia. Am Rev Respir Dis 118:997, 1978.

205. Lapinski EM, Flakas ED, Taylor BC: An evaluation of some methods for culturing sputum from patients with bronchitis and emphysema. Am Rev Respir Dis 89:760, 1964.

206. Pirtle JK, Monroe PW, Smalley TK, et al: Diagnostic and therapeutic advantages of serial quantitative cultures of fresh sputum in acute bacterial pneumonia. Am Rev Respir Dis 100:831, 1969.

3

207. Bartlett JG, Finegold SM: Bacteriology of expectorated sputum with quantitative culture and wash technique compared to transtracheal aspirates. Am Rev Respir Dis *117*:1019, 1978.

208. Bermann SZ, Mathison DA, Stevenson DD, et al: Transtracheal aspiration studies in asthmatic patients in relapse with "infective" asthma and in subjects without respiratory disease. J Allergy Clin Immunol *56*:206, 1975.

209. Wallace RJ Jr: (Another) New technique for an old disease: The protected brush catheter and bacterial pneumonia. Chest *81*:532, 1982.

210. Teague RB, Wallace RJ Jr, Awe RJ: The use of quantitative sterile brush culture and gram stain analysis in the diagnosis of lower respiratory tract infection. Chest *79*:157, 1981.

211. Flatauer FE, Chabalko JJ, Wolinsky E: Fiberoptic bronchoscopy in bacteriologic assessment of lower respiratory tract secretions: Importance of microscopic examination. JAMA *244*:2427, 1980.

212. Kalinske RW, Parker RH, Brandt D, et al: Diagnostic usefulness and safety of transtracheal aspiration. N Engl J Med *276*:604, 1967.

213. Hahn HH, Beaty HN: Transtracheal aspiration in the evaluation of patients with pneumonia. Ann Intern Med *72*:183, 1970.

214. Ries K, Levison ME, Kaye D: Transtracheal aspiration in pulmonary infection. Arch Intern Med *133*:453, 1974.

215. Bartlett JG, Rosenblatt JE, Finegold SM: Percutaneous transtracheal aspiration in the diagnosis of anaerobic pulmonary infection. Ann Intern Med *79*:535, 1973.

216. Pecora DV: A comparison of transtracheal aspiration with other methods of determining the bacterial flora of the lower respiratory tract. N Engl J Med *269*:664, 1963.

217. Bartlett JG: Diagnostic accuracy of transtracheal aspiration bacteriologic studies. Am Rev Respir Dis *115*:777, 1977.

218. Bjerkestraud G, Digranes A, Schreiner A: Bacteriological findings in transtracheal aspirates from patients with chronic bronchitis and bronchiectasis. Scand J Respir Dis *56*:201, 1975.

219. Fossieck BE Jr, Parker RH, Cohen MH, et al: Fiberoptic bronchoscopy and culture of bacteria from the lower respiratory tract. Chest *72*:5, 1977.

220. Peltier P, Martin M, Barrier J, et al: Guided transtracheal distal pulmonary brushing-washing: Diagnosing acute pneumonia in high risk patients. Br Med J *284*:147, 1982.

221. Spencer CD, Beaty HN: Complications of transtracheal aspiration. N Engl J Med *286*:304, 1972.

222. Unger KM, Moser KM: Fatal complication of transtracheal aspiration: A report of two cases. Arch Intern Med *132*:437, 1973.

223. Shim C, Fine N, Fernandez R, et al: Cardiac arrhythmias resulting from tracheal suctioning. Ann Intern Med *71*:1149, 1969.

224. Marx GF, Steen SN, Arkins RE, et al: Clinical Anesthesia Conference: Endotracheal Suction and Death. NY State J Med *68*:565, 1968.

225. Thiede WH, Banaszak EF: Selective bronchial catheterization. N Engl J Med *286*:526, 1972.

226. Repsher LH: The diagnostic potential of endobronchial brush biopsy. Chest *63*:650, 1973.

227. Finley R, Kieff, E, Thomsen S, et al: Bronchial brushing in the diagnosis of pulmonary disease in patients at risk for opportunistic infection. Am Rev Respir Dis *109*:379, 1974.

228. Repsher LH, Schröter G, Hammond WS: Diagnosis of *Pneumocystis carinii* pneumonitis by means of endobronchial brush biopsy. N Engl J Med *287*:340, 1972.

229. Matthay RA, Farmer WC, Odero D: Diagnostic fibreoptic bronchoscopy in the immunocompromised host with pulmonary infiltrates. Thorax *32*:539, 1977.

230. Jett JR, Cortese DA, Dines DE: The value of bronchoscopy in the diagnosis of mycobacterial disease: A five year experience. Chest *80*:575, 1981.

231. Wimberley N, Faling LJ, Bartlett JG: Uncontaminated lower airway secretions for bacterial culture. Am Rev Respir Dis *119*:337, 1979.

232. Joshi JH, Wang K-P, DeJongh CA, et al: A comparative evaluation of 2 fiberoptic bronchoscopy catheters: The plugged telescoping catheter versus the single sheathed nonplugged catheter. Am Rev Respir Dis *126*:860, 1982.

233. Hayes DA, McCarthy LC, Friedman M: Evaluation of two bronchofiberscopic methods of culturing the lower respiratory tract. Am Rev Respir Dis *122*:319, 1980.

234. Higuchi JH, Coalson JJ, Johanson WG Jr: Bacteriologic diagnosis of nosocomial pneumonias in primates: Usefulness of the protected specimen brush. Am Rev Respir Dis *125*:53, 1982.

235. Halperin SA, Suratt PM, Gwaltney JM Jr, et al: Bacterial cultures of the lower respiratory tract in normal volunteers with and without experimental rhinovirus infection using a plugged double catheter system. Am Rev Respir Dis *125*:678, 1982.

236. Bordelon JY Jr, Legrand P, Gewin WC, et al: The telescoping plugged catheter in suspected anaerobic infections: A controlled series. Am Rev Respir Dis *128*:465, 1983.

237. Wimberley NW, Bass JB Jr, Boyd BW, et al: Use of a bronchoscopic protected catheter brush for the diagnosis of pulmonary infections. Chest *81*:556, 1982.

238. Springmeyer SC, Silvestri RC, Sale GE, et al: The role of transbronchial biopsy for the diagnosis of diffuse pneumonias in immunocompromised marrow transplant recipients. Am Rev Respir Dis *126*:763, 1982.

239. Hopkin JM, Turney JH, Young JA, et al: Rapid diagnosis of obscure pneumonia in immunosuppressed renal patients by cytology of alveolar lavage fluid. Lancet *2*:299, 1983.

240. Zavala DC, Schoell JE: Ultra-thin needle aspiration of the lung in infectious and malignant disease. Am Rev Respir Dis *123*:125, 1981.

241. Bhatt ON, Miller R, Le Riche J, et al: Aspiration biopsy in pulmonary opportunistic infections. Acta Cytol *21*:206, 1977.

242. Castellino RA, Blank N: Etiologic diagnosis of focal pulmonary infection in immunocompromised patients by fluoroscopically guided percutaneous needle aspiration. Radiology *132*:563, 1979.

243. Gibney RTN, Man GCW, King EG, et al: Aspiration biopsy in the diagnosis of pulmonary disease. Chest *80*:300, 1981.

244. Linnemann CC: Lung punctures. Chest *78*:1, 1980.

245. Palmer DL, Davidson M, Lusk R: Needle aspiration of the lung in complex pneumonias. Chest *78*:16, 1980.

246. Toledo-Pereyra LH, De Meester TR, Kinealey A, et al: The benefits of open lung biopsy in patients with previous non-diagnostic transbronchial lung biopsy: A guide to appropriate therapy. Chest *77*:647, 1980.

247. Jaffe JP, Maki GD: Lung biopsy in immunocompromised patients: One institution's experience and an approach to management of pulmonary disease in the compromised host. Cancer *48*:1144, 1981.

248. Haverkos HW, Dowling JN, Pasculle AW, et al: Diagnosis of pneumonitis in immunocompromised patients by open lung biopsy. Cancer *52*:1093, 1983.

249. Manson-Bahr PH: Manson's Tropical Diseases. A Manual of the Diseases of Warm Climates. 16th ed. London, Baillière, Tindall, and Cassell, 1966.

250. Joyner CR Jr, Herman RJ, Reid JM: Reflected ultrasound in the detection and localization of pleural effusion. JAMA *200*:399, 1967.

251. Viikeri M, Jääskeläinen J, Tähti E: Ultrasonic examination of pleural thickenings and calcifications in occupational asbestosis. Dis Chest *54*:17, 1968.

252. Viikeri M: Ultrasound examination of pleural plaques: Experimental, pathologic and clinical studies. Acta Radiol (Suppl) *301*:7, 1970.

253. Sandweiss DA, Hanson JC, Gosink BB, et al: Ultrasound in diagnosis, localization, and treatment of loculated pleural empyema. Ann Intern Med *82*:50, 1975.

254. Janik JS, Nagaraj HS, Groff DB: Thoracoscopic evaluation of intrathoracic lesions in children. J Thorac Cardiovasc Surg *83*:408, 1982.

255. Van Heerden JA, Laufenberg HJ Jr: Simplified thoracentesis. Mayo Clin Proc *43*:311, 1968.

256. Epstein RL: Constituents of sputum: A simple method. Ann Intern Med *77*:259, 1972.

257. Sheffner AL: The reduction *in vitro* in viscosity of mucoprotein solutions by a new mucolytic agent. *N*-acetyl-L-cysteine. Ann NY Acad Sci *106*:298, 1963.

258. Lorian V, Lacasse ML: *N*-acetyl-L-cysteine sputum homogenization and its mechanism of action on isolation of tubercle bacilli. Dis Chest *51*:275, 1967.

259. Wilson MM: Fluorescence microscopy in examination of smears for *Mycobacterium tuberculosis*. Am Rev Tuberc *65*:709, 1952.

260. Chakravarty SC, Sandhu RS: Incidence of bronchopulmonary candidiasis in patients treated with antibiotics. Acta Tuberc Scand *44*:152, 1964.

261. Baum GL: The significance of *Candida albicans* in human sputum. N Engl J Med *263*:70, 1960.

262. Gernez-Rieux C, Biguet P, Capron A, et al: Étude de la flore mycologique des bronches par examen des sécrétions bronchiques prélevées sous bronchoscope chez 1120 malades, de 1956 à 1964. (Fungus studies of bronchial secretions obtained at bronchoscopy in 1120 patients from 1956 to 1964.) Rev Tuberc *28*:439, 1964.

263. Overholt EL, Tigertt WD, Kadull PJ, et al: An analysis of forty-two cases of laboratory-acquired tularemia: Treament with broad spectrum antibiotics. Am J Med *30*:785, 1961.

264. Johnson JE, Kadull PJ: Laboratory-acquired Q fever: A report of 50 cases. Am J Med *41*:391, 1966.

265. Johnson JE III, Perry JE, Fekety FR, et al: Laboratory-acquired coccidioidomycosis: A report of 210 cases. Ann Intern Med *60*:941, 1964.

266. Murray JF, Howard D: Laboratory-acquired histoplasmosis. Am Rev Respir Dis *89*:631, 1964.

267. Goodwin RA Jr, Snell JD, Hubbard WW, et al: Early chronic pulmonary histoplasmosis. Am Rev Respir Dis *93*:47, 1966.

268. Edwards LB, Acquaviva FA, Livesay VT, et al: An atlas of sensitivity to tuberculin, PPD-B, and histoplasmin in the United States. Am Rev Respir Dis *99*:1, 1969.

269. Evans S, Brobst M: Bronchitis, pneumonitis and pneumonia in University of Wisconsin students. N Engl J Med 265:401, 1961.

270. Tunevall G, Ohlson M, Svedmyr A, et al: Aetiologic agents in respiratory illness. Occurrence of bacteria and of serologic reactions against viruses and bacteria in acute respiratory illness. Acta Med Scand 174:237, 1963.

271. George RB, Ziskind MM, Rasch JR, et al: Mycoplasma and adenovirus pneumonias. Comparison with other atypical pneumonias in a military population. Ann Intern Med 65:931, 1966.

272. Griffin JP, Crawford YE: Mycoplasma pneumoniae in primary atypical pneumonia. JAMA 193:1011, 1965.

273. Forsyth BR, Bloom HH, Johnson KM, et al: Etiology of primary atypical pneumonia in a military population. JAMA 191:364, 1965.

274. Rytel MW: Primary atypical pneumonia: Current concepts. Am J Med Sci 247:84, 1964.

275. Hilleman MR, Flatley FJ, Anderson SA, et al: Distribution and significance of Asian and other influenza antibodies in the human population. N Engl J Med 258:969, 1958.

276. Hayslett J, McCarroll J, Brady E, et al: Endemic influenza. I. Serologic evidence of continuing and subclinical infection in disparate populations in the post-pandemic period. Am Rev Respir Dis 85:1, 1962.

277. Salvin SB: Current concepts of diagnostic serology and skin hypersensitivity in the mycoses. Am J Med 27:97, 1959.

278. Buechner HA, Seabury JH, Campbell, CC, et al: The current status of serologic, immunologic and skin tests in the diagnosis of pulmonary mycoses. Report of the committee on fungus diseases and subcommittee on criteria for clinical diagnosis—American College of Chest Physicians. Chest 63:259, 1973.

279. Richert JH, Campbell CC: The significance of skin and serologic tests in the diagnosis of pulmonary residuals of histoplasmosis: A review of 123 cases. Am Rev Respir Dis 86:381, 1962.

280. Buechner HA: Clinical aspects of fungus diseases of the lungs including laboratory diagnosis and treatment. In Banyai AL, Gordon BL (eds): Advances in Cardiopulmonary Diseases. Vol 3. Chicago, Yearbook Medical Publishers, 1966, p 123.

281. Walter JE: The significance of antibodies in chronic histoplasmosis by immunoelectrophoretic and complement fixation tests. Am Rev Respir Dis 99:50, 1969.

282. Scalarone GM, Levine HB, Pappagianis D, et al: Spherulin as a complement-fixing antigen in human coccidioidomycosis. Am Rev Respir Dis 110:324, 1974.

283. Jones RD, Sarosi GA, Parker JD, et al: The complement-fixation test in extracutaneous sporotrichosis. Ann Intern Med 71:913, 1969.

284. Rosner F, Gabriel FD, Taschdjian CL, et al: Serologic diagnosis of systemic candidiasis in patients with acute leukemia. Am J Med 51:54, 1971.

285. Remington JS, Gaines JD, Gilmer MA: Demonstration of Candida precipitins in human sera by counterimmunoelectrophoresis. Lancet 1:413, 1972.

286. Preisler HD, Hasenclever HF, Levitan AA, et al: Serologic diagnosis of disseminated candidiasis in patients with acute leukemia. Ann Intern Med 70:19, 1969.

287. Goodman JS, Kaufman L, Koenig MG: Diagnosis of cryptococcal meningitis: Value of immunologic detection of cryptococcal antigen. N Engl J Med 285:434, 1971.

288. Miller LH, Brown HW: The serologic diagnosis of parasitic infections in medical practice. Ann Intern Med 71:983, 1969.

289. Beverley JKA: A new look at infectious diseases: Toxoplasmosis. Br Med J 2:475, 1973.

290. Leading article: Hydatid disease. Br Med J 4:448, 1970.

291. Kagan IG, Osimani JJ, Varela JC, et al: Evaluation of intradermal and serologic tests for the diagnosis of hydatid disease. Am J Trop Med Hyg 15:172, 1966.

292. Vogel H, Widelock D, Fuerst HT: A microflocculation test for trichinosis. J Infect Dis 100:40, 1957.

293. Liu C: Studies on primary atypical pneumonia. I. Localization, isolation, and cultivation of a virus in chick embryos. J Exp Med 106:455, 1957.

294. Leading article: Diagnostic value of fluorescent antibodies. Br Med J 4:375, 1967.

295. Goodburn GM, Marmion BP, Kendall EJC: Infection with Eaton's primary atypical pneumonic agent in England. Br Med J 1:1266, 1963.

296. Clyde WA Jr, Denny FW, Dingle JH: Fluorescent-stainable antibodies to the Eaton agent in human primary atypical pneumonia transmission studies. J Clin Invest 40:1638, 1961.

297. Lynch HJ Jr, Plexico KL: A rapid method for screening sputums for Histoplasma capsulatum employing the fluorescent-antibody technic. N Engl J Med 266:811, 1962.

298. Carski TR, Cozad, GC, Larsh HW: Detection of Histoplasma capsulatum in sputum by means of fluorescent antibody staining. Am J Clin Pathol 37:465, 1962.

299. Gray KG, MacFarlane DE, Sommerville RG: Direct immunofluores-

300. Furcolow ML, Hewell B, Nelson WE: Quantitative studies of the tuberculin reaction. III. Tuberculin sensitivity in relation to active tuberculosis. Am Rev Tuberc 45:504, 1942.

301. Allen AR, Harmon RWJ, Klacsan LJ, et al: Accuracy of the confirmatory diagnosis of tuberculosis. Am J Med 22:904, 1957.

302. Nash DR, Douglass JE: Anergy in active tuberculosis: A comparison between positive and negative, and an evaluation of 5 TU and 250 TU skin test doses. Chest 77:32, 1980.

303. Comstock GW, Furcolow ML, Greenberg RL, et al: The tuberculin skin test: A statement by the Committee on Diagnostic Skin Testing, American Thoracic Society. Am Rev Respir Dis 104:769, 1971.

304. Egsmose T: The effect of an exorbitant intracutaneous dose of 200 micrograms PPD tuberculin compared with 0.02 micrograms PPD tuberculin. Am Rev Respir Dis 102:35, 1970.

305. Badger TL: Tuberculosis. N Engl J Med 261:30, 131, 1959.

306. Browder AA, Griffon AL: Tuberculin tine tests on medical wards. Am Rev Respir Dis 105:299, 1972.

307. Katz J, Kunotsky S, Krasnitz A: Variation in sensitivity to tuberculin. Am Rev Respir Dis 106:202, 1972.

308. National Tuberculosis Association: Diagnostic Standards and Classification of Tuberculosis. New York, National Tuberculosis Association, 1969, pp 61–63.

309. Fine MH, Furcolow ML, Chick EW, et al: Tuberculin skin test reactions. Effects of revised classification on comparative evaluations. Am Rev Respir Dis 106:752, 1972.

310. Edwards LB, Acquaviva FA, Livesay VT: Identification of tuberculous infected. Dual tests and density of reaction. Am Rev Respir Dis 108:1334, 1973.

311. Schachter EN: Tuberculin negative tuberculosis. Am Rev Respir Dis 106:587, 1972.

312. Erdtmann FJ, Dixon KE, Llewellyn CH: Skin testing for tuberculosis: Antigen and observer variability. JAMA 28:479, 1974.

313. Rhoades ER, Bryant RE: The influence of local factors on the reaction to tuberculin. Chest 77:190, 1980.

314. Hyde L: Clinical significance of the tuberculin skin test. Am Rev Respir Dis 105:453, 1972.

315. Parish HJ, O'Brien RA: The heat-stability and "tenacity" of tuberculin. Br Med J 1:1018, 1935.

316. Waaler H, Guld J, Magnus K, et al: Adsorption of tuberculin to glass. Bull WHO 19:783, 1958.

317. Marks J: Adsorption of tuberculin as a source of error in Mantoux tests. Tubercle 45:62, 1964

318. Zack MB, Fulkerson LL, Stein E: Clinical evaluation of persons positive to stabilized tuberculin but negative to nonstabilized tuberculin. Chest 60:437, 1971.

319. Landi S, Held HR, Tseng MC: Disparity of potency between stabilized and nonstabilized dilute tuberculin solutions. Am Rev Respir Dis 104:385, 1971.

320. Holden M, Dubin MR, Diamond PH: Frequency of negative intermediate-strength tuberculin sensitivity in patients with active tuberculosis. N Engl J Med 285:1506, 1971.

321. Wijsmuller G, Termini J: The tuberculin test. Effects of storage and method of delivery on reaction size. Am Rev Respir Dis 107:267, 1973.

322. Magnusson M, Guld J, Magnus K, et al: Diluents for stabilization of tuberculin. Bull WHO 19:799, 1958.

323. Leading article: Tuberculin anergy. Br Med J 4:573, 1970.

324. Battershill JH: Cutaneous testing in the elderly patient with tuberculosis. Chest 77:188, 1980.

325. Woodruff CE, Chapman PT: Tuberculin sensitivity in elderly patients. Am Rev Respir Dis 104:261, 1971.

326. National Tuberculosis Association: Diagnostic Standards and Classification of Tuberculosis. New York, National Tuberculosis Association, 1969, p 68.

327. Reichman LB, O'Day R: The influence of a history of a previous test on the prevalence and size of reactions to tuberculin. Am Rev Respir Dis 119:587, 1979.

328. Atuk NO, Hunt EH: Serial tuberculin testing and isoniazid therapy in general hospital employees. JAMA 218:1795, 1971.

329. Smith DT, Johnston WW: The problem of the "boost" effect in tuberculin skin testing. Am Rev Respir Dis 106:118, 1972.

330. Miller SD, Jones HE: Correlation of lymphocyte transformation with tuberculin skin-test sensitivity. Am Rev Respir Dis 107:530, 1973.

331. Thompson NJ, Glassroth JL, Snider, DE Jr, et al: The booster phenomenon in serial tuberculin testing. Am Rev Respir Dis 119:587, 1979.

332. Bass, JB Jr, Serio RA: The use of repeat skin tests to eliminate the booster phenomenon in serial tuberculin testing. Am Rev Respir Dis 123:394, 1981.

333. Valenti WM, Andrews BA, Presley BA, et al: Absence of the booster phenomenon in serial tuberculin skin testing. Am Rev Respir Dis 125:323, 1982.

3

334. Nilsson BS, Magnusson M: Comparison of the biologic activity of tuberculins by the use of lymphocyte cultures. Am Rev Respir Dis 108:565, 1973.

335. Smith JA, Reichman LB: Lymphocyte transformation. An aid in the diagnosis of tuberculosis in patients with nonreactive skin tests. Am Rev Respir Dis 106:194, 1972.

336. Heilman DH, Thornton C, Baetz B: A method for quantitating blastogenesis by tuberculins in cultures of human blood lymphocytes. Am Rev Respir Dis 101:569, 1970.

337. Chaparas SD, Sheagren JN, DeMeo A, et al: Correlation of human skin reactivity with lymphocyte transformation induced by mycobacterial antigens and histoplasmin. Am Rev Respir Dis 101:67, 1970.

338. Kane R, MacVandiviere H: The significance of multiple simultaneous tuberculin skin-testing in the prediction of various mycobacterial infections in the host. Am Rev Respir Dis 105:296, 1972.

339. Woodruff CE, Chapman PT, Howard WL, et al: Quantitative tests with old tuberculin in sanatorium practice. Am Rev Respir Dis 98:270, 1968.

340. Howard WL, Klopfenstein MD, Steininger WJ, et al: The loss of tuberculin sensitivity in certain patients with active pulmonary tuberculosis. Chest 57:530, 1970.

341. Hsu KHK: Diagnostic skin test for mycobacterial infections in man. Chest 64:1973.

342. Zack MB, Fulkerson LL, Hartshorne G, et al: Clinical evaluation of stabilized and nonstabilized PPD-B in patients with group III atypical mycobacteria. Chest 63:348, 1972.

343. Buchanan TM, Brooks GF, Brachman PS: The tularemia skin test; 325 skin tests in 210 persons. Serologic correlation and review of the literature. Ann Intern Med 74:336, 1971.

344. Chick EW: Pulmonary fungal infections simulating and misdiagnosed as other diseases. Am Rev Respir Dis 85:702, 1962.

345. Heiner DC: Influence of skin testing on the serologic diagnosis of tuberculosis and histoplasmosis. J Dis Child 98:673, 1959.

346. McDearman SC, Young JM: The development of positive serologic tests with Histoplasma capsulatum antigens following single histoplasmin skin tests. Am J Clin Pathol 34:434, 1960.

347. Stevens DA, Levine HB, TenEyck DR: Dermal sensitivity to different doses of spherulin and coccidioidin. Chest 65:530, 1974.

348. Levine HB, Gonzalez-Ochoa A, Ten Eyck DR: Dermal sensitivity to Coccidioides immitis. A comparison of responses elicited in man by spherulin and coccidioidin. Am Rev Respir Dis 107:379, 1973.

349. Burgi H, Wiesmann U, Richterich R, et al: New objective criteria for inflammation in bronchial secretions. Br Med J 2:654, 1968.

350. Carr DT, Power MH: Clinical value of measurements of concentration of protein in pleural fluid. N Engl J Med 259:926, 1958.

351. Light RW, MacGregor MI, Luchsinger PC, et al: Pleural effusions: The diagnostic separation of transudates and exudates. Ann Intern Med 77:507, 1972.

352. Glenert: Sugar levels in pleural effusions of different etiologies. Acta Tuberc Scand 42:222, 1962.

353. Light RW, Ball WC Jr: Glucose and amylase in pleural effusions. JAMA 225:257, 1973.

354. Barber LM, Mazzadi L, Deakins DD, et al: Glucose level in pleural fluid as a diagnostic aid. Dis Chest 31:680, 1957.

355. Carr DT, Power MH: Pleural fluid glucose with special reference to its concentration in rheumatoid pleurisy with effusion. Dis Chest 37:321, 1960.

356. Carr DT, Mayne JG: Pleurisy with effusion in rheumatoid arthritis, with reference to the low concentration of glucose in pleural fluid. Am Rev Respir Dis 85:345, 1962.

357. Schools GS, Mikklesen WM: Rheumatoid pleuritis. Arthritis Rheum 5:369, 1962.

358. Lillington GA, Carr DT, Mayne JG: Rheumatoid pleurisy with effusion. Arch Intern Med 128:764, 1971.

359. Berger HW, Maher G: Decreased glucose concentration in malignant pleural effusions. Am Rev Respir Dis 103:427, 1971.

360. Carr DT and McGuckin WF: Chemistry of pleural effusions. Biochem Clin 4:283, 1963.

361. Vianna NJ: Nontuberculous bacterial emphysema in patients with and without underlying diseases. JAMA 215:69, 1971.

362. Russakoff AH, LeMaistre CA, Dewlett HJ: An evaluation of the pleural fluid glucose determination. Am Rev Respir Dis 85:220, 1962.

363. Dodson WH, Hollingsworth JW: Pleural effusion in rheumatoid arthritis. Impaired transport of glucose. N Engl J Med 275:1337, 1966.

364. Good JT Jr, Taryle DA, Maulitz RM, et al: The diagnostic value of pleural fluid pH. Chest 78:55, 1980.

365. Funahashi A, Sarkar TK, Kory RC: Measurements of respiratory gases and pH of pleural fluid. Am Rev Respir Dis 108:1266, 1973.

366. Light RW, MacGregor MI, Ball WC Jr, et al: Diagnostic significance of pleural fluid pH and Pco₂. Chest 64:591, 1973.

367. Leuallen EC, Carr DJ: Pleural effusion. A statistical study of 436 patients. N Engl J Med 252:79, 1955.

368. Roy PH, Carr DT, Payne WS: The problem of chylothorax. Mayo Clin Proc 42:457, 1967.

369. Hammarsten JF, Honska WL Jr, Limes BJ: Pleural fluid amylase in pancreatitis and other diseases. Am Rev Respir Dis 79:606, 1959.

370. Goldman M, Goldman G, Fleischner FG: Pleural-fluid amylase in acute pancreatitis. N Engl J Med 266:715, 1962.

371. Bittar EE: Amylase activity in hemothorax associated with pancreatitis. Arch Intern Med 109:601, 1962.

372. Kaye MD: Pleuropulmonary complications of pancreatitis. Thorax 23:297, 1968.

373. Abbott OA, Mansour KA, Logan WD Jr, et al: Atraumatic so-called "spontaneous" rupture of the esophagus. A review of 47 personal cases with comments on a new method of surgical therapy. J Thorac Cardiovasc Surg 59:67, 1970.

374. Sherr HP, Light RW, Merson MH, et al: Origin of pleural fluid amylase in esophageal rupture. Ann Intern Med 76:985, 1972.

375. Hunder GG, McDuffie FC, Hepper NGG: Pleural fluid complement in systemic lupus erythematosus and rheumatoid arthritis. Ann Intern Med 76:357, 1972.

376. Tacquet A, Biserte F, Havez R, et al: Biochemical criteria in the diagnosis of pleural mesothelioma. Lille Med 10:146, 1965.

377. Harington JS, Wagner JC, Smith M: The detection of hyaluronic acid in pleural fluids of cases with diffuse pleural mesotheliomas. Br J Exp Pathol 44:81, 1963.

378. Klockars M, Pettersson T, Riska H, et al: Pleural fluid lysozyme in human disease. Arch Intern Med 139:73, 1979.

379. Hilman BC: Limitations of countercurrent immunoelectrophoresis (CIE) in the diagnosis of empyema. Chest 78:866, 1980.

380. Holsclaw DS Jr, Schaffer DA: Counterimmunoelectrophoresis in the diagnosis of Hemophilus influenzae pleural effusion. Chest 78:867, 1980.

381. Naiman HL, Albritton WL: Counterimmunoelectrophoresis in the diagnosis of acute infection. J Infect Dis 142:524, 1980.

382. Unger KM, Raber M, Bedrossian CW, et al: Analysis of pleural effusions using automated flow cytometry. Cancer 52:873, 1983.

383. Savage AM: Gas liquid chromatography: From taxonomy to diagnosis. Chest 77:506, 1980.

384. Jenkinson SG, Banschbach MW: Radioimmunoassay determinations of prostaglandin E in pleural effusions of varying causes. Am Rev Respir Dis 126:21, 1982.

385. Miller ME, Rørth M, Parving HH, et al: pH effect on erythropoietin response to hypoxia. N Engl J Med 288:706, 1973.

386. Douglas RG Jr, Alford RH, Cate TR, et al: The leukocyte response during viral respiratory illness in man. Ann Intern Med 64:521, 1966.

387. Park BH, Fikrig SM, Smithwick EM: Infection and nitroblue-tetrazolium reduction by neutrophils: A diagnostic aid. Lancet 2:532, 1968.

388. Matula G, Paterson PY: Spontaneous in vitro reduction of nitroblue tetrazolium by neutrophils of adult patients with bacterial infection. N Engl J Med 285:311, 1971.

389. Steigbigel RT, Johnson PK, Remington JS: The nitroblue tetrazolium reduction test versus conventional hematology in the diagnosis of bacterial infection. N Engl J Med 290:235, 1974.

390. Segal AW, Trustey SF, Levi AJ: Re-evaluation of nitroblue-tetrazolium test. Lancet 2:879, 1973.

391. Soonattrakul W, Andersen BR: Diagnostic accuracy of the nitroblue tetrazolium test. Arch Intern Med 132:529, 1973.

392. Spodick DH: Electrocardiographic studies in pulmonary disease. I. Electrocardiographic abnormalities in diffuse lung disease. II. Establishment of criteria for the electrocardiographic inference of diffuse lung disease. Circulation 20:1067, 1959.

393. Permutt S: Pulmonary function testing and the prevention of pulmonary disease (editorial). Chest 74:608, 1978.

394. Bunn AE, Vermaak J C, De Kock MA: A comprehensive on-line computerised lung function screening test. Respiration 37:42, 1979.

395. Cary J, Huseby J, Culver B, et al: Variability in interpretation of pulmonary function tests. Chest 76:389, 1979.

396. Hogg J C, Macklem PT, Thurlbeck WM: Site and nature of airway obstruction in chronic obstructive lung disease. N Engl J Med 278:1355, 1968.

397. Macklem PT, Mead J: Resistance of central and peripheral airways measured by a retrograde catheter. J Appl Physiol 22:395, 1967.

398. Becklake MR, Permutt S: Evaluation of tests of lung function for "screening" for early detection of chronic obstructive lung disease. In Macklem PT, Permutt S (eds): The Lung in Transition Between Health and Disease. Lung Biology in Health and Disease. New York, Marcel Dekker, 1979.

399. Buist AS, Ghezzo NR, Anthonisen RM, et al: Relationship between the single-breath N₂ test and age, sex and smoking habit in three North American cities. Am Rev Respir Dis 120:305, 1979.

400. Hudgel D, Petty T, Baidwan B, et al: A community pulmonary disease screening effort—"Denver Lung Days." Chest 74:619, 1978.

401. Dosman JA, Cotton DJ: Interpretation of tests of early lung dysfunction. Chest 79:261, 1981.

402. Macklem P, Becklake M: Is screening for chronic limitation of airflow desirable? Chest 74:607, 1978.
403. Solomon D: Clinical significance of pulmonary function tests: Are small airway tests helpful in the detection of early airflow obstruction? Chest 74:567, 1978.
404. Van de Woestijne KP: Are the small airways really quiet? Eur J Respir Dis 63:19, 1982.
405. Gelb F, Williams J, Zamel N: Spirometry: FEV$_1$ vs FEF 25–75%. Chest 84:473, 1983.
406. Racineux J, Peslin R, Hannhart B: Sensitivity of forced expiration indices to induced changes in peripheral airway resistance. J Appl Physiol 50:15, 1981.
407. Lam S, Abboud R, Chan-Yeung M: Use of maximal expiratory flow-volume curves with air and helium-oxygen in the detection of ventilatory abnormalities in population surveys. Am Rev Respir Dis 123:234, 1981.
408. Hubert H, Fabsitz R, Feinleib M, et al: Genetic and environmental influences on pulmonary function in adult twins. Am Rev Respir Dis 125:409, 1982.
409. Webster M, Lorimer G, Man S, et al: Pulmonary function in identical twins: Comparison of nonsmokers and smokers. Am Rev Respir Dis 119:223, 1979.
410. Sobol BJ, Sobol PG: Percent of predicted as the limit of normal in pulmonary function testing: A statistically valid approach. Thorax 34:1, 1979.
411. Crapo R, Morris A, Clayton P, et al: Lung volumes in healthy nonsmoking adults. Bull Eur Physiopathol Resp 18:419, 1982.
412. Statement on Spirometry. Chest 83:547, 1983.
413. Hurwitz S, Allen J, Liben A: Lung function in young adults: Evidence for differences in the chronological age at which various functions start to decline. Thorax 35:615, 1980.
414. Schoenberg J, Beck G, Bouhuys A: Growth and decay of pulmonary function in healthy blacks and whites. Respir Physiol 33:367, 1978.
415. Bande J, Clement J, Van de Woestijne K: The influence of smoking habits and body weight on vital capacity and FEV$_1$ in male air force personnel: A longitudinal and cross-sectional analysis. Am Rev Respir Dis 122:781, 1980.
416. Woolcock AJ, Colman MH, Blackburn CRB: Factors affecting normal values for ventilatory lung function. Am Rev Respir Dis 106:692, 1972.
417. Dugdale AE, Bolton JM, Ganendran A: Respiratory function among Malaysian aboriginals. Thorax 26:740, 1971.
418. Yokoyama T, Mitsufuji M: Statistical representation of the ventilatory capacity of 2,247 healthy Japanese adults. Chest 61:655, 1972.
419. Wall M, Olson D, Bonn B, et al: Lung function in North American Indian children—reference standards for spirometry maximal expiratory flow volume curves, and peak expiratory flow. Am Rev Respir Dis 125:158, 1982.
420. Lam K, Pang S, Allan W, et al: Predictive nomograms for forced expiratory volume, forced vital capacity and peak expiratory flow rate in Chinese adults and children. Br J Dis Chest 77:390, 1983.
421. Huang S, White D, Douglas N, et al: Respiratory function in normal Chinese: Comparison with Caucasians. Respiration 46:265, 1984.
422. Pennock B, Rogers R, McCaffree DR: Changes in measured spirometric indices—what is significant? Chest 80:97, 1981.
423. Hutchison DCS, Barter CE, Martelli NA: Errors in the measurement of vital capacity. A comparison of three methods in normal subjects and in patients with pulmonary emphysema. Thorax 28:584, 1973.
424. Hughes J, Hutchinson D: Errors in the estimation of vital capacity from expiratory flow-volume curves in pulmonary emphysema. Br J Dis Chest 76:279, 1982.
425. Goldman HI, Becklake MR: Respiratory function tests: Normal values at median altitudes and the prediction of normal results. Am Rev Tuberc 79:457, 1959.
426. Knudson R, Lebowitz M, Holberg C, et al: Changes in the normal maximal expiratory flow volume curve with growth and aging. Am Rev Respir Dis 127:725, 1983.
427. ACCP Scientific Section Recommendations: The determination of static lung volumes. Report of the Section on Respiratory Pathophysiology. Chest 86:471, 1984.
428. Heldt G, Peters M: A simplified method to determine functional residual capacity during mechanical ventilation. Chest 74:492, 1978.
429. Pino J, Teculescu D: Validity of total lung capacity determination by the single-breath nitrogen technique. Eur J Respir Dis 61:265, 1980.
430. Krumpe P, MacDannald J, Finley T, et al: Use of an acoustic helium analyzer for measuring lung volumes. J Appl Physiol 50:203, 1981.
431. Begin P, Peslin R: Plethysmographic measurements of thoracic gas volume. Back to the assumptions. Bull Eur Physiopathol Resp 19:247, 1983.
432. Paré PD: Breaking Boyle's law. Am Rev Respir Dis 119:684, 1979.
433. Habib M, Engel L: Influence of the panting technique on the plethysmographic measurement of the thoracic gas volume. Am Rev Respir Dis 117:265, 1978.
434. Brown R, Hoppin F Jr, Ingram R Jr, et al: Influence of abdominal gas on the Boyle's law determination of thoracic gas volume. J Appl Physiol 44:469, 1978.
435. Rodenstein D, Goncette L, Stanescu D: Extrathoracic airways changes during plethysmographic measurements of lung volume. Respir Physiol 52:217, 1983.
436. Rodenstein D, Stanescu D, Francis C: Demonstration of failure of body plethysmography in airway obstruction. J Appl Physiol 52:949, 1982.
437. Rodenstein D, Stanescu D: Reassessment of lung volume measurement by helium dilution and by body plethysmography in chronic airflow obstruction. Am Rev Respir Dis 126:1040, 1982.
438. Shore S, Milic-Emili J, Martin J: Reassessment of body plethysmographic technique for the measurement of thoracic gas volume in asthmatics. Am Rev Respir Dis 126:515, 1982.
439. Stanescu D, Rodenstein D, Cauberghs M, et al: Failure of body plethysmography in bronchial asthma. J Appl Physiol 52:939, 1982.
440. Knudson R, Knudson D: Frequency dependent phase and amplitude differences between simulated mouth and pleural pressures during panting. Demonstration with a mechanical model. Chest 86:589, 1984.
441. Paré PD, Coppin CA: Errors in the measurement of total lung capacity in patients with chronic obstructive pulmonary disease. Thorax 38:468, 1983.
442. Rodenstein D, Stanescu D: Frequency dependence of plethysmographic volume in healthy and asthmatic subjects. J Appl Physiol 54:159, 1983.
443. Bohadana A, Peslin R, Hannhart B, et al: Influence of panting frequency on plethysmographic measurements of thoracic gas volume. J Appl Physiol 52:739, 1982.
444. Shore S, Huk O, Mannix S, et al: Effect of panting frequency on the plethysmographic determination of thoracic gas volume in chronic obstructive pulmonary disease. Am Rev Respir Dis 128:54, 1983.
445. Begin P, Peslin R: Influence of panting frequency on thoracic gas volume measurements in chronic obstructive pulmonary disease. Am Rev Respir Dis 130:121, 1984.
446. Brown R, Ingram R Jr, McFadden E Jr: Problems in the plethysmographic assessment of changes in total lung capacity in asthma. Am Rev Respir Dis 118:685, 1978.
447. Garcia J, Hunninghake G, Nugent K: Thoracic gas volume measurement: Increased variability in patients with obstructive ventilatory defects. Chest 85:272, 1984.
448. Barnhard HJ, Pierce JA, Joyce JW, et al: Roentgenographic determination of total lung capacity. A new method evaluated in health, emphysema and congestive heart failure. Am J Med 28:51, 1960.
449. Loyd HM, String ST, DuBois AB: Radiographic and plethysmographic determination of total lung capacity. Radiology 86:7, 1966.
450. Harris TR, Pratt PC, Kilburn KH: Total lung capacity measured by roentgenograms. Am J Med 50:756, 1971.
451. Nicklaus TM, Watanabe S, Mitchell MM, et al: Roentgenologic, physiologic and structural estimations of the total lung capacity in normal and emphysematous subjects. Am J Med 42:547, 1967.
452. Pierce R, Brown D, Holmes M, et al: Estimation of lung volumes from chest radiographs using shape information. Thorax 34:726, 1979.
453. O'Brien R, Drizd T: Roentgenographic determination of total lung capacity: Normal values from a national population survey. Am Rev Respir Dis 128:949, 1983.
454. Thurlbeck WM: Post-mortem lung volumes. Thorax 34:735, 1979.
455. Sackner J, Nixon A, Davis B, et al: Noninvasive measurement of ventilation during exercise using a respiratory inductive plethysmograph. I. Am Rev Respir Dis 122:867, 1980.
456. Spier S, England S: The respiratory inductive plethysmograph—Bands versus Jerkins. Am Rev Respir Dis 127:784, 1983.
457. Cohn M, Rao A, Broudy M, et al: The respiratory inductive plethysmograph: A new non-invasive monitor of respiration. Bull Eur Physiopathol Respir 18:643, 1982.
458. Guyatt A, McBride M, Meanock C: Evaluation of the respiratory inductive plethysmograph in man. Eur J Respir Dis 64:81, 1983.
459. Tobin J, Jenouri G, Lind B, et al: Validation of respiratory inductive plethysmography in patients with pulmonary disease. Chest 83:615, 1983.
460. Chadha T, Watson H, Birch S, et al: Validation of respiratory inductive plethysmography using different calibration procedures. Am Rev Respir Dis 125:644, 1982.
461. Sackner M, Rao A, Birch S, et al: Assessment of time-volume and flow-volume components of forced vital capacity. Chest 82:272, 1982.
462. Sackner M, Rao A, Birch S, et al: Assessment of density dependent flow-volume parameters in nonsmokers and smokers. Measurement with spirometry, body plethysmography and respiratory inductive plethysmography. Chest 82:137, 1982.
463. Peslin R, Bohadana A, Hannhart B, et al: Comparison of various

3

methods for reading maximal expiratory flow-volume curves. Am Rev Respir Dis *119*:271, 1979.

464. Ferris B Jr, Speizer F, Bishop G, et al: Spirometry for an epidemiologic study: Deriving optimum summary statistics for each subject. Bull Eur Physiopathol Respir *14*:145, 1978.

465. Medical Section, American Thoracic Society of the American Lung Association: ATS Statement, Snowbird Workshop on Standardization of Spirometry. Am Rev Respir Dis *119*:831, 1979.

466. Suratt P, Hooe D, Owens D, et al: Effect of maximal versus submaximal expiratory effort on spirometric values. Respiration *42*:233, 1981.

467. Shaw A, Fisher J: Reproducibility of the flow-volume loop (correspondence). Thorax *35*:480, 1980.

468. Whitaker C, Chinn D, Lee W: Statistical reliability of indices derived from the closing volume and flow volume traces. Bull Eur Physiopathol Respir *14*:237, 1978.

469. Ferris BG: Epidemiology standardization project. Am Rev Respir Dis *118* (Part 2):1, 1978.

470. Lam S, Abboud R, Chan-Yeung M: Use of maximal expiratory flow-volume curve with air and helium-oxygen in the detection of ventilatory abnormalities in population surveys. Am Rev Respir Dis *123*:234, 1981.

471. Rossoff L, Csima A, Zamel N: Reproducibility of maximum expiratory flow in severe chronic obstructive pulmonary disease. Bull Eur Physiopathol Respir *15*:1129, 1979.

472. Knudson RJ, Lebowitz MD: Maximal mid-expiratory flow (FEF 25–75%): Normal limits and assessment of sensitivity. Am Rev Respir Dis *117*:609, 1978.

473. Quanjer PH: Standardized lung function testing. Bull Eur Physiopathol Respir *19*:1, 1983.

474. Sourk R, Nugent K: Bronchodilator testing—Confidence intervals derived from placebo inhalations. Am Rev Respir Dis *128*:153, 1983.

475. Light RW, Conrad SA, George RB: Clinical significance of pulmonary function tests: The one best test for evaluating the effects of bronchodilator therapy. Chest *72*:512, 1977.

476. Paré PD, Lawson LM, Brooks LA: Patterns of response to inhaled bronchodilators in asthmatics. Am Rev Respir Dis *127*:680, 1983.

477. Girard M, Light W: Should the FVC be considered in evaluating response to bronchodilator? Chest *84*:87, 1983.

478. Ramsdell J, Tisi G: Determination of bronchodilation in the clinical pulmonary function laboratory—role in changes in static lung volumes. Chest *76*:622, 1979.

479. Despas PJ, Leroux M, Macklem PT: Site of airway obstruction in asthma as determined by measuring maximal expiratory flow breathing air and a helium-oxygen mixture. J Clin Invest *51*:3235, 1972.

480. Hutcheon M, Griffin P, Levison H, et al: Volume of isoflow. A new test in detection of mild abnormalities of lung mechanics. Am Rev Respir Dis *110*:458, 1974.

481. Teculescu D, Bohadana A, Peslin R, et al: One-second forced expiratory volume and density dependence in early airflow limitation. Respiration *44*:433, 1983.

482. Knudson R, Bloom W, Lantenborn T, et al: Assessment of air vs. helium-oxygen flow-volume curves as an epidemiologic screening test. Chest *86*:419, 1984.

483. Teculescu D, Pino J, Sadoul P: Cigarette smoking and density-dependence of maximal expiratory flow in asymptomatic men. Am Rev Respir Dis *122*:651, 1980.

484. Spiro S, Bierman C, Petheram I: Reproducibility of flow rates measured with low density gas mixtures in exercise-induced bronchospasm. Thorax *36*:852, 1981.

485. Berend N, Nelson N, Rutland J, et al: The maximum expiratory flow-volume curve with air and a low-density gas mixture—an analysis of subject and observer variability. Chest *80*:23, 1981.

486. Li K, Tan L, Chong P, et al: Between-technician variation in the measurement of spirometry with air and helium. Am Rev Respir Dis *124*:196, 1981.

487. Dull W, Secker-Walker R: Helium-oxygen flow volume curves in young healthy adults. Respiration *38*:18, 1979.

488. Loveland M, Corbin R, Ducic S, et al: Evaluation of the analysis and variability of the helium response. Bull Eur Physiopathol Respir *14*:551, 1978.

489. Teculescu D, Pino J, Peslin R: Composite flow-volume curves matched at total lung capacity in the study of density dependence of maximal expiratory flows. Lung *159*:127, 1981.

490. Zeck R, Solliday N, Celic L, et al: Variability of the volume of isoflow. Chest *79*:269, 1981.

491. MacDonald J, Cole T: The flow-volume loop: Reproducibility of air- and helium-based tests in normal subjects. Thorax *35*:64, 1980.

492. Bogaard J, Verheijen-Breemhaar L, Stam H: Density-dependence of flow-volume curves: Limitations and applicability. Eur J Respir Dis *63*:89, 1982.

493. Mink S, Wood L: How does HeO$_2$ increase maximum expiratory flow in human lungs? J Clin Invest *66*:720, 1980.

494. Castille R, Hyatt R, Rodarte J: Determinants of maximal expiratory flow and density dependence in normal humans. J Appl Physiol *49*:897, 1980.

495. Paré PD, Brooks LA, et al: Density dependence of maximum expiratory flow and its correlation with small airway pathology in smokers. Am Rev Respir Dis *131*:521, 1985.

496. Lavelle T Jr, Rotman H, Weg J: Isoflow-volume curves in the diagnosis of upper airway obstruction. Am Rev Respir Dis *117*:845, 1978.

497. Castile R, Mead J, Jackson A, et al: Effects of posture on flow-volume curve configuration in normal humans. J Appl Physiol *53*:1175, 1982.

498. Mead J: Analysis of the configuration of maximum expiratory flow-volume curves. J Appl Physiol *44*:156, 1978.

499. Jansen M, Peslin R, Bohadana A, et al: Usefulness of forced expiration slope ratios for detecting mild airway abnormalities. Am Rev Respir Dis *122*:221, 1980.

500. Jordanoglou J, Hadjistavrou C, Tatsis G, et al: Total effective time of the forced expirogram in disease: Sources of error and a correction factor. Thorax *37*:304, 1982.

501. Vermaak J, Bunn A, deKock M: A new lung function index. The area under the maximum expiratory flow-volume curve. Respiration *37*:61, 1979.

502. Wall M, Misley M, Dickerson D: Partial expiratory flow-volume curves in young children. Am Rev Respir Dis *129*:557, 1984.

503. Yernault J-C, De Troyer A, Rodenstein D: Sex and age differences in intrathoracic airways mechanics in normal man. J Appl Physiol *46*:556, 1979.

504. Aldrich T, Arora N, Rochester D: The influence of airway obstruction and respiratory muscle strength on maximal voluntary ventilation in lung disease. Am Rev Respir Dis *126*:195, 1982.

505. Lavietese M, Clifford E, Silverstein D, et al: Relationship of static respiratory muscle pressure and maximum voluntary ventilation in normal subjects. Respiration *38*:121, 1979.

506. Martin B, Thomas C: Variation among normal persons in short-term ventilatory capacity. Respiration *43*:23, 1982.

507. Kraemer R, Wiese G, Albertini M, et al: Elastic behaviour of the lungs in healthy children determined by means of an exponential function. Respir Physiol *52*:229, 1983.

508. Colebatch H, Ng C, Nikov N: Use of an exponential function for elastic recoil. J Appl Physiol *46*:387, 1979.

509. Gibson G, Pride N, Davis J, et al: Exponential description of the static pressure-volume curve of normal and diseased lungs. Am Rev Respir Dis *120*:799, 1979.

510. Knudson R, Kaltenborn W: Evaluation of lung elastic recoil by exponential curve analysis. Respir Physiol *46*:29, 1981.

511. Colebatch H, Greaves I, Ng C: Exponential analysis of elastic recoil and aging in healthy males and females. J Appl Physiol *47*:683, 1979.

512. Yernault J, Noseda A, Van Muylem A, et al: Variability in lung elasticity measurements in normal humans. Rev Respir Dis *128*:816, 1983.

513. McCuaig C, Vessal S, Coppin C, et al: Variability in measurements of pressure volume curves in normal subjects. Am Rev Respir Dis *131*:656, 1985.

514. Paré PD, Brooks LA, Bates J, et al: Exponential analysis of the lung pressure volume curve as a predictor of pulmonary emphysema. Am Rev Respir Dis *126*:54, 1982.

515. Berend N, Skoog C, Thurlbeck W: Exponential analysis of lobar pressure-volume characteristics. Thorax *36*:452, 1981.

516. Haber P, Colebatch H, Ng C, et al: Alveolar size as a determinant of pulmonary distensibility in mammalian lungs. J Appl Physiol *54*:837, 1983.

517. McFadden ER Jr, Lyons HA: Airway resistance and uneven ventilation in bronchial asthma. J Appl Physiol *25*:365, 1968.

518. Ingram RH Jr, Schilder DP: Association of a decrease in dynamic compliance with a change in gas distribution. J Appl Physiol *23*:911, 1967.

519. Woolcock AJ, Vincent NJ, Macklem PT: Frequency dependence of compliance as a test for obstruction in the small airways. J Clin Invest *48*:1097, 1969.

520. Cutillo A, Renzetti A Jr: Mechanical behaviour of the respiratory system as a function of frequency in health and disease. Bull Eur Physiopathol Respir *19*:293, 1983.

521. Bates DV, Macklem PT, Christie RV: Respiratory Function in Disease; An Introduction to the Integrated Study of the Lung. 2nd ed. Philadelphia, WB Saunders, 1971.

522. Mead J, Whittenberger JL: Physical properties of human lungs measured during spontaneous respiration. J Appl Physiol *5*:779, 1953.

523. Von Neergaard, Wirz K: Die Messung der Stromunswiederstande in den alemvegen des Menschen, Insbesondere bei Asthma und Emphysem. Z Klin Med 51-82, 1927.

524. Lisboa C, Ross W, Jardim J, et al: Pulmonary pressure-flow curves measured by a data-averaging circuit. J Appl Physiol *47*:621, 1979.

525. Clement J, Landser P, Van de Woestijne K: Total resistance and reactance in patients with respiratory complaints with and without airways obstruction. Chest 83:215, 1983.

526. Landser F, Clement J, Van de Woestijne K: Normal values of total respiratory resistance and reactance determined by forced oscillations—influence of smoking. Chest 81:586, 1982.

527. Bhansali P, Irvin C, Dempsey J, et al: Human pulmonary resistance: Effect of frequency and gas physical properties. J Appl Physiol 47:161, 1979.

528. Petro W, Nieding G, Boll W, et al: Determination of respiratory resistance by an oscillation method. Studies of long-term and short-term variability and dependence upon lung volume and compliance. Respiration 42:243, 1981.

529. Fowler W: Lung function studies. II. The respiratory dead space. Am J Physiol 154:405, 1948.

530. Engel L: Intraregional ventilation distribution. Bull Eur Physiopathol Respir 18:181, 1982.

531. Comroe J, Fowler W: Lung function studies. VI. Detection of uneven alveolar ventilation during a single-breath of oxygen: A new test of pulmonary disease. Am J Med 10:408, 1951.

532. Cormier Y, Belanger J: The role of gas exchange in phase IV of the single-breath nitrogen test. Am Rev Respir Dis 125:396, 1982.

533. Nichol G, Michels D, Guy H: Phase V of the single-breath washout test. J Appl Physiol 52:34, 1982.

534. Leblanc P, Ruff F, Milic-Emili J: Effects of age and body position on "airway closure" in man. J Appl Physiol 28:448, 1970.

535. McCarthy DS, Spencer R, Greene R, et al: Measurement of "closing volume" as a simple and sensitive test for early detection of small airway disease. Am J Med 52:747, 1972.

536. Green M, Travis DM, Mead J: A simple measurement of phase IV ("closing volume") using a critical orifice helium analyzer. J Appl Physiol 33:827, 1972.

537. Anthonisen NR, Danson J, Robertson PC, et al: Airway closure as a function of age. Respir Physiol 8:58, 1969–70.

538. Berend N, Skoog C, Thurlbeck W: Single-breath nitrogen test in excised human lungs. J Appl Physiol 51:1568, 1981.

539. Buist A, Ross B: Predicted values for closing volumes using a modified single-breath nitrogen test. Am Rev Respir Dis 107:744, 1973.

540. Buist A, Ross B: Quantitative analysis of the alveolar plateau in the diagnosis of early airway obstruction. Am Rev Respir Dis 108:1078, 1973.

541. Darling RC, Cournand A, Mansfield JS, et al: Studies on the intrapulmonary mixture of gases. I. Nitrogen elimination from blood and body tissues during high oxygen breathing. J Clin Invest 19:591, 1940.

542. Meneely GR, Kaltreider NL: The volume of the lung determined by helium dilution. Description of the method and comparison with other procedures. J Clin Invest 28:129, 1949.

543. Bates DV, Christie RV: Intrapulmonary mixing of helium in health and in emphysema. Clin Sci 9:17, 1950.

544. Krogh A, Krogh M: On the rate of diffusion of carbonic oxide into the lungs of man. Scand Arch Physiol 23:236, 1910.

545. Krogh M: The diffusion of gases through the lungs of man. J Physiol (Lond) 49:271, 1914.

546. Forster RE, Fowler WS, Bates DV, et al: The absorption of carbon monoxide by the lungs during breathholding. J Clin Invest 33:1135, 1954.

547. Ogilvie CM, Forster RE, Blakemore WS, et al: A standardized breath holding technique for the clinical measurement of the diffusing capacity of the lung for carbon monoxide. J Clin Invest 36:1, 1957.

548. Russell N, Bagg L, Dobrzynski J: Clinical assessment of a rebreathing method for measuring pulmonary gas transfer. Thorax 38:212, 1983.

549. Graham B, Mink J, Cotton D: Improved accuracy and precision of single-breath CO diffusing capacity measurements. J Appl Physiol 55:1306, 1981.

550. Cotton D, Newth C, Portner P, et al: Measurement of single-breath CO diffusing capacity by continuous rapid CO analysis in man. J Appl Physiol 46:1149, 1979.

551. Jones RS, Meade F: Pulmonary diffusing capacity. An improved single-breath method. Lancet 1:94, 1960.

552. Gaensler EA, Smith AA: Attachment for automated single breath diffusing capacity. Chest 63:136, 1973.

553. Make B, Miller A, Epler G, et al: Single breath diffusing capacity in the industrial setting. Chest 82:351, 1982.

554. Graham B, Mink J, Cotton D: Overestimation of the single-breath carbon monoxide diffusing capacity in patients with air-flow obstruction. Rev Respir Dis 129:403, 1984.

555. Newth C, Cotton D, Nadel J: Pulmonary diffusing capacity measured at multiple intervals during a single exhalation in man. J Appl Physiol 43:617, 1977.

556. Siegler D, Zorab P: The influence of lung volume on gas transfer in scoliosis. Br J Dis Chest 76:44, 1982.

557. Ayers L, Ginsberg M, Fein J, et al: Diffusing capacity, specific diffusing capacity and interpretation of diffusion defects. West J Med 123:255, 1975.

558. Crapo R, Morris A: Standardized single breath normal values for carbon monoxide diffusing capacity. Rev Respir Dis 123:185, 1981.

559. Ogilvie CM, Forster RE: Single-breath transfer factor 25 years on. A reappraisal. Thorax 38:1, 1983.

560. Finley T, Engelman E, Packer B, et al: Use of the R.C. time constant for CO in the measurement of diffusing capacity. Am Rev Respir Dis 109:682, 1974.

561. Davies N: Does the lung work? 4. What does the transfer of carbon monoxide mean? Br J Dis Chest 76:105, 1982.

562. Bates DV, Woolf CR, Paul GI: Chronic bronchitis: A report on the first two stages of the coordinated study of chronic bronchitis in the Department of Veterans Affairs, Canada. Med Ser J Can 18:211, 1962.

563. Weinberger SE, Johnson TS, Weiss ST: Clinical significance of pulmonary function tests—use and interpretation of the single-breath diffusing capacity. Chest 78:483, 1980.

564. Crapo J, Crapo R: Comparison of total lung diffusion capacity and the membrane component of diffusion capacity as determined by physiologic and morphometric techniques. Respir Physiol 51:183, 1983.

565. Harris E, Whitlock R: Fractional carbon monoxide uptake and "diffusing capacity" in models of pulmonary maldistribution. Bull Eur Physiopathol Respir 19:427, 1983.

566. Harris E, Whitlock R: Prediction equations for fractional CO uptake derived from 50 healthy subjects. Bull Eur Physiopathol Respir 19:433, 1983.

567. Mohsenifar Z, Tashkin D: Effect of carboxyhemoglobin on the single breath diffusing capacity: Derivation of an empirical correction factor. Respiration 37:185, 1979.

568. Cotes J, Dabbs J, Elwood P, et al: Iron-deficiency anemia: Its effect on transfer factor for the lung (diffusing capacity) and ventilation and cardiac frequency during sub-maximal exercise. Clin Sci 42:325, 1972.

569. Mohsenifar Z, Brown H, Schnitzer B, et al: The effect of abnormal levels of hematocrit on the single breath diffusing capacity. Lung 160:325, 1982.

570. Greening A, Patel K, Goolden A: Carbon monoxide diffusing capacity in polycythaemia rubra vera. Thorax 37:528, 1982.

571. Riepl G: Effects of abnormal hemoglobin concentration in human blood on membrane diffusing capacity of the lung and on pulmonary capillary blood volume. Respiration 36:10, 1978.

572. Dinakara P, Blumenthal WS, Johnston RF, et al: The effect of anemia on pulmonary diffusing capacity with derivation of a correction equation. Am Rev Respir Dis 102:965, 1970.

573. Fisher J, Cerny F: Characteristics of adjustment of lung diffusing capacity to work. J Appl Physiol 52:1124, 1982.

574. Cotton D, Mink J, Graham B: Effect of high negative inspiratory pressure on single-breath CO diffusing capacity. Respir Physiol 54:19, 1983.

575. Nemery B, Piret L, Brasseur L, et al: Effect of nitroglycerin on D_L of normal subjects at rest and during exercise. J Appl Physiol 52:851, 1982.

576. Miller A, Thornton JC, Warshaw R, et al: Single breath diffusing capacity in a representative sample of the population of Michigan, a large industrial state. Predicted values, lower limits of normal, and frequencies of abnormality by smoking history. Am Rev Respir Dis 127:270, 1983.

577. Hallenberg C, Holden W, Menzel T, et al: The clinical usefulness of a screening test to detect static pulmonary blood using a multiple breath analysis of diffusing capacity. Am Rev Respir Dis 119:349, 1979.

578. Sanderson DR, Dawson B, Wang JK: Bronchospirometry during diagnostic bronchoscopy. Chest 60:225, 1971.

579. Lopata M, Lourenco R: Evaluation of respiratory control. Clin Chest Med 1:33, 1980.

580. Cherniack N: Applied cardiopulmonary physiology. The clinical assessment of the chemical regulation of ventilation. Chest 70:274, 1976.

581. Derenne J, Macklem P, Roussos C: State of the Art. The respiratory muscles. Mechanics, control and pathophysiology. Part II. Am Rev Respir Dis 118:373, 1978.

582. Cherniack N, Dempsey J, Fencl V, et al: Workshop on assessment of respiratory control in humans. 1. Methods of measurement of ventilatory responses to hypoxia and hypercapnia. Am Rev Respir Dis 115:177, 1977.

583. Rebuck A, Slutsky A: Measurement of ventilatory responses to hypercapnia and hypoxia. In Hornbein TF, Lenfant C (eds): Regulation of Breathing—Part II. Lung Biology in Health and Disease. New York, Marcel Dekker, 1981, p 745.

584. Read D: A clinical method for assessing the ventilatory response to carbon dioxide. Aust Ann Med 16:20, 1967.

3

585. Milic-Emili J: Clinical methods for assessing the ventilatory response to carbon dioxide and hypoxia. *In* Macklem PT (ed): Medical Intelligence—Current Concepts—New tests to assess lung function. N Engl J Med 293:865, 1975.

586. Sullivan T, Yu P: Reproducibility of CO_2 response curves with 10 minutes separating each rebreathing test. Am Rev Respir Dis 129:23, 1984.

587. Rebuck AS, Read J: Patterns of ventilatory response to carbon dioxide during recovery from severe asthma. Clin Sci 41:13, 1971.

588. Arkinstall WW, Nirmel K, Klissouras V, et al: Genetic differences in the ventilatory response to inhaled CO_2. J Appl Physiol 36:6, 1974.

589. Douglas N, White D, Weil J, et al: Effect of breathing route on ventilation and ventilatory drive. Respir Physiol 51:209, 1983.

590. McBride BJ, Whitelaw WA: A physiological stimulus to upper airway receptors in humans. J Appl Physiol 51:1189, 1981.

591. Hirshman C, McCullough R, Weil J: Normal values for hypoxic and hypercapnic ventilatory drives in man. J Appl Physiol 38:1095, 1975.

592. Rebuck AS, Campbell EJM: A clinical method for assessing the ventilatory response to hypoxia. Am Rev Resp Dis 109:345, 1974.

593. Easton P, Slykerman L, Anthonisen N: Does the hypoxic ventilatory response measurement (Ve/SaO$_2$) overestimate the ventilatory response to sustained hypoxia? (Abstract.) Am Rev Respir Dis 129:A237, 1984.

594. Shaw R, Schonfeld S, Whitcomb M: Progressive and transient hypoxic ventilatory drive tests in healthy subjects. Am Rev Respir Dis 126:37, 1982.

595. Patakas D, Kakavelas H, Louridas G: Respiratory chemosensitivity evaluated by respiratory drive and breath holding. Respiration 40:256, 1980.

596. Whitelaw W, Derenne JP, Milic-Emili J: Occlusion pressure as a measure of respiratory centre output in conscious man. Respir Physiol 23:181, 1975.

597. Ward S, Agleh K, Poon C-S: Breath-to-breath monitoring of inspiratory occlusion pressures in humans. J Appl Physiol 51:520, 1981.

598. Grassino A, Derenne J, Almirall J, et al: Configuration of the chest wall and occlusion pressures in awake humans. J Appl Physiol 50:134, 1981.

599. Marazzini L, Cavestri R, Gori D, et al: Difference between mouth and esophageal occlusion pressure during CO_2 rebreathing in chronic obstructive pulmonary disease. Am Rev Respir Dis 118:1027, 1978.

600. Milic-Emili J, Whitelaw W, Grassino A: Measurement and testing of respiratory drive. *In* Hornbein TF, Lenfant C (eds): Regulation of Breathing, Part II. Lung Biology in Health and Disease. New York, Marcel Dekker, 1981, p 675.

601. Zackon H, Despas P, Anthonisen N: Occlusion pressure responses in asthma and chronic obstructive pulmonary disease. Am Rev Respir Dis 114:917, 1976.

602. Milic-Emili J: Recent advances in clinical assessment of control of breathing. Lung 160:1, 1982.

603. Black LF, Hyatt RE: Maximal respiratory pressures: Normal values and relationship to age and sex. Am Rev Resp Dis 99:696, 1969.

604. Ringqvist T: The ventilatory capacity in healthy subjects: An analysis of causal factors with special reference to the respiratory forces. Scand J Clin Lab Invest 18 (Suppl 88):5, 1966.

605. Smyth R, Chapman K, Rebuck A: Maximal inspiratory and expiratory pressures in adolescents: Normal values. Chest 86:568, 1984.

606. Leech J, Ghezzo H, Stevens D, et al: Respiratory pressure and function in young adults. Am Rev Respir Dis 128:17, 1983.

607. Wilson S, Cooke N, Edwards R, et al: Predicted normal values for maximal respiratory pressure in Caucasian adults and children. Thorax 39:535, 1984.

608. Loh L, Goldman M, Newsom D: The assessment of diaphragm function. Medicine 56:165, 1977.

609. Gibson G, Clark E, Pride N: Static transdiaphragmatic pressures in normal subjects and in patients with chronic hyperinflation. Am Rev Respir Dis 124:685, 1981.

610. Vanmeenen M, Demedts M, Vaerenbergh H, et al: Transdiaphragmatic, esophageal and gastric pressures during maximal static inspiratory and expiratory efforts in young subjects: Effects of maneuver and sex. Eur J Respir Dis 65:216, 1984.

611. Lisboa C, Contreras G, Pertuze J, et al: Inspiratory muscle function in diaphragmatic hemiparalysis. Am Rev Respir Dis 131:A327, 1985.

612. Nickerson B, Keens T: Measuring ventilatory muscle endurance in humans as sustainable inspiratory pressure. J Appl Physiol 52:768, 1982.

613. Martyn JB, Moreno RH, Paré PD, et al: Two minute incremental loading as a test of inspiratory muscle performance. Am Rev Respir Dis 131:A329, 1985.

614. Gross D, Grassino A, Ross W, et al: Electromyogram pattern of diaphragmatic fatigue. J Appl Physiol 46:1, 1979.

615. Bellemare F, Grassino A: Effect of pressure and timing of contraction on human diaphragm fatigue. J Appl Physiol 53:1190, 1982.

616. Weiss S, Robb G, Blumgart H: The velocity of blood flow in health and disease as measured by the effect of histamine on the minute vessels. Am Heart J 4:664, 1929.

617. Weiss S, Robb G, Ellis L: The systemic effects of histamine in man with special reference to the responses of the cardiovascular system. Arch Intern Med 49:360, 1932.

618. Curry J: Comparative action of acetyl-beta-methylcholine and histamine on the respiratory tract in normals, patients with hay fever and subjects with bronchial asthma. J Clin Invest 26:430, 1947.

619. Tiffeneau R: L'hyperexcitabilite acetylcholinique du poumon: Critere physio-pharmacodynamique de la maladie asthmatique. Presse Med 63:227, 1955.

620. Van der Straeten M: Introduction, to Symposium on Bronchial Hyperreactivity, Ghent, 1980. Eur J Respir Dis (Suppl 117)63:1, 1982.

621. Chai H, Farr RS, Froehlich LA, et al: Standardization of bronchial inhalation challenge procedures. J Allergy Clin Immunol 56:323, 1975.

622. Cockcroft D, Killian D, Mellon J, et al: Bronchial reactivity to inhaled histamine. A method and clinical survey. Clin Allergy 7:235, 1977.

623. Juniper EF, Frith PA, Dunnett C, et al: Reproducibility and comparison of response to inhaled histamine and methacholine. Thorax 33:705, 1978.

624. Cockcroft D, Berscheid B, Murdock K: Measurement of responsiveness to inhaled histamine using FEV_1: Comparison of PC_{20} and threshold. Thorax 38:523, 1983.

625. Lam S, Wong R, Yeung M: Nonspecific bronchial reactivity in occupational asthma. J Allergy Clin Immunol 63:28, 1979.

626. Orehek J, Gayrard P, Smith A, et al: Airway response to carbachol in normal and asthmatic subjects. Distinction between bronchial sensitivity and reactivity. Am Rev Respir Dis 115:937, 1977.

627. Yan K, Salome C, Woodcock A: Rapid method for measurement of bronchial responsiveness. Thorax 38:760, 1983.

628. Michoud M-C, Ghezzo H. Amyot R: A comparison of pulmonary function tests used for bronchial challenges. Bull Eur Physiopathol Respir 18:609, 1982.

629. Dehaut P, Rachiele A, Martin R, et al: Histamine dose-response curves in asthma: Reproducibility and sensitivity of different indices to assess response. Thorax 38:516, 1983.

630. Ryan G, Bolovitch M, Obminski G, et al: Standardization of inhalation provocation tests: Influence of nebulizer output, particle size, and the method of inhalation. J Allergy Clin Immunol 67:156, 1931.

631. Juniper E, Syty-Golda M, Hargreave F: Histamine inhalation tests: Inhalation of aerosol via a facemask versus a valve box with mouthpiece. Thorax 39:556, 1984.

632. Cockcroft DW, Berscheid BA: Effect of pH on bronchial response to inhaled histamine. Thorax 37:133, 1982.

633. Cockcroft D, Berscheid B: Standardization of inhalation provocation tests. Chest 82:572, 1982.

634. Hargreave F, Ryan G, Thomson N, et al: Bronchial responsiveness to histamine or methacholine in asthma measurement and clinical significance. J Allergy Clin Immunol 68:347, 1981.

635. Thomson N, Roberts R, Bandouvakis J, et al: Comparison of bronchial responses to prostaglandin F2-alpha and methacholine. J Allergy Clin Immunol 68:392, 1981.

636. Salome C, Schoeffel R, Woolcock A: Comparison of bronchial reactivity to histamine and methacholine in asthmatics. Clin Allergy 10:541, 1980.

637. Lowhagen O, Lindholm N: Short-term and long-term variation in bronchial response to histamine in asthmatic patients. Eur J Respir Dis 64:466, 1983.

638. Juniper E, Frith P, Hargreave F: Long-term stability of bronchial responsiveness to histamine. Thorax 37:288, 1982.

639. Ryan G, Dolovich MB, Roberts RS, et al: Standardization of inhalation provocation tests: Two techniques of aerosol generation and inhalation compared. Am Rev Respir Dis 123:195, 1981.

640. Malo JL, Pineau L, Cartier A, et al: Reference values of the provocative concentrations of methacholine that cause 6% and 20% changes in forced expiratory volume in one second in a normal population. Am Rev Respir Dis 128:8, 1983.

641. Orehek J: The concept of airway "sensitivity" and "reactivity." Eur J Respir Dis (Suppl 131) 64:27, 1983.

642. Eiser N: Calculation of data. Eur J Resp Dis (Suppl 131) 64:241, 1983.

643. Walters E, Davies P, Smith A: Measurement of bronchial reactivity: A question of interpretation. Thorax 36:960, 1981.

644. Beaupre A, Malo J: Histamine dose-response curves in asthma: Relevance of the distinction between PC_{20} and reactivity in characterizing clinical state. Thorax 36:731, 1981.

645. Shapiro G, Furukawa C, Pierson W, et al: Methacholine bronchial challenge in children. J Allergy Clin Immunol 69:365, 1982.

646. Henry R, Mellis C, South R, et al: Comparison of peak expiratory flow rate and forced expiratory volume in one second in histamine challenge studies in children. Br J Dis Chest 76:167, 1982.

647. Cockcroft D, Ruffin R, Frith P, et al: Determinants of allergen-induced asthma: Dose of allergen, circulating IGE antibody concentration and bronchial responsiveness to inhaled histamine. Am Rev Respir Dis 120:1053, 1979.

648. Deal E, McFadden E, Ingram R, et al: Hyperpnea and heat flux: Initial reaction sequence in exercise-induced asthma. J Appl Physiol 46:476, 1979.

649. O'Byrne P, Ryan G, Morris M, et al: Asthma induced by cold air and its relation to non-specific bronchial responsiveness to methacholine. Am Rev Respir Dis 125:281, 1982.

650. Anderson S, Schoeffel R, Finney M: Evaluation of ultrasonically nebulized solutions for provocation testing in patients with asthma. Thorax 38:284, 1983.

651. Haslam RH, Freigang B: Cough syncope mimicking epilepsy in asthmatic children. Can J Neurol Sci 12:45, 1985.

652. Becklake MR: Organic or functional impairment: Overall perspective. Am Rev Respir Dis 129:896, 1984.

653. Adelman M, Haponik EF, Bleecker ER, et al: Cryptogenic hemoptysis: Clinical features, bronchoscopic findings, and natural history in 67 patients. Ann Intern Med 102:829, 1985.

654. Heimer D, Bar-Ziv J, Scharf SM: Fiberoptic bronchoscopy in patients with hemoptysis and nonlocalizing chest roentgenograms. Arch Intern Med 145:1427, 1985.

655. Remy J, Lemaitre L, Lafitte JJ, et al: Massive hemoptysis of pulmonary arterial origin: Diagnosis and treatment. Am J Roentgenol 143:963, 1984.

656. Shim CS, Williams MH Jr: Relationship of wheezing to the severity of obstruction in asthma. Arch Intern Med 143:890, 1983.

657. Baughman RP, Loudon RG: Quantitation of wheezing in acute asthma. Chest 86:718, 1984.

658. Galko B, Grossman RF, Day A, et al: Hypertrophic pulmonary osteoarthropathy in four patients with interstitial pulmonary disease. Chest 88:94, 1985.

659. Braude S, Kennedy H, Hodson M, et al: Hypertrophic osteoarthropathy in cystic fibrosis. Br Med J 288:822, 1984.

660. Prakash UB: The use of the pediatric fiberoptic bronchoscope in adults. Rev Respir Dis 132:715, 1985.

661. Naidich DP, Lee J-J, Garay SM, et al: Comparison of CT and fiberoptic bronchoscopy in the evaluation of bronchial disease. AJR 148:1, 1987.

662. Geckler RW, McAllister CK, Gremillion DH, et al: Clinical value of paired sputum and transtracheal aspirates in the initial management of pneumonia. Chest 87:631, 1985.

663. Torzillo PJ, McWilliam DB, Young IH, et al: Use of protected telescoping brush system in the management of bacterial pulmonary infection in intubated patients. Br J Dis Chest 79:125, 1985.

664. Villers D, Derriennic M, Raffi F, et al: Reliability of the bronchoscopic protected catheter brush in intubated and ventilated patients. Chest 88:527, 1985.

665. DeMaria AA Jr, Westmoreland BF, Sharbrough FW: EEG in cough syncope. Neurology, 34:371, 1984.

3

4

C H A P T E R

Roentgenologic Signs in the Diagnosis of Chest Disease

The integration of information obtained from systematic interpretation of the chest roentgenogram and careful analysis of the clinical status of the patient yields a high degree of diagnostic accuracy in most chest diseases. However, although the final assessment must take into account the patient's history, physical examination, laboratory tests, and pulmonary function studies, the roentgenologist should glean as much information as possible from an objective assessment of the roentgenogram *before* attempting clinical correlation. A roentgenographic pattern of disease may be sufficiently distinctive that an etiologic diagnosis can be made with reasonable certainty on that evidence alone; confirmation will depend upon whether the roentgenologic conclusions and the clinical picture can be reconciled. Thus, a systematic approach to roentgenologic interpretation is of cardinal importance. Appreciation of signs such as the size, number, and density of pulmonary lesions, their homogeneity, sharpness of definition, and anatomic location and distribution, as well as the presence or absence of cavitation or calcification, is needed for an understanding of the pathogenesis of the disease and leads to a reasonable differential diagnosis.

The roentgenographic characteristics of specific disease entities are given in the relevant chapters. This chapter describes *basic roentgen signs* as they indicate the *fundamental nature* of disease. It is subdivided into three major sections: increased roentgenographic density, decreased roentgenographic density, and diseases of the pleura.

Since a knowledge of the pathogenesis and pathology of a disease process is necessary to an understanding of the roentgenographic images it creates, wherever possible we relate the signs to their gross and microscopic morphologic characteristics and to the mechanisms of these changes (Fig. 4–1).

LUNG DISEASES THAT INCREASE ROENTGENOGRAPHIC DENSITY

The various anatomic structures of the lung can be considered to comprise two functional units, that concerned with *conduction* (bronchi, blood vessels, and lymphatics), and that concerned with *gaseous exchange* (acini, or lung parenchyma, made up of peripheral air spaces, accompanying vessels, and extravascular interstitial tissue). Excluding the vascular system, it is obvious that all pulmonary disease that increases density in the lung periphery involves change in one or both of two components, the air spaces and extravascular interstitial tissue. Although most diseases that affect the acinus so as to produce an increase in roentgenograph density involve *both* the air spaces and interstitial tissue to a variable extent, it is helpful to divide these diseases into three general groups, depending upon which component is *predominantly* affected:

1. *Air spaces.* The air may be replaced by liquids, cells, or a combination of the two (consolidation) or absorbed and not replaced (atelectasis).
2. *Interstitial tissues.*
3. *Combined air spaces and interstitial tissues.*

PREDOMINANTLY AIR-SPACE DISEASE

Parenchymal Consolidation

In this situation the air within the acinus is *replaced*, usually by a substance of unit density consisting of liquids, cells, or a combination of the two (Fig. 4–2). Typically, many contiguous acini are involved, producing an opacity of homogeneous density varying in size from a few centimeters to a whole lobe. Sometimes, however, *individual shadows* approximately 7 mm in diameter can be identified that coincide roughly with the size and configuration of single acini and are a distinctive feature of air-space consolidation.

THE ACINAR SHADOW

Aschoff,[1] in 1924 was the first to report the distinctive roentgenographic appearance that he interpreted as a single acinus consolidated by tuberculous inflammatory exudate and granulation tissue; he likened it to a rosette and termed it the acinonodose lesion. Since the acinus is a unit of parenchymal structure approximately 7 mm in diameter (*see* page 29, Chapter 1), it can be assumed that replacing its air with a substance of unit density would result in a roentgenographic shadow approximately 7 mm in diameter, fairly well circumscribed, and with a slightly irregular contour (Fig. 4–3). Although we feel that the acinus should be accepted as the basic unit of lung structure for roentgenologic description, this does not imply that *individual* acinar shadows must be identified roentgenographically for a pulmonary shadow to qualify as an air-space filling disease; in fact, this is the exception rather than the rule. In an experimental study in which silicone rubber compound was injected into peripheral air spaces by micropuncture, Raskin and Herman[2, 3] showed rapid dissemination of the medium throughout the secondary lobule via interacinar ducts, with little respect for acinar boundaries; although a few individual acini could be identified, the only border limiting dissemination of the injected material was the connective tissue septum of the secondary lobule. As we pointed out previously, however, such limitation of dispersion would apply only in areas containing secondary lobules and not in central lung areas, where one of the commonest diseases to consolidate air spaces—pulmonary edema—has its major effects. Why only certain diseases (for example, bronchogenic spread of tuberculosis) and not others (undoubtedly the majority) appear to respect acinar boundaries is not

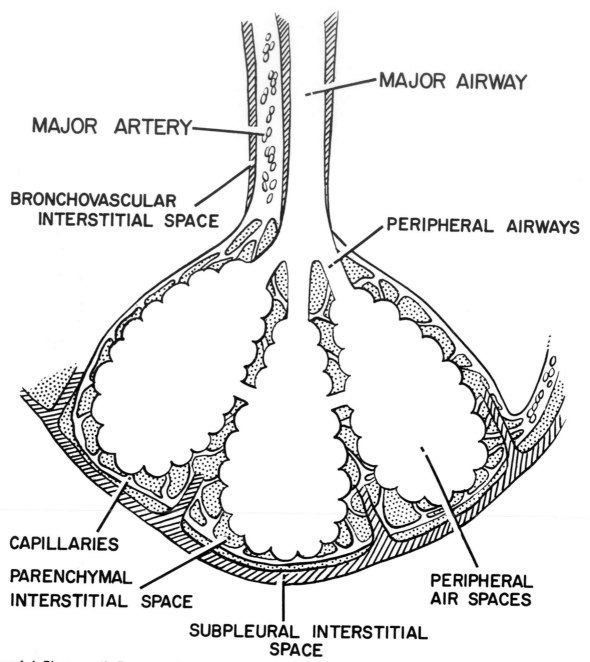

Figure 4–1. Diagrammatic Representation of the Lung. This diagram depicts the components of the lung that are involved in the majority of pulmonary diseases—the large and small airways, the peripheral air spaces (including communicating channels), the arteries, veins, and capillaries, and the bronchovascular, subpleural, and parenchymal interstitial space. Throughout the chapter this diagram of the normal lung is reproduced alongside diagrams depicting disturbances in morphology.

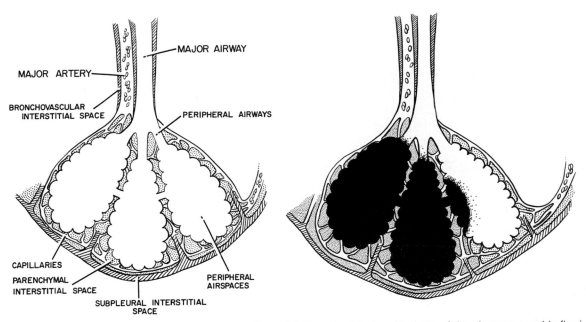

Figure 4–2. The Lung Diagram: Peripheral Air-space Consolidation. Exudate has filled two of the air spaces and is flowing into the third via pores of Kohn. Volume is unaffected, and the airways are patent. The parenchymal interstitial tissue is increased in amount around the consolidated air spaces.

known; the viscosity of the consolidating medium probably plays a part. The inflammatory edema caused by some organisms—*Streptococcus pneumoniae*, for example—is of low viscosity and therefore spreads readily via interalveolar pores, whereas that of others—such as *Mycobacterium tuberculosis*—may be of sufficient viscosity to prevent such ready dissemination. Although viscosity of the medium employed by Raskin and Herman was not reported, obviously it was low enough to permit passage of the medium through interacinar ducts measuring about 200μm in diameter.[3] The suspension used by Gamsu and his colleagues[4] (tantalum, 100 grams; neutral medium, 50 ml; distilled water, 50 ml) was of 550 centipoises' viscosity, high enough to opacify individual acinar units; a mosaic of spherical acinar structures was maintained until immediately before coalescence. Results similar to those of the Gamsu study were obtained by Lui and associates,[5] whose injection material was barium sulfate mixed with gelatin (a modification of Schlesinger mass).[6] Although we feel that the viscosity of the filling medium must play a significant role, Gamsu and his colleagues suggested two other mechanisms by which liquid might remain localized to an acinus for some time without passing into surrounding parenchyma: (1) in normal lungs, resistance to flow is considerably higher in collateral channels than in peripheral airways,[7] a difference that would tend to account for retention of fluid in peripheral airways within the acinus; and (2) the terminal bronchiole, being situated at the outlet of the acinus, is the narrowest portion of the entire bronchial tree[8] and as such would tend to resist passage of fluid.

Roentgenologic Criteria of Air-Space Disease

The currently accepted roentgenographic criteria of air-space disease are listed in Table 4–1. These signs are closely related and depend upon displacement of air from the acinus by either intrinsic or extrinsic means. Accumulation of edema, hemorrhage, or tissue elements within the acinar air-spaces exemplifies the intrinsic mechanism, whereas massive encroachment upon the distal air spaces by certain expanding interstitial disorders explains the extrinsic pathogenesis. Both of these mechanisms can appear in an almost pure form, exemplified respectively by idiopathic pulmonary

Table 4–1. Conventional Roentgenographic and CT Criteria of Air-space Disease*

CRITERIA	CONVENTIONAL RADIOGRAPH	CT
Air-space nodule (ASN)	typical	not typical
Coalescence	yes	yes
Segmental/nonsegmental	yes	yes
Poor margination	yes	yes
Air bronchogram	yes	yes
Air bronchiologram	in ASN	no
Air alveologram	in ASN	no
Rapid/slow evolution	yes	yes
Minimal atelectasis	yes	yes

*The air-space nodule (ASN), exemplified by the acinar opacity, is seen in its most typical form on conventional roentgenograms. CT spatial resolution does not permit identification of the characteristic air bronchiologram and air alveologram of the ASN with certainty. Both techniques display other criteria with equal facility.

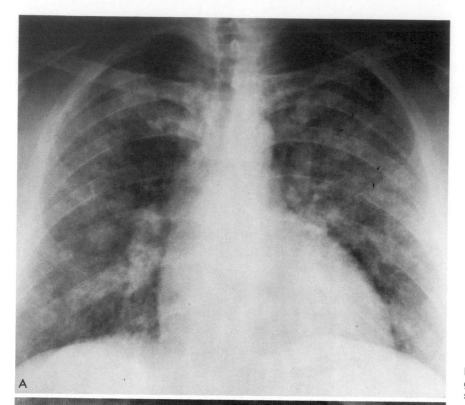

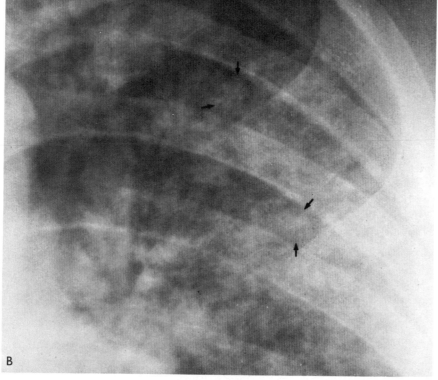

Figure 4–3. Idiopathic Pulmonary Hemorrhage. A posteroanterior roentgenogram of the chest (*A*) reveals extensive airspace consolidation throughout both lungs, confluent in many areas but patchy in others, permitting identification of individual acinar shadows (*B-arrows* in *B*).

Illustration continued on opposite page

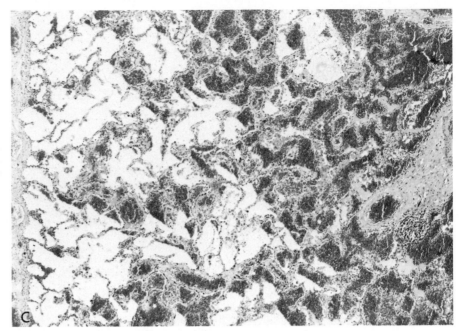

Figure 4–3 *Continued. C,* Photomicrographs show the alveoli to be filled with blood, uniformly on the right and focally on the left. (× 40.)

hemorrhage and lymphoma. On the other hand, there are cases in which both the interstitium and air spaces are involved simultaneously, in which case either an air space or interstitial pattern can predominate. For example, certain interstitial pneumonias, such as the early form of fibrosing alveolitis (desquamative interstitial pneumonia), are associated with both thickened alveolar septa and alveolar filling, accounting for the variable roentgenographic appearance of these types of diseases.

THE AIR-SPACE NODULE

The presence of a nodular lesion in air-space disease has been recognized for some time, but unfortunately the nomenclature has been confusing: various names have been proposed, including the acinar shadow,[10] acinar opacity, peribronchiolar nodule,[11] and alveolar nodule. Because of these semantic difficulties, coupled with the fact that we now recognize three varieties of these nodules, an all-encompassing term such as the "air-space nodule" is recommended.

The classic *acinar nodule* shows three features (Fig. 4–4): (1) a nodular shape measuring 4 to 10 mm in diameter; (2) poor margination, although the lesion remains discrete enough to permit individual identification; and (3) multiple small radiolucencies within its confines caused by air within bronchioles and alveoli. Although the presence of nodular lesions in air-space–filling disorders is undoubted, debate continues as to whether the opacities represent actual acini or merely shadows that closely resemble acini. This question cannot be easily resolved because of the obvious difficulty in obtaining precise radiologic/pathologic correlation in a clinical setting. Nevertheless, the identification of

such nodular opacities constitutes convincing evidence of an air-space–filling process.

The *subacinar nodule* (Fig. 4–4) possesses the same general characteristics as the acinar opacity except that many more radiolucencies are visible within it; thus the two are distinguished by quantitative features. Invariably, the subacinar nodule is dispersed against a background of minute (less than 1 mm) opacities descriptively termed "stippling,"[12] "granularity,"[13] or "ground-glass."[14] The recognition of the subacinar pattern and its significance as a sign of distal air-space disorders are not widely appreciated. The pattern may be mistaken for a fine reticular or micronodular pattern of interstitial disease (see page 553), although the confusion can be diminished by "standing back" from the film and identifying both the trees (subacinar nodules) and the forest (background stippling).

The *spokewheel nodule* (Fig. 4–4), the third and least frequent variety, measures 4 to 10 mm in diameter and shows a central, relatively large lucency from which smaller, linear radiolucencies radiate peripherally.[15] The genesis of this pattern is uncertain; correlative radiologic/bronchographic studies suggest that the opacity may result from tangentially imaged and summated small bronchioles (Fig. 4–4). Conceivably, the central lucency of the spoke is caused by air within terminal bronchioles viewed end-on, while the radiating spokes are air-containing bronchioles seen tangentially.

These nodular opacities can be easily identified on CT; however, they do not conform precisely to the criteria of an air-space nodule since air bronchiolograms and air alveolograms are not seen, a deficiency caused by the decreased spatial resolution of CT relative to conventional roentgenography.[16] As a result, the air-space nodule cannot be reliably

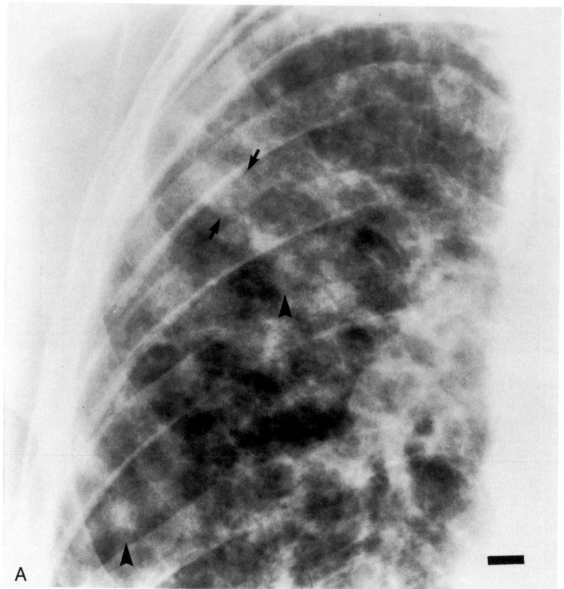

Figure 4–4. Varieties of Air-space Nodules. *A*, A detail view of the right lung from a PA chest roentgenogram of a patient with biopsy-proved bronchioalveolar cell carcinoma. The acinar nodule (*arrowheads*) is characterized by poor margination, nodular shape, 4 to 10 mm size, and intranodular radiolucencies caused by air within bronchioles and alveoli. Confluence of several acinar nodules creates a larger air-space opacity (*between arrows*). Bar represents 1 cm.

Illustration continued on opposite page

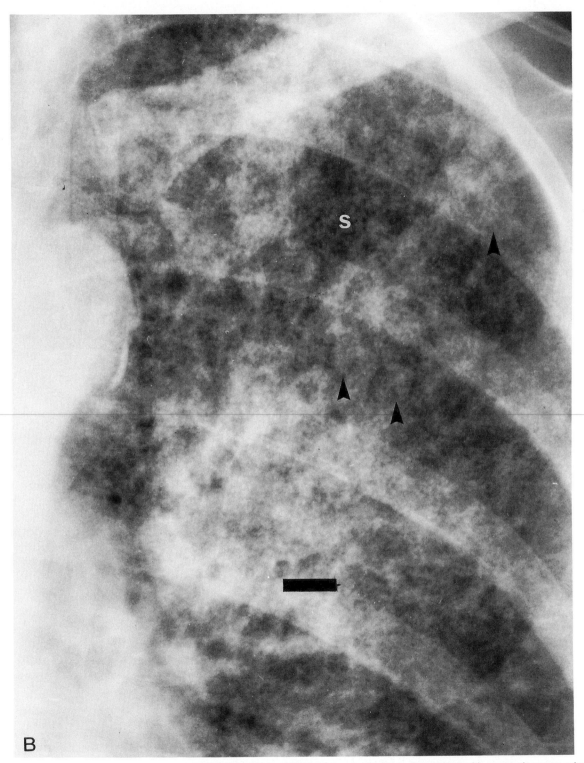

Figure 4–4 *Continued. B,* A detail view of the left lung from a PA chest roentgenogram of a patient with acute air-space edema. The subacinar nodule (*arrowheads*) differs from the acinar nodules depicted in *A* by the presence within it of more radiolucencies. Concomitant background stippling (S) is a prominent feature. Bar represents 1 cm.

Illustration continued on following page

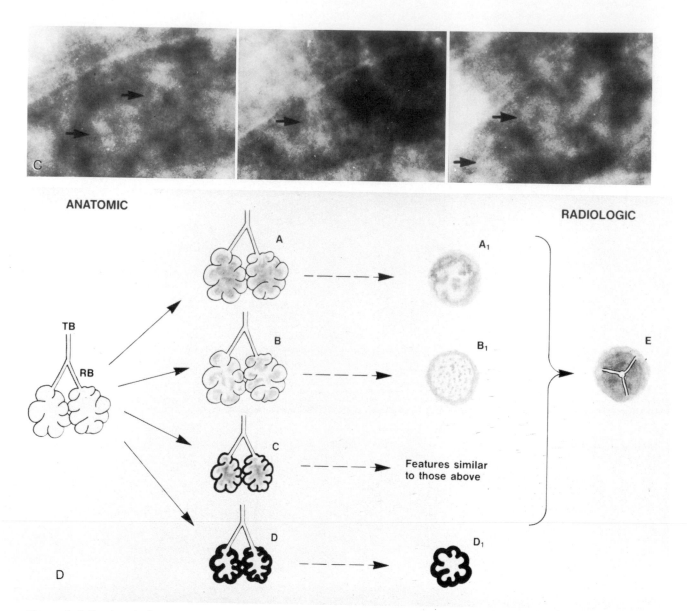

Figure 4–4 *Continued. C,* A closeup of the right lung from PA chest roentgenograms of three patients with different diseases: bronchogenic spread of tuberculosis (*left*), alveolar cell carcinoma (*middle*), and *Pneumocystis carinii* pneumonia (*right*). The spokewheel nodule (*arrows*) measures 4 to 10 mm in diameter and is composed of a central radiolucency with smaller linear lucencies (spokes) radiating to the periphery. *D,* A schematic representation of the pathogenesis of air-space nodules. The normal acinus consists of all parenchyma distal to the terminal bronchiole (TB) including respiratory bronchioles (RB) and other distal elements. Complete (*A*) or incomplete (*B*) filling of the acinus results in the roentgenographic perception of acinar (A_1) or subacinar (B_1) opacities. Mural thickening of alveolar septa with "spillover" into the alveolar spaces (*C*) shows similar features. Diffuse thickening of the alveolar septa with encroachment upon alveolar gas, resulting in microatelectasis (*D*), is the probable cause of an opacity that closely simulates the air-space nodule (D_1). Tangential x-ray projection of an opacified acinus is the probable explanation of the spokewheel nodule (*E*). (From Genereux GP: Med Radiogr Photogr *61:*2, 1985.)

distinguished from a homogeneous interstitial nodule of similar size and shape. On CT, the subacinar pattern possesses a bubbly appearance, closely simulating interstitial reticulation. In all other respects, CT scans are capable of defining the characteristic signs of an air-space–filling process (see Figure 4–6).

Obviously, identification of an air-space opacity establishes the *anatomic location* of the disease process, *not* its mechanism of production, and extends the differential diagnosis to a multitude of diseases of varying pathogenesis. The common causes of diffuse air-space disease include (1) alveolar edema, either cardiogenic or permeability in type, (2) the inflammatory exudate associated with an acute infection, (3) bleeding into the acini from any cause, (4) aspiration of blood or lipid, (5) neoplastic infiltration, most commonly from bronchioloalveolar cell carcinoma or locally invasive lymphoma, (6) idiopathic conditions such as alveolar proteinosis, and (7) certain chronic interstitial processes typified by the early stages of fibrosing alveolitis (desquamative interstitial pneumonia).

In summary: (1) *Air within an acinus may be replaced by fluid or cells, either completely or incompletely, resulting respectively in an acinar or subacinar opacity (Fig. 4–4).* (2) *Mural thickening of alveolar septa with a concomitant "spillover" of fluid or cells into the alveolar spaces results in similar features (Fig. 4–5).* (3) *It is possible that diffuse thickening of alveolar septa alone with encroachment upon the alveolar gas can cause an opacity that closely simulates a true air-space nodule.* (4) *Tangential x-ray projection of the pathologic acinus is the likely explanation for the spokewheel configuration.*

COALESCENCE

Air in the distal air spaces may be partly or completely replaced by a variety of transudates, exudates, desquamated or proliferated epithelial cells, or the deposition of calcific material.[17] Fluid in particular can disseminate rapidly through collateral pathways of the lung into adjacent air spaces, coalescing as it proceeds.[11] Since all areas of the lung are seldom affected simultaneously and to the same degree, the result is a spreading, irregular

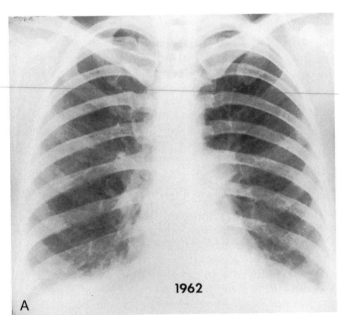

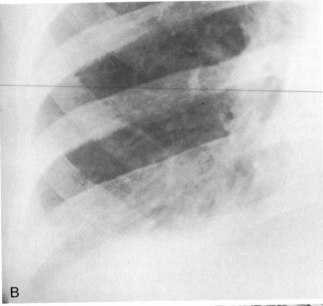

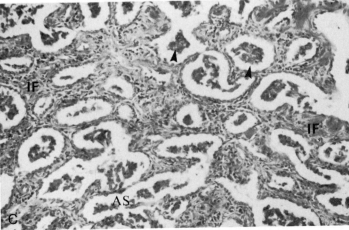

Figure 4–5 Thickening of Alveolar Septa with Concomitant Air-space Filling. A posteroanterior chest roentgenogram (*A*) and a closeup of the right lower lung zone (*B*) reveal features consistent with an air-space filling process although opacity is inhomogeneous; an air bronchogram is suggested. A photomicrograph (*C*) from this patient demonstrates the "spillover" phenomenon associated with some interstitial diseases. Revised alveolar spaces (AS) are partly filled with macrophages (*arrowheads*). Note that the dominant histopathology is interstitial and is characterized by an infiltration of chronic inflammatory cells and fibrosis (IF). Features are consistent with the desquamative phase of fibrosing alveolitis.

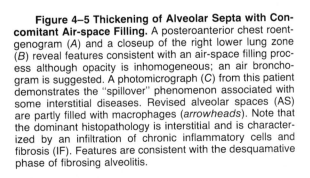

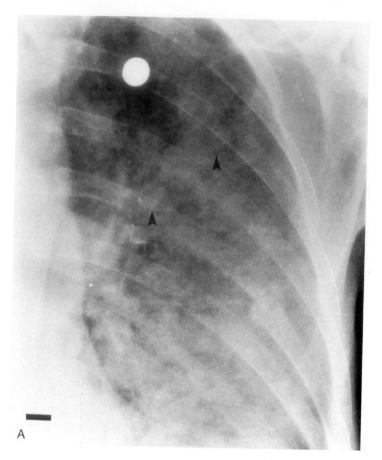

Figure 4–6. Interstitial Lung Disease Simulating Air-space Disease. *A,* A closeup of the left upper lobe from a PA chest roentgenogram of a patient with metastatic calcinosis associated with chronic renal insufficiency. Multiple subacinar nodules (*arrowheads*), coalescence, and a faint air bronchogram are present against a background of fine reticulation or stippling. Features are those of a primary air-space process.

Illustration continued on opposite page

wave of consolidation with ill-defined borders.[18] Large and small bronchi tend to remain air containing and become surrounded by a sea of fluid. Similar events in nearby or remote acini eventually replace major areas of parenchyma with homogeneous nonsegmental consolidation.

DISTRIBUTION CHARACTERISTICS

A characteristic feature of diseases associated with air-space consolidation is failure to respect segmental boundaries. In widely disseminated disease, such as acute pulmonary edema, lack of segmental distribution is not unexpected. Even in localized disease, however, intersegmental spread occurs; for example, in acute pneumococcal pneumonia, infection is propagated centrifugally via channels of collateral ventilation. Since segmental boundaries do not impede the passage of gas or liquid via these channels, the exudate of acute air-space pneumonia can spread throughout the lung periphery. Consequently, such diseases are *nonsegmental* in distribution, an observation of importance in establishing the pathogenesis of the disease process and thereby in suggesting an etiologic diagnosis (Fig. 4–6). By contrast, processes that are propagated via the vascular or tracheobronchial tree usually display a striking *segmental* distribution. For instance, aspiration of lipid (Fig. 4–7) characteristically results in consolidation of multiple segments, the particular areas of lung involved being largely dependent on the patient's position at the time of aspiration. Large pleural-based pulmonary infarcts also reveal segmental distribution characteristics.

MARGINATION

The edge characteristics of air-space–filling processes often show poor margination.[18] This feature is a consequence of the spreading and coalescing wave of consolidation that partly fills acinar components in a serrated fashion so that the x-ray beam fails to detect a sharp border between involved and uninvolved parenchyma. The clearest example of this phenomenon is the "butterfly" or "bat's wing" appearance of acute air-space edema or hemorrhage. However, in acute diplococcal or *Klebsiella* pneumonia, because the infection is propagated by centrifugal spread, the advancing margin of consolidation is sometimes fairly smooth and sharply defined.

THE AIR BRONCHOGRAM

Consolidation of lung parenchyma, with little or no involvement of conducting airways, creates another important roentgenographic sign. In acute air-space pneumonia, for example, consolidation usually begins in subpleural parenchyma, the exudate rapidly spreading centrifugally to surround

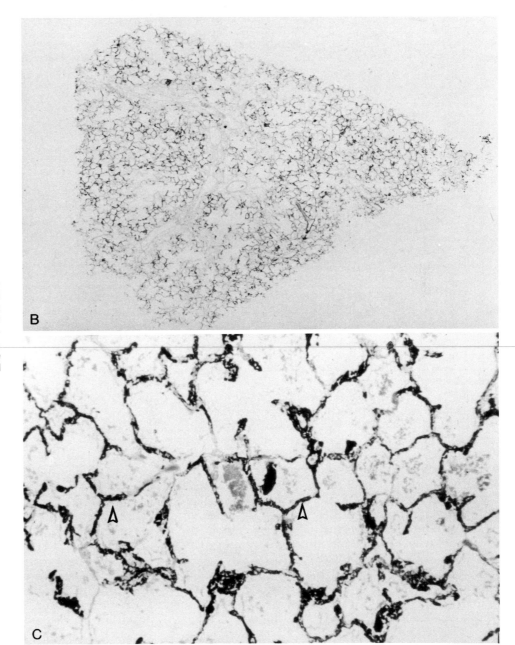

Figure 4–6 *Continued*. However, low power (*B*) and high power (*C*) histologic sections obtained at autopsy reveal a normal complement of alveolar septa that are diffusely although minimally thickened by interstitial calcification (dark linear staining material, *arrowheads*). The air spaces are normal. (From Genereux GP: Med Radiogr Photogr *61*:2, 1985.)

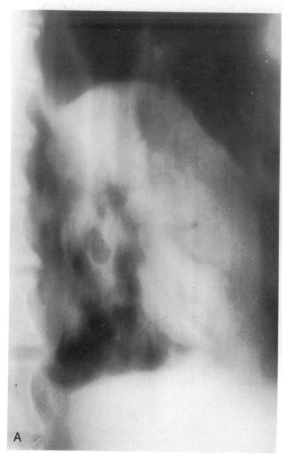

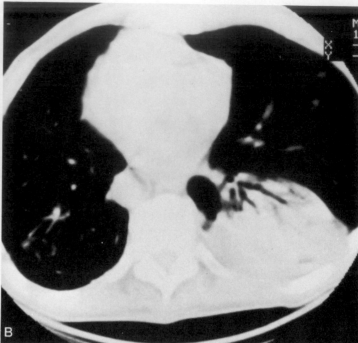

Figure 4–7. Multisegmental Consolidation of the Left Lower Lobe Caused by Aspiration of Lipid. A conventional linear tomogram (*A*) and transverse CT scan (*B*) demonstrate segmental consolidation of the left lower lobe associated with a prominent air bronchogram. Similar areas of consolidation were present in the posterior portions of both upper lobes. The patient is an elderly man with situs inversus who ingested large quantities of mineral oil for chronic constipation. The sputum contained abundant free and intracellular Sudan-III positive material.

bronchi as it advances toward the hilum. Since the consolidation is entirely parenchymal, air in the bronchi is not displaced. This produces contrast between the air within the bronchial tree and the surrounding airless parenchyma, so that the normally invisible bronchial air column becomes roentgenographically visible (Fig. 4–8). This invaluable sign was described originally by Fleischner[19, 20] in 1927 and was aptly named the *air bronchogram* sign by Felson.[21] Two situations must exist for an air bronchogram to be identified: the airways must be air containing (the bronchus cannot be completely occluded at its origin), and surrounding lung parenchyma must be of markedly reduced air content or *airless*. Since the parenchyma may be airless when its air has been replaced by liquid or tissue (consolidation) or when it has been absorbed and not replaced (atelectasis), an air bronchogram may be seen in either circumstance *but only when the supplying bronchus is not occluded*. As discussed further on, four mechanisms can result in atelectasis, the commonest being obstruction of a supplying bronchus; in such circumstances, an air bronchogram cannot exist since the distal parenchyma no longer communicates with the mouth. In the other three types of atelectasis—relaxation, cicatrization, and adhesive—bronchi are not obstructed, and since the parenchyma surrounding air-containing bronchi is of reduced air content or airless, an air broncho-

gram is anticipated. For example, the collapsed lung behind a large pneumothorax (relaxation atelectasis) invariably shows an air bronchogram; in fact, its absence indicates central bronchial obstruction associated with the pneumothorax. Similarly, both bronchiectasis and radiation fibrosis—varieties of cicatrization atelectasis—often are associated with air bronchograms. In fact, "pure" interstitial lung disease of sufficient severity (e.g., talc granulomatosis accompanying longstanding intravenous drug abuse) can be associated with a prominent air bronchogram (Fig. 4–8), an observation that has been illustrated by Reed and Madewell in a radiologic/pathologic correlative study.[22] Finally, the adhesive atelectasis that occurs in acute radiaton pneumonitis and hyaline membrane disease nearly always is associated with an air bronchogram. It is important to recognize that although an air bronchogram is an almost invariable finding in air-space consolidation from whatever cause, it is *not* restricted to this state.

Most diseases associated with air-space consolidation show this sign, although in some—for example, pulmonary infarction—it may be only temporary because of early filling of airways by blood or exudate.

In summary, regardless of its etiology, any pathologic process associated with an air bronchogram must fulfill three criteria: (1) it must be anatomically situated within

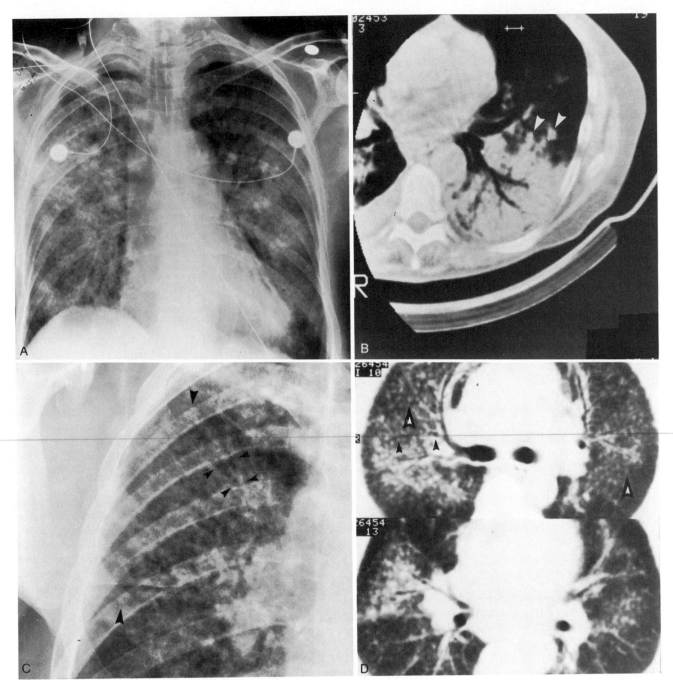

Figure 4–8. An Air Bronchogram Associated with Diffuse Lung Disease. *A*, A conventional anteroposterior chest roentgenogram of this elderly woman with idiopathic pulmonary hemorrhage shows coalescent, poorly marginated, nonsegmental opacities involving both lungs somewhat asymmetrically. Distribution on the left is of a "bat's-wing" variety. Multiple isolated and confluent nodular opacities and air bronchograms are seen. *B*, A CT scan through the left lower zone reveals confluent, poorly defined consolidation in the lower lobe and lingula. A prominent air bronchogram is present. Several opacities (*arrowheads*) conform in size to acinar nodules but do not show the typical intra-acinar features of air-containing bronchioles and alveoli. Slight volume loss is present in the lower lobe. CT density is in the +65 to +75 HU range. *C*, A closeup of the right lung from a posteroanterior chest roentgenogram of a patient with sarcoidosis: multiple nodular opacities (*arrowheads*) essentially indistinguishable from subacinar shadows are seen. Confluence of many such nodules accounts for faint air bronchogram formation (*small arrowheads*). Hilar lymph nodes are enlarged. *D*, CT scans through the upper lobes (*top*) and the middle lobe/lingula (*bottom*) of the same patient show a prominent air bronchogram (*small arrowheads*) throughout the lung medulla. Multiple isolated and confluent small nodular opacities (*arrowheads*) are present. The lobulated contour of the hila confirms the presence of lymph node enlargement. (From Genereux GP: Med Radiogr Photogr *61*:2, 1985.)

lung parenchyma; (2) *the parenchyma must be completely or almost completely airless as a result of consolidation or atelectasis or both*; and (3) *the lumen of the bronchus leading to the affected parenchyma must be patent.*

AIR BRONCHIOLOGRAM AND AIR ALVEOLOGRAM

The identification of minute radiolucencies within air-space consolidation, best exemplified in the air-space nodule, is an important sign and relates histopathologically to incompletely filled bronchioles and alveoli (air bronchiologram and air alveologram respectively). Clearly, neither of these microscopic structures is normally visible on conventional roentgenograms, but when the acinus becomes partly consolidated, some of these smaller units are rendered visible. Thus, the demonstration of such radiolucencies is analogous to an air bronchogram and carries the same pathogenetic implications. Despite what the term air alveologram might suggest—the depiction of air within an alveolus—such is clearly impossible: there are at least 300 million of these structures in the human lung, the inevitable conclusion being that their visibility must result from the air content of a multitude of alveoli within the acinus.

TIME FACTOR

The rapidity with which consolidation resolves can be of great importance as a sign of air-space disease. Thus, an air-space pattern that clears over a period of hours or a couple of days is certain evidence of pulmonary edema or hemorrhage. By contrast, air-space disease that persists over time, sometimes for weeks or months, is usually caused by infection, aspiration, bronchioloalveolar cell carcinoma, lymphoma, or idiopathic conditions such as alveolar proteinosis.

ABSENCE OF ATELECTASIS

In distal air-space consolidation, maintenance of lung volume is understandable when one considers its pathogenesis. In the first place, air in the acini is replaced by an equal or almost equal quantity of liquid or tissue. Second, since the process is predominantly parenchymal, airways leading to affected portions of lung remain patent; thus, there is no reason for collapse to occur before exudate fills the air spaces. Again, there are occasional exceptions to this rule; for example, in pulmonary infarction, volume is often diminished by causes other than airway obstruction, possibly surfactant deficit.

EXPERIMENTAL CORRELATION: SIMULATION OF AIR-SPACE DISEASE

There is now abundant evidence from experimental,[23, 24] postmortem,[25] and bronchographic

studies to substantiate the concepts underlying the roentgenographic air-space nodule. If a formalin-inflated lung is injected with a barium-gelatin mixture via the bronchial tree and then radiographed, appropriate areas for further study can be delineated (Fig. 4–9). This type of preparation shows many shadows that are remarkably similar to air-space nodules observed in a clinical setting, including the highly characteristic small radiolucencies within the injected medium. Serial sectioning followed by radiography (Fig. 4–9) and paper mounting of the slice permits precise photomicrographic/radiographic correlation: in these circumstances, the barium-gelatin mixture in the well-formed nodular opacities (Fig. 4–9) is entirely intraacinar, the radiolucencies representing unfilled, air-containing terminal airways. In areas where a subacinar pattern is perceived, there is only a quantitative difference in the degree of filling of the nodules so that air bronchiologram and air alveologram formation is more prominent.

The genesis of the infrequently identified spokewheel nodule is uncertain. Correlative radiographic/bronchographic studies (Fig. 4–9) suggest that the opacity may result from tangentially imaged and summated small bronchioles. As suggested previously, the central lucency of the spoke could be accounted for by air within terminal bronchioles (end-on air bronchiologram), whereas the radiating spokes are profiled by smaller air-containing bronchioles.

Parenchymal Atelectasis

In its pure form atelectasis may be regarded conceptually as the antithesis of consolidation: in the former, air is absorbed and not replaced, and in the latter, air is replaced by liquid or cells of approximately equal volume. Thus, from a roentgenologic point of view, the major difference is one of volume: in consolidation, volume is normal; in atelectasis, it is reduced.

The terminology of pulmonary atelectasis is controversial. Etymologically, the word is derived from the Greek words *ateles* (incomplete) and *ektasis* (stretching). The interpretation placed on this by the semantic purist is that "incomplete stretching" is necessarily neonatal and cannot be applied to a state that develops after full inflation has occurred. We prefer to use the word in its broad sense—to denote *diminished air within the lung associated with reduced lung volume.* This definition simply implies loss of volume, not increase in roentgenographic density. A fairly common form of atelectasis occurs in the postoperative period, when collapse of acinar units may be so extensive that it results in significant venoarterial shunting, but roentgenographic evidence shows only diaphragmatic elevation. Diament and Palmer,[26] who measured arterial blood gases during 100 per cent oxygen breathing in 23 patients

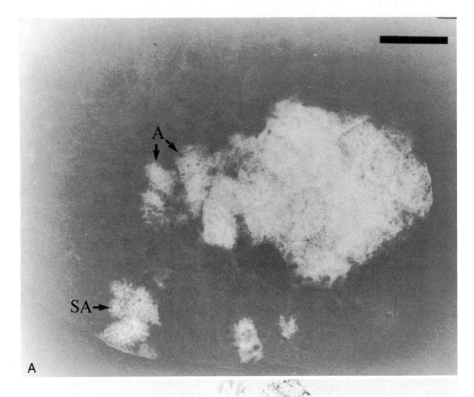

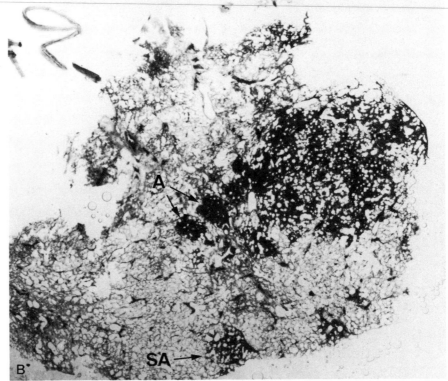

Figure 4–9. Simulation of Air-space Disease. *A*, A roentgenogram of a lung specimen following injection of a barium/gelatin mixture reveals nodular opacities similar to clinical acinar (*A*) and subacinar (SA) nodules. Note that the former differ from the latter only in the number of perceived radiolucencies within them. Bar denotes 1 cm. *B*, Similar opacities can be identified on a roentgenogram of a thin slice of the specimen.

Illustration continued on following page

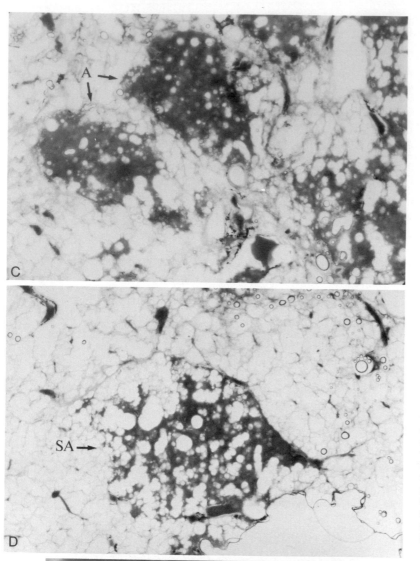

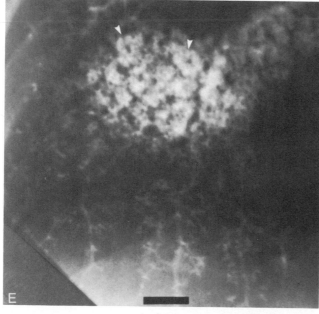

Figure 4–9 *Continued. C* and *D*, Photomicrographs (2 × magnification) of a paper-mounted section of the specimen in *B* show the radiolucencies in the acinar (*A*) and subacinar (*SA*) nodules to be caused by unfilled, air-containing respiratory bronchioles and alveoli. The two nodular opacities are similar, differing only quantitatively in the amount of air replaced by the barium/gelatin mixture. *E*, In an overfilled clinical bronchogram, filling does not extend beyond the millimeter pattern, indicating that contrast medium had not penetrated farther than the respiratory bronchiole. Some nodules (*arrowheads*) possess a relatively large central radiolucency from which linear radiolucencies emanate (spokewheel appearance). This presentation conceivably relates to axial imaging of air-containing respiratory bronchioles. Bar denotes 1 cm. (From Genereux GP: Med Radiogr Photogr *61*:2, 1985.)

before and after surgery, showed a mean true shunt of 12 per cent during the postoperative period. In a correlation of the degree of shunting with roentgenographic appearances postoperatively, venoarterial shunt averaged 7 per cent in 12 patients with completely normal chest roentgenograms, 13 per cent in 5 patients whose chest roentgenograms showed no more than basal linear opacities, and 19 per cent in 6 patients whose roentgenograms revealed segmental collapse. In this series of patients, the important group from the point of view of the present discussion is the first—patients with physiologic evidence of significant atelectasis but no roentgenographic changes. Of a similar nature but different etiology is the loss of volume that occurs in a lobe whose blood supply has been interrupted by thromboembolism. This may be accompanied by considerable volume loss of the affected lobe or segment and manifested by diaphragmatic elevation and fissure displacement but no increase in roentgenographic density; in fact, density may be reduced because of the oligemia resulting from arterial obstruction. These two examples indicate the importance of *regarding atelectasis as a process in which the only direct roentgenographic sign is loss of lung volume, and it is in this context that "atelectasis" is used throughout this book.*

Since we have described atelectasis essentially in terms of lung volume, it is important to consider the mechanisms that keep the lung expanded. Alterations in these mechanisms provide a suitable basis for classifying atelectasis. However, the lesions are varied and depend upon prevailing circumstances. These will be considered, and the roentgenographic abnormalities will be described in the light of these principles.

MAINTENANCE OF LUNG VOLUME

As described in Chapter 1 (*see* page 56), the lung has a natural tendency to collapse and does so when removed from the chest. While the lungs are in the thoracic cavity, this tendency is opposed by the chest wall, and at the resting respiratory position (FRC) the tendency for the lung to collapse and for the chest wall to expand are equal and opposite. When the thorax contains a space-occupying process (e.g., pneumothorax), the lung retracts and its volume decreases; this is *passive or relaxation atelectasis.* A similar mechanism exists at the edge of a local space-occupying lesion within the lung; because of its inherent elastic recoil properties, the parenchyma for some distance contiguous with the mass or cyst is reduced in volume. Although this mechanism of volume loss has been termed compression atelectasis, from a conceptual point of view we consider it preferable to regard it as a variant of passive or relaxation atelectasis.

In a static system, the volume attained by the lung depends upon the balance between the applied force and the opposing elastic forces, generally termed compliance or change in volume per unit change in pressure. It follows that when the lung is stiffer than normal, that is, when compliance is decreased, lung volume is decreased. This classically occurs with pulmonary fibrosis and is called *cicatrization atelectasis.* The pressure-volume behavior also depends upon the forces acting at the air-tissue interface of the alveolar wall. As alveoli diminish in volume, the surface tension of the interface is diminished by the "alveolar lining fluid," or surfactant. When the action of surfactant is interfered with, as may occur in the respiratory distress syndrome or after bypass surgery, there may be widespread collapse of alveoli. This type of atelectasis has been referred to as microatelectasis or nonobstructive atelectasis, but we shall refer to it as *adhesive atelectasis.*

The most common form of atelectasis, and the most complex, is caused by the resorption of gas from the alveoli, as may occur in acute bronchial obstruction. Since we have classified other forms of atelectasis on the basis of mechanism rather than etiology, this type of atelectasis is best termed *resorption atelectasis.*

RESORPTION ATELECTASIS

This occurs when communications between alveoli and trachea are obstructed (Figure 4–10). The mechanism of resorption is simple: the partial pressure of gases is lower in mixed venous blood than in alveolar air; as blood passes through the alveolar capillaries, the partial pressures of its gases equilibrate with alveolar pressure. The alveoli diminish in volume corresponding to the quantity of oxygen absorbed, their pressure remaining atmospheric; consequently, the partial pressures of carbon dioxide and nitrogen in the alveoli rise relative to capillary blood, and both gases diffuse into blood to maintain equilibrium. Thus alveolar volume is further reduced, with a consequent rise in the alveolar-capillary blood Po_2 gradient; oxygen diffuses into capillary blood, and this cycle is repeated until all alveolar gas is absorbed. In a previously healthy lobe, all air will have disappeared after 18 to 24 hours.[27] Since oxygen is absorbed selectively much more rapidly than nitrogen, when a lobe is filled with oxygen at the moment of occlusion (a situation that might pertain during anesthesia), collapse occurs much more rapidly and should be roentgenographically apparent within an hour (Fig. 4–11).[28] In fact, Rahn[29] has shown that the rate at which a lung collapses after an airway is blocked is 60 times faster when oxygen rather than air is breathed. In a recent study in our laboratories, Stein and his colleagues[30] obstructed the lobar bronchi of dogs with a balloon catheter following 100 per cent oxygen breathing for 5 min. The affected lobe became airless in 5 min or less; in fact, continuous cinefluorography of the events in one dog showed unequivocally that opacity in the obstructed lobe

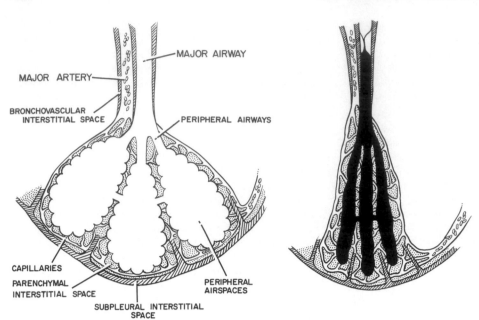

Figure 4–10. The Lung Diagram: Resorption Atelectasis. The major airway is obstructed, and the peripheral airways and air spaces are airless and collapsed.

was increased after three respiratory cycles! These facts are of considerable clinical significance: as pointed out by Fletcher and Avery,[31] total pulmonary opacification may be observed roentgenographically in some infants ventilated with 80 to 100 per cent oxygen; they suggest that this may be caused by rapid oxygen resorption during respiratory arrest. To substantiate their suspicion they occluded the endotracheal tube in a puppy that had breathed 100 per cent oxygen for 25 to 50 min: the lungs became completely gas-free in 3 to 5 min. The same effect may be observed in both infants and adults in whom malposition of endotracheal tubes has caused bronchial occlusion, and it is vital that the physician be aware of the exceptional rapidity with which an obstructed lung or lobe can collapse in such circumstances. Similarly, collapse may occur very rapidly when a one-way valve allows air to escape from a lobe but prevents its entrance. Coulter[27] produced total lobar collapse in 49 min after inserting such a valve in a dog's bronchus, and Henry and Miscall[32] observed complete lobar atelectasis in a human subject within a few minutes of his assuming the supine position because a mobile bronchial tumor impacted at the orifice of a bronchus and acted as a one-way valve.

It is important to realize that *resorption atelectasis* is not the inevitable or only accompaniment of bronchial obstruction, nor is obstruction of a major bronchus the only cause of resorption atelectasis. The effect of obstruction of the airways depends upon the site and extent of bronchial or bronchiolar obstruction, the pre-existing condition of the lung tissue, and collateral air drift. This last feature is so important that it deserves special mention.

COLLATERAL AIR DRIFT

Collateral ventilation and collateral air drift are the terms used to describe ventilation of alveoli other than by direct airway connections. Four potential routes have been identified (*see* page 35): (1) *The pores of Kohn*, which are circular or oval discontinuities in alveolar walls. (2) *The canals of Lambert*, which are epithelium-lined tubules between preterminal bronchioles and surrounding alveoli. (3) *Direct airway anastomoses*, consisting of tubular structures ranging from 80 to 200 μm in diameter, which have been described in both dog[33] and human[3] lungs. And (4), direct communications between adjacent acini at the level of alveolar sacs.[34] It is not known which of these routes is the most important in humans, but it is clear that considerable collateral ventilation can occur, even from upper to lower lobes. Of particular importance is the possibility of air trapping in collaterally ventilated lung (Fig. 4–12). The analysis by Brown and his associates[35] of 160 children with foreign bodies in the tracheobronchial tree supplied useful information in this regard; "obstructive overinflation" was by far the commonest roentgenographic finding, being present in 109 patients (68.1 per cent); collapse was the presenting roentgenographic finding in only 22 (13.8 per cent). This large discrepancy between the number of cases of overinflation and of atelectasis is almost certainly attributable to collateral air drift. The observation that overinflation occurs distal to bronchial atresia indicates the remarkable potency of collateral ventilation.[36] In fact, it has been implicated in the pathogenesis of emphysema,[36–39] in which case the airway obstruction is situated in distal bronchioles.

Customarily, collateral air drift has been regarded as occurring readily between lobar segments but not between pulmonary lobes; such a conclusion seems obvious in view of the fissures separating the lobes and the impossibility of air passing across the pleural space. However, in a study at necropsy of eight normal and eight emphysematous excised human lungs in which the resistance of collateral

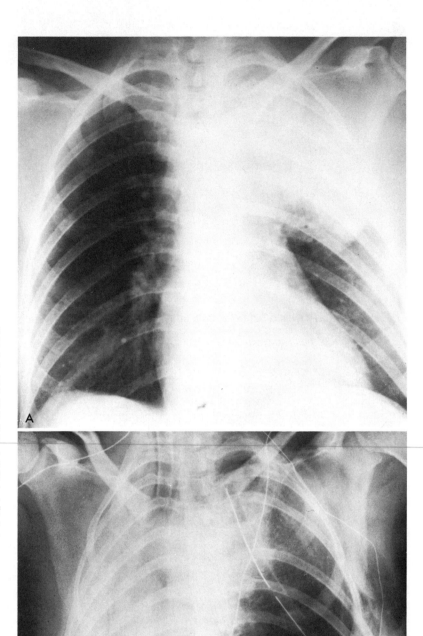

Figure 4–11. Acute Atelectasis of the Right Lung: Influence of Contained Gas on Rapidity of Collapse. *A,* The initial roentgenogram of this 44-year-old man reveals a large mass in the left upper lobe that proved on biopsy to be adenocarcinoma; at thoracotomy, the lesion was unresectable. Shortly after his return to the recovery room, the patient appeared to be suffering considerable respiratory distress: a roentgenogram (*B*) showed complete collapse of the right lung associated with marked shift of the mediastinum into the right hemithorax. Bronchoscopy revealed a large mucous plug in the right main stem bronchus and this was removed; 3 hours later the right lung had completely re-expanded. The rapidity with which the right lung underwent collapse resulted from the presence within it of 100 per cent oxygen or other readily miscible anesthetic gas at the time the bronchial occlusion occurred.

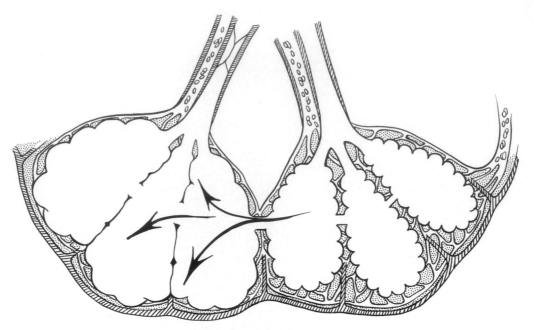

Figure 4–12. The Lung Diagram: Collateral Ventilation Associated with Air Trapping. The airway on the left is obstructed, that on the right patent; the parenchyma distal to the obstructed airway is being ventilated by collateral air drift. The diagram depicts a situation in which air enters the obstructed segment more easily than it leaves, thus resulting in air trapping.

channels was measured, Hogg and his associates[7] found the fissures between upper and lower lobes complete in only three normal lungs and one emphysematous lung. Thus collateral drift occurred between these two lobes in five of the eight normal lungs and in seven of the eight emphysematous lungs. It was shown further that air could flow through collateral channels between lobes throughout their whole volume range. These findings, based on physiologic studies, confirm the anatomic observations made by Kent and Blades in 1942[40] that the fissures rarely are complete in human lungs; they found *major* defects in interlobar fissures in 30 per cent of the lungs they dissected.

Similarly, in their study of 100 fixed and inflated lung specimens (50 right and 50 left lungs), Raasch and his colleagues[42] found considerable variation in the frequency with which the three fissures were complete. In the right lung, fusion of lung parenchyma (incomplete fissure) was found between the lower and upper lobes in 70 per cent of cases, whereas fusion between the lower and middle lobes was observed in only 47 per cent; in addition, fusion between the lower and upper lobes was commonly more extensive than between the lower and middle lobes. However, incompleteness of the minor fissure was far more common than in any portion of either major fissure: of the 50 right lungs examined, extensive fusion was present in 88 per cent of cases, especially medially; thus, fusion is more common and usually more extensive between the middle and upper lobe (across the minor fissure) than between the middle and lower lobe (across the major fissure). In the left lung, fusion between the lower and upper lobes was somewhat less frequent than on the right: 40 per cent of cases showed an incomplete fissure between the lower lobe and the superior part of the upper lobe, and 46 per cent between the lower lobe and lingula.

These observations are of obvious importance in the assessment of roentgenographic signs when an endobronchial mass in a lobar bronchus appears to occlude its lumen completely; in one of our patients a bronchial carcinoid tumor at the origin of the left lower lobe bronchus prevented passage of bronchographic contrast material, but the lower lobe was air containing although slightly reduced in volume.

If collateral air drift is such a potent force in preventing parenchymal collapse, under what circumstances does collapse occur? This depends chiefly upon the site of bronchial obstruction. If the obstruction is in a lobar bronchus, the development of atelectasis is readily explained by the absence of a parenchymal bridge from the involved lobe to a contiguous lobe; if the obstruction is in a segmental or subsegmental bronchus, collapse must be caused by some influence *preventing* collateral air drift[36]— probably inflammatory exudate. Fleischner[41] confirmed the existence of alveolar exudate in his two cases of "platelike" atelectasis.

Even excluding the effect of collateral air drift, the end result of bronchial obstruction is not necessarily a collapsed lobe. For example, "obstructive pneumonitis" may lead to consolidation severe enough to limit loss of volume (Fig. 4–13). Although the opacity that develops distal to an obstructing endobronchial lesion is often described by the term obstructive pneumonitis, it is emphasized that the pathologic counterpart is actually a combination of atelectasis, bronchiectasis with mucous plugging, and true parenchymal inflammation. In the major-

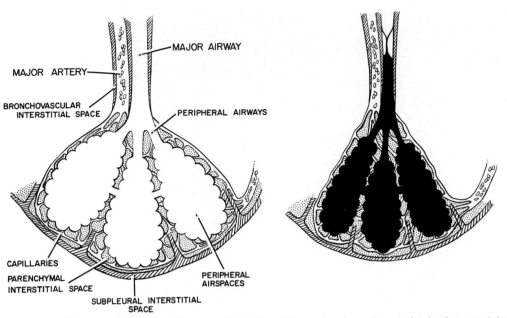

Figure 4–13. The Lung Diagram: Obstructive Pneumonitis. Although the major airway is completely obstructed, loss of volume of the peripheral air spaces is only moderate; accumulated fluid and alveolar macrophages within the air space have prevented the complete collapse depicted in Figure 4–10.

ity of cases, the inflammation is not caused by bacterial infection but by retention of normal epithelial secretions distal to the point of obstruction. Thus, in parenchyma that has been recently obstructed, the principal histologic finding is filling of alveolar air spaces by an eosinophilic proteinaceous fluid containing scattered macrophages (Fig. 4–14A); the polymorphonuclear leukocytes and necrosis that would be expected in infection are not evident. In later stages, the fluid is less conspicuous and in its place are numerous foamy macrophages (Fig. 4–14B); although there is still no evidence of an acute inflammatory cellular response, the alveolar interstitium is frequently thickened by a combination of fibrous tissue and a lymphocytic infiltrate. In longstanding cases, the interstitial fibrosis and chronic inflammation become more prominent, with a concomitant decrease in air-space consolidation. When infection does occur distal to a bronchial obstruction, it is almost always superimposed on these underlying noninfectious parenchymal changes. It is emphasized that *in most cases, it is not possible to determine whether or not infection is present from the roentgenologic findings alone.* Nevertheless, the characteristic roentgenographic picture of "obstructive pneumonitis" should immediately alert the physician to the presence of an obstructing endobronchial lesion (Fig. 4–15).

Another variable is intra-alveolar edema. Since intrapleural pressure represents the balance of forces between inward recoil of the lung and the position of the chest wall, it becomes more negative when air is resorbed and collapse results. This negative pressure is transmitted to the interstitial space of the lungs, and when of sufficient magnitude it increases hydrostatic pressure, pulling fluid from the vascular bed. In experiments on dogs in our laboratories, Stein and his colleagues[30] selectively produced atelectasis of each pulmonary lobe following a period of 100 per cent oxygen breathing; when the lobe was completely airless, the animal was sacrificed, frozen whole, and sectioned in a transverse axial or coronal plane. Planimetric volume determinations of the collapsed and contralateral lobes showed approximately 50 per cent reduction in the former; and in three animals the wet weight–dry weight ratios were $7 \pm$ in the collapsed lobes and $5 \pm$ in the normal lobes. Hemoglobin concentrations were higher in tissue from collapsed lobes than from contralateral lobes, suggesting that the increase in wet weight–dry weight ratio was probably due more to sequestration of blood (largely intravascular) than to accumulation of edema fluid. These investigators thus showed that acute bronchial obstruction rapidly renders an oxygen-filled lobe airless, not only from gas absorption but also from air replacement by edema fluid and blood drawn into the air space and interstitial compartments.

Such fluid exudation and sequestration of blood occur to some extent in all cases of acute obstructive atelectasis. Although assessment of volumetric reduction necessarily is rough, it might reasonably be estimated that 24 to 48 hours after complete bronchial occlusion in a patient breathing room air the volume of a pulmonary lobe seldom is reduced more than 50 per cent. Since a completely collapsed lung (as in total pneumothorax, for example) occupies a volume no larger than a man's fist, obviously a large amount of fluid must exude into the substance of a lobe before its volume is reduced by only 50 per cent. This accumulation of sterile edema fluid and blood behind a bronchial obstruction is euphemistically termed "drowned

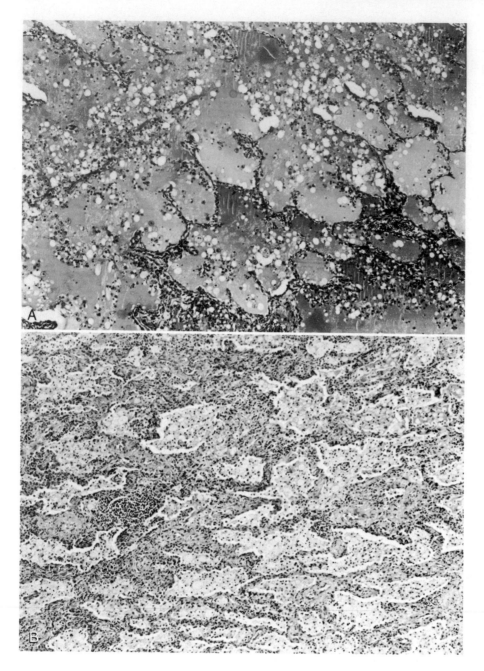

Figure 4–14. Obstructive Pneumonitis. *A*, Early obstructive pneumonitis showing alveoli filled with proteinaceous fluid and occasional macrophages. *B*, Later stage, with absence of fluid and numerous intra-alveolar foamy macrophages. Moderate interstitial fibrosis and chronic inflammation are also present.

lung" (Fig. 4–15) although the bulk of the accumulated liquid probably is blood rather than water (edema). If the obstruction persists and the obstructed lobe remains sterile, volumetric readjustment occurs within the hemithorax whereby other compensatory processes try to restore normal volume. As these other mechanisms play an increasingly important role in restoring pleural pressure to normal levels, excess edema fluid and blood within the "drowned lobe" gradually are reabsorbed, and eventually the lobe occupies the smallest possible volume. The result is chronic uncomplicated atelectasis. The collapsed lobe may be so small that it is almost invisible roentgenographically, and then the diagnostician must rely heavily on evidence of compensatory phenomena.

Resorption atelectasis may occur in the absence of occlusion of a major bronchus but cannot develop unless there is interruption of communication between alveoli and a major airway. Perhaps the best example is lower lobe bronchiectasis consequent upon childhood bronchopulmonary infection. Sufficient obliterative and stenosing bronchitis and bronchiolitis results so as to render ventilation through normal channels inadequate. Collateral ventilation may be interfered with in two ways: the pathways leading to the channels for collateral ventilation may be obliterated or narrowed, and the parenchymal disease may be sufficiently extensive to interfere with the collateral channels themselves. In this situation permanent atelectasis ensues and, together with bronchial infection, results in bron-

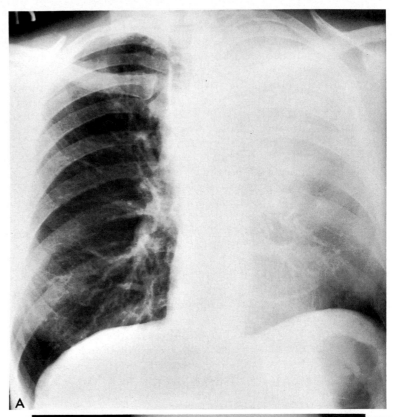

Figure 4–15. Obstructive Pneumonitis—Left Upper Lobe. Posteroanterior (*A*) and lateral (*B*) roentgenograms reveal homogeneous opacification of the left upper lobe; there is no air bronchogram. The chief fissure (*arrow*) is not displaced forward, and the only signs indicating loss of volume are slight mediastinal shift and hemidiaphragmatic elevation. Collapse was prevented by the accumulation of fluid and alveolar macrophages within distal air spaces and chronic inflammatory cells and fibrous tissue within the interstitium—obstructive pneumonitis. Squamous cell carcinoma.

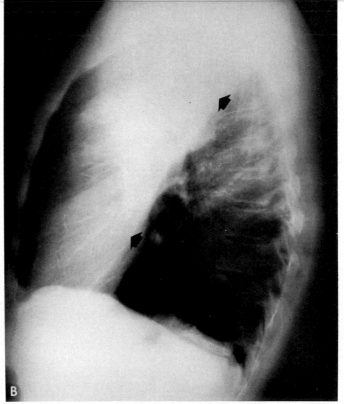

chiectasis. This, of course is an oversimplification; since the chain of events leading to irreversible bronchiectasis doubtless also would result in fibrosis, the mechanisms underlying the development of bronchiectasis relate to both resorption and cicatrization. In addition, it must be borne in mind that the results of bronchial and bronchiolar obliteration vary considerably; at the other extreme from bronchiectasis are air trapping, overinflation, and emphysema.

Thus, a wide variety of lesions may be present in resorption atelectasis caused by peripheral airway obstruction, and roentgenographic density generally is less uniform than when a major airway is obstructed. Another difference is apparent between resorption atelectasis produced by central obstruction and by peripheral obstruction. In the latter, an air bronchogram will be seen if there is sufficient parenchymal collapse, since the obstruction is peripheral to the major bronchial tree (Fig. 4–16). Resorption atelectasis due to peripheral airway disease is sometimes referred to as "nonobstructive atelectasis" because the major airways are not occluded; this term is both confusing and incorrect and is best avoided.

Resorption atelectasis may result from reversible bronchial obstruction; in such cases, when the obstruction is removed the lung reinflates—a situation illustrated by postoperative resorption atelectasis due to bronchial obstruction by a mucous plug.

In summary, it is important to recognize that *parenchymal atelectasis may be present without major bronchial obstruction*. In cases of chronic atelectasis as in bronchiectasis, the pathogenetic mechanisms are fairly well understood; when collapse is acute and temporary, as in the postoperative state, a complex group of forces appears to operate whose precise nature we do not fully comprehend but in which surfactant deficit likely plays a prominent role.

PASSIVE ATELECTASIS

This term (*synonym:* relaxation atelectasis) denotes pulmonary collapse in the presence of pneumothorax or hydrothorax (Fig. 4–17). Provided the pleural space is free (i.e., without adhesions), collapse of any portion of lung is proportional to the amount of air or fluid in the adjacent pleural space. In upright human beings, the tendency for air to pass to the upper portion of the pleural space results in a relatively greater degree of collapse of upper lobe tissue than of lower. This is particularly important when diagnostic pneumothorax is used to differentiate the intra- or extrapulmonary location of a lesion in the base of the hemithorax; separation of the base of the lung from the diaphragm requires induction of a very large pneumothorax when the patient is erect, but is achieved easily when he or she is recumbent or preferably in the Trendelenburg position. For the same reason, identification

of tiny pneumothoraces, particularly in infants, is easier with the patient in the lateral decubitus position, using a horizontal roentgen beam.

It might be thought logical that shrinkage of a lung to half its normal projected area would double roentgenologic density. That this is not so is illustrated by the difficulty commonly experienced in identifying the lung edge in any case of spontaneous pneumothorax, even of moderate degree (Fig. 4–17). As a lung shrinks under pneumothorax, its density does not increase notably until its projected area is reduced to about one-tenth its normal area at total lung capacity.[9] The probable explanation for this anomalous situation is twofold: first, the reduction in lung volume is approximately balanced by reduction in blood content, net roentgenographic density being altered only slightly; and second, air in the pleural space both anteriorly and posteriorly serves as a nonabsorbing medium, contributing to the overall radiolucency of the roentgenographic image. It is important that the physician be aware of this unusual facet of density change in the passive atelectasis of pneumothorax; it constitutes a likely diagnostic pitfall for the unwary.

The pulmonary collapse that occurs in association with total pneumothorax presents a unique opportunity for appreciating how small a volume the lung may occupy when its parenchyma is completely airless. A lung whose volume at total lung capacity approximates 3.5 liters may shrink to no larger than a man's fist (Fig. 4–18). Even when pneumothorax-induced collapse is total, however, the lung mass is not completely airless—the lobar and larger segmental bronchi are sufficiently stable structurally to resist collapse; therefore, they remain air-filled and, although reduced in caliber, should be apparent as an air bronchogram (Fig. 4–18). For obvious reasons it is essential that this sign be sought carefully in any case of total or almost total pneumothorax; absence of an air bronchogram should immediately arouse suspicion of an endobronchial obstruction.[43] It is clear that, in such circumstances, the lung will not re-expand no matter how rigorous the therapeutic maneuvers to reduce the pneumothorax; the burden is on the roentgenologist to recognize this sign so that remedial steps can be taken to remove the bronchial obstruction bronchoscopically. It should also be apparent that the response of the lung to a large pleural effusion will be similar to that of a pneumothorax of the same volume: the lung undergoes passive atelectasis which, if complete, should be associated with an identifiable air bronchogram (Fig. 4–19).

So-called "compression" or "mantle" atelectasis, formerly classified separately, differs so little from passive atelectasis that it does not warrant a separate category. The term has been used to designate parenchymal collapse contiguous to a space-occupying mass within the thorax (Fig. 4–20) and therefore local rather than general atelectasis as in pneumothorax. Any intrathoracic space-occupying

Text continued on page 487

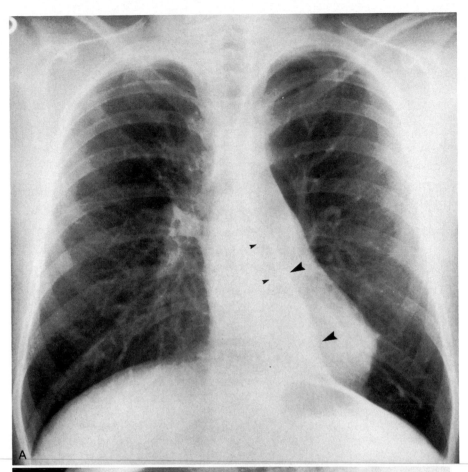

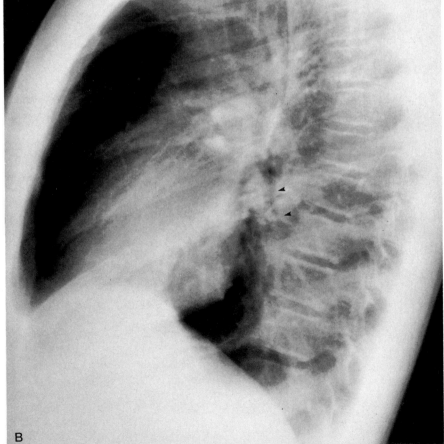

Figure 4–16. Effects of Peripheral Obstruction. Conventional posteroanterior *(A)* and lateral *(B)* chest roentgenograms disclose a triangular homogeneous opacity *(large arrowheads)* behind the heart. A faint central air bronchogram *(small arrowheads)* is present.
Illustration continued on following page

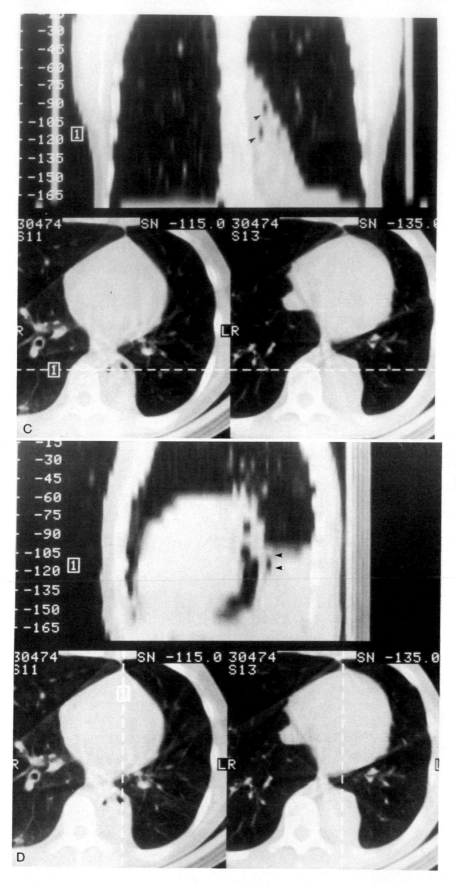

Figure 4–16 *Continued* Coronal (*C*) and sagittal (*D*) CT reformations (*top*) and representative transverse images (*bottom*) reveal the typical features of left lower lobe atelectasis caused by obstruction of multiple peripheral airways and destruction of lung parenchyma. The larger central airways (*arrowheads*) are patent. The patient is a young woman with severe bronchiectasis.

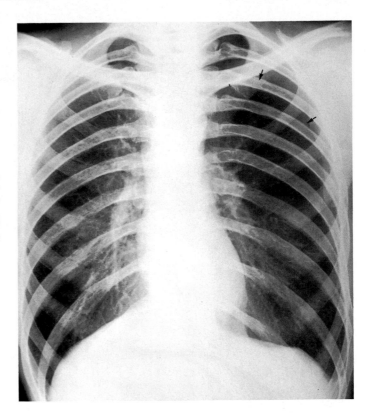

Figure 4–17. Spontaneous Pneumothorax. A posteroanterior roentgenogram reveals a small left pneumothorax (*arrows* point to the visceral pleural line). Although the left lung is partly collapsed, the left hemithorax is more radiolucent than the right. *See* text. Note increased size of left hemithorax as a result of the removal of the influence of the lung's elastic recoil on the chest wall.

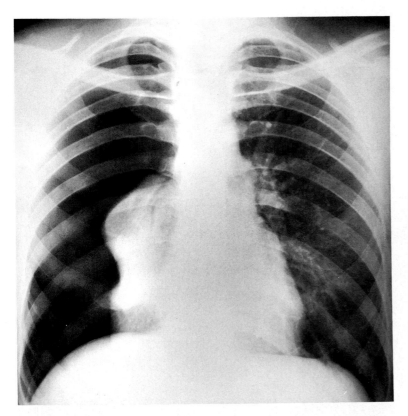

Figure 4–18. Pneumothorax with Total Pulmonary Collapse. A posteroanterior roentgenogram following spontaneous pneumothorax reveals the small volume occupied by a whole lung when totally collapsed. The well-defined air bronchogram indicates airway patency.

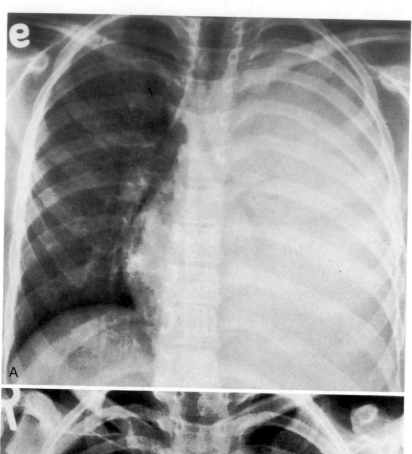

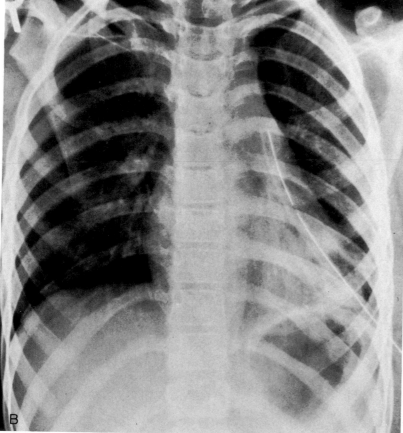

Figure 4–19. Relaxation Atelectasis in the Presence of a Massive Pleural Effusion. *A*, An air bronchogram is clearly visible within the opacity caused by a massive left pleural effusion, analogous to the atelectasis that accompanies a large pneumothorax. *B*, Shortly following the insertion of a chest tube and removal of the fluid, the lung had almost completely reinflated.

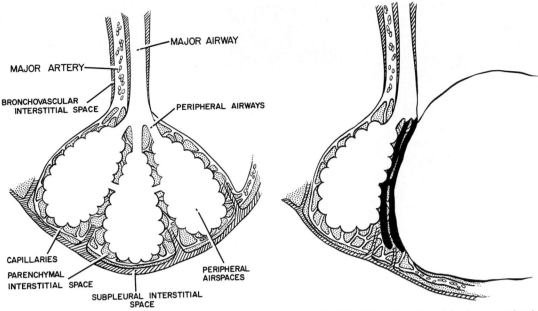

Figure 4–20. The Lung Diagram: Compression Atelectasis. A large "bulla" situated on the right has permitted relaxation of contiguous parenchyma resulting in total air-space collapse.

process—for example, a bronchogenic cyst or peripheral neoplasm—induces airlessness of a thin layer of contiguous lung parenchyma; although this could reasonably be regarded as "compression," the lung's elastic recoil properties render a concept of "relaxation" more logical. Thus we prefer to regard this process as a form of passive atelectasis.

The pathologist is accustomed to seeing a thin zone of collapsed lung adjacent to a pulmonary mass; in most cases, however, the airless lung is contiguous to tissue of identical density, and roentgenographic differentiation of the basic lesion from adjacent collapsed tissue often is impossible. Only when the loss of volume occurs contiguous to a zone of relative radiolucency, such as a bulla or bleb, is the atelectatic lung recognizable as a distinct shadow of increased density. Even then the wall of a bulla, however large, may be no more than a hairline shadow, indicating the extremely small volume of completely collapsed lung parenchyma. Generally speaking, therefore, atelectasis of this type is seldom of roentgenologic significance as a cause of increased density.

An unusual and more frequently recognized form of atelectasis has been described recently under the name *rounded or helical atelectasis.*[48, 49, 381] On conventional roentgenograms, the lesion presents as a fairly homogeneous, ill-defined, pleural-based opacity that measures up to 6 or 7 cm in diameter, most commonly although not exclusively (Fig. 4–21A) situated in the posterior portion of a lower lobe. The bronchovascular bundles in the vicinity of the mass are gathered together in a curvilinear fashion as they pass toward the mass, simulating the tail of a comet. Lateral tomography (or more precisely tomography designed to profile the lesion optimally) or bronchography shows the broncho-

vascular bundles curving toward and converging on one margin of the mass (Fig. 4–21B). Lung parenchyma below or lateral to the mass may be strikingly oligemic. The CT appearance is highly variable. As described by Doyle and Lawler,[50] the typical appearance consists of a rounded mass measuring 4 to 7 cm located subpleurally, usually in a lower lobe; the mass is densest at its periphery whereas the more central (hilar) aspect shows an air bronchogram. Contiguous pleural thickening due to fibrosis is invariably present. Hilgenberg and Mark[51] have shown that subpleural fat may be identified within the mass (Fig. 4–21C), a feature that undoubtedly reflects chronicity and therefore will not be seen in all cases; however, it is our opinion that this finding is highly suggestive of rounded atelectasis and that its presence strongly militates against other more serious conditions, such as infectious or neoplastic subpleural masses. Vessels and bronchi curve into the lesion (Fig. 4–21D), resulting in a blurred central margin, the basis for the "comet tail" sign. Lung parenchyma adjacent to the mass is hyperinflated and oligemic. Pleural invaginations can occasionally be visible as radiolucent areas within the atelectatic lung, simulating cavitation. Felson (personal communication) likened the festooned CT appearance of the vessels to an octopus and Proto (also in personal communication) to a ureteral stone basket (Fig. 4–21E). Some workers[52] believe that the roentgenographic appearances on both conventional films and CT are sufficiently characteristic that neither biopsy nor further investigative procedures are necessary to exclude more ominous disease; however, Greyson-Fleg[53] has described a patient with the typical roentgenographic features of rounded atelectasis, which on subsequent biopsy proved to be an infiltrating, poorly differentiated

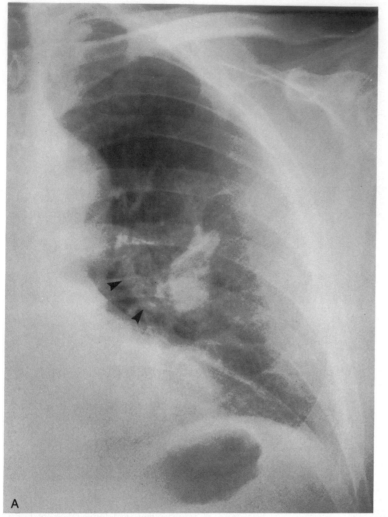

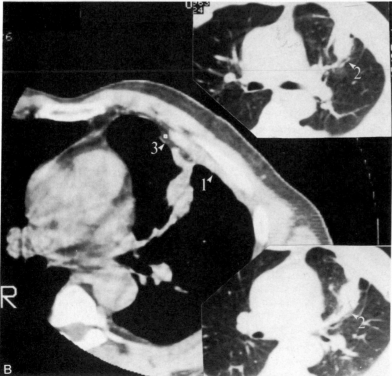

Figure 4–21. Roentgenographic Features of Round (Helical) Atelectasis. *A,* Detail view of the left lung from a conventional posteroanterior roentgenogram reveals a triangular opacity in the left upper lobe. Note the curvilinear course of pulmonary vessels (*arrowheads*) as they relate to the inferior aspect of the lesion. *B,* A CT scan shows an elongated mass in the lingula. Features that are characteristic of round atelectasis include focal pleural thickening (1), curvilinear displacement of vessels and bronchi into the mass (2, inset), and subpleural fat (3).

Illustration continued on opposite page

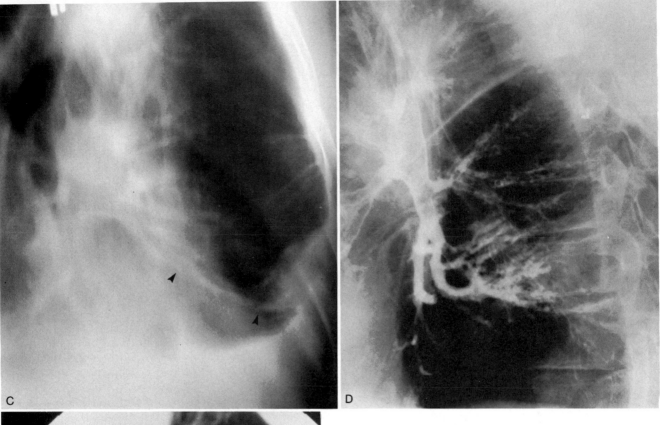

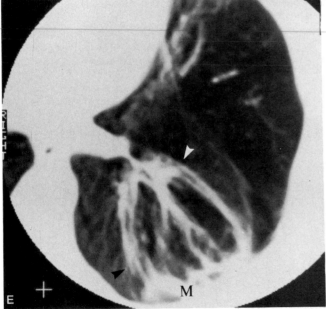

Figure 4–21 *Continued. C,* A conventional oblique tomogram shows typical curvilinear displacement of the bronchovascular bundles (*arrowheads*) as they converge on the inferior margin of the subpleural mass ("comet tail" sign). The parenchyma caudad to the mass is characteristically oligemic. *D,* In another patient, a bronchogram reveals the typical deformity of bronchovascular bundles. The parenchyma is oligemic caudally. *E,* A CT scan of the lower lobe of the patient depicted in *D* discloses multiple vessels and bronchi (*arrowheads*) displaced in a curvilinear fashion toward the mass (M). This CT appearance has been likened to the tentacles of an octopus or to a ureteral stone basket.

carcinoma (probably bronchioloalveolar cell carcinoma). It was concluded that the carcinoma probably abutted a zone of rounded atelectasis and that the benign nature of such lesions cannot always be guaranteed from their roentgenographic appearances. From a practical point of view, however, such an event must be exceptional, and careful roentgenographic follow-up rather than TTNA or thoracotomy is probably the best course of action in these patients.

The pathogenesis of this condition is uncertain. It has been hypothesized that initially a pleural effusion floats the lower lobe upward, compressing it into a finger-like projection[381, 382]; this atelectatic lung parenchyma then becomes adherent to the parietal pleural through fibrin deposition, and, as the pleural fluid recedes, the central part of the collapsed lung reinflates while the peripheral part remains atelectatic and tends to roll into a ball. We consider it more likely that the majority of cases are caused by pleural fibrosis which contracts as it develops, resulting in compression of contiguous lung parenchyma. In a number of patients on whom thoracotomy has been performed for a mistaken diagnosis of cancer, the collapsed pulmonary parenchyma has re-expanded following the decortication of the region of pleural fibrosis; as a consequence, it is reasonable to regard this form of atelectasis as the passive or relaxation type.

ADHESIVE ATELECTASIS

This term describes alveolar collapse in the presence of patent airway connections and, thus, is true "nonobstructive" atelectasis. The condition is controversial and poorly understood. The best examples are the respiratory distress syndrome of newborn infants and acute radiation pneumonitis (Fig. 4–22). In both conditions atelectasis may be a prominent feature and may be related, at least in part, to an inactivation or absence of surfactant. Clements[44] showed that surfactant reduces the surface tension of an alveolus as its surface area or volume decreases. In other words, it protects against collapse in that the critical closing pressure of alveoli occurs at a lower volume and distending pressure. Absence of surfactant has been reported in studies of atelectatic lungs, with[45] and without[46] associated pneumonia. In many conditions in which hyaline membranes form within the alveoli—for example, acute radiation pneumonitis, influenza, rheumatic fever, and uremia—the conversion of plasminogen into the fibrinolytic enzyme plasmin may be interrupted; similarly, inhibition of plasminogen activator is the presumed cause of atelectasis in hyaline membrane disease of neonates.[47]

It is likely that adhesive ("nonobstuctive") atelectasis also plays a part in loss of volume postoperatively and accounts for the marked arteriovenous shunting that may occur even when chest roentgenograms are relatively normal.

The frequency with which patients who have undergone cardiac bypass surgery develop a left lower lobe opacity in the postoperative period is truly astounding and to the best of our knowledge has never been adequately explained; the opacity is characteristically homogeneous except for an air bronchogram that is invariably present. Although signs of atelectasis are seldom convincing, partly as a result of the technical quality of the examination (AP projection, supine position at the patient's bedside), we have assumed that the combination of airlessness of the lower lobe and an air bronchogram indicates that "nonobstructive" atelectasis is the likely morphology and that surfactant deficit is the probable etiology. Characteristically, patients do not manifest signs or symptoms of acute pneumonia, thus more or less excluding that diagnosis. Beckmann and his colleagues[54] have suggested that a common cause of nonuniform pulmonary artery perfusion on pulmonary angiograms is compression of the left lower lobe arteries by an enlarged heart, an effect that is accentuated by gravity in the supine position. Although their article refers specifically to a false diagnosis of pulmonary embolism that might occur as a result of such compression, we wonder

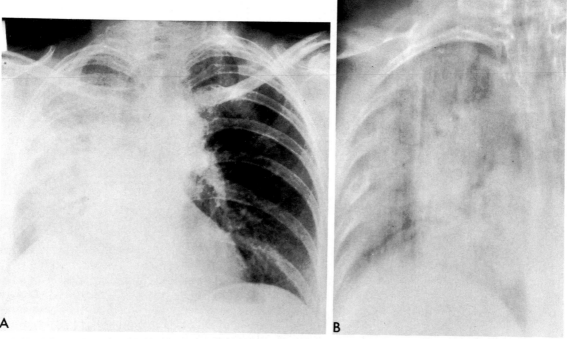

Figure 4–22. Adhesive Atelectasis in Acute Radiation Pneumonitis. *A*, A posteroanterior roentgenogram reveals severe loss of volume of the right lung associated with marked mediastinal shift and hemidiaphragmatic elevation; the density is rather granular (the oblique shadow across the left upper lung is an artifact). A well-defined air bronchogram (seen to better advantage on the anteroposterior tomogram—*B*) indicates major airway patency.

whether the same mechanism might not be operative in the pathogenesis of adhesive atelectasis postoperatively; since pulmonary artery perfusion is necessary for the production of surfactant by alveolar type II cells, hypoperfusion could conceivably result in surfactant deficit.

A Detroit group[55] undertook a retrospective and prospective analysis of chest roentgenograms of patients following coronary artery bypass surgery, particularly with reference to the effects of topical cooling of the heart with ice on the incidence of left lower lobe abnormality during the postoperative period: of 40 patients who were operated upon without topical cooling, 13 (32.5 per cent) developed a left lower lobe opacity; by contrast, of 162 patients who were operated upon with ice cooling of the heart, 111 (69 per cent) developed a left lower lobe opacity. The investigators attribute this increased incidence to the effect of ice cooling on the phrenic nerve, the result being paresis or actual paralysis of the left hemidiaphragm and resultant left lower lobe abnormality, presumably as a result of retained secretions. Although the difference in the incidence of left lower lobe abnormality in the two groups is highly significant, we are not at all convinced that altered diaphragmatic motion would result in the extensive lower lobe opacity usually observed; in addition, the elevation of the left hemidiaphragm that would be a necessary concomitant of paralysis is seldom if ever a notable finding in these patients. As a result, we continue to regard the abnormality as a form of adhesive atelectasis.

Various other pathologic processes occur concomitantly with adhesive atelectasis. These may be related to the causal agent, such as congestion, edema, or hemorrhage, or to the hyaline membrane that forms in cases of radiation pneumonitis. Edema is sometimes a prominent feature of the respiratory distress syndrome. Thus, the roentgenographic density of affected lung may be greater than anticipated from reduction in lung volume alone. Since the process is peripheral, an air bronchogram will be present (Fig. 4–23).

CICATRIZATION ATELECTASIS

Some may object to the inclusion of loss of lung volume caused by fibrosis as a type of atelectasis, but we believe this entity is best described here. Further, diffuse idiopathic pulmonary fibrosis is best considered as a diffuse collapse of air spaces with proximal bronchiolectasis. Thus, cicatrization is a useful concept, although we readily admit that multifarious factors affect lung volume in most examples of this condition. The pathologic process is one of fibrosis with resultant cicatrization; the former may or may not be associated with parenchymal destruction, but in either event it results in loss of volume of the affected portion of lung. Not only is air per unit lung volume decreased, but, also, tissue per unit lung volume is increased, thus increasing roentgenographic density. The roentgenologic signs depend upon whether the process is local or general.

Localized disease is best exemplified by chronic

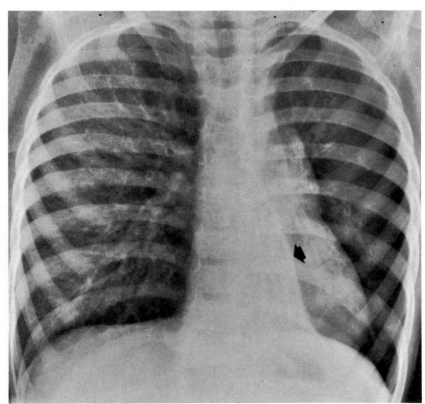

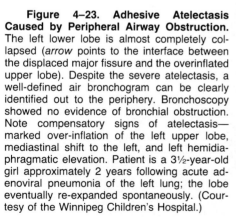

Figure 4–23. Adhesive Atelectasis Caused by Peripheral Airway Obstruction. The left lower lobe is almost completely collapsed (*arrow* points to the interface between the displaced major fissure and the overinflated upper lobe). Despite the severe atelectasis, a well-defined air bronchogram can be clearly identified out to the periphery. Bronchoscopy showed no evidence of bronchial obstruction. Note compensatory signs of atelectasis—marked over-inflation of the left upper lobe, mediastinal shift to the left, and left hemidiaphragmatic elevation. Patient is a 3½-year-old girl approximately 2 years following acute adenoviral pneumonia of the left lung; the lobe eventually re-expanded spontaneously. (Courtesy of the Winnipeg Children's Hospital.)

infection, often granulomatous in nature, and epitomized by longstanding fibrocaseous tuberculosis. In essence, it is a chronic "nonobstructive" atelectasis in which the destruction of lung parenchyma is followed by fibrosis and progressive loss of volume through cicatrization (Fig. 4–24). The peripheral bronchi and bronchioles are usually destroyed along with the parenchyma, so that resorption atelectasis also occurs; the more proximal bronchi become dilated, so that the morphologic picture is one of chronic bronchiectasis and parenchymal scarring. The roentgenologic signs are as might be expected (Fig. 4–25): a segment or lobe occupying a volume smaller than normal, with a density rendered inhomogeneous by dilated, air-containing bronchi (often better demonstrated by tomography), and with irregular thickened strands extending from the collapsed segment to the hilum. The compensatory signs of chronic loss of volume are usually evident: local mediastinal shift, frequently manifested by a sharp deviation of the trachea when segments of the upper lobe are involved, displacement of the hilum (which may be severe in upper lobe disease), and compensatory overinflation of the remainder of the affected lung. The loss of volume may be so severe as to render the collapsed lung almost invisible on standard posteroanterior chest roentgenograms, particularly if involvement of apical or apical-posterior segments of an upper lobe results in incorporation of the shadow of the collapsed lung into that of the mediastinum; in such circumstances, the diagnostician must rely on compensatory signs of pulmonary collapse.

Generalized fibrotic disease of the lungs also may be associated with loss of volume (Fig. 4–26). In chronic interstitial pulmonary fibrosis, for example, involvement of the interstitial space results in widespread reduction in the volume of air-containing parenchyma (Fig. 4–27); this may be evidenced roentgenologically by elevation of the diaphragm and overall reduction in lung size. In our experience, this gradual reduction in thoracic volume in cases of diffuse interstitial disease is a useful indicator of the fibrotic nature of the pathologic process (Fig. 4–28).

Other diseases associated with pulmonary fibrosis may produce entirely different roentgenographic patterns (Fig. 4–29). For example, the fibrotic stage of pulmonary sarcoidosis may be accompanied by severe compensatory overinflation or even emphysema, while the end-stage lung of eosinophilic granuloma is frequently accompanied by a picture of pulmonary overinflation. Similarly, in silicosis, conglomerate masses in upper lung zones, caused by the coalescence of individual fibrotic lesions, induce severe overinflation in the lower zones (Fig. 4–30).

In summary, atelectasis may occur by means of four mechanisms which, in any given situation, may operate independently or in combination.

1. *Resorption atelectasis* occurs when communications between the trachea and alveoli are obstructed; the obstruction may be in a major bronchus or in multiple small bronchi or bronchioles.

2. *Passive (relaxation) atelectasis* denotes loss of volume accompanying an intrathoracic space-occupying process, particularly pneumothorax or hydrothorax. Atelectasis contiguous to a local space-occupying process such as a pulmonary mass or bulla is of the same nature and does not warrant the separate designation of compression atelectasis.

3. *Adhesive atelectasis* (nonobstructive or microatelectasis) is related to a complex group of forces, of which abnormality of surfactant is probably the

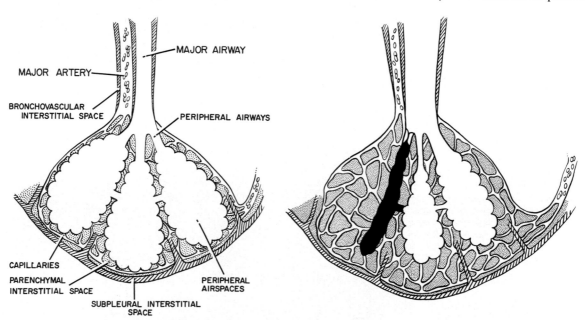

Figure 4–24. The Lung Diagram: Local Cicatrization Atelectasis. The interstitial space is increased in amount and density (fibrosis). The left air space is totally obliterated while those to the right show different degrees of loss of volume. The major airway is dilated (bronchiectasis), as is the peripheral airway on the right (bronchiolectasis).

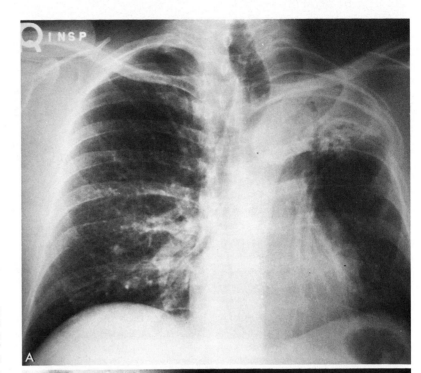

Figure 4–25. Local Cicatrization Atelectasis: Postirradiation Fibrosis. One and one-half years previously, this 48-year-old man was found to have inoperable squamous cell carcinoma of the left upper lobe, for which he had received an intensive course of cobalt therapy. *A*, A posteroanterior roentgenogram reveals considerable loss of volume of the left upper lung, with displacement of the trachea to the left, approximation of the left upper ribs, and elevation of the left hilum. *B*, A magnified view shows a prominent air bronchogram in an otherwise homogeneous opacity.

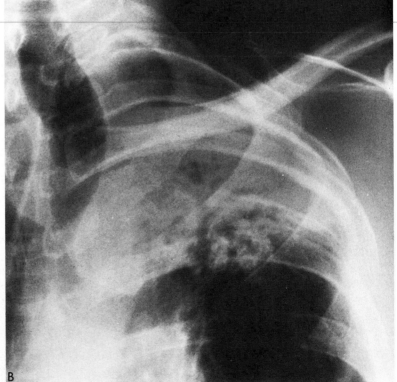

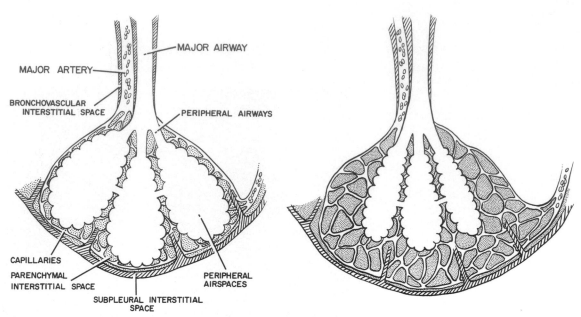

Figure 4–26. The Lung Diagram: General Cicatrization Atelectasis. There is a marked increase in interstitial tissue with uniform reduction in the volume of all air spaces as a result of cicatrization. The dilatation of the major airway seen in local cicatrization atelectasis is not a prominent part of the picture, although peripheral airway dilatation may occur.

most common. As with passive and cicatrization atelectasis, this form of collapse is associated with patent large airway communications.

4. *Cicatrization atelectasis* designates volume loss resulting from local or general pulmonary fibrosis.

ROENTGENOLOGIC SIGNS OF ATELECTASIS

The roentgenologic signs of atelectasis may be both *direct* and *indirect*, the latter consisting chiefly of compensatory phenomena.

DIRECT SIGNS

Displacement of Interlobar Fissures. We define atelectasis simply as loss of lung volume. Accordingly, the only *direct* sign is *displacement of interlobar fissures*. Although local increase in density is a common manifestation of pulmonary atelectasis, it is not essential to the definition and therefore cannot be construed as a direct sign. In addition, displacement of the fissures that form the boundary of a collapsed lobe is one of the most dependable and easily recognized signs of atelectasis (Fig. 4–31). For each lobe, the position and configuration of the displaced fissures are predictable for a given loss of volume; these factors are considered later in relation to patterns of lobar and segmental collapse.

INDIRECT SIGNS

Local Increase in Density. This is undoubtedly the most important indirect sign of atelectasis and is caused by airless lung. The volume of an airless

lobe or segment depends not only upon which order of bronchus is obstructed, but also upon the amount of sequestered blood and edema fluid, either sterile or infected, within the obstructed parenchyma.

The chief indirect roentgenologic signs of atelectasis, other than local opacity, are those processes that compensate for the reduction in intrapleural pressure—diaphragmatic elevation, mediastinal shift, approximation of ribs, and overinflation of the remainder of the lung (Fig. 4–32). The part played by each compensatory mechanism in any given situation is somewhat unpredictable, although predominance is dictated largely by the anatomic position of the collapsed lobe; all four mechanisms may operate fairly equally, or one or two may predominate to the exclusion of others. Two general rules deserve emphasis. (1) Displacement of the diaphragm and mediastinum is maximal contiguous to the major collapse; for example, lower lobe collapse tends to elevate the posterior more than the anterior portion of the hemidiaphragm and to displace the inferior more than the superior mediastinum. Conversely, upper lobe collapse is associated with upper mediastinal displacement, often with little hemidiaphragmatic elevation. (2) The more acute the atelectasis, the greater the predominance of diaphragmatic and mediastinal displacement (Fig. 4–32); the more chronic the collapse, the more will compensatory overinflation predominate (Fig. 4–31).

Until recently it has been inferred that the visceral pleura covering a collapsed lobe remains intimately related to the parietal pleura no matter how complete the collapse. The study by Stein and his colleagues[30] confirmed maintenance of the relationship in the presence of acute lobar collapse,

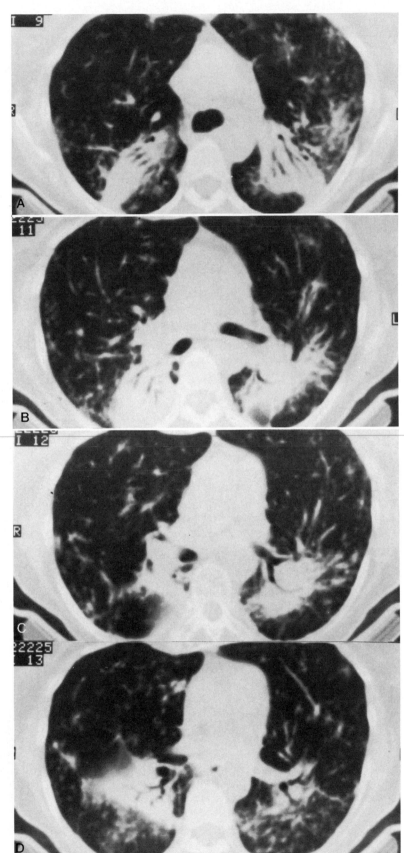

Figure 4–27. Chronic Interstitial Pulmonary Fibrosis Associated with Reduction in Lung Volume. Sequential transverse CT scan (*A* to *D*) reveal broad areas of parenchymal consolidation in the perihilar regions of the upper and lower lobes bilaterally. A prominent air bronchogram is present. The hila are elevated and displaced posteriorly by the fibrotic process. The distribution and characteristics of the parenchymal consolidation are typical of Stage IV sarcoidosis. Middle-aged woman.

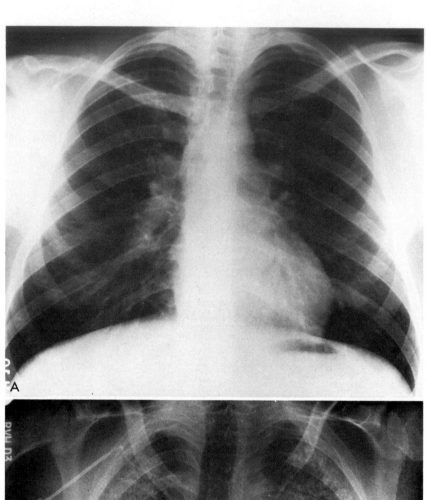

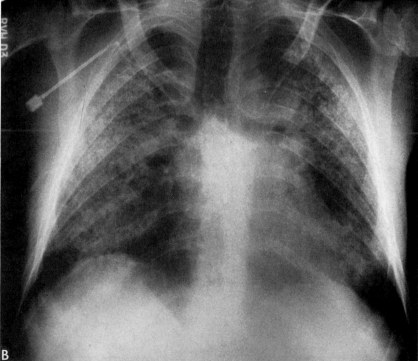

Figure 4–28. General Cicatrization Atelectasis Secondary to Talcosis in a Heroin Addict. At the time of the normal chest roentgenogram illustrated in A, this 19-year-old white man had been taking drugs (both heroin and methadone) intravenously for over 2 years. Six years later, a roentgenogram (B) reveals diffuse interstitial disease throughout both lungs associated with severe loss of lung volume as evidenced by elevation of the diaphragm and smallness of the thoracic cage. This represents diffuse interstitial fibrosis caused by intravenously injected talc.

but it is now known from CT studies that the visceral pleural surface can sometimes retract inward from the parietal pleura toward the hilum (*see further on*).

Elevation of the Hemidiaphragm. As already stated, hemidiaphragmatic elevation is always a more prominent feature of lower than of upper lobe collapse (compare Figure 4–32*A* and *B*). In the lower lung zones, elevation tends to occur in the area contiguous to the lobe involved—posterior elevation in lower lobe collapse and anterior elevation in middle lobe or lingular collapse (although, in the latter two situations, diaphragmatic displacement is seldom severe). When assessing diaphragmatic elevation, one should take into consideration possible variations in the relationship of the two hemidiaphragms. Although the right dome normally is approximately half an interspace higher than the left, Felson,[21] who reviewed the chest roentgenograms of 500 normal subjects, recorded a deviation from the normal relationship in 11 per cent: in 9 per cent, the two were level or the left was higher than the right, and in 2 per cent the right hemidiaphragm was more than 3 cm higher than the left. When attaching significance to diaphragmatic elevation, the influence of subphrenic disease must not be disregarded; although atelectasis secondary to airway obstruction is a common complication during the postoperative period after laparotomy, it should be borne in mind that diaphragmatic elevation may result directly from "splinting" secondary to abdominal pain or subphrenic infection.

Mediastinal Displacement. The normal mediastinum is a surprisingly mobile structure and reacts promptly to differences in pressure between the two halves of the thorax (Fig. 4–32). The anterior and middle mediastinal compartments are less stable than the posterior and, therefore, shift to a greater extent. The degree of shift is usually greatest in the region of major pulmonary collapse; thus tracheal and upper mediastinal displacement is a feature of upper lobe collapse and may be negligible when the lower lobes are involved; in the latter instance, the inferior mediastinum undergoes the greatest displacement. (However, Kattan and his coworkers[56] have drawn attention to a triangular opacity sometimes apparent in the right superior paramediastinal zone in cases of atelectasis of the right lower lobe, which they attribute to the displacement of the upper anterior mediastinum to the right. We also have noted similar displacement of the anterior mediastinal triangle and line to the *left* in some patients with left lower lobe atelectasis.) As with the diaphragm, normal variations in configuration of the mediastinum should be recognized; this is less of a problem with the trachea and upper mediastinum than with the heart, since the trachea is consistently a midline structure. The amount of cardiac silhouette that projects to the right of the spine varies in normal subjects, however, and a central position of the heart does not necessarily indicate displacement.

Compensatory Overinflation. Overinflation of the remainder of the ipsilateral lung is one of the most important and reliable indirect signs of atelectasis (Fig. 4–31). It seldom occurs rapidly and, in the early stages of lobar collapse, usually is of less diagnostic help than the other compensatory phenomena, such as diaphragmatic elevation and mediastinal displacement. As the period of collapse

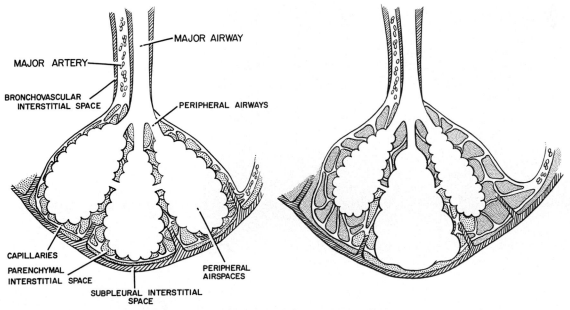

Figure 4–29. The Lung Diagram: Cicatricial Atelectasis with Compensatory Overinflation. The interstitial tissue around the left and right air spaces is increased in amount and density, resulting in loss of volume of the air spaces. The central air space is surrounded by normal interstitial tissue and has overinflated to compensate for adjacent loss of volume.

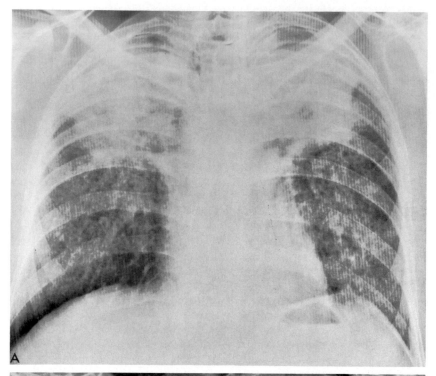

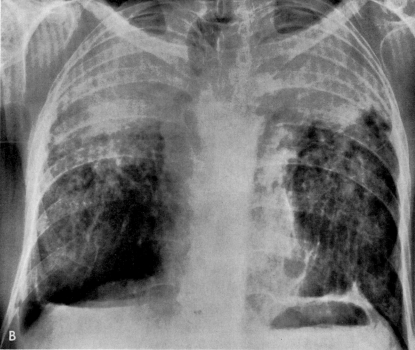

Figure 4–30. Cicatrization Atelectasis with Compensatory Overinflation. *A,* A posteroanterior roentgenogram shows massive consolidation of both upper lobes associated with a diffuse nodular pattern throughout the lower half of both lungs. Proved silicosis with advanced conglomeration (progressive massive fibrosis). *B,* Two years later, the conglomerate shadows have increased in size while the nodular pattern in the lower lungs has diminished markedly in extent and in some areas has virtually disappeared. The silicotic nodules have become incorporated into the conglomerate shadows, leaving behind markedly overinflated parenchyma.

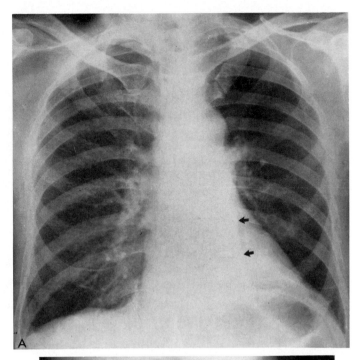

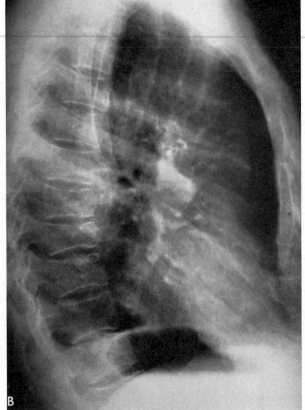

Figure 4–31. Atelectasis of the Left Lower Lobe. *A,* A posteroanterior roentgenogram shows a triangular shadow of homogeneous density in the inferomedial portion of the left hemithorax. Its lateral margin (*arrows*) represents the interface between the collapsed left lower lobe and overinflated left upper lobe. Indirect signs of atelectasis include increased radiolucency of the left upper lobe compared with the right upper lobe, redistribution of vascular markings, and elevation of the left hemidiaphragm. The mediastinum shows little or no shift. *B,* In lateral projection, the shadow is barely visible as an area of increased density situated in the posterior costophrenic sulcus, but its presence is indicated by the loss of visibility of the posterior portion of the left hemidiaphragm (the silhouette sign).

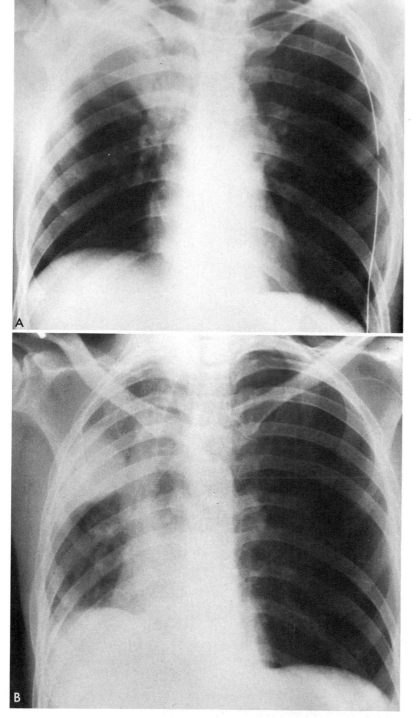

Figure 4–32. Roentgenologic Signs of Atelectasis. *A,* A roentgenogram of the chest in anteroposterior projection, supine position, reveals a homogeneous shadow in the upper portion of the right hemithorax; its concave lower margin is formed by the upward displaced horizontal fissure; the right hemidiaphragm is slightly elevated. Atelectasis of the right upper lobe (24 hours postoperative for the thoracoabdominal repair of hiatus hernia). *B,* Twenty-four hours later, the right upper lobe collapse is clearing, but the diaphragmatic elevation has increased and the mediastinum has shifted markedly to the right; note the approximation of ribs. These signs indicate acute obstruction of the right intermediate bronchus with progressing collapse of the middle and lower lobes, undoubtedly caused by a mucous plug displaced from the upper lobe bronchus.

Illustration continued on opposite page

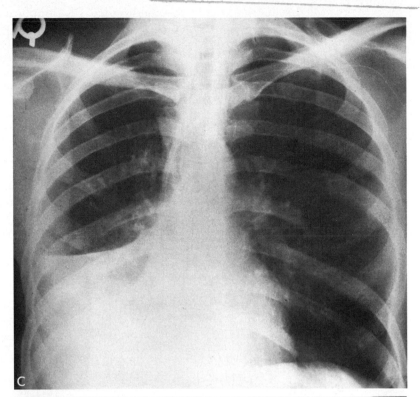

Figure 4–32 *Continued.* Twenty-four hours later, PA (*C*) and lateral (*D*) views reveal the right middle and lower lobes to be virtually airless; the right upper lobe has completely re-expanded. The roughly horizontal interface in *C* is the major fissure, not the minor as might intuitively be thought: in the lateral projection, note that the upper portion of the major fissure has swung downward to a roughly horizontal position (*arrows*), thus making it tangential to the x-ray beam and creating the sharp interface in PA projection. Following this examination, a mucous plug was removed from the intermediate bronchus bronchoscopically.

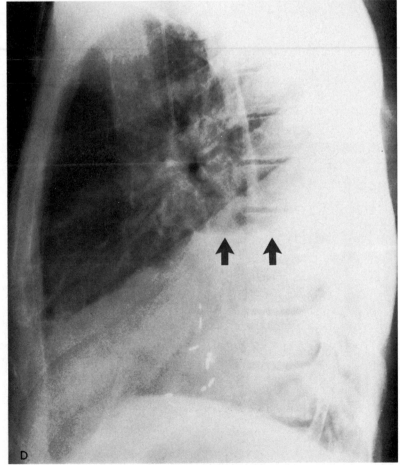

lengthens, however, overinflation becomes more prominent and the diaphragmatic and mediastinal changes regress. The degree to which the lung can be overinflated without its functional capabilities being significantly affected is truly remarkable. In one of our patients, a young woman whose entire left lung and right lower and middle lobes were removed because of severe bronchiectasis, the remaining right upper lobe overinflated and filled the whole thorax (Fig. 4–33); her pulmonary function, though obviously impaired, was approximately what might be predicted for one fifth the normal complement of pulmonary tissue.

Roentgenologic evidence of compensatory overinflation may be extremely subtle. It may be difficult to estimate the increase in lung translucency resulting from the greater air-blood ratio, but appreciation may be enhanced by viewing the roent-genogram from a distance of several feet or through minification lenses. Clearly, more reliable evidence for overinflation is supplied by the *alteration in vascular markings* resultant upon the increased lung volume (Fig. 4–31);[57] the vessels are more widely spaced and sparser than in the normal contralateral lung. As emphasized by Simon,[58] appreciation of vascular redistribution may be facilitated by full lung tomography. The densitometric capabilities combined with the transverse display of the pulmonary vessels make CT an ideal examination technique for the combined detection of increased lung translucency and the vascular spatial redistribution phenomenon.

When only a relatively small volume of one lung is collapsed, compensatory overinflation is usually restricted to the remainder of that lung, at least insofar as is apparent roentgraphically. When

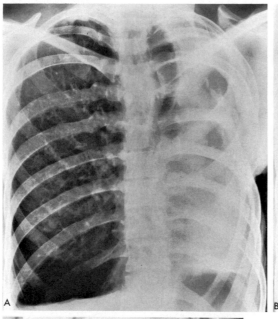

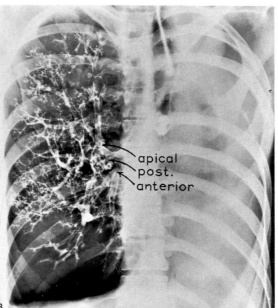

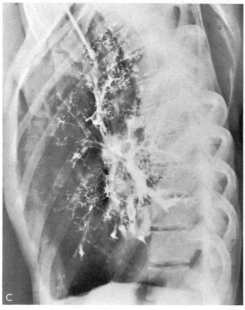

Figure 4–33. Compensatory Overinflation: The One-lobe Thorax. Over a span of several years, thoracotomy was performed on this 28-year-old woman on three different occasions for advanced incapacitating bronchiectasis: on the first, the left lower lobe and lingula were removed; on the second, the left upper lobe; and on the third, the right middle and lower lobes. At the time of each thoracotomy, the bronchial tree was found to be normal bronchographically in those areas subsequently affected. A right bronchogram (*B* and *C*) reveals only three segmental bronchi of the right upper lobe, at least one of which shows moderately advanced bronchiectasis. *See* text.

greater amounts of one lung become atelectatic, the tendency is greater for overinflation to involve the contralateral lung; this may progress to the stage in which the opposite lung displaces the mediastinum either generally or locally. These local displacements occur in the three weakest areas of the mediastinum, where the two lungs are separated only by loose connective tissue:[59] (1) the anterior mediastinal compartment, at the level of the first three or four costal cartilages, limited anteriorly by the sternum and posteriorly by the great vessels; (2) the posterosuperior mediastinum, at the level of the third to fifth thoracic vertebrae, limited anteriorly by the esophagus and trachea and posteriorly by the vertebral column (the supra-aortic triangle); and (3) the posteroinferior mediastinum, limited anteriorly by the heart and posteriorly by the vertebral column and aorta (the retrocardiac space, or space of Holzknecht). Roentgenologic appreciation of anterior mediastinal displacement is usually easy, through identification of the displaced anterior junction line; the curvilinear opacity of the apposed pleural surfaces is usually visible on a posteroanterior roentgenogram, protruding into the involved hemithorax; in lateral projection the anterior mediastinum appears exceptionally radiolucent and increased in depth. Appreciation of displacement of the posterior mediastinal weak areas may be more difficult; these portions of the mediastinal septum normally form the posterior junction line and azygoesophageal recess interface, and recognition of their displacement to one side may be facilitated by overpenetrated sagittal projections, tomography, or opacification of the esophagus with barium.

The term "mediastinal herniation" commonly is used to refer to mediastinal displacement by overinflated lung compensating for atelectasis of the whole or part of the contralateral lung. We dislike the term "herniation" in this context, since it is defined as displacement of a viscus from one chamber into another through a defect or hiatus in the intervening septum. In this condition the mediastinum is intact: the effects that collapse and compensatory overinflation have on this structure constitute displacement, either local or general, and should be differentiated from herniation.[59]

An interesting although very uncommon sign of atelectasis is the "shifting granuloma":[375] a pulmonary nodule whose position shifts from one examination to another is almost certainly related to loss of volume of either the lobe in which the nodule is situated or in a contiguous lobe; it thus represents an internal marker of atelecteasis. Of a similar nature is the nodule or mass that disappears from one examination to another as a result of being surrounded by airless lung in an atelectatic lobe (Fig. 4–34).

When an entire lung becomes atelectatic consequent upon obstruction of a main bronchus, the resultant loss of volume of the hemithorax must be compensated for largely by overinflation of the contralateral lung (similar to the situation after pneumonectomy) (Fig. 4–33). The mediastinal shift may be large; since the mediastinum is less stable anteriorly than elsewhere, the anterior septum is rotated laterally and posteriorly, the normal lung overinflating to such an extent that it occupies the whole anterior portion of the thorax. Thus the heart and the collapsed lung are displaced into the posterior portion of the ipsilateral hemithorax. In such circumstances the roentgenologic appearance in lateral projection is distinctive.[60] Depth and radiolucency of the retrosternal air space are increased, the heart and great vessels are displaced posteriorly, and there is a general increase in density posteroinferiorly (Fig. 4–33); the margin of the collapsed lung may be sharply delineated where it comes in contact with the opposite overinflated lung. As emphasized by Lubert and Krause,[60] such an appearance enhances differentiation of massive collapse from massive unilateral pneumonic consolidation or pleural effusion (Fig. 4–35).

Displacement of the Hila. The hila are often involved in the redistribution of anatomic structures within the thorax in the presence of atelectasis, and such displacement constitutes an invaluable sign. It occurs more predictably in collapse of the upper than of the lower lobes and usually is more marked the more chronic the atelectasis (for example, chronic scarring of the upper lobes as a result of tuberculosis commonly engenders severe upward displacement of the ipsilateral hilum—Fig. 4–36). Downward displacement of the hila, in cases of lower lobe atelectasis, is seldom so clearly appreciated. Downward displacement of only the left hilum, however, is more readily apparent, particularly if it brings the left hilum level with the right—an almost invariably significant sign, seen in only 3 per cent of normal subjects.[21] Whalen and Lane[61] have stressed the importance of assessing the position of the air columns of the trachea and major bronchi in lateral projection as an indication of collapse. They point out that on a well-aligned lateral roentgenogram of the chest, the trachea, both main bronchi, and both upper lobe bronchi are in vertical alignment, and that any alteration in this relationship should be considered abnormal. Since the upper lobes are situated mainly anteriorly, atelectasis of these lobes will displace their respective main bronchi forward; similarly, with atelectatic lower lobes, the posterior position of these lobes will displace their major bronchi backward (Fig. 4–37). We have seen this sign repeatedly in cases of lower lobe collapse but seldom very clearly when the upper lobes are affected. Posterior displacement of the left upper lobe bronchus also may result from distention of the left superior pulmonary vein (Fig. 4–38) in cases of left atrial and pulmonary venous hypertension,[62] and occasionally from a prominent but normal common left pulmonary venous confluence; it is of obvious importance to

Text continued on page 511

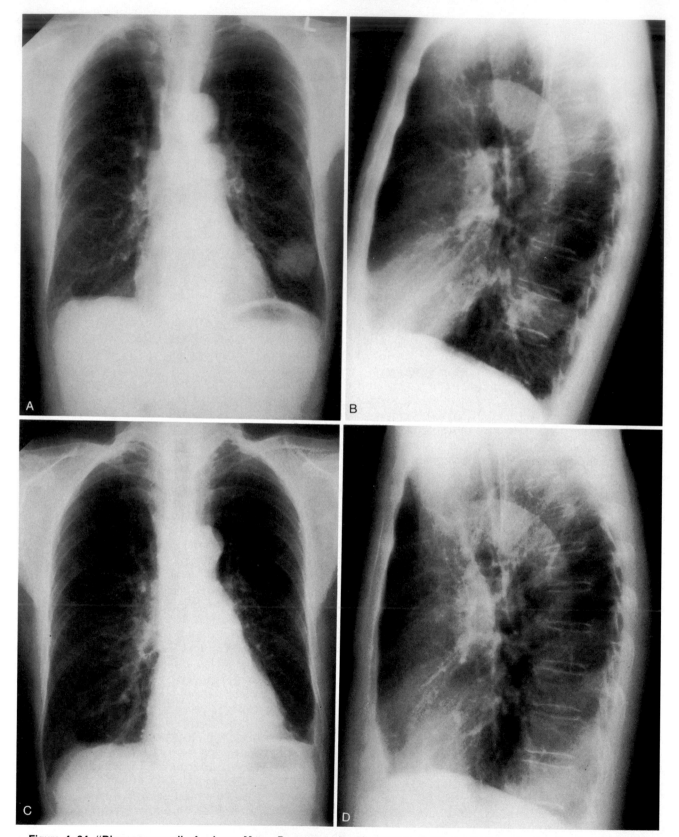

Figure 4–34. "Disappearance" of a Lung Mass. Posteroanterior (A) and lateral (B) roentgenograms reveal a 5 cm mass in the posterior portion of the left lower lobe. Several days later, similar projections (C and D) show the mass to have disappeared. In the interval, the left lower lobe has undergone total atelectasis as a result of bronchial compression by metastatic lymph nodes, and the mass has become invisible because of surrounding airless parenchyma.

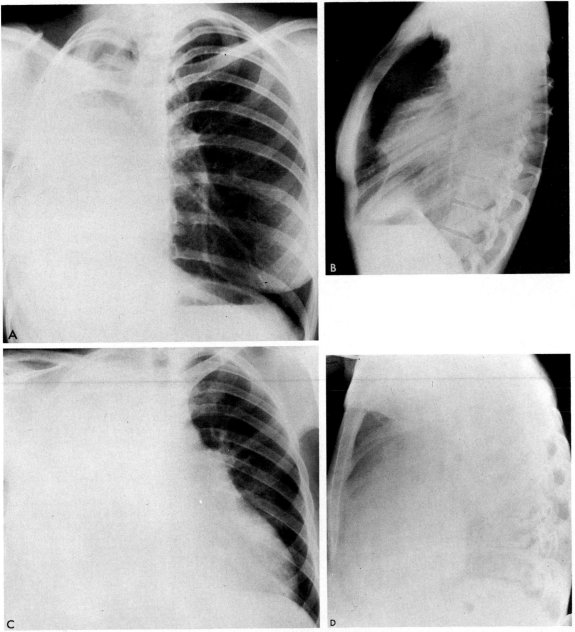

Figure 4–35. Comparison of Massive Collapse and Massive Pleural Effusion. Roentgenograms of the chest in posteroanterior and lateral projections (*A* and *B*) of a patient whose right lung has been removed (analogous to total right pulmonary collapse) reveals marked shift of the mediastinum into the posterior portion of the right hemithorax, with herniation of the overinflated left lung across the midline into the anterior right chest (note the clear retrosternal space). In *C* and *D* (roentgenograms of another patient), a massive right pleural effusion has resulted in a shift of the mediastinum to the left; in lateral projection opacity of the thorax is more or less homogeneous (the uniform filter effect). Compare the appearance of the retrosternal space in the two patients.

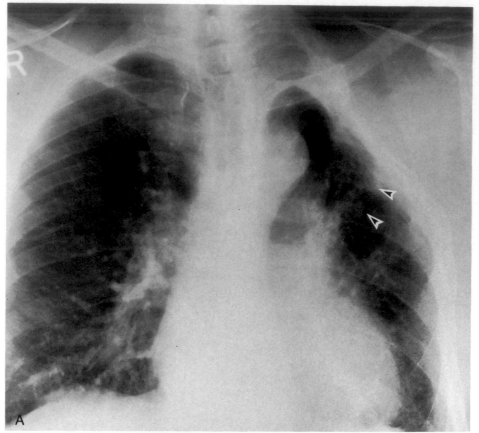

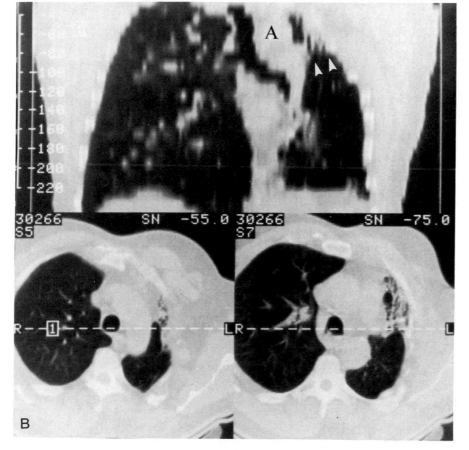

Figure 4–36. Unilateral Hilar Elevation Caused by Chronic Left Upper Lobe Fibrosis. *A,* Posteroanterior chest roentgenogram of a 50-year-old man with prior tuberculosis and thoracoplasty discloses an elevated and outwardly displaced left hilum. An inhomogeneous opacity containing an air bronchogram (*arrowheads*) extends from the hilum to the left rib deformity. The features are consistent with severe left upper lobe atelectasis and bronchiectasis caused by tuberculosis. Note the para-aortic radiolucency caused by the superior segment of the lower lobe intruding between and separating the atelectatic lobe and the arch of the aorta (the Luftsichel). Coronal (*B*) and sagittal (*C*) CT reformations (*top*) with transverse images (*bottom*) show severe left upper atelectasis (*arrowheads*) due to bronchiectasis. (*A* indicates the aortic arch.) *D,* Transverse CT scans show the dilated bronchi (*arrowheads*) within the collapsed lobe. Note that the over-expanded superior segment of the lower lobe has insinuated itself between the atelectatic lobe and the aortic arch (*white arrowhead*), accounting for the features described in *A.* The peaked appearance of the atelectasis posteriorly is possibly attributable to fusion (incompleteness) of the fissure between the upper and lower lobe (*large arrowhead*).

Illustration continued on opposite page

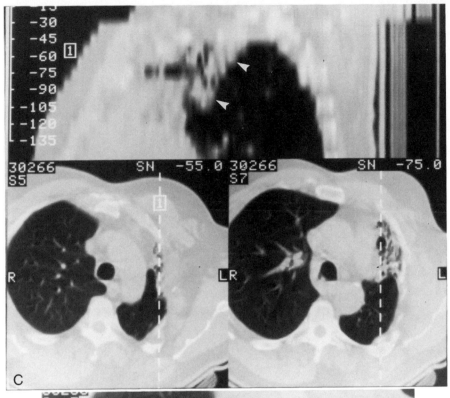

Figure 4–36 *Continued*

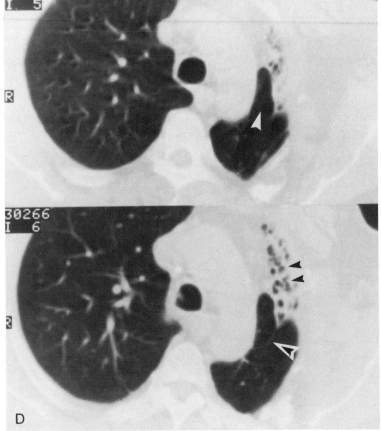

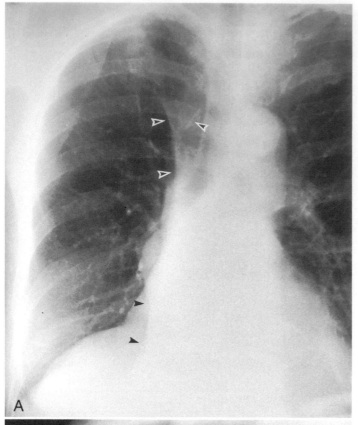

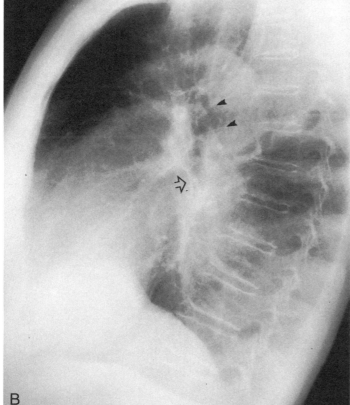

Figure 4–37. Posterior Displacement of the Intermediate and Lower Lobe Bronchi Associated with Atelectasis of the Right Lower Lobe. *A,* In posteroanterior projection, the right lower lobe is collapsed and airless (*small arrowheads* point to the interface between the downward-displaced major fissure and the overinflated right upper lobe). The anterior junction line and mediastinal triangle (*arrowheads*) are displaced to the right (upper triangle sign). Note that the right interlobar artery is no longer visible because of silhouetting by the airless lower lobe. *B,* In lateral projection, collapse of the lower lobe is manifested by a vague triangular opacity overlying the lower thoracic vertebrae, and by posterior displacement of the air column of the intermediate and right lower lobe bronchi (*arrowheads*). Normally, the lower lobe bronchus is aligned with the tracheal air column, slightly in front of the anterior wall of the left lower lobe bronchus (*open arrow*).

Illustration continued on opposite page

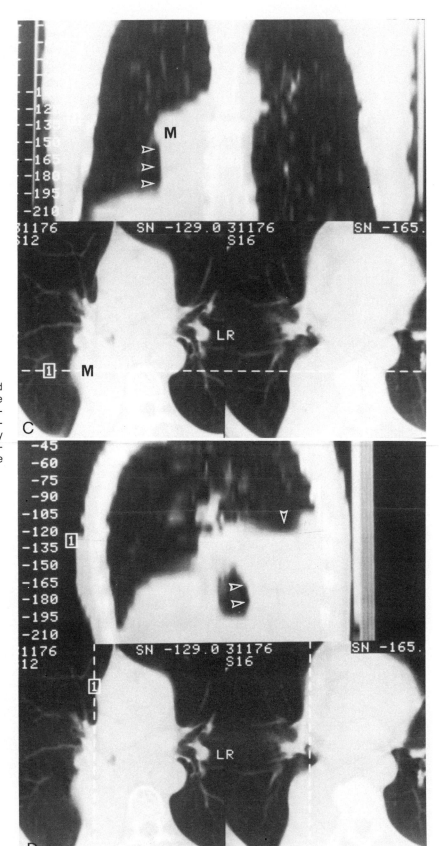

Figure 4–37 *Continued.* Coronal (*C*) and sagittal (*D*) CT reformations (*top*) with appropriate transverse images (*bottom*) identify the downward (*single arrowhead*), posterior (*two arrowheads*), and medial (*three arrowheads*) deformity of the major fissure. Centrally obstructing bronchogenic carcinoma (M) is the cause of the atelectasis in this 55-year-old man.

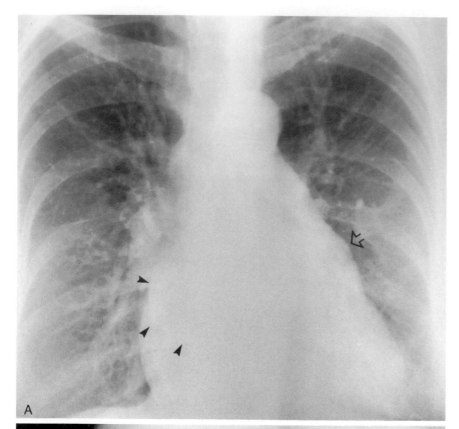

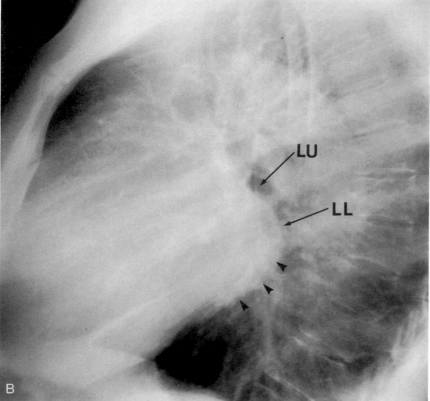

Figure 4–38. Posterior Displacement of the Left Main and Lower Lobe Bronchi in Postcapillary Pulmonary Venous Hypertension. Conventional posteroanterior (*A*) and lateral (*B*) chest roentgenograms disclose an abnormal cardiac silhouette consistent with right ventricular enlargement; the left atrium (*three arrowheads*) and left atrial appendage (*open arrow*) are also enlarged. The left upper lobe (LU) and lower lobe (LL) bronchi are displaced posteriorly; this feature is usually caused by enlargement of the left superior pulmonary vein or confluence rather than by the left atrium *per se*. Note the flow redistribution into the arteries and veins of the upper lobes, loss of the normal right hilar concavity, and lack of definition of the lower zone vasculature, features indicative of postcapillary (venous) hypertension. The patient is a 47-year-old women with mitral stenosis.

distinguish such displacement from that caused by lower lobe atelectasis.

Of equal importance to displacement of the hila as a sign of atelectasis is the *redistribution* of vascular shadows that form these structures. The right hilum normally possesses a concave lateral aspect formed by the superior pulmonary vein above and the descending pulmonary artery below. Simon[58] showed that collapse of the right upper lobe rotates the superior pulmonary vein medially, flattening the right hilar concavity. However, note that the concavity can also be flattened by distention of the superior pulmonary vein in cases of severe pulmonary venous hypertension.

A cardinal sign of lower lobe collapse is loss of visibility of the interlobar artery; since the lung parenchyma adjacent to the artery is airless, the air-tissue interface is lost and the vessel becomes invisible. This sign is particularly valuable on the left side, where pleural effusion sometimes creates a triangular shadow in the posterior paravertebral zone that simulates total left lower lobe collapse. Preservation of the shadow of the interlobar artery establishes the pleural origin of the opacity, whereas its obliteration indicates lobar collapse.

Changes in the Chest Wall. Approximation of the ribs is, in our experience, the least dependable of all compensatory signs of atelectasis. Even a slight degree of rotation of the patient at the time of roentgenography may produce an asymmetry of the two sides of the rib cage that renders assessment of abnormal approximation difficult or even hazardous. The difficulty may be compounded further by alterations in rib angulation, produced by even minor degrees of scoliosis. Although approximation of ribs as a sign of smallness of a hemithorax may be of some value in cases of chronic loss of volume, we feel that it should not be relied upon too heavily as an accurate indicator of reduction in hemithoracic volume in cases of acute lobar collapse.

Absence of an Air Bronchogram. For the most part, *resorption atelectasis* cannot be present if air is visible in the bronchial tree. If bronchial obstruction is severe enough to cause absorption of air from the parenchyma of the affected lobe, it also must cause absorption of gas from the bronchial tree. Particularly when pneumonitis behind the obstruction is so severe that consolidation exceeds atelectasis, absence of an air bronchogram is a roentgenologic sign of vital importance, since it may be the only aid to differentiating between an obstruction by a bronchogenic carcinoma and a consolidative process such as simple bacterial pneumonia. There are rare exceptions to this (e.g., an endobronchial lesion causing retention of secretions and peripheral pneumonitis but incomplete obstruction of the bronchial lumen), but the true nature of the underlying pathologic process should become evident either when the lesion completely obstructs the bronchus or when serial roentgenograms reveal nonresolution of the pneumonia despite appropri-

atc therapy. Another exception to the general rule is acute confluent bronchopneumonia, such as from *Staphylococcus aureus*, in which a lobe or segment becomes homogeneously opaque and the bronchi are filled with inflammatory exudate; obviously an air bronchogram would not be anticipated.

The preceding statements apply only to atelectasis produced by resorption and not by the other three mechanisms (passive, adhesive, and cicatrization). In the first two particularly, an air bronchogram is virtually always present. In fact, absence of an air bronchogram—for example, in a lung collapsed behind a pneumothorax—indicates endobronchial obstruction in addition to the passive atelectasis, a fact that must promptly be brought to the attention of the referring physician or surgeon, since attempts at lung expansion by draining the pneumothorax will be futile.

In summary, the roentgenologic signs of atelectasis are:

A. *Direct:*
  1. Displacement of interlobar fissures.
B. *Indirect:*
  1. Local increase in density.
  2. Elevation of the hemidiaphragm.
  3. Displacement of the mediastinum.
  4. Compensatory overinflation.
  5. Displacement of hila.
  6. Approximation of ribs.
  7. Absence of an air bronchogram (in cases of resorption atelectasis only).
  8. Absence of visibility of the interlobar artery (in cases of lower lobe atelectasis only).

Patterns of Lobar and Segmental Atelectasis

Roentgenologists are indebted to Robbins and Hale[63–69] for clarifying for the first time the varied roentgenographic patterns of lobar and total pulmonary collapse. Later, Lubert and Krause[70–72] depicted patterns of collapse most lucidly in line drawings and three-dimensional models. The CT characteristics of lobar collapse have been described by several authors.[383, 384] In the descriptions that follow we have borrowed freely from the publications of these workers, our findings having been fundamentally similar to their observations.

As discussed earlier in this section, the roentgenographic pattern of atelectasis may be influenced by several variables. For example, pre-existing disease within the involved lobe or elsewhere in the lungs, a relatively fixed thoracic cage or mediastinum, pleural adhesions, pleural fluid, or pneumothorax, alone or in various combinations, alters the "typical" roentgenographic pattern. These variables are not discussed here; the patterns described are those that typically occur in collapse of previously normal lung tissue.

Since the degree of collapse of a lobe is governed largely by the amount of fluid and cells it contains, the resultant roentgenographic image varies from a consolidated lobe in which there is only minimal loss of volume to a state of total lobar collapse; therefore, the anatomicospatial relationships in each lobe are described from a state of normal volume through all stages to total atelectasis.

Provided the pleural space is intact (i.e., no pneumothorax or hydrothorax), certain basic characteristics are common to all forms of lobar atelectasis. It is important to realize that, regardless of the severity of collapse, the visceral pleura covering the affected lobe generally continues to relate intimately to the parietal pleura; in other words, the visceral pleural surface usually attempts to maintain contact with the parietal pleura over either the convex or mediastinal surface of the hemithorax (Figs. 4–39A and B). There are noteworthy exceptions to this rule; occasionally in lower lobe atelectasis (Fig. 4–39C) and frequently in severe middle lobe atelectasis (Fig. 4–39D), the convex pleural contact may be lost as the lobe foreshortens in a triangular fashion toward the hilum. Maintenance of visceral and parietal pleural contiguity with the mediastinum is generally maintained, although in severe middle lobe atelectasis even this relationship may be lost. In the majority of instances, however, maintenance of contiguity of pleural surfaces restricts movement hilarward; since the medial aspect of the lobe is relatively fixed at the hilum, the form that the atelectatic lobe must adopt is limited. The resultant shape is partly affected by the semirigid components of the lung (bronchi, arteries, and veins), which can be crowded together in very close apposition in one plane but have a limited capacity to foreshorten. As depicted by Lubert and Krause,[70] any pulmonary lobe in its fully inflated state may be likened to a pyramid with its apex at the hilum and its base contiguous with the parietal pleura; as the lobe loses volume, two surfaces of the pyramid approximate, the end result of total atelectasis being a flattened triangle or triangular "pancake" whose apex and base tend to maintain contiguity with the hilum and parietal pleura, respectively.

Lubert and Krause[72] emphasized that the roentgenologist must not be misled by lack of correlation between what he or she recognizes as spatial readjustment roentgenographically and what the surgeon or pathologist finds at thoracotomy or necropsy—in the latter situations, pneumothorax dissipates all anatomicospatial relationships in the intact thorax. This rare aspect of roentgenologic-pathologic correlation is notoriously inaccurate. The exception is chronic atelectasis associated with severe fibrosis, in which circumstance the location and shape of the affected lobe are not likely to change on opening the thorax.

TOTAL PULMONARY ATELECTASIS

When an entire lung collapses because of obstruction of a main bronchus, the compensatory phenomena are identical in character to those that develop with less severe pulmonary collapse but obviously are greater in degree and in some respects less readily apparent (Fig. 4–40). Elevation of the ipsilateral hemidiaphragm is recognizable only on the left side, the stomach bubble indicating its position. The hemithorax usually evidences retraction. It is on the mediastinum, however, that the most important effect is exerted by the net difference in pressure between the two halves of the thorax. As the normal contralateral lung overinflates, the whole mediastinum moves to the affected side, the greatest shift occurring anteriorly, where the mediastinum is most mobile. As the overinflated lung moves across the midline, it displaces the heart, aorta, and collapsed lung posteriorly. The resultant roentgenologic signs in lateral projection were clearly defined by Lubert and Krause.[60] Depth and radiolucency of the retrosternal air space are increased, with a general increase in roentgenographic density in the posterior portion of the thorax (Fig. 4–40); if the overinflated normal lung has rotated sufficiently so as to come in contact with the collapsed lung, the interface between the two may become evident. In posteroanterior projection, the uniform opacity caused by the superimposed cardiovascular structures and collapsed lung is interrupted by the radiolucency of overinflated contralateral lung that has passed across the midline of the thorax. The margin of the overinflated lung is usually visible extending into the involved hemithorax.

Lubert and Krause[60] emphasized the importance of assessing the retrosternal space in lateral projection to differentiate complete pulmonary collapse from massive pulmonary consolidation or massive pleural effusion (Fig. 4–35). In the latter conditions the anterior mediastinum is little altered in appearance, although its density may be increased; in total unilateral collapse the anterior mediastinum is increased not only in depth but also in radiolucency. These investigators refer to the "uniform-filter effect" observed in total pulmonary consolidation and massive pleural effusion, in which x-rays passing through the thorax in lateral projection are absorbed uniformly, preventing identification of a specific roentgenographic shadow.

LOBAR ATELECTASIS

The patterns created by atelectasis of the right and left upper lobes differ and therefore are described separately; the lower lobes have almost identical patterns and are considered together.

Right Upper Lobe. The minor fissure and the upper half of the major fissure approximate by shifting upward and forward, respectively (Fig. 4–41). Both fissures become gently curved as seen on lateral projection, the minor fissure assuming a concave configuration inferiorly whereas the major fissure may be convex, concave, or flat;[73] the minor fissure shows roughly the same curvature in pos-

Text continued on page 519

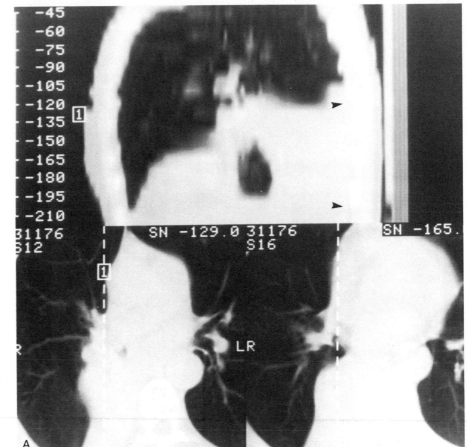

Figure 4–39. Relationship Between the Visceral and Parietal Pleura in the Presence of Atelectasis. *A,* A sagittal CT reformation (*top*) and representative transverse images (*bottom*) of a patient with right lower lobe atelectasis caused by a central obstructing pulmonary carcinoma: contiguity of the visceral and parietal pleura is maintained over the convex (posterior) surface of the lobe (*arrowheads*). *B,* A sagittal CT reformation (*top*) and representative transverse images (*bottom*) in left upper lobe atelectasis: visceral and parietal pleural contiguity is maintained anteriorly (*arrowheads*); the upper lobe bronchus is occluded by an adenocarcinoma.

Illustration continued on following page

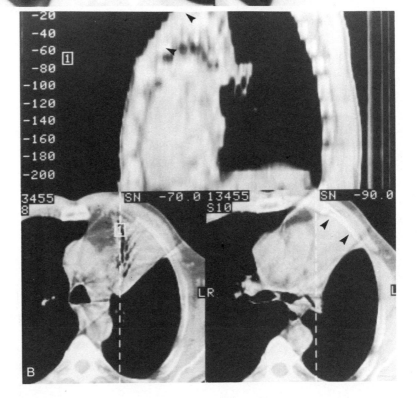

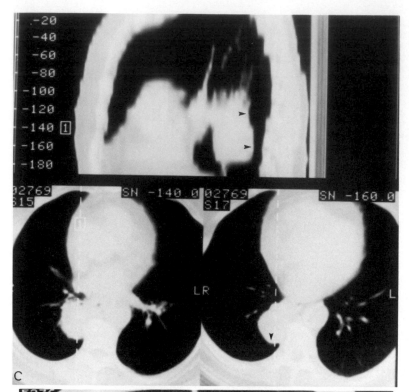

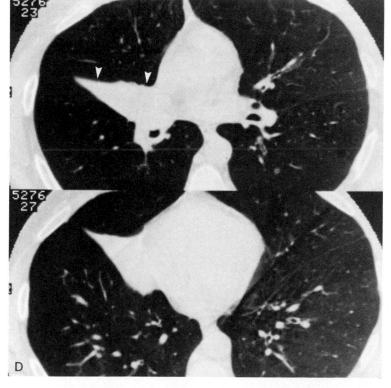

Figure 4–39 *Continued. C,* In contrast to these two cases, a sagittal CT reformation (*top*) and representative transverse images (*bottom*) in a patient with right lower lobe atelectasis reveal the visceral pleura (*arrowheads*) to have lost all contact with the parietal pleura of the posterior chest wall but not the mediastinum. Similarly, transverse CT scans (*D*) of a patient with right middle lobe atelectasis (*arrowheads*) show the visceral pleura over the convex (anterior) surface of the lobe to have lost contact with the parietal pleura; however, a thin linear opacity is still visible between the lateral point of the collapsed lobe and the chest wall, which conceivably could be caused by either contact between the upper and lower lobes or airless lung at the extreme periphery of the middle lobe. Loss of contiguity between the visceral and parietal pleura over the convex surface of a lobe is most apt to occur with atelectasis of the middle lobe, occasionally in a lower lobe, and rarely if ever in an upper lobe.

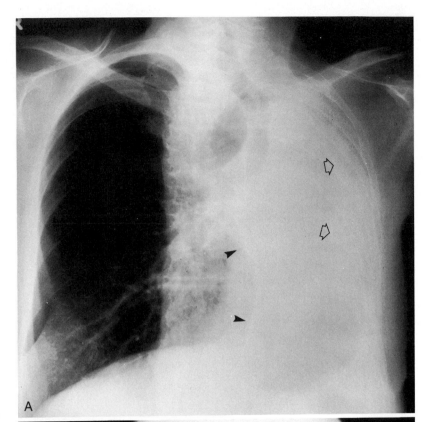

Figure 4–40. Total Atelectasis of the Left Lung. Conventional posteroanterior (*A*) and lateral (*B*) chest roentgenograms disclose an opaque and shrunken left hemithorax. The right lung is markedly overinflated and has displaced the mediastinum to the left both posteriorly (*arrowheads*) and anteriorly (*open arrows*). The cardiac silhouette is obscured except for its anterior surface that is clearly visible in lateral projection; curvilinear calcification in the upper left hemithorax identifies the aortic arch.

Illustration continued on following page

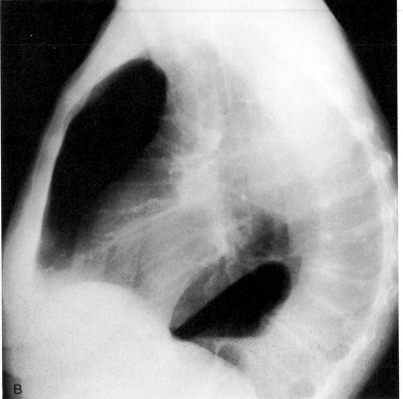

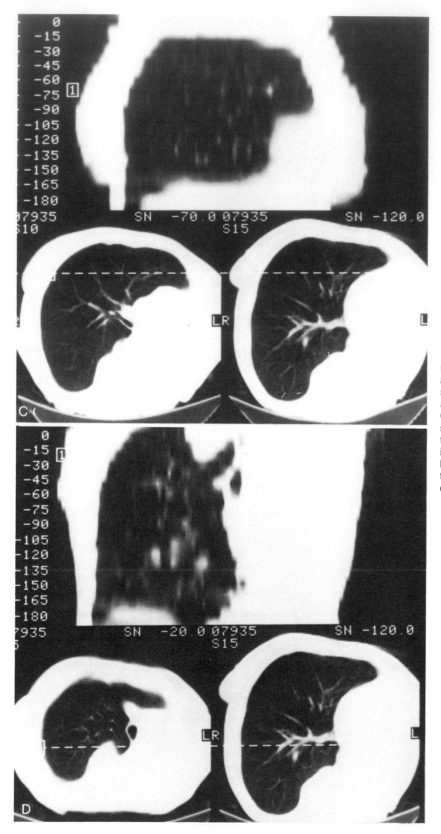

Figure 4–40 *Continued. C,* A coronal CT reformation (*top*) and transverse CT images (*bottom*) through the anterior mediastinum demonstrate the marked overinflation of the right lung as it intrudes into the left hemithorax. *D,* A coronal CT reformation (*top*) and appropriate transverse scans (*bottom*) through the posterior mediastinum show the overinflated lower lobe intruding into the left hemithorax above and below the right hilum. The patient is a 73-year-old woman with total atelectasis of the left lung due to a centrally obstructing pulmonary carcinoma.

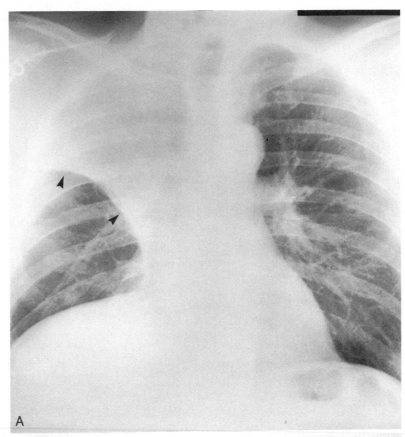

A

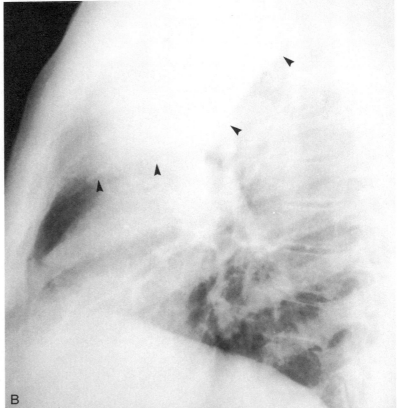

B

Figure 4–41. Right Upper Lobe Atelectasis (Moderate). Conventional posteroanterior (*A*) and lateral (*B*) roentgenograms reveal a homogeneous opacity (*arrowheads*) occupying the anterosuperior portion of the right hemithorax. In lateral projection the opacity is sharply defined on its posterior and anteroinferior margins. The right hemidiaphragm is elevated and there is slight displacement of the trachea to the right.

Illustration continued on following page

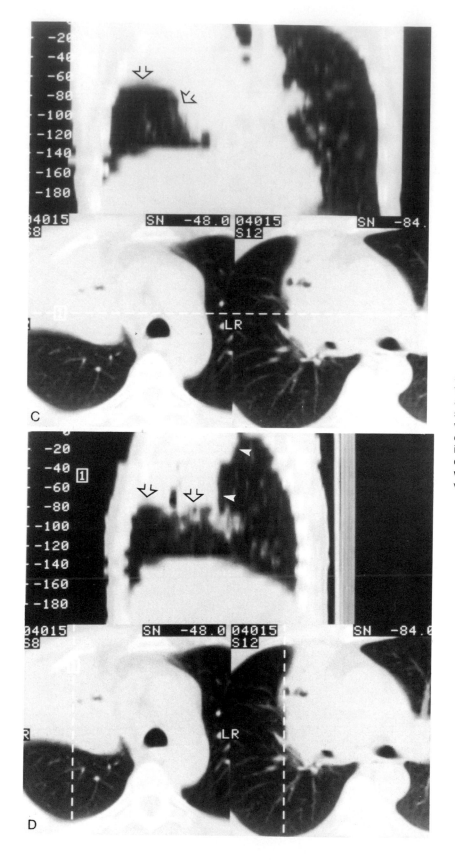

Figure 4–41 *Continued.* Coronal (*C*) and sagittal (*D*) reformations (*top*) with appropriate transverse CT images (*bottom*) show the typical appearance of right upper lobe atelectasis: the superior portion of the major fissure moves forward (*arrowheads*) while the minor fissure is displaced superiorly (*open arrows*). The patient is a 51-year-old man with a large squamous cell carcinoma in the right upper lobe; the atelectasis was caused by bronchial compression from involved lymph nodes.

teroanterior projection. As volume diminishes further, the visceral pleural surface sweeps upward over the apex of the hemithorax, so that the lobe comes to occupy a flattened position contiguous with the superior mediastinum. When completely collapsed, its volume is so small that in posteroanterior projection its shadow creates no more than a slight widening of the superior mediastinum (Fig. 4–42). In lateral projection, the collapsed lobe may appear as an indistinctly defined triangular shadow with its apex at the hilum and its base contiguous with the parietal pleura just posterior to the extreme apex of the hemithorax ("the mediastinal wedge"). The collapsed lobe is usually contiguous with the mediastinum so that no air shadow separates them; occasionally, however, overinflated lower lobe is interposed between the mediastinum and the medial edge of the atelectatic upper lobe, a feature seen much more often with left upper lobe atelectasis (*see* further on).

A sign sometimes associated with right[74] or left upper lobe atelectasis is the "juxtaphrenic peak." This sign consists of a small, sharply defined triangular opacity that projects upward from the medial half of the hemidiaphragm at or near the highest point of the dome (Fig. 4–43). Kattan and his colleagues[74] believe that the peak may be related to upward displacement of the diaphragmatic component of the pulmonary ligament. Raasch and his associates[75] showed that this feature may result from extrapleural fat drawn into a reoriented major fissure or from stretched basilar lung scars. Khoury and colleagues[73] identified an inferior accessory fissure as an additional cause of this configuration. We have seen classic peaks in patients *without* appreciable atelectasis, for example in a patient with acute diplococcal pneumonia, and in the presence of generalized pulmonary overinflation due to atopic asthma.

Left Upper Lobe. The major difference between collapse of the left and right upper lobes is the absence of a minor fissure on the left, on which side all lung tissue anterior to the major fissure is involved (Fig. 4–44). This fissure, which is slightly more vertical than the chief fissure on the right, is displaced forward in a plane roughly parallel to the anterior chest wall, a relationship depicted particularly well on lateral roentgenograms (Fig. 4–45). As volume loss increases, the fissure moves further anteriorly and medially, until on lateral projection the shadow of the lobe is no more than a broad linear opacity contiguous with and parallel to the anterior chest wall (Fig. 4–46). The contiguity of the collapsed lobe with the anterior mediastinum obliterates the left cardiac border in frontal projection (the "silhouette sign"). The apical segment tends to move downward and forward, the space it vacates being occupied by the overinflated superior bronchopulmonary segment of the lower lobe; the apex of the hemithorax thus contains aerated lung (Fig. 4–46).[76] Sometimes the overinflated superior

bronchopulmonary segment of the lower lobe inserts itself medially between the apex of the atelectatic upper lobe and the mediastinum, creating a sharp interface with the medial edge of the collapsed lobe. This feature, termed the "Luftsichel" in the German literature,[77] is more often seen on the left than on the right.[73] Computed tomographic assessment of the atelectatic lobe in such circumstance almost invariably shows a triangular or peaked appearance to the posteromedial fissural surface between the atelectatic upper lobe and the hyperexpanded lower lobe (Fig. 4–47). Khoury and his associates[73] identified this configuration in five of six patients with left upper lobe atelectasis, leading them to conclude that the V-shaped major fissure deformity was the usual pattern on CT scans (Fig. 4–48); however, a straight-bordered pattern characteristic of Luftsichel was seen in only one of their six patients. The precise nature of this deformity is uncertain; however, we are of the opinion that the sign is related to upper and lower lobar parenchymal fusion occasioned by incompleteness of the major fissure since the peak always occurs in the same anatomic location where fusion is most apt to occur (*see* page 161). The "mediastinal wedge" produced by the triangular opacity extending from the collapsed parenchyma to the hilum is often difficult to identify but may be seen on a lateral tomogram. If atelectasis becomes complete, the lower end of the chief fissure swings upward anteriorly to produce the final result of a triangular opacity, with its apex at the hilum and its base contiguous with the parietal pleura at the apex of the hemithorax (in a position somewhat more anterior than seen in total right upper lobe collapse).

Shift of the superior mediastinum as a compensatory phenomenon is usually more marked in left than in right upper lobe collapse, probably because of the former's larger volume. Displacement of the mediastinal septum to the left by the overinflated right lung may separate the collapsed left upper lobe from the anterior chest wall and produce an exceptionally radiolucent retrosternal space as viewed in lateral projection, with a sharp line of definition between the right lung and the collapsed left upper lobe.

Right Middle Lobe. The diagnosis of atelectasis of the right middle lobe is one of the easiest to make on a lateral roentgenogram and one of the most difficult on posteroanterior projection (Fig. 4–49). With progressive loss of volume, the minor fissure and the lower half of the major fissure approximate and are almost in contact when collapse is complete (Fig. 4–50). The resultant triangular "pancake" of tissue has its apex at the hilum and its base apparently contiguous to the parietal pleura over the anterolateral convexity of the thorax. As indicated, CT may demonstrate that this is largely spurious since the visceral pleura can be retracted almost completely from the anterior chest wall (Fig. 4–49). In lateral projection, middle lobe

Text continued on page 529

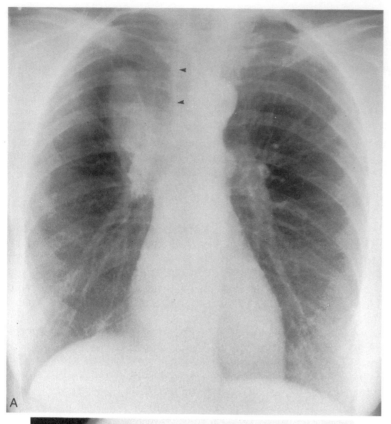

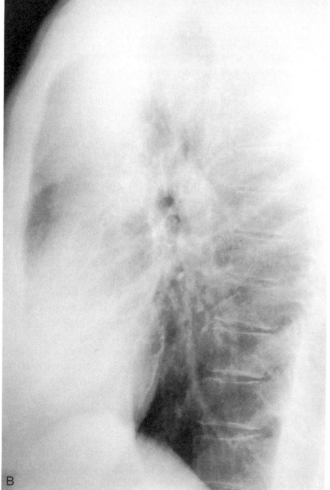

Figure 4–42. Right Upper Lobe Atelectasis (Severe). Posteroanterior (*A*) and lateral (*B*) chest roentgenograms disclose a reduction in volume of the right hemithorax, elevation of the right hemidiaphragm, and a peaked appearance to the superomedial contour of the right hemidiaphragm. The trachea is displaced minimally to the right but the tracheal stripe is maintained (*arrowheads*). Note the slight lucency immediately lateral to the trachea. An opacity is present that extends from an elevated right hilum superiorly toward the apex of the right lung.

Illustration continued on opposite page

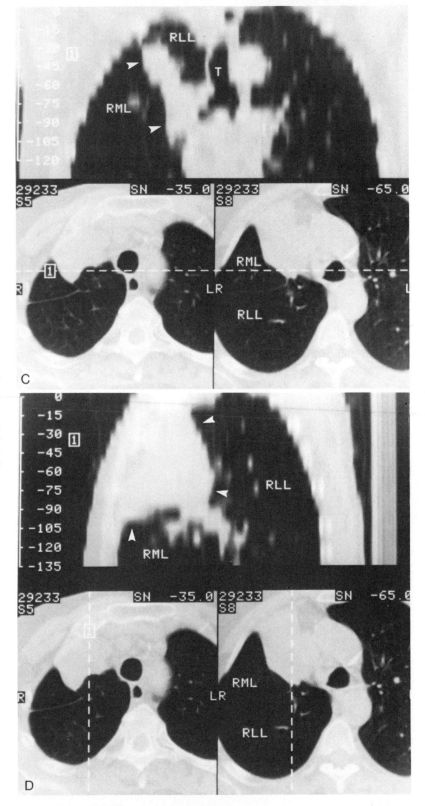

Figure 4–42 *Continued.* Coronal (*C*) and sagittal (*D*) CT reformations (*top*) with appropriate axial images (*bottom*) disclose the typical triangular configuration of severe right upper lobe atelectasis (*arrowheads*). The superior segment of the right lower lobe (RLL) has expanded to fill the apex of the hemithorax; a small tongue of this segment is situated between the trachea (T) and the collapsed lobe, representing a right-sided Luftsichel. The right middle lobe (RML) abuts the anteromedial and inferior surface of the atelectatic lobe. The patient is a 68-year-old woman with severe right upper lobe atelectasis caused by a central squamous cell carcinoma.

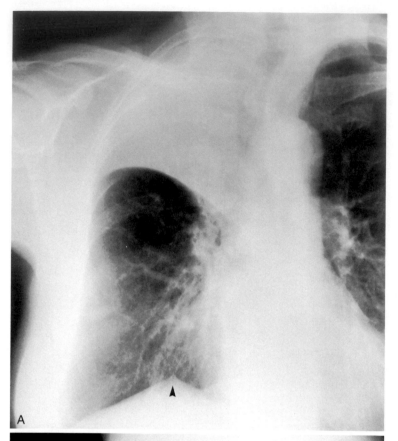

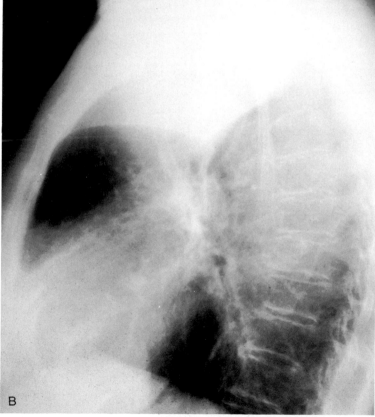

Figure 4–43. The Juxtaphrenic Peak in Upper Lobe Atelectasis. Posteroanterior (*A*) and lateral (*B*) chest roentgenograms in a patient with right upper lobe atelectasis show the normally smooth contour of the right hemidiaphragm to be interrupted by a triangular opacity (*arrowhead*), apex pointing cephalad. This juxtaphrenic peak has been variously attributed to reorientation of the pulmonary ligament or major fissure and to stretched basilar lung scars. Intrusion of diaphragmatic fat into the deformity has been shown in some instances.

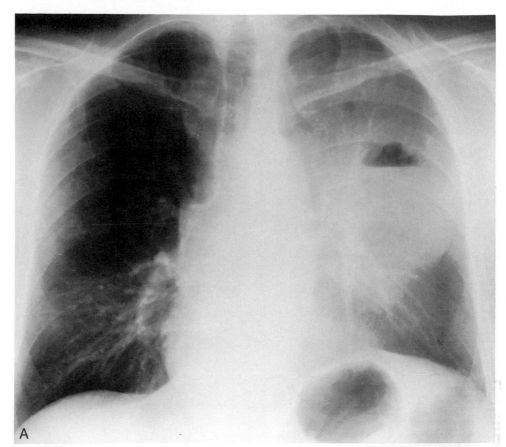

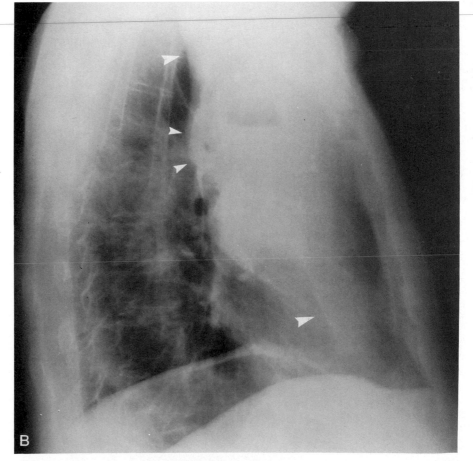

Figure 4–44. Left Upper Lobe Atelectasis, Obstructive Pneumonitis, and Lung Abscess. Posteroanterior (*A*) and lateral (*B*) roentgenograms reveal an extensive opacity over the left hemithorax caused by atelectasis of the upper lobe. Note the anterior displacement of the major fissure (*large arrowheads*). A fluid level is present in the superoposterior portion of the lobe, representing an abscess associated with obstructive pneumonia. Note the convex posterior bulge (*small arrowheads*) in the major fissure caused by the mass effect of the abscess.

Illustration continued on following page

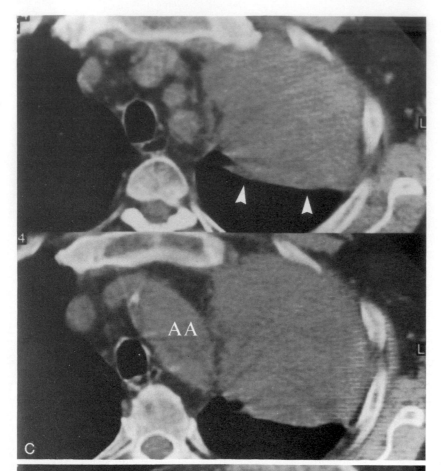

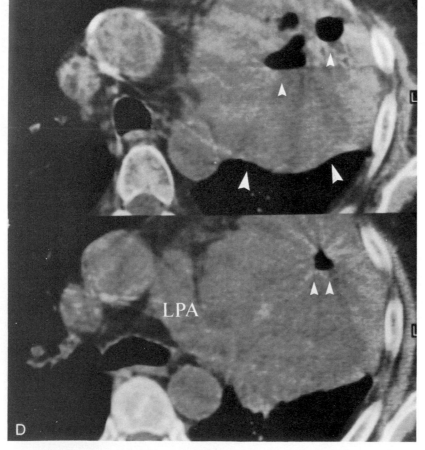

Figure 4–44 *Continued.* Transverse CT scans (*C* and *D*) through the aortic arch (*AA*) and left pulmonary artery (*LPA*) demonstrate massive consolidation of the upper lobe (*large arrowheads*); the abscess is clearly seen (*small arrowheads*). Squamous cell carcinoma, left upper lobe bronchus.

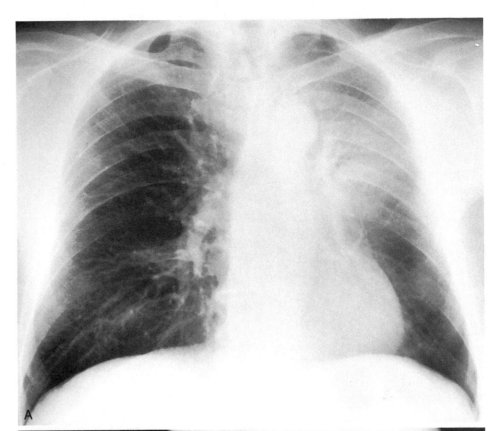

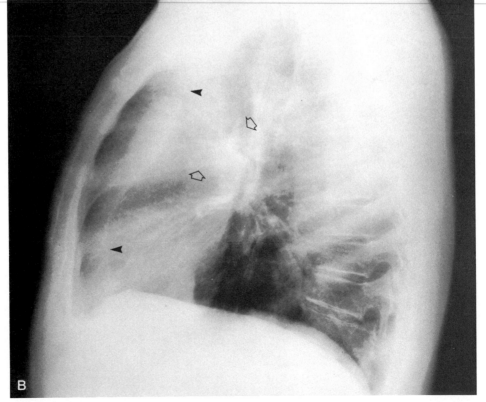

Figure 4–45. Severe Left Upper Lobe Atelectasis. Posterior (*A*) and lateral (*B*) chest roentgenograms reveal the medial-to-lateral decrease in roentgenographic density characteristic of severe left upper lobe atelectasis. A faint air bronchogram is present. On the lateral projection, the serpentine interface between the collapsed upper lobe and overinflated lower lobe (*arrowheads*) relates closely to the anterior chest margin; a vague mediastinal wedge is seen extending upward and forward from the hilum (*arrows*). Note the clarity with which the posterior portion of the aortic arch can be seen.

Illustration continued on following page

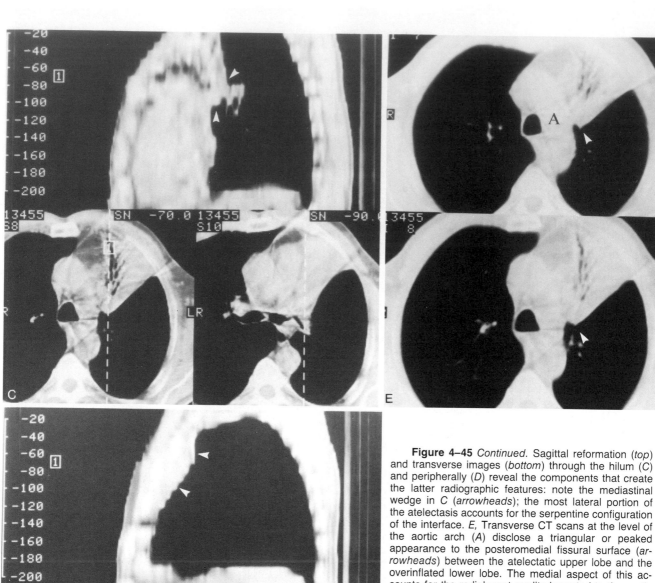

Figure 4–45 *Continued.* Sagittal reformation (*top*) and transverse images (*bottom*) through the hilum (*C*) and peripherally (*D*) reveal the components that create the latter radiographic features: note the mediastinal wedge in *C* (*arrowheads*); the most lateral portion of the atelectasis accounts for the serpentine configuration of the interface. *E,* Transverse CT scans at the level of the aortic arch (*A*) disclose a triangular or peaked appearance to the posteromedial fissural surface (*arrowheads*) between the atelectatic upper lobe and the overinflated lower lobe. The medial aspect of this accounts for the radiolucent quality imparted to the aortic arch on the conventional PA view (the Luftsichel). The patient is a 61-year-old woman with left upper lobe atelectasis caused by a central obstructing bronchogenic carcinoma.

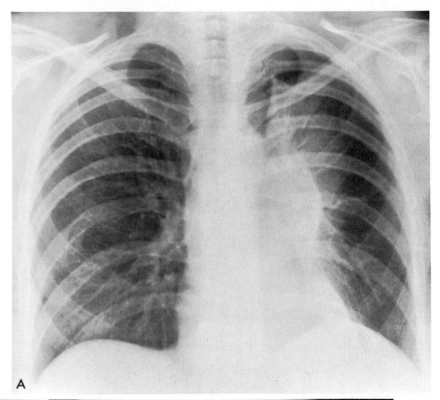

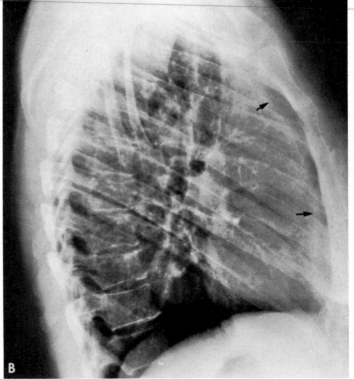

Figure 4–46. Atelectasis of the Left Upper Lobe (Severe). The homogeneous shadow created by the almost complete collapse of the left upper lobe occupies the anteromedial portion of the left hemithorax contiguous to the mediastinum. *A,* In posteroanterior projection, the apex of the hemithorax is occupied by the overinflated lower lobe. *B,* In lateral projection, the chief fissure has swept far anteriorly and can be identified as a rather indistinctly defined shadow of increased density paralleling the anterior chest wall (*arrows*). The "mediastinal wedge" can be only vaguely distinguished.

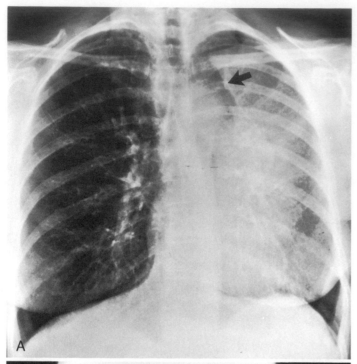

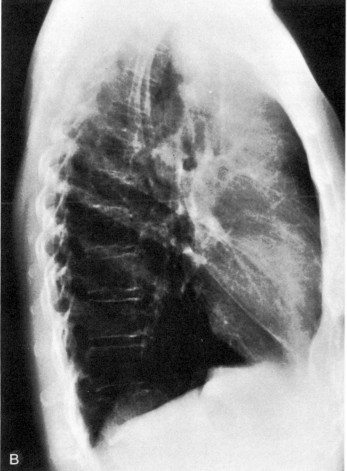

Figure 4–47. Left Upper Lobe Atelectasis with Luftsichel. Posteroanterior (*A*) and lateral (*B*) roentgenograms reveal a common configuration of left upper lobe atelectasis; note the sharp air-tissue interface (*arrow*) representing the tongue of overinflated lower lobe inserted between the mediastinum and airless upper lobe.

Illustration continued on opposite page

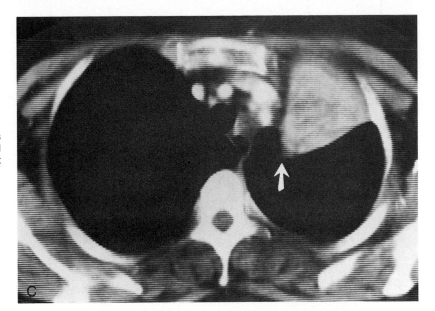

Figure 4–47 *Continued. C,* A CT scan shows a V-shaped posterior extremity of the collapsed lobe, an *arrow* pointing along the interface that creates Luftsichel.

atelectasis appears as a broad linear opacity, at times no more than 2 or 3 mm wide. As Heitzman has emphasized in personal communication, should the thinnest portion of the collapsed lobe be situated some distance from the hilum, thus creating an hourglass configuration, a central mass should be sought as the cause of the atelectasis.

In posteroanterior projection there may be no discernible increase in density, the only evidence of disease being obliteration of part of the right cardiac border (the silhouette sign) owing to contiguity of the right atrium with the medial bronchopulmonary segment of the collapsed lobe. The inability to detect right middle lobe atelectasis in some patients on posteroanterior projection is caused by the obliquity of the collapsed lobe in a superoinferior plane and the thickness of the collapsed lobe itself. The obliquity that the collapsed lobe assumes is variable, undoubtedly related in large measure to the fixation of the lobe at the hilum. In lateral projection, the lobe is sometimes almost horizontal in orientation, whereas on other occasions it may run obliquely, at times paralleling the plane of the major fissure. The horizontal and sharp oblique patterns of middle lobe atelectasis have been described by Raasch and his associates[75] as "tipped up" and "tipped down" (Fig. 4–49). Severe atelectasis of the right middle lobe in the tipped down position may be insufficiently thick to cause a discernible roentgenographic shadow in PA projection. When the patient assumes a lordotic position or the middle lobe collapses in a tipped up direction, the downward displaced minor fissure becomes oriented in a plane parallel to the roentgen beam on PA projection, so that the atelectatic lobe appears as a thin, "sail-like" or triangular opacity; the apex of this opacity is directed away from the hilum whereas the base abuts the right cardiac border.

The CT depiction of right middle lobe atelectasis is characteristic and consists of a broad trian-

gular or trapezoidal opacity with the apex directed toward the hilum. The anterior margin of the collapsed lobe tends to retract hilarward while the overinflated right upper lobe parenchyma intrudes anteromedially. In the tipped up pattern, the collapsed lobe tends to parallel the plane of the x-ray beam; consequently, the atelectasis is usually identified as a broad opacity on only one or two of the CT scans. By contrast, in the tipped down position the triangular configuration is much smaller but is identified on three or four scans. In both varieties of right middle lobe atelectasis, contiguity with a portion or all of the cardiac silhouette is maintained, although unusual configurations of these more typical patterns may result from pleural adhesions.[78, 79]

Lower Lobes. The configuration adopted by the lower lobes in the presence of atelectasis is modified by the fulcrum-like effect exerted on the lung by the hilum and pulmonary ligament,[79] the fissures approximating in such a manner that the upper half of the major fissure swings downward and the lower half backward (Fig. 4–51). This displacement is best appreciated in lateral projection when the lobe is only partly atelectatic and the major fissure is tangential to the x-ray beam and thus visible as a well-defined interface (Fig. 4–52). During its downward displacement, the upper half of the fissure usually becomes clearly evident in posteroanterior projection as a well-defined interface extending obliquely downward and laterally from the region of the hilum (Fig. 4–52).[80, 81] As collapse progresses, the lobe moves posteromedially to occupy a position in the posterior costophrenic gutter and medial costovertebral angle. Since the flat surface of the triangular "pancake" lies against the mediastinum, the thickness of tissue traversed by the roentgen beam in lateral projection may be insufficient to cast a shadow; indeed, when atelectasis is severe the only abnormal feature may be a subtle increase in the radiographic density of the

Text continued on page 534

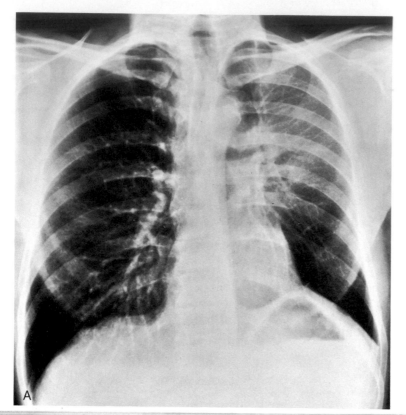

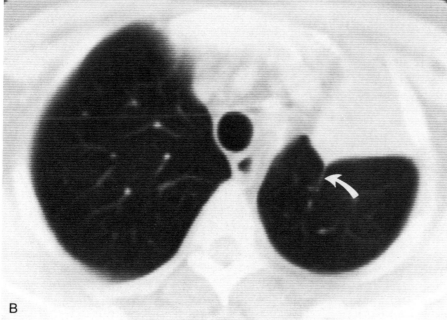

Figure 4–48. Left Upper Lobe Atelectasis with Luftsichel and Tag. In this example of left upper lobe atelectasis (A), the posterior extremity of the collapsed lobe on CT (B) possesses a broad V configuration so that the Luftsichel viewed on the PA roentgenogram is less sharp than in Figure 4–47. Note also the thin linear opacity (arrow) extending posteriorly from the peak; this is thought to represent a pleural reflection.

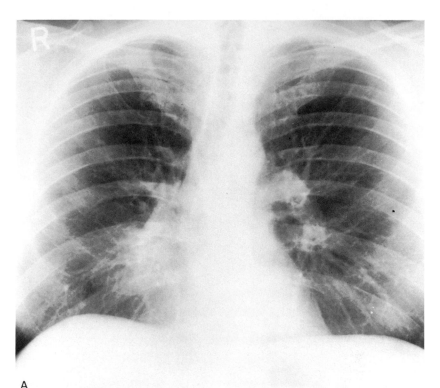

A

Figure 4–49. Right Middle Lobe Atelectasis. A posterior roentgenogram (A) reveals a vague opacity in the right lower hemithorax obliterating the right cardiac border, whereas a lateral projection of the same patient (B) shows the characteristic triangular opacity of middle lobe atelectasis. Note the convex inferior configuration of the major fissure at the hilum (*arrowheads*) indicative of an underlying mass. The opacity of the middle lobe possesses a sharp oblique orientation downward, constituting the "tipped-down" pattern of middle lobe atelectasis.

Illustration continued on following page

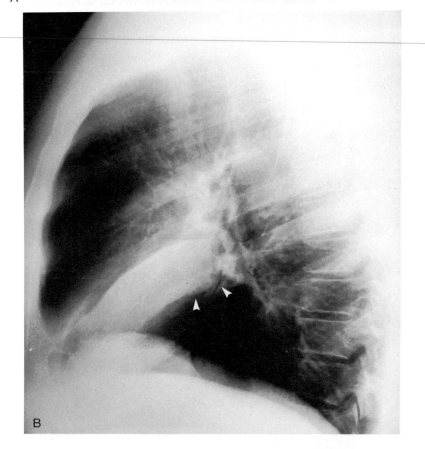

B

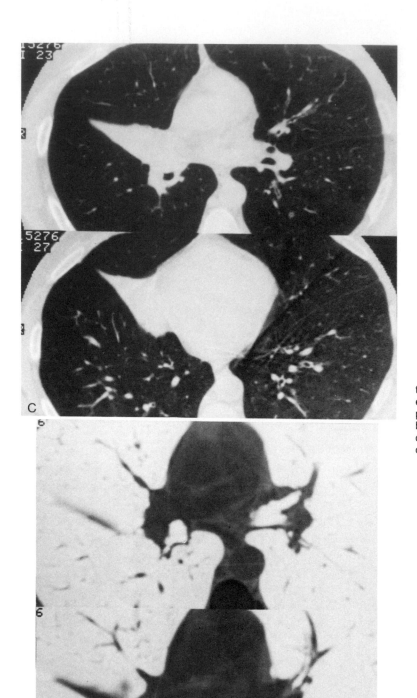

Figure 4–49 *Continued. C,* CT scans show the typical triangular opacity with its apex pointing peripherally. Contiguity between the visceral and parietal pleura over the anterolateral aspect of the lobe has been lost. *D,* CT scans through the middle lobe bronchus demonstrate an endo- and exophytic obstructing bronchogenic carcinoma (*arrowheads*).

Illustration continued on opposite page

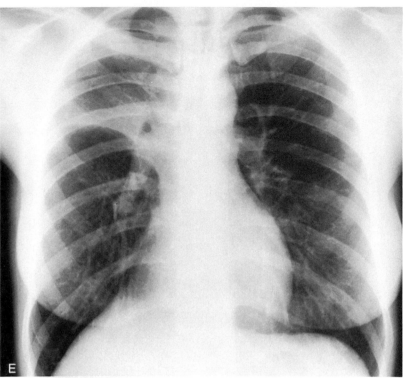

Figure 4–49 *Continued. E* and *F* are conventional posteroanterior and lateral roentgenograms of another patient with an obstructing middle lobe carcinoid tumor: the atelectatic middle lobe is in a "tipped-up" configuration, a pattern that closely simulates anterior segmental disease of the right upper lobe.

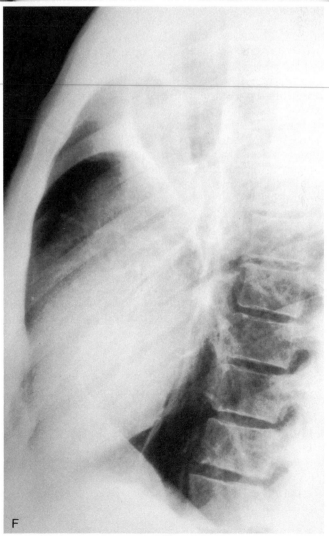

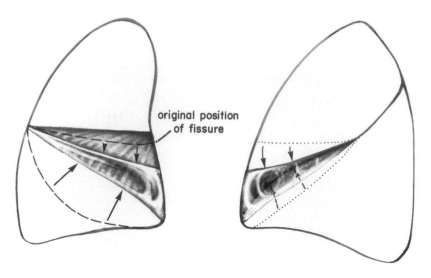

original position
of fissure

Figure 4–50. Patterns of Lobar Collapse: Right Middle Lobe. *See* text for description.

lower thoracic vertebrae (Fig. 4–53) (normally, the vertebrae become relatively more radiolucent from above downward). The "mediastinal wedge" (consisting of the conducting tissues) may be apparent as a narrow triangular band of increased density extending downward and posteriorly from the hilum. In frontal projection, provided that exposure factors ensure adequate penetration of the heart, the collapsed lobe should be plainly visible as a diminutive triangular or rounded opacity in the costovertebral angle.[79]

These varying appearances are thought to be the result of the different forms that the pulmonary ligament may assume: when the ligament is complete, the lung is tethered to the mediastinum and hemidiaphragm so that the atelectatic lobe maintains a close relationship to both, accounting for the triangular configuration. On the other hand, when the ligament is incomplete, the base of the lobe is not adherent to the hemidiaphragm and consequently the shape that the collapsed lobe assumes is dependent primarily on the mediastinal attachment; as a result, the lobe assumes a more rounded configuration.[79] As noted previously, the interlobar artery is not identifiable because of obscuration by surrounding airless lung; therefore, a localized convex bulge in the expected location of the interlobar artery should suggest an underlying central mass.

COMBINED LOBAR ATELECTASIS

Since involvement of the two lobes of the left lung results in total pulmonary collapse, atelectasis of two lobes simultaneously produces a distinctive roentgenographic pattern only in the right lung.

Combined Right Middle and Lower Lobe Atelectasis. The major and minor fissures are displaced downward and backward so that the resultant opacity occupies the posteroinferior portion of the hemithorax. Lubert and Krause[72] stated that on a posteroanterior roentgenogram the density created by the collapsed lobes completely obliterates the shadow of the right dome of the diaphragm and may possess an upper surface that is concave or convex upward. Thus, this condition easily may be confused with pleural effusion (either "typical" or infrapulmonary in configuration).

Combined Right Upper and Middle Lobe Atelectasis (Fig. 4–54). Because of the independent and even remote origin of the lobar bronchi of these lobes, such an occurrence must be uncommon, although Lubert and Krause[72] stated they had seen it "more frequently than might be anticipated." Again, because of the independent bronchial origins, multiple etiologies or a single etiology operating at two anatomic locations must be invoked to explain coincidental involvement. Although these workers claim to have seen combined lesions in association with primary and metastatic neoplasms and inflammatory disease, they considered that mucous plugs were probably a direct, contributing etiologic factor in most cases. A study of 17 patients with combined right upper and middle lobe disease[385] revealed pus or mucous plugs in the lobar bronchi in nine and bronchogenic carcinoma in four different presentations in the other eight. In three of these eight patients a carcinoma arising from the right upper lobe bronchus had led to obstructive pneumonitis of this lobe, which, because of an incomplete horizontal fissure, had extended into the right middle lobe. In another three in whom carcinoma had originated in the upper lobe bronchus, enlarged lymph nodes due to metastases had occluded the middle lobe bronchus. In one an upper lobe primary neoplasm had spread intraluminally to the middle lobe bronchus, with subsequent occlusion and atelectasis. The eighth patient had a primary upper lobe carcinoma and unrelated bronchiectasis of the middle lobe. The only example of this condition that we have seen was an asthmatic child with a chronic right middle lobe syndrome in whom a mucous plug had caused atelectasis of the

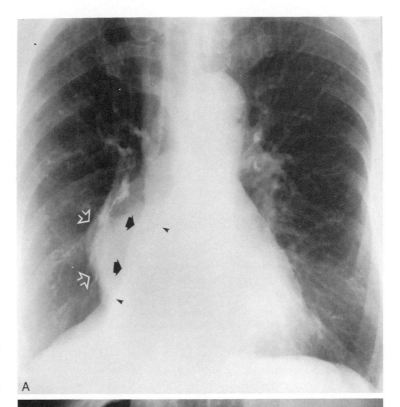

Figure 4–51. Right Lower Lobe Atelectasis. Conventional posteroanterior (*A*) and lateral (*B*) chest roentgenograms disclose an abnormal configuration to the right cardiac and mediastinal silhouette: in frontal projection, there is a triple density effect consisting of right hilar mass (*open arrows*), the right cardiac border (*closed arrows*), and the posterior surface of an atelectatic lower lobe (*small arrowheads*). The configuration of the right hilar vasculature is diminutive compared with the left as a result of incorporation of the interlobar artery within the atelectatic lobe. In lateral projection, the superior portion of the major fissure (*arrowheads*) is displaced downward, and a large mass (*M*) is present in the right hilum.

Illustration continued on following page

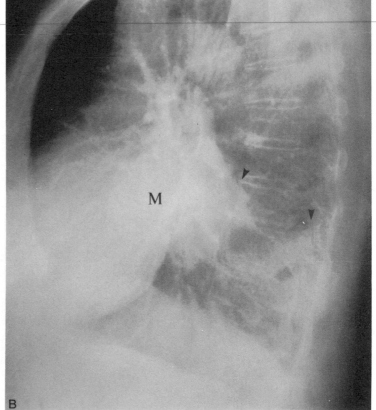

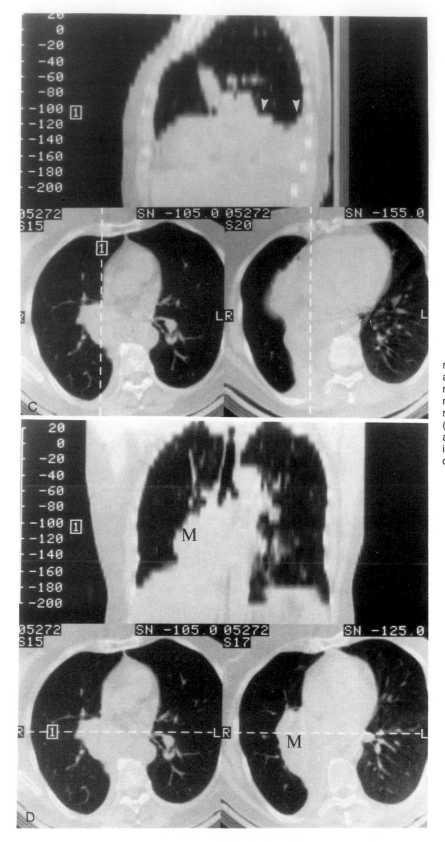

Figure 4–51 *Continued. C,* A sagittal CT reformation (*top*) with appropriate transverse images (*bottom*) illustrate the downward-displaced major fissure (*arrowheads*). Coronal CT reformations (*top*) through the hilum (*D*) and posteriorly (*E*) with representative transverse images (*bottom*) reveal the hilar mass (*M*) and posterior atelectatic component (*arrowheads*). The patient is a 65-year-old woman with squamous cell carcinoma.

Illustration continued on opposite page

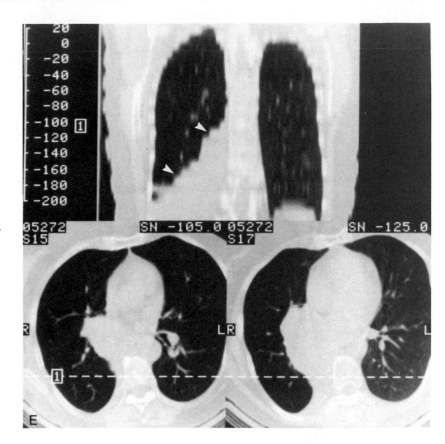

Figure 4–51 *Continued.*

"SEGMENTAL ATELECTASIS"

right upper lobe (Fig. 4–54); the roentgenographic pattern produced by this combined lesion was identical to that of left upper lobe collapse.

"SEGMENTAL ATELECTASIS"

These words have been placed in quotation marks to emphasize the fact that the term is probably a misnomer, at least in a pure sense. The reasons for the semantic inaccuracy are relatively simple. We have already seen that collateral channels can exert a potent force in ventilating alveoli other than by direct airway connections. Since collateral channels exist in profusion within segments, obstruction of a segmental or subsegmental bronchus cannot result in collapse unless some influence is present that prevents collateral air drift. In fact, provided there is no infection, the presence of a complete obstruction in a segmental bronchus over a long period of time often results in overinflation of distal parenchyma rather than collapse. When an opacity is present distal to an obstructed segmental bronchus, the influence that prevents collateral air drift in the majority of cases is inflammatory exudate, so that in effect the pathologic process is one of pneumonia. Since the pneumonia has developed as a consequence of obstruction of a segmental bronchus, the correct appellation is "obstructive pneumonitis." Thus, a homogeneous opacity that conforms to the anatomic distribution of a bronchopulmonary segment and in which no air bronchogram is identifiable should immediately alert the physician to the presence of an obstructing endobronchial lesion, associated with pneumonia (Fig. 4–55). Obviously, the caveat regarding the use of the term segmental atelectasis applies equally to subsegments although, as will be discussed later, it is conceivable that linear opacities commonly observed in the lung bases could be caused by subsegmental atelectasis in which collapse of alveoli resulted from surfactant deficit (plate atelectasis).

As might be anticipated, the opacity resulting from segmental or subsegmental obstructive pneumonitis depends not only upon the original volume of lung parenchyma affected but also upon the volume of inflammatory tissue that has replaced it. Thus, the shadow can vary from a large conical opacity in which there is very little loss of volume to little more than a broad linear opacity in which atelectasis has predominated. Regardless of the severity of the loss of volume, however, it is recommended that the term segmental atelectasis be struck from our descriptive vocabulary and that we employ terminology that more accurately reflects the true nature of an important pathologic process.

PREDOMINANTLY INTERSTITIAL DISEASE

This heading covers the multitude of pulmonary diseases characterized by predominant involve-

Text continued on page 545

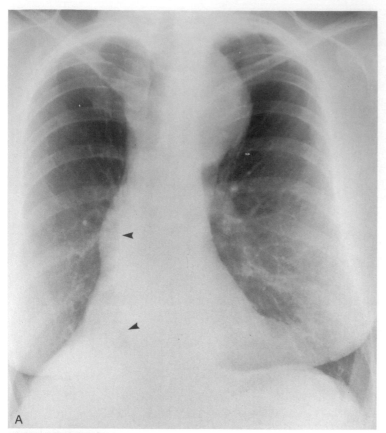

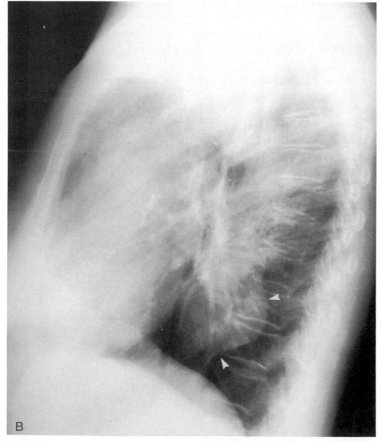

Figure 4–52. Right Lower Lobe Atelectasis. Posteroanterior (*A*) and lateral (*B*) chest roentgenograms of a 65-year-old woman reveal an aortic arch aneurysm that was confirmed by angiography. The right hemithorax is somewhat smaller than the left, and the mediastinum is displaced slightly to the right. An opacity is visible (*arrowheads*) behind the heart extending from approximately the level of the hilum to a point slightly above the right hemidiaphragm. The right hilum is diminished in size, and the right interlobar artery cannot be identified because of incorporation into the opacity of the collapsed lobe. In lateral projection, a sharply defined opacity (*arrowheads*) extends from the inferior aspect of the hilum to a point a few centimeters above the right hemidiaphragm.

Illustration continued on opposite page

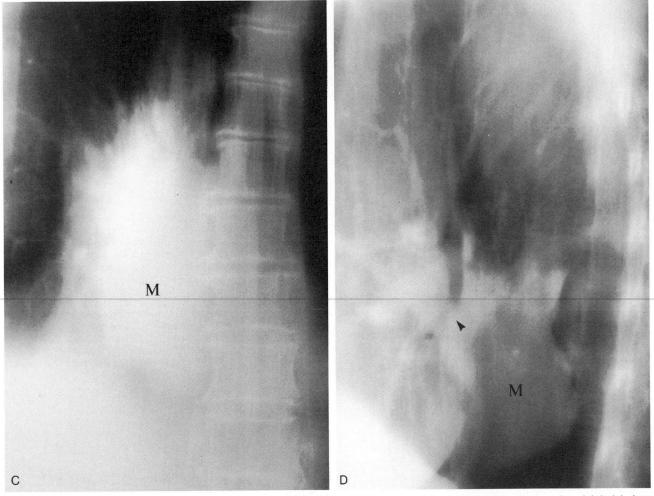

Figure 4–52 *Continued.* Conventional anteroposterior (*C*) and 55° right posterior oblique (*D*) tomograms reveal a sightly lobulated opacity (*M*) in the right paraspinal region; its superior margin is poorly defined and there is air-containing lung between the opacity and the right hemidiaphragm. The right lower lobe bronchus is occluded at or near its orifice (*arrowhead*).

Illustration continued on following page

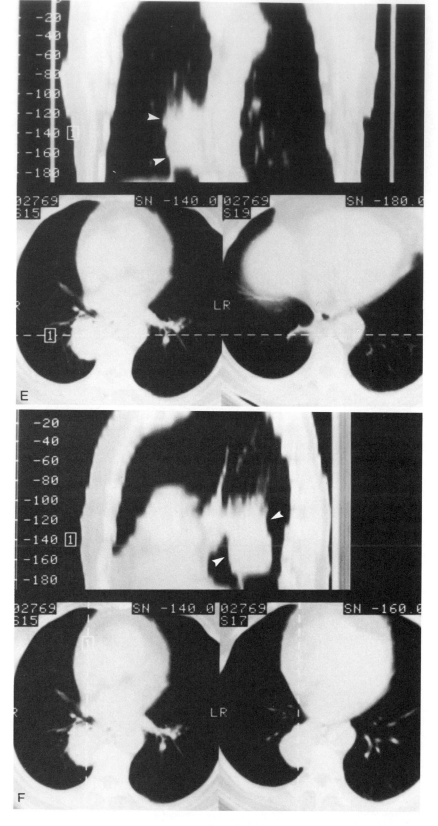

Figure 4–52 *Continued.* Coronary (*E*) and sagittal (*F*) CT reformations (*top*) with representative transverse images (*bottom*) show a markedly shrunken right lower lobe (*arrowheads*) that has retracted away from the posterior chest wall toward the hilum. Note that there is air-containing lung between the lobe and the right hemidiaphragm in front of and behind the mediastinal component of the pulmonary ligament. This uncommon "ball-like" appearance of right lower lobe atelectasis is thought to result from incompleteness of the diaphragmatic component of the pulmonary ligament, allowing the lobe to retract superiorly.

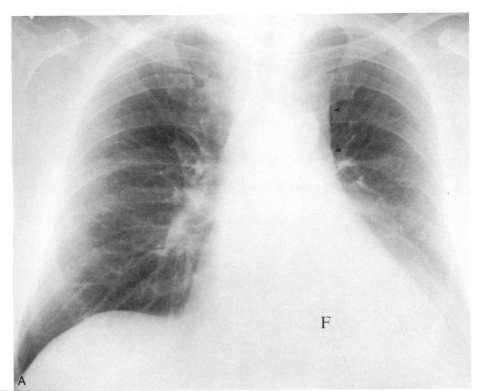

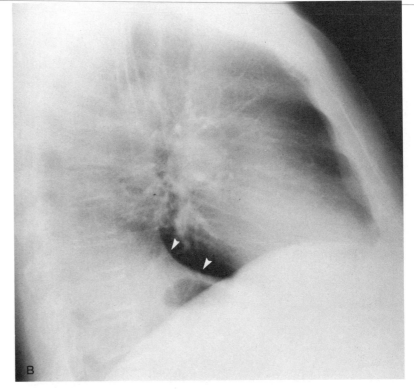

Figure 4–53. Left Lower Lobe Atelectasis. Conventional posteroanterior (*A*) and lateral (*B*) roentgenograms disclose an opacity behind the heart on the left. The left hemidiaphragm is elevated as indicated by the position of the gas-filled gastric fundus (*F*), although the diaphragm itself is obscured. The anterior mediastinal triangle is displaced to the left (*small arrowheads*). In lateral projection, the lower thoracic vertebrae are more opaque than normal, and the major fissure is displaced posteriorly (*arrowheads*).

Illustration continued on following page

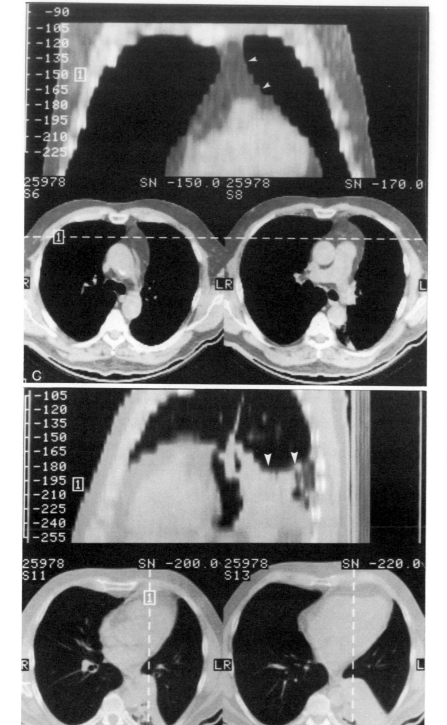

Figure 4–53 *Continued. C*, A coronal CT reformation (*top*) with representative transverse images (*bottom*) shows the displacement of the anterior mediastinal triangle to the left (*arrowheads*). *D*, A sagittal CT reformation (*top*) with appropriate transverse images (*bottom*) discloses a sharp demarcation between the atelectatic lower lobe and the hyperexpanded upper lobe (*arrowheads*). Note that the lobe has relocated posteromedially following rotation in a clockwise fashion around the hilum and pulmonary ligament. The patient is a 63-year-old man with squamous cell carcinoma of the left lower lobe bronchus.

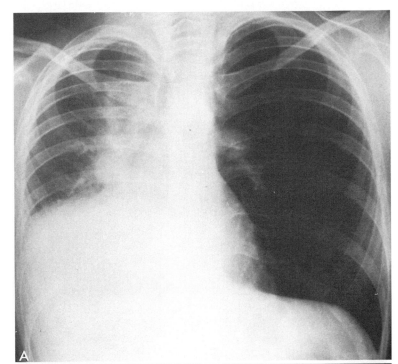

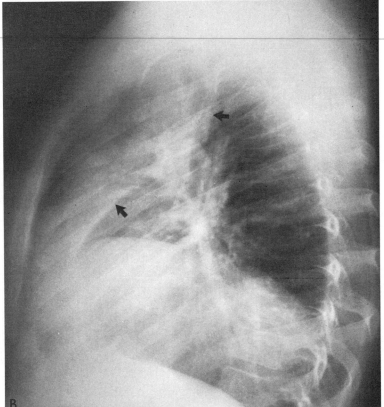

Figure 4–54. Atelectasis of the Right Upper and Middle Lobes Combined. Posteroanterior (*A*) and lateral (*B*) roentgenograms reveal a pattern of collapse that is virtually identical to the one seen in the left upper lobe (compare Figure 4–45). The collapsed lobes relate to the anteromedial aspect of the hemithorax; thus, in lateral projection (*B*), the major fissure is seen to be displaced forward (*arrows*). The apex of the right hemithorax is occupied by the overdistended lower lobe. Compensatory signs of diaphragmatic elevation and mediastinal shift are readily apparent. The patient is a 12-year-old boy with spasmodic asthma; a mucous plug impacted in the right upper lobe bronchus was coughed up spontaneously; the right middle lobe collapse was chronic and irreversible (chronic "right middle lobe syndrome") as revealed in follow-up roentgenograms *C* and *D* (*arrows* in *D*).

Illustration continued on following page

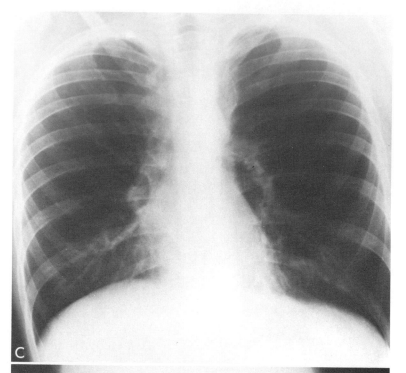

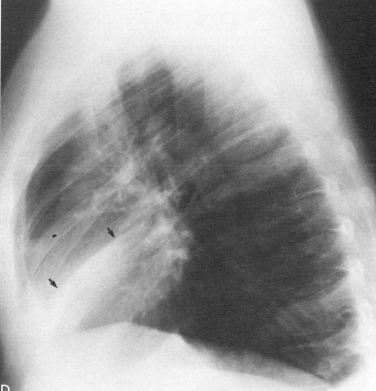

Figure 4–54 *Continued*

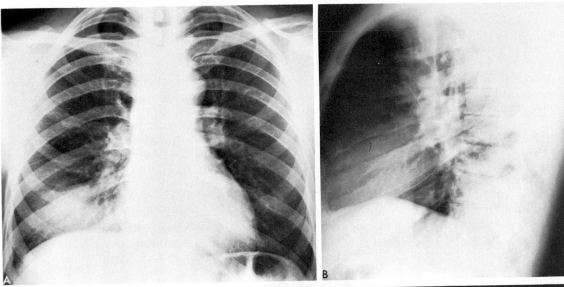

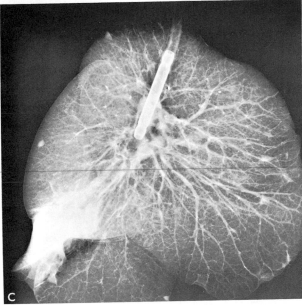

Figure 4–55. Segmental Atelectasis and Consolidation, Posterior Basal Segment, Right Lower Lobe. Posteroanterior (A) and lateral (B) roentgenograms reveal a homogeneous opacity localized to the posterior bronchopulmonary segment of the right lower lobe; no air bronchogram is present. The process is both consolidative and atelectatic, the latter evidenced by posterior displacement of the major fissure. A lateral roentgenogram of the resected lung (C) shows the precise segmental nature of the disease; as a result of preoperative chemotherapy, the bronchial obstruction had been partly relieved so that the operative specimen shows a well-defined air bronchogram. Squamous cell carcinoma of the posterior basal bronchus.

ment of the interstitial tissues of the lung. Conceptually, these diseases are the antithesis of the alveolar consolidative processes, in that *alveolar air is largely preserved and it is the tissues surrounding the air spaces that are increased in volume.* An enormous number of diseases can produce predominantly interstitial involvement of the lungs. The roentgenographic pattern may be so distinctive that in some cases a diagnosis can be strongly suggested on the basis of these appearances alone. In others, the diagnosis may be suggested when roentgenographic changes are considered in relation to the history or to evidence supplied by special roentgenographic procedures, laboratory findings, or pulmonary function values. In the majority, however, architectural disturbance is so similar that a definitive diagnosis cannot be made without recourse to histologic examination of tissue removed at biopsy.[82, 83]

Concepts of Roentgenologic Anatomy

It will be recalled that the lung parenchyma is sharply demarcated from the connective tissues of the bronchovascular tree, the interlobular septa, and the pleura by a limiting membrane.[84] This membrane is composed of dense elastic tissue and collagen that merges into the elastic fibers of alveolar walls. The blood vessels, nerves, and lymphatics lie in this compartment of loose connective tissue, called the *perivascular (or axial) interstitial space.* In addition, there is a small interstitial space in the walls of the alveoli themselves; this is referred to as the *parenchymal (or acinar) interstitial space,* in keeping with our use of the term "parenchyma" to denote the gas-exchanging part of the lung.

The *axial interstitial space* consists of the sheath of loose connective tissue around the bronchoarterial bundles that form the visible lung markings. This interstitial sheath extends out to the terminal bronchioles, beyond which the airways are intimately related to the parenchyma. A similar sheath exists around the venous radicals within the lung, and this interstitial space is continuous with the peripheral interlobular septa that contain the veins and lymphatics that drain the peripheral parenchyma; it is also continuous with the subpleural interstitial space. The *parenchymal (acinar) interstitial space* lies between the alveolar and capillary basement membranes. This small space contains elastic and collagen fibers as well as a number of connective tissue and inflammatory cells (*see* page 21).

Since interstitial diseases of the lung usually affect both "compartments" to some degree, it might be argued that their subdivision is arbitrary and of little practical importance. From a roentgenologic point of view, however, we have found their distinction to be of some value, chiefly because their individual involvement usually produces distinguishable roentgenographic patterns and different diagnostic considerations. For example, one of the common abnormalities affecting the interstitial tissues of the lung is pulmonary edema. In studies of rapidly frozen dog lungs in which pulmonary ve-

nous pressures were raised by graded levels, Staub and his colleagues[85] showed a definite sequence of fluid accumulation in various compartments of the lung (Fig. 4–56). Fluid appeared first in the interstitial connective tissue compartment around the large blood vessels and airways; thickening of the alveolar wall followed, but it was not until the interstitial compartment was well filled that alveolar edema appeared; alveolar filling occurred independently and rapidly in individual alveoli. It is this anatomic localization in the perivascular and lobular interstitium that produces the typical roentgenographic pattern of loss of the normal sharp definition of the pulmonary vascular markings and thickening of the interlobular septa (B lines of Kerley) (Fig. 4–57). Edema fluid that accumulates in the *parenchymal* interstitial tissues in these circumstances usually produces little or no discernible roentgenographic change. The pattern of roentgenologic abnormality in such instances shows predominantly perivascular interstitial tissue involvement. A similar distribution of disease occurs in lymphangitic spread of carcinoma,[86] some pneumoconioses,[87] and interstitial lymphoma (Fig. 4–58).[88]

It is probable that the same statement can be made about other types of interstitial disease in

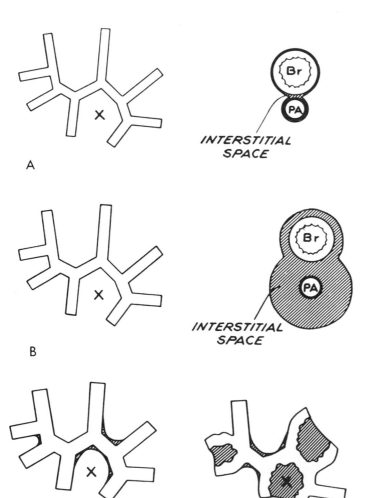

Figure 4–56. Schematic Representation of the Sequence of Fluid Accumulation in Acute Pulmonary Edema. *A*, Normal lung (alveolar wall and alveoli on the left, bronchovascular bundle on the right); *B*, interstitial edema in which fluid accumulated preferentially in the loose interstitial space around the conducting blood vessels and airways without affecting the alveolar walls; *C*, early alveolar edema showing loose interstitial spaces filled and fluid overflowing into alveoli, preferentially at the corners at which the curvature is greatest; *D*, alveolar flooding in which individual alveoli have reached a critical configuration at which existing inflation pressure can no longer maintain stability and the alveolar gas volume rapidly passes to a new configuration with much reduced curvature. (Slightly modified from Staub NE, Nagano H, Pearce ML: J Appl Physiol 22:227, 1967, with permission.)

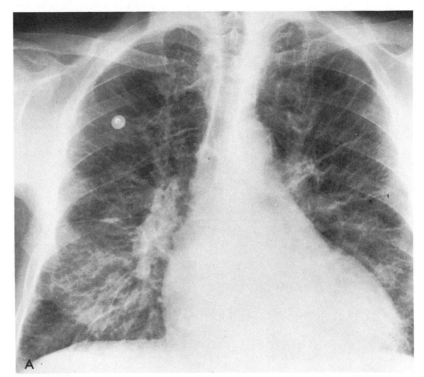

Figure 4–57. Interstitial Pulmonary Edema.
Posteroanterior (A) and lateral (B) roentgenograms
reveal multiple linear opacities throughout both
lungs, seen to better advantage in magnified views
of the right lower (C) and left upper (D) lungs.
These lines consist of a combination of long septal
lines (Kerley A), predominantly in the midlung
zones (arrows in B and D), and shorter peripheral
septal lines (Kerley B). In lateral projection (B), the
interlobar fissures are very prominent (arrows),
representing subpleural edema. Twenty-four hours
later (E), the edema in the subpleural interstitium
had cleared completely.

Illustration continued on following page

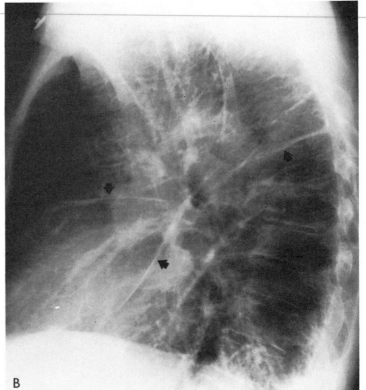

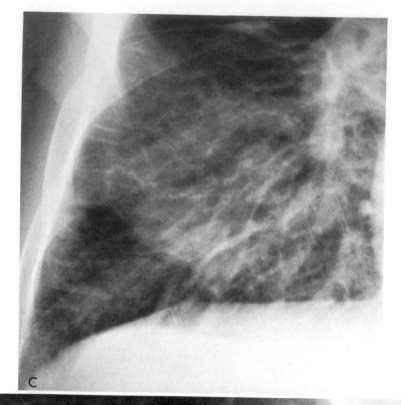

C

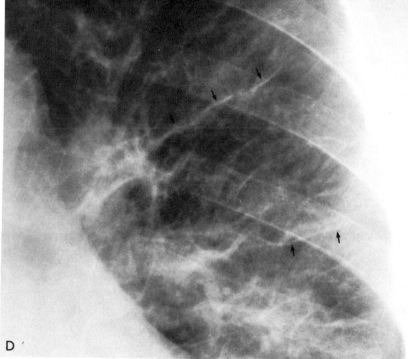

D

Figure 4–57 *Continued*
Illustration continued on opposite page

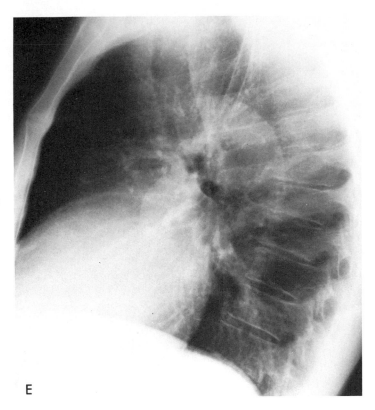

Figure 4–57 *Continued*

E

which the alveolar wall is widened without much associated distortion of lung architecture. Since the number of alveoli in the human lung ranges from 300 to 600 million,[89] it is most unlikely that an increase in the wall thickness of these tiny structures could produce individually identifiable roentgenographic opacities. As with interstitial pulmonary edema that widens the alveolar wall, it is probable that such an abnormality can result in a ground-glass opacity over the lungs, although we acknowledge that minor involvement may be associated with a normal chest roentgenogram.[15] Resolution of this perceptual uncertainty can be achieved by using the increased densitometric capability of CT.[17]

Generalized interstitial diseases may affect all parenchymal elements to varying degrees, although involvement of the interstitium is predominant. For example, in desquamative interstitial pneumonitis (fibrosing alveolitis), the morphologic picture is not one of simple thickening of alveolar walls with maintenance of pulmonary architecture but also of an abundance of macrophages within the alveoli; thus, the disease affects both interstitium and air spaces. In its advanced stages the disease obliterates alveoli and dilates bronchioles proximal to obliterated acini, resulting in severe disorganization of lung architecture characteristic of the so-called honeycomb pattern and end-stage lung (*see* later on).

The concept of predominance is important. Those who criticize the logic of dividing diffuse lung disease into interstitial and air-space patterns[90] state that histologically the majority of diseases affect both anatomic compartments to some degree

and that their distinction is therefore arbitrary. This is perhaps true, but we submit that the division is nevertheless valid if one accepts the concept of *predominant* involvement: an acinar pattern indicates *predominant* involvement of the parenchymal air spaces, and a nodular or reticular pattern indicates *predominant* involvement of the interstitium. Bearing this in mind, pattern recognition becomes a logical and useful technique in roentgenologic interpretation.

Roentgenographic Patterns of Diffuse Interstitial Disease

Confusion in the interpretation of diffuse lung disease is not surprising—not only are the patterns numerous and extremely varied but also until recently our knowledge suffered from a lack of accurate roentgenologic/pathologic correlation. Genereux[91] has recently detailed the morphologic basis for the four fundamental interstitial patterns and, although the specific etiology cannot be firmly established without histologic examination, broad categories of disease entities can now be appropriately suggested by the roentgenologist.

Much of the confusion concerning diffuse interstitial lung disease has arisen because of doubt over precisely what is seen and what can be seen on a chest roentgenogram. For example, it might be logical to assume that a network of opacities forming a reticular pattern should be produced by linear accumulations of tissue within the lung; or, conversely, that a nodular pattern should be produced

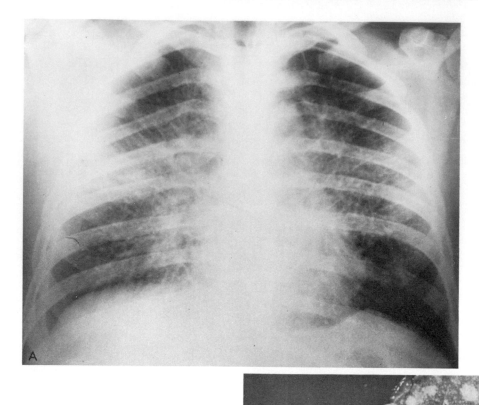

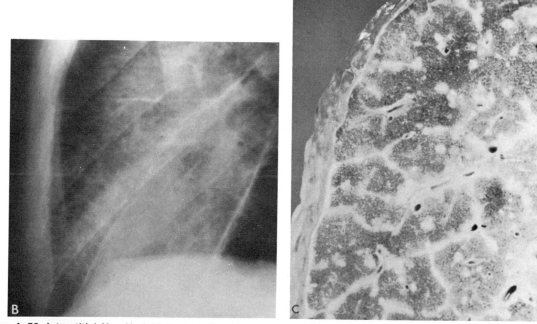

Figure 4–58. Interstitial Non-Hodgkin's Lymphoma. *A,* A posteroanterior roentgenogram reveals extensive involvement of both lungs by a rather coarse reticular pattern. The severity of interstitial abnormality is reflected in a loss of definition of vascular markings throughout both lungs, reminiscent of severe interstitial edema. *B,* A magnified view of the retrosternal area from a lateral roentgenogram reveals a coarse network of linear opacities, many of which are oriented perpendicular to the plane of the sternum in the form of septal lines. *C,* A photograph of the anterior portion of the lung removed at necropsy and sliced in a sagittal plane reveals extensive thickening of the interlobular septa and perivascular interstitial tissues. The patient was an 18-year-old male with non-Hodgkin's lymphoma.

by multiple nodular lesions throughout the lungs. Clearly, such an assumption is only partly valid; the roentgenographic effect of *superimposition* of many layers of opacities within the lungs is poorly understood, but there is little doubt that superimposition creates largely unpredictable variations in pattern. This raises one of the most fascinating issues of the interpretation of diffuse lung disease—the controversial question of summation of images (precise superimposition of identical shadows in the direction of the roentgen beam). The principle of summation has been invoked by many to explain the roentgenographic visibility of multiple shadows which, individually, would be too small to cast a roentgenographic shadow—for example, the lesions of miliary tuberculosis. However, studies carried out by Resink[92] strongly suggest that summation of shadows is not the method by which multiple subliminal opacities (below the limit of roentgenologic visibility) become supraliminal (roentgenologically visible); in fact, Resink believes that in such circumstances individual shadows become visible *only when they are not summated.* Genereux[91] studied the question of summation using household sponges and garden seeds. An artificial reticular or reticulonodular pattern was created by radiographing various layers of water-impregnated, frozen household sponges (Fig. 4–59), and it was shown that some of the "cysts" visible with two layers of sponges could also be identified, basically unchanged, with six or eight layers. However, in some areas the pattern was not faithfully reproduced, and it was concluded that it represents a summation effect caused by the superimposition of the various layers. We and others[93, 94] are therefore of the opinion that this radiographic pattern is determined by factors that are both nonsummated (lesions closest to the film)[92] and summated (lesions more removed from the film). A synthetic nodular pattern (Fig. 4–59) also can be created by dispersing garden peas in various layers and differing concentrations in a plastic mold. Radiographs of this model show that peas measuring 5 to 7 mm can be individually identified, but when superimposition causes several peas to be nearly perfectly aligned, the roentgenogram shows only a single nodular opacity; however, the latter differs qualitatively from the single nodule in that it is radiographically more opaque. Implicit to this observation is the phenomenon of subtraction due to superimposition—i.e., at least one of the nodules has been deleted from the true number forming the summated images.[25] Thus, like a reticular pattern, a nodular pattern can represent either a true or a summated image. Superimposition of small nodules, simulated by clustered millet seeds, can cause an apparent reduction in the size of the individual nodules and in the formation of curvilinear and nodular opacities (i.e., false reticulonodularity) (Fig. 4–59).

One other facet of this problem deserves mention. The four basic roentgenographic patterns of interstitial disease are reticular, nodular, reticulonodular, and linear. Although reticular and nodular patterns exist in pure forms, it is probable that most interstitial diseases show a mixed reticulonodular architecture. In some, the pattern may begin as reticular and be transformed into a relatively pure nodular pattern as the disease progresses; such a transformation has been emphasized by Wholey and associates in fibrosing alveolitis and interstitial pulmonary fibrosis.[82] Similarly, it is logical that in a reticular network, particularly if it is coarse, many linear densities will be seen *en face* and thus appear as a reticular pattern roentgenographically, but many must be seen on end and thus simulate nodules. This dual roentgenographic pattern produced by purely reticular disease was emphasized by Stolberg and his coworkers, who studied it in pulmonary Hodgkin's disease.[88] Because of this obvious visual effect, it might appear logical to designate all these diseases "reticulonodular"; however, as is shown later on, the distinction between reticular and nodular diseases not only possesses certain morphologic significance but also may be important in relation to the effects each may exert on pulmonary function.

Although recognizing these several problems in the field of diffuse interstitial lung disease, nevertheless it is tempting to devise a classification based on recognizable roentgenographic patterns of disease. The following is not a detailed description of specific disease processes but rather a descriptive classification of *patterns* of disease; in each instance an attempt is made to relate roentgenographic pattern to morphology.

Before discussing specific roentgenographic manifestations of diffuse interstitial lung diseases, we shall indicate the roentgenologic changes common to all and without which the purely interstitial site of involvement should be doubted. Since the disease is anatomically interstitial, the acini remain air-containing, although their volume may be reduced by such effects as cicatrization. Therefore, *diffuse interstitial disease must be of inhomogeneous roentgenographic density*; in most cases this feature alone distinguishes interstitial from air-space disease. Secondly, and for the same reason, the airways seldom are involved significantly so that, by and large, there is nothing to prevent air from reaching the lung parenchyma. Therefore, *volume reduction due to airway obstruction is not a feature of interstitial disease.*

McLoud and her colleagues[95] have devised a new scheme for a semiquantitative description of diffuse infiltrative lung diseases that uses the terminology of the International Labor Office for describing the pneumoconioses. They use the designations p, q, r to describe the various sizes of rounded opacities (corresponding to our nodular pattern) and s, t, u to categorize irregular opacities (corresponding to our reticular pattern). In addition, they included a third group of opacities called x, y, z corresponding to reticulonodular patterns,

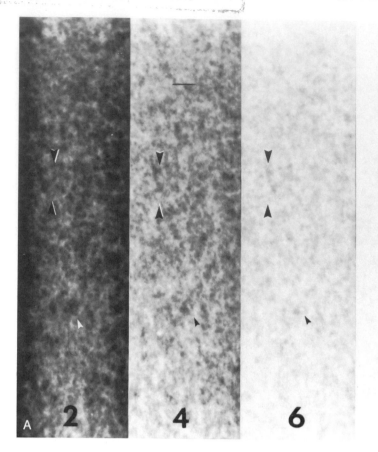

Figure 4–59. Experimental Basis for Reticulonodular and Nodular Patterns. In *A*, artificial reticular and reticulonodular patterns have been created by radiographing layers of water-impregnated, frozen household sponges. The radiographic factors were constant for the various layers, accounting for over- and underpenetration at 2 and 8 layer levels respectively. Note that despite superimposition, the basic pattern formed with a small number of sponges persists at the 6-sponge level (*between arrowheads*), although the superimposition diminishes clarity of the pattern (*small arrowheads*).

Illustration continued on opposite page

and "ground glass" to describe alveolar patterns. We agree that this classification provides an understandable and quantifiable system of communication and a tool for teaching, clinical research, and epidemiologic studies, but we believe that the more traditional nomenclature satisfies the usual clinical requirements and prefer to recognize four basic roentgenographic patterns of interstitial disease: (1) reticular, (2) nodular, (3) reticulonodular, and (4) linear. These patterns, correlated with their CT equivalents, are listed in Table 4–2.

RETICULAR PATTERN

This consists of a network of curvilinear opacities, conceptually a series of rings surrounding spaces of air density. The precise pattern of reticulation depends upon several variables; the two most important are the degree of thickening of the interstitial space and the effect that the interstitial involvement exerts on parenchymal air spaces. It is useful to describe a reticular pattern according to the size of the "net"; accordingly, the terms fine, medium, and coarse, although arbitrary, are in wide use and appear to be generally acceptable. *Fine* reticulation simulates a very fine mesh (e.g., as in a nylon stocking) (Fig. 4–60); this pattern, also sometimes referred to as a ground-glass pattern, is easily overlooked or confused with either subacinar stippling or interstitial micronodularity (*see* further on). At the opposite end of the spectrum, *coarse* reticulation is characterized by large cystic spaces, 1 cm

or more in diameter, ringed by soft tissue (Fig. 4–61). Between these two extremes lies *medium* reticulation (Fig. 4–62), characterized by 3 to 10 mm cystic spaces. The designation "honeycomb" pattern

Table 4–2. Patterns of Interstitial Disease: Conventional Roentgenographic and CT Appearance*

PATTERN	CONVENTIONAL ROENTGENOGRAPHY	CT
Reticular		
Fine	yes	groundglass micronodular
Medium	yes	yes
Coarse	yes	yes
Nodular		
Micronodular	yes	groundglass micronodular
Small	yes	yes
Medium	yes	yes
Large	yes	yes
Reticulonodular	yes	yes
Linear		
Bronchoarterial	yes	yes or nodular
Venous	yes	yes or nodular
Interlobar		
A	yes	yes
B	yes	yes

*Spatial resolution on CT scanning devices is insufficient to depict a fine reticular or micronodular pattern. Both these patterns are displayed on CT as a focal or diffuse ground-glass opacity, with or without an accompanying granular appearance. Branching tubular opacities on conventional roentgenograms may be identified as such on CT or as end-on nodular shadows.

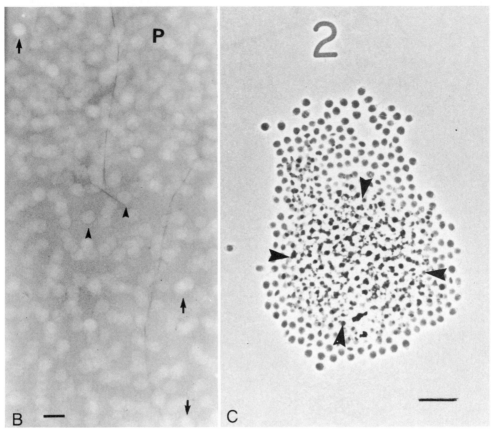

Figure 4–59 *Continued. B* is a radiograph of garden peas (P) imbedded in a plastic mold; approximately twice the number of peas are present in the upper half of the radiograph as in the lower half. Close visual correlation of the actual model (not shown) and the radiograph showed that the nodular pattern results from a single pea (*arrowheads*) or from the precise superimposition of several peas on one another (*arrows*). With superimposition, however, the nodule is more opaque. Dark lines transecting the specimen represent crack artifacts. Bar denotes 1 cm. *C* is a xeroradiograph of millet seeds in an attempt to simulate a miliary pattern. The seeds are clustered toward the center of the sample (*between arrowheads*). Although a single "miliary" nodule is visible, nodular opacities in the central area are perceived as being smaller and radiographically denser. Increased numbers and superimposition of small nodules create a curvilinear and nodular quality to the pattern, i.e., reticulonodularity. Bar denotes 1 cm. (From Genereux GP: Med Radiogr Photogr *61*:2, 1985.)

should be reserved for cystic spaces in the medium and coarse categories.

On CT, fine reticulation (Fig. 4–63) is manifested by an amorphous ground-glass opacity or as micronodularity (usually a fine granular pattern). The latter is uncommon and is invariably dispersed against a background of an amorphous opacity. Medium and coarse reticulation correlates closely with conventional roentgenograms (Fig. 4–63); indeed, CT often portrays these gross changes more clearly.[96, 97]

The reticular pattern results from an increase in the amount of tissue in the interstitial space of the lung, both axial and parenchymal, but whether involvement of the parenchymal interstitium *alone* produces roentgenographically demonstrable reticulation is somewhat controversial. Consider for a moment the geometry, dimensions, and morphology of the respiratory zone of the lung (*see* page 17): the adult lung contains approximately 300 × 10[6] alveoli whose walls in some areas are extremely thin (0.15 micron) and in thick areas measure no more than 1.0 micron in width. A pathologic process that uniformly thickens the wall of the alveoli by a

factor of 5 could cause a uniform haze over the lungs on a conventional chest roentgenogram, but we feel that it is highly unlikely that opacities would be created that would be individually identifiable as a fine reticular pattern. In this example, of course, we are visualizing a process that uniformly thickens alveolar walls with tissue of unit density (e.g., cellular infiltration). By contrast, consider a situation in which alveolar walls have been thickened by a substance of greater than unit density; for example, a contrast medium. An excellent example of roentgenologic/morphologic correlation has been provided by studies of the reaction that occurs in interstitial tissues after lymphangiography. Fraimow and colleagues,[99] who obtained pulmonary tissue by biopsy within 12 hours after the lymphatic injection of Ethiodol, found lipid droplets widely distributed throughout the pulmonary capillary bed, corresponding to a fine granular stippling observed throughout both lungs roentgenographically. Biopsy specimens obtained the day after lymphangiography revealed a smaller but still appreciable amount of lipid material in the parenchymal interstitial space, but no longer exclusively in the capil-

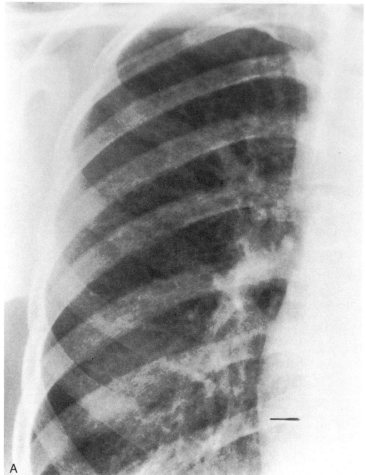

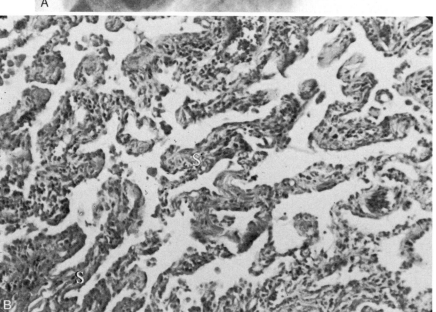

Figure 4–60. Reticular Interstitial Pattern. *A*, Detail view of the right lung from a PA chest roentgenogram reveals a fine reticulation similar to a nylon stocking; the appearance suggests diffuse interstitial lung disease without major distortion of lung architecture. Bar denotes 1 cm. *B*, A histologic section of a biopsy specimen reveals diffuse alveolar septal thickening (*S*) with infiltration of chronic inflammatory cells and fibrosis. Cystic spaces are not evident in this portion of the biopsy. These features are consistent with fibrosing alveolitis. (From Genereux GP: Med Radiogr Photogr *61*:2, 1985.)

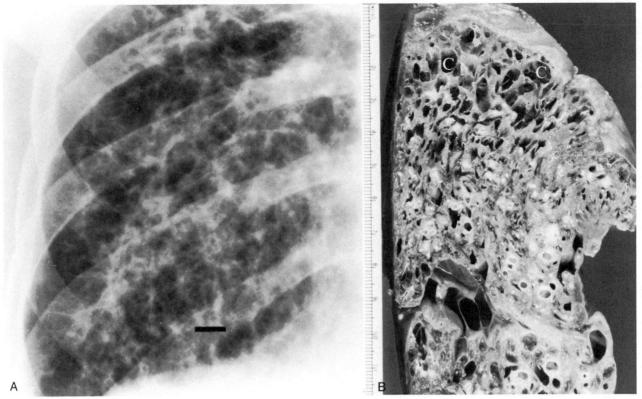

Figure 4–61. Reticular Interstitial Pattern (Honeycomb Lung). *A*, A closeup of the right lower lung zone from a PA chest roentgenogram shows a coarse reticulation, many of the cystic spaces exceeding 1 cm in diameter. Bar denotes 1 cm. *B*, An uninflated section of lung from the same patient at autopsy reveals gross disorganization of architecture characteristic of the end-stage lung. Note the variable size of the cystic spaces (*C*). The patient is a young male adult with eosinophilic granuloma. (From Genereux GP: Med Radiogr Photogr *61*:2, 1985.)

lary bed (much of it having passed into the extra-vascular interstitial tissues and, to a lesser extent, into the alveoli). In our experience and that of others,[98] roentgenograms at this stage may show a fine reticular pattern, sometimes revealed only on roentgenographically magnified images (Fig. 4–64). It is noteworthy that in the 20 patients studied by Fraimow and his associates,[99] the average diffusing capacity had decreased from 21.2 to 15.9 two hours after the injection, at a time when capillaries were blocked by oil embolism; gradual but incomplete improvement in diffusing capacity occurred over the next 24 hours, an effect that these researchers interpret as secondary, probably caused by the membrane component of the diffusion. Thus, these studies showed correlation between morphologic, roentgenologic, and functional abnormalities resultant upon lymphangiography. Despite the foregoing, we remain ambivalent regarding the relative roles played by the axial and parenchymal interstitial spaces in the production of a roentgenographic reticular pattern; when the parenchymal interstitium is involved predominantly, it is possible that summation is the mechanism by which abnormal images are produced.

The observation that different roentgenographic patterns of reticulation indicate different degrees of severity of interstitial replacement fos-

tered the concept of the *end-stage lung*.[100] The idea of an end-stage organ, implying a nonspecific pathogenetic, pathologic, and roentgenologic entity, has been widely accepted in chronic renal and liver disease. However, it is not generally appreciated that a similar situation prevails in the lungs, wherein many causes of diffuse lung disease, originally histologically distinct, can converge toward an appearance lacking specificity by both roentgenologic and pathologic criteria following longstanding and persistent activity. It is our feeling that this situation is best described radiologically by a noncommital designation such as the end-stage lung.

The fundamental underlying pathologic foundation is the fact that the lungs, like most other organs, can respond in only a relatively limited and stereotyped manner to a variety of insults, particularly during the chronic, reparative phase of a given disease. The concept of diffuse lung disease converging toward a final common end result is illustrated in Figure 4–65: only three of a large list of possible disorders have been depicted although the principle applies equally to the majority of other causes of diffuse lung disease, particularly those with a primary impact on the interstitium. In general, both vertical and horizontal factors influence this evolution. The *vertical* factors represent the gamut of diseases now capable of diffusely damag-

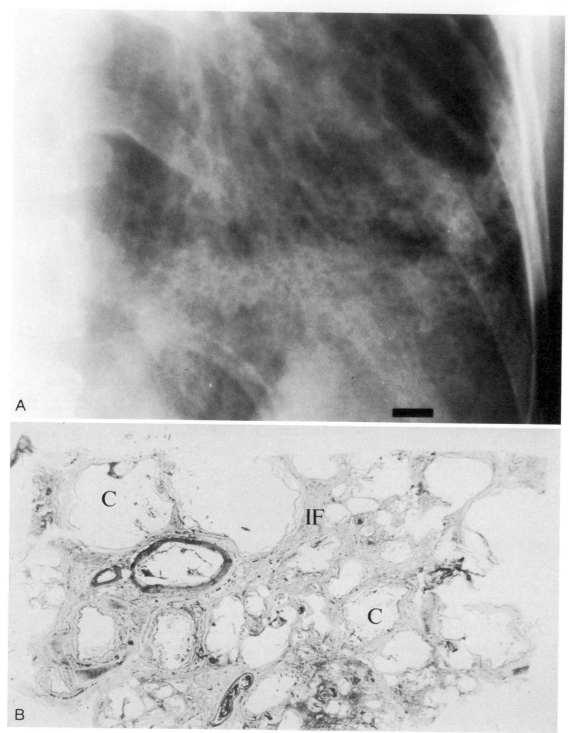

Figure 4–62. Reticular Interstitial Pattern. *A*, Detail view of the left lower lung zone from a PA chest roentgenogram reveals a medium reticular pattern characterized by multiple radiolucencies surrounded by curvilinear opacities. Bar denotes 1 cm. *B*, A histologic section of the left lower lobe obtained at autopsy demonstrates extensive fibrosis (*IF*) surrounding cystic spaces of variable size (*C*). Bar denotes 1 cm. The patient is a young woman with progressive systemic sclerosis. (From Genereux GP: Med Radiogr Photogr *61*:2, 1985.)

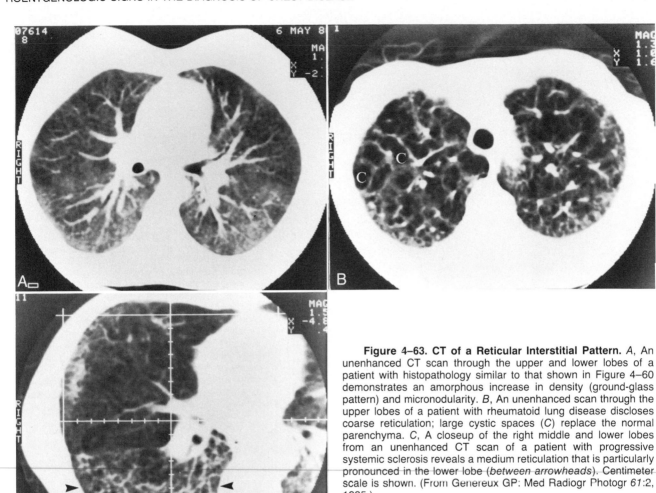

Figure 4–63. CT of a Reticular Interstitial Pattern. *A,* An unenhanced CT scan through the upper and lower lobes of a patient with histopathology similar to that shown in Figure 4–60 demonstrates an amorphous increase in density (ground-glass pattern) and micronodularity. *B,* An unenhanced scan through the upper lobes of a patient with rheumatoid lung disease discloses coarse reticulation; large cystic spaces (*C*) replace the normal parenchyma. *C,* A closeup of the right middle and lower lobes from an unenhanced CT scan of a patient with progressive systemic sclerosis reveals a medium reticulation that is particularly pronounced in the lower lobe (*between arrowheads*). Centimeter scale is shown. (From Genereux GP: Med Radiogr Photogr 61:2, 1985.)

ing the lungs, conservatively estimated at more than 250. However, it should be realized that each one of these has a *horizontal* component, which is influenced by the virulence of a particular disease, time, continuous or repeated exposure to the etiologic agent, or modifying factors such as therapy or complications. The process may be stopped or reversed at any point so that an end-stage appearance is not inevitable. However, these favorable results can be expected only if the horizontal components are altered either spontaneously or by therapeutic manipulation early in the course of a given disease, before irrevocable destruction has occurred.

It is stressed that the particular appearance to be described implies *only that a state of severe, irreversible, and chronic pathologic change has occurred; it should not be concluded that the patient is in imminent danger of terminal respiratory insufficiency.* Thus, the definition as herein applied is entirely morphologic and does not necessarily connote common physiologic abnormalities. Nevertheless, it is true that most patients who manifest the roentgenologic and path-

ologic features described subsequently will display a restrictive pattern on pulmonary function testing.

The end-stage lung is characterized pathologically by certain common features (Table 4–3). Grossly, the pleural surfaces are irregularly nodular and thickened, imparting a "bosselated"[101] or "hobnailed"[102] appearance caused by the presence of numerous subpleural cystic spaces that are invariably ringed by fibrotic tissue. The lungs may be shrunken, firm, and noncrepitant (Fig. 4–66A), or they may be enlarged when emphysematous change prevails (Fig. 4–66B). On cut section, the cystic spaces can be identified both subpleurally and deeper within the parenchyma. Throughout the lungs, cysts are irregular in both distribution and size, ranging in diameter from 1 mm to more than 2.5 cm; they are usually contiguous, superficially resembling a honeycomb in appearance. The walls of the cystic areas also vary in thickness and are composed of a mixture of different types of soft tissue elements.[93, 94, 103–109] Many cysts may be partly or completely filled with mucus.

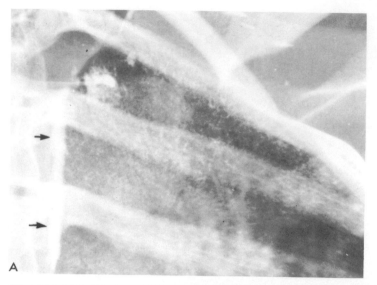

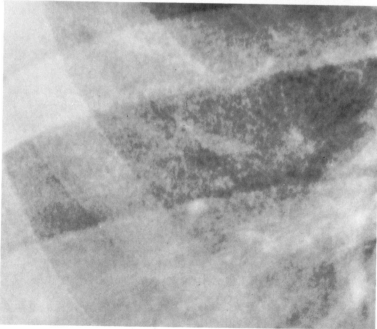

Figure 4–64. The Reticulonodular Pattern. *A,* A magnified view of the apex of the left upper lobe approximately 1½ hours following the injection of 7 ml of Lipiodol into the lymphatics of each leg reveals a fine network of shadows of high density. This network is caused by the presence of contrast medium in the microvascular circulation of the lung. The thoracic duct can be identified on the left *(arrows).* Twenty-four hours later a fine stippled pattern is present throughout both lungs, distributed diffusely and evenly; this pattern is so fine that it is barely visible on a standard roentgenogram, but with primary and secondary magnification (B) reveals itself as a fine reticular pattern (the nodular component is thought to be due to viewing line shadows on end).

Microscopically, the end-stage lung is characterized by (a) thickening of the alveolar septa due to chronic inflammatory cell infiltration or fibrosis or both (Fig. 4–67), (b) dissolution of the alveolar septa, resulting in enlargement of the alveolar spaces (alveolar simplification), (c) dilatation of the terminal and respiratory bronchioles, (d) smooth muscle proliferation in the septa and around the bronchioles and lymphatics (Fig. 4–67), (e) proliferation and degenerative changes in the arterioles and venules, (f) obliteration of the microvascular (capillary) circulation, (g) hypertrophy of the bronchial artery, with precapillary anastamoses to the pulmonary circulation, (h) air-space and interstitial foci of lipid-laden histiocytes (endogenous lipid pneumonitis), (i) osseous metaplasia of the mesenchymal tissue (Fig. 4–67), and (j) proliferative changes in the bronchiolar and alveolar epithelium,

ranging from hyperplasia to metaplasia and occasionally neoplasia (Fig. 4–67).[103–105, 110–120] The process is seldom uniform throughout the lungs, either grossly or microscopically, so areas of relatively uninvolved or normal lung tissue may persist. The latter are occasionally of diagnostic importance, since they can reveal early histologic evidence of the original process, thereby permitting an etiologic diagnosis to be made or at least suggested.

The pathogenesis of the cystic spaces has now been reasonably well established (Fig. 4–68) and is related to the deposition of foreign material, irrespective of its nature, within the interstitium (Fig. 4–68). Correlative studies have shown that most cysts are related to bronchiolectasia and alveolar septal dissolution with lumen enlargement. Obliteration of the microvascular circulation, with resultant ischemia, promotes the rupture of septa. Certain

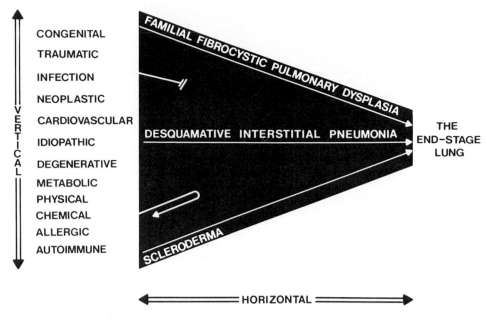

Figure 4–65. Evolutionary Trends in Diffuse Lung Disease. A general pathologic classification of disease is listed in the vertical column. A large number of specific disorders may be included under each of these broad categories, but only three are included in the diagram. The horizontal factors can influence the pathogenicity of each disease in a different manner (see text). There is a distinct tendency for all disorders to telescope toward a final common appearance, the end-stage lung (ESL). The process may cease (———//) or reverse (⇄) before irreparable damage has occurred. (Reprinted from Genereux GP: Radiology 116:279, 1975.)

interstitial diseases show a predilection for involvement of the lower lobes and, by increasing lung weight, may create additional tension and rupture of mid and upper zone alveolar septa already damaged by concurrent inflammation and fibrosis. In this regard, the mechanism is analogous to that proposed for the development and upper zonal predominance of cystic spaces in centrilobular emphysema, in which increased stress resulting from a more negative pleural pressure and the weight of the lung is thought to favor the anatomic bias displayed by the cysts.[120] Thus, in end-stage lung, the cystic spaces may be larger in the upper than in the lower zones (Fig. 4–69). Bronchiolar stenosis or obliteration, augmented by collateral air drift, results in the third type of cystic spaces, obstructive emphysema.

Usually, several of these pathologic criteria are present simultaneously, a fact that has created considerable confusion in terminology. Table 4–3 lists some of the synonyms used by various authors to describe widespread severe parenchymal damage resulting from diffuse lung disease. In many instances, it was these workers' opinions that each pathologic abnormality represented a separate and distinct entity; however, close scrutiny of the morphologic descriptions in these reports suggests that the terminology employed usually reflected quantitative rather than qualitative pathologic differences. For example, when the fibrotic component is dominant and the specific cause cannot be ascertained, the terms usual interstitial pneumonia,[94] Hamman-Rich syndrome,[102, 103, 115] idiopathic pulmonary fibrosis,[108] or fibrosing alveolitis[114] have been employed. By contrast, when the cystic spaces are very extensive, the terms honeycomb lung[103, 106, 107] and bronchiolar emphysema[121–123] are likely to be used. Some

have been so impressed by the smooth muscle proliferation that the terms muscular cirrhosis of the lung[93, 108] and pulmonary muscular hyperplasia,[124, 125] with or without bronchiolectasis,[93, 108, 126] have been coined as appropriate descriptors.

The conventional chest roentgenogram reveals a lung volume that is decreased, normal, or increased, depending upon which of the various pathologic features predominates (Table 4–3). For example, when fibrosis is dominant, the lungs are typically shrunken and poorly inflated (Fig. 4–70), whereas when obstructive bronchiolar phenomena have been in effect, lungs tend to have a large volume, as in some cases of eosinophilic granuloma, sarcoidosis, or pulmonary leiomyomatosis (Fig. 4–70). The reticular or reticulonodular pattern characteristically involves most portions of both lungs, although often not symmetrically, either from side-to-side or from lobe-to-lobe within one lung. Cystic spaces are surrounded by a rim of soft tissue that varies in thickness, and the cysts themselves vary considerably in size, the most frequent and characteristic being less than 1 cm in diameter whereas the largest may be 2.5 cm or more. When these spaces become filled with fluid or cellular material, a distal air-space pattern ensues, masking even pronounced reticulation which is the hallmark of predominant interstitial disease. The pleura may show thickening due to fibrosis, edema, or calcification, while rupture of subpleural cysts into the pleural cavity can result in spontaneous pneumothorax. Cardiovascular changes indicative of pulmonary arterial hypertension and cor pulmonale are apt to be present at this stage. In some instances, metaplastic foci of bone develop in more severely damaged areas of the lung, giving rise to calcific nodules 1 to 3 mm in size (Fig. 4–71). In rare

Table 4–3. The End-stage Lung

TERMINOLOGY	PATHOLOGY	RADIOLOGY
Usual interstitial pneumonia	*Gross*	*Lung Volume*
The honeycomb lung	Firm, shrunken, or enlarged	Decreased, normal, or increased
Hamman-Rich syndrome	Thickened, nodular pleura	*Interstitial Pattern*
"Chronic" Hamman-Rich syndrome	Cystic spaces	Reticular or reticulonodular
Idiopathic pulmonary fibrosis	Edema, pneumonia	Medium or coarse
Diffuse pulmonary fibrosis	*Microscopic*	Asymmetric involvement
Fibrosing alveolitis (preferred)	Thickened alveolar septa	Chronic
Muscular cirrhosis of the lung	Cystic spaces	*Pleural Thickening*
Pulmonary muscular hyperplasia	Bronchiolectasia	*Cor Pulmonale*
Pulmonary muscular hyperplasia with	Smooth muscle hyperplasia	*Other*
bronchiolectasia	Vascular sclerosis	Lymph node enlargement
Bronchiolar emphysema	Lipid degeneration	Pneumothorax
	Osseous metaplasia	Calcific nodules
	Bronchopulmonary anastomoses	Scar carcinoma
	Epithelial proliferation	

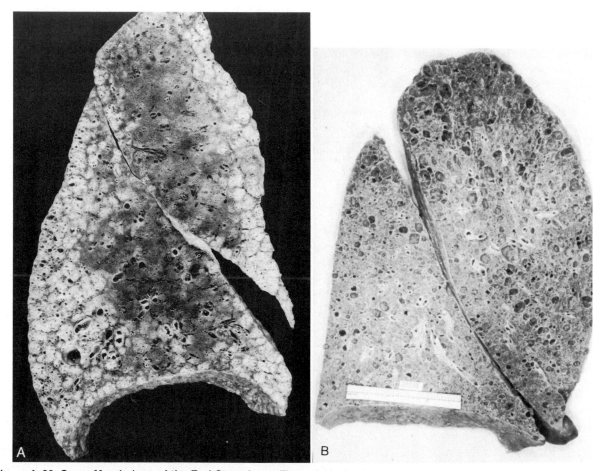

Figure 4–66. Gross Morphology of the End-Stage Lung. The variable appearance of the gross morphology is exemplified in these two patients with end-stage fibrosing alveolitis (*A*) and idiopathic leiomyomatosis (*B*). The lung can be firm, shrunken, and noncrepitant as in the fibrotic pattern in *A* or enlarged when emphysematous changes prevail as in *B*. The common features include an irregularly nodular and thickened pleural surface and the presence of numerous subpleural and central cystic spaces. (*B* reprinted from Genereux GP: Radiology *116*:279, 1975.)

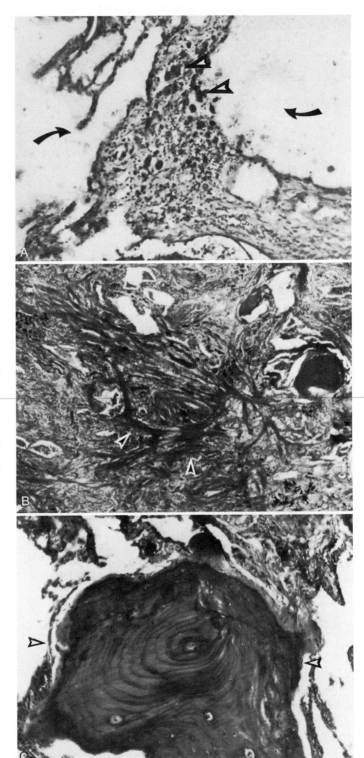

Figure 4–67. Microscopic Morphology of the End-Stage Lung. *A,* A histologic section of lung from a patient with eosinophilic granuloma reveals distortion and thickening of alveolar septa by an inflammatory cellular reaction and fibrosis, resulting in rupture of alveolar septa (*curved arrows*) and "alveolar simplification." Extensive deposits of lipid material representing endogenous lipid pneumonitis are visible in the interstitium (*arrowheads*). End-stage fibrosing alveolitis can be manifested by smooth muscle hyperplasia (*arrowheads*) (*B*), osseous metaplasia (*arrowheads*) (*C*), and a spectrum of epithelial cellular proliferation (*D*): bronchiolar epithelial hyperplasia (*top left*), Type II cell hyperplasia (*top right*), squamous metaplasia (*bottom right*), and bronchioloalveolar cell carcinoma (*bottom left*).

Illustration continued on following page

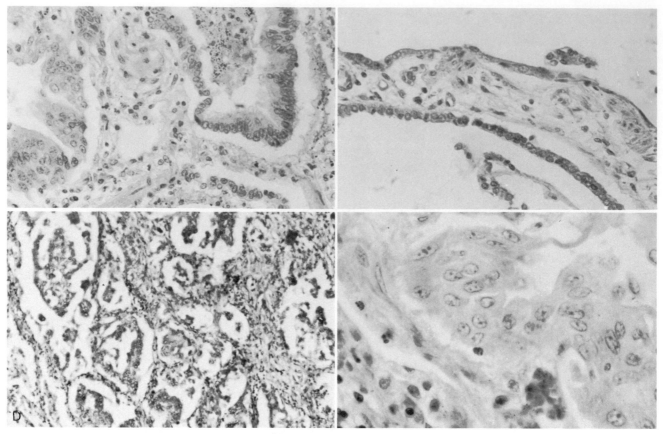

Figure 4–67 *Continued*

instances, carcinoma may develop, appearing as either a nodular mass or as an area of air-space consolidation (Fig. 4–71*B*).

Medium reticulation, as herein defined, is characterized by cystic spaces ranging in diameter from 3 to 10 mm; although the term "honeycomb" is not our preferred descriptive appellation for this pattern, we suggest that if it must be used, it be restricted to these size criteria. To the best of our knowledge, the term was coined to describe the roentgenographic pattern seen in the late stages of

eosinophilic granuloma, in which air-containing cystic spaces 3 to 10 mm in diameter are surrounded by thick walls. Undoubtedly, the term honeycomb is overused; although it has gained some popularity in recent years and has been applied to a great variety of roentgenographic patterns (too many in our estimation), we feel it should be reserved for an appearance that bees might have a reasonable expectation of recognizing! This position is in direct conflict with that of Friedman,[13] who states that "use of the term in radiology is derived from its appli-

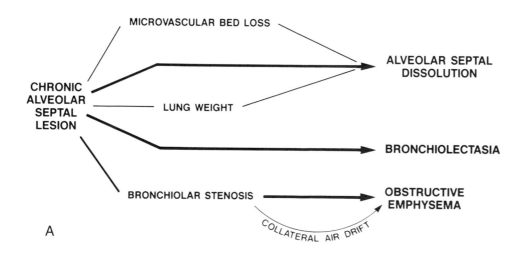

Figure 4–68. Pathogenesis of Cystic Spaces in the End-Stage Lung. *A,* Three features—alveolar wall dissolution, bronchiolectasia, and obstructive emphysema—characterize the cystic spaces, facilitated by a chronic alveolar septal lesion augmented by ischemia, bronchiolar stenosis, and increased lung weight.

Illustration continued on opposite page

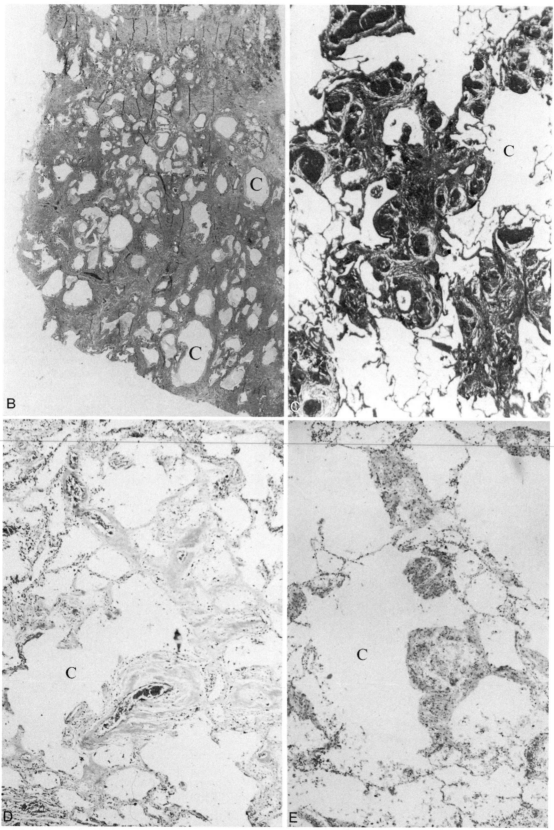

Figure 4–68 *Continued* Microscopic cystic spaces (*C*) resulting from alveolar simplification are illustrated in patients with fibrosing alveolitis (*B*), sarcoidosis (*C*), amyloidosis (*D*), and idiopathic leiomyomatosis (*E*). The presence and not the type of alveolar septal lesion is sufficient to cause this type of cyst. (From Genereux GP: Med Radiogr Photogr *61*:2, 1985.)

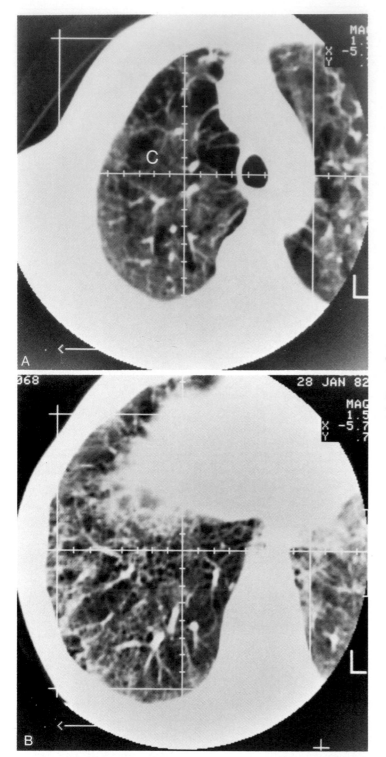

Figure 4–69. Influence of Lung Stress on Cyst Size in the End-Stage Lung. In this patient with rheumatoid lung disease, CT scans of the right lung reveal the average cyst (*C*) in the upper lobe (*A*) to be larger than that in the lower lobe (*B*) as a result of increased stress on upper zone parenchyma from the more negative intrapleural pressure and increased lung weight at the base where fibrosis is most marked. Centimeter scale is depicted. (From Genereux GP: Med Radiogr Photogr *61*:2, 1985.)

cation in pathology, not apiculture." Perhaps true, but what we are looking at is a roentgenogram, not a histologic section: to follow Friedman's recommendation that the term should be employed to describe focal lucencies of *any* size seems to sink us still deeper into a semantic morass of little utility.

The roentgenographic pattern of honeycombing may be produced by a number of diseases, including eosinophilic granuloma, fibrosing alveo-litis (idiopathic pulmonary fibrosis), rheumatoid lung, pulmonary lymphangiomyomatosis, progressive systemic sclerosis, asbestosis, chronic interstitial fungal infections, and occasionally end-stage sarcoidosis. Anatomic predominance of the pattern aids considerably in the differential diagnosis; for example, eosinophilic granuloma and sarcoidosis often show a predilection for the upper lung zones, whereas the remainder of the diseases just listed tend to a lower zonal predominance. It is clear from this short list that restriction of the term honeycomb lung to the pattern described here reduces the diagnostic possibilities to relatively few diseases, especially if one takes into account anatomic bias. We submit that this is the only way to bring some order to the confusion that surrounds diffuse interstitial lung disease.

NODULAR PATTERN

A nodular pattern is produced when spherical lesions accumulate within the interstitium. The interstitial nodule differs fundamentally from its airspace counterpart in that it is homogeneous, well-circumscribed, and of variable size. The last-named feature permits further subdivision—micronodular

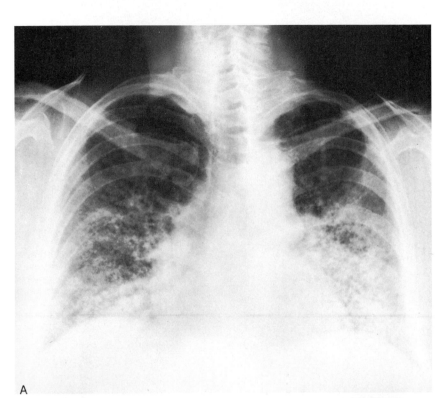

Figure 4–70. Roentgenographic Features of the End-Stage Lung. Posteroanterior (*A*) and lateral (*B*) chest roentgenograms demonstrate a diffuse, medium reticular pattern, more marked in the lower zones, particularly the left. Overall lung volume is diminished. In this middle-aged man with severe fibrosing alveolitis, the heart is moderately enlarged as are the main and hilar pulmonary arteries, indicating the presence of pulmonary arterial hypertension and cor pulmonale.

Illustration continued on following page

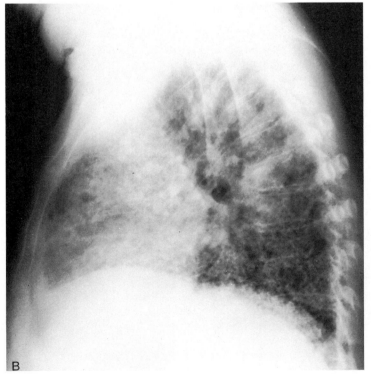

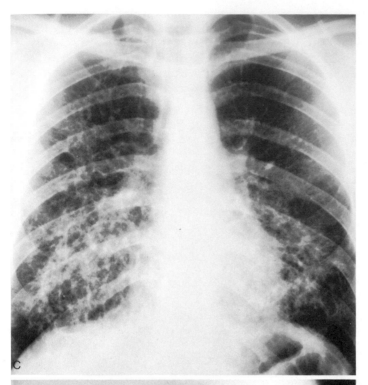

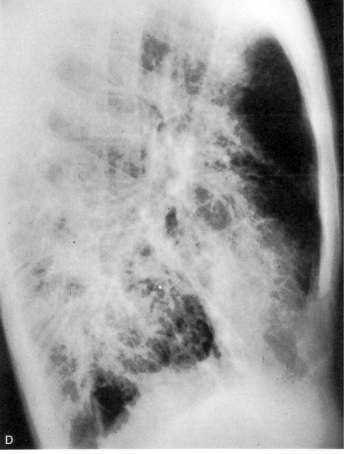

Figure 4–70 *Continued.* In another young man with end-stage lung caused by eosinophilic granuloma, posteroanterior (*C*) and lateral (*D*) chest roentgenograms show a coarse reticular pattern; distribution throughout the lungs is asymmetric, the lower lobes being more prominently involved than the upper and the right lung more than the left. This basal anatomic predominance is uncommon in histiocytosis X in which upper lung zones are usually more severely involved. Overall lung volume is increased. (From Genereux GP: Radiology *116*:279, 1975.)

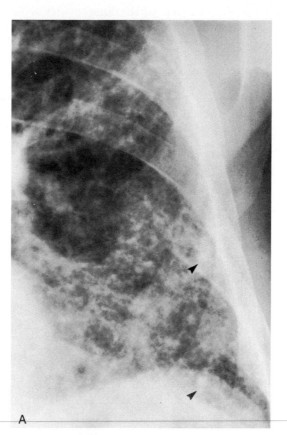

Figure 4–71. Unusual Roentgenographic Features of the End-Stage Lung. *A*, A closeup of the left lower lung zone from a posteroanterior chest roentgenogram reveals multiple nodules ranging in size from 1 to 3 mm; some of the nodules are opaque enough to suggest the presence of calcification (*arrowheads*). Metaplastic foci of bone were identified on the lung biopsy specimen (*see* Figure 4–67C). The patient was a middle-aged man with fibrosing alveolitis. *B*, In another man with end-stage fibrosing alveolitis, a posteroanterior chest roentgenogram demonstrates a large, inhomogeneous area of air-space consolidation in the right upper lobe, medium-to-coarse reticulation throughout both lungs, right hilar node enlargement, and chronic cor pulmonale. At autopsy, the upper lobe consolidation was found to be caused by bronchioloalveolar carcinoma and the hilar node enlargement by metastases. (From Genereux GP: Radiology *116*:279, 1975.)

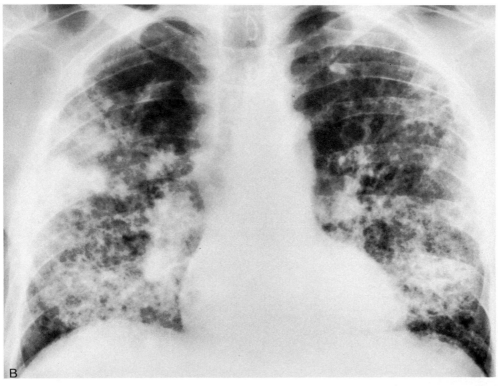

(less than 1 mm), small (1 to 3 mm), medium (3 to 5 mm), and large (5 to 10 mm or more).

Nodular interstitial disease of the lungs is perhaps best epitomized by hematogenous infection such as miliary tuberculosis (Fig. 4–72). Since the infecting organism reaches the lung via the circulation and is trapped in the capillary sieve, it must be purely interstitial in location (at least early in its course; as the infection spreads, it may involve acinar air spaces). As the tubercles grow, they create a micronodular or small nodular pattern. Early

disseminated hematogenous carcinomatosis can have an identical appearance. The interstitial location of these hematogenous diseases is clearly established by the pathogenesis, but many other diseases of widely differing pathogenesis exert their earliest morphologic change in the interstitial space. For example, intravenous injection of talc particles associated with drug abuse (Fig. 4–72) and certain inhalation diseases such as silicosis[128] are characterized by the formation of discrete nodular lesions within the interstitial space. Similarly, sarcoidosis

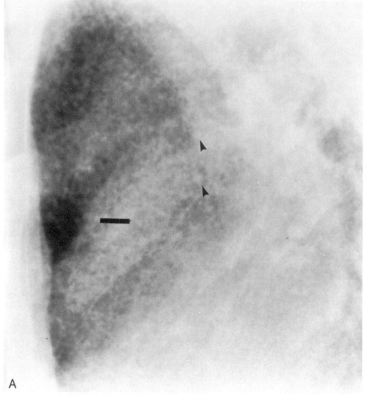

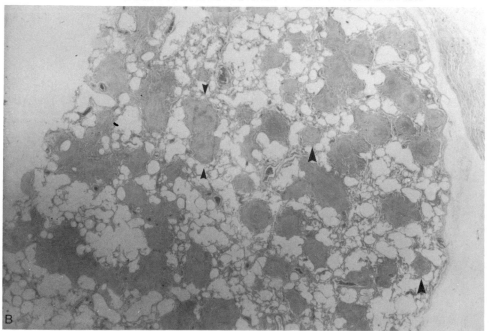

Figure 4–72. Nodular Interstitial Patterns. *A*, In a patient with miliary tuberculosis, a detail view of the retrosternal lung from a lateral chest roentgenogram shows isolated and confluent small nodular opacities; some of the nodules are denser (whiter) (*arrowheads*) than others, presumably as a result of summation. Bar denotes 1 cm. *B*, A histologic section of the biopsy specimen from this patient discloses isolated (*single arrowheads*) and confluent (*between arrowheads*) caseating granulomas.

Illustration continued on opposite page

may be associated with multiple, well-defined nodular shadows throughout the interstitium, ranging in diameter from 1 to 10 mm.[129]

Occasionally, a nodular pattern of diffuse interstitial lung disease, particularly the micronodular variety, can be confused with the subacinar pattern of air-space disease, best exemplified by alveolar microlithiasis.[130] The latter is characteized roentgenographically by tiny, discrete nodular opacities and subacinar nodules widely distributed throughout the lungs; however, the minute "calcispherites" are located entirely within the alveoli.

On CT, small, medium, and large nodules can be readily identified (Fig. 4–73),[25] whereas micronodularity creates an amorphous opacity or fine granularity[15] indistinguishable from the CT pattern of fine reticulation (Fig. 4–73B).

RETICULONODULAR PATTERN

Although a curvilinear network throughout the interstitial tissues usually presents roentgenographically as a reticular pattern, orientation of some linear opacities parallel to the x-ray beam sometimes suggests a nodular component in addition to the reticular (Fig. 4–74). Although in any given situation a reticulonodular pattern can be produced by this mechanism, it can also result from an admixture of nodular deposits and diffuse curvilinear thickening throughout the interstitium—for example, in

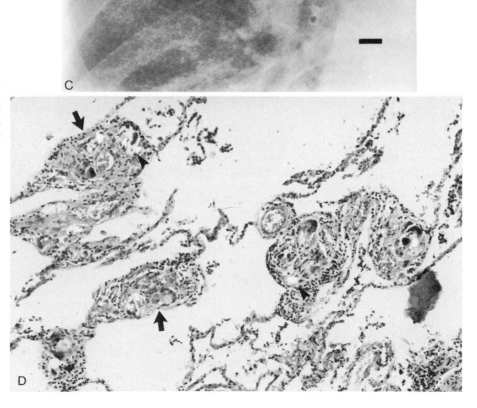

Figure 4–72 *Continued.* C, In a patient with intravenous talc-induced granulomatosis, a detail view of the right lung from a PA chest roentgenogram reveals innumerable micronodules measuring less than 1 mm in diameter. This pattern can be confused with subacinar stippling (compare with Figure 4–4B), but the absence of subacinar nodules is an important differentiating point. Bar denotes 1 cm. *D,* A histologic section of lung from the patient in *C* reveals isolated and coalescent noncaseating interstitial granulomas (*arrows*). Polarized light revealed optically active talc particles (*arrowheads*) in the granulomas. (From Genereux GP: Med Radiogr Photogr *61:*2, 1985.)

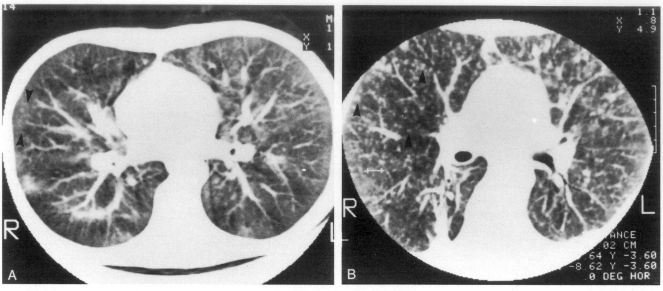

Figure 4–73. CT of Nodular Interstitial Patterns. *A,* A CT scan through the lower lobes of a patient with intravenous talc-induced pulmonary granulomatosis shows a diffuse, amorphous increase in CT density (ground-glass pattern). Superimposed micronodularity is suggested in some areas (*between arrowheads*). *B* is a CT scan of a middle-aged woman with miliary tuberculosis; small nodular opacities (*arrowheads*) are widely distributed throughout both lungs. Bar denotes 1 cm. (From Genereux GP: Med Radiogr Photogr *61*:2, 1985.)

sarcoidosis (Fig. 4–74). The CT depiction of reticulonodularity reflects the pattern seen on conventional roentgenograms.

LINEAR PATTERN

A linear pattern results from thickening in or around the bronchoarterial bundles, the perivenous interstitium, or the interlobular septa (Kerley A and B lines) (Fig. 4–75); sometimes all three areas are involved simultaneously. Septal lines effectively restrict the diagnostic considerations to hydrostatic interstitial edema and lymphangitic malignancy, usually with simultaneous involvement of bronchoarterial and perivenous spaces. When the linear pattern is localized to the bronchoarterial sheaths, diagnostic implications are different and include conditions such as cystic fibrosis, bronchiectasis, atopic asthma, dysproteinemia, and the "increased markings" variety of emphysema. Diffuse pleonemia (e.g., in left-to-right cardiac shunts) occasionally can be confused with diffuse linear or nodular disease by increasing the visibility of fully distended and recruited small intrapulmonary vessels. However, disproportionate dilatation of arteries in relation to bronchi in the perihilar regions (arteries are normally only slightly larger than contiguous bronchi) and the increased size of pulmonary veins usually permit roentgenographic distinction.

On CT, the bronchoarterial and perivenous bundles in the upper and to a lesser degree the lower lobes tend to be oriented perpendicular to the transverse plane of the scan; as a consequence, thickening of these structures is exquisitely demonstrable. However, the tomographic quality of the study, coupled with the plane of the scan, mandates

that the thickening is portrayed either as well-defined, lobulated nodular opacities or as tubular branching opacities (Fig. 4–76). Kerley A and B lines (Fig. 4–76) are seen in their characteristic central and peripheral locations as haphazardly arranged, thin, sharply marginated linear opacities or, when viewed end-on, as small nodules.

Based on Weibel's division of the interstitial space into three compartments, axial, parenchymal, and peripheral, Bergin and Müller[386] have recently attempted to correlate CT appearances with the distribution of disease in 44 patients with proven interstitial lung disease; they found that specific entities tend to involve predominant compartments and that CT demonstration of differential involvement can be useful in limiting diagnostic possibilities.

MODIFYING INFLUENCES

Certain secondary effects sometimes produced by diffuse interstitial disease may considerably modify the basic roentgenographic pattern. For example, emphysema, either secondary to bronchiolar obstruction or compensatory to pulmonary fibrosis, may distort the pulmonary architecture and render the original disease pattern unrecognizable: the combination of conglomerate shadows and emphysema in advanced silicosis exemplifies this situation. Similarly, cicatrization produced by diffuse interstitial fibrosis may reduce lung volume severely, with resultant crowding of the reticular markings. Such modifying influences usually occur in relation to fairly definite etiologic and pathogenetic circumstances and, therefore, may help one differentiate the many diseases in which the interstitium is diffusely affected.

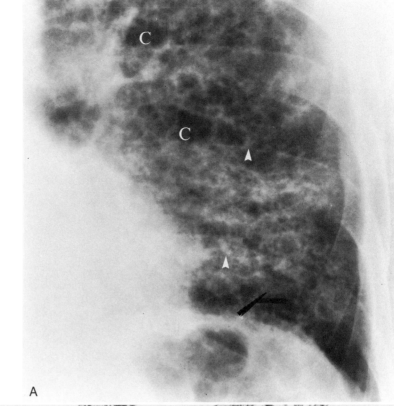

Figure 4–74. Reticulonodular Interstitial Patterns. *A,* A detail view of the left lower lung zone from a PA chest roentgenogram of a young man with end-stage lung caused by fibrosing alveolitis shows apparent nodulation (*arrowheads*) and cystic spaces (*C*). *B,* A representative histologic section of lung from this patient at autopsy discloses typical features of end-stage lung; no true nodules are seen. The pseudonodulation seen on the roentgenogram apparently results from tangential projection of the x-ray beam along the path of the curvilinear opacities (*between arrowheads*).

Illustration continued on following page

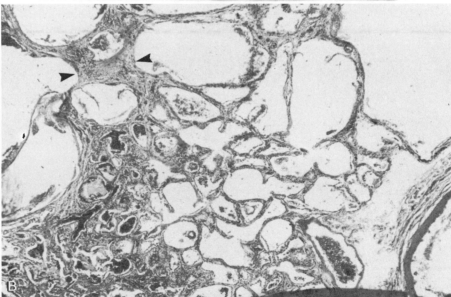

CT Densitometry in Diffuse Lung Disease

Diffuse lung disease implies an acute or chronic increase in roentgenographic density caused by an abnormal accumulation of fluid, cells, or other tissue elements within the air spaces or interstitium or both. The word *diffuse* connotes involvement of most portions of both lungs, although the abnormality need not be symmetric on the two sides or uniform throughout the various lobes on one side.[15] With computed tomography, disorders that fulfill these criteria can be designated high-density lung disease, in contrast to those disorders, also diffuse, that fall under the terminologic umbrella chronic obstructive pulmonary disease, and that can be called low-density lung disease—specifically, atopic asthma and emphysema.

In most clinical situations of high-density lung disease, densitometric analysis is both unnecessary and inaccurate. For example, in patients with well-defined medium or coarse reticular patterns, the morphologic features are clear-cut, whereas CT

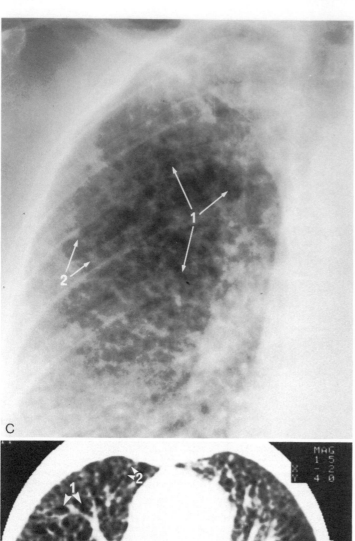

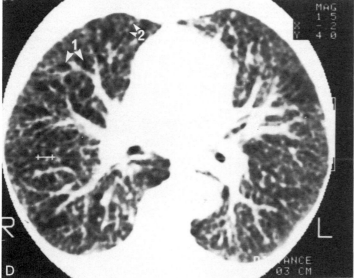

Figure 4–74 *Continued. C,* In another patient with sarcoidosis, a detail view of the right upper lung zone from a PA chest roentgenogram reveals multiple nodular opacities (*2*) interspersed against a background of cystic spaces (*1*), resulting in a reticulonodular pattern. *D,* A CT scan through the midportion of the lungs in this patient discloses both reticular (*1*) and nodular (*2*) components of the interstitial abnormality. Bar denotes 1 cm. (From Genereux GP: Med Radiogr Photogr *61*:1, 1985.)

attenuation values may be abnormally low as a result of nearby cystic emphysematous spaces (partial volume effect). However, in selected instances CT densitometry can play a useful role in predicting the underlying pathology:[387] we have used attenuation values to identify pulmonary calcinosis associated with chronic renal insufficiency (+80 to +120 HU), pulmonary hemorrhage (+60 to +80 HU), exogenous lipid pneumonia (−20 to −50 HU), and the conglomerate opacity associated with intravenous drug abuse (+146 to +180 HU).[16] We have also studied six patients whose conventional chest roentgenograms were either normal (two subjects) or borderline abnormal (four subjects); the carbon monoxide diffusing capacity was slightly diminished in five patients and normal in one; other pulmonary function tests were normal. Biopsy material from these patients revealed alveolar septal thickening attributable to fibrosing alveolitis (usual interstitial pneumonia in four patients and desquamative interstitial pneumonia in two). The CT scan confirmed the presence of diffuse lung disease by showing a diffuse ground-glass opacity in all six patients and the additional finding of micronodularity in one. Objective confirmation of this visual impression was obtained from abnormal attenuation coefficient gradients using a methodology described elsewhere.[131]

It is our belief that CT densitometry has a limited role to play in the evaluation of the diffusely abnormal chest; however, in certain selected conditions, the procedure has proved definitive in predicting the correct pathology. In an experimental CT study on dogs, Wandtke and his colleagues concluded that disruption of normal density gradients may be an indicator of early lung disease.[388]

COMBINED AIR-SPACE AND INTERSTITIAL DISEASE

In many pulmonary diseases, the roentgenologic and pathologic changes include a *combination* of the three basic abnormalities: consolidation, atelectasis, and interstitial disease. The commonest combinations are interstitial disease and air-space consolidation, and all three combined.

The pattern created by combined air-space consolidation and interstitial disease is best exemplified by pulmonary edema, secondary to pulmonary venous hypertension. The roentgenographic manifestations of interstitial involvement are largely those of a change in the perivascular interstitial sheath—edema fluid within the sheath increasing the size and reducing the definition of lung markings (Fig. 4–77). The roentgenographic manifestations of parenchymal consolidation, produced by edema fluid within the acini, consist of a few discrete and several confluent "fluffy" opacities characteristic of air space–filling processes (Fig. 4–77). This combination is also characteristic of certain diffuse infectious diseases of the lungs, notably by *Pneumocystis carinii* and cytomegalovirus: these two infections are characterized at the outset by diffuse interstitial pneumonitis whose roentgenographic pattern may be indistinguishable from interstitial edema of cardiac

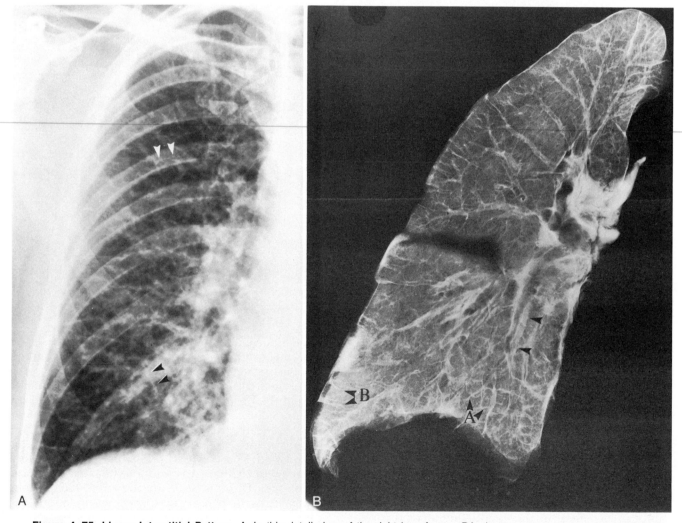

Figure 4–75. Linear Interstitial Pattern. *A,* In this detail view of the right lung from a PA chest roentgenogram of a patient with interstitial edema, there are thickening and loss of definition of the bronchovascular bundles; Kerley A and B lines are visible (*arrowheads*). *B,* A sliced, inflated postmortem specimen from another patient with interstitial edema reveals enlargement of the bronchovascular bundles (*arrowheads*) and both A lines (*A*) and B lines (*B*).

Illustration continued on following page

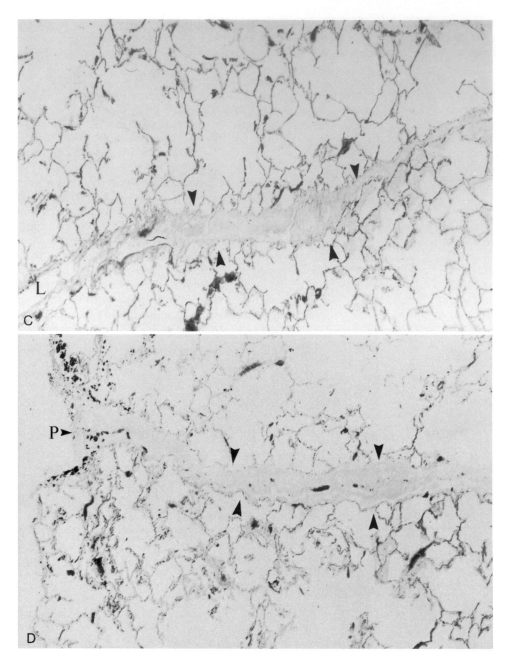

Figure 4–75 *Continued*. Histologic sections show thickening (*arrowheads*) of the deep (*C*) and peripheral (*D*) interlobular septa caused by edema. Although the lymphatics (*L*) are distended, the roentgenographic demonstration of Kerley lines is related chiefly to a combination of edematous widening of the septa and the maintenance of surrounding aerated lung (note the absence of edema within the alveoli). Visceral pleura (*P*) is shown on the left. (From Genereux GP: Med Radiogr Photogr *61*:2, 1985.)

origin; the disease then spreads into parenchymal air spaces, producing widespread alveolar consolidation. Another example of combined involvement of this type is acute pneumonitis of *Mycoplasma* or viral etiology. This infection tends to be local rather than general in distribution and characteristically causes acute interstitial inflammation, creating a pattern early in its course of fine-to-medium reticulation in segmental distribution. This "pure" interstitial involvement is often of short duration, the inflammatory reaction soon extending into parenchymal air spaces and resulting in consolidation. Since involvement of the conducting airways is relatively insignificant, loss of volume is negligible in the acute stage of the disease.

The entity of combined air-space consolidation, atelectasis, and interstitial disease is best exemplified

by acute bronchopneumonia, for example, of staphylococcal origin (Fig. 4–78). The infection primarily involves bronchial and bronchiolar walls and produces acute bronchitis and bronchiolitis with distention of the bronchovascular interstitial sheath by an inflammatory exudate. Intraluminal mucopurulent material leads to irregular airway obstruction, resulting in focal areas of air-space collapse. Adjacent areas of lung parenchyma may show no abnormality or may overinflate to compensate for the focal atelectasis. Dissemination of the infection peripherally leads to patchy air-space consolidation; because of this mechanism of spread, the involvement is necessarily segmental. The resultant roentgenographic pattern of changes depicts the interstitial involvement, irregular zones of peripheral air-space consolidation, peripheral air-space collapse, and normal or overinflated parenchyma. Depending upon the degree of consolidation, volume loss in the segment may be slight or moderate; overall density is inhomogeneous as a result of the foci of normal or overinflated parenchyma.

There are infrequent exceptions to this typical roentgenographic pattern. For example, when the organism is highly virulent, involvement of the parenchymal air spaces may be so extensive that consolidation is confluent. If such consolidation occurs so rapidly that loss of volume is negligible, it may be impossible to distinguish this form of pneumonia from obstructive pneumonitis except through response to antibiotic therapy.

Numerous other diseases may produce a similar pattern of combined involvement. Examples include chronic bronchiectasis (which on purely roentgenographic grounds may be indistinguishable from acute bronchopneumonia) and chronic aspiration pneumonia (such as might result from esophageal stenosis).

GENERAL SIGNS IN DISEASES THAT INCREASE ROENTGENOGRAPHIC DENSITY

In addition to the basic signs already described, several others may aid in determining the nature of a pathologic process within the lungs. The signs are described in general terms only, the intention being to indicate the mechanisms by which they are

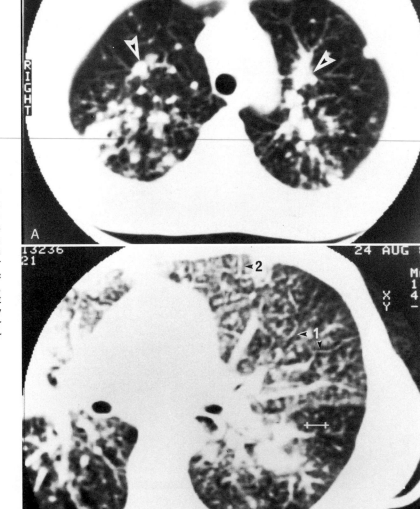

Figure 4–76. CT of Linear Interstitial Pattern. *A*, A CT scan through the upper lobes of a patient whose chest roentgenogram (not shown) revealed thickened bronchovascular bundles caused by sarcoidosis: the linearity observed on the roentgenogram is represented on the CT scan by nodular thickening of the bronchovascular bundles (*arrowheads*) owing to tomographic quality and the transverse plane of the scan. *B*, A CT scan through the left midlung of a patient with lymphocytic interstitial pneumonitis clearly shows Kerley A lines (*1*) and B lines (*2*). Bar denotes 1 cm. (From Genereux GP: Med Radiogr Photogr *61*:2, 1985.)

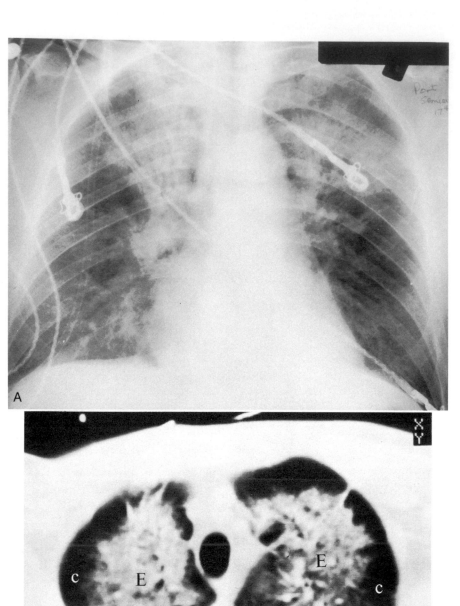

Figure 4–77. Combined Air-space and Interstitial Disease. *A,* An anteroposterior chest roentgenogram of a patient with pulmonary venous hypertension shows a bat's-wing distribution of airspace consolidation in the upper lobes. The lower zone bronchovascular bundles and veins are poorly defined. The heart is slightly enlarged, as are the hila. *B,* A CT scan through the upper lobes shows a striking central accumulation of edema fluid (*E*), the peripheral portions of the lungs being spared laterally and anteriorly (*c*). Except for the possible effect of the supine position in this bedridden patient following a myocardial infarction, the upper lobe predominance of the edema is unexplained. (From Genereux GP: J Can Assoc Radiol *36*:88, 1985.)

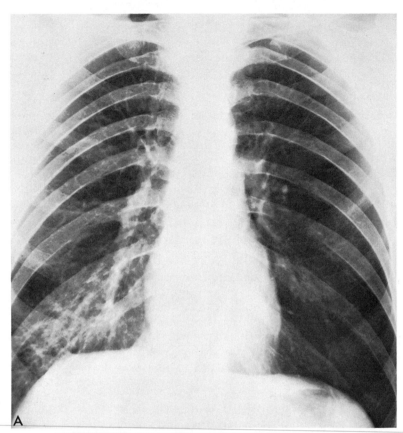

Figure 4–78. Bronchopneumonia, Right Lower Lobe. Posteroanterior (*A*) and lateral (*B*) roentgenograms reveal patchy consolidations of the anterior and lateral basal segments of the right lower lobe. Posterior bowing of the chief fissure (*arrow*) indicates some degree of loss of volume. The inhomogeneous nature of the disease suggests combined air-space consolidation, focal atelectasis, and focal compensatory overinflation.

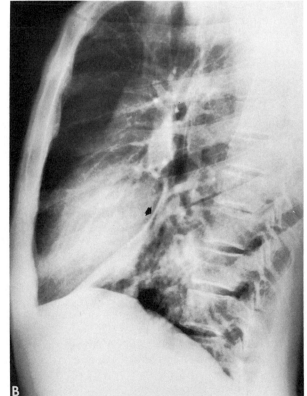

produced and the significance of each in roentgenologic interpretation. The following signs are discussed.

(1) Characteristics of the border of a pulmonary lesion
(2) Change in position of interlobar fissures
(3) Cavitation
(4) Calcification and ossification
(5) Bullae and cysts
(6) Change in size or position of intrathoracic lesions
(7) Distribution of disease within the lungs (anatomic bias)
(8) Roentgenologic localization of pulmonary disease (the "silhouette sign")
(9) The time factor in roentgenologic diagnosis

Characteristics of the Border of a Pulmonary Lesion

The sharpness of definition of a consolidative process within the lungs gives some indication of the nature of its marginal tissues. Acute air-space pneumonia (e.g., from *Streptococcus pneumoniae*) that has extended to an interlobar pleural surface has a sharply defined contour along that border; where it does not abut against a fissure its margin is less distinct (Fig. 4–79), since it is formed by a spreading zone of confluent acinar lesions. Regardless of the etiology and extent of acinar consolidation, the margin between consolidated lung and contiguous air-containing parenchyma has the same definitive character, whether the lesion is a small focus of exudative tuberculosis or a massive consolidation produced by *Klebsiella pneumoniae*. The margin of an organized fibrotic granulomatous lesion generally will be sharply defined, whereas the margin of an infiltrative cancer tends to be indistinct and fuzzy.

As statements of fact, these observations stand up to fairly close scrutiny; roentgenographic assessment of the margin of a pulmonary lesion coincides reasonably accurately with the morphologic appearance of the junction of consolidated tissue and normal lung parenchyma. Unfortunately, what is seen is an anatomic border, not the nature of the cells forming the border. In an analysis of 155 solitary lung lesions, Bateson[132] found that 58 of 80 primary carcinomas (73.5 per cent) had indistinctly defined margins and the remaining 22 were well defined; of 20 lesions of infectious etiology, 15 had ill-defined margins and 5 were well defined; only the 40 mixed tumors and other benign lesions had sharply defined margins in all cases. It may be concluded, therefore, that although the sharpness of definition of a pulmonary opacity gives *some* indication of its nature, it cannot be a sign of *absolute* value in distinguishing benign from malignant lesions (Fig. 4–80).

The *smoothness of contour* (as distinct from nodularity or lobulation) has a significance in many respects similar to that of sharpness of definition. In general, smoothness of contour suggests benignity, and nodularity or lobulation indicates malignancy (Fig. 4–80). Of 100 solitary circumscribed pulmonary carcinomas studied by Bateson,[133] 29 had well-defined margins and *all* of these were lobulated. Probably the "umbilication" or notching of the border of a solitary pulmonary nodule described by Rigler[134] as a sign of malignancy is merely a manifestation of lobulation. Unfortunately, umbilication is not an infallible sign of malignancy, since in our experience and that of others[135] it is present in a significant number of inflammatory nodules; for example, Drevvatne and Frimann-Dahl[135] found umbilication in 16 of 22 cases of tuberculoma.

"Satellite lesions" might be included here since they are closely related to the margins of a pulmonary lesion. They are small, punctate opacities in close proximity to a larger lesion, usually a solitary peripheral nodule, and are thought to suggest an infectious nature of a parenchymal lesion, particularly of tuberculous etiology (Fig. 4–80D). Satellite lesions were observed in 9.8 per cent of 52 reported cases of tuberculoma[136] and in 10 of 122 patients with tuberculosis.[137] However, in the latter series satellite lesions were found in 3 of 280 cases of primary carcinoma—an admittedly very low incidence but one that belies the validity of assuming an infectious origin for a peripheral lesion on the strength of satellite lesions.

The contour of an opacity that relates to the pleura, either over the convexity of the thorax or contiguous to the mediastinum or diaphragm, can provide a useful clue to whether the process is intra- or extrapulmonary in origin. A mass that originates within the pleural space or extrapleurally displaces the pleura and underlying lung inward such that the angle formed by the margins of the mass and the chest wall is obtuse; by contrast, an intrapulmonary mass tends to relate to contiguous pleura with an acute angle. It should be obvious that these general rules apply when such lesions are viewed tangentially; when viewed *en face*, the extrapleural mass will be indistinctly defined because of the obtuse angle of its margins, whereas an intrapulmonary mass will tend to be more sharply defined. As with all other roentgenologic signs, the "extrapleural" sign is fallible: occasionally an extrapleural mass relates to the lung with an acute angle and an intrapulmonary mass with an obtuse angle, but there is no doubt that these are the exceptions to the rule.

Change in Position of Interlobar Fissures

Displacement of fissures toward a zone of increased density constitutes the only direct sign of atelectasis. An equally valuable but less frequent sign is displacement of interlobar fissures in the opposite direction from the involved lobe—in other

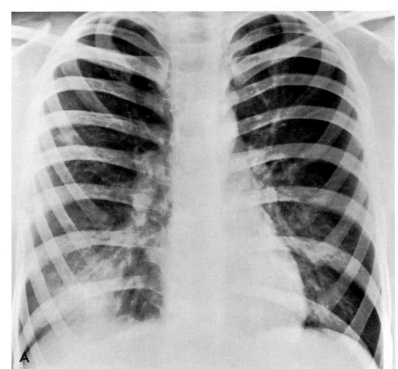

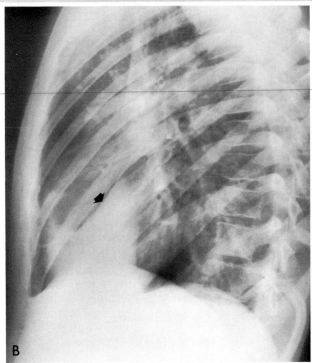

Figure 4–79. Acute Air-space Pneumonia. Posteroanterior (*A*) and lateral (*B*) roentgenograms reveal consolidation of the anterior basal zone of the right lower lobe; the shadow is homogeneous except for an air bronchogram (visualized in *A*). Where the consolidation abuts against the chief fissure (*arrow*), it is sharply defined, but its definition posteriorly, medially, and laterally is less sharp because of the spreading nature of the inflammatory reaction. A small area of parenchymal consolidation is also visible in the medial segment of the middle lobe in *B*, possibly representing spread via collateral channels across a parenchymal bridge (incomplete fissure).

words, bulging of the fissures. Clearly, this is evidence of expansion of the involved lobe; since diseases of increased density capable of increasing the volume of a lobe are relatively few, recognition of such displacement frequently permits specific etiologic diagnosis.

Bulging of fissures occurs most commonly in acute infections of the lung in which the virulence of the organism produces an abundant exudate; the commonest of these are pneumonia caused by *Klebsiella pneumoniae* (Friedländer's pneumonia),[138] *Streptococcus pneumoniae*, *Mycobacterium tuberculosis*, and *Yersinia pestis* (plague pneumonia). Acute lung abscess often expands a lobe, particularly when air trapping by a check-valve mechanism in the communicating airway distends the abscess cavity (a causative mechanism that may operate early in the course of acute Friedländer's pneumonia) (Fig. 4–81).

In addition to the acute pneumonias, any space-

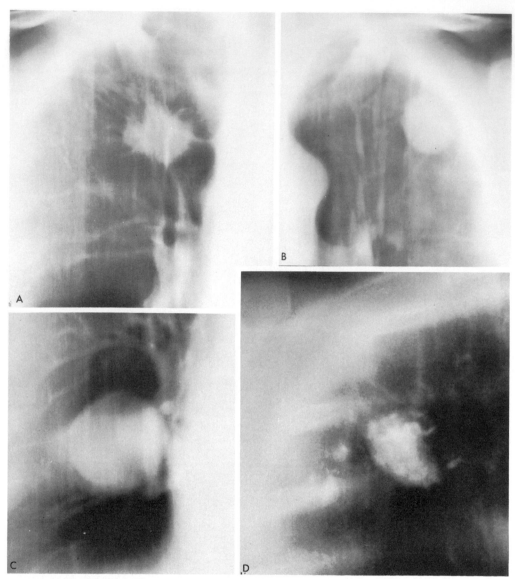

Figure 4–80. Characteristics of the Border of Four Different Pulmonary Nodules Observed Tomographically. *A*, Shaggy, lobulated border of a primary adenocarcinoma; *B*, a smooth, nonlobulated contour of a primary adenocarcinoma; *C*, a smooth, nonlobulated border of a solitary metastasis from embryonal carcinoma of the testis; *D*, a sharply defined, somewhat lobulated contour of a histoplasmoma, with several satellite lesions situated laterally; both the larger nodule and the satellite lesions are calcified.

occupying mass within a lobe may displace a fissure if the lesion occupies significant volume or if it is contiguous to the fissure: peripheral pulmonary carcinoma is perhaps the most common of these masses (Fig. 4–82).

The interlobar fissures are ordinarily an efficient barrier to the interlobar spread of parenchymal disease. A few diseases, however, have a propensity for crossing pleural boundaries, thus creating a sign invaluable to differential diagnosis. Undoubtedly the commonest cause of pleural transgression is mycotic or actinomycotic infection of the lungs, particularly the latter: these organisms pass not only across interlobar fissures but also across the visceral and parietal pleural layers over the convexity of the lung, and they may incite abscesses and osteomyelitis in the chest wall. Pulmonary tuberculosis, particularly in children, may transgress pleural boundaries; pulmonary carci-

noma rarely does so. One caveat to the unwary: these statements apply to complete interlobar fissures; the frequency with which fissures are incomplete (*see* page 159) introduces a situation that may cause confusion—the extension of a pathologic process from one lobe to a contiguous lobe through a parenchymal bridge (Fig. 4–79). In such circumstances, involvement of contiguous lobes need not imply transgression of interlobar fissures and thus extends the differential diagnosis.

Cavitation

The word "cavity" can be defined as a gas-containing space within the lung surrounded by a wall whose thickness is greater than 1 mm and usually irregular in contour (a gas-containing space possessing a wall 1 mm or less in thickness constitutes a bulla). The presence of a fluid level is not necessary to the definition, nor is size of the cavity. The terms "cavity" and "abscess" are not synonymous; an intrapulmonary abscess without communication with the bronchial tree is roentgenographically opaque; only when the abscess cavity communicates with the bronchial tree, allowing air to replace necrotic material, should "cavity" be applied.

The great majority of pulmonary cavities are caused by tissue necrosis and the expulsion of necrotic material into the bronchial tree. Exceptions are uncommon: for example, rupture of a bronchogenic cyst or an echinococcus cyst whose contents were originally fluid rather than necrotic tissue; or infection of an existing cystic space, such as a bulla. The mechanism by which necrosis occurs varies according to the underlying disease. In infectious

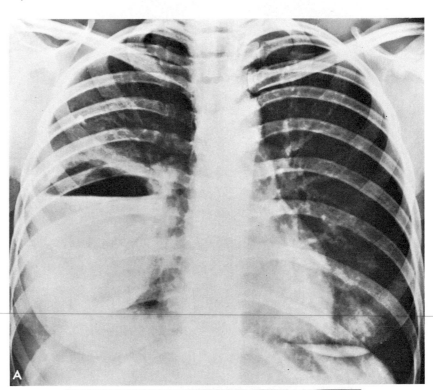

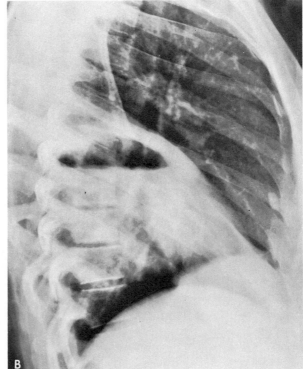

Figure 4–81. Bulging of Interlobar Fissures: Acute Staphylococcal Lung Abscess. Roentgenograms in posteroanterior (A) and lateral (B) projection reveal a large abscess in the right lower lobe producing upward bulging of the major fissure.

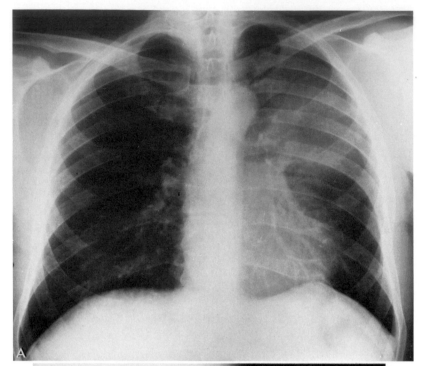

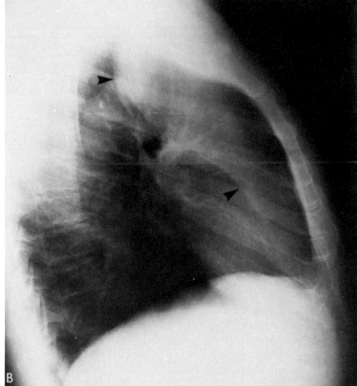

Figure 4–82. Bulging of Interlobar Fissures: Bronchogenic Carcinoma. Roentgenograms in posteroanterior (*A*) and lateral (*B*) projection reveal obliteration of much of the left border of the heart; the opacity is homogeneous and does not contain an air bronchogram. Anterior displacement of the chief fissure (*arrowheads*) and elevation of the left hemidiaphragm indicate considerable loss of volume. The lower half of the chief fissure is concave posteriorly, the upper half convex posteriorly. This bulging of the upper portion of the fissure is caused by a large peripheral bronchogenic carcinoma. Metastatic lymph nodes from this neoplasm produced upper lobe bronchial obstruction and atelectasis.

processes such as acute staphylococcal pneumonia, bacterial toxins and enzymes released by dead or dying leukocytes may lead directly to tissue death; the necrosis of neoplasms probably is related at least partly to deficient blood supply, although the very small size (not exceeding 1 cm in diameter) of some neoplasms that undergo cavitation suggests another mechanism, perhaps delayed hypersensitivity reaction. In septic emboli it is likely that both vascular deficiency and bacterial toxins are operative.

The roentgenographic demonstration of pulmonary cavitation may be simple or exceedingly difficult. If the cavity contains fluid, as is frequently the case, the identification of a fluid level is clearly pathognomonic; should there be doubt as to the presence of this level on standard roentgenograms exposed with the patient erect, lateral decubitus projection with a horizontal x-ray beam may be helpful by demonstrating alteration in the position of the fluid. A major difficulty in diagnosis may present when cavities are small or are situated either among an inhomogeneous group of opacities or in anatomic regions ordinarily difficult to see, such as the paramediastinal zones. In these latter circumstances, conventional or computed tomography may be essential to confirm the diagnosis or, perhaps

more commonly, to identify cavitary disease that was not even remotely suspected on plain roentgenography.

Although the nature of cavity formation within specific disease groups varies considerably, in most cases the general patterns give some indication of the underlying etiology (Fig. 4–83). The roentgenographic features that should be noted in any case of cavitary lung disease include the thickness of the cavity wall, the smoothness or irregularity of its inner lining, the presence and character of its contents, whether lesions are solitary or multiple, and, when multiple, the number that have cavitated. The following examples indicate prevailing patterns; in each category there are occasional exceptions to the general rule.

Cavity Wall. This is usually thick in acute lung abscess (Fig. 4–84), primary (Fig. 4–85) and metastatic carcinoma, and Wegener's granulomatosis (Fig. 4–86), and is usually thin in infected bullae and posttraumatic cysts. From a study of 65 solitary cavities in the lung designed to evaluate diagnostic implications of cavity wall thickness, Woodring and his colleagues[141] found that all lesions in which the thickest part of the cavity wall was 1 mm were benign; of the lesions whose thickest measurement

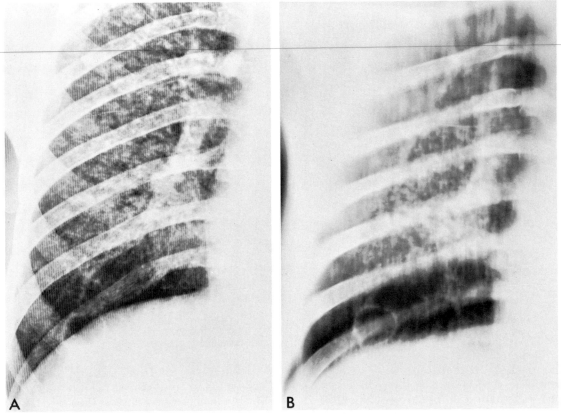

Figure 4–83. Tuberculous Lung Abscess with Bronchogenic Spread. A posteroanterior roentgenogram (A) and anteroposterior tomogram (B) of the right lung reveal a well-defined thin-walled cavity in the base of the right lower lobe. As expected, only the erect study (A) shows an air-fluid level (the tomogram was performed in the supine position). Multiple poorly defined shadows possessing the typical characteristics of acinar lesions can be identified throughout much of the right lung, representing bronchogenic spread from the tuberculous cavity. This combination of changes constitutes almost certain evidence of a tuberculous etiology. (Courtesy of the Montreal Chest Hospital Center.)

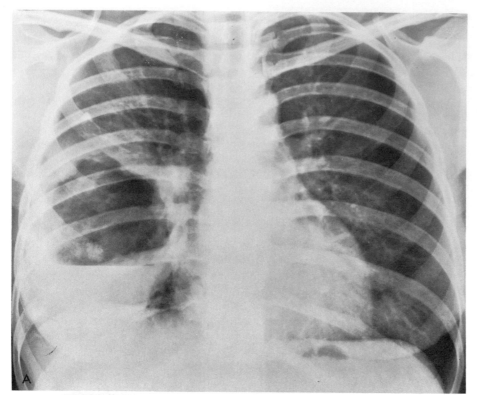

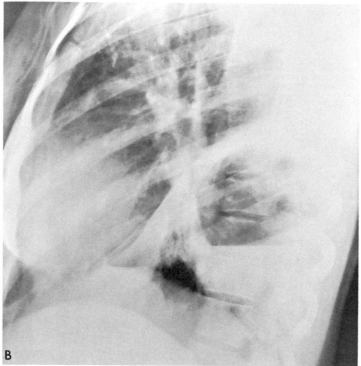

Figure 4–84. Acute Staphylococcal Lung Abscess. Roentgenograms in posteroanterior (A) and lateral (B) projection reveal a huge cavity in the right lower lobe. The thickness of its wall and shaggy irregular nature of its inner lining suggest an acute lung abscess.

was 4 mm or less, 92 per cent were benign; of cavities that were 5 to 15 mm in their thickest part, benign and malignant lesions were equally divided; when the cavity wall was over 15 mm in thickness, 92 per cent of lesions were malignant. These investigators concluded that measurement of the thickest part of a cavity wall provides a more reliable indication of benignancy or malignancy than measurement of the thinnest part.

Character of Inner Lining. This is usually irregular and nodular in carcinoma (Fig. 4–85), shaggy in acute lung abscess (Fig. 4–81), and smooth in most other cavitary lesions.

Nature of Contents. In the majority of cases the contents are liquid, with no distinctive characteristics. With few exceptions (to which reference is made further on), a fluid level within a pulmonary cavity is distinct, an observation employed by Caruso and Berk to differentiate left lower lobe cavities from the stomach bubble; in the latter, the fluid level tends to be fuzzy and irregular because of the character of gastric contents.[139] However, the validity of this sign has been questioned by Mettler and Ghahremani,[140] who contend that the fuzzy appearance of a fluid level depends on the alignment of the x-ray beam in relation to the surface of the fluid rather than on the chemical composition of the liquid; on the basis of the evidence presented and our own experience, we are inclined to favor the latter interpretation. Obviously, fluid levels that are visible on conventional chest roentgenograms obtained in the erect position on fixed equipment

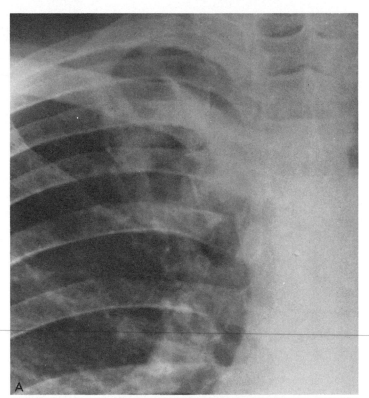

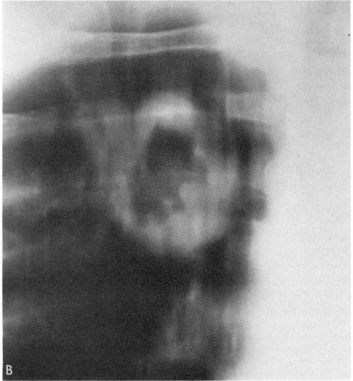

Figure 4–85. Cavitating Pulmonary Carcinoma. Views of the upper half of the right lung from a posteroanterior roentgenogram (A) and an anteroposterior tomogram (B) reveal a rather poorly defined cavitating mass. The thickness of the wall and irregular nodular character of the inner lining are highly suggestive of bronchogenic carcinoma. Proved squamous cell cancer.

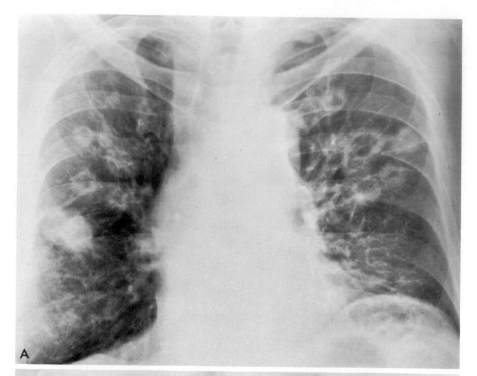

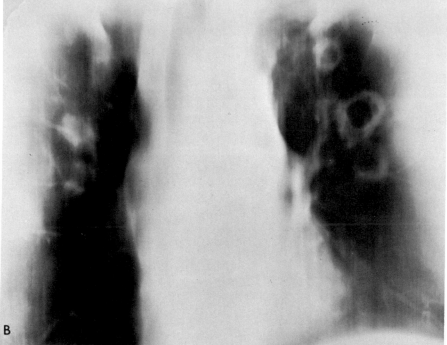

Figure 4–86. Multiple Cavities in Wegener's Granulomatosis. A postero-anterior roentgenogram (*A*) and an anteroposterior tomogram (*B*) show multiple thick-walled cavities scattered throughout both lungs but predominantly in the upper zones. The lesions range from 1.5 to 3 cm and are rather thick-walled. At least three lesions show no evidence of cavitation.

within a department should be perfectly horizontal and parallel to the upper or lower borders of the film (this rule clearly does not apply to roentgenograms exposed with mobile apparatus at a patient's bedside); however, very occasionally a fluid level may be tilted slightly from the horizontal, a peculiarity that has been explained by Jackson and Stark[146] as being caused by displacement of the fluid by cardiac pulsation. These investigators fluoroscoped one of three patients with hydropneumothorax in which the fluid interface was tilted and found that

the interface "seesawed" synchronously with the heart beat.

In contrast to the usually flat, smooth character of fluid levels, in certain diseases the contents may be so typical as to be diagnostic; for example, the intracavitary fungus ball (mycetoma—Fig. 4–87) or blood clot (Fig. 4–88), both of which may form freely mobile intracavitary masses; or the collapsed membranes of a ruptured echinococcus cyst, which float on top of the fluid within the cyst and create the characteristic "water-lily" sign[142] or the "sign of the camalote" (a water plant found in South American rivers) (Fig. 4–89).[143]

A rare but characteristic intracavitary mass is that associated with massive pulmonary gangrene, in which extensive necrosis of lung tissue occurs in cases of acute Friedländer's or pneumococcal pneumonia; irregular pieces of sloughed lung parenchyma float like icebergs in the cavity fluid (Fig. 4–90).[144]

Multiplicity of Lesions. Some cavitary disease is characteristically solitary—for example, primary pulmonary carcinoma, acute lung abscess, and post-traumatic lung cyst; other diseases are characteristically multiple—for example, metastatic neoplasm, Wegener's granulomatosis,[145] and acute pyemic abscesses.

We will mention briefly simulation of cavities—an uncommon occurrence. At necropsy some cavitary lesions visible on premortem roentgenograms are found to contain no air and to have no communication with the bronchial tree. Histologically, the center of such lesions is necrotic, and it is assumed that some histochemical change has occurred in this necrotic material whereby its lipid content is sufficiently high to cause a relatively radiolucent shadow roentgenographically, thus simulating cavitation (Fig. 4–91). Although this phenomenon is generally regarded as a feature of granulomas,[147] unquestionably pseudocavitation should *not* be regarded as an unequivocal sign of benignancy: examples have been reported in multiple pulmonary metastases,[148] and we have seen one case in which a solitary lesion containing a central radiolucency proved to be bronchioloalveolar carcinoma contiguous with a fibrocaseous granuloma. It has been our experience also that lobulation of a nodular opacity can create a false intranodular radiolucency, particularly on conventional tomography; a tomographic section must pass through the center of a lesion rather than its periphery before the presence of cavitation can be stated with certainty.

Calcification and Ossification

Intrathoracic *calcification* is an important parameter of pulmonary disease. In the majority of cases it is dystrophic (calcium deposition in damaged or dead cells or tissue); less commonly, it is metastatic (calcification of vital tissues). Although the latter is frequent in cases of severe hypercalcemia, presumably because of the relatively alkaline pH of lung tissue, it is seldom roentgenographically visible. In addition to the simple tissue deposition of calcium, lamellar bone can also be identified roentgenographically or pathologically in some cases, and then the term *ossification* should be employed.

Both the distribution and character of calcification should be noted, since each has diagnostic significance. It is convenient to consider intratho-

Text continued on page 592

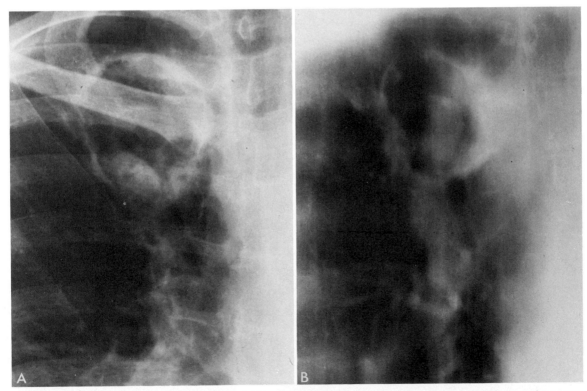

Figure 4–87. Intracavitary Fungus Ball (Mycetoma). Views of the upper half of the right lung from a posteroanterior roentgenogram (*A*) and an anteroposterior tomogram (*B*) reveal a rather thin-walled but irregular cavity in the paramediastinal zone. Situated within it is a smooth oblong shadow of homogeneous density whose relationships to the wall of the cavity change from the erect (*A*) to the supine (*B*) positions. The cavity was of tuberculous etiology but the loose body was composed mainly of mycelial threads characteristic of *Aspergillus*.

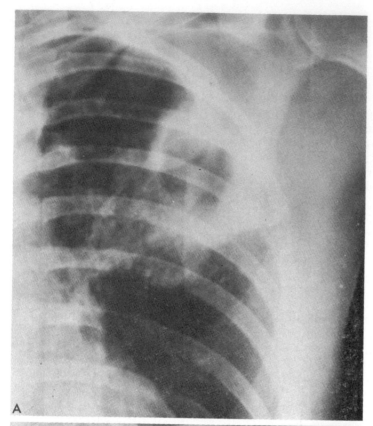

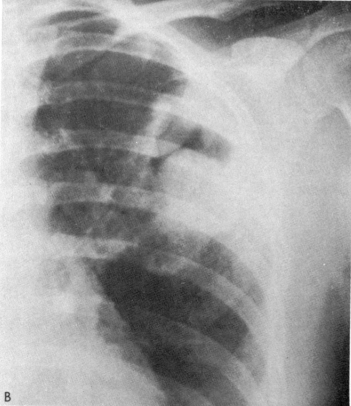

Figure 4–88. Rapid Development of an Intracavitary Foreign Body (Blood Clot). Shortly before the roentgenogram illustrated in *A*, this 30-year-old woman suffered a massive hemoptysis. The roentgenogram reveals a large, thick-walled, air-containing cavity in the left upper lobe; there is no evidence of fluid or other foreign material within the cavity. Six hours later (*B*), a large, fairly smooth mass appeared within the cavity, lying in its dependent portion. Following a second massive hemoptysis, an emergency left upper lobectomy was performed. The specimen showed a large blood clot within a tuberculous cavity.

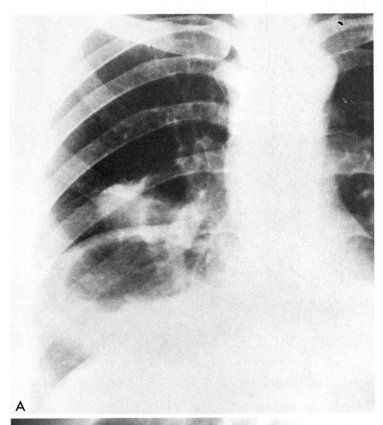

Figure 4–89. Hydatid Cyst with Bronchial Communication. Posteroanterior (*A*) and lateral (*B*) roentgenograms reveal a large mass in the right middle lobe and a smaller mass in the superior segment of the right lower lobe; the middle lobe mass contains a large central cavity with a prominent air-fluid level, the latter possessing an irregular, lumpy configuration caused by floating membranes from a collapsed echinococcal endocyst (the water lily sign or sign of the camalote.) (Courtesy of the Jean Talon Hospital, Montreal.)

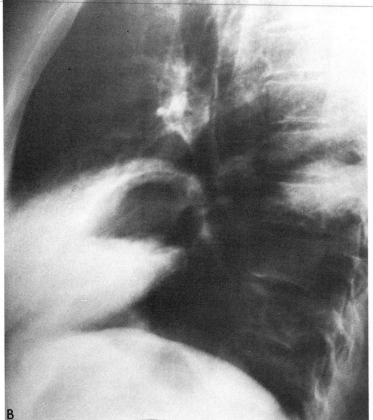

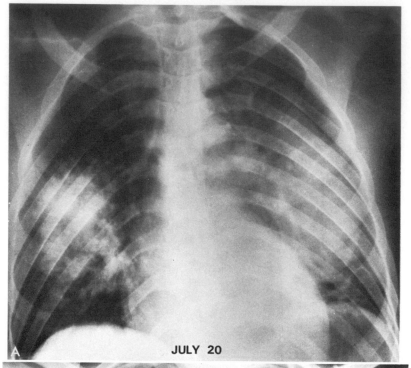

JULY 20

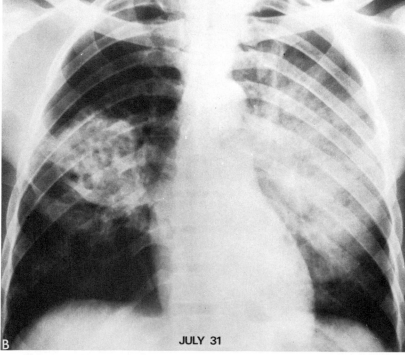

JULY 31

Figure 4–90. Acute Lung Gangrene in Klebsiella Pneumonia. The patient is a 37-year-old man. On admission to the hospital, an antero-posterior roentgenogram in the supine position (A) revealed massive air-space consolidation throughout much of the left lung and the midportion of the right lung. He was exceedingly ill and required assisted ventilation. *K. pneumoniae* was grown from the sputum; blood cultures were negative. Although 11 days later his clinical condition had improved somewhat, a roentgenogram (B) revealed a change in the texture of the consolidation in that its homogeneity was disturbed by a multitude of poorly defined air-containing spaces, better visualized in the right than the left lung. This represents the earliest roentgenologic sign of acute lung gangrene.

Illustration continued on opposite page

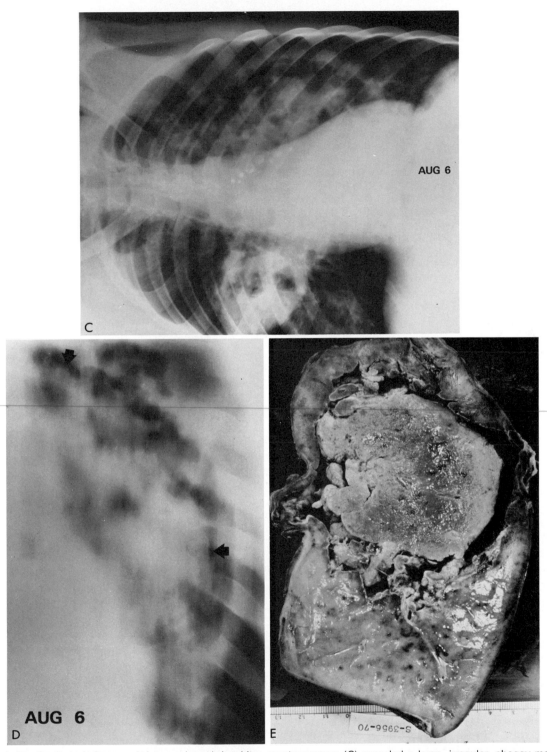

Figure 4–90. *Continued.* One week later, a lateral decubitus roentgenogram (*C*) revealed a large, irregular, shaggy mass within a huge cavity in the left lung, indicated to better advantage in an anteroposterior tomogram (*arrows* in *D*). The left lower lobe was resected and the specimen (*E*) showed a large necrotic mass lying within a huge cavity and completely separated from the cavity walls. (From Knight L, Fraser RG, Robson HG: Can Med Assoc J *112*:196, 1975.)

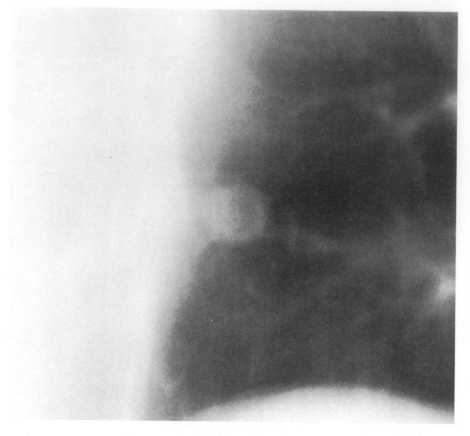

Figure 4–91. Pseudocavitation in a Solitary Pulmonary Nodule. A detail view of the right lower lobe from a conventional linear tomogram in AP projection reveals a solitary nodule measuring 15 mm in diameter. The central portion is relatively radiolucent compared with the periphery, although its density is slightly greater than would be expected if it were air. This effect has been attributed to an accumulation of lipid-containing macrophages, presumably secondary to necrosis. Although the greater-than-air density usually permits distinction from true cavitation, such is not always possible. Of importance is the fact that the pseudocavitation does not permit distinction of the benign or malignant character of a nodule.

racic calcification or ossification under five headings, depending on its anatomic location and distribution: local parenchymal, widespread parenchymal, lymph nodal, pleural, and other.

LOCAL PARENCHYMAL CALCIFICATION OR OSSIFICATION

The commonest form of pulmonary calcification is the single, often densely calcified focus, situated anywhere in the lungs and representing calcification of a healed primary granulomatous lesion. It is most frequently caused by histoplasmosis,[149] less often tuberculosis, occasionally coccidioidomycosis, and rarely blastomycosis (Fig. 4–92).[149] This Ghon lesion is usually part of a duo (the Ranke complex), the other component being calcification of a hilar or mediastinal drainage lymph node. Calcification in the pulmonary lesion is usually homogeneous, whereas that in the lymph node generally consists of scattered punctate deposits. Salzman[149] states that pulmonary calcifications are found in about one third of patients who react to the histoplasmin test but in only one tenth of those with a positive reaction to tuberculin testing. Identification of the Ranke complex fairly conclusively establishes previous infection by one of the two commonest causative organisms. Deciding upon the correct etiology may be aided by the roentgenographic demonstration of multiple punctate calcifications within the spleen, which are almost always due to histoplasmosis.[159]

Although calcification nearly always is associated with healing of the infectious process, it does not necessarily indicate that the lesion is inactive; reactivation may occur in contiguous parenchyma, especially in tuberculosis although seldom in histoplasmosis.

Calcification within *solitary pulmonary nodules* is a useful indicator of the nature of these perplexing lesions. Most importantly, it is the most reliable single piece of evidence that a lesion is benign.[151] Exceptions to this general rule are rare but must be borne in mind. (1) Most important from a differential diagnostic point of view is the isolated instance of a peripheral primary carcinoma engulfing an existing calcified granuloma, in which case the calcification is usually eccentric. (2) A solitary metastasis from osteogenic sarcoma or chondrosarcoma (Fig. 4–93), true ossification occurring in the neoplastic osteoid tissue. (3) The very rare instance of a primary peripheral squamous cell[389] or papillary adenocarcinoma or metastatic papillary adenocarcinoma which, because of psammomatous or dystrophic calcification, presents as a diffusely calcified solitary nodule.[152] (4) Rare cases of carcinoid tumor and metastatic mucinous adenocarcinoma of the colon. The statement regarding the benign nature of calcified nodules refers to *calcium roentgenographically demonstrable in vivo;* roentgenography *in vitro* of surgically excised specimens shows calcification of malignant neoplasms in 10 to 15 per cent of cases.[153]

The character of the calcification within a solitary pulmonary nodule may be a reliable indicator of the lesion's etiology. For example, a small central *nidus* (Fig. 4–94) is the sign of a granulomatous lesion in most cases but also occurs in some hamartomas; *lamination* is almost pathognomonic of a granuloma, usually histoplasmoma, and is the most reliable sign of a benign lesion; *"popcorn-ball"* calcification is characteristic of hamartoma; and *multiple punctate foci* throughout a lesion may be seen in either granulomas or hamartomas (Fig. 4–95).[151] In the investigation of solitary pulmonary nodules, both conventional tomography and CT can some-

times permit identification of calcification not seen or only suggested on plain roentgenograms. Recently, however, dual-energy digital radiography has been shown to be a highly reliable quantitative technique in the assessment of the calcium content of pulmonary nodules (Fig. 4–96).[376] Preliminary investigations indicate that in distinguishing benign from malignant lesions on the basis of calcium content, the accuracy of dual-energy was in all instances comparable and in some instances superior to that of conventional radiography, conventional tomography, and CT. Of practical impor-

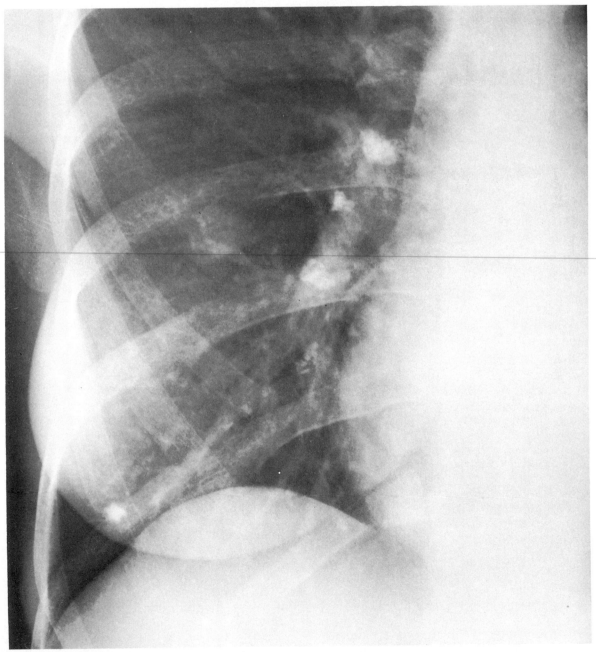

Figure 4–92. The Ranke Complex. A view of the lower half of the right lung from a posteroanterior roentgenogram reveals a solitary, densely calcified nodule just above the right costophrenic sulcus (the Ghon lesion); the calcification is homogeneous although irregular. Situated in the right hilum are three or four lymph nodes containing scattered punctate calcium deposits. The solitary nodule in the right midlung proved to be metastatic adenocarcinoma of the uterus.

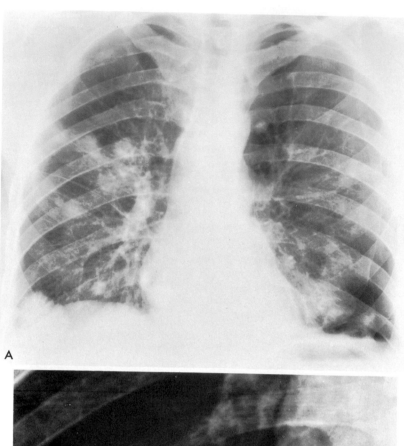

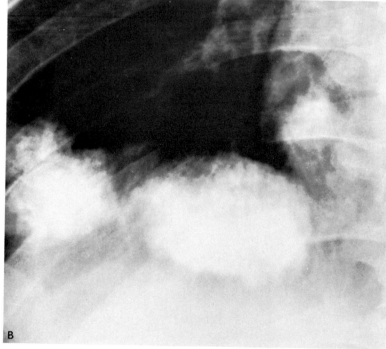

Figure 4–93. Calcified Metastases from Osteogenic Sarcoma. A posteroanterior (A) roentgenogram reveals multiple nodular shadows throughout both longs, varying considerably in size. A spontaneous pneumothorax is present on the left, a remarkably frequent complication of metastatic osteogenic sarcoma. A detailed view of the lower right lung from an overexposed roentgenogram (B) reveals extensive calcification (? ossification) of the two largest metastatic lesions.

tance is that this accuracy could be easily and conveniently achieved with one modest radiation exposure and with no more expenditure of technologists' time than required to perform a routine examination on a conventional dedicated chest unit.

A rare form of local parenchymal calcification occurs when a solitary calcified focus, commonly the result of histoplasmosis, moves by some unknown mechanism from adjacent parenchyma or lymph node into the lumen of a bronchus (Fig. 4–97). Appropriately termed broncholiths, these

foci can produce segmental or subsegmental bronchial obstruction and may occasion hemoptysis. A case has been reported in which a broncholith situated in the left hilum was observed on a follow-up roentgenogram obtained 2 weeks later to have shifted to the right hilum via the major bronchi.[154]

An exceedingly rare condition is nephrobronchial fistula associated with nephrolithiasis; in the case reported the renal calculi passed through the fistula into the bronchial tree (nephrobroncholithiasis) and occasioned the usual symptoms of broncholithiasis–cough, hemoptysis, and expectoration of calculi.[155]

DIFFUSE PARENCHYMAL CALCIFICATION OR OSSIFICATION

This form may be caused by several conditions, but the pattern in each is usually distinctive. For example, the tiny punctate "calcispherytes" of alveolar microlithiasis present a unique, virtually unmistakable roentgenographic image. Multiple nodular foci of calcification or ossification occur in various conditions, including silicosis,[390] mitral stenosis (Fig. 4–98)[156, 157] and other diseases associated with elevated left atrial pressure such as idiopathic hypertrophic subaortic stenosis,[158] and certain healed disseminated infectious diseases such as tuberculosis,[149, 159] histoplasmosis, and varicella pneumonitis (Fig. 4–99).[160, 161] The multiple ossifications of mitral stenosis usually can be differentiated from the calcifications of healed infectious disease by their size (the former measure up to 8 mm in diameter, whereas calcifications seldom exceed 2 to 3 mm) and occasionally by bony trabeculae. Pulmonary interstitial ossification is a rare condition; the roentgenographic pattern is one of branching shadows of calcific density extending along the bronchovascular distribution of the interstitial space;[162] it has been described in association with fibrosing alveolitis (Fig. 4–100),[163, 164] long-term busulfan therapy,[165] longstanding chronic pulmonary "congestion,"[166] and as idiopathic in origin.[167]

Extensive metastatic pulmonary calcification may occur in cases of longstanding hypercalcemia associated with chronic renal disease and secondary hyperparathyroidism (Fig. 4–101),[168] and in other diseases such as diffuse myelomatosis in which the serum calcium level is chronically elevated.[169] Metabolic factors etiologically related to this type of calcification are increased serum calcium and phosphate and impaired renal function.[149] Metastatic calcification is especially common in patients undergoing maintenance hemodialysis, in which case its extent usually reflects the length of the patient's survival,[170, 171] or in patients with hyperphosphatemia being treated with a dialysate high in calcium.[172] Parfitt[173] has postulated that the acidosis that occurs in the intervals between dialysis leaches calcium from bone and that this is deposited in soft tissue during the alkalosis that develops by the end of dialysis. Metastatic calcification has been observed occasionally in the absence of supersaturation of extracellular fluid with calcium and phosphate ions.[174]

Both morphologically and roentgenographically, metastatic calcification shows remarkable predilection for apical and subapical lung zones, a feature readily attributable to regional differences in the physiology of the lung.[175] As West has pointed out, a much higher ventilation/perfusion ratio exists

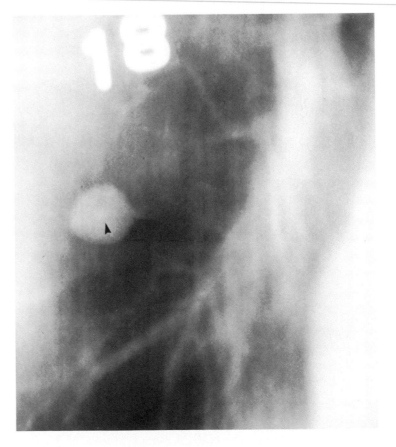

Figure 4–94. Central Calcification in a Tuberculous Granuloma. A conventional linear tomogram in AP projection reveals a 2 cm, well-defined nodule in the anterior portion of the middle lobe. A small central nidus of calcification (*arrowhead*) is seen within the nodule, confirmed by lateral tomograms (not shown). The presence of central calcification sometimes requires tomography in both AP and lateral projection for confirmation. The patient is a 29-year-old man with a pathologically documented tuberculous granuloma.

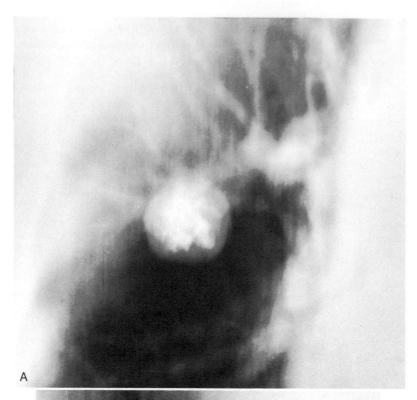

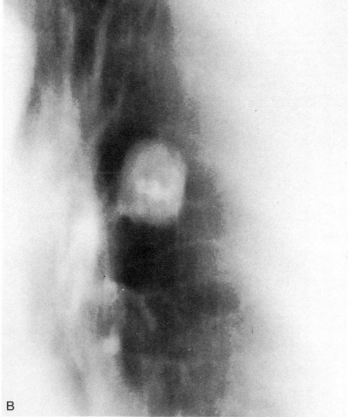

Figure 4–95. Calcification in Pulmonary Hamartomas. *A*, A conventional linear tomogram in AP projection shows a 3 cm, well-defined nodule in the anterior segment of the right upper lobe. The lesion contains a large central area of so-called "popcorn ball" calcification characteristic of hamartoma (presumptive diagnosis in this 52-year-old man). *B*, In another patient, a linear tomogram demonstrates a similar 3 cm, sharply defined nodule in the left upper lobe, in this case with nodular calcification. Histologic features following resection were typical of hamartoma; 60-year asymptomatic man.

at the apex than at the base of the lung, the local milieu at the apex containing a higher Po_2, a lower Pco_2, and a higher pH.[377] West states that at the apex of the normal lung the pH is roughly 7.50, compared with 7.39 at the base; the relative alkalinity at the apex favors calcium deposition. However, when calcium/phosphate metabolism is severely deranged, metastatic calcification may be so diffuse as to resemble severe air-space pulmonary edema.[177] The calcific nature of the pulmonary opacities can be readily confirmed by scanning with bone imaging agents such as ^{99m}Tc diphosphonate;[178] diffuse uptake of ^{67}gallium has also been observed.[179]

Although deposition of calcium salts is usually rather diffuse, whether localized to apical zones or general throughout the lungs, an unusual form has been reported in which large nodules within the lungs became calcified as a result of metabolic abnormalities occasioned by chronic renal failure.[180] Despite the foregoing, it is probable that few pa-

tients in whom calcium is demonstrable in the lungs at necropsy show evidence of its presence during life on conventional roentgenograms. However, dual-energy digital radiography has recently been shown to be a highly effective technique for the demonstration of increased levels of calcium in both lung parenchyma and myocardium in dialysis patients with end-stage renal disease, at a stage when conventional roentgenograms reveal no abnormality.[391]

LYMPH NODE CALCIFICATION

This form of calcification is usually amorphous and irregularly distributed throughout the node (Fig. 4–92). It results most commonly from healed granulomatous infection, usually tuberculosis or histoplasmosis, and constitutes part of the Ranke complex. Although calcified hilar or mediastinal lymph nodes are usually an incidental finding of little or

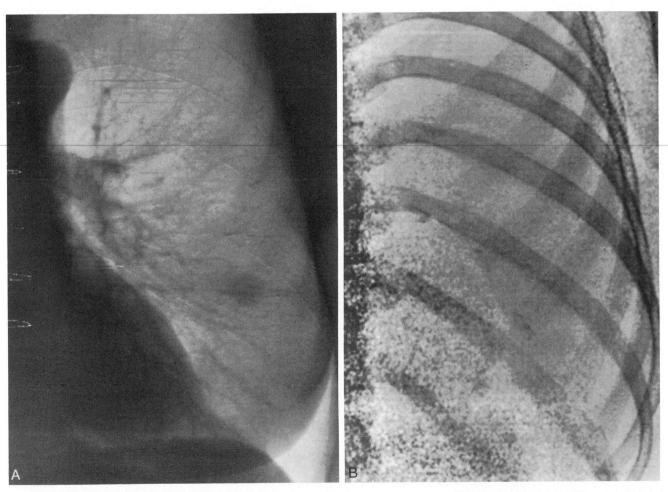

Figure 4–96. Evaluation of the Calcium Content of Solitary Pulmonary Nodules by Dual-energy Digital Radiography. A digital image of the left lower lobe with bones subtracted (*A*) reveals a solitary pulmonary nodule of soft tissue density. On a bone image (soft tissues subtracted) (*B*), the lesion is no longer visible and thus is not calcified. Proved adenocarcinoma. Compare these appearances with images of the right lower lobe of a different patient who had had a right mastectomy several years previously: the nodule on the soft tissue image (*C*) looks much the same as the nodule in *A*; however, on the bone image (*D*), a calcification is visible (*arrow*) that measures about 6 mm less than the nodule in *C*, indicating that the latter possesses a central calcified nidus. Presumed histoplasmoma (being followed).

Illustration continued on following page

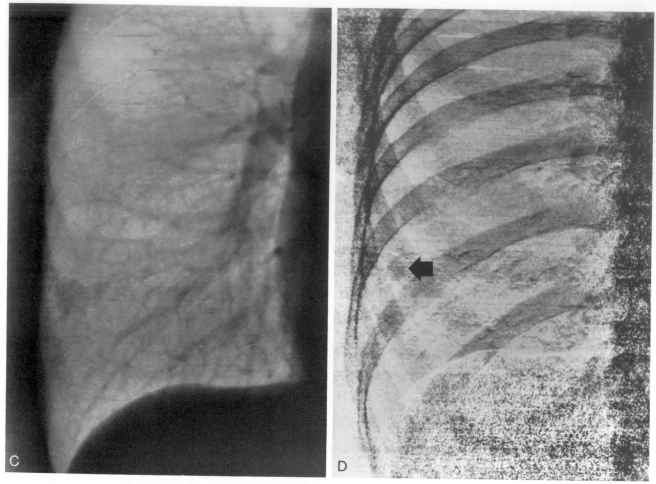

Figure 4–96 *Continued*

no clinical significance, they may erode a contiguous airway (broncholith), causing hemoptysis and chronic cough.

"Eggshell" calcification is uncommon; it consists of a ring of calcification around the periphery of a lymph node and occurs most typically in silicosis and coal workers' pneumoconiosis. This subject has been reviewed by Gross and his colleagues,[181] who list the following criteria for the diagnosis of egg-shell calcification.

1. Shell-like calcifications up to 2 mm thick in the peripheral zone of at least two lymph nodes.
2. The calcifications may be solid or broken.
3. In at least one of the lymph nodes, the ringlike shadow must be complete.
4. The central part of the lymph node may show additional calcifications.
5. One of the affected lymph nodes must be at least 1 cm in its greatest diameter.

The bronchopulmonary nodes are affected most frequently, but involvement of mediastinal and even retroperitoneal nodes has been described.[182] Eggshell calcification is almost diagnostic of either silicosis or coal workers' pneumoconiosis; other rare causes include sarcoidosis, following irradiation of

Hodgkin's lymph nodes, blastomycosis, histoplasmosis, progressive systemic sclerosis, and amyloidosis.[181] Gross and associates[181] describe two cases of sarcoidosis and were able to find 11 cases reported in the literature; we have seen three cases (Fig. 4–102).

PLEURAL CALCIFICATION (OR OSSIFICATION)

Pleural calcification is most often the result of a remote hemothorax, pyothorax, or tuberculous effusion and commonly is associated with thickening of the pleura over the entire lung surface. The calcification may be in the form of a broad continuous sheet (Fig. 4–103) or of multiple discrete plaques. It usually extends from about the level of the midthorax posteriorly, around the lateral lung margin in a generally inferior direction, roughly paralleling the chief fissure (Fig. 4–104). The calcium may be deposited on the inner surface of the thickened pleura, either visceral or parietal; if only the former is calcified, a thick tissue layer of unit density exists between the calcium and the thoracic wall (Fig. 4–105). CT studies have shown that extrapleural fat may be deposited adjacent to the thickened parietal pleura, so the assumption that

Text continued on page 608

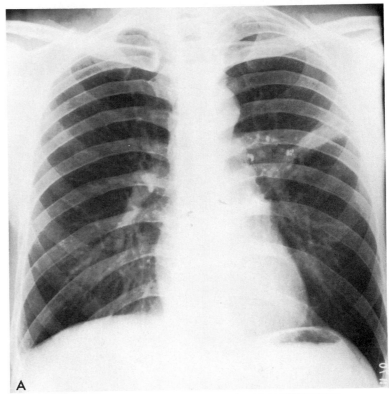

Figure 4–97. Broncholith Associated with Focal Atelectasis and Pneumonitis, Left Upper Lobe. A broad band shadow can be seen in both the posteroanterior roentgenogram (*A*) and the anteroposterior tomogram (*B*), extending in a roughly horizontal plane from the lateral aspect of the left hilum to the axillary visceral pleura. The shadow is of variegated density, suggesting the presence of air within dilated airways. The calcific density at the medial aspect of the shadow is a broncholith that is partially obstructing the affected bronchus. Presumed histoplasmosis.

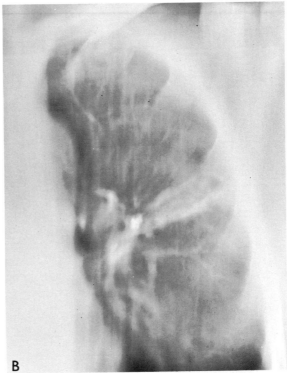

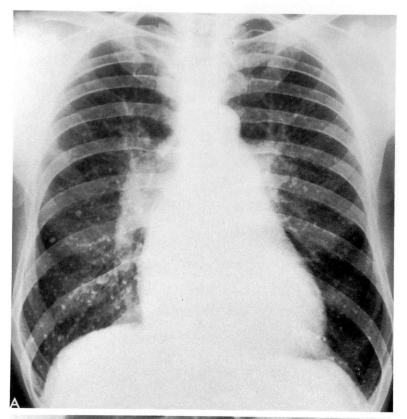

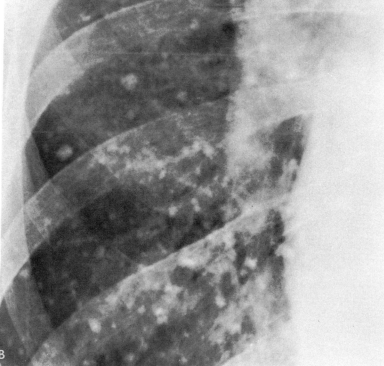

Figure 4–98. Pulmonary Ossification in Mitral Stenosis. A posteroanterior roentgenogram (*A*) of a 46-year-old man with longstanding mitral stenosis and severe pulmonary arterial hypertension reveals multiple, densely calcified nodular shadows ranging in diameter from 1 to 5 mm, situated predominantly in the lower half of the right lung (*B*). Lesions of this type and localization are highly suggestive (if not diagnostic) of longstanding mitral stenosis. They should not be confused with hemosiderosis.

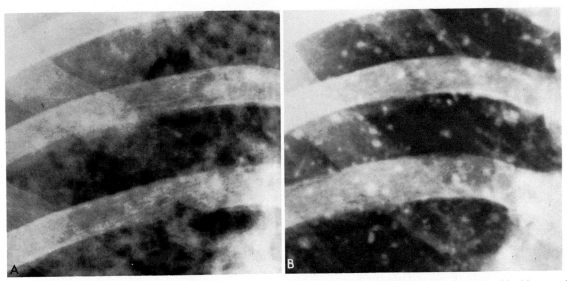

Figure 4–99. Multiple Punctate Calcifications Following Acute Varicella-Zoster Pneumonia. In 1962, this 28-year-old woman developed widespread air-space pneumonia in association with classic cutaneous chickenpox. A chest roentgenogram revealed generalized patchy acinar consolidation, seen to advantage in a magnified view of the right midlung zone (*A*). Eight years later, a posteroanterior roentgenogram (*B*) revealed multiple tiny punctate calcifications throughout both lungs. (Courtesy of Dr. Max Palayew, Jewish General Hospital, Montreal.)

Figure 4–100. Interstitial Calcification (Ossification) Associated with Fibrosing Alveolitis. A posteroanterior chest roentgenogram discloses a nodular and reticulonodular pattern throughout both lungs with considerable lower zonal predominance. Many of the nodular opacities in the left lower lobe (*arrowheads*) are of sufficient density to suggest calcification. Biopsy of the left lung in this 72-year-old man disclosed mature bone related to extensive fibrosing alveolitis.

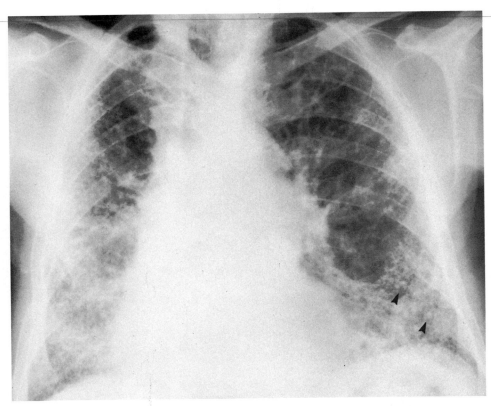

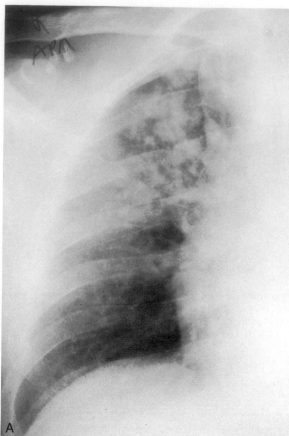

Figure 4–101. Metastatic Pulmonary Calcification Associated with Chronic Renal Insufficiency. *A,* Detail view of the right lung from an AP chest roentgenogram reveals extensive opacities with air-space-filling qualities. The left lung was similarly involved. *B,* CT scans of the right upper lobe with wide (*left*) and narrow (*right*) windows show the consolidation to represent calcinosis (compare the CT density of lung with that of the regional bones). This upper zonal predominance of metastatic calcification is characteristic. (From Genereux GP: Sem Roentgen *19*:211, 1984.)

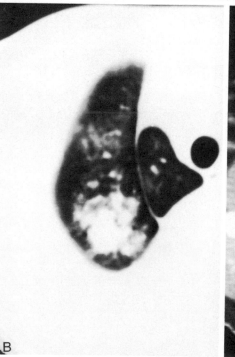

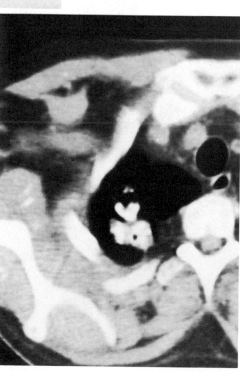

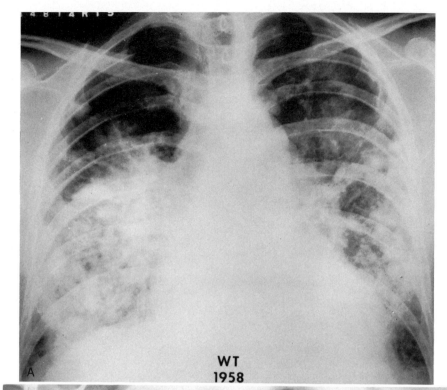

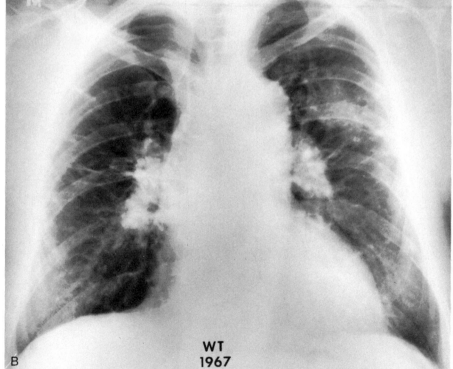

Figure 4–102. "Eggshell" Calcification in Sarcoidosis. *A*, A posteroanterior chest roentgenogram discloses multiple nodular opacities and large coalescent areas of consolidation. The hilar and mediastinal nodes are enlarged, and there is moderate cardiomegaly. An open lung biopsy from the left upper lobe revealed noncaseating granulomas consistent with sarcoidosis. *B*, A posteroanterior chest roentgenogram 8 years later shows remarkable resolution of the parenchymal opacities except for isolated areas such as the left upper lobe; however, the hila are still enlarged and abnormally contoured.

Illustration continued on following page

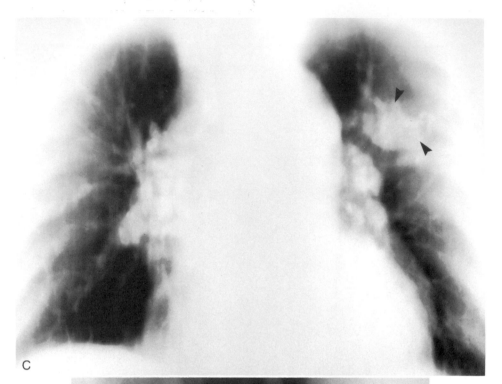

C

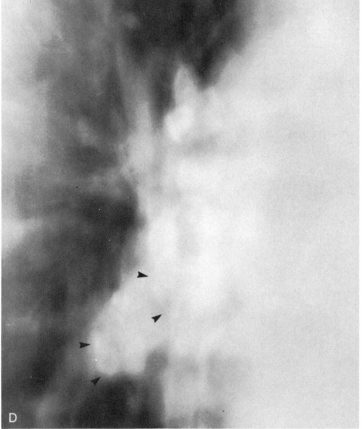

D

Figure 4–102 *Continued. C,* A full lung tomogram demonstrates bilateral hilar calcification; calcium is also present in the parenchymal lesion in the upper lobe (*arrowheads*). *D,* A detail view of the right hilum from an anteroposterior tomogram discloses calcification in a curvilinear configuration (*arrowheads*) in the periphery of enlarged lymph nodes—so-called eggshell calcification. Central, amorphous calcific deposits are also present in some of the enlarged nodes.

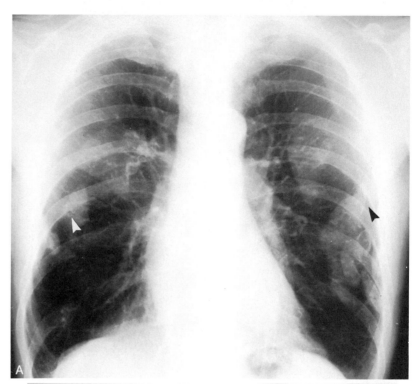

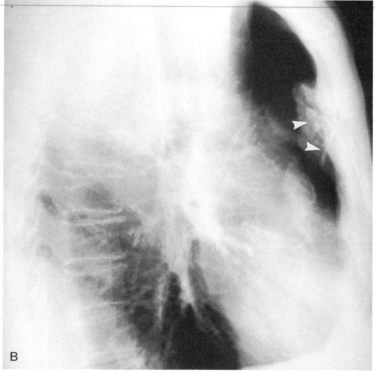

Figure 4–103. Pleural Calcification. Postero-anterior (*A*) and lateral (*B*) chest roentgenograms reveal numerous peripheral masses or plaques bilaterally with roentgenographic characteristics of pleural or extrapleural lesions. The plaques are congregated along the midaxillary and anterior portions of the thorax; many contain linear or mottled calcifications (*arrowheads*). This appearance is virtually diagnostic of asbestos-related pleural disease. The patient is a 55-year-old man with a history of exposure to asbestos for 5 years some 30 years previously.

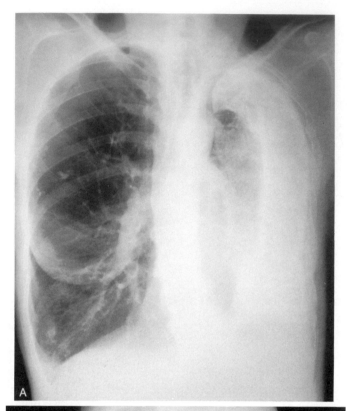

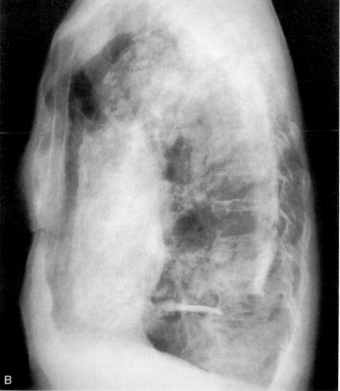

Figure 4–104. Pleural Fibrosis and Calcification (Calcific Fibrothorax). Posteroanterior (*A*) and lateral (*B*) chest roentgenograms reveal a "candy stick"-shaped, thick calcific rind separated by a broad band of intervening soft tissue. The most lateral portion of the calcification relates closely to hypertrophied ribs.

Illustration continued on opposite page

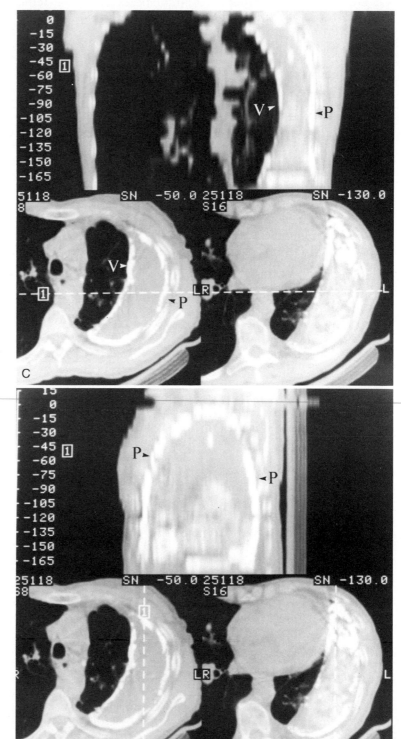

Figure 4–104 *Continued.* Coronal (*C*) and sagittal (*D*) CT reformations (*top*) with appropriate axial CT scans (*bottom*) illustrate a thick mantle of calcification delineating the visceral (*V*) and parietal (*P*) pleura; the tissue between the pleural layers is both fibrous and calcific in nature. The patient is a middle-aged woman with a history of previous tuberculous empyema.

the pleura is markedly thickened due to fibrosis or calcification is not always valid (Fig. 4–105). Hypertrophic enlargement of the ribs adjacent to chronic, calcified pleural empyemas is a common occurrence.

Pleural calcification of an entirely different form is now recognized as a manifestation of the silicatoses, including asbestosis and talcosis.[183, 184] Kiviluoto,[185] in central Finland, found pleural thickening of unusual type in 126 of 39,000 chest roentgenograms. Although none of these patients had a history of occupational exposure to dust, all but eight were living or had lived close to two open anthophyllite (asbestos) mines. Similarly, in 59 of 166 cases (35 per cent) of uncomplicated asbestosis studied by Oosthuizen and Theron in South Africa,[186] roentgenography showed calcific pleural plaques unassociated with detectable changes in the lungs. The roentgenologic characteristics are sufficiently different from calcification secondary to empyema or hemothorax that there should be no difficulty in differentiating the two. The calcification usually forms in plaques, commonly along the diaphragm, and with extensive thickening of the pleura in some cases; it invariably occurs in the parietal pleura, whereas when secondary to pyothorax or hemothorax it may be confined to the visceral pleura. It is most often bilateral and seldom unilateral. The mediastinal pleura may be involved, but calcification of the interlobar pleura has not been observed.[185] It is of interest that in Kiviluoto's series there was a very low incidence of pulmonary fibrosis and there were no reported cases of pulmonary carcinoma (asbestosis is one of the few pneumoconioses in which the incidence of bronchogenic and pleural neoplasm is known to be increased). It appears that only a very short exposure to asbestos is necessary for the development of pleural fibrosis. Sargent and his colleagues[187] described two cases of calcified diaphragmatic pleural plaques without evidence of other pleural or pulmonary disease that developed 19 and 22 years after brief exposure (exposure times were 11 and 8 months, respectively). Thus it seems clear that roentgenologic detection of diaphragmatic pleural calcification, especially if bilateral, almost invariably indicates previous exposure to asbestos dust.

Kiviluoto[185] postulated that calcification in cases of asbestosis is caused by mechanical irritation of the parietal pleura. He suggested that respiratory movements cause the protruding ends of asbestos fibers implanted near the visceral pleura to scratch the parietal pleura, producing small hemorrhages that subsequently calcify. To the best of our knowledge, this hypothesis has been neither supported nor refuted by more recent investigation.

CALCIFICATION OR OSSIFICATION IN OTHER SITES

Calcification or ossification of the cartilages of the trachea and major bronchi appears to be a physiologic concomitant of aging (Fig. 4–106); cu-

riously, it is far more common in elderly women than in men.[149] It also may appear in younger patients with hypercalcemia and hyperphosphatemia. In contrast to this innocuous calcification of degenerative or metastatic origin is the rare condition, of unknown etiology, known as tracheobronchopathia osteochondroplastica: nodules or spicules of cartilage and bone develop in the submucosa of the trachea and bronchi[188–192] and may occasion symptoms of chronic obstructive pulmonary disease.

Calcification of the walls of the central pulmonary arteries occurs in a high percentage of patients with severe longstanding pulmonary arterial hypertension, particularly those with a left-to-right shunt. The calcification may be localized to the main pulmonary artery or may extend into the major hilar and even lobar branches;[193] the arteries invariably are severely dilated. Somewhat similar is the calcification that occurs in the walls of pulmonary artery aneurysms; this extremely rare local dilatation of unknown origin chiefly affects the main pulmonary artery or its hilar branches. Even rarer is calcification of the pulmonary arteries in association with an organized thrombus: one case has been reported in which a cylindrical, branching, V-shaped calcification was detected in a hilar pulmonary artery approximately 30 years after pulmonary embolization;[194] the nature of the shadow was proved at necropsy.

Bullae and Cysts

Bullae are air-containing spaces within the lung parenchyma that measure more than 1 cm in diameter when distended and that have a wall thickness of less than 1 mm. Since they occur occasionally as a complication of consolidative lung diseases, they may considerably modify the roentgenographic appearances.

Apart from their common occurrence in emphysema (discussed later in this chapter), bullae may develop as a complication of acute staphylococcal pneumonia, particularly in infants and children (Fig. 4–107), and are familiarly known as pneumatoceles. Their pathogenesis is believed to relate either to check-valve obstruction of a small bronchus or bronchiole, distending the lung distal to the obstruction in the form of a coalescent cystic space, or to local necrosis of a bronchial wall and distention outward from this point. Such a lesion in a child with acute pneumonia is virtually pathognomonic of staphylococcal etiology; it occurs frequently, having been found in 34 of a series of 75 cases of staphylococcal pneumonia.[195] In adults, bulla formation is uncommon in pneumonia but may occur in other diseases, both local and general (apart from emphysema). In a review of causes of multiple, thin-walled cystic lesions of the lung, Godwin and his colleagues[200] include the following conditions: bronchopulmonary dysplasia and Wilson-Mikity syndrome; cystic adenomatoid malformation of the

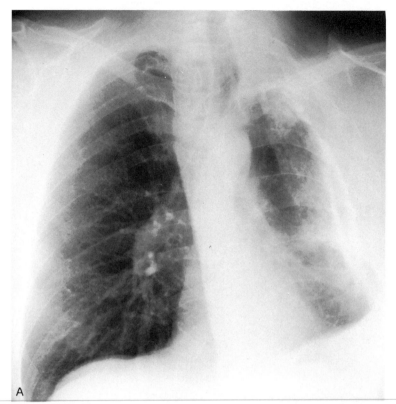

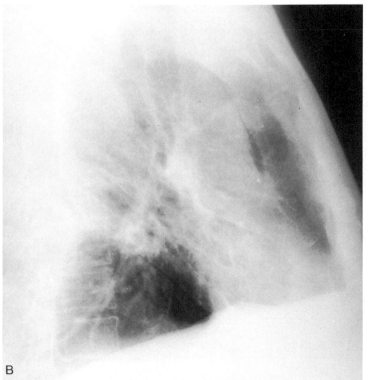

Figure 4–105. Pleural Fibrosis, Calcification, and Chronic Bronchopleural Fistula. Posteroanterior (*A*) and lateral (*B*) chest roentgenograms reveal extensive calcification that circumscribes the anterolateral, lateral, and posterolateral portions of the left lung. In the PA projection, two calcific stripes are separated by a gas-containing cavity; note also the separation between the lateral calcification and the underlying hypertrophied ribs.

Illustration continued on following page

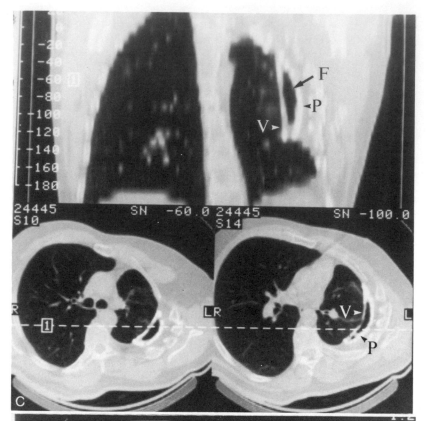

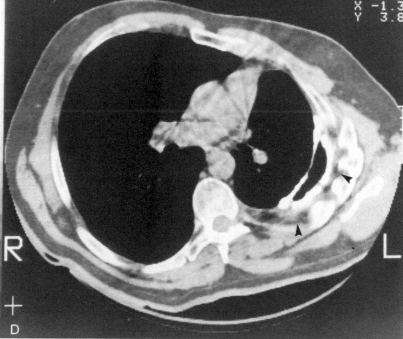

Figure 4–105 *Continued. C*, A coronal CT reformation (*top*) with appropriate axial CT scans (*bottom*) demonstrates thick calcification in both visceral (*V*) and parietal (*P*) pleural layers, separated by a gas-containing cavity that represents a bronchopleural fistula (*F*). *D*, On a CT scan with different window settings, it can be seen that although there is a fibrous component to the thickened parietal pleura, most of the extraparietal thickening is composed of fat (*arrowheads*). Hypertrophic changes are present in the ribs overlying the fibrocalcific pleura (compare with the contralateral ribs). The patient is a 61-year-old man with a previous history of tuberculous empyema.

lung; bullous emphysema; cystic bronchiectasis; fungal and tuberculous infection; staphylococcal and gram-negative pneumonia (pneumatoceles); parasitic diseases; septic pulmonary emboli; cavitating hematogenous metastases; pulmonary spread of laryngeal papillomatosis; Hodgkin's disease; necrobiotic nodules of rheumatoid arthritis; Wegener's granulomatosis; sarcoidosis; histiocytosis X; and traumatic lung cysts. Note that many of these conditions represent true cavitation, although their common denominator is an air-containing cystic space with a relatively thin wall.

The roentgenographic manifestations of bullae and blebs are considered in more detail later.

Change in Size or Position of Intrathoracic Lesions

The effects of changes in intrathoracic pressure on the size and configuration of vascular lesions within the lungs constitute an invaluable sign in the diagnosis of these lesions.[196–199] Application of the Valsalva and Mueller maneuvers not only aids in the differentiation of vascular and solid lesions of the lung parenchyma or an azygos vein from an enlarged azygos lymph node (although we prefer comparison of roentgenograms exposed in the erect and recumbent positions for this differentiation) but also may help in sorting out the confusing shadows that form the hila. Tomography facilitates assessment in most cases.[196]

The decision whether an intrathoracic mass in the periphery of the thorax is intrapulmonary or extrapulmonary is of obvious importance to diagnosis. Although such differentiation is readily provided by CT, useful information may be gained with simpler roentgenologic techniques. Consider, for example, a mass in the posterior thoracic gutter contiguous to the visceral pleura. On chest roentgenograms exposed in full inspiration and full expiration, two possibilities exist: (1) if the mass shows no change in its relationship to contiguous ribs, it must arise from thoracic wall tissues; and (2) if the relationship alters, the mass must be pleural or intrapulmonary. The same information may be gained by roentgenography in different body positions—the relationship of the intrapulmonary mass to contiguous ribs or vertebrae usually changes on roentgenograms exposed in the erect, supine, and lateral decubitus positions (Fig. 4–108) but does not alter when the lesion arises in the thoracic wall or paravertebral tissues (Fig. 4–109).

The *change in shape* of an intrathoracic mass with variations in intrathoracic pressure and body position may indicate that its contents are liquid rather than solid. For example, a "spring-water" cyst in the anterior mediastinum may undergo a change in contour from inspiration to expiration or from erect to supine position, whereas a solid teratoma or other tumor remains unchanged. This sign has been used by Gramiak and Koerner[201] to identify the fluid nature of subpleural lipomas.

Although these roentgenographic techniques are simple and relatively cost-effective, it is probable that most of the conditions discussed would be evaluated nowadays by CT, a technique that admit-

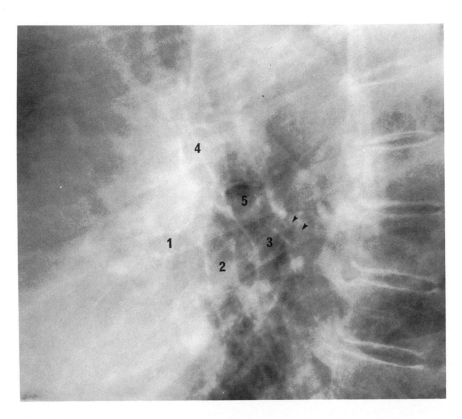

Figure 4–106. Calcification of the Cartilages of the Trachea and Major Bronchi. A detail view from a conventional lateral chest roentgenogram reveals calcification within the cartilages of the trachea and major bronchi, permitting enhanced perception of the middle lobe bronchus (*1*), the anterior and posterior walls of the right (*2*) and left (*3*) lower lobe bronchi, and the orifices of the right (*4*) and left (*5*) upper lobe bronchi. Note the clarity with which the superior segmental bronchus of the left lower lobe is seen (*arrowheads*). The patient is an elderly woman.

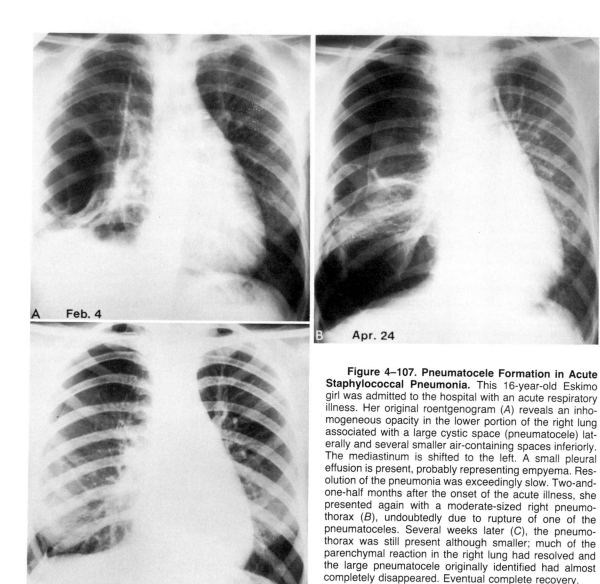

Figure 4–107. Pneumatocele Formation in Acute Staphylococcal Pneumonia. This 16-year-old Eskimo girl was admitted to the hospital with an acute respiratory illness. Her original roentgenogram (*A*) reveals an inhomogeneous opacity in the lower portion of the right lung associated with a large cystic space (pneumatocele) laterally and several smaller air-containing spaces inferiorly. The mediastinum is shifted to the left. A small pleural effusion is present, probably representing empyema. Resolution of the pneumonia was exceedingly slow. Two-and-one-half months after the onset of the acute illness, she presented again with a moderate-sized right pneumothorax (*B*), undoubtedly due to rupture of one of the pneumatoceles. Several weeks later (*C*), the pneumothorax was still present although smaller; much of the parenchymal reaction in the right lung had resolved and the large pneumatocele originally identified had almost completely disappeared. Eventual complete recovery.

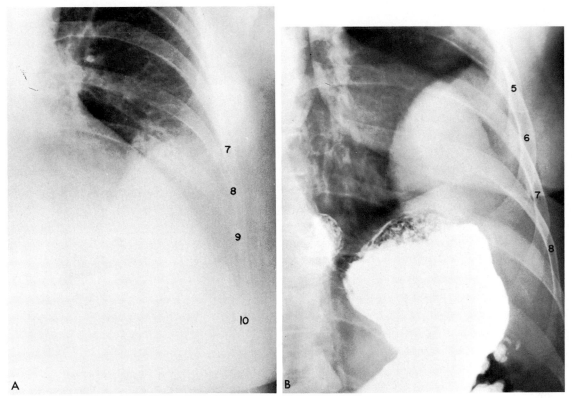

Figure 4–108. Change in Position of Intrathoracic Masses. A view of the lower half of the left hemithorax from a posteroanterior roentgenogram exposed in the erect position (*A*) reveals a rather poorly defined homogeneous mass lying in the posterior portion of the thorax contiguous to the diaphragm and lateral chest wall; in this body position, it relates to the axillary portion of ribs seven to ten. A view of the same area with the patient in the prone position (*B*) shows the mass to relate to the axillary portion of ribs five to eight. Such movement establishes the fact that mass is not attached to the rib cage. At thoracotomy, the mass was found to arise from the costal surface of the visceral pleura to which it was attached by a long pedicle. Pathologic diagnosis—solitary (localized) fibrous tumor of the pleura.

tedly would provide more complete information about their morphologic nature.

Distribution of Disease Within the Lungs (Anatomic Bias)

For several reasons, some known and others obscure, many lung diseases tend to develop only in certain anatomic locations. Knowledge of such anatomic bias is of obvious diagnostic importance; the following selected examples indicate how this sign can be used in differential diagnosis.

Aspiration pneumonia is a typical example in which the influence of gravity largely establishes the anatomic distribution of disease (Fig. 4–110). If aspiration occurs when the patient is supine (during the postoperative period, for instance), the upper lobes are involved more often than the lower[202] and their posterior portions more frequently than their anterior; conversely, if aspiration occurs when the patient is erect, involvement of the lower lobes predominates.[203] Whether the patient is recumbent or erect, aspiration occurs more readily into the right than left lung because of the more direct origin of the right main bronchus from the trachea.

Gravity also plays a significant role in the pathogenesis of pneumococcal pneumonia. In an ingen-

ious series of experiments on dogs, Robertson and Hamburger[204] showed that the anatomic site in which pneumonia developed could be controlled by altering the position of a dog's thorax so that bacteria-laden exudate flowed into specific segments under the influence of gravity. That this effect is operative in humans is lent support by the tendency of acute air-space pneumonia to occur predominantly in the posterior portions of lobes.[205, 206]

The important influence exerted by gravity on the hemodynamics of the pulmonary circulation has received much attention in recent years. It is dealt with in detail in the section concerning the pulmonary vasculature (*see* Chapter 10).

Pulmonary infarction occurs much more frequently in lower than in upper lobes. Fleischner[207] reported only 10 per cent infarcts in the upper lobes but stated that whereas this figure may accurately reflect postmortem incidence, it probably is lower in those who survive infarction. This anatomic bias undoubtedly reflects the disparity in blood flow to the base and apex of the lung in erect humans, amounting to approximately 5 to 1. For the same reason, metastatic lesions occur more frequently in lower lobes; a solitary mass in an upper lobe is unlikely to be metastatic. This preponderance of metastatic neoplastic involvement of lower lobes in

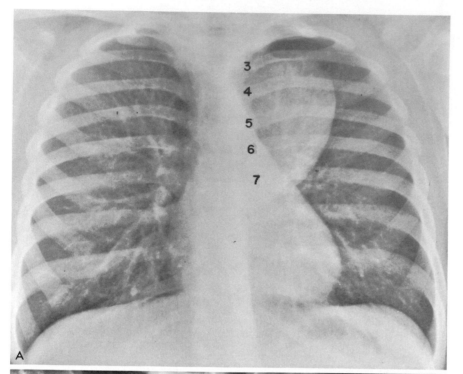

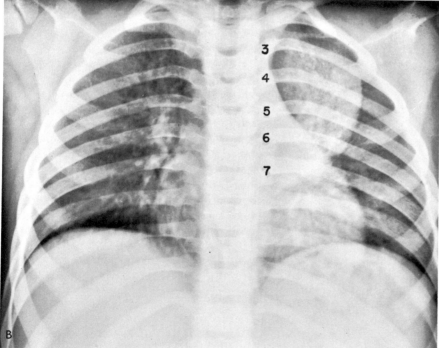

Figure 4–109. Lack of Change in Position of Intrathoracic Lesions. On both a posteroanterior roentgenogram exposed in the erect position (A) and an anteroposterior roentgenogram exposed in the supine position (B), a large, smooth, partly calcified mass can be identified in the posterior paravertebral gutter; in both body positions, it bears a constant relationship to ribs three to seven, indicating fixation to the bony thorax or contiguous tissues.

Illustration continued on opposite page

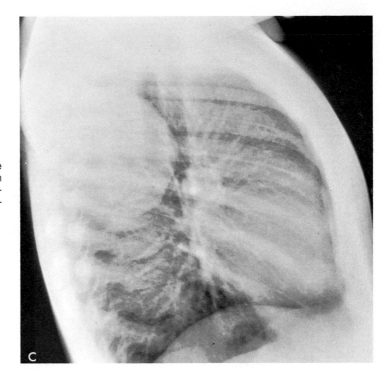

Figure 4–109 *Continued.* In lateral projection (*C*), the position of the mass is well illustrated. The patient is an asymptomatic 5-year-old boy. Pathologic diagnosis—well differentiated juvenile ganglioneuroma. (Courtesy of the Montreal Children's Hospital.)

patients in whom metastases are developing reflects the longer duration in the erect posture (the average adult spends only one third of his or her time recumbent in bed); in bedridden patients, metastatic deposits do not show the usual anatomic bias and in fact may predominate in upper zones (Fig. 4–111).

In contrast to the bias for lower lung zones displayed by metastatic neoplasms, primary pulmonary carcinoma has an unexplained predilection for upper lung zones. In 250 cases analyzed by Garland,[208] the ratio of upper to lower lobe origin was approximately 2.5 to 1. Such predilection shown by primary and metastatic neoplasms for a specific anatomic zone can be of obvious value in their differentiation. Cavitary carcinoma similarly shows a strong anatomic bias for the upper lobes; of 8 cases of roentgenographically apparent cavitation in 80 cases of pulmonary carcinoma,[209] 7 were in the upper lobes and 1 in the apex of a lower lobe. Clearly, such anatomic distribution does not assist in differentiation from cavitary tuberculosis. It has been postulated by West[378] that the greater tendency for lesions in upper lung zones to undergo cavitation is attributable to the stresses to which the lungs are subject: such stresses are three to four times greater at the apex of the lung than at the base, creating a situation conducive to cavitation.

Pulmonary tuberculosis provides a singular opportunity to employ anatomic bias in differential diagnosis. In postprimary tuberculosis in adults, susceptibility of the apical and posterior bronchopulmonary segments of the upper lobes and the superior segment of the lower lobes is well recognized; these three segments were involved in *all* 100 cases in one series,[210] and in whole (93 per cent) or in part (3.4 per cent) of 500 patients with cavitary tuberculosis in another.[211] These segments of lung, termed "the upper lung" in the former[210] and "the vulnerable portions" of lung in the latter,[211] are characterized by a high $\dot{V}/\dot{Q}$ ratio and relatively high P_{O_2} levels, favoring growth of mycobacteria. The rarity with which the anterior bronchopulmonary segment of an upper lobe is affected *to the exclusion* of other segments is sufficient to make the diagnosis of postprimary tuberculosis in this area extremely unlikely (only 1 case was reported in the series of 100 cases).[210]

Tuberculosis of the lower lung zones, of which 94 examples were reported by Segarra and associates,[212] is said to be present in 0.5 to 4.0 per cent of patients admitted to sanatoria in the United States. The majority of cases (72 per cent) reported by Segarra and associates[212] were in young women.

In contrast, *primary tuberculosis* shows an opposite anatomic bias. In the 90 children studied by Frostad,[213] involvement greatly predominated in the anterior segments of the right lung, both in the upper and middle lobes. (However, Weber and colleagues[214] found no significant differences between anterior and posterior segmental involvement in their 83 child patients.) The reasons for this difference in anatomic distribution in primary and postprimary tuberculosis are not clear.

Pulmonary sequestration occurs almost exclusively in the lower lobes, most commonly in the posterior basilar bronchopulmonary segment, and more commonly on the left side than the right.[215, 216] According to Witten and associates,[217] only three cases of intralobar bronchopulmonary sequestration in the

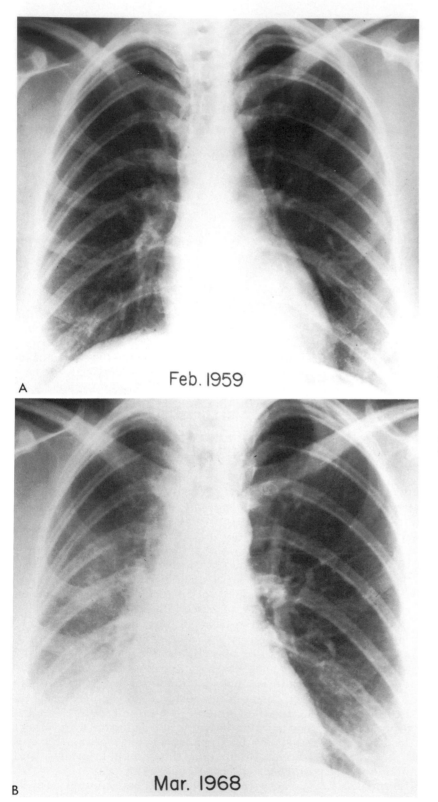

Feb. 1959

A

Mar. 1968

B

Figure 4–110. Anatomic Bias in Disease: Exogenous Lipid Pneumonia. In 1959, a roentgenogram (*A*) of this 20-year-old woman was within normal limits although the volume of the right hemithorax might have been slightly less than that of the left. Ten years later (*B*), there had developed a diffuse increase in opacity and loss of volume of the right lung; the pattern suggested combined air-space and interstitial disease of some form.

Illustration continued on opposite page

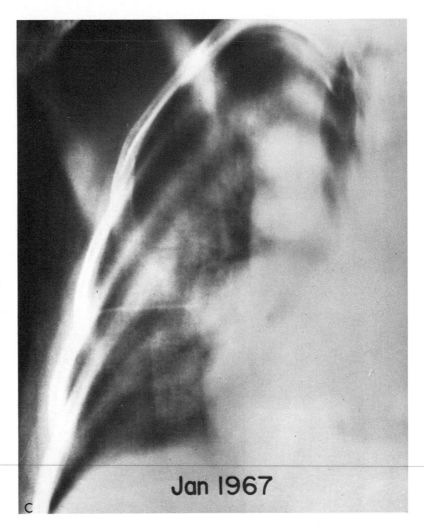

Figure 4–110 *Continued.* The left lung was perfectly clear. A tomogram of the right lung obtained in 1967 (*C*) reveals a well-defined air bronchogram, indicating airlessness of the surrounding parenchyma. On biopsy, the lung was found to harbor much lipid material within both air spaces and interstitial tissues. This mentally retarded, epileptic woman was asymptomatic except for severe constipation, for which she was given 1 to 2 oz of mineral oil each day; she spent most of her time in bed, almost always lying on her right side.

Jan 1967

C

upper lobes had been reported in the literature by 1962 (they described three additional cases). Intrapulmonary bronchogenic cysts have a similar but lesser predilection for the lower lobes; two thirds of 32 cases reported by Rogers and Osmer[218] were so located.

Diffuse lung disease frequently shows an anatomic bias, a factor that may be important to differential diagnosis. For example, the ground-glass opacity and reticulation of asbestosis typically is of basal distribution.[219, 220] Chronic idiopathic interstitial fibrosis and interstitial fibrosis of progressive systemic sclerosis frequently are predominantly basal in distribution, particularly in the early stages. Conversely, upper lobe predilection is shown by silicosis, sarcoidosis, eosinophilic granuloma, and the conglomerate shadows of complicated silicosis and coal workers' pneumoconiosis.

Roentgenologic Localization of Pulmonary Disease (The Silhouette Sign)

The anatomic location of the great majority of pulmonary diseases that increase local density can be established precisely from posteroanterior and lateral roentgenograms. When doubt exists, fluo-

roscopic examination, oblique or stereoscopic roentgenography, or tomography, can be employed. In two situations, however, it may be difficult to locate disease precisely: when multiple segments of both lungs are involved, with resultant confusion of superimposed shadows in lateral projection; and when only an anteroposterior projection of the chest is available for evaluation (for example, in the immediate postoperative period or when a patient is too ill for standard roentgenography). In these circumstances, the "silhouette sign"[221] is useful. Felson and Felson[221] credited Dunham with first reference to this invaluable roentgenographic sign in the mid 1930s. Since then many writers have emphasized its value in localizing pulmonary disease.[221–232] The mediastinal and diaphragmatic contours are rendered roentgenographically visible by their contrast with contiguous air-containing lung. When an opacity is situated in any portion of lung adjacent to a mediastinal or diaphragmatic border, that border can no longer be seen roentgenographically (Fig. 4–112). The corollary is that an opacity within the lungs that does *not* obliterate the mediastinal or diaphragmatic contour cannot be situated within lung contiguous to these structures (Fig. 4–113). Clearly, this sign is apparent only when structures have been adequately penetrated; for example, in an underpenetrated roentgenogram, massive consolidation of the right lower lobe prevents identification of the right border of the heart, merely because the flux of roentgen rays is of insufficient penetration to reproduce the heart shadow through the massive lower lobe density—despite the presence of air-containing lung contiguous to the heart. The silhouette sign is perhaps of greatest use in the differentiation of middle lobe and lingular disease from lower lobe disease, but in many other sites it may show the precise anatomic location—for example, obliteration of the aortic knuckle on the left side by airlessness of the apical-posterior segment of the left upper lobe, obliteration of the ascending arch of the aorta and of the superior vena cava by consolidation of the anterior bronchopulmonary segment of the right upper lobe, or obliteration of

the posterior paraspinal line by contiguous airless lung in the left posterior gutter.

Although this sign is used chiefly to localize pulmonary disease, we have found it almost as useful for identifying disease processes. For example, on a posteroanterior roentgenogram the increased density produced by total collapse of the right middle lobe may be negligible and in fact impossible to appreciate subjectively; however, the silhouette sign invariably accompanies such collapse (apparent as loss of sharp definition of the right heart border) and should permit a categorical statement that there is disease in the right middle lobe (a lateral or lordotic projection will be confirmatory); an uncommon exception to this rule is severe pectus excavatum, which occasionally is associated with loss of definition of the right heart border. It may be very difficult to identify the shadow of

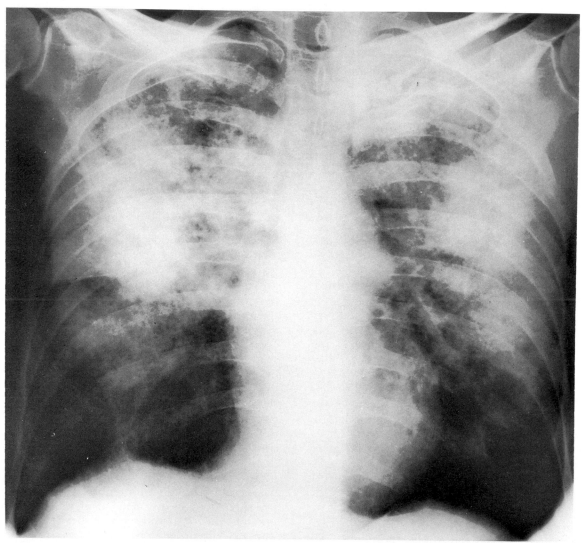

Figure 4–111. Anatomic Bias in Pulmonary Metastases. An anteroposterior roentgenogram of this 59-year-old man reveals extensive disease affecting predominantly the upper two thirds of both lungs. Although there is some superimposed acute pneumonia, most of the opacities are due to metastases from a primary carcinoma of the colon. The unusual anatomic distribution of metastases in this patient was related to two factors: (1) emphysema affecting predominantly both lower lung zones; and (2) a recumbent position necessitated by long-standing quadriplegia.

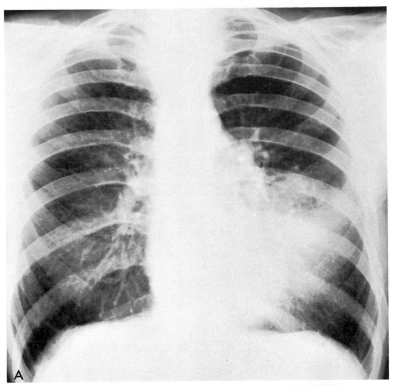

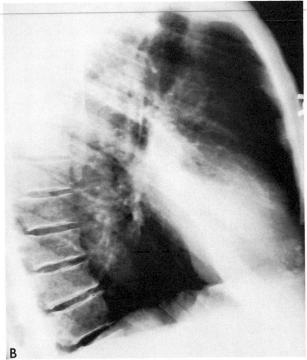

Figure 4–112. The Silhouette Sign. Posteroanterior (*A*) and lateral (*B*) roentgenograms reveal obliteration of the left heart border by a shadow of homogeneous density situated within the lingula; such obliteration inevitably indicates lingular disease (provided there is adequate roentgenographic exposure). Squamous cell carcinoma of the lingular bronchus with distal obstructive pneumonitis.

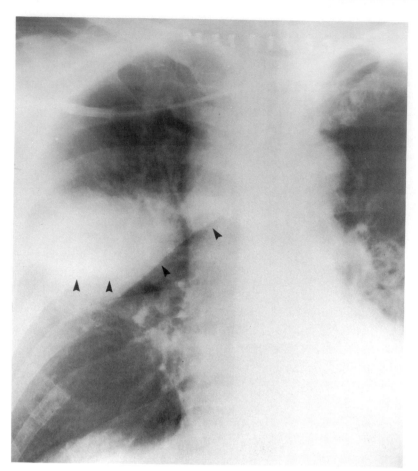

Figure 4–113. Application of the Silhouette Sign for Disease Localization. A detail view of the right hemithorax from an anteroposterior chest roentgenogram demonstrates an area of air-space consolidation in the right lung caused by acute bacterial pneumonia. The process does not obliterate any portion of the right mediastinal contour and is sharply delineated by the superomedial portion of the right major fisssure (*oblique arrowheads*) and the lateral aspect of the minor fissure (*vertical arrowheads*). These three features thus localize the pneumonia to the posterior and lateral portions of the right upper lobe.

minor consolidation or atelectasis in a posterior basal segment of a lower lobe as an area of increased density, but invisibility of the posterior portion of the hemidiaphragm in lateral projection often permits identification of disease in that segment.

The physical basis underlying production of the silhouette sign was questioned by Tuddenham,[233] who stated that obliteration of a portion of the mediastinal or diaphragmatic contour occurs *not* because of the contiguity of the disease process to the involved border but because the shape and configuration of airless lung are identical to that of the obliterated structure. Thus, if a volume of lung in the right lower lobe had a surface identical to the contour of the right border of the heart, consolidation of this lung tissue would obliterate the right heart border—provided that the two were exactly superimposed in posteroanterior projection. Tuddenham feels that this does not occur in the human thorax because the distribution of bronchopulmonary segments prevents such volumetric consolidation. In an attempt to assess the validity of the two theories (air replacement and summation), Kattan and his colleagues[234] recently carried out experiments with a number of different substances and found that the air replacement theory was the most plausible explanation for the phenomenon, al-

though they admitted that both theories are potentially valid.

To recapitulate, the *silhouette sign* is an extremely valuable roentgenologic sign in both localizing and identifying local pulmonary disease. It can best be defined in the words of Felson,[21] who is to be commended for emphasizing its importance in roentgenologic diagnosis. *"An intrathoracic lesion touching a border of the heart or aorta will obliterate that border on the roentgenogram; an intrathoracic lesion not anatomically contiguous with a border of the heart or aorta will not obliterate the border."*

Mention should be made of two other roentgen signs described by Felson:[235] "hilus overlay" and "hilus bifurcation." The former sign permits differentiation of true cardiomegaly from large anterior mediastinal masses that mimic cardiac enlargement; in the presence of an anterior mediastinal mass, the hilum is projected medial to the lateral border of the mass, and in cardiomegaly the hilum is displaced laterally. The "hilus bifurcation sign" is meant to differentiate hilar masses from vascular structures in cases of hilar enlargement: if vessels are seen to arise directly from the hilar shadow, the enlargement is vascular; if they appear to arise medial to the lateral aspect of the hilar shadow, the enlargement is caused by an extravascular mass. We have not found either sign of much value in roentgenographic assessment.

The Time Factor in Roentgenologic Diagnosis

In clinical practice, situations occur relatively frequently in which a lack of specific roentgenologic signs precludes positive diagnosis. In both acute and chronic lung diseases, roentgenographic signs may overlap so that only differential diagnostic possibilities can be suggested at the first examination; if the diagnosis cannot be established by the integrated clinical evidence and results of laboratory and pulmonary function tests, serial films showing changes over the subsequent days, weeks, or months often provide valuable clues. A few examples illustrate the importance of assessing time relationships in roentgenologic diagnosis.

Acute pneumonia caused by *Streptococcus pneumoniae* or *Mycoplasma pneumoniae* organisms sometimes can be differentiated by their characteristic roentgenographic patterns. If this is not possible immediately, changes evidenced in roentgenograms over the next few days sometimes permit distinction, even without antibiotic therapy (progressive changes despite penicillin therapy might suggest a *Mycoplasma* etiology, indicating the need for administration of a more efficacious antibiotic). The progress of changes after pulmonary embolism allows significant deductions concerning the underlying pathologic process: consolidation that clears fairly rapidly within 4 to 7 days indicates pulmonary hemorrhage without necrosis; persistence of the opacity with progressive retraction and loss of volume supports an assumption of infarction with tissue death. The rapidity with which diffuse interstitial pulmonary edema may appear and disappear (often within hours) allows immediate differentiation from irreversible interstitial disease, which it may otherwise closely mimic. Finally, it is surprising how frequently a small area of parenchymal consolidation in an upper lobe, roentgenographically typical of exudative tuberculosis, disappears in a few days, indicating a less significant etiology.

In all these examples it is preferable to be able to suggest the correct diagnosis at the time of the first roentgenogram, so that treatment can be instituted immediately. When this is impossible, however, and clinical and laboratory evidence is inconclusive, the observation of progressive changes in serial roentgenograms draws attention not only to the need for the discontinuation of useless therapy in the face of an erroneous diagnosis, but also for the institution of suitable treatment when the true nature of the process becomes known.

It is not only in the field of acute pulmonary disease that the time relationship is important. Growth characteristics of peripheral pulmonary nodules have been studied a great deal in recent

years. The "doubling time"* hypothesis developed by Collins and associates[236] and extended by others[237–242] has increased our knowledge of the natural history of pulmonary carcinoma. For example, in a study of 218 pulmonary nodules, of which 177 were malignant and 41 benign, Nathan and his colleagues[237] concluded that virtually all nodules with a doubling time of 7 days or less are benign; if metastatic choriocarcinoma, testicular neoplasms, and osteogenic sarcoma can be eliminated (generally relatively simple by the time pulmonary metastases appear), the doubling time for benign lesions can be increased to 11 days. At the other end of the scale, almost all nodules whose volume doubles in 465 days or more are benign (Fig. 4–114). Perhaps the growth rate principle is most useful in assessing solitary nodules in patients over 40 years of age, when the incidence of malignancy increases significantly. In this age group, Nathan and associates found that nearly all solitary nodules that doubled in less than 37 days were benign, and that the longest doubling time of 72 malignant nodules was 200 days. It seems, therefore, that pulmonary nodules whose rate of growth falls outside these "benign" limits should be considered malignant.

Clearly, the doubling time hypothesis yields a more accurate assessment of the underlying nature of disease than does simple increase in size. Since benign lesions such as hamartoma,[243, 244] histoplasmoma, and certain others may grow slowly, increase in size *per se* should not be the sole consideration in deciding therapy for a pulmonary nodule.

The conclusions reached from these and other similar studies are of great diagnostic importance. They are considered in detail in Chapter 8; it suffices here to stress the value of applying the growth rate principle to the roentgenologic assessment of peripheral pulmonary nodules.

LINE SHADOWS

A linear opacity (*synonyms:* line shadow, linear shadow, band shadow) is defined in our glossary as "a shadow resembling a line; hence, any elongated opacity of approximately uniform width." The normal substratum of all chest roentgenograms is formed by line shadows—the vascular markings and interlobar fissures; the roentgenologic appearance of these is described in Chapter 1. The present section describes the many line shadows of varied etiology, seen from time to time in roentgenograms of the chest, which can be grouped most appropriately under this descriptive umbrella. Primary and

---

*"Doubling" refers to *volume*, not diameter. Assuming a nodule to be spherical, multiply its diameter by 1.25 to obtain the diameter of a sphere whose volume is double; e.g., the volume of a nodule 2 cm in diameter is doubled by the time its diameter reaches 2.5 cm.

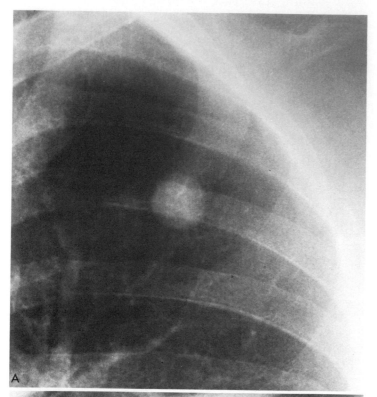

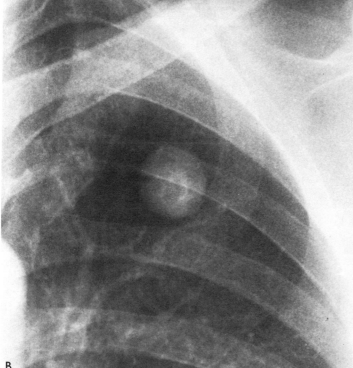

Figure 4–114. Solitary Nodule: Enlarging Histoplas-moma. In 1969 (*A*), a solitary nodule in the left upper lobe of this 61-year-old asymptomatic man measured 17 mm in diameter; it was sharply circumscribed and showed no convincing evidence of calcification. Two years later (*B*), the diameter of the lesion had reached 21 mm, representing almost a doubling of volume.

Illustration continued on opposite page

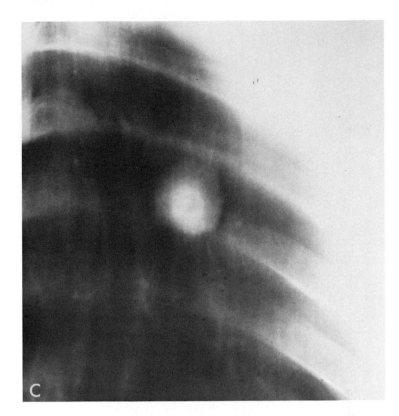

Figure 4–114 *Continued.* Tomography at that time (*C*) showed a large central nidus of calcification. Despite the extensive central calcification, the lesion was resected; organisms consistent with *Histoplasma capsulatum* were identified histologically.

secondary abnormalities of the pulmonary vasculature form a comprehensive topic in their own right and are considered in detail in Chapter 10.

Linear opacities on a chest roentgenogram fall into six different categories on the basis of pathogenesis:

1. Septal lines.
2. Tubular shadows (bronchial wall shadows).
3. Linear opacities extending from peripheral parenchymal lesions to the hila or visceral pleura.
4. Parenchymal scarring.
5. Line shadows of pleural origin.
6. Horizontal or obliquely oriented linear opacities of unknown nature.

SEPTAL LINES

In 1933, Kerley[245] described certain linear shadows in the chest roentgenogram that he ascribed to engorged lymphatics. In 1951, he further categorized three patterns of linear change, which he designated "A" lines, "B" lines, and "C" lines.[246–248] Our knowledge of the pathogenesis and morphology of these lines has increased tremendously in recent years, but Kerley's valuable contribution in first drawing attention to their roentgenologic importance is still recognized by the eponymous designations "Kerley A," "Kerley B," and "Kerley C" lines.

Kerley A lines are straight or almost straight linear opacities, seldom more than 1 mm thick and 2 to 6 cm long, within the lung substance; their course bears no definite relationship to the anatomic distribution of bronchoarterial bundles (Fig. 4–115). Unlike Kerley B lines, they never extend to the visceral pleura, although their medial extension is usually to a hilum. Trapnell[249] originally thought they were produced by anastomotic lymph channels crossing from perivenous to peribronchial locations, most being approximately midway between hilum and pleura and none more peripherally. More recently, however, in a radiologic-pathologic correlative study, he revised this interpretation slightly by showing positive correlation between roentgenographic A lines and sheets of connective tissue deep within the lung in which run both veins and anastomotic lymphatics.[250] The major difference in his more recent interpretation of the pathologic basis of Kerley A lines appears to lie chiefly in the contribution of the lymphatics: he showed histologically that the lymphatics contribute one tenth or less to the thickness of the line shadow, and in certain conditions such as pulmonary edema they may be invisible. As with Kerley B lines, the visibility of A lines depends upon the accumulation of abnormal amounts of edema fluid or other tissue within the perilymphatic connective tissue, and not distention of the lymphatics themselves; in the absence of such accumulation, the deep septa are not roentgenographically visible. Depending upon the disease process that causes them, they may be reversible (as in pulmonary edema) or irreversible (as in pneumoconiosis or lymphangitic carcinoma). A point of anatomic interest is that the distribution of Kerley A lines, as distinct from that of bronchoar-

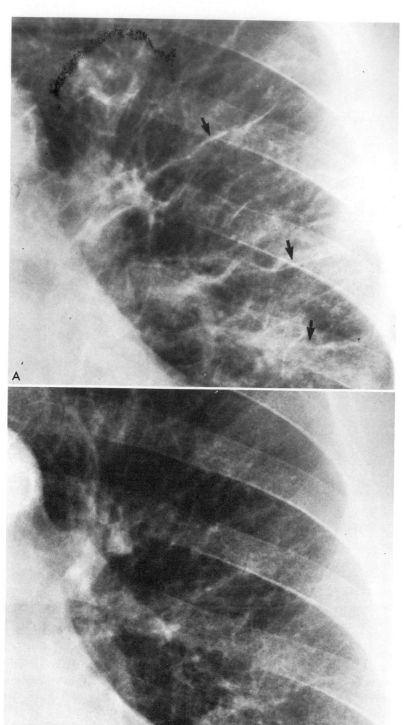

Figure 4–115. Line Shadows: Kerley A Lines. A view of the left lung from a posteroanterior roentgenogram (*A*) reveals a coarse network of linear strands widely distributed throughout the lung. Several long line shadows measuring up to 4 cm in length can be identified in the central zone approximately midway between the axillary lung margin and the heart (*arrows*); the orientation of these lines does not conform to the distribution of bronchovascular bundles. These are Kerley A lines and represent edema of central pulmonary septa. A roentgenogram made several days later (*B*) shows complete clearing. Cardiac decompensation.

terial bundles, corresponds to the remoteness of venous from arterial trunks within the lung.

Kerley B lines are less than 2 cm long (shorter than A lines). In contrast to A lines, which lie in the substance of the lungs, B lines are in the periphery; they are short and straight, seldom more than 1 mm thick, and lie roughly perpendicular to the pleural surface (Fig. 4–116). Their outer ends invariably abut against the visceral pleura, although this relationship may not be apparent on posteroan-

terior roentgenograms. Care is needed to avoid mistaking small vascular shadows in the lung periphery for Kerley B lines; the former branch, a characteristic never seen with the latter. B lines are caused by increased fluid or tissue in the interlobular septa of the lungs, chiefly in the perilymphatic interstitial tissue (*see* Figure 4–57, page 547). (It is unlikely that lymphatic engorgement *per se* can produce a roentgenographically visible shadow.) Because of their anatomic location they are sometimes referred to as "septal lines." Their pathogenesis varies widely: one of the commonest causes is interstitial pulmonary edema secondary to pulmonary venous hypertension (as in mitral stenosis or left ventricular failure). In such circumstances the influence of gravity on pulmonary hemodynamics gives rise to interlobular septal edema in the lower portions of the lungs and not in the upper; thus, line shadows are seen to best advantage just above the costophrenic angles on posteroanterior and oblique roentgenograms. When the edema is transient, septal lines appear and disappear sporadically with each episode of decompensation; with repeated insults of this character, or in the presence of chronic and severe pulmonary venous hypertension, fibrosis within the interlobular septa gives rise to permanent, irreversible B lines.

In diseases whose pathogenesis is other than edema, the anatomic distribution of B lines may be entirely different. For example, in pneumoconiosis,[246–248, 252] sarcoidosis,[253] lymphangitic carcinomatosis,[254] lipid pneumonia,[255] and lymphoma (*see* Figure 4–58, page 550),[256] in which gravity does not influence hemodynamics, septal lines may be visible anywhere in the lung periphery where septa normally occur—along most of the axillary portion of the lung up to the apex and in the retrosternal space[257] (although retrosternal B lines may be observed occasionally in some patients with severe interstitial edema).

Kerley C Lines, are reputed to be caused by engorgement of pleural lymphatics, but we do not believe that a single layer of lymphatics projected *en face* could conceivably cast a roentgenographic shadow, an opinion to which Trapnell[249] subscribes. Rather, it is likely that the fine network of interlacing linear shadows sometimes seen in cases of interstitial pulmonary edema is caused by the superimposition of many Kerley B lines in the anterior and posterior portions of the lungs (Fig. 4–117), an explanation strongly supported by the roentgenologic-pathologic correlation obtained by Heitzman and associates.[258] Such a network of shadows is almost certainly a manifestation of severe interlobular edema rather than separate and distinct anatomic involvement of lymphatic channels.

TUBULAR SHADOWS (BRONCHIAL WALL SHADOWS)

The air column of the trachea, main bronchi, right intermediate bronchus, and left lower lobe bronchus normally is visible on well-exposed roentgenograms. Where these structures are in contact with air-containing parenchyma their walls also are visible, their thickness being sufficient to cast a roentgenographic shadow. Beyond the immediate confines of the hilar shadows, however, neither the bronchial walls nor their air columns should be visible normally (except when viewed end-on—*see* further on); thus, when tubular shadows are iden-

tified outside the hilar limits they constitute a definite sign of disease. Tubular shadows are double-line shadows that may be parallel or slightly tapered as they proceed distally, and always follow the bronchovascular distribution; they may branch in a manner typical of the bronchial tree. When one of the paired lines is contiguous with a vessel it casts no roentgenographic shadow, but identification of a single line paralleling a vessel has the same significance as a tubular shadow.

The commonest cause of tubular shadows is bronchiectasis (Fig. 4–118), in which the line shadows are roughly parallel and measure 1 mm or slightly more in width. The width of the air column separating them depends upon the severity of the bronchial dilatation. Since chronic bronchiectasis is often associated with atelectasis, multiple tubular shadows may be crowded together with little air-containing parenchyma separating them. Morphologically, these line shadows are caused by a combination of thickened bronchial walls and peribronchial fibrosis and alveolar collapse. When bronchiectatic segments become filled with retained mucus or pus, their tubular appearance is transformed into homogeneous, bandlike opacities, which Simon[259] termed the "gloved-finger" shadow (Fig. 4–119). Of a similar nature but more proximal in the bronchial

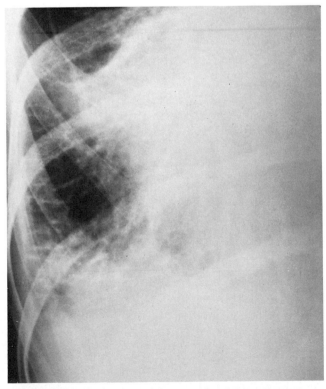

Figure 4–116. Line Shadows: Septal (Kerley B) Lines. A magnified view of the lower portion of the right lung from a posteroanterior roentgenogram reveals several line shadows approximately 1 cm in length oriented in a horizontal plane perpendicular to the axillary pleura (there is a small pleural effusion as well). These are Kerley B lines, caused by edema of the interlobular septa.

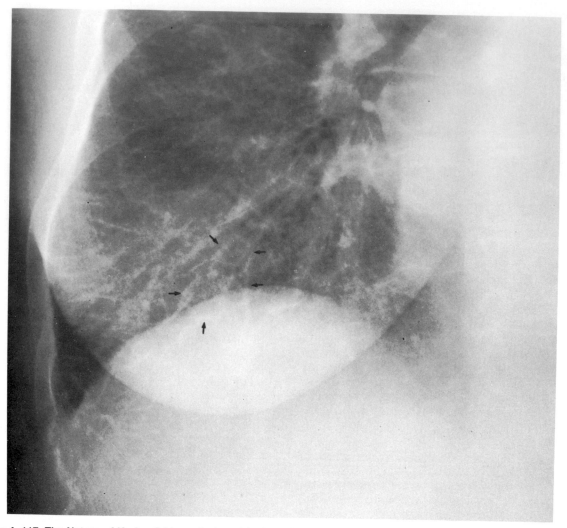

Figure 4–117. The Nature of Kerley C Lines. A view of the lower half of the right lung from a posteroanterior roentgenogram reveals numerous septal (Kerley B) lines in the axillary lung zone. In addition, at least three or four roughly circular ring shadows (*arrows*) can be seen in the midlung zone, representing the boundaries of secondary lobules thickened by edema fluid. These Kerley C lines are thus another manifestation of septal edema and are no more than Kerley B lines perceived *en face*.

tree are the mucous plugs of mucoid impaction or hypersensitivity bronchopulmonary aspergillosis; these vary from a broad linear shadow to a Y or V configuration, depending on the length of airway involved and whether a bronchial bifurcation is affected.

In 1960, Hodson and Trickey[260] drew attention to the frequency with which tubular shadows are seen in the lungs of children with bronchial asthma, identifying them in 121 (64 per cent) of 190 such patients. The patients were divided into three groups: those with chronic infectious asthma (26), with purely allergic asthma (58), and with asthma of mixed etiology (106). The researchers identified bronchial walls in 88 per cent of those with infectious or mixed etiology asthma but in only 9 per cent of those with the allergic type, and therefore they related bronchial wall thickening in asthma to chronic infection (Fig. 4–120). In a series of 22 patients who died of status asthmaticus, Cardell[261]

described the histologic changes in the bronchi of those in whom there was an infective factor as infiltration of the walls with eosinophils, lymphocytes, plasma cells, and a thick peribronchial cuff of fibrous tissue containing many abnormal capillaries; in those in whom the asthma was purely allergic in type, there was little or no peribronchial fibrosis, and the cellular infiltrate was almost entirely eosinophilic. From the reproductions in Cardell's article it is not clear whether the airways whose histologic changes he describes are of the same order as those that create tubular shadows roentgenographically; they appear to be much more peripheral and probably are bronchioles.

In one other group of patients tubular shadows are of unknown nature and pathogenesis. Most commonly they are seen as isolated shadows in the right lower lobe of adult patients of any age; their walls may be parallel, as in bronchiectasis, or may taper in much the same fashion as a normal bronchus. Colloquially referred to by the British as "tram lines," in our experience they occur most often in cases of chronic bronchitis; Bates and his colleagues[262] reported seeing them in 45 per cent of 185 patients with this disease. However, in describing the roentgenographic changes of chronic bronchitis, Simon[263] attributed such isolated tubular shadows to an accompanying bronchiectasis and has stated that in chronic bronchitic patients in Britain tram lines are rarely seen roentgenographically.

The differences between Simon and ourselves in finding tram lines in patients with chronic bronchitis have understandably caused us some concern and may be related to different criteria of recognition, since thin line shadows can often be identified in the medial third of the lungs and may confuse interpretation. A more reliable and more easily recognizable sign of bronchial wall thickening would help eradicate the inconsistency in reporting this abnormality; such a sign may be the "end-on" bronchial shadows roentgenographically identifiable in the parahilar zones of a large percentage of subjects (Fig. 4–121). These bronchi represent segmental or subsegmental bronchi in the anterior bronchopulmonary segment of an upper lobe or the superior bronchopulmonary segment of a lower lobe. They range in diameter from 3 to 7 mm and thus represent different stages in bronchial subdivision. In a review of the posteroanterior roentgenograms of 200 individuals in the United Kingdom (100 normal

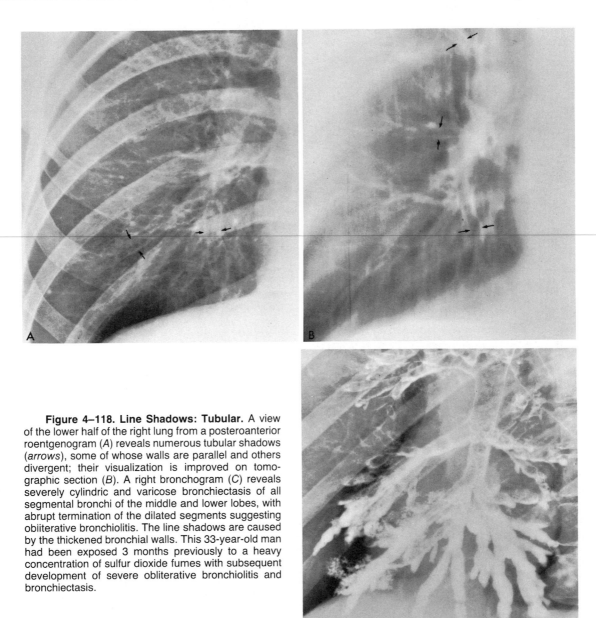

Figure 4–118. Line Shadows: Tubular. A view of the lower half of the right lung from a posteroanterior roentgenogram (A) reveals numerous tubular shadows (arrows), some of whose walls are parallel and others divergent; their visualization is improved on tomographic section (B). A right bronchogram (C) reveals severely cylindric and varicose bronchiectasis of all segmental bronchi of the middle and lower lobes, with abrupt termination of the dilated segments suggesting obliterative bronchiolitis. The line shadows are caused by the thickened bronchial walls. This 33-year-old man had been exposed 3 months previously to a heavy concentration of sulfur dioxide fumes with subsequent development of severe obliterative bronchiolitis and bronchiectasis.

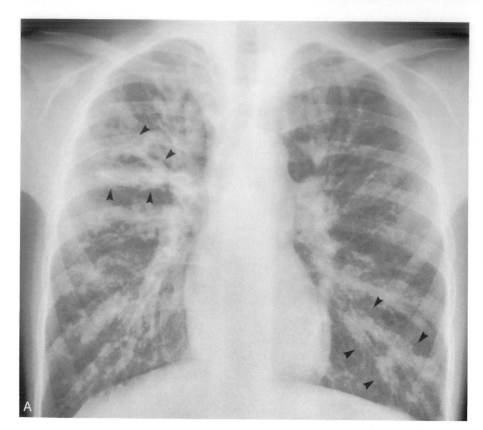

Flgure 4–119. Cystic Fibrosis, Bronchiectasis, and Mucoid Impaction (Bronchocele Formation). *A,* A posteroanterior chest roentgenogram reveals numerous tubular, branching opacities (*arrowheads*), most numerous in the right upper and left lower lobes. End-on bronchi in the perihilar regions are slightly dilated and have thickened walls.

Illustration continued on opposite page

subjects and 100 patients with chronic obstructive pulmonary disease), we identified end-on bronchi in 160 (80 per cent). Roentgenographic visibility of the wall of an air-containing tube within the lungs viewed perpendicular to its longitudinal axis (i.e., *en face*) depends upon the absorptive power of its tissue "in tangent" (Fig. 4–122); since the image of the tangential wall thickness fades off at the margins, loss of definition precludes accurate appreciation of total wall thickness. In contrast, when the same tube is viewed end-on, a substantially greater amount of tissue is traversed by the x-ray beam, particularly at its periphery, thus reducing the effect of subliminal absorption.

To assess whether thickening of the walls of bronchi seen end-on reliably distinguishes the patient with chronic bronchitis from the normal subject, we studied the roentgenograms of 300 persons—roughly equal numbers of patients with established chronic obstructive pulmonary disease and age-matched asymptomatic subjects with normal standard pulmonary function tests. Obje. ive measurement of bronchial wall thickness and subjective assessment of thickening provided suggestive but not conclusive evidence for the presence of chronic bronchitis. The chief potential for error lay in the absence of wall thickening in patients with clinically established chronic bronchitis (false negatives); we are still of the opinion that convincing evidence of bronchial wall thickening constitutes a reliable sign of chronic bronchial disease, usually

chronic bronchitis. More is said of this study in the chapter on obstructive airway disease.

LINEAR OPACITIES EXTENDING FROM PERIPHERAL PARENCHYMAL LESIONS TO THE HILA OR VISCERAL PLEURA

Line shadows of varying width are often visible extending from a peripheral parenchymal opacity to the hilum. Usually they are uneven in width and their course may be interrupted for varying distances. Their conformity to the pattern of vascular distribution establishes their anatomic location within bronchovascular bundles. Such communicating strands have been described in both infectious and neoplastic processes. For example, in active cavitary tuberculosis the connecting line shadows are produced by an admixture of tubercles, fibrous tissue, thickened lymphatics, and thickened bronchial walls; when tuberculosis becomes chronic and productive, fibrosis is histologically more predominant. In some cases of a peripheral mass or nodule, line shadows extend to the hilum; since the sign may be present in both infectious and neoplastic lesions, it is of no value in differential diagnosis.

When a parenchymal mass of almost any etiology is situated near the periphery of the lung, a line shadow is sometimes visible extending from the mass to the visceral pleura, commonly with a local indrawing of the pleura (Fig. 4–123). Rigler[264] observed this sign in 20 of 25 cases of alveolar cell

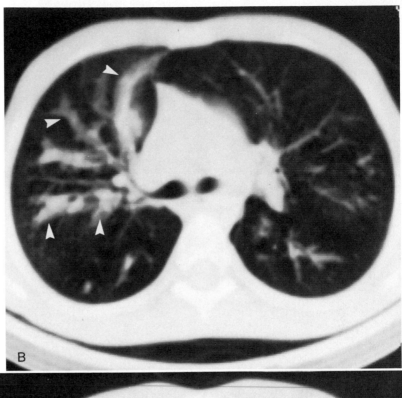

Figure 4–119 *Continued.* Transverse CT scans through the carina (*B*) and the lower lobes (*C*) reveal tubular, branching opacities (*arrowheads*) in the anterior and posterior segments of the right upper lobe and the anterior and lateral segments of the left lower lobe. The branched opacities are typical of mucoid impaction (bronchoceles) in association with cystic fibrosis.

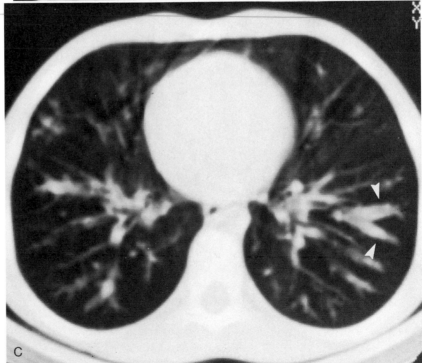

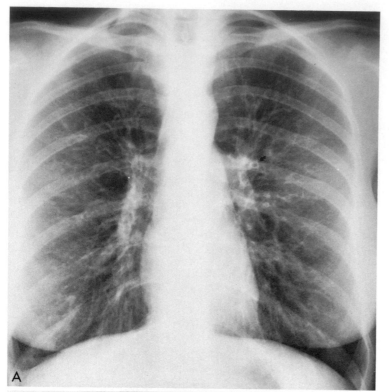

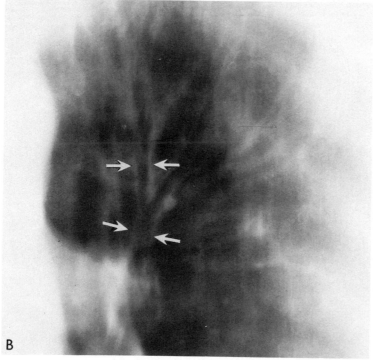

Figure 4–120. Line Shadows Caused by Thickened Bronchial Walls: Tram Lines. A posteroanterior roentgenogram (*A*) reveals prominent markings throughout both lungs. In the left upper zone, parallel or slightly tapering line shadows can be identified in the bronchial distribution of the left upper lobe, seen to better advantage on the anteroposterior tomogram in *B* (*arrows*).

Illustration continued on opposite page

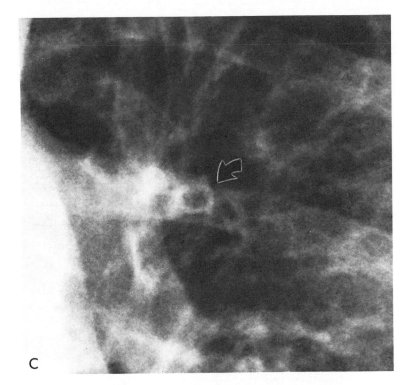

Figure 4–120 *Continued.* These "tram lines" represent thickened bronchial walls, an abnormality more easily appreciated by viewing a bronchus end-on, as in the magnified view of the left parahilar area in *C* (*arrow*). The patient is a 17-year-old girl with chronic infectious asthma.

C

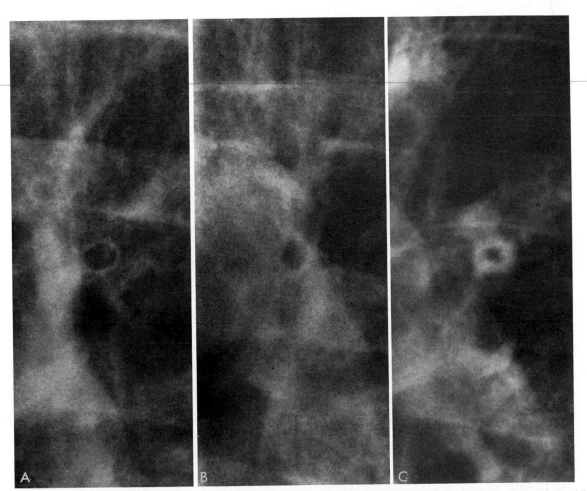

A   B   C

Figure 4–121. Bronchial Wall Thickening as Assessed from Parahilar Bronchi Viewed End-on. Views of the left parahilar zone from posteroanterior roentgenograms of three different patients, showing a normal bronchus (*A*), a bronchus with moderate wall thickening (*B*), and a bronchus with marked wall thickening (*C*). (From Fraser RG, Fraser RS, Renner JW, et al: Radiology *120*:1, 1976.

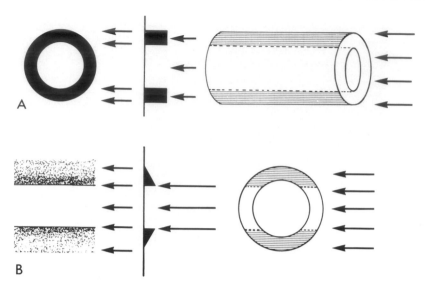

Figure 4–122. Diagram of a hollow tube viewed (*A*) in cross section (end on), and (*B*) in tangent (longitudinally). *See* text. (From Fraser RG, Fraser RS, Renner JW, et al: Radiology *120*:1, 1976.)

carcinoma and felt that its presence was highly suggestive of that diagnosis; he stated further that, although such lines may occur occasionally in cases of peripheral adenocarcinoma, he had not observed them in squamous cell cancer. This experience is in contrast to ours and that of others.[127, 265] For example, of 18 patients with the so-called "tail sign" studied by Webb,[127] 9 had benign disease (granulomas of varying etiology); of the nine cancers, five were bronchioloalveolar, two adenocarcinoma, one squamous cell carcinoma, and one metastatic carcinoma of the colon. In a more extensive study, Hill[265] concluded that the tail sign (and its related signs, the "rabbit ears" sign and "participating tail" sign) are entirely nonspecific features of peripherally located pulmonary lesions and cannot be used to differentiate a benign from a malignant lesion. We further believe that the variations on the tail sign just referred to serve little or no useful purpose from a diagnostic point of view.

PARENCHYMAL SCARRING

A segment of lung that was the site of infectious disease and has undergone healing through fibrosis may present as a linear shadow. Again, the width of the shadow largely depends upon the amount of lung originally involved. Healed upper lobe postprimary tuberculosis is a common example of this type of linear shadow (Fig. 4–124). Several shadows may be fairly closely grouped, commonly extending from the hilum to the visceral pleural surface and diverging slightly toward the periphery. In many cases there is compensatory overinflation of adjacent lung parenchyma.

The line shadow created by healed pulmonary infarction represents fibrous scarring secondary to lung necrosis. These linear shadows always extend to a pleural surface, and Reid has suggested[266] that this relationship is caused, at least in part, by an

indrawing of the pleura by the scar (Figs. 4–125 and 4–126). According to Fleischner and his colleagues,[267] shadows of healed infarction often terminate in a nodular rounded extremity at the pleural surface, a finding probably related to the indrawn pleura as described by Reid.

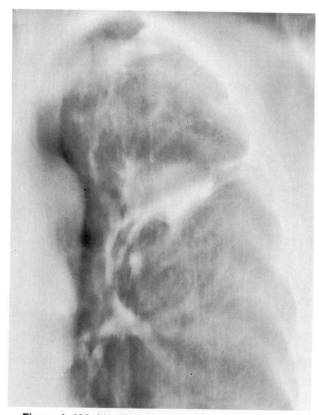

Figure 4–123. Line Shadows: Communication Between a Peripheral Mass and the Visceral Pleura. A view of the upper half of the left lung from an anteroposterior tomogram reveals a rather indistinctly defined homogeneous mass lying in the midlung zone. A prominent line shadow extends from the lateral margin of the mass to the pleura, resulting in a V-shaped deformity of the pleura caused by indrawing. Proved exudative histoplasmosis.

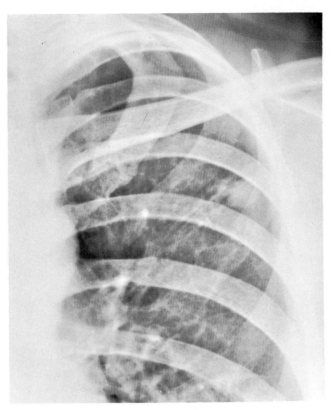

Figure 4–124. Line Shadows: Healed Pulmonary Tuberculosis. A view of the upper half of the left lung of a posteroanterior roentgenogram reveals a well-defined nodular shadow in the axillary lung zone. Line shadows of uneven width can be seen to extend both centrally and peripherally from the lesion. Presumed scarring.

LINE SHADOWS OF PLEURAL ORIGIN

In addition to the normal interlobar fissure lines and those that occur sporadically in anomalous locations, such as the azygos fissure, some line shadows that originate in the pleura constitute important direct or indirect signs of disease. Roentgenographic visibility of fissures not normally seen in a particular projection may be important evidence of otherwise invisible disease. For example, when a lower lobe loses volume, the upper portion of the major fissure sweeps downward and medially and at a certain stage becomes visible on posteroanterior roentgenograms as an obliquely oriented shadow extending inferiorly and laterally from the lateral aspect of the mediastinum above the hilum, across the shadow of the hilum, to end near the lateral costophrenic sulcus. This evidence of atelectasis may be present even when the density in the lower lobe is not increased.

Thickening of an interlobar fissure, especially if more or less uniform, is caused more often by "pleural" edema than by pleural effusion. Since the pleural connective tissue layer is continuous with the interlobular septa, it is reasonable to assume that when edema fluid accumulates in the latter sites—Kerley B lines—it might also collect in the subpleural space (*see* Figure 4–57, page 547). In such circumstances, it not only thickens the interlobar fissures but also widens the pleural layer along the lung's convex surface.

Fibrous pleural thickening over the anterior or posterior lung surfaces occasionally gives rise to rather broad linear opacities usually situated near the lung bases (Fig. 4–127). These line shadows tend to appear rather "stringy" and commonly are oriented in a horizontal or oblique plane—not unlike the scars of old pulmonary infarction. Their true nature is usually apparent from their association with other signs of pleural fibrosis (such as obliteration of the costophrenic angle) or by the minimal change in their relationship to contiguous ribs during respiration.

Another important indicator of disease is the visceral pleural line in pneumothorax; recognition of this line is of paramount importance in the diagnosis of that condition. Of a similar nature is the "double" pleural line seen along either side of the mediastinum in cases of mediastinal emphysema (Fig. 4–128); the line shadow is created by the combined thicknesses of parietal and visceral pleura dislocated laterally by mediastinal gas.

In response to loss of volume in one lung, the contralateral lung commonly undergoes compensatory overinflation, and its anterior portion, together with the anterior junction line, shifts into the affected hemithorax; the combined thickness of the visceral and parietal pleural surfaces of the two lungs creates a curved line shadow that is visible over the medial half of the affected lung in posteroanterior projection. As was pointed out in the section on atelectasis, this line may be a major indicator of unilateral loss of lung volume.

HORIZONTAL OR OBLIQUELY ORIENTED LINEAR OPACITIES OF UNKNOWN NATURE

Few would dispute the statement that of all pathologic linear opacities observed on chest roentgenograms, by far the most common are those that tend to occur in the lung bases and that for many years have traditionally been called "platelike atelectasis" (*synonyms*: plate atelectasis, platter atelectasis, discoid atelectasis). Despite the frequency of these lines as a sign of pulmonary disease, their precise pathogenesis remains shrouded in mystery. These linear opacities of unit density range in thickness from 1 to 3 mm and in length from 4 to 10 cm and are situated anatomically in the mid and lower lung zones, most commonly the latter (Fig. 4–129). Although usually oriented in a roughly horizontal plane, they may be obliquely oriented depending upon the zone of lung affected, and in midlung zones particularly may be angled more than 45 degrees to the horizontal. They may be single or multiple, unilateral or bilateral.

Plate atelectasis was originally described by Fleischner[268] in 1936 and has come to bear the

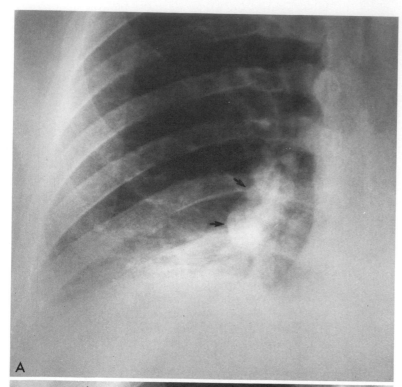

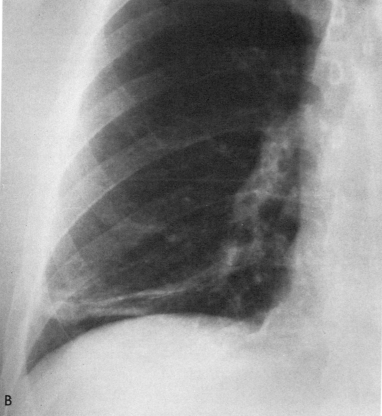

Figure 4–125. Linear Scarring Secondary to Pulmonary Embolism. Two days before the roentgenogram illustrated in A, this 33-year-old man had experienced a sudden onset of right chest pain and hemoptysis. This view of the right lung in anteroposterior projection reveals bulging of the right interlobar artery (*arrows*), "knuckling" of this vessel, a poorly defined opacity in the right lower lobe, and elevation of the right hemidiaphragm. This combination of changes is highly suggestive of pulmonary embolism and infarction. Ten days later, a detail view of the right lower zone (B) demonstrated a horizontally oriented linear opacity at the right base which subsequently underwent little change in appearance over the next several months. Presumed scar secondary to infarction.

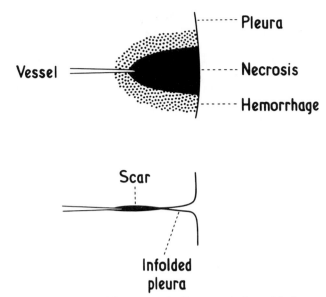

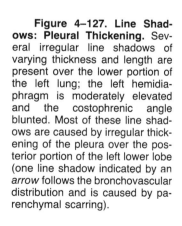

Figure 4–126. Diagrammatic Representation of Indrawn Pleura. Possible mechanism of the production of a line shadow with a pleural component, specifically following an infarct. (Reprinted from Br. J. Radiol, *43*:327, 1970, with permission of Dr. Lynne Reid and the editor.)

eponymous designation "Fleischner's lines." Despite the frequency with which these lines are observed, it has proved exceedingly difficult to determine their precise morphologic nature, either because the pathologist is unaware of their presence or because the lesion rarely is found in lungs examined at necropsy. Recently, however, Westcott and Cole[269] carried out a detailed roentgenologic/ pathologic correlative study of 10 patients on whom a linear opacity characteristic of plate atelectasis was present on their last antemortem roentgenogram and who subsequently were autopsied. All 10 revealed pathologic evidence of peripheral subpleural linear collapse combined with invagination of overlying pleura. The atelectasis was either deep to incomplete fissures or extended to pre-existing pleural clefts, but in either case the surface of the lung appeared folded in at the site of linear atelectasis. This frequent association with congenital pleural clefts, identations, scars, and incomplete fissures suggested to the researchers that plate atelectasis may develop preferentially at sites of pre-existing pleural invagination. The bronchi supplying the areas of atelectasis showed neither obstruc-

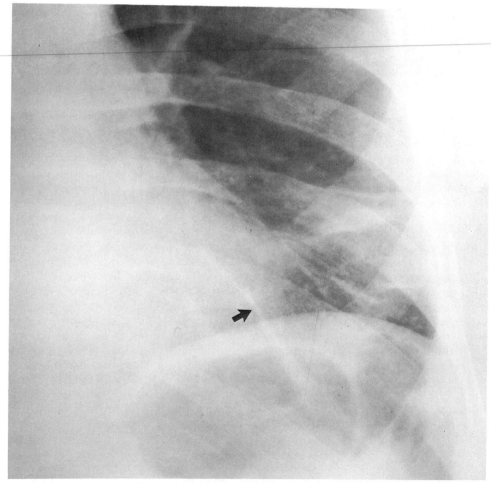

Figure 4–127. Line Shadows: Pleural Thickening. Several irregular line shadows of varying thickness and length are present over the lower portion of the left lung; the left hemidiaphragm is moderately elevated and the costophrenic angle blunted. Most of these line shadows are caused by irregular thickening of the pleura over the posterior portion of the left lower lobe (one line shadow indicated by an *arrow* follows the bronchovascular distribution and is caused by parenchymal scarring).

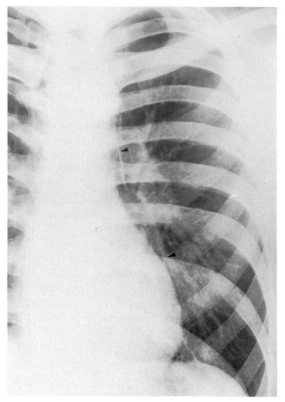

Figure 4–128. LIne Shadows: The Pleural Line in Medias-tinal Emphysema. A thin, continuous line shadow is present along the left border of the cardiovascular silhouette extending from just above the aortic knob to the left hemidiaphragm (*arrow-heads*). This represents the combined thickness of the visceral and parietal pleural membranes separated off the mediastinum by an accumulation of mediastinal gas. Spontaneous pneumome-diastinum of unknown etiology; uneventful recovery.

they also commonly showed "alveolitis," inflamma-tory exudate lying within the alveoli and alveolar walls. We suspect that the latter changes were inti-mately involved in the pathogenesis of the process, although Westcott and Cole[269] found alveolitis or edema in only 4 of their 10 cases. The pathogenesis of this unusual condition appears to be influenced most by an absence of collateral air drift and a deficiency of surfactant; which of these mechanisms is operative in individual cases is conjectural.

These linear opacities are almost invariably associated with diseases that diminish diaphragmatic excursion, but it is doubtful whether this factor *per se* is solely responsible. A frequent contributing factor is intra-abdominal disease, usually inflam-matory. After abdominal surgery, for example, it is probable that a complex group of changes combine to produce basal linear opacities: (a) restriction of diaphragmatic excursion diminishes ventilation of the lungs, especially in the bases; (b) coughing is inhibited by the pain and discomfort it engenders, resulting in accumulation of bronchial secretions in the dependent portions of the lungs and obstruction of small airways; and (c) stagnation of secretions encourages the development of pneumonia, with the resulting inflammatory exudate obstructing the channels of interalveolar communication. The re-sult is focal pneumonitis and atelectasis.

It is important to recognize that the postoper-ative clinical setting just described is commonly accompanied by an entirely different group of path-ologic conditions—those associated with pulmonary thromboembolism (Fig. 4–130). In the late 1960s, Simon[272, 273] attributed horizontally or obliquely ori-ented linear opacities in the mid and lower lung zones to thrombosed arteries or veins, more com-monly the latter. Bronchography and tomography, performed simultaneously in a few patients, failed to show any relationship between the lines and the bronchial tree. His evidence for the vascular nature of these opacities was both inferential and di-rect—inferential because the direction taken by the linear opacity was identical to that followed by a pulmonary vein, particularly the position of its me-dial extremity (which coincided with the left atrium), and direct because the position of the line shadow related to that of the vein in subsequent angiography. In recent years, in many cases we have observed line shadows whose anatomic distribution was similar to that reported by Simon; the major clues to their nature are their anatomic position (which shows little or no relationship to broncho-vascular distribution) and the position of their me-dial extremity (which coincides with the left atrium). They range in thickness from 2 to 10 mm, and, in our experience, just as frequently follow the distri-bution of a major upper lobe vein as of veins draining the middle or lower zones. These shadows cannot be caused purely by thrombus within the vein itself: since the density of thrombus is identical to that of fluid blood, the roentgenographic shad-

tion nor rearrangement, confirming our previous assertions that the process does not represent ob-structive atelectasis. Of considerable interest was the observation that in 9 of the 10 patients, prominent interlobular septa were observed either within or bordering the linear atelectasis, a finding that may go part way in explaining the absence of collateral air drift in the pathogenesis of the atelectasis. Al-though 6 of the 10 patients manifested pathologic evidence of acute pulmonary embolism, Westcott and Cole contended that there was no evidence that the atelectasis directly represented thrombosed ves-sels or infarcts. The linear opacities were caused by atelectasis alone in six patients, atelectasis associated with edema in three, and atelectasis combined with "alveolitis" in one.

Fleischner and his colleagues[270, 271] described the typical gross appearance of plate atelectasis as a grayish-blue linear band of collapsed lung slightly depressed below the pleural surface. In their cases, the small bronchi and bronchioles leading to the collapsed zone showed inflammatory changes of varying degrees of severity and often contained mucous plugs. In personal communication, Fleis-chner stated that not only were the alveoli collapsed,

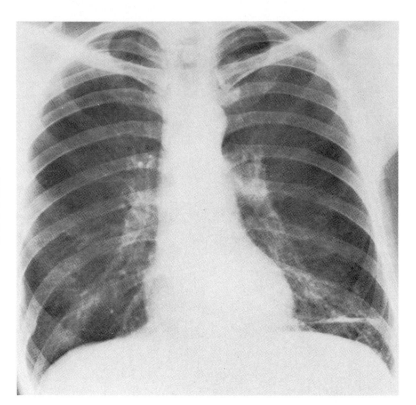

Figure 4–129. Line Shadows: Platelike Atelectasis. A posteroanterior roentgenogram reveals a line shadow measuring 3 mm in width and 9 cm in length situated in a plane just above the left hemidiaphragm and roughly horizontal in position; the left hemidiaphragm is slightly elevated. The shadow was barely visible in lateral projection. Two days postoperative laparotomy; the line had disappeared 4 days later.

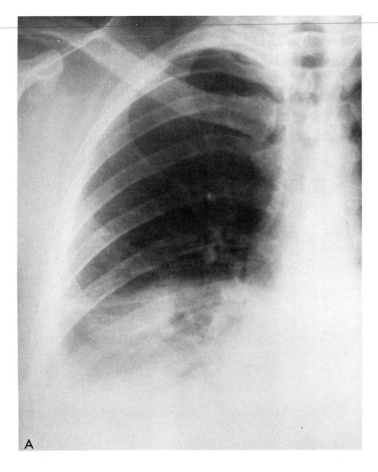

A

Figure 4–130. Line Shadows Following Pulmonary Infarction. A view of the right lung from a posteroanterior roentgenogram (*A*) reveals a large, indistinct opacity in the right lower lobe associated with elevation of the right hemidiaphragm and a small right pleural effusion. Both the clinical presentation and the presence of perfusion defects in other portions of the lungs on lung scan supported the diagnosis of pulmonary embolism and infarction.

Illustration continued on following page

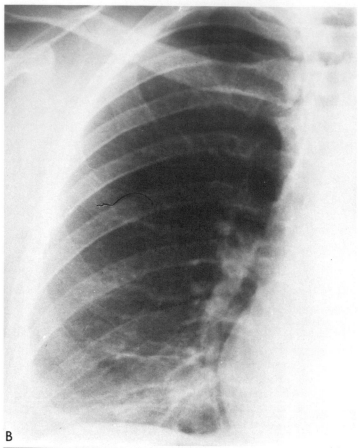

B

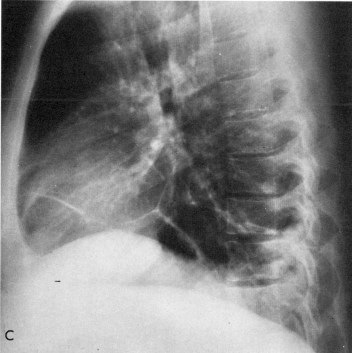

C

Figure 4–130 *Continued*. Nine days later, posteroanterior (*B*) and lateral (*C*) roentgenograms showed two well-defined linear opacities, one in the right middle lobe and the other in the right lower lobe (seen to best advantage in *C*). The anterior extremity of the lower lobe opacity relates to the major fissure and is associated with local posterior displacement of the fissure. It is suggested that this opacity represents a pulmonary vessel (? vein) with reaction in contiguous parenchyma. Both linear opacities had disappeared 3 weeks later. In *C*, the residual opacity from the infarct can be seen in the region of the posterior gutter.

ows of thrombus and vein should be identical. Although pathologic confirmation appears singularly difficult to obtain in these cases, it seems reasonable to suggest that the process is rendered visible by a combination of edema, hemorrhage, and perhaps atelectasis and fibrosis in lung parenchyma surrounding the vein.

Despite the foregoing, the evidence provided by Westcott and Cole[269] appears sufficiently convincing to warrant continued use of the term plate atelectasis as an entity. However, we feel that taking all facts into consideration, including our own personal observations over the past several years, evidence is now strong enough that the presence of these linear opacities on a chest roentgenogram should alert the referring physician or surgeon to the *possibility* of thromboembolic disease, despite the fact that in many of these cases the patients' clinical histories give no hint of an acute thromboembolic episode apart from their being in a postoperative period or confined to bed for other reasons.

LUNG DISEASES THAT DECREASE ROENTGENOGRAPHIC DENSITY

The lung diseases that cause a decrease in roentgenographic density (increase in translucency) can be considered appropriately in the same manner as diseases that increase density, but as their antithesis. Just as density may be increased by a combination of changes in the relative amounts of air, blood, and interstitial tissue, so may decreased density result from alteration of these three elements in the opposite direction. In both groups of diseases, one component seldom is altered to the exclusion of the others, but it is useful to subdivide the diseases on the basis of predominant modification of each component, individually and combined.

It is emphasized that here we are dealing with the diseases of the *lung* that cause reduced roentgenographic density and not of the thorax as a whole. Any assessment of chest roentgenograms must take into consideration the contribution that abnormalities of *extrapulmonary tissue* might make to reduced density. Thus, certain pleural diseases (e.g., pneumothorax) and some congenital and acquired abnormalities of the chest wall (e.g., congenital absence of the pectoral muscles (Fig. 4–131), mastectomy, poliomyelitis, and other neuromuscular disorders that affect one side of the thorax) produce unilateral radiolucency that easily might be mistaken for pulmonary disease unless this possibility is continuously borne in mind.

In the discussion on lung density in Chapter 1 it was pointed out that, for all practical purposes, assessment of changes in lung density must be purely subjective, except when roentgen densitometry or computed tomography[274] is employed. In diseases of increased density, assessment may be relatively simple, since the variation in density from normal lung to consolidated lung approximates a factor of 10—from the average density of lung parenchyma (0.08 gram/ml) to that of consolidated lung (1.0 gram/ml). By contrast, the reduction from normal lung density in diseases that increase translucency may be very slight, probably amounting to no more with 0.01 or 0.02 gram per ml. Thus we are faced with the apparent paradox of trying to classify a group of diseases on the basis of a roentgenologic sign that at best is extremely subtle. The reasons by which this approach may be justified are twofold.

1. In *generalized* diseases of the lung characterized by diffuse pulmonary overinflation (for example, diffuse emphysema), general reduction in density or "increased translucency" traditionally is cited as a reliable roentgenologic sign of these diseases. In fact, the validity of this sign is questionable. For many reasons, of which the most cogent is the wide variation in exposure factors that characterizes much chest roentgenography, the impression of increased translucency is not only unreliable as a sign of overinflation but also may be false, particularly in healthy young men with a large total lung capacity. In such situations reliance must be placed on the *secondary signs* that are an integral part of these diseases; then, recognition of the overall pattern of roentgenographic change permits the *inference* that lung density must be reduced, allowing inclusion in this broad category of disease. Such reasoning appears somewhat artificial but does focus attention on those signs that are of greatest diagnostic reliability rather than on one we have found undependable.

2. In *localized* diseases that reduce roentgenographic density (for example, lobar emphysema or a large bulla), the story is entirely different. These conditions provide a region of lung in which the density change can be compared with that in the remainder of the same lung or the opposite lung, thereby supplying the dependable criterion of contrast. Thus, this group of local diseases can be classified according to absolute change in density, an advantage lacking in generalized disease. This is not to imply that secondary signs are not as valuable in local as in general disease; as is shown, signs of overinflation and of alteration in vasculature play an integral role in the diagnosis and differential diagnosis of all diseases characterized by reduced density.

Accepting that diseases that reduce density are characterized by an altered ratio of the three components of air, blood, and interstitial tissue, four combinations of changes can reduce lung density.

Increased Air but Unchanged Blood and Tissue (Fig. 4–132). This group of diseases is exemplified by obstructive overinflation without lung destruction. It may be either *local* (e.g., compensatory overinflation secondary to pulmonary resection or atelectasis) or *general* (e.g., spasmodic asthma).

Increased Air with Decreased Blood and Tis-

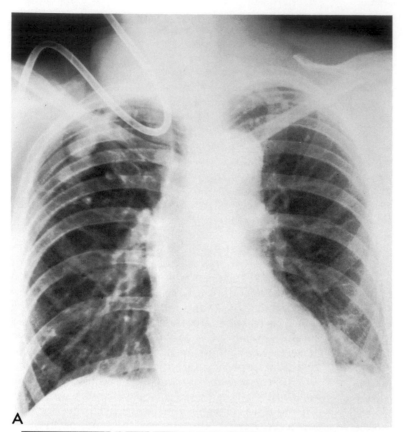

A

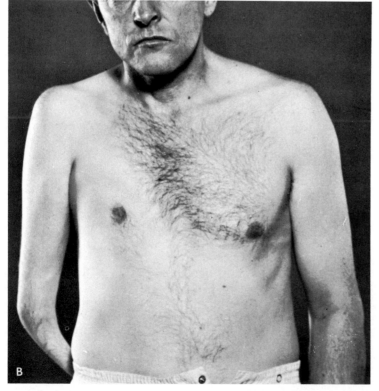

B

Figure 4–131. Unilateral Hyperlucency: Congenital Absence of the Musculature of the Right Shoulder Girdle. A posteroanterior roentgenogram (*A*) reveals a marked asymmetry of radiolucency of the two lungs. Fairly extensive nodular scarring of the right upper lobe is associated with moderate upward displacement of the right hilum, indicating considerable loss of volume of the right upper lobe. However, the loss of volume was considered insufficient to account for compensatory overinflation of the middle and lower lobes of a degree that would explain the difference in radiolucency. A considerable disparity in thickness of the supraclavicular soft tissues (and of the axillary folds) suggested an anomaly of the thoracic wall. A photograph of the patient (*B*) shows marked underdevelopment of the musculature of the right shoulder and chest wall, associated with phocomelia of the right arm.

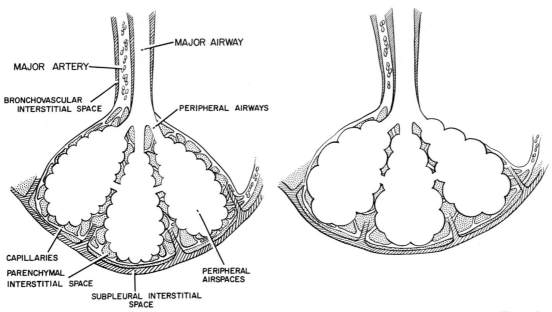

Figure 4–132. The Lung Diagram: Increase in the Amount of Air, Blood, and Tissue Being Unchanged. The only abnormality depicted is an increase in the size of the peripheral air spaces.

sue **(Fig. 4–133).** This group is epitomized by diffuse emphysema; not only are the lungs overdistended but also the capillary bed is reduced and alveolar walls are dissipated. Bullae and thin-walled cysts are examples of local diseases within this category.

Normal Amount of Air but Decreased Blood (and Tissue) (Fig. 4–134). This group is characterized by lack of pulmonary overinflation but reduced quantities of blood and tissue. *Local* diseases include lobar or unilateral emphysema and pulmonary embolism without infarction. (However, in both these conditions the volume of air also may be reduced,

in the former because of incomplete maturation of lung parenchyma and in the latter because of surfactant deficit.) The generalized abnormalities include diseases characterized by diminished pulmonary artery flow (e.g., tetralogy of Fallot) and those affecting the peripheral vascular system (e.g., primary pulmonary hypertension and multiple peripheral pulmonary emboli).

Reduction in All Three Components (Fig. 4–135). This condition is rare and probably relates to only one abnormality or variants thereof—unilateral pulmonary artery agenesis. Usually the lung is reduced in volume and derives its vascular supply

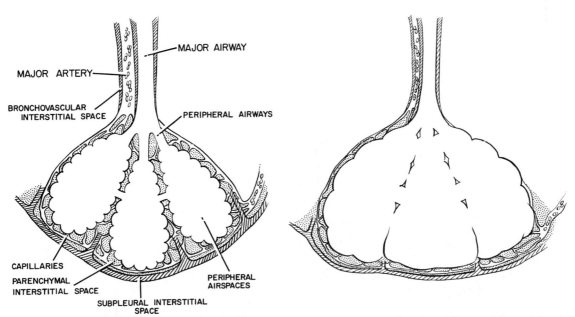

Figure 4–133. The Lung Diagram: Increase in Air with Concomitant Reduction in Blood and Tissue. The peripheral air spaces are markedly dilated, with dissolution of their walls. The major artery and vein are reduced in caliber and the capillaries greatly diminished in number.

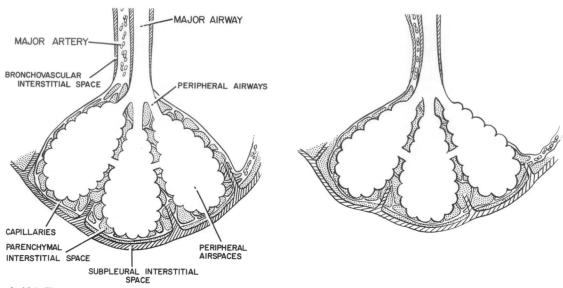

Figure 4–134. The Lung Diagram: Normal Air, Diminished Blood and Tissue. The peripheral air spaces are normal in size, but the major artery and vein are reduced in caliber and the capillaries diminished in number.

solely from the systemic circulation; the resultant density is usually but not always reduced.[275]

On the basis of these concepts and using the roentgenologic signs to be described, one can fairly confidently diagnose most cases of pulmonary disease that decrease density. In the following section no attempt is made to describe roentgenologic characteristics of individual disease entities; specific affections will be cited only to illustrate points under discussion.

ROENTGENOLOGIC SIGNS

Alteration in Lung Volume

With the exception of the reduction in lung volume that occurs in unilateral pulmonary artery agenesis, unilateral or lobar emphysema (Swyer-James syndrome), partly obstructing endobronchial lesions, and pulmonary embolism without infarction, all such lung diseases *in which lung volume is altered* are characterized by *overinflation*. Before considering the roentgenologic signs of overinflation, it is well to review briefly the mechanisms that keep the lung expanded and the alterations in these mechanisms that increase lung volume.

As described in Chapter 1 (*see* page 56), the lung has a natural tendency to collapse and does so when removed from the chest. This tendency stems from its inherent elastic recoil properties, which are partly related to collagenous and elastic fibers that impart an elastic quality similar to that of a coil spring, and partly to alveolar surface tension. When

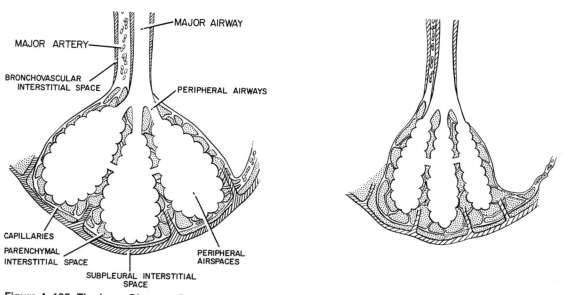

Figure 4–135. The Lung Diagram: Decrease in Air, Blood, and Tissue. All elements of the lung are diminished.

the lung's elastic properties are deranged, as in emphysema, the organ inflates beyond its normal maximal volume; this constitutes *overinflation*. Similarly, the lung's compliance—the change in volume per unit change in pressure—is increased; in other words, a given pressure will produce a greater volume change than in normal lung. It is important to recognize that this loss of elastic recoil is the major if not the only factor that permits the lung to overinflate. The loss of recoil may be irreversible, as in emphysema, or temporary and reversible, as in spasmodic asthma; in any event, *unequivocal roentgenographic evidence of pulmonary overinflation implies loss of elastic recoil*.

The roentgenologic signs of overinflation depend upon whether the process is *general* or *local*.

GENERAL EXCESS OF AIR IN THE LUNGS

Signs to be observed include changes in the diaphragm, the retrosternal space, and the cardio-vascular silhouette (Fig. 4–136); by far the most important of these is the diaphragm. At total lung capacity the diaphragm is depressed, often to the level of the seventh rib anteriorly and the eleventh interspace or twelfth rib posteriorly in the severe overinflation of diffuse emphysema; the normal "dome" configuration is flattened, particularly as viewed in lateral projection. The severity of flattening may be of value in differential diagnosis, being invariably most marked in emphysema; the overinflation of emphysema may render the diaphragmatic contour actually concave rather than convex upward (Fig. 4–136), a sign we have seen only occasionally in other than destructive lung disease. In asthma the upper surface is nearly always convex (this applies in adults only—severe air trapping in infants and children may be associated with remarkable depression of diaphragmatic domes; Fig. 4–137). The low position of the diaphragm increases the angle of the costophrenic sinuses, sometimes almost to a right angle. Costophrenic muscle

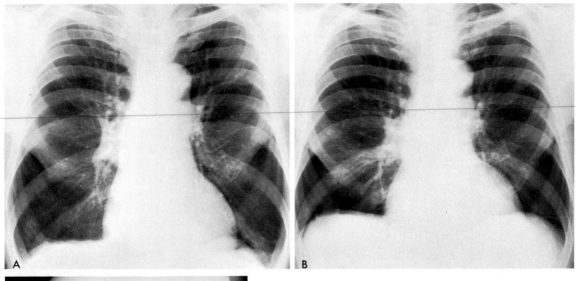

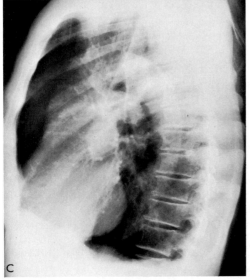

Figure 4–136. Diffuse Emphysema. Posteroanterior roentgenograms of the chest in inspiration (*A*) and expiration (*B*) reveal a low position and somewhat flattened contour of both hemidiaphragms; excursion of the diaphragm from TLC to RV is reduced. In lateral projection (*C*), the superior aspect of the diaphragm is concave rather than convex and the retrosternal air space somewhat deepened. The lungs are generally oligemic.

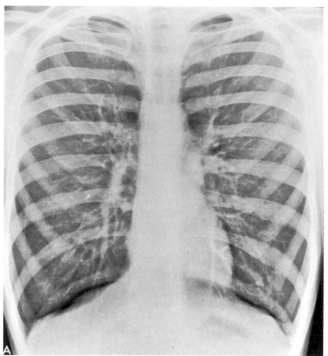

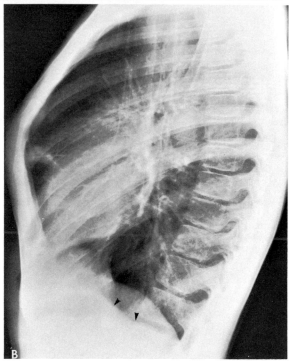

Figure 4–137. Overinflation in Spasmodic Asthma. Postero-anterior (*A*) and lateral (*B*) roentgenograms of the chest of a 14-year-old boy with longstanding spasmodic asthma reveal a low position and flattened contour of both hemidiaphragms. In lateral projection, one hemidiaphragm can be seen to possess a concave superior surface (*arrowheads*). The retrosternal air space is markedly deepened and the sternum bowed anteriorly.

slips, extending from the diaphragm to the posterior and posterolateral ribs, may be prominent, but these are seen occasionally in normal adults who have taken an exceptionally deep breath and, therefore, should not necessarily be regarded as a sign of great importance.

In a study designed to test the accuracy of a variety of measurements from posteroanterior and lateral roentgenograms in discriminating normal and overinflated lungs, Thomson and his colleagues[379] found that the best criterion was obtained

from the sum of the height of each diaphragmatic dome, measured in PA projection from a line extending from the costophrenic to the costovertebral angle, and in lateral projection from the posterior to the anterior costophrenic sulcus. It was of interest in this preliminary study that some commonly used roentgenologic criteria of pulmonary overinflation, such as the anterior rib count and the distance from the ascending aorta to the sternum (*see* further on), were poor discriminants of normal and overinflated lungs.

Limited diaphragmatic excursion during respiration is a reliable sign of air trapping, particularly but not exclusively in emphysema. Whereas the average range of diaphragmatic excursion in normal subjects is 3 to 4 cm, the range in emphysema may be no more than 1 to 2 cm (Fig. 4–136).[58] In assessing local and general air trapping, Greenspan and his colleagues[276] use a 1-second forced expiratory roentgenogram (FEV_1) in addition to films exposed at TLC and RV: in over 200 subjects studied, local air trapping was identified in 16, 12 of whom had a normal spirogram; in 9 patients, trapping was detectable only on the FEV_1 roentgenogram. FEV_1 roentgenography is more difficult to perform and more time-consuming than untimed expiratory roentgenography, but it does provide more accurate information about air trapping: it is important to recognize that, *given sufficient time*, a patient with extensive emphysema will move his or her diaphragm on expiration through a range very similar to normal.

Identification in lateral projection of separation of the cardiovascular structures from the sternum indicates increase in the depth of the retrosternal air space and is a sign that has been employed by some[277] to indicate overinflation; however, as mentioned earlier, we have found it a poor discriminant of normal and overinflated lungs.

Alteration in the size and contour of the thoracic cage is a variable and usually undependable sign of excess air in the lungs. Although the barrel-shaped chest is commonly regarded as indicative of emphysema, often its roentgenologic expression as an increase in the anteroposterior diameter of the chest is inconspicuous. Both anterior bowing of the sternum and increased thoracic kyphosis are unreliable roentgenologic signs in assessment of excess air in the lungs.[278]

When the diaphragm is depressed the heart tends to be elongated, narrow, and central in position. This long vertical configuration of the cardiovascular contour is of little value as a roentgenologic sign, but it creates difficulty in the assessment of cardiac enlargement when pulmonary hypertension has given rise to right ventricular hypertrophy and cor pulmonale. An interesting paradox concerns the variation in cardiac diameter from inspiration to expiration in certain diseases characterized by severe air trapping and general overinflation. In normal subjects the cardiovascular shadow narrows during inspiration and widens during expiration; in acute spasmodic asthma, acute bronchiolitis of infants,[279] and diffuse emphysema,[21] paradoxic enlargement during inspiration and diminution during expiration are said to occur.

LOCAL EXCESS OF AIR

Overinflation of a segment or of one or more lobes, the remainder of the lungs being normal, occurs in two quite different sets of circumstances:

with and without air trapping; distinction between the two is of major diagnostic importance.

Overinflation *with air trapping* results from obstruction of the egress of air from affected lung parenchyma. In our experience, it has few causes—for example, lobar emphysema in infants (Fig. 4–138)[280–282] and congenital atresia of the apicoposterior segmental bronchus of the left upper lobe (Fig. 4–139).[283, 284] Although overinflation of lung distal to an endobronchial lesion as a result of check-valve obstruction is frequently cited as an important sign in the early diagnosis of bronchogenic neoplasm, in our experience and that of others[285–288] it is in fact a rare manifestation.[134] For example, in the Mayo Clinic study of the roentgenographic patterns of 600 cases of bronchogenic carcinoma,[285–288] overinflation of lung parenchyma distal to a partly obstructing endobronchial lesion was not seen in any case. *In our experience, the volume of lung behind a partly obstructing endobronchial lesion is almost invariably reduced at TLC.* Overinflation of the lung at TLC must be distinguished from air trapping on expiration, a vital distinction considered in greater detail subsequently.

Overinflation *without air trapping* is a compensatory process: parts of the lung assume a larger volume than normal in response to loss of volume elsewhere in the thorax. This may occur after surgical removal of lung tissue (Fig. 4–140) or as a result of atelectasis or parenchymal scarring, but in any event the remaining lung contains more than its normal complement of air. Since there is no airway obstruction, the roentgenologic signs are different from those of conditions in which air trapping plays a significant role. Thus it is important to consider the roentgenologic signs of local excess of air under two headings, static and dynamic, according to the presence or absence of airway obstruction.

Static Signs. By "static" is implied the changes apparent on standard roentgenograms exposed at total lung capacity.

1. *Alteration in lung density*: The fact that the excess of air is local permits comparison with normal density in the remainder of the lung or in the contralateral lung; thus, in contrast to those diseases with generalized excess of air, altered density is a significant and reliable sign. The increased translucency is caused chiefly by an increase in air in relation to blood content; blood flow to the affected lung is normal or reduced, the only difference being that, in the latter circumstances, translucency is even more increased. In the case of a partly obstructing endobronchial lesion, the situation is somewhat different: as discussed earlier, our experience dictates that the volume of lung behind a partly obstructing endobronchial lesion is almost invariably reduced, not increased, at TLC. Despite this smaller volume, however, the density of affected parenchyma typically is *less* than that of the opposite lung rather than greater as might be anticipated. This is caused

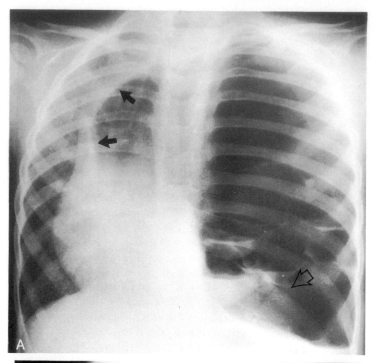

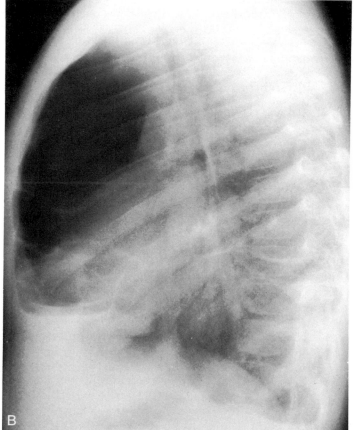

Figure 4–138. Neonatal Lobar Hyperinflation. Anteroposterior (*A*) and lateral (*B*) chest roentgenograms disclose a markedly overinflated and hyperlucent left upper lobe displacing the mediastinum into the right hemithorax, particularly anteriorly (*arrows*). The left lower lobe (*open arrow*) is severely compressed and displaced posteromedially.

by a reduction in perfusion (oligemia), resulting from hypoxic vasoconstriction in response to alveolar hypoventilation. The overall effect is an increase in translucency despite the reduction in volume.

2. *Alteration in volume:* The volume of the affected lung depends entirely upon whether the excess of air is compensatory (secondary to resection or atelectasis) or caused by airway obstruction. Since compensatory overinflation is the expansion of lung tissue beyond its normal volume to fill a limited space, the volume that the expanded lung tissue occupies cannot exceed the volume for which it compensates. When the alteration in the lung volume results from bronchial obstruction, however, the volume of affected lung may be normal, less than normal, or greater than normal. Conditions in which volume is greater than normal include atresia of the apical posterior bronchus of the left upper lobe and neonatal lobar emphysema; as already stated, a partly obstructing endobronchial lesion is usually associated with lung volume that is less than normal (Fig. 4–141).

The main roentgenologic sign of increased volume is displacement of structures contiguous to overinflated lung, the degree varying with the amount and location of affected lung tissue: if in a lower lobe, the hemidiaphragm may be depressed and the mediastinum shifted to the contralateral side; if in an upper lobe, the mediastinum may be displaced and the thoracic cage expanded; if a whole lung is involved, the hemithorax in general is enlarged, the diaphragm is depressed, the mediastinum shifted, and the thoracic cage enlarged. One of the more reliable signs of *lobar* overinflation is outward bulging of the interlobar fissure.

3. *Alteration in vascular pattern:* The linear markings throughout the affected lung are splayed out in a distribution consistent with the extent of overinflation, and their angles of bifurcation are increased. Provided blood flow is maintained at normal or almost normal levels, vessel caliber is little altered.

Dynamic Signs. By "dynamic" is implied changes that occur during respiration; they are most readily apparent on fluoroscopy, although many of the signs may be seen equally clearly on roentgenograms exposed during full inspiration and maximal expiration.

When local increase in translucency is caused by *compensatory overinflation*, during expiration the volume of the overinflated lobe decreases proportionately with the normal lung tissue: airway ob-

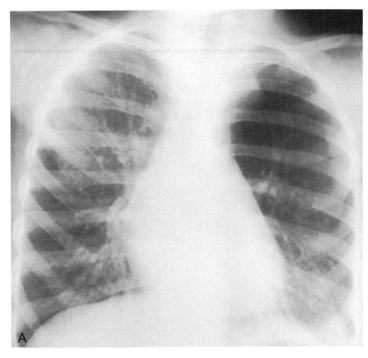

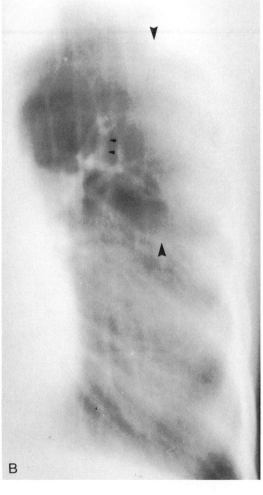

Figure 4–139. Congenital Bronchial Atresia of the Left Upper Lobe. *A,* A conventional posteroanterior chest roentgenogram demonstrates a striking translucency of the upper two thirds of the left lung; the mediastinum is displaced slightly to the right. *B,* A full chest tomogram reveals oligemia of the left upper lobe associated with a reduction in the normal tomographic background-veil phenomenon indicating decreased small vessel perfusion (*between large arrowheads*). A bifurcating band-like opacity (*small arrowheads*) represents the branched form of mucoid impaction.

Illustration continued on following page

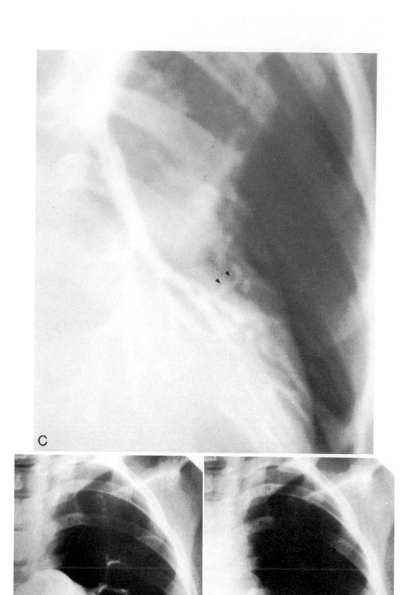

C

D ARTERIAL　　　　VENOUS

Figure 4–139 *Continued. C,* A selective left bronchogram demonstrates downward displacement of left upper lobe bronchi; subsegmental branches (*arrowheads*) originate from what was ultimately shown to be the posterior segmental bronchus of the upper lobe. *D,* A pulmonary angiogram in AP projection during the arterial and venous phases shows that the bifurcating opacity in *B* is not part of the vascular tree.

Illustration continued on opposite page

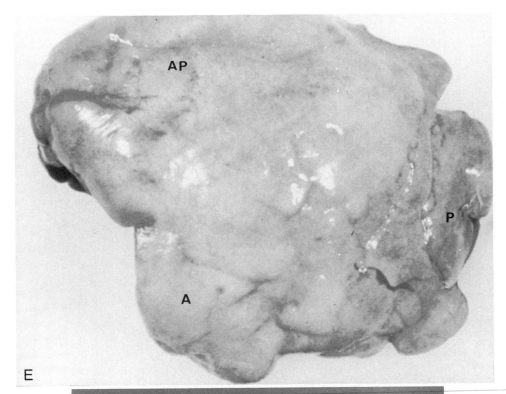

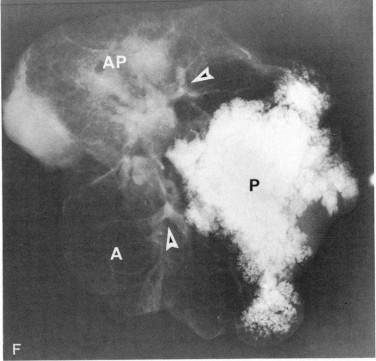

Figure 4–139 *Continued. E,* The resected left upper lobe specimen viewed from the lateral aspect shows the apical (*AP*) and anterior (*A*) segments to remain hyperinflated while the posterior (*P*) segment has collapsed normally. The specimen was inflated and barium injected into the only patent bronchus (the posterior segmental bronchus); the lung was sectioned in the sagittal plane and radiographed (*F*). Marked destructive emphysema is seen in the apical and anterior segments (more severe in the latter). The atretic bronchi (*arrowheads*) are filled with mucus. (From Genereux GP: J Can Assoc Radiol *22*:71, 1971.)

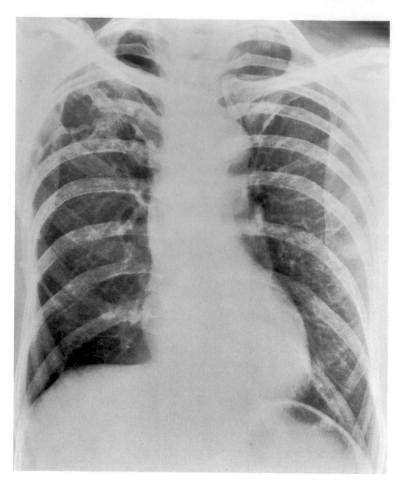

Figure 4–140. Overinflation without Air Trapping: Compensatory to Lobectomy. The right hemithorax is more radiolucent than the left because of overinflation of the right upper and middle lobes following resection of the lower lobe for pulmonary carcinoma. Note the redistribution of vascular markings. The nodule in the left lung is a metastasis.

struction being absent, the affected lung parenchyma deflates normally. Since the overinflated lung tissue contains more air than normal at total lung capacity, it still contains a greater than normal complement of air at residual volume and, therefore, is still relatively more translucent.

In the presence of partial airway obstruction, regardless of whether distal lung parenchyma is overinflated or underinflated, roentgenologic signs are vastly different from those seen in compensatory overinflation. During expiration, air is trapped within the affected lung parenchyma and volume changes little, whereas the remainder of the lung deflates normally. The roentgenologic signs depend upon both the volume and the anatomic location of affected lung: since during expiration there is negligible change in the amount of air within the obstructed lung parenchyma, density is little altered and the contrast between affected areas and normally deflated lung is maximally accentuated at residual volume (Figs. 4–142 and 4–143). Since the overinflated parenchyma occupies space within the hemithorax, contiguous structures are displaced away from the affected lobe during expiration: the mediastinum shifts toward the contralateral side and elevation of the hemidiaphragm is restricted. Distribution of the vascular pattern throughout the overinflated lobe changes little. Those dynamic changes are particularly impressive fluoroscopically: when the patient breathes deeply and rapidly, the mediastinum swings like a pendulum, away from the lesion during expiration and back to the midline during inspiration; the extent of diaphragmatic excursion and of reduction in size of the thoracic cage are diminished on the ipsilateral side.

It cannot be overemphasized that evidence of local excess of air may be extremely subtle on roentgenograms exposed at full inspiration (Fig. 4–142); when such changes are even remotely suspected, the dynamics should be studied.

Alteration in Vasculature

Just as overinflation may reflect abnormality of the conducting airways of the lung, so may alteration in the vascular pattern indicate abnormality of perfusion. Vascular loss may be central or peripheral, in the former instance produced by vascular obstruction (for example, pulmonary artery thrombosis) and in the latter by peripheral vascular obliteration (for example, emphysema or multiple peripheral pulmonary emboli).

Like overinflation, alteration in lung vasculature may be either general or local; since the roentgenologic signs differ somewhat, it is desirable to describe them separately.

GENERAL REDUCTION IN VASCULATURE

Diffuse pulmonary oligemia is characterized by a reduction in caliber of the arterial tree throughout the lungs. As pointed out in Chapter 1, appreciation of such vascular change is a subjective process based on a thorough familiarity with the normal. Although such an assessment admittedly is subject to observer error, to our knowledge it has not been replaced by any method that provides an accurate, objective evaluation, with the possible exception of roentgen densitometry and computed tomography. In an observer error study of proved pulmonary overvascularity and undervascularity,[392] the former was detected with significantly greater accuracy than the latter; this experiment dealt with children only, but it is probable that similar results would obtain

in adult patients. As previously emphasized, undervascularity is more readily appreciated on full lung tomograms than on plain roentgenograms.[289–291]

Since reduction in the size of peripheral vessels constitutes the main criterion of diagnosis of all diseases in this category, reliance must be placed on secondary signs for their differentiation. There are two ancillary signs of major importance: *the size and configuration of the central hilar vessels* and *the presence or absence of general pulmonary overinflation*. The following examples serve to indicate how these signs may be useful in differential diagnosis. Three combinations of changes are possible:

1. *Small peripheral vessels; no overinflation; normal or small hila*. This combination indicates reduced pulmonary blood flow from central causes and is virtually pathognomonic of cardiac disease, usually

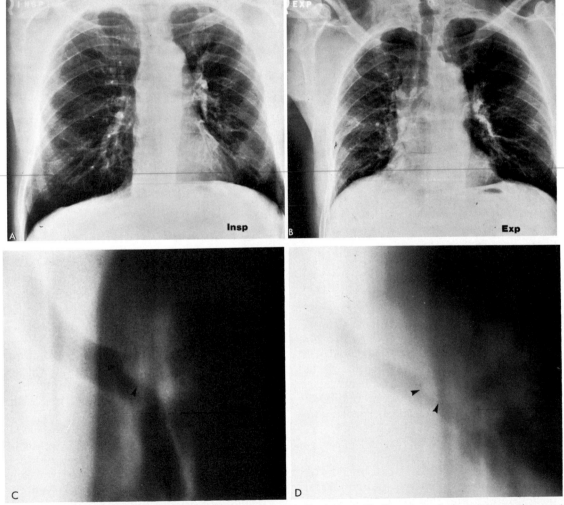

Figure 4–141. Small Cell Carcinoma, Left Main Bronchus, with Expiratory Air Trapping. *A,* A posteroanterior roentgenogram exposed at full inspiration reveals decreased size of the left lung compared with the right; the left hemidiaphragm is moderately elevated and the mediastinum is shifted to the left. Despite this loss of volume, no opacities can be identified in the left lung to suggest collapse or airlessness. Left lower lobe vessels are obviously smaller than corresponding vessels on the right, indicating reduced perfusion. *B,* A roentgenogram exposed at maximal expiration reveals little change in the volume of the left lung from inspiration, indicating air trapping; by contrast, the right hemidiaphragm has elevated considerably and the mediastinum has swung to the right, indicating good air flow from the right lung. Tomograms of the left main bronchus in inspiration (*C*) and expiration (*D*) reveal a smooth, well-defined soft tissue mass protruding into the air column of the bronchus near its bifurcation (*arrowheads*): the caliber of the bronchial air column is markedly reduced on expiration.

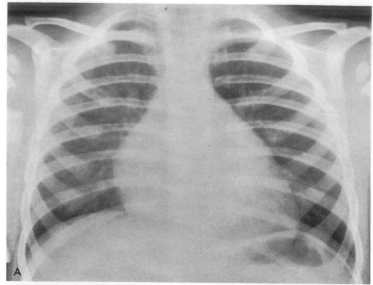

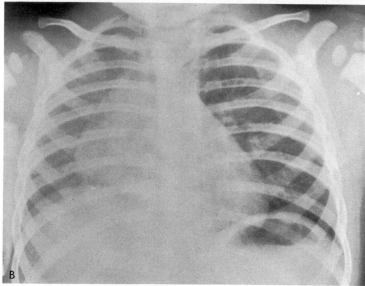

Figure 4–142. Value of Inspiratory-Expiratory Roentgenography in the Assessment of Bronchial Obstruction. *A,* A roentgenogram in full inspiration (TLC) of an 11-month-old girl with sudden onset of dyspnea. No abnormalities are apparent. *B,* At full expiration (RV), the volume of the left hemithorax has changed little from the inspiratory roentgenogram, and the mediastinum has shifted markedly to the right. The findings are those of obstruction of the left main bronchus (a crayon was removed bronchoscopically). Fluoroscopy would have shown the mediastinal swing to excellent advantage but would have provided no more information than can be gleaned from these static roentgenograms.

congenital (Fig. 4–144). Such anomalies as the tetralogy of Fallot, Ebstein's anomaly, and occasionally, isolated pulmonic stenosis are associated with a reduced pulmonary artery blood flow manifested roentgenographically by small peripheral vessels and hila. The same combination is seen occasionally in certain acquired conditions such as cardiac tamponade and inferior vena caval obstruction.[292]

2. *Small peripheral vessels; no overinflation; enlarged hilar pulmonary arteries.* This combination may result from peripheral or central causes. The *peripheral* conditions include primary pulmonary arterial hypertension,[293] multiple peripheral emboli, and pulmonary hypertension secondary to chronic schistosomiasis.[294] In each of these the major changes apparent roentgenographically are the consequence of pulmonary arterial hypertension and consist of enlargement of the hilar pulmonary arteries and diminution of the peripheral vessels (Fig. 4–145). The commonest cause of *central* origin is

massive pulmonary artery embolism without infarction.[295, 296] In this situation the reduction in peripheral pulmonary artery flow results from mechanical obstruction in the large hilar vessels, the latter being ballooned out by thrombus within them; severe cardiac enlargement caused by acute cor pulmonale is usually present (Fig. 4–146).

3. *Small peripheral vessels; general pulmonary overinflation; normal or enlarged hilar pulmonary arteries.* This combination is virtually pathognomonic of diffuse emphysema (Fig. 4–147).[297–299] Since diffuse overinflation may also occur in spasmodic asthma, recognition of peripheral vascular deficiency is important in the differentiation of these two conditions. (Roentgenographic differentiation may be facilitated by full lung tomography.[289]) Enlargement of the hilar pulmonary arteries may be present but is not essential to the diagnosis; it indicates pulmonary arterial hypertension resulting from chronically increased vascular resistance and usually is

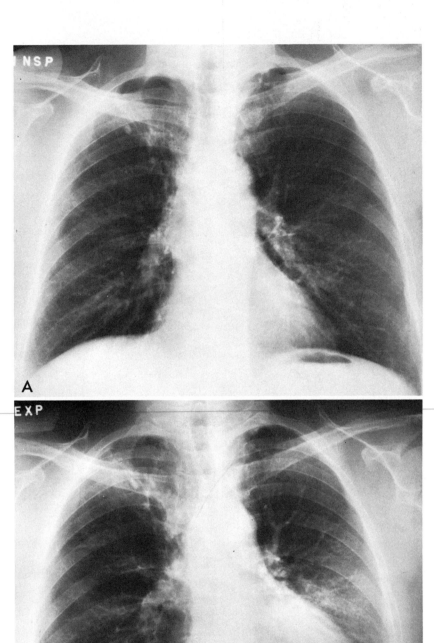

Figure 4–143. Expiratory Air Trapping Caused by Endobronchial Obstruction. A posteroanterior roentgenogram exposed at full inspiration (A) shows both the volume and density of the right lung to be less than that of the left; vessel markings are smaller throughout. Anatomic structures in the right hilum are somewhat obscured. On expiration (B), the left hemidiaphragm has elevated normally while the right has maintained its inspiratory position; the mediastinum has shifted to the left. The small volume and relative oligemia of the right lung on inspiration associated with air trapping on expiration indicate an obstructing lesion in the right main bronchus. This 40-year-old woman had a 4-month history of low-grade fever, cough, retrosternal pain, tightness in the chest, and yellow sputum; coughing brought on wheezing. Physical examination demonstrated rales and muffled breath sounds over the right upper zone and a general wheeze over the whole thorax. Bronchoscopy revealed granulation tissue piled up in the right main stem bronchus, almost occluding the right upper lobe bronchus and extending up onto the tracheal wall. *M. tuberculosis* was identified on smear and culture.

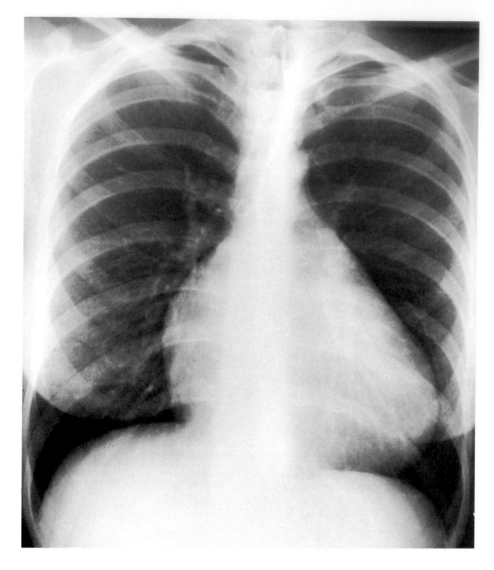

Figure 4–144. Diffuse Oligemia without Overinflation: Ebstein's Anomaly. The peripheral pulmonary markings are diminished in caliber, and the hila are diminutive; the lungs are not overinflated. The contour of the markedly enlarged heart is consistent with Ebstein's anomaly. Proved case.

seen only in the late stages of emphysema. In such circumstances, the rapid tapering of pulmonary vessels distally is accentuated by the hilar enlargement.

LOCAL REDUCTION IN VASCULATURE

The same three combinations of changes apply as in general reduction in vasculature; the major difference lies in their effects on pulmonary hemodynamics. In the following examples the affected portion of lung may be segmental, lobar, or multilobar:

1. *Small peripheral vessels; normal or subnormal inflation; normal or small hilum.* This combination is epitomized by lobar or unilateral hyperlucent lung, variously known by the eponyms Swyer-James syndrome[300] and Macleod's syndrome (Fig. 4–148).[303] This unique abnormality is characterized by normal or slightly reduced lung volume at total lung capacity, severe airway obstruction during expiration, greatly reduced circulation (oligemia), and a diminutive hilum.[301, 302] The increased vascular

resistance in affected areas results in a redistribution of blood flow to the contralateral lung or unaffected lobes. Pathogenetically it is believed to be related to acute bronchiolitis during infancy,[302, 303] since the volume of the lung in adulthood is related, at least partly, to the age at which bronchiolar damage occurred.

Roentgenographic changes identical to those of Swyer-James syndrome may result from a clinically more important situation. Consider an endobronchial lesion incompletely obstructing the lumen of a main bronchus (Fig. 4–141): the reduced ventilation of distal parenchyma results in local hypoxia, which leads to reflex vasoconstriction and consequent reduced perfusion of affected bronchopulmonary segments. Contrary to common belief and teaching, the volume of affected lung generally is reduced rather than increased. Since the endobronchial lesion invariably causes expiratory air trapping, it may be extremely difficult roentgenologically to differentiate this combination of changes from the less significant Swyer-James syndrome. Therefore, whenever this combination of changes is present, it

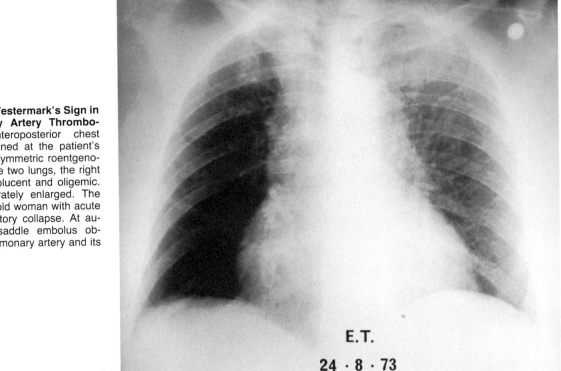

Figure 4–145. Westermark's Sign in Massive Pulmonary Artery Thromboembolism. An anteroposterior chest roentgenogram obtained at the patient's bedside discloses asymmetric roentgenographic density of the two lungs, the right being markedly radiolucent and oligemic. The heart is moderately enlarged. The patient is a 69-year-old woman with acute dyspnea and circulatory collapse. At autopsy, a massive saddle embolus obstructed the right pulmonary artery and its two major branches.

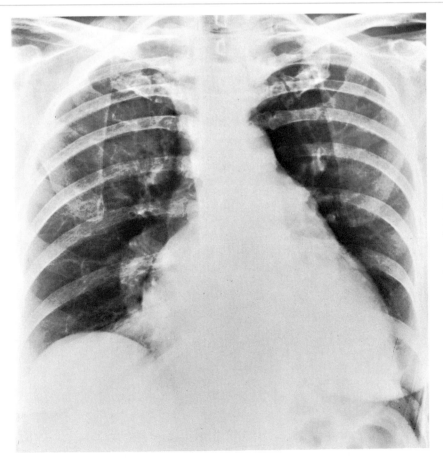

Figure 4–146. Diffuse Oligemia without Overinflation: Massive Pulmonary Artery Thromboembolism without Infarction. Marked oligemia of both lungs is associated with moderate enlargement of both hila and rapid tapering of the pulmonary arteries as they proceed distally. The cardiac contour is typical of cor pulmonale. There is no overinflation.

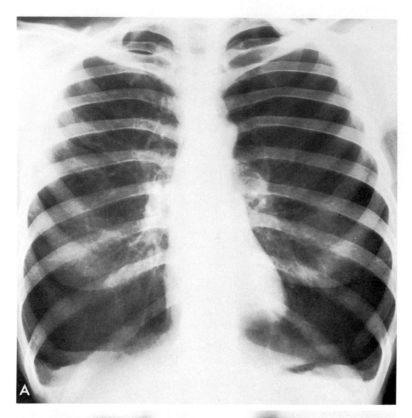

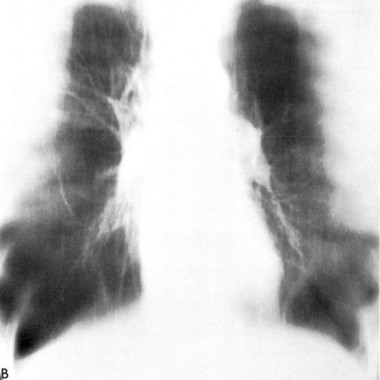

Figure 4–147. Diffuse Oligemia with Generalized Overinflation: Emphysema. The peripheral vasculature of the lungs is markedly diminished as revealed in both the posteroanterior roentgenogram (A) and the anteroposterior tomogram (B). Despite the severe oligemia, the hilar pulmonary arteries are not enlarged. The lungs are severely overinflated.

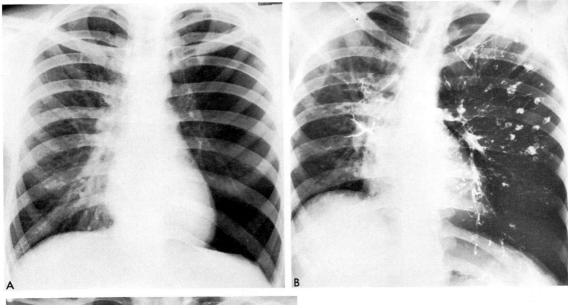

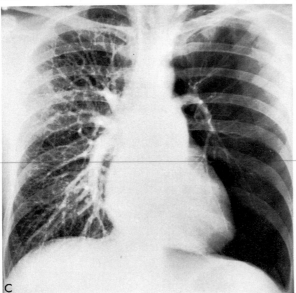

Figure 4–148. Unilateral Hyperlucent Lung: Swyer-James or Macleod's Syndrome. A postero-anterior roentgenogram exposed at TLC (*A*) reveals a marked discrepancy in the radiolucency of the two lungs, the left showing severe oligemia. The left hilar shadow is diminutive. The left lung appears to be of approximately normal volume compared with the right. An anteroposterior roentgenogram at RV following bronchography (*B*) demonstrates severe air trapping in the left lung, little change in volume having occurred from TLC. Since deflation of the right lung is normal, the mediastinum has swung sharply to the right. The bronchial tree shows less bronchiectasis than is generally the case, although there is filling of numerous large spaces typical of emphysema. In the pulmonary angiogram (*C*), the discrepancy of blood flow to the two lungs is readily apparent; note that the left pulmonary artery is present although diminutive (differentiation from congenital absence of the left pulmonary artery).

is imperative to exclude an endobronchial lesion (preferably by bronchoscopy).

The site of vasoconstriction in response to hypoxia has been clarified by Allison and Stanbook[307] from studies on greyhound dogs. In response to hypoxia in an exteriorized lobe, arteriography revealed vasoconstriction that was maximal in vessels 0.3 mm in diameter in which a 19 per cent reduction in diameter was observed. No significant change in caliber occurred in vessels exceeding 2 mm in diameter. Reversal of the vascular response occurred promptly upon withdrawal of the hypoxic stimulus. In another study[308] it was observed that in patients with local hypoventilation as a result of a partly obstructing endobronchial lesion, hypoxic vasoconstriction may be strikingly prolonged following removal of the bronchial obstruction; and further, that the interval for return of blood flow to normal levels is probably related directly to the duration of the initial airway obstruction. The precise mechanism for this phenomenon is unclear.

A picture somewhat similar to that produced by Swyer-James syndrome or a partly obstructing endobronchial lesion may be seen in patients with unilateral pulmonary artery agenesis, in which the pulmonary artery is interrupted in the region of the hilum so that the lung is devoid of pulmonary artery perfusion.[275, 304–306] On plain roentgenographic study, the two may be distinguished by the virtual absence of a hilar shadow in pulmonary artery agenesis and a diminutive hilar shadow in Macleod's syndrome; also in the former there is no expiratory airway obstruction. In pulmonary artery agenesis, linear markings throughout the affected lung are caused by a greatly increased bronchial arterial circulation; those through the contralateral lung are often enlarged (pulmonary plethora or pleonemia) as a result of associated intracardiac left-

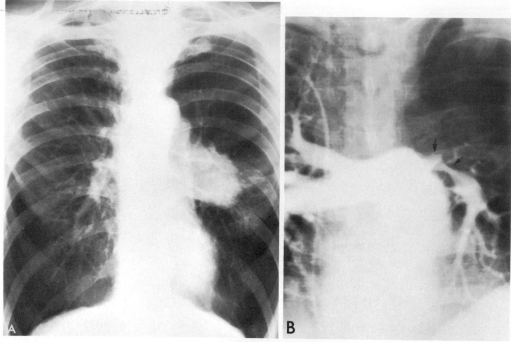

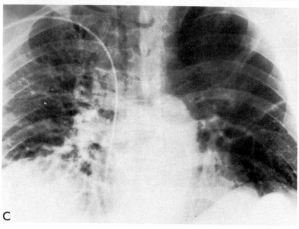

Figure 4–149. Unilateral Pulmonary Oligemia: Compression of Hilar Pulmonary Arteries by Bronchogenic Carcinoma. A posteroanterior roentgenogram (*A*) reveals discrepancy in the radiolucency of the two lungs, the left being oligemic and comparatively more radiolucent. The large hilar mass proved to be primary squamous cell carcinoma. This patient did not have a pulmonary angiogram, but an angiogram on another patient showing a similar hilar mass (but less reproducible changes on standard roentgenography) reveals the effects on the pulmonary circulation to be anticipated in such a situation: in the arterial phase (*B*), there is marked narrowing and distortion of the main pulmonary artery and its interlobar branch (*arrows*); the upper lobe arteries are completely occluded. In the late capillary and early venous phase (*C*), opacification of the vasculature of the left lung is markedly reduced compared with the right, and there is delayed flow through the lower lobe arteries.

to-right shunts. Pulmonary arteriography accurately differentiates the two if standard roentgenographic techniques leave the diagnosis in doubt.

Fouché and D'Silva[309] induced unilateral miliary emboli of pulmonary arteries in animals and produced a roentgenographic effect similar to that of Swyer-James syndrome; however, airway obstruction was absent, a sign which differentiates these two conditions. A similar combination of roentgenographic changes occurs sometimes in humans when pulmonary arterial flow has been reduced by compression or obstruction of a pulmonary artery by a contiguous compressive or invasive process (Fig. 4–149). Generally speaking, however, such a process results in enlargement or increase in density of the involved hilum.

2. *Small peripheral vessels; normal or subnormal lung volume; enlarged hilar pulmonary arteries (or an enlarged hilum).* This combination is nearly always caused by unilateral pulmonary artery embolism without infarction (Fig. 4–150). The occluding embolus almost invariably leads to enlargement of the involved artery.[310] Since bronchial obstruction is not a feature, there is no overinflation—on the contrary, lung volume may be reduced. A similar roentgenographic picture may be produced by obstruction of a pulmonary artery by invasive neoplasm: the hilar enlargement is caused by the original lesion rather than by a distended vessel, although the overall roentgenographic appearance may be the same. Jacques and Barclay[311] described identical roentgenographic changes in sarcomatous replacement of the lumen of the pulmonary artery.

3. *Small peripheral vessels; overinflation; normal hilar pulmonary arteries.* This combination is distinctive of local emphysema. The roentgenographic

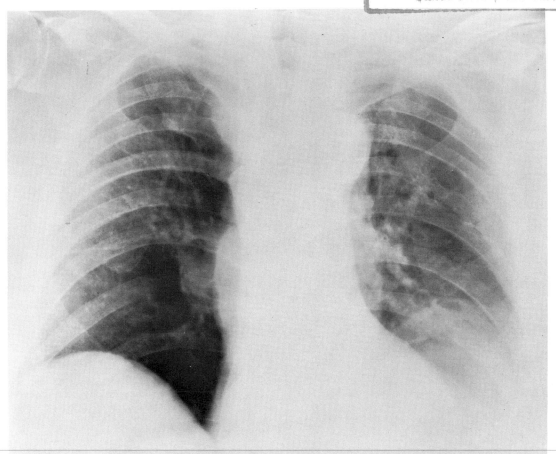

Figure 4–150. Lobar Oligemia without Overinflation: Thromboembolism without Infarction. Anteroposterior roentgenogram exposed in the supine position demonstrates marked increase in the radiolucency of the lower half of the right lung. The vascular markings are diminished in caliber and the descending branch of the right pulmonary artery is dilated and sharply defined; this vessel tapers rapidly as it proceeds distally. Lobar oligemia as a result of thromboembolism without infarction constitutes Westermark's sign.

appearance of the vascular deficiency of emphysema is often local rather than general; in one study, 13 of 26 patients with established emphysema had predominantly local involvement.[289] The lower or upper lobes or almost any combination of individual lobes may be predominantly affected (Fig. 4–151). The involved portions of lung show a combination of overinflation and severely diminished peripheral vasculature; less involved areas tend to be pleonemic as a result of redistribution of blood to them caused by the increased resistance to pulmonary blood flow in emphysematous areas. Since the lack of increase in vascular resistance in uninvolved lung prevents the development of pulmonary artery hypertension, the hilar pulmonary arteries do not enlarge.

Pulmonary Air Cysts

This term is used for all thin-walled air-containing intrapulmonary spaces that are roentgenologically visible, regardless of their pathogenesis. Although their clinical significance varies widely, it is useful to group these lesions under one heading for roentgenologic description. One of the most important distinctions to be made is whether an air cyst is a solitary abnormality in otherwise healthy lung or part of generalized pulmonary disease: the implications in terms of the effects on pulmonary function, which are of obvious importance, have been covered in detail by Bates and his coauthors.[312]

A pulmonary air cyst (bulla or bleb) is an air-containing space ranging in size from 1 cm in diameter to the volume of a whole hemithorax and possessing a smooth wall of minimal thickness (1 mm or less). The space may be unilocular or separated into several compartments by thin septa (Fig. 4–152). It may arise *de novo*, when surrounding lung tissue is normal, or may occur secondary to other disease, usually infectious and commonly associated with much parenchymal scarring (Fig. 4–153); in the latter circumstances the cyst is associated with a variable amount of disease in adjacent parenchyma. Secondary signs may be present, depending upon the size of the cyst; for example, when a huge bulla occupies most of the volume of one hemithorax (Fig. 4–154), signs of air trapping are apparent during deep breathing—the mediastinum is displaced to the side of the normal lung

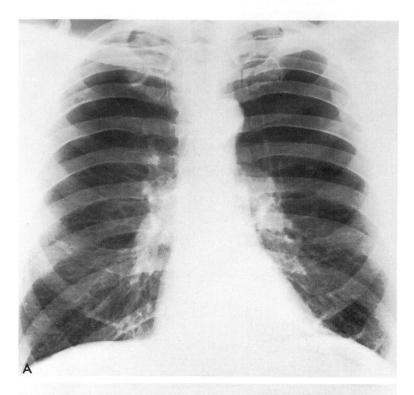

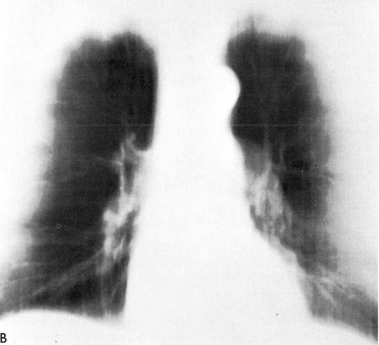

Figure 4–151. Lobar Oligemia with Overinflation: Pulmonary Emphysema (Local). A posteroanterior roentgenogram (*A*) reveals a marked reduction in the vascularity of both upper lung zones. An anteroposterior tomogram (*B*) shows the upper lobe oligemia to excellent advantage; note that "grayness" of the lower half of the left lung is greater than the corresponding area of the right lung, indicating greater microvascular perfusion of the left lower lobe than of the right. Since vascular resistance in the lower lung zones is normal, blood has been redistributed from the upper to the lower lobes so that pulmonary arterial hypertension has not developed.

during expiration, and ipsilateral hemidiaphragmatic excursion and movements of the thoracic wall are restricted. When an air cyst occupies most of one lobe, lobar expansion may be apparent, with outward bulging of the interlobar fissure. Cysts are characteristically avascular, an observation that may be facilitated by tomographic examination, particularly with small lesions. Although seldom indicated, angiography[313] and bronchography are useful in showing displacement of pulmonary vessels and the bronchial tree around the cyst. These roentgenologic signs conform to the physiologic observations that pulmonary air cysts are poorly ventilated and unperfused.[313] Studies of the mechanical properties of pulmonary cysts and bullae[314] have shown that, during expiration, the cysts inflate while the rest of the lung deflates (Fig. 4–153), a paradox attributed to their high compliance and to air flow restriction by small deficiencies in the walls of the bullae occasioned by loss of alveolar tissue. When the air cyst is filled, these communications are compressed, resulting in permanent inflation.

The specific characteristics of individual forms of pulmonary air cysts are discussed in detail in Chapter 11. A brief outline of the nomenclature used and of the general characteristics of each lesion is presented here.

Pulmonary air cysts may be *congenital* or *acquired*. The congenital type includes bronchogenic cysts whose fluid contents have been expelled, and "congenital cystic disease" of the lung;[315] air cysts as part of intralobar pulmonary sequestration also should qualify as disease of congenital origin. Acquired disease includes the two common types of pulmonary air cysts, *blebs* and *bullae*. Blebs seldom exceed 1 cm in diameter; they are either immediately subpleural or intrapleural and most frequently develop over the lung apices. They are equivalent to the type 1 bullae described by Reid;[316] they characteristically have a narrow neck and usually contain only gas, without evidence of alveolar remnants or blood vessels. The mechanism of their development has been attributed to the dissection of air from a ruptured alveolus, through interstitial tissue into the thin fibrous layer of visceral pleura, where it accumulates in the form of a cyst;[317, 318] however, they basically represent paraseptal emphysema. These lesions are usually regarded as the major cause of spontaneous pneumothorax. *Bullae*, which are intrapulmonary structures, are usually attributed to excessive rupture of alveolar walls; they are equivalent to the type 3 bullae described by Reid.[316] Bullae appear to affect upper and lower lobes equally and may develop in the absence of generalized emphysema. Their walls are composed of compressed parenchymal tissue,[317] and strands of emphysematous lung and intact blood vessels are pathologically identifiable within many of these lesions. The role played by bronchial or bronchiolar obstruction in the pathogenesis of these structures is not clear, although check-valve obstruction probably is operative in at least some cases; for example, the development of bullae in decompression workers has been repeatedly attributed to bronchiolar obstruction.[319–321] Some bullae develop as a sequela of lung abscess, of either tuberculous or staphylo-

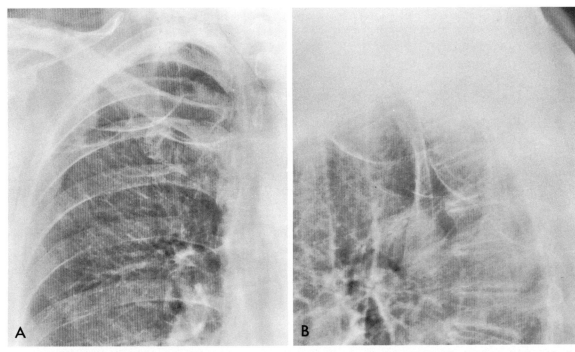

Figure 4–152. Bullae or Blebs. View of the upper half of the right lung in posteroanterior (*A*) and lateral (*B*) projections reveal several cystic spaces in the lung apex sharply separated from contiguous lung by curvilinear, hairline shadows. The appearance suggests multiple blebs or bullae rather than a single space separated into compartments by thin septa.

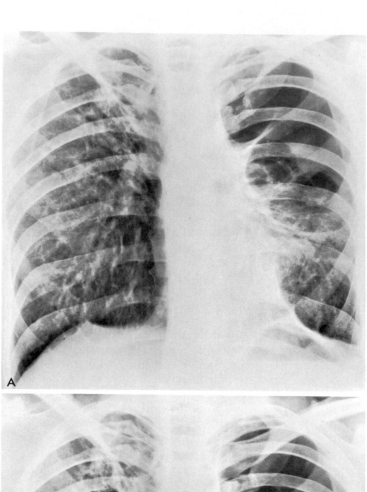

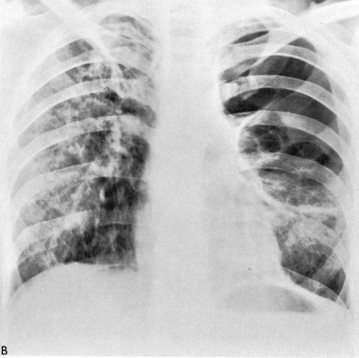

Figure 4–153. Bulla Formation Associated with Pulmonary Scarring. A posteroanterior roentgenogram exposed at TLC (*A*) demonstrates a large, well-defined cystic space occupying the upper half of the left hemithorax, sharply demarcated from contiguous lung. There is extensive bilateral parenchymal disease due to chronic fibroproductive tuberculosis. A roentgenogram exposed at RV (*B*) reveals marked air trapping within the pneumatocele; in fact, by actual measurement, the space is larger at RV than at TLC. *See* text. (Courtesy of the Montreal Chest Hospital Center.)

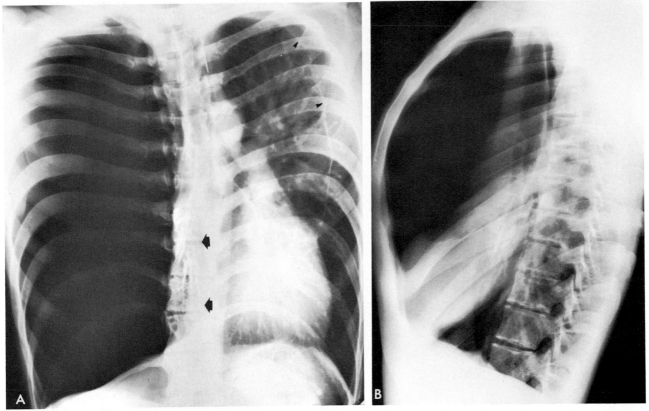

Figure 4–154. Huge Bulla. An anteroposterior roentgenogram of the chest following bronchography reveals a huge air sac completely filling and overdistending the right hemithorax and extending across the anterior mediastinal septum almost as far as the left axillary pleura (the line shadow indicated by *arrowheads* is formed by four layers of pleura). The right lung is compressed into a small nubbin of tissue situated in the midline; note the markedly crowded right bronchial tree (*thick arrows*). In lateral projection (*B*), herniation of the pneumatocele across the anterior mediastinal septum has resulted in marked increase in depth of the retrosternal air space and posterior displacement of the heart and major vessels.

coccal etiology; resolution of acute pneumonia surrounding the abscess leaves a thin-walled cystic space that is indistinguishable from a bulla arising *de novo* in otherwise healthy lung. (It has been suggested that direct communication between post-abscess bullae and the bronchial tree permits opacification of these structures with bronchographic contrast media, whereas bullae of other origins do not communicate;[322] we have observed this communication after acute lung abscess in two cases [Fig. 4–155]). Post-traumatic pneumatoceles resulting from lung tissue laceration associated with non-penetrating chest trauma may present as typical thin-walled air cysts,[323] with or without an air-fluid level. Although rare, bronchial carcinoma mimicking a thin-walled cyst[324] points up the hazard in dismissing every cystic pulmonary lesion as inconsequential.

Finally, bullae frequently occur as a manifestation of diffuse pulmonary emphysema. The cysts are characteristically very thin-walled, frequently are small, and usually are distributed widely throughout the subpleural zone.

ROENTGENOLOGIC SIGNS OF PLEURAL DISEASE

Since effusion is by far the commonest and most important abnormality affecting the pleura, it is worthwhile to review briefly the forces that govern the formation and absorption of fluid in the normal pleural space (*see* Chapter 1, page 175, for more detailed discussion of the normal physiology of the pleura). In health, fluid is formed at the parietal pleura and absorbed at the visceral pleura. Transudation and absorption depend primarily upon a balance between hydrostatic pressure, which forces fluid out of the capillaries, and osmotic pressure of blood, which draws tissue fluid into capillaries. Since colloid osmotic pressure and pleural pressure exert an equal effect on both pleural surfaces, the only difference in the forces acting on the parietal and visceral pleura is that hydrostatic pressure is systemic in the pareital pleural capillaries (approximately 30 cm H_2O) and pulmonary in the visceral pleural capillaries (approximately 11 cm H_2O). The net effect is a driving pressure of 9 cm H_2O from

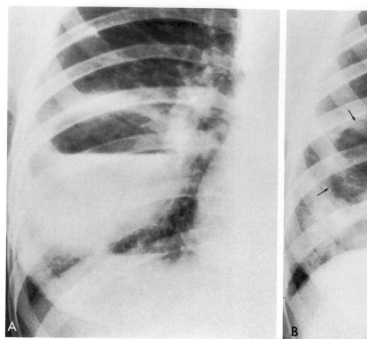

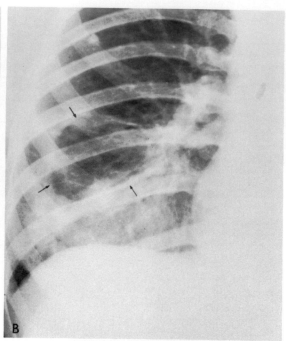

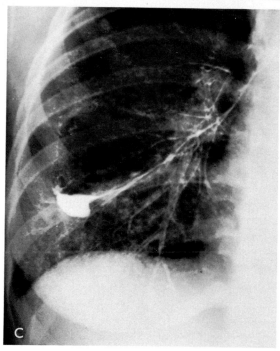

Figure 4–155. Communication with the Bronchial Tree of a Solitary Postinflammatory Bulla. A view of the lower portion of the right lung from a posteroanterior roentgenogram (*A*) reveals a large, thick-walled abscess containing a prominent air-fluid level (heavy growth of *Staphylococcus aureus* from the sputum). One month later (*B*), most of the pneumonia had resolved, leaving a thin-walled bulla as a residuum (*arrows*). A bronchogram performed at this time (*C*) shows contrast medium forming an air-fluid level within the bulla.

the parietal pleural capillaries to the pleura and of 10 cm H_2O from the pleura to the visceral pleural capillaries. Thus, normal pleural dynamics insure that the accumulation of pleural fluid is prevented by an osmotic-hydrostatic pressure gradient.[325]

Despite this usually effective combination of forces, physiologically occurring pleural fluid is identifiable roentgenographically in a significant percentage of normal healthy humans. Using their modification of the lateral decubitus projection with a horizontal x-ray beam, Müller and Löfstedt[326] identified pleural fluid in 15 of 120 healthy adults (12.5 per cent). They performed thoracentesis on

some of these subjects and concluded that the smallest amount of fluid identifiable by this technique was 3 to 5 ml; the largest amount found was 15 ml. In a later study of 300 healthy adults (163 women and 137 men), Hessén,[327] who used a similar technique, found conclusive evidence of roentgenologically demonstrable fluid in 12 healthy adults (4.0 per cent) and suggestive evidence in an additional 19 (6.3 per cent). The thickness of the fluid layer ranged from 1 to 10 mm and averaged 5 mm. Fluid was identified unilaterally in some subjects and bilaterally in others, and in some the amount varied from one examination to another. It was often observed during repeated examinations of the same subjects, suggesting to Hessén that such a fluid accumulation was an inherent feature of the individual's physiologic status. It is of interest that in 92 women studied a few days postpartum, he showed convincing evidence of pleural fluid in 21 (22.8 per cent) and the possiblity of fluid in another 14 (15 per cent). Moskowitz and his colleagues extended these obsevations in a study of cadavers;[328] they injected 5 ml increments of saline or plasma into the pleural space and showed that even 5 ml of fluid were clearly visible on roentgenograms exposed in the unmodified lateral decubitus position; increasing amounts caused a stepladder increase in density.

The studies by Müller and Löfstedt[326] and Hessén[327] were carried out on healthy adults: in an attempt to estimate the incidence and amount of fluid that might be roentgenographically visible in the pleural space of healthy infants and children, Eklöf and Törngren[329] studied 115 asymptomatic subjects (55 boys and 60 girls) ranging in age from 7 days to 18 years (mean 6.4 years), none of whom evidenced thoracic disease. Roentgenography was performed by the standard lateral decubitus technique, not the modified technique described by Müller and Löfstedt. Pleural fluid (maximal thickness, 1.5 to 2.0 mm) was demonstrated in five subjects (4.3 per cent), three boys and two girls; the fluid was right-sided only in two, left-sided only in two, and bilateral in one. Re-examination of four of these five children 5 years later again demonstrated a small amount of fluid, essentially unchanged from the earlier examination.

These studies are of obvious practical importance insofar as they indicate that small amounts of pleural fluid may be demonstrated roentgenographically in the absence of disease; thus, they point up a potential source of error in the diagnosis of clinically significant pleural effusion.

Reported figures for the amount of pleural fluid required for roentgenographic demonstration in the erect subject range from 250 to 600 ml.[330–332] Rigler[333] was the first to suggest that smaller quantities—as little as 100 ml—could be shown by roentgenography in the lateral decubitus position, and there is no doubt that his development led to improved accuracy in the roentgenologic diagnosis of plcural cffusion. The later studies described previously reduced this figure still further—to 5 to 15 ml—and it seems reasonable to accept the latter figures as the amount of fluid demonstrable with special roentgenographic techniques.

ROENTGENOLOGIC SIGNS OF PLEURAL EFFUSION

Typical Arrangement of Free Pleural Fluid

It will be recalled from the discussion on the physiology of the pleura that the negative pressure within the pleural cavity represents the difference between the elastic forces of the chest wall and of the lungs. Lung tissue has a natural tendency to recoil but is prevented from doing so beyond a certain point by the chest wall's tendency to expand outward with an equal, opposite force. Thus, in the normal state, intimate contact between the visceral and parietal pleural surfaces is maintained. When a buffer medium (e.g., liquid or gas) is introduced into the pleural space, the lung can recoil inward toward its fixed moorings at the hilum, the amount of retraction depending upon the quantity of buffer. The site of retraction depends upon the position of the buffer medium within the pleural space, as illustrated by the different effects of hydrothorax and pneumothorax: in the upright subject, the effect of gravity causes gas to rise and liquid to fall in the pleural space. The different manner in which the lung responds to these two buffer media is purely a matter of anatomic location—in the former instance the upper portions of the lung retract, and in the latter the lower portions. The different roentgenographic appearances of the two media are owing to the fact that one is radiopaque and the other radiolucent; for example, if a roentgenogram was taken of a patient with a pleural effusion of 1 liter, in a 90 degree head down position, the form of the lung would be *roughly* the same as if 1 liter of gas was present and the patient was erect (Fig. 4–156). The lung tends to maintain its traditional shape at all stages of collapse, a characteristic termed by Fleischner[334] the "form elasticity" of the lung. When pneumothorax is present or the thoracic cage is opened (thoracotomy or necropsy), the shape of the lung in its completely collapsed state is a miniature replica of its shape in the fully distended form (*see* Figure 4–18, page 485). The effect is the same when pleural effusion or pneumothorax is present, except that the collapse may be local rather than general.

These two influences—gravity and elastic recoil—are the major forces that control the arrangement of free fluid in the pleural space.[327, 334] Fluid gravitates first to the base of the hemithorax, where it comes to lie between the inferior surface of the lung and the hemidiaphragm (Fig. 4–157)—particularly posteriorly, where the pleural sinus is deepest. With increasing amounts, the fluid spills out into the costophrenic sinuses posteriorly, laterally, and eventually anteriorly; with further accumulation, it spreads upward in mantle-like fashion around the convexity of the lung, tapering gradually as it assumes a higher position in the thorax.

On the basis of this description, it is easy to construct the typical roentgenographic appearance of pleural effusion. Consider the hypothetic situation of a "moderate" pleural effusion (1000 ml) (Fig. 4–158): such an amount of fluid will completely obscure the hemidiaphragm and the costophrenic sinuses and will extend upward around the anterior, lateral, and posterior thoracic wall, to about the midportion of the hemithorax. Since the

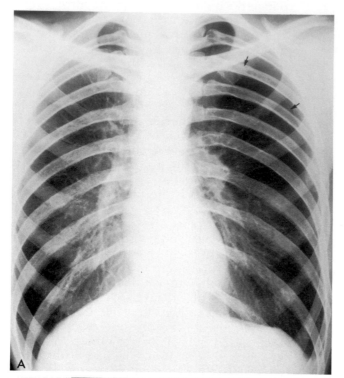

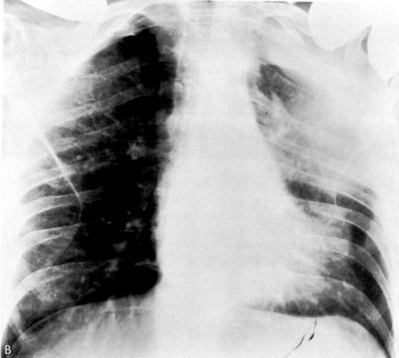

Figure 4–156. Similarity in the Effects on the Lung of Pneumothorax and Hydrothorax. *A,* A posteroanterior roentgenogram of the chest (erect position) of a patient with a small pneumothorax reveals partial collapse of the upper and midportions of the lung (visceral pleural line at *arrows*). *B,* The roentgenogram of another patient with a moderate pleural effusion on whom roentgenography was carried out in a 45-degree Trendelenburg position. The effects on the lung in these two situations are almost identical.

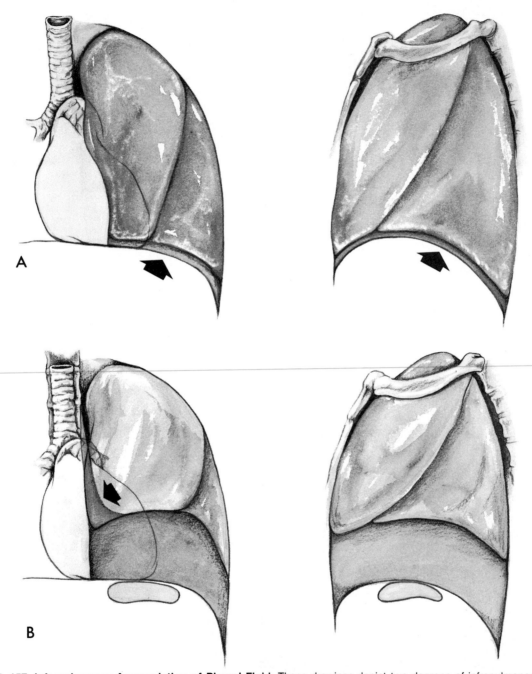

Figure 4–157. Infrapulmonary Accumulation of Pleural Fluid. These drawings depict two degrees of infrapulmonary effusion: in *A*, the situation is "typical" in that it represents the *usual* anatomic location of small amounts of fluid (up to 500 ml); in *B*, the amount of fluid is large (e.g., 1500 ml) and the local infrapulmonary accumulation thus "atypical." *See* text.

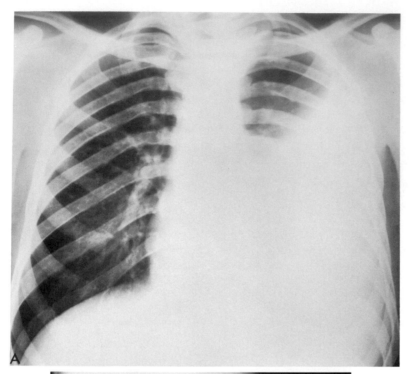

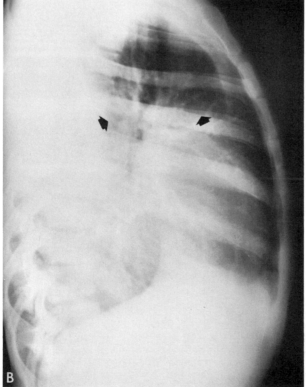

Figure 4–158. Large Pleural Effusion: Typical Arrangement. Posteroanterior (A) and lateral (B) roentgenograms exposed in the erect position demonstrate uniform opacification of the lower two thirds of the left hemithorax. The upper level of the fluid is meniscus-shaped in both posteroanterior and lateral projection (*arrows* on B). Note that only the right hemidiaphragm is visualized in lateral projection, the left being obscured by fluid (the silhouette sign).

mediastinal surface of the lung possesses relatively less elastic recoil because of its fixation at the hilum and pulmonary ligament, less fluid accumulates along this surface than around the convexity. Thus, in posteroanterior projection, the density of the fluid is high laterally and curves gently downward and medially, with a smooth meniscus-shaped upper border, to terminate along the midcardiac border. In lateral projection, since the fluid has ascended along the anterior and posterior thoracic wall to roughly an equal extent, the upper surface of the fluid density will be semicircular, being high anteriorly and posteriorly and curving smoothly downward to its lowest point in the midaxillary line. Comparison of the maximal height of the fluid density in the posteroanterior and lateral projections will show that this height is identical posteriorly, laterally, and anteriorly (Fig. 4–188)—that is, the top of the fluid accumulation is *horizontal*; the meniscus shape is caused by the fact that the layer of fluid is of insufficient depth to cast a discernible shadow when viewed *en face*. This typical configuration was excellently reproduced roentgenographically by Fleischner,[334] who constructed paraffin wax models in the shape of half a hollow truncated cone. An ingenious experiment with a Plexiglas phantom

designed by Khomiakov and Fedorova[335] yielded identical roentgenographic results, as did the studies of Davis and his colleagues with plaster.[336] The interested reader is directed to these three articles for lucid illustrations of the roentgenographic appearance of pleural effusion.

Since the distribution of fluid within the free pleural space tends to obey the law of gravity, and since the lung tends to maintain its shape as it diminishes in size, the first place fluid accumulates in the erect patient is between the inferior surface of the lower lobe and the diaphragm: in effect, the lung is "floating" on a layer of fluid (Fig. 4–157). If the amount of fluid is small it may occupy only this position without spilling over into the costophrenic sinuses—not even the most dependent sinus posteriorly (Fig. 4–159). In such circumstances the configuration of the hemidiaphragm is maintained and the appearance on posteroanterior and lateral roentgenograms suggests no more than slight elevation of that hemidiaphragm. This has been illustrated by Collins and his associates,[337] who infused successive aliquots of 25 ml of saline into the pleural space of five erect cadavers. They reported that as little as 25 ml was detectable—as evidenced by elevation of the apparent level of the hemidia-

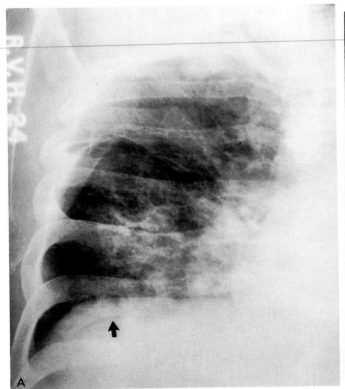
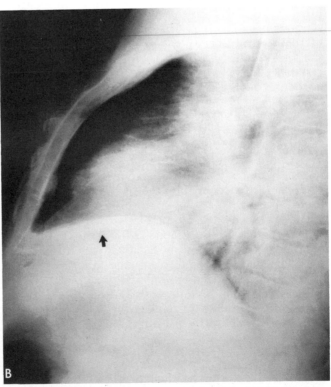

Figure 4–159. Infrapulmonary Pleural Effusion Associated with Pneumoperitoneum. Views of the right hemithorax from posteroanterior (A) and lateral (B) roentgenograms (exposed in the erect position postmortem) demonstrate a thin line of air density (*arrow*) situated approximately 1 cm below the base of the right lung, roughly parallel to the right hemidiaphragm. Since this gas is situated within the peritoneal space, it outlines the undersurface of the right hemidiaphragm, indicating the presence of a layer of fluid approximately 1 cm in thickness between the diaphragm and the undersurface of the right lung. By multiplying the anteroposterior and lateral dimensions of the right hemidiaphragm by the thickness of fluid (1 cm), it was estimated that the amount of fluid in the pleural space was approximately 400 ml. At necropsy, the right pleural space was found to contain 450 ml. This study demonstrates the large quantity of fluid that may accumulate in an infrapulmonary location without producing convincing roentgenologic evidence of its presence.

phragm—although their illustrations suggest to us that the evidence was provided more by a separation of the "pseudohemidiaphragm" from the stomach bubble. Bearing in mind the individual variation in the height of the diaphragm in normal subjecs, it is readily apparent that small accumulations of fluid in the pleural space easily can be missed roentgenologically. Only if the physician is alert to the possibility of a small pleural effusion can the diagnosis be confirmed by roentgenography in the lateral decubitus position with a horizontal x-ray beam. Thus, as Hessén[327] emphasized, "infrapulmonary" is the *usual* (*not* atypical) distribution in the free pleural space (although it would be reasonable to consider the infrapulmonary accumulation of large amounts of fluid paradoxic or atypical; this subject is dealt with in the section on atypical arrangement of pleural fluid). Sometimes a subpulmonic effusion not apparent on full inspiration may become evident on a roentgenogram exposed in full expiration, owing to a lateral shift of the apex of the dome.

When the amount of fluid in the infrapulmonary pleural space reaches a certain level, it spills over into the posterior costophrenic sinus and obliterates that sinus as viewed in lateral roentgenographic projection. The normally sharp costophrenic angle is obliterated by a shallow, homogeneous shadow whose upper surface is meniscus-shaped. As a result of pleural capillarity, the shadow inevitably is associated with increased width of the pleural line up the posterior thoracic wall: this represents the earliest roentgenographic manifestation of the typical mantle distribution. Such a roentgenographic appearance–pseudodiaphragmatic elevation due to subpulmonic localization, with or without obliteration of the posterior costophrenic sulcus—may be unaccompanied by other discernible evidence of pleural effusion; for example, a posteroanterior roentgenogram may reveal a normally sharp lateral costophrenic angle. Since the evidence supplied by blunting of the posterior costophrenic sinus may be subtle, lateral roentgenograms of excellent technical quality are necessary.

With increasing amounts of fluid, the roentgenologic signs develop in predictable fashion: obliteration of the lateral and eventually anterior costophrenic sulci, and extension of fluid up the chest wall in its usual mantle distribution. Fluid that occupies a costophrenic sulcus on full inspiration characteristically shifts to a subpulmonic location on full expiration.

Of some importance in the roentgenologic manifestations of pleural effusion is the pattern that develops when the major interlobar fissures are incomplete medially.[338] In such circumstances, fluid that extends into the major fissures creates a sharp concave line, medial to which the lung is of normal or almost normal lucency and peripheral to which the fluid creates a uniform opacity.

The effects on the thorax as a whole of the accumulation of large amounts of fluid in the pleural space depend largely upon the condition of the ipsilateral lung. Even small amounts of fluid produce "relaxation" atelectasis of contiguous lung, in much the same manner as when air is the buffer medium in pneumothorax. When pleural effusion is massive, collapse of the ipsilateral lung may be almost complete. Despite severe atelectasis, however, the overall effect of a massive effusion almost invariably is that of a space-occupying process, with enlargement of the ipsilateral hemithorax, displacement of the mediastinum to the contralateral side, and severe depression and flattening of the ipsilateral hemidiaphragm; in fact, the hemidiaphragm may be depressed so severely as to be concave superiorly (Fig. 4–160).[339] When one hemithorax is totally opacified, appreciation of the balance of forces between the two sides of the thorax is of obvious importance. If the mediastinum shows no shift and the hemidiaphragm is only slightly depressed, the presence of disease within the ipsilateral lung can be stated with absolute certainty (Fig. 4–161); the conclusion that *must* be reached is that the balance of forces between effusion (a space-occupying process) and parenchymal disease (which reduces volume) ensures that the volume of the hemithorax is not greater than normal. The possibility of an obstructing endobronchial lesion (e.g., bronchogenic carcinoma with pleural metastases) is obvious: in fact, total opacification of one hemithorax without mediastinal or diaphragmatic displacement is highly suggestive of bronchogenic cancer with pleural metastases. (Exceptions are uncommon—for example, extensive mesothelioma.)

Atypical Distribution of Free Pleural Fluid

The typical arrangement of fluid in the free pleural space requires that the underlying lung be free of disease and thus capable of preserving its shape even while recoiling from the chest wall—that is, it maintains its "form elasticity." An alteration in this uniform recoiling tendency is the influence by which most if not all atypical arrangements of pleural fluid can be explained (excluding the restriction of free movement occasioned by pleural adhesions and fibrosis). It has been suggested[334, 340, 341] that parenchymal disease, particularly atelectasis, in any portion of the lung modifies the retractility of that portion of the lung locally so that pleural fluid is attracted to it. Zidulka and his colleagues[342] found that lobar collapse in dogs is associated with a local pleural pressure around the collapsed lobe that is more negative than that surrounding the uncollapsed lobes. Extending this study to a radiographic investigation in dogs, Rigby and his associates[341] produced atelectasis of selected lobes and studied the distribution of fluid injected into the pleural space: they found that when lower lobes were collapsed, fluid tended to move to the area of maximal parenchymal distortion where negative pleural pressure was greatest. However, in the presence of upper lobe collapse, free pleural fluid tended to

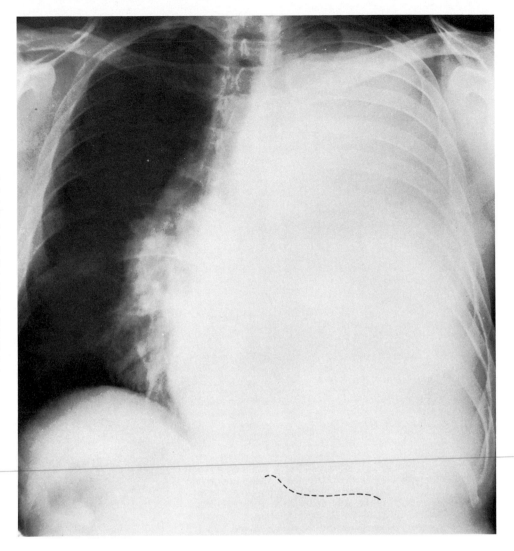

Figure 4–160. Massive Effusion, Underlying Lung Normal. A posteroanterior roentgenogram reveals total opacification of the left hemithorax by a massive pleural effusion. The mediastinum is displaced to the right. The stomach bubble (*dotted line*) is displaced far inferiorly and its upper surface is concave rather than convex, suggesting that the hemidiaphragm possesses the same contour. A faint air bronchogram can be visualized through the fluid in the medial portion of the left lung; the underlying lung was normal. Pleural metastases from carcinoma of the maxillary antrum.

remain in its "typical" location in an infrapulmonary position.

Regardless of the mechanism whereby fluid accumulates in atypical locations within the pleural space, there is little doubt that in the majority of cases it relates to underlying pulmonary disease. Thus, the major roentgenologic significance of atypical pleural effusion is that it *alerts the physician to the presence of both parenchymal and pleural disease.*

The roentgenographic appearance of atypical pleural fluid accumulation in disease affecting individual lobes has been described in detail.[327, 334] One example will illustrate the variations produced. In *lower lobe disease*, fluid tends to accumulate posteromedially. In posteroanterior projection, the opacity tends to be higher on the mediastinal than on the axillary border, its upper surface curving downward and laterally toward the lateral costophrenic sulcus (simulating the shadow of combined atelectasis and consolidation of the right middle and lower lobes). In lateral projection, the upper border of the density roughly parallels the major fissure, beginning high in the thorax posteriorly and curving downward and anteriorly, toward the anterior costophrenic gutter, which may be clear and sharp (Fig. 4–162).

Since roentgenography in other than the erect position will detect any change in distribution of *free* pleural fluid, examination in the supine or, preferably, lateral decubitus position will show displacement of the fluid over the posterior or lateral pleural space, respectively. The nature of these unusual opacities can thus be clarified in questionable cases (e.g., an effusion simulating lower lobe consolidation). In addition, these procedures permit clearer identification and more accurate assessment of the underlying parenchymal disease.

Some physicians contend that the removal of fluid by thoracentesis in cases of combined parenchymal and pleural disease permits better perception of the diseased lung under the effusion. In fact, this procedure is seldom productive from a roentgenologic point of view (although obviously advantageous in providing fluid for pathologic and biochemical examination). The reasons for this lack should be obvious in the light of the foregoing discussions: since atelectasis usually is present, the removal of fluid accentuates the forces that are

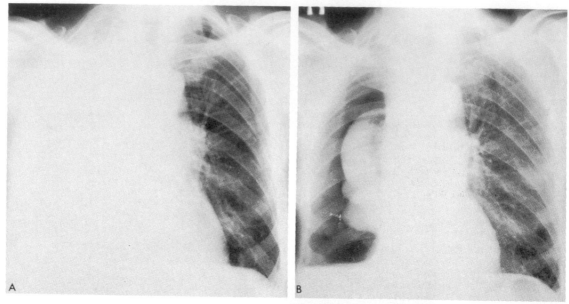

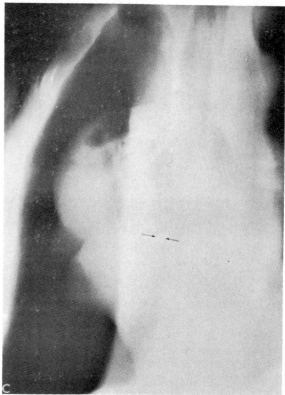

Figure 4–161. Massive Pleural Effusion Associated with Obstructive Atelectasis of the Underlying Lung. A posteroanterior roentgenogram (*A*) shows total opacification of the right hemithorax; in contrast to the situation in Figure 4–160, the mediastinum is central in position. Following removal of almost all the fluid and replacement with an equal quantity of air (without air replacement, the patient became severely dyspneic), the right lung (*B*) can be seen to be totally collapsed and airless (with the exception of small quantities of air in the upper lobe); the configuration of the collapsed lung resembles the profile of a face whose nose is the right middle lobe and chin the right lower lobe. In such a situation, the absence of an air bronchogram constitutes absolute evidence of endobronchial obstruction. An anteroposterior tomogram (*C*) confirms the airlessness of the right middle and lower lobes and reveals the intermediate stem bronchus to be obstructed at its distal end (*arrows*). At thoracotomy, stenosis of the intermediate stem bronchus was found to be caused by compression by enlarged lymph nodes replaced by adenocarcinoma.

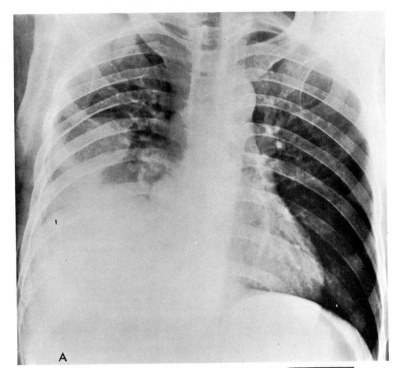

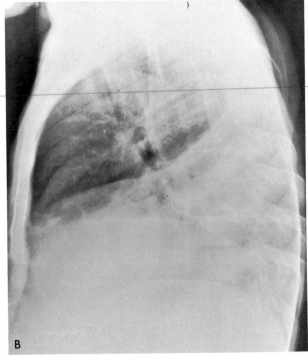

Figure 4–162. Right Pleural Effusion, Atypical Accumulation. A moderate-sized right pleural effusion identified on posteroanterior (*A*) and lateral (*B*) roentgenograms does not possess typical meniscus-shaped upper border in either projection; it is high posteriorly and low anteriorly so as to simulate consolidation of the middle and lower lobes (particularly as visualized in lateral projection). Right lower lobe pneumonia with effusion.

trying to compensate for the parenchymal collapse. Thus the mediastinum and diaphragm are shifted further toward the affected side, so that fluid remaining in the pleural space will still accumulate around and obscure the underlying diseased parenchyma. Thus, supine and lateral decubitus roentgenography is clearly superior for assessing parenchymal disease.

There is disagreement whether *infrapulmonary pleural effusion* (*synonyms:* subpulmonic. diaphragmatic) should be considered atypical, since, as

already discussed, this is the site where effusion first accumulates "normally." Usually, increasing amounts of fluid spill over into the costophrenic sulci and produce the roentgenologic signs described. However, for reasons as yet incompletely understood, fluid sometimes continues to accumulate in an infrapulmonary location without spilling into the costophrenic sulci or extending up the chest wall, producing a roentgenographic configuration in the erect subject that closely simulates diaphragmatic elevation (thus the designation

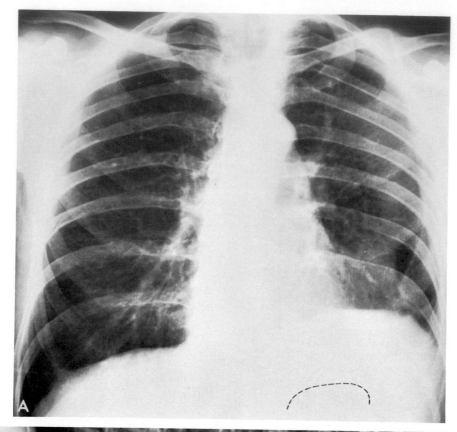

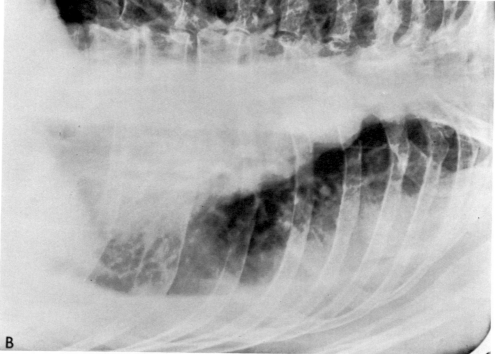

Figure 4–163. Infrapulmonary Pleural Effusion. A posteroanterior roentgenogram exposed in the erect position (*A*) shows a high left pseudodiaphragm whose peak is more laterally situated than that of a normal hemidiaphragm. It is situated several centimeters from the stomach bubble (*dotted line*). The costophrenic sulcus is sharp. A roentgenogram exposed in the left lateral decubitus position with a horizontal x-ray beam (*B*) shows the fluid to have extended along the axillary lung zone.

Illustration continued on opposite page

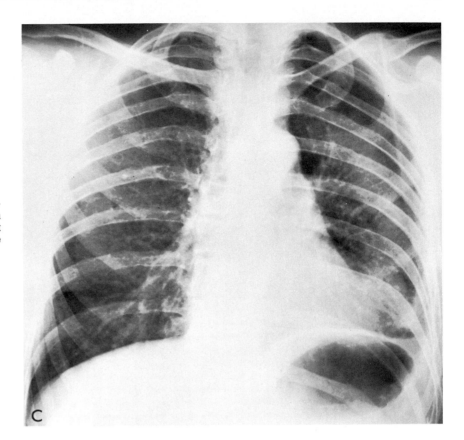

Figure 4–163 *Continued*. Following removal of approximately 1000 ml of fluid, a posteroanterior roentgenogram in the erect position (*C*) shows normal apposition of the gastric air bubble to the left hemidiaphragm.

"pseudodiaphragmatic contour") (Fig. 4–157). Infrapulmonary pleural effusion occurs in such multifarious conditions (inflammatory, cardiovascular, traumatic, neoplastic, and renal[327, 334, 343–345]) that it is difficult to cite a specific pathogenetic mechanism. Similarly, the nature and specific gravity of the fluid seem to possess no real significance, since the effusion may be either an exudate or a transudate. "Encapsulation" secondary to fibrous pleural adhesions plays no part in the pathogenesis, since appropriate positioning of the patient invariably shows the fluid spread over the free pleural space. The explanation proposed by Fleischner[334] was that infrapulmonary effusion develops in precisely the same manner as atypical accumulation of fluid elsewhere in the pleural space—as a result of local changes in contiguous lung that modify its recoil tendency. However, this hypothesis does not coincide with the experimental studies of Rigby and his colleagues,[341] who found that when lungs were normally aerated fluid remained in a subpulmonic location, even when 2000 ml was present; only when the lower lobe was collapsed did fluid assume an atypical position.

Some roentgenologic characteristics are common to most cases of infrapulmonary effusion,[327, 334, 343–347] and any combination of these warrants confirmatory roentgenographic study in lateral decubitus position. All these signs refer to changes observed on posteroanterior and lateral roentgenograms of the erect patient.

1. Infrapulmonary accumulation may be unilateral or bilateral; when unilateral, it occurs more commonly on the right.[343]

2. In posteroanterior projection (Fig. 4–163) the peak of the pseudodiaphragmatic configuration is lateral to that of the normal hemidiaphragm, being situated near the junction of the middle and lateral thirds rather than near the center, and slopes down sharply toward the lateral costophrenic recess.

3. On the left side, the pseudodiaphragmatic contour is separated farther than normal from the gastric air bubble (Fig. 4–163); the diaphragm and the bubble normally are in contact or at least are within 1 cm of each other, although it is important to view the relationship in both PA and lateral projection. Care is also needed to detect interposition of the spleen or the left lobe of the liver and to exclude the presence of gross ascites, which can occasionally simulate subpulmonic effusion.[348] Incidentally, the distinction between pleural and intra-abdominal fluid collections can sometimes be difficult on CT, but Teplick and his colleagues[349] have described a sign that accomplishes this readily and accurately: called the interface sign, it consists of CT evidence of a hazy interface between the fluid and liver or spleen in the presence of pleural effusion and a sharp interface that is characteristic of ascites.

4. Both the lateral and the posterior costophrenic sulci may be sharp and clear (Fig. 4–164), although in many cases the posterior gutter appears

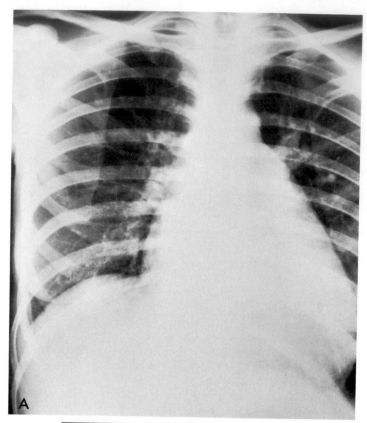

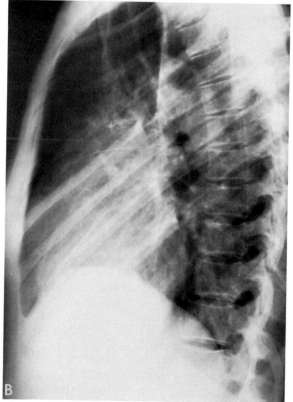

Figure 4–164. Infrapulmonary Pleural Effusion. Posteroanterior (*A*) and lateral (*B*) roentgenograms show what appears to be a high right hemidiaphragm; both the lateral and posterior costophrenic sulci are sharp, although minimal thickening of the pleural line immediately above the lateral sulcus suggests that the shadow may be caused by an infrapulmonary effusion. This suspicion is heightened by the characteristic configuration of the shadow in lateral projection: its anterior portion ascends abruptly and in almost a straight line to the region of the chief fissure; a "dome" configuration is present posterior to this point. The major fissure is slightly thickened by fluid.

blunted because fluid has spilled over into it. We disagree with Peterson's statement[344] that the posterior gutter is obliterated *without exception:* we have seen several patients with substantial subpulmonic effusions in whom lateral chest roentgenograms of excellent technical quality have shown a normally sharp posterior costophrenic recess. The anterior costophrenic gutter is invariably clear.

5. In lateral projection (Fig. 4–164) a characteristic configuration is frequently seen anteriorly where the convex upper margin of the fluid meets the major fissure. In many cases the contour anterior to the fissure is flattened, this segment descending abruptly to the costophrenic angle. A small amount of fluid is usually apparent in the lower end of the chief fissure where it joins the infrapulmonary collection.

6. In posteroanterior projection, a thin, triangular opacity may be observed in the left paramediastinal zone, with its apex approximately halfway up the mediastinum and its base contiguous to the pseudodiaphragmatic contour inferiorly (Fig. 4–165). This shadow, which represents mediastinal extension of the infrapulmonary fluid collection, was observed in 8 of 39 patients in one study;[343] since it is situated posteriorly, it obliterates or causes an apparent widening of the left para-spinal line.[343a] It must not be mistaken for left lower lobe atelectasis which it closely resembles (identification of the left interlobar artery permits ready distinction).

7. Fluoroscopic examination usually reveals no impairment of diaphragmatic excursion during respiration. The pseudodiaphragmatic contour may pulsate synchronously with cardiac pulsation, fluid waves being propagated from the heart toward the lateral chest wall. Fleischner[334] demonstrated this electrokymographically.

Finally, both fluoroscopy and roentgenography in frontal projection with the patient tilted to one side may show the infrapulmonary fluid spilling over into the lateral costophrenic sulcus. This maneuver, originally described by Hessén,[327] is confirmatory when other roentgenographic findings are inconclusive. In any event, lateral decubitus roentgenography with a horizontal beam should be performed in all cases, both to confirm the diagnosis and to permit assessment of the quantity of fluid more accurately than is possible with the patient erect. Sonography can also be useful in identifying subpulmonic collections of fluid, but, as pointed out by Connell and his associates,[393] the examination should be carried out in the erect rather than the supine position; in fact, they report a patient in whom a subpulmonic effusion, clearly identified in the erect position, could not be seen at all with the patient supine. Signs by which subpulmonic pleural effusion can be distinguished from subphrenic fluid accumulation on CT have recently been described by Federle and his colleagues.[394]

Loculation of Pleural Fluid

Loculated or encysted pleural effusions may occur anywhere in the pleural space, either between parietal and visceral pleura over the periphery of the lung or between visceral layers in the interlobar septa. Encapsulation is caused by adhesions between contiguous pleural surfaces and, therefore, tends to occur during or following episodes of pleuritis—often pyothorax or hemothorax. Over the convexity of the thorax the loculated effusion appears as a smooth, sharply demarcated, homogeneous opacity protruding into the hemithorax and compressing contiguous lung (Fig. 4–166). Fluoroscopic examination with subsequent roentgenography in tangential projection helps establish their precise location for subsequent diagnostic or therapeutic thoracentesis, but ultrasonography or CT is a superior technique for this purpose. Ultrasonography not only assesses the amount of fluid loculated in a pleural pocket and indicates the precise anatomic point for thoracentesis but also simplifies the procedure: special aspiration transducers are applied, through which the needle is inserted directly into the specified site. CT scanning is distinctly advantageous in distinguishing pleural from pulmonary lesions, especially when complex combined disease is present;[352] when combined with contrast enhancement, it may also be of value in differentiating empyema from a peripheral pulmonary abscess.[353–355] Mediastinal encysted effusions are uncommon in our experience; they may be situated anteriorly or posteriorly in various locations.[356]

Interlobar loculated effusions are typically elliptical when viewed tangentially, and their extremities blend imperceptibly with the interlobar fissure. In some conditions, particularly cardiac decompensation, the effusion may simulate a mass roentgenographically and be misdiagnosed as a pulmonary neoplasm (Fig. 4–167);[350, 351] however, its distinctive configuration in either posteroanterior or lateral projection should establish the diagnosis. These fluid accumulations tend to absorb spontaneously when the heart failure is relieved and, therefore, have acquired the epithet "vanishing tumor" (*synonyms:* "phantom tumor," "pseudo-tumor").[357] In one series[357] the effusion was localized to the right horizontal fissure in 78 per cent of the 41 cases.

It is sometimes difficult to differentiate encapsulated fluid in the lower half of the major fissure from atelectasis or combined atelectasis and consolidation of the right middle lobe. Three points should be borne in mind in this differentiation: (1) If the minor fissure is visible as a separate shadow, the diagnosis of encapsulated fluid is certain. (2) Encapsulated fluid tends not to obscure the right heart border, whereas middle lobe atelectasis almost invariably does (silhouette sign). (3) In lateral projection, loculated effusion usually is shown to have a bulging surface on one or both sides, but when

Text continued on page 682

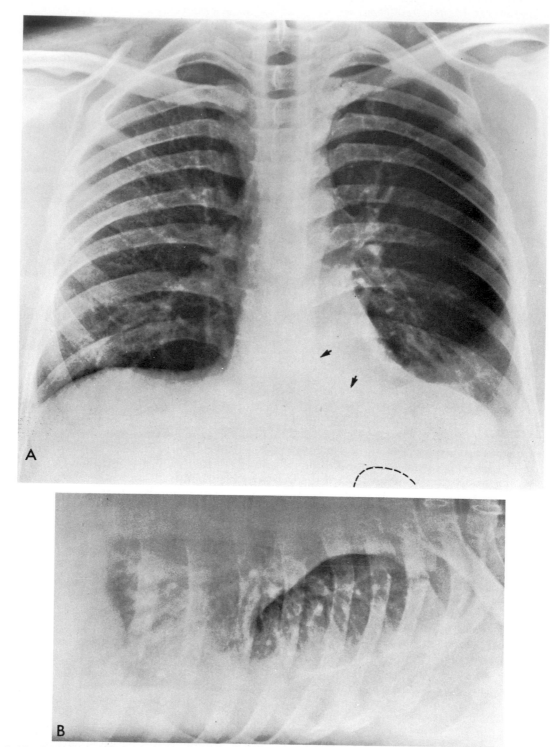

Figure 4–165. Bilateral Infrapulmonary Pleural Effusion. In posteroanterior projection (*A*), the "hemidiaphragms" are at the same level. This roentgenogram conceivably could be interpreted as normal except for three changes which suggest that there is bilateral infrapulmonary effusion: (1) the cardiac shadow is too short, suggesting that its lower portion may be enveloped by fluid; (2) the stomach bubble (*dotted line*) is situated several centimeters from the left "hemidiaphragm"; (3) a triangular shadow of homogeneous density can be identified in the posterior costovertebral angle (*arrows*), suggesting upward extension of fluid along the posterior mediastinal septum. Confirmation of bilateral infrapulmonary effusion was obtained by roentgenography in the lateral decubitus position with a horizontal x-ray beam (the left side is illustrated in *B*).

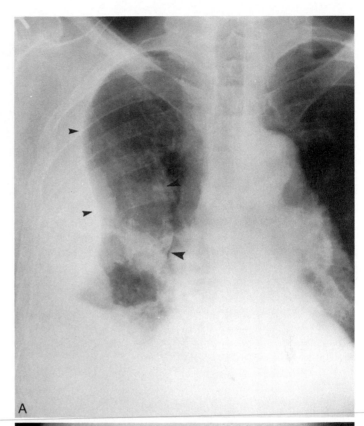

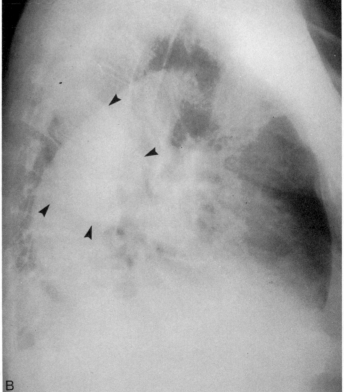

Figure 4–166. Loculated Pleural Effusion. Detail views of the right hemithorax from posteroanterior (*A*) and lateral (*B*) roentgenograms demonstrate a serpentine opacity that relates to the lateral *(small arrowheads)* and posterior interlobar *(large arrowheads)* pleura.

Illustration continued on following page

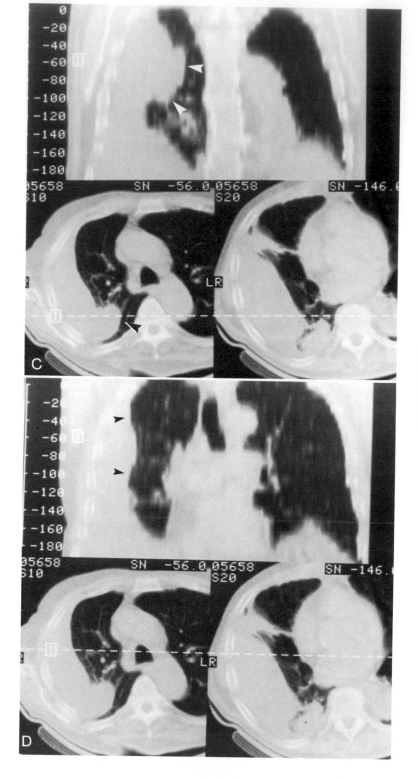

Figure 4–166 *Continued*. Coronal CT reformations (*top*) through the opacity posteriorly (*C*) and anteriorly (*D*) with appropriate axial CT images (*bottom*) reveal the contributions to the features shown in *A* and *B* by the posterior interlobar (*large arrowheads*) and lateral (*small arrowheads*) components of the encapsulated empyema.

Illustration continued on opposite page

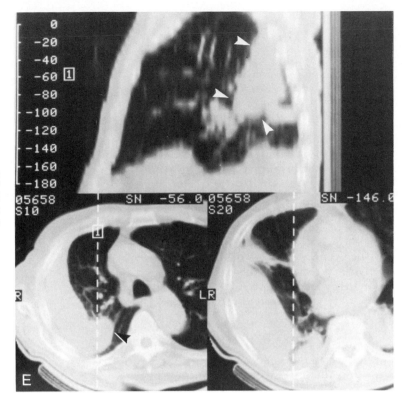

Figure 4–166 *Continued. E, A sagittal reformation (top)* with axial CT images *(bottom)* through the posterior interlobar component *(arrowheads)* shows the typical configuration of an interlobar effusion. The patient is an 81-year-old man with chest pain and cough following an episode of right lower lobe pneumonia.

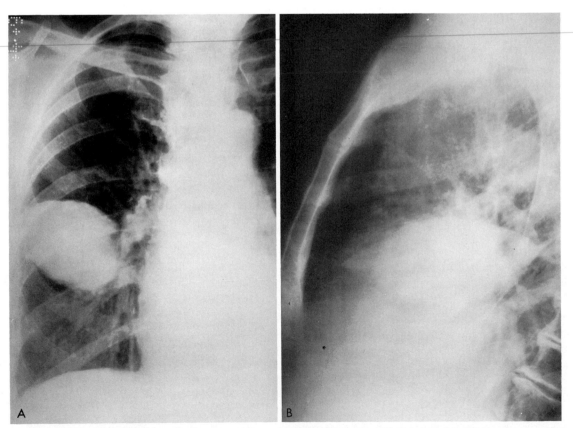

Figure 4–167. Pleural Effusion Localized to the Horizontal Fissure. A view of the right hemithorax from a posteroanterior roentgenogram (*A*) reveals a sharply circumscribed opacity of homogeneous density in the right midlung zone. In lateral projection (*B*), the true nature of the opacity can be appreciated: the mass is elliptical in shape, its pointed extremities being situated anteriorly and posteriorly in keeping with the position of the minor fissure. This unusual collection of pleural fluid developed during a recent episode of cardiac decompensation. With appropriate therapy, it disappeared completely in 3 weeks; thus the designation "vanishing tumor."

the right middle lobe is diseased the borders of the shadow tend to be straight or slightly concave.

ROENTGENOLOGIC SIGNS OF PLEURAL THICKENING

Pleural Fibrosis

Thickening of the pleural line over the convexity of the thorax and occasionally in the interlobar fissures is fairly common and is familiar to all roentgenologists. The thickness of the pleural line may increase to 1 to 10 mm, usually after an episode of pleuritis and almost exclusively as a result of fibrosis of the visceral pleural surface. The major exception is the pleural plaque formation characteristic of asbestos-related disease that occurs exclusively on the parietal pleura; this subject is considered in detail in the chapter on inhalational lung disease. Severe thickening may markedly restrict pulmonary expansion, in which case surgical removal of the "peel" may be curative. Although sometimes local, pleural fibrosis is more often uniform over the whole lung surface, presenting as a thin line of unit density separating air-containing lung from contiguous ribs. The costophrenic recesses often are partly or completely obliterated, particularly laterally, and roentgenography in the lateral decubitus position may be necessary to differentiate such old fibrous thickening from a small pleural effusion; in cases of pleural thickening, however, the blunted costophrenic angle usually is sharply angulated rather than meniscus-shaped, and often the two can be distinguished on this evidence alone.

A curved shadow of unit density frequently is identified in the apex of one or both lungs, in the concavity formed by the first and second ribs (Fig. 4–168). Euphemistically called the "apical cap," it is sometimes ascribed to tuberculosis,[358] despite evidence to the contrary in at least one study.[359] Renner and his colleagues[360] studied the visceral pleura and subpleural parenchyma of 113 left lungs obtained

at necropsy; premortem roentgenograms of 104 were available for correlation. In no case was there histologic evidence of tuberculosis. The commonest pathologic finding (in 20.3 per cent of cases) was nonspecific fibrous scarring of apical lung parenchyma, which merged with the visceral pleura. Calcification (and occasionally ossification) was present in some cases and anthracotic pigment deposition in all. Roentgenologic-pathologic correlation showed a surprising incidence of false-negative and false-positive roentgenologic interpretations, which were considerably more frequent with minor degrees of subpleural scarring. The frequency of scarring observed pathologically increased significantly with age. An extensive review of the subject by McLoud and her associates[361] listed the following causes of unilateral or bilateral apical caps.

1. Tuberculosis and extrapleural abscesses extending from the neck.
2. Postirradiation fibrosis after mantle therapy for Hodgkin's disease, or supraclavicular radiation in the treatment of breast carcinoma.
3. Lymphoma extending from the neck into the mediastinum; superior sulcus bronchogenic carcinoma; and metastases.
4. Traumatic abnormalities, including extrapleural dissection of blood from a ruptured aorta, fractures of the ribs or spine, or hemorrhage secondary to subclavian line placement.
5. Vascular causes, including coarctation of the aorta with dilated collateral vessels over the apex and fistula formation between the subclavian artery and vein.
6. Miscellaneous causes, including mediastinal lipomatosis with subcostal fat extending over the apices.

The subject of pleural calcification has been discussed in a previous section (*see* page 598).

Pleural Neoplasms

These are discussed in detail in the chapter on the pleura, and the present section is concerned only with two roentgenologic signs sometimes of value in distinguishing between diseases that arise in the lung and in the pleura. *Local mesothelial*

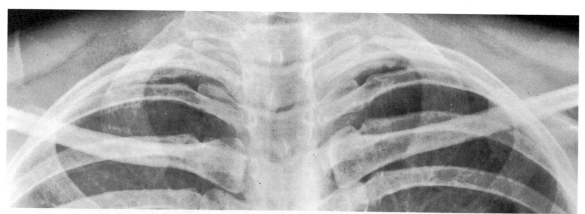

Figure 4–168. Apical Pleural Thickening. A view of the apical zones from a posteroanterior roentgenogram reveals irregular symmetric thickening of the apical pleura. The irregularity serves to differentiate this thickening from companion shadows of the ribs.

neoplasms may arise from either the parietal or visceral pleural surface, over the convexity of the lung, or from an interlobar fissure. Neoplasms that arise from a fissure may simulate an intrapulmonary nodule or an encapsulated interlobar effusion; in either case, CT should help establish the true nature of the lesion. When they arise from the convexity of the lung these solitary tumors may be either sessile or pedunculated,[362, 363] but in either event they almost invariably form an obtuse angle with the chest wall when viewed in profile; this obtuse angle usually distinguishes these lesions from those that arise within the lung parenchyma, which tend to form an acute angle with the chest wall. *Diffuse mesothelial neoplasms*, which usually are highly malignant, are commonly accompanied by pleural effusion. Even when the effusion is massive, however, there tends to be little displacement of the mediastinum away from the affected hemithorax.[364] The reasons for this are twofold: in some cases it may result from "compression" of lung by extensive neoplastic involvement of the pleural surface; in others, it occurs when neoplastic invasion of the mediastinal surface of the lung has caused bronchial occlusion, resulting in atelectasis. Regardless of the mechanism, the lack of displacement is important to the roentgenologic diagnosis of this highly malignant lesion—although it should be borne in mind that a similar picture may be produced by primary bronchogenic carcinoma with obstructive atelectasis and metastatic pleural effusion.

ROENTGENOLOGIC SIGNS OF PNEUMOTHORAX

The discussion earlier in this section on the influence on underlying lung of a buffer medium within the pleural space applies as well to pneumothorax as to hydrothorax. The only difference is in the manner in which gravity affects the media: air rises to the apex of the hemithorax and causes relaxation atelectasis of the upper portion of the lung; fluid falls to the bottom of the hemithorax and permits relaxation of the lower lobe. When pneumothorax is present, the weight of the lung in its gaseous surroundings causes it to drop to its most dependent position, slung by its fixed attachment at the pulmonary ligament. For this reason, a pneumothorax must be large to produce complete collapse of the lung, including its lower lobe.

A roentgenologic diagnosis of pneumothorax can be made only on identification of the visceral pleural line. Since the lung is partly collapsed by the pneumothorax, it might be anticipated that its density would be increased and that this altered density, compared with that of the normal lung, should be sufficient to suggest the diagnosis; in fact, this is not so. Dornhorst and Pierce[205] were the first to point out that, as the lung progressively collapses with increasing size of the pneumothorax, blood flow through it diminishes; therefore the ratio of air and blood is not materially altered and the overall density of the collapsing lung is not changed (Fig. 4–169). Undoubtedly the gas in the pleural space anterior and posterior to the collapsed lung makes an important contribution to overall lucency, but, regardless of the mechanism involved, the empiric observation made by Dornhorst and Pierce is valid: roentgenographic density of a collapsing lung changes little until volume is greatly reduced.

The visceral pleural line is usually fairly readily identifiable, even on roentgenograms exposed at total lung capacity. When pneumothorax is strongly suspected clinically but a pleural line is not identified (possibly obscured by an overlying rib), gas in the pleural space can be detected by either of two procedures: (1) Roentgenography in the erect position in full expiration (the rationale being that lung volume is reduced although the volume of gas in the pleural space is constant, thereby providing a smaller surface of visceral pleura in contact with air). (2) Roentgenography in the lateral decubitus position with a horizontal x-ray beam; the rationale here is obvious—air rises to the highest point in the hemithorax and is more clearly visible over the lateral chest wall than over the apex, where confluence of overlying bony shadows may obscure fine linear shadows. The value of this technique in the recognition and evaluation of pneumothorax in young infants has been emphasized by MacEwan and his colleagues.[365]

In the majority of clinical settings, patients with suspected pneumothorax will be radiographed in the erect position, in which case air rises to the apex of the hemithorax and causes collapse of the upper portion of the lung. When patients must be examined in the supine position, as is so often the case with today's proliferation of intensive care units, gas within the pleural space rises to the highest point in the hemithorax, which is in the vicinity of the diaphragm. Depending on the size of the pneumothorax, the result can be an exceptionally deep radiolucent costophrenic sulcus,[366] a lucency over the right or left upper quadrant,[367] or a much sharper than normal appearance of the hemidiaphragm, with or without the presence of a visceral pleural line visible above the hemidiaphragm.[368] The whole subject of the radiographic anatomy of pneumothorax in the supine patient has recently been beautifully reviewed by Tocino[369] and by Tocino and her colleagues.[370] A subpulmonic location of gas also has been reported as an occasional manifestation of spontaneous pneumothorax in erect patients with chronic obstructive pulmonary disease,[371] and following penetrating injury to the thorax.[372]

Inspiration-expiration roentgenography may be employed to advantage in the assessment of the size of the pleural defect in spontaneous pneumothorax. If the defect is closed or very small, the expiratory roentgenogram will show a marked

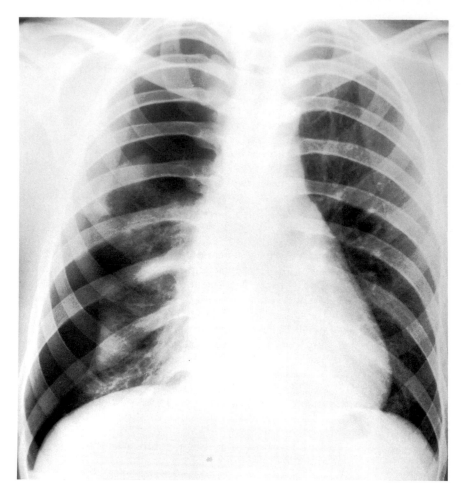

Figure 4–169. Effect of Pneumothorax on Lung Density. A posteroanterior roentgenogram reveals a moderate right pneumothorax; despite the fact that the right lung has been reduced in volume by approximately 50 per cent, its density (except in local areas) differs little from that of the left lung. *See* text.

change in volume of the ipsilateral lung because air has been expired via the tracheobronchial tree (Fig. 4–170); if the defect is open, volume change in the ipsilateral lung will be minimal (Fig. 4–171), since communication persists between the pleural space and the lung parenchyma. Such information should help referring physicians or surgeons decide whether insertion of a chest tube is necessary.

Small pleural blebs, the commonest cause of spontaneous pneumothorax, may be more easily identified by tomography—especially when the lung is partially collapsed, in which case the blebs tend to collapse less than the normal surrounding parenchyma. Fibrous adhesions between the visceral and parietal pleural layers in the region of blebs are an important prognostic sign, since they tend to "hold the communication open" and thereby prevent spontaneous re-expansion.

Although for most practical clinical purposes it usually suffices to designate the size of a pneumothorax as small, medium, or large, two methods have been described recently by which the size of a pneumothorax can be more precisely quantified.[373, 374]

Hydropneumothorax should be immediately apparent on roentgenograms exposed in the erect position, by dint of the almost invariable air-fluid level. Encapsulated hydropneumothorax may occur as single or multiple loculated collections, some of which may contain air-fluid levels. Roentgenography of a patient in various body positions sometimes shows the passage of fluid from one apparently loculated space into another, evidencing their communication.

"Tension" Pneumothorax and Hydrothorax

On the evidence supplied by roentgenograms of the chest at total lung capacity, the detection of increased pressure in a pneumothorax may be exceedingly difficult, especially if the pneumothorax is complete and collapse of the ipsilateral lung total. Shift of the mediastinum away from the side of a pneumothorax of any size is inevitable, pressure in the contralateral (normal) hemithorax being relatively more negative; such a shift must not be mistaken for evidence of "tension" pneumothorax. In fact, the term tension is semantically inaccurate. For the volume of a pneumothorax to increase, air must flow from the lung parenchyma (where pressure is atmospheric) through the pleural defect and into the pleural space; obviously such flow cannot occur if pleural pressure is greater than atmospheric, or under tension. Thus, for a pneumothorax to increase in volume, pressure within the pleural space must be relatively negative *during inspiration:*

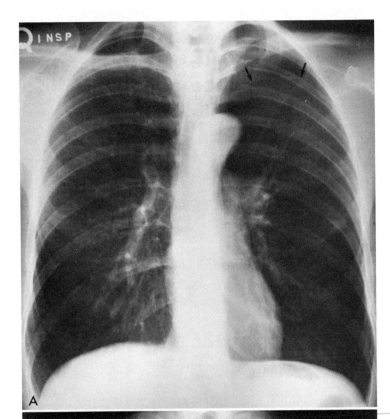

Figure 4–170. Inspiratory-Expiratory Roentgenograms in Spontaneous Pneumothorax Showing Large Reduction in Lung Volume on Expiration. A posteroanterior roentgenogram exposed at full inspiration (*A*) shows a 10 per cent left pneumothorax (the visceral pleural surface is indicated by *arrows*). On expiration (*B*), the volume of the left lung has diminished markedly, suggesting that its air has been expelled via the tracheobronchial tree and that the pleural defect therefore must be either closed or exceedingly small. The possibility that air was escaping from the lung *into* the pleural space (thus enlarging the pneumothorax) was excluded by exposing a third film at TLC which had an appearance identical to that in *A*.

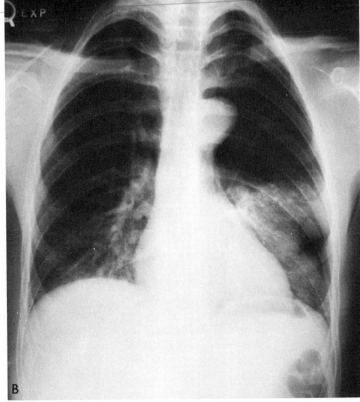

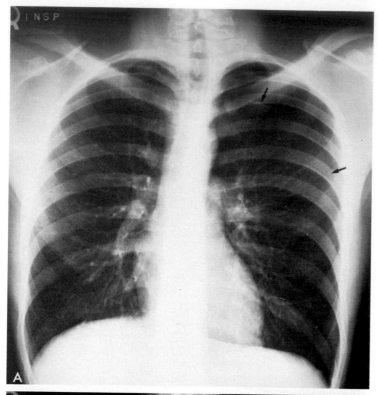

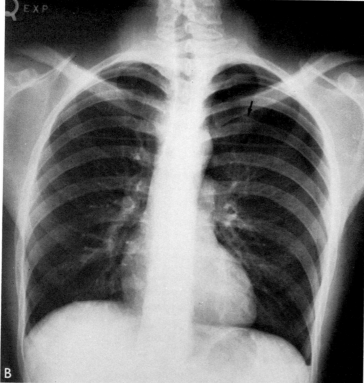

Figure 4–171. Inspiratory-Expiratory Roentgenograms in Spontaneous Pneumothorax Showing Little Change in Lung Volume on Expiration. A posteroanterior roentgenogram exposed at full inspiration (*A*) shows a 10 to 15 per cent left pneumothorax (the visceral pleura is indicated by *arrows*). On expiration (*B*), the volume of the pneumothorax and of the left lung have reduced roughly proportionately, suggesting that equilibrium is present between the two compartments and that the pleural defect thus is open. Contrast with Figure 4–170.

if a check-valve mechanism exists, allowing air to enter the pleural space during inspiration but preventing its egress during expiration, pressure within the pleural space will be positive only during the latter phase of respiration. Thus the correct term is *expiratory* tension pneumothorax. If the pleural defect is closed or very small, as air is absorbed from the pleural space the ipsilateral pleural pressure becomes negative and the mediastinum moves back to the midline (although mediastinal swing may still be apparent fluoroscopically—toward the side of the pneumothorax during inspiration and away during expiration). If the pleural defect is open and operates as a check-valve mechanism— expiratory tension pneumothorax—the roentgenologic findings may be identical apart from more severe contralateral mediastinal shift and ipsilateral hemidiaphragmatic depression. On fluoroscopic examination, however, the situation should be clear: the increased tension prevents mediastinal shift toward the side of the pneumothorax on inspiration and may severely restrict inflation of the normal lung, constituting what may be the major cause of respiratory difficulty. For the same reason, movement of the ipsilateral hemidiaphragm is markedly restricted during respiration. This combination of changes, *when viewed fluoroscopically*, should prompt the diagnosis of expiratory tension pneumothorax. Assessment of the presence or absence of tension

on plain roentgenograms is highly unreliable and, in fact, tension pneumothorax should be regarded as a clinical state characterized by cardiorespiratory embarrassment.

Tension hydrothorax, although rare, constitutes as much of a danger as expiratory tension pneumothorax—perhaps more so, since the possibility of its occurrence is not generally recognized. Rabinov and his colleagues[380] reported a case of a 23-year-old woman with metastatic undifferentiated carcinoma in whom massive pleural effusion increased greatly and rapidly and caused severe dyspnea and eventual collapse. At thoracotomy, serosanguineous fluid spurted to a height of about 25 cm; several liters were removed. The explanation suggested by the investigators for this unusual circumstance seems reasonable: serum albumin was severely diminished, amounting to 1.4 grams per dl, and the protein content of the pleural fluid was 4.8 grams per dl; thus, the colloid osmotic pressure difference between blood and pleural space was reversed, creating an alteration of pleural space dynamics that favored massive accumulation of fluid. Although such a set of circumstances must be rare, it is well to bear the possibility in mind in any patient with a massive pleural effusion, disproportionately increasing symptoms, and progressive deterioration in condition.

REFERENCES

1. Aschoff L: *In* Lectures on Pathology. New York, Hoeber, 1924, pp 42–43, 53–57.
2. Raskin SP, Herman PG: A new experimental model to study flow patterns in the distal airways (abstract). Invest Radiol 8:263, 1973.
3. Anderson JB, Jaspersen W: Demonstration of intersegmental respiratory bronchioles in normal human lungs. Eur J Respir Dis 61:337, 1980.
4. Gamsu G, Thurlbeck WM, Macklem PT, et al: Roentgenographic appearance of the human pulmonary acinus. Invest Radiol 6:171, 1971.
5. Lui YM, Taylor JR, Zylak CJ: Roentgen-anatomical correlation in the individual human pulmonary acinus. Radiology 109:1, 1973.
6. Schlesinger MJ: New radiopaque mass for vascular injection. Lab Invest 6:1, 1957.
7. Hogg JC, Macklem PT, Thurlbeck WM: The resistance of collateral channels in excised human lungs. J Clin Invest 48:421, 1969.
8. Loeshcke H: Die Morphologie des normalen und emphysemetosen Acinus der Lung. Beitr Z Pathol Anat 68:213, 1921.
9. Dornhorst AC, Pierce JW: Pulmonary collapse and consolidation: The role of collapse in the production of lung field shadows and the significance of segments in inflammatory lung disease. J Fac Radiol 5:276, 1954.
10. Fraser RG, Pare JAP: Diagnosis of Diseases of the Chest. Ed 2, Vol I. Philadelphia, WB Saunders, 1977, p 344.
11. Recaverren S, Benton C, Gall EA: Pathology of acute alveolar diseases of the lung. Semin Roentgenol 2:22, 1967.
12. Ziskind MM, Weill H, Payzant AR: The recognition and significance of acinus-filling processes of the lung. Am Rev Respir Dis 87:551, 1963.
13. Friedman PG: The concept of alveolar and interstitial disease. *In* Potchen EJ (ed): Current Concepts in Radiology. St. Louis, CV Mosby, 1972, pp 64–106.
14. McLoud TC: Diffuse infiltrative lung disease. *In* Putman CE (ed): Pulmonary Diagnosis, Imaging, and Other Techniques. New York, Appleton-Century-Crofts, 1981, pp 125–153.
15. Genereux GP: Radiographic patterns in diffuse lung disease with experimental/pathologic correlation. Paper delivered at Fleischner Society Postgraduate Course. Williamstown, VA, 1971.
16. Genereux GP: CT of acute and chronic distal airspace (alveolar) disease. Semin Roentgenol 19:211, 1984.
17. Katzenstein AL, Askin BF: Surgical pathology of non-neoplastic lung disease. *In* Bennington JL (ed): Major Problems in Pathology. Philadelphia, WB Saunders, 1982, pp 9–42.
18. Reed JC, Madewell JE: The air bronchogram in interstitial disease of the lungs. A radiological-pathological correlation. Radiology 116:1, 1975.
19. Fleischner FG: The visible bronchial tree: A roentgen sign in pneumonic and other pulmonary consolidations. Radiology 50:184, 1948.
20. Fleischner FG: Der sichtbare Bronchialbaum, ein differentialdiagnostisches Symptom im Röntgenbild der Pneumonie. Fortschr Roentgenstr 36:319, 1927.
21. Felson B: Chest Roentgenology. Philadelphia, WB Saunders, 1973.
22. Reed JC, Madewell JE: The air bronchogram in interstitial disease of the lungs. A radiological-pathological correlation. Radiology 116:1, 1975.
23. Lui YM, Taylor JR, Zylak CJ: Roentgen-anatomical correlation of the individual human pulmonary acinus. Radiology 109:1, 1973.
24. Gamsu G, Thurlbeck WM, Macklem PT, et al: Peripheral bronchographic morphology in the normal lung. Invest Radiol 6:171, 1971.
25. Heitzman ER: The Lung: Radiologic-pathologic correlations. St. Louis, CV Mosby, 1984, pp 70–105.
26. Diament ML, Palmer KNV: Venous arterial pulmonary shunting as the principal cause of postoperative hypoxemia. Lancet 1:15, 1967.
27. Coulter WW Jr: Experimental massive pulmonary collapse. Dis Chest 18:146, 1950.
28. Lansing AM: Radiological changes in pulmonary atelectasis. Arch Surg 90:52, 1965.
29. Rahn H: The role of N_2 gas in various biological processes, with particular reference to the lung. Harvey Lect 55:173, 1960.
30. Stein LA, McLoud TC, Vidal JJ, et al: Acute lobar collapse in canine lungs. Invest Radiol 11:518, 1976.
31. Fletcher BD, Avery ME: The effects of airway occlusion after oxygen breathing on the lungs of newborn infants: Radiologic demonstration in the experimental animal. Radiology 109:655, 1973.
32. Henry WJ, Miscall L: Rapidly reversible atelectasis due to change in position. J Thorac Cardiovasc Surg 41:686, 1961.
33. Martin HB: Respiratory bronchioles as the pathway for collateral ventilation. J Appl Physiol 21:1443, 1966.
34. Boyden EA: Structure of the pulmonary acinus in a child of six years and eight months. Am J Anat 132:275, 1971.
35. Brown B StJ, Ma H, Dunbar JS, et al: Foreign bodies in the tracheobronchial tree in childhood. J Can Assoc Radiol 14:158, 1963.
36. Culiner MM, Reich SB: Collateral ventilation and localized emphysema. Am J Roentgenol 85:246, 1961.
37. Reich SB, Abouav J: Interalveolar air drift. Radiology 85:80, 1965.
38. McLean KH: The histology of generalized pulmonary emphysema. I. The genesis of the early centrolobular lesion: Focal emphysema. Australas Ann Med 6:124, 1957.
39. McLean KH: The pathogenesis of pulmonary emphysema. Am J Med 25:62, 1958.
40. Kent EM, Blades B: The surgical anatomy of the pulmonary lobes. J Thorac Surg 12:18, 1942.
41. Fleischner FG: Linear shadows in the lung field. *In* Rabin CB (ed): Roentgenology of the Chest. Springfield, IL, Charles C Thomas, 1958.
42. Raasch BN, Carsky EW, Lane EJ, et al: Radiographic anatomy of the interlobar fissures: A study of 100 specimens. Am J Roentgenol 138:1043, 1982.
43. Nelson SW: Large pneumothorax and associated massive collapse of the homolateral lung due to intrabronchial obstruction: A case report. Radiology 68:411, 1957.
44. Clements JA: Surface phenomena in relation to pulmonary function. Physiologist 5:11, 1962.
45. Sutnick AI, Soloff LA: Atelectasis with pneumonia. A pathophysiologic study. Ann Intern Med 60:39, 1964.
46. Sutnick AI, Soloff LA: Surface tension reducing activity in the normal and atelectic human lung. Am J Med 35:31, 1963.
47. Lieberman JA: A unified concept and critical review of pulmonary hyaline membrane formation. Am J Med 35:443, 1963.
48. Schneider HJ, Felson B, Gonzalez LL: Rounded atelectasis. Am J Roentgenol 134:225, 1980.
49. Cho S-R, Henry DA, Beachley MC, et al: Round (helical) atelectasis. Br J Radiol 54:643, 1981.
50. Doyle TC, Lawler GA: CT features of rounded atelectasis of the lung. Am J Roentgenol 143:225, 1984.
51. Hilgenberg AD, Mark EJ: Case records of the Massachusetts General Hospital. N Engl J Med 308:1466, 1983.
52. Geremia G, Mintzer RA: An unusual case of rounded atelectasis. Chest 86:485, 1984.
53. Greyson-Fleg RT: Lung biopsy in rounded atelectasis (letter). Am J Roentgenol 144:1316, 1985.
54. Beckmann CF, Levin DC, Ulreich S: Cardiomegaly as a cause of nonuniform pulmonary artery perfusion. Am J Roentgenol 129:661, 1977.
55. Benjamin JJ, Cascade PN, Rubenfire M, et al: Left lower lobe atelectasis and consolidation following cardiac surgery: The effect of topical cooling on the phrenic nerve. Radiology 142:11, 1982.
56. Kattan KR: Upper mediastinal changes in lower lobe collapse. Semin Roentgenol 15:183, 1980.
57. Cranz HJ, Pribam HFW: The pulmonary vessels in the diagnosis of lobar collapse. Am J Roentgenol 94:665, 1965.
58. Simon G: Principles of Chest X-ray Diagnosis. 3rd ed. London, Butterworth, 1971.
59. Lodin H: Mediastinal herniation and displacement studied by transversal tomography. Acta Radiol 48:337, 1957.
60. Lubert M, Krause GR: Total unilateral pulmonary collapse: A study of the roentgen appearance in the lateral view. Radiology 67:175, 1956.
61. Whalen JP, Lane EJ Jr: Bronchial rearrangements in pulmonary collapse as seen on the lateral radiograph. Radiology 93:285, 1969.
62. Lane EJ Jr, Whalen JP: A new sign of left atrial enlargement: Posterior displacement of the left bronchial tree. Radiology 93:279, 1969.

63. Robbins LL, Hale CH: Roentgen appearance of lobar and segmental collapse of the lung; Preliminary report. Radiology 44:107, 1945.
64. Robbins LL, Hale CH, Merrill OE: Roentgen appearance of lobar and segmental collapse of the lung; Technic of examination. Radiology 44:471, 1945.
65. Robbins LL, Hale CH: The roentgen appearance of lobar and segmental collapse of the lung. II. The normal chest as it pertains to collapse. Radiology 44:543, 1945.
66. Robbins LL, Hale CH: The roentgen appearance of lobar and segmental collapse of the lung. III. Collapse of an entire lung or the major part thereof. Radiology 45:23, 1945.
67. Robbins LL, Hale CH: The roentgen appearance of lobar and segmental collapse of the lung. IV. Collapse of the lower lobes. Radiology 45:120, 1945.
68. Robbins LL, Hale CH: The roentgen appearance of lobar and segmental collapse of the lung. V. Collapse of the right middle lobe. Radiology 45:260, 1945.
69. Robbins LL, Hale CH: The roentgen appearance of lobar and segmental collapse of the lung. VI. Collapse of the upper lobes. Radiology 45:347, 1945.
70. Lubert M, Krause GR: Patterns of lobar collapse as observed radiographically. Radiology 56:165, 1951.
71. Krause GR, Lubert M: Cross anatomico-spatial changes occurring in lobar collapse; A demonstration by means of three-dimensional plastic models. Am J Roentgenol 79:258, 1958.
72. Lubert M, Krause GR: Further observations on lobar collapse. Radiol Clin North Am 1:331, 1963.
73. Khoury MB, Godwin JD, Halvorsen RA Jr, et al: CT of obstructive lobar collapse. Invest Radiol 20:708, 1985.
74. Kattan KR, Eyler WR, Felson B: The juxtaphrenic peak in upper lobe collapse. Semin Roentgenol 15:187, 1980.
75. Raasch BN, Heitzman ER, Carsky EW, et al: A computed tomographic study of bronchopulmonary collapse. Radiographics 4:195, 1984.
76. Zdansky E: Bemerkung zur atelektatischen retraktion des linken oberlappens. (Atelectatic retraction of the left upper lobe.) Fortschr Roentgenstr 100:725, 1964.
77. Webber M, Davies P: The Luftsichel: An old sign in upper lobe collapse. Clin Radiol 32:271, 1981.
78. Naidich DP, McCauley DI, Khouri NF, et al: Computed tomography of lobar collapse: 1. Endobronchial obstruction. J Comput Assist Tomogr 7:745, 1983.
79. Cohen BA, Rabinowitz JG, Mendleson DS: The pulmonary ligament. Radiol Clin North Am 22:659, 1984.
80. Fisher MS: Significance of a visible major fissure on the frontal chest radiograph. Am J Roentgenol 137:577, 1981.
81. Friedman PJ: Radiology of the superior segment of the lower lobe. A regional perspective, introducing the B6 bronchus sign. Radiology 144:15, 1982.
82. Wholey MH, Good CA, McDonald JR: Disseminated indeterminate pulmonary disease: Value of lung biopsy. Radiology 71:651, 1958.
83. Gould DM, Dalrymple GV: A radiological analysis of disseminated lung disease. Am J Med Sci 238:621, 1959.
84. von Hayek H: The Human Lung. New York, Hafner Publishing Company, 1960.
85. Staub NC, Nagano H, Pearce ML: Pulmonary edema in dogs, especially the sequence of fluid accumulation in lungs. J Appl Physiol 22:227, 1967.
86. Levin B: Subpleural interlobular lymphectasis reflecting metastatic carcinoma. Radiology 72:682, 1959.
87. Trapnell DH: Septal lines in pneumoconiosis. Br J Radiol 37:805, 1964.
88. Stolberg HO, Patt NL, MacEwen KF, et al: Hodgkin's disease of the lung: Roentgenologic-pathologic correlation. Am J Roentgenol 92:96, 1964.
89. Angus GE, Thurlbeck WM: Number of alveoli in the human lung. J Appl Physiol 32:483, 1972.
90. Felson B: A new look at pattern recognition of diffuse pulmonary disease. Am J Roentgenol 133:183, 1979.
91. Genereux GP: Pattern recognition in diffuse lung disease. A review of theory and practice. Med Radiogr Photogr 61:2, 1985.
92. Resink JEJ: Is a roentgenogram of fine structures a summation image or a real picture? Acta Radiol 32:391, 1949.
93. Kuisk H, Sanchez JS: Diffuse bronchiolectasis with muscular hyperplasia ("muscular cirrhosis of the lung"). Relationship to chronic form of Hamman-Rich syndrome. Am J Roentgenol 96:979, 1966.
94. Liebow AA, Carrington CB: The interstitial pneumonias. In Simon M, Potchen EJ, LeMay M (eds): Frontiers of Pulmonary Radiology. New York, Grune & Stratton, 1969, pp 102–141.
95. McLoud TC, Carrington CB, Gaensler EA: Diffuse infiltrative lung disease: A new scheme for description. Radiology 149:353, 1983.
96. Nakata H, Kimoto T, Nakayama T, et al: Diffuse peripheral lung disease: Evaluation by high-resolution computed tomography. Radiology 157:181, 1985.
97. Burgen CJ, Muller NL: CT in the diagnosis of interstitial lung disease. Am J Roentgenol 145:505, 1985.
98. Bron M, Baum S, Abrams HL: Oil embolism in lymphangiography: Incidence, manifestations, and mechanism. Radiology 80:194, 1963.
99. Fraimow W, Wallace S, Lewis P, et al: Changes in pulmonary function due to lymphangiography. Radiology 85:231, 1965.
100. Genereux GP: The end-stage lung. Pathogenesis, pathology, and radiology. Radiology 116:279, 1975.
101. Jerry LM, Ritchie AC: Bronchiolar emphysema. A report of a necropsied case of diffuse bronciolectasis and review of the literature. Can Med Assoc J 90:964, 1964.
102. Kuisk H, Sanchez JS: Diffuse bronchiolectasis with muscular hyperplasia ("muscular cirrhosis of the lung"). Relationship to chronic form of Hamman-Rich syndrome. Am J Roentgenol 96:979, 1966.
103. Anderson AE Jr, Foraker AG: Morphological aspects of interstitial pulmonary fibrosis. Arch Pathol 70:79, 1960.
104. Beams AJ, Harmos O: Diffuse progressive interstitial fibrosis of the lungs. Am J Med 7:425, 1949.
105. Felson B: Disseminated interstitial diseases of the lung. In Simon M, Potchen EJ, LeMay M (eds): Frontiers of Pulmonary Radiology. New York, Grune & Stratton, 1969, pp 154–173.
106. Heppleston AG: The pathology of honeycomb lung. Thorax 11:77, 1956.
107. Koch B: Familial fibrocystic pulmonary dysplasia: Observations in one family. Can Med Assoc J 92:801, 1965.
108. Kuisk H, Sanchez JS: Desquamative interstitial pneumonia and idiopathic diffuse pulmonary fibrosis. With their advanced final stages as "muscular cirrhosis of the lung" (diffuse bronchiolectasis with muscular hyperplasia). Fibrosing alveolitis. Am J Roentgenol 107:258, 1969.
109. Smith KV: Chronic diffuse interstitial pneumonia and diffuse interstitial pulmonary fibrosis. Med J Aust 48:244, 1961.
110. Fraser RG, Paré JAP: Diagnosis of Diseases of the Chest: An Integrated Study Based on the Abnormal Roentgenogram. Philadelphia, WB Saunders, 1970, pp 240–255.
111. Genereux GP: Lipids in the lungs: Radiologic-pathologic correlation. J Can Assoc Radiol 21:2, 1970.
112. Genereux GP: Peripheral Interstitial Pneumonitis, Fibrosis, and Ossification of the Elderly. Presented at the 35th Annual Meeting of the Canadian Association of Radiologists, Toronto, January, 1972.
113. Genereux GP, Merriman JE: Desquamative interstitial pneumonia: Progression to the end-stage lung and the unusual complication of alveolar cell carcinoma (case report). J Can Assoc Radiol 24:144, 1973.
114. MacKay IR, Ritchie B: Diffuse fibrosing alveolitis (diffuse interstitial fibrosis of the lungs): Two cases with autoimmune features. Thorax 20:200, 1965.
115. Mendeloff J: Disseminated nodular pulmonary ossification in the Hamman-Rich lung. Am Rev Respir Dis 103:269, 1971.
116. Meyer EC, Liebow AA: Relationship of interstitial pneumonia honeycombing and atypical epithelial proliferation to cancer of the lung. Cancer 18:322, 1965.
117. Reingold IM, Mizunoue GS: Idiopathic disseminated pulmonary ossification. Chest 40:543, 1961.
118. Scadding JG, Hinson KFW: Duffuse fibrosing alveolitis (diffuse interstitial fibrosis of the lungs). Correlation of histology at biopsy with prognosis. Thorax 22:291, 1967.
119. Teskuk H, Ikeda RM: Pulmonary carcinoma originating in chronic diffuse interstitial fibrosis of the lung. Chest 57:386, 1970.
120. Wells HG, Dunlap CE: Disseminated ossification of the lungs. Arch Pathol 35:420, 1943.
121. Bower GC: So-called bronchiolar emphysema. Its relationship to diffuse pulmonary fibrosis and pulmonary emphysema. Am Rev Respir Dis 95:1049, 1967.
122. Bryk D, Mori K: Bronchiolar emphysema. Am J Roentgenol 94:660, 1965.
123. Jerry LM, Ritchie AC: Bronciolar emphysema. A report of a necropsied case of diffuse bronchiolectasis and review of the literature. Can Med Assoc J 90:964, 1964.
124. Sheft DJ, Moskowitz H: Pulmonary muscular hyperplasia. Am J Roentgenol 93:836, 1965.
125. Thomas MP, Storer J, Goodsit E, et al: Pulmonary muscular hyperplasia. A report of functional data in three cases with a brief review of the literature. Chest 51:1, 1967.
126. Christoforidis AJ, Nelson SW, Pratt PC: Bronchiolar dilatation associated with muscular hyperplasia: Polycystic lung. Am J Roentgenol 92:513, 1964.
127. Webb WR: The pleural tail sign. Radiology 127:309, 1978.
128. Gough J, Wentworth JE: The use of thin sections of entire organs in morbid anatomical studies. J Roy Micr Soc 69:231, 1949.
129. Ellis K, Renthal G: Pulmonary sarcoidosis: Roentgenographic observations on course of disease. Am J Roentgenol 88:1070, 1962.
130. Sosman MC, Dodd GD, Jones WD, et al: The familial occurrence of pulmonary alveolar microlithiasis. Am J Roentgenol 77:947, 1957.

4

131. Genereux GP: Computed tomography and the lung: Review of anatomic and densitometric features with their clinical application. J Can Assoc Radiol 36:88, 1985.

132. Bateson EM: An analysis of 155 solitary lung lesions illustrating the differential diagnosis of mixed tumours of the lung. Clin Radiol 16:51, 1965.

133. Bateson EM: The solitary circumscribed bronchogenic carcinoma: A radiological study of 100 cases. Br J Radiol 37:598, 1964.

134. Rigler LG: The roentgen signs of carcinoma of the lung. Am J Roentgenol 74:415, 1955.

135. Drevvatne T, Frimann-Dahl J: Peripheral bronchial carcinomas: A radiological and pathological study. Br J Radiol 34:180, 1961.

136. Bleyer JM, Marks JH: Tuberculomas and hamartomas of the lung: Comparative study of 66 proved cases. Am J Roentgenol 77:1013, 1957.

137. Steele JD: The Solitary Pulmonary Nodule. Springfield, IL, Charles C Thomas, 1964.

138. Holmes RB: Friedländer's pneumonia. Am J Roentgenol 75:728, 1956.

139. Caruso RD, Berk RN: The fuzzy fluid level sign. Radiology 98:369, 1971.

140. Mettler FA, Ghahremani GG: The fuzzy fluid level sign: Reappraisal of its cause and diagnostic value. Radiology 105:509, 1972.

141. Woodring JH, Fried M, Chuang VP: Solitary cavities of the lung: Diagnostic implications of cavity wall thickness. Am J Roentgenol 135:1269, 1980.

142. Bloomfield JA: Protean radiological manifestations of hydatid infestation. Australas Radiol 10:330, 1966.

143. Fainsinger MH: Pulmonary hydatid disease: The sign of the camalote. S Afr Med J 23:723, 1949.

144. Danner PK, McFarland DR, Felson B: Massive pulmonary gangrene. Am J Roentgenol 103:548, 1968.

145. Klein EW, Griffin JP: Coccidioidomycosis (diagnosis outside the Sonoran Zone): The roentgen features of acute multiple pulmonary cavities. Am J Roentgenol 94:653, 1965.

146. Jackson H, Stark P: Tilted air-fluid interfaces on chest radiographs. Am J Roentgenol 144:37, 1985.

147. Bancks N, Zornoza J: Pseudocavitary granulomas of the lung. Am J Roentgenol 127:251, 1976.

148. Curran JD, MacCarthy JMT: Cavitating pulmonary metastases. Case report. J Fac Radiol 10:166, 1959.

149. Salzman E: Lung Calcifications in X-ray Diagnosis. Springfield, IL, Charles C Thomas, 1968.

150. Serviansky B, Schwarz J: Calcified intrathoracic lesions caused by histoplasmosis and tuberculosis. Am J Roentgenol 77:1034, 1957.

151. Good CA: The solitary pulmonary nodule: A problem of management. Radiol Clin North Am 1:429, 1963.

152. London SB, Winter WJ: Calcification within carcinoma of the lung: Report of a case with isolated pulmonary nodule. Arch Intern Med 94:161, 1954.

153. O'Keefe ME Jr, Good CA, McDonald JR: Calcification in solitary nodules of the lung. Am J Roentgenol 77:1023, 1957.

154. Slasky BS, Lerberg DB, Herbert DL: The wandering broncholith. J Can Assoc Radiol 32:173, 1981.

155. Gordonson J, Sargent EN: Nephrobroncholithiasis: Report of a case secondary to renal lithiasis with a nephrobronchial fistula. Am J Roentgenol 110:701, 1970.

156. Whitaker W, Black A, Warrack AJN: Pulmonary ossification in patients with mitral stenosis. J Fac Radiol 7:29, 1955.

157. Galloway RW, Epstein EJ, Coulshed N: Pulmonary ossific nodules in mitral valve disease. Br Heart J 23:297, 1961.

158. Buja LM, Roberts WC: Pulmonary parenchymal ossific nodules in idiopathic hypertrophic subaortic stenosis. Am J Cardiol 25:710, 1970.

159. Katz S, Stanton J, McCormick G: Miliary calcification of the lungs after treated miliary tuberculosis. N Engl J Med 253:135, 1955.

160. Abrahams EW, Evans C, Knyvett AF, et al: Varicella pneumonia: A possible cause of subsequent pulmonary calcification. Med J Aust 2:781, 1964.

161. Knyvett AF: Pulmonary calcifications following varicella. Am Rev Resp Dis 92:210, 1965.

162. Fisher E, Frühformen der verästelten Lungenverknöcherungen. (Early stages of branching pulmonary ossification.) Fortschr Roentgenstr 86:455, 1957.

163. Mendeloff J: Disseminated nodular pulmonary ossification in the Hamman-Rich lung. Am Rev Respir Dis 103:269, 1971.

164. Genereux G: Personal communication, 1973.

165. Kuplic JB, Higley CS, Niewoehner DE: Pulmonary ossification associated with long-term busulfan therapy in chronic myeloid leukemia. Case report. Am Rev Respir Dis 106:759, 1972.

166. Jacobs AN, Neitzschman HR, Nice CM Jr: Metaplastic bone formation in the lung. Am J Roentgenol 118:344, 1973.

167. Green JD, Harle TS, Greenberg SD, et al: Disseminated pulmonary ossification. A case report with demonstration of electron microscopic features. Am Rev Respir Dis 101:293, 1970.

168. Mootz JR, Sagel SS, Roberts TH: Roentgenographic manifestations of pulmonary calcifications: A rare cause of respiratory failure in chronic renal disease. Radiology 107:55, 1973.

169. Kempf K, Capesius P, Mugel JL: Un cas de calcinose pulmonaire au cours d'une myélomatose diffuse. J Radiol Electrol Med Nucl 53:861, 1972.

170. Johnson C, Graham CB, Curtis FK: Roentgenographic manifestations of chronic renal disease treated by periodic hemodialysis. Am J Roentgenol 101:915, 1967.

171. Parfitt AM, Massry SG, Winfield AC, et al: Disordered calcium and phosphorus metabolism during maintenance hemodialysis. Correlation of clinical, roentgenographic and biochemical changes. Am J Med 51:319, 1971.

172. Boner G, Jacob ET, Pevzner S, et al: Diffuse calcification of lungs in a patient on maintenance hemodialysis. Isr J Med Sci 7:1182, 1971.

173. Parfitt AM: Soft-tissue calcification in uremia. Arch Intern Med 124:544, 1969.

174. Neff M, Yalcin S, Gupta S, et al: Extensive metastatic calcification of the lung in an azotemic patient. Am J Med 56:103, 1974.

175. Jost RG, Sagel SS: Metastatic calcification in the lung apex. Am J Roentgenol 133:1188, 1979.

176. Friedman PJ: Editorial: Radiologic reporting: Describing the lungs and pleura. Am J Roentgenol 140:1030, 1983.

177. Firooznia H, Pudlowski R, Golimbu C, et al: Diffuse interstitial calcification of the lungs in chromic renal failure mimicking pulmonary edema. Am J Roentgenol 129:1130, 1977.

178. Rosenthal DI, Chandler HL, Azizi F, et al: Uptake of bone imaging agents by diffuse pulmonary metastatic calcification. Am J Roentgenol 129:871, 1977.

179. Auerbach JM, Ho J: Gallium-67 uptake in the lung associated with metastatic calcification. Am J Roentgenol 136:605, 1981.

180. Chinn DH, Gamsu G, Webb WR, et al: Calcified pulmonary nodules in chronic renal failure. Am J Roentgenol 137:402, 1981.

181. Gross BH, Schneider HJ, Proto AV: Eggshell calcification of lymph nodes: An update. Am J Roentgenol 135:1265, 1980.

182. Bellini F, Ghislandi E: "Egg-shell" calcifications at extrahilar sites in a silicotuberculotic patient. Med Lav 51:600, 1960.

183. Lawson JP: Pleural calcification as a sign of asbestosis: A report of three cases. Clin Radiol 14:414, 1963.

184. Schneider L, Wimpfheimer F: Multiple progressive calcific pleural plaque formation: A sign of silicatosis. JAMA 189:328, 1964.

185. Kiviluoto R: Pleural calcification as a roentgenologic sign of non-occupational edemic anthophyllite-asbestosis. Acta Radiol (Suppl) 194, 1960.

186. Oosthuizen SF, Theron CP: Correlation between the radiographic and pathological findings in silicosis. Med Proc 10:337, 1964.

187. Sargent EN, Jacobson G, Wilkinson EE: Diaphragmatic pleural calcification following short occupational exposure to asbestos. Am J Roentgenol 115:473, 1972.

188. Whitehouse G: Tracheopathia osteoplastica: Case report. Br J Radiol 41:701, 1968.

189. Baird RB, McCartney JN: Tracheopathia osteoplastica. Thorax 21:321, 1966.

190. Dalgaard JB: Tracheopathia chondro-osteoplastica. A case elucidating the problems concerning development and ossification of elastic cartilage. Acta Pathol Microbiol Scand 24:118, 1947.

191. Carr DT, Olsen AM: Tracheopathia osteoplastica. JAMA 155:1563, 1954.

192. Bowen DAL: Tracheopathia osteoplastica. J Clin Pathol 12:435, 1959.

193. Mallamo JT, Baum RS, Simon AL: Diffuse pulmonary artery calcifications in a case of Eisenmenger's syndrome. Radiology 99:549, 1971.

194. McAlister WH, Blatt E: Calcified pulmonary artery thrombus. Am J Roentgenol 87:908, 1962.

195. Williams JR, Bonte FJ: Pulmonary changes in nonpenetrating thoracic trauma. Texas State J 59:27, 1963.

196. Amundsen P: Planigraphy in Möller and Valsalva experiments. Acta Radiol 40:387, 1953.

197. Steinberg I, Finby N: Roentgen manifestations of pulmonary arteriovenous fistula: Diagnosis and treatment of four new cases. Am J Roentgenol 78:234, 1957.

198. van de Weyer KH: Zur Roentgendiagnostik arteriovenoser Lungenfisteln. (The roentgen diagnosis of pulmonary arteriovenous fistulas.) Fortschr Roentgenstr 102:393, 1965.

199. Poller S, Wholey MH: Pulmonary varix: Evaluation by selective pulmonary angiography. Radiology 86:1078, 1966.

200. Godwin JD, Webb WR, Savoca CJ, et al: Review: Multiple, thin-walled cystic lesions of the lung. Am J Roentgenol 135:593, 1980.

201. Gramiak R, Koerner HJ: A roentgen diagnostic observation in subpleural lipoma. Am J Roentgenol 98:465, 1966.
202. Baker GL, Heublein GW: Postoperative aspiration pneumonitis. Am J Roentgenol 80:42, 1958.
203. Brown BJ, Ma H, Dunbar JS, et al: Foreign bodies in the tracheobronchial tree in childhood. J Can Assoc Radiol 14:158, 1963.
204. Robertson OH, Hamburger M: Studies on the pathogenesis of experimental pneumococcus pneumonia in dogs. II. Secondary pulmonary lesions. Their production by intratracheal and intrabronchial injection of fluid pneumonic exudate. J Exp Med 72:275, 1940.
205. Dornhorst AC, Pierce JW: Pulmonary collapse and consolidation: The role of collapse in the production of lung field shadows and the significance of segments in inflammatory lung disease. J Fac Radiol 5:276, 1954.
206. Fraser RG, Wortzman G: Acute pneumococcal lobar pneumonia: The signficance of non-segmental distribution. J Can Assoc Radiol 10:37, 1959.
207. Fleischner FG: Roentgenology of the pulmonary infarct. Semin Roentgenol 2:61, 1967.
208. Garland LH: Bronchial carcinoma. Lobar distribution of lesions in 250 cases. Calif Med 94:7, 1961.
209. Rutishauser M: Die maligne Lungencaverne. (The malignant pulmonary cavity.) Schweiz Med Wochenschr 95:349, 1965.
210. Lentino W, Jacobson HG, Poppel MH: Segmental localization of upper lobe tuberculosis: The rarity of anterior involvement. Am J Roentgenol 78:1042, 1957.
211. Poppius H, Thomander K: Segmentary distribution of cavities: A radiologic study of 500 consecutive cases of cavernous pulmonary tuberculosis. Ann Med Int Fenn 46:113, 1957.
212. Segarra F, Sherman DS, Rodriguez-Aguero J: Lower lung field tuberculosis. Am Rev Respir Dis 87:37, 1963.
213. Frostad S: Segmental atelectasis in children with primary tuberculosis. Am Rev Respir Dis 79:597, 1959.
214. Weber L, Bird KT, Janower ML: Primary tuberculosis in childhood with particular emphasis on changes affecting the tracheobronchial tree. Am J Roentgenol 103:123, 1968.
215. Ranniger K, Valvasorri GE: Angiographic diagnosis of intralobar pulmonary sequestration. Am J Roentgenol 92:540, 1964.
216. Kilman JW, Battersby JS, Taybi H, et al: Pulmonary sequestration. Arch Surg 90:648, 1965.
217. Witten DM, Clagett OT, Woolner LB: Intralobar bronchopulmonary sequestration involving the upper lobes. J Thorac Cardiovasc Surg 43:523, 1962.
218. Rogers LF, Osmer JC: Bronchogenic cyst: A review of 46 cases. Am J Roentgenol 91:273, 1964.
219. Hurwitz M: Roentgenologic aspects of asbestosis. Am J Roentgenol 85:256, 1961.
220. Smith KW: Pulmonary disability in asbestos workers. Arch Industr Health 12:198, 1955.
221. Felson B, Felson H: Localization of intrathoracic lesions by means of the postero-anterior roentgenogram: The silhouette sign. Radiology 55:363, 1950.
222. Temple HL, Evans JA: The bronchopulmonary segments. Am J Roentgenol 63:26, 1950.
223. Kane IJ: Segmental localization of pulmonary disease on the postero-anterior chest roentgenogram. Radiology 59:229, 1952.
224. Hodson CJ: The localization of pulmonary collapse-consolidation. J Fac Radiol 8:41, 1956.
225. Robbins LL, Hale CH: Roentgen appearance of lobar and segmental collapse of the lung: Preliminary report. Radiology 44:107, 1945.
226. Robbins LL, Hale CH, Merrill OE: Roentgen appearance of lobar and segmental collapse of the lung: Technic of examination. Radiology 44:471, 1945.
227. Robbins LL, Hale CH: The roentgen appearance of lobar and segmental collapse of the lung. II. The normal chest as it pertains to collapse. Radiology 44:543, 1945.
228. Robbins LL, Hale CH: The roentgen appearance of lobar and segmental collapse of the lung. III. Collapse of an entire lung or the major part thereof. Radiology 45:23, 1945.
229. Robbins LL, Hale CH: The roentgen appearance of lobar and segmental collapse of the lung. IV. Collapse of the lower lobes. Radiology 45:120, 1945.
230. Robbins LL, Hale CH: The roentgen appearance of lobar and segmental collapse of the lung. V. Collapse of the right middle lobe. Radiology 45:260, 1945.
231. Robbins LL, Hale CH: The roentgen appearance of lobar and segmental collapse of the lung. VI. Collapse of the upper lobes. Radiology 45:347, 1945.
232. Lubert M, Krause GR: Patterns of lobar collapse as observed radiographically. Radiology 56:165, 1951.
233. Tuddenham WJ: Problems of perception in chest roentgenology: Facts and fallacies. Radiol Clin North Am 1:277, 1963.
234. Kattan KR, Felson B, Eyre JT: The silhouette sign revisited experimentally. Appl Radiol May/June:114, 1984.
235. Felson B: More chest roentgen signs and how to teach them. (Annual oration in memory of L. Henry Garland, M.D., 1903–1966.) Radiology 90:429, 1968.
236. Collins VP, Loeffler RK, Tivey H: Observations on growth rates of human tumors. Am J Roentgenol 76:988, 1956.
237. Nathan MH, Collins VP, Adams RA: Differentiation of benign and malignant pulmonary nodules by growth rate. Radiology 79:221, 1962.
238. Weiss W, Boucot KR, Cooper DA: The survival of men with measurable proved lung cancer in relation to growth rate. Am J Roentgenol 98:404, 1966.
239. Rigler LG: A roentgen study of the evolution of carcinoma of the lung. J Thorac Surg 34:283, 1957.
240. Spratt JS Jr, Spjut HJ, Roper CL: The frequency distribution of the rates of growth and the estimated duration of primary pulmonary carcinomas. Cancer 16:687, 1963.
241. Garland LH, Coulson W, Wollin E: The rate of growth and apparent duration of untreated primary bronchial carcinoma. Cancer 16:694, 1963.
242. Garland LH: The rate of growth and natural duration of primary bronchial cancer. Am J Roentgenol 96:604, 1966.
243. Jensen KG, Schiødt T: Growth conditions of hamartoma of the lung: A study based on 22 cases operated on after radiographic observation for from one to 18 years. Thorax 13:233, 1958.
244. Weisel W, Glicklich M, Landis FB: Pulmonary hamartoma, an enlarging neoplasm. Arch Surg 71:128, 1955.
245. Kerley P: Radiology in heart disease. Br Med J 2:594, 1933.
246. Twining EW (revised by Kerley P): Respiratory system. In Shanks SC, Kerley P (eds): A Textbook of X-Ray Diagnosis. 2nd ed, Vol II. Philadelphia, WB Saunders, 1951, p 414.
247. Kerley P: In Shanks SC, Kerley P (eds): A Textbook of X-Ray Diagnosis. 2nd ed, Vol II. Philadelphia, WB Saunders, 1951, p 241.
248. Kerley P: In Shanks SC, Kerley P (eds): A Textbook of X-Ray Diagnosis. 2nd ed, Vol II. Philadelphia, WB Saunders, 1951, p 404.
249. Trapnell DH: The peripheral lymphatics of the lung. Br J Radiol 36:660, 1963.
250. Trapnell DH: The differential diagnosis of linear shadows in chest radiographs. Radiol Clin North Am 11:77, 1973.
251. Fleischner FG, Reiner L: Linear x-ray shadows in acquired pulmonary hemosiderosis and congestion. N Engl J Med 250:900, 1954.
252. Trapnell DH: Septal lines in pneumoconiosis. Br J Radiol 37:805, 1964.
253. Trapnell DH: Septal lines in sarcoidosis. Br J Radiol 37:811, 1964.
254. Levin B: Subpleural interlobular lymphectasia reflecting metastatic carcinoma. Radiology 72:682, 1959.
255. Brody JS, Levin B: Interlobular septal thickening in lipid pneumonia. Am J Roentgenol 88:1061, 1962.
256. Stolberg HO, Patt N, MacEwen KF, et al: Hodgkin's disease of the lung: Roentgenologic/pathologic correlation. Am J Roentgenol 92:96, 1964.
257. Reid L: The connective tissue septa in the adult human lung. Thorax 14:138, 1959.
258. Heitzman ER, Ziter FM Jr, Makarian B, et al: Kerley's interlobular septal lines: Roentgen pathologic correlation. Am J Roentgenol 100:578, 1967.
259. Simon G: Principles of Chest X-ray Diagnosis. 3rd ed. London, Butterworth, 1971.
260. Hodson CJ, Trickey SE: Bronchial wall thickening in asthma. Clin Radiol 11:183, 1960.
261. Cardell BS: Pathological findings in deaths from asthma. Int Arch Allergy Appl Immunol 9:189, 1956.
262. Bates DV, Gordon CA, Paul GI, et al: Chronic bronchitis: Report on the third and fourth stages of the co-ordinated study of chronic bronchitis in the Department of Veterans Affairs, Canada. Med Serv J Can 22:5, 1966.
263. Simon G: Chronic bronchitis and emphysema: A symposium. III. Pathological findings and radiological changes in chronic bronchitis and emphysema. (b) Radiological changes in chronic bronchitis. Br J Radiol 32:292, 1959.
264. Rigler LG: Personal communication, 1965.
265. Hill CA: "Tail" signs associated with pulmonary lesions: Critical reappraisal. Am J Roentgenol 139:311, 1982.
266. Reid L: Quoted by Simon G, as a personal communication. Br J Radiol 43:327, 1970.
267. Fleischner F, Hampton AO, Castleman B: Linear shadows in the lung (interlobar pleuritis, atelectasis and healed infarction). Am J Roentgenol 46:610, 1941.
268. Fleischner F: Uber das Wesen der basalan horizontalen Schattenstreifen im Lungenfeld. Wien Arch Inn Med 28:461, 1936.
269. Westcott JL, Cole S: Plate atelectasis. Radiology 155:1, 1985.
270. Fleischner F, Hampton AO, Castleman B: Linear shadows in the lung (interlobar pleuritis, atelectasis and healed infarction). Am J Roentgenol 46:610, 1941.
271. Fleischner FG: Personal communication, 1967.

4

272. Simon G: The cause and significance of some long line shadows in the chest radiograph. Proc R Soc Med 58:861, 1965.

273. Simon G: Further observations on the long line shadows across a lower zone of the lung. Br J Radiol 43:327, 1970.

274. Rosenblum LJ, Mauceri RA, Wellenstein DE, et al: Computed tomography of the lung. Radiology 129:521, 1978.

275. Sherrick DW, Kincaid OW, DuShane JW: Agenesis of a main branch of the pulmonary artery. Am J Roentgenol 87:917, 1962.

276. Greenspan RH, Sagel S, McMahon J, et al: Timed expiratory chest films in the detection of air-trapping (abstract). Invest Radiol 8:264, 1973.

277. Sutinen S, Christoforidis AJ, Klugh GA, et al: Roentgenologic criteria for the recognition of nonsymptomatic pulmonary emphysema: Correlation between roentgenologic findings and pulmonary pathology. Am Rev Respir Dis 91:69, 1965.

278. Christie RV: Emphysema of the lungs. Br Med J 1:105, 1944.

279. Munk J, Lederer KT: Inspiratory widening of the heart shadow: A fluoroscopic sign in acute obstructive laryngo-tracheitis. Br J Radiol 27:294, 1954.

280. Reid JM, Barclay RS, Stevenson JG, et al: Congenital obstructive lobar emphysema. Dis Chest 49:359, 1966.

281. Franken EA, Buehl I: Infantile lobar emphysema; Report of two cases with the usual roentgenographic manifestation. Am J Roentgenol 98:354, 1966.

282. Staple TW, Hudson HH, Hartman AF Jr, et al: The angiographic findings in four cases of infantile lobar emphysema. Am J Roentgenol 97:195, 1966.

283. Simon G, Reid L: Atresia of an apical bronchus of the left upper lobe—report of three cases. Br J Dis Chest 57:126, 1963.

284. Waddell JA, Simon G, Reid L: Bronchial atresia of the left upper lobe. Thorax 20:214, 1965.

285. Lehar TJ, Carr DT, Miller WE, et al: Roentgenographic appearance of bronchogenic adenocarcinoma. Am Rev Resp Dis 96:245, 1967.

286. Byrd RB, Miller WE, Carr DT, et al: The roentgenographic appearance of squamous cell carcinoma of the bronchus. Mayo Clin Proc 43:327, 1968.

287. Byrd RB, Miller WE, Carr DT, et al: The roentgenographic appearance of large cell carcinoma of the bronchus. Mayo Clin Proc 43:333, 1968.

288. Byrd RB, Miller WE, Carr DT, et al: The roentgenographic appearance of small cell carcinoma of the bronchus. Mayo Clin Proc 43:337, 1968.

288a. Arnois D-C, Silverman FN, Turner ME: The radiographic evaluation of pulmonary vasculature in children with congenital cardiovascular disease. Radiology 72:689, 1959.

289. Fraser RG, Bates DV: Body section roentgenography in the evaluation and differentiation of chronic hypertrophic emphysema and asthma. Am J Roentgenol 82:39, 1959.

290. Michelson E, Salik JO: The vascular pattern of the lung as seen on routine and tomographic studies. Radiology 73:511, 1959.

291. Wojtowicz J: Some tomographic criteria for an evaluation of the pulmonary circulation. Acta Radiol (Diagn) 2:215, 1964.

292. Templeton AW, Garotto LJ: Acquired extracardiac causes of pulmonary ischemia. Dis Chest 51:166, 1967.

293. Yu PN: Primary pulmonary hypertension: Report of six cases and review of literature. Ann Intern Med 49:1138, 1958.

294. Farid Z, Greer JW, Ishak KG, et al: Chronic pulmonary schistosomiasis. Am Rev Respir Dis 79:119, 1959.

295. Keating DR: Thrombosis of pulmonary arteries. Am J Surg 90:447, 1955.

296. Ball KP, Goodwin JF, Harrison CV: Massive thrombotic occlusion of the large pulmonary arteries. Circulation 14:766, 1956.

297. Reid JA, Heard BE: The capillary network of normal and emphysematous human lungs studied by injections of India ink. Thorax 18:201, 1963.

298. Laws JW, Heard BE: Emphysema and the chest film: A retrospective radiological and pathological study. Br J Radiol 35:750, 1962.

299. Scarrow GD: The pulmonary angiogram in chronic bronchitis and emphysema. Clin Radiol 17:54, 1966.

300. Swyer PR, James GCW: A case of unilateral pulmonary emphysema. Thorax 8:133, 1953.

301. Margolin HN, Rosenberg LS, Felson B, et al: Idiopathic unilateral hyperlucent lung: A roentgenologic syndrome. Am J Roentgenol 82:63, 1959.

302. Reid L, Simon G: Unilateral lung transradiancy. Thorax 17:230, 1962.

303. MacLeod WM: Abnormal transradiancy of one lung. Thorax 9:147, 1954.

304. Elder JC, Brofman BL, Kohn PM, et al: Unilateral pulmonary artery absence or hypoplasia. Radiographic and cardiopulmonary studies in five patients. Circulation 17:557, 1958.

305. Vaughan BF: Syndromes associated with hypoplasia or aplasia of one pulmonary artery. J Fac Radiol 9:161, 1958.

306. Kieffer SA, Amplatz K, Anderson RC, et al: Proximal interruption of a pulmonary artery: Roentgen features and surgical correction. Am J Roentgenol 95:592, 1965.

307. Allison DJ, Stanbrook HS: A radiologic and physiologic investigation into hypoxic pulmonary vasoconstriction in the dog. George Simon Memorial Fellowship Award, No 3, 1979, p 178.

308. Chiorazzi N, Weiss HS, Margouleff D, et al: Long-term pulmonary blood flow alterations following relief of partial bronchial obstruction. Am J Med 56:559, 1974.

309. Fouché RF, D'Silva JL: Hypertransradiancy of one lung field and its experimental production by unilateral miliary embolisation of pulmonary arteries in cats. Clin Radiol 11:100, 1960.

310. Fleischner FG: Unilateral pulmonary embolism with increased compensatory circulation through the unoccluded lung: Roentgen observations. Radiology 73:591, 1959.

311. Jacques JE, Barclay R: The solid sarcomatous pulmonary artery. Br J Dis Chest 54:217, 1960.

312. Bates DV, Macklem PT, Christie RV: Respiratory Function in Disease; An introduction to the Integrated Study of Lung. 2nd ed. Philadelphia, WB Saunders, 1971.

313. Laurenzi GA, Turino GM, Fishman AP: Bullous disease of the lung. Am J Med 32:361, 1962.

314. Ting EY, Klopstock R, Lyons HA: Mechanical properties of pulmonary cysts and bullae. Am Rev Respir Dis 87:538, 1963.

315. Minnis JF Jr: Congenital cystic disease of the lung in infancy: Successful lobectomy in a one-day-old infant. J Thorac Cardiovasc Surg 43:262, 1962.

316. Reid L: The Pathology of Emphysema. London, Lloyd-Luke (Medical Books) Ltd, 1967.

317. Grimes OF, Farber SM: Air cysts of the lung. Surg Gynecol Obstet 113:720, 1961.

318. Feraru F, Morrow CS: Surgery of subpleural blebs: Indications and contraindications. Am Rev Respir Dis 79:577, 1959.

319. Davidson JK: Pulmonary changes in decompression sickness: Some observations on compressed air workers at the Clyde Tunnel. Clin Radiol 15:106, 1964.

320. Golding FC, Griffiths P, Hempleman HV, et al: Decompression sickness during construction of the Dartford Tunnel. Br J Industr Med 17:167, 1960.

321. Collins JJ Jr: An unusual case of air embolism precipitated by decompression. N Engl J Med 266:595, 1962.

322. Flaherty RA, Keegan JM, Sturtevant HN: Post-pneumonic pulmonary pneumatoceles. Radiology 74:50, 1960.

323. Fagan CJ: Traumatic lung cyst. Am J Roentgenol 97:186, 1966.

324. Peabody JW Jr, Rupnick EJ, Hanner JM: Bronchial carcinoma masquerading as a thin-walled cyst. Am J Roentgenol 77:1051, 1957.

325. Agostoni E, Mead J: Statics of the respiratory system. In Fenn WO, Rahn H (eds): Handbook of Physiology; Section 3, Respiration. Vol I. Washington, DC, American Physiological Society, 1964, pp 387–409.

326. Müller R, Löfstedt S: The reaction of the pleura in primary tuberculosis of the lungs. Acta Med Scand 122:105, 1945.

327. Hessén, I: Roentgen examination of pleural fluid: A study of the localization of free effusion: The potentialities of diagnosing minimal quantities of fluid and its existence under physiological conditions. Acta Radiol (Suppl) 86, 1951.

328. Moskowitz H, Platt RT, Schachar R, et al: Roentgen visualization of minute pleural effusion: An experimental study to determine the minimum amount of pleural fluid visible on a radiograph. Radiology 109:33, 1973.

329. Eklöf O, Törngren A: Pleural fluid in healthy children. Acta Radiol Diag 11:346, 1971.

330. Ganter G: Über die Druckverhältnisse in der Pleurahöhle und ihren Einfluss auf Langerung und Form von Pleuraegüsse. (Pressure in the pleural cavity.) Dtsch Arch Klin Med 141:68, 1922–1923.

331. Bowen A: Quantitative roentgen diagnosis of pleural effusions. Radiology 17:520, 1931.

332. Kaunitz J: Landmarks in simple pleural effusions. JAMA 113:1312, 1939.

333. Rigler LG: Roentgen diagnosis of small pleural effusion: A new roentgenographic position. JAMA 96:104, 1931.

334. Fleischner FG: Atypical arrangement of free pleural effusion. Radiol Clin North Am 1:347, 1963.

335. Khomiakov YS, Fedorova RG: (Relation of the roentgenological picture of the upper limit of shadows of exudates in the free pleural cavity to the nature of exudates and the retractile capacity of the lung.) Vestn Rentgen Radiol 37:8, 1962.

336. Davis S, Gardner F, Ovist G: The shape of a pleural effusion. Br Med J 1:436, 1963.

337. Collins JD, Burwell D, Furmanski S, et al: Minimal detectable pleural effusions: A roentgen pathology model. Radiology 105:51, 1972.

338. Dandy WE Jr: Incomplete pulmonary interlobar fissure sign. Radiology 128:21, 1978.

339. Mulvey RB: The effect of pleural fluid on the diaphragm. Radiology 84:1080, 1965.

340. Hinson KFW, Kuper SWA: The diagnosis of lung cancer by examination of sputum. Thorax 18:350, 1963.
341. Rigby M, Zylak CJ, Wood LDH: The effect of lobar atelectasis on pleural fluid distribution in dogs. Radiology 136:603, 1980.
342. Zidulka A, Nadler S, Antonisen NR: Pleural pressure with lobar obstruction in dogs. Respir Physiol 26:239, 1976.
343. Dunbar JS, Favreau M: Infrapulmonary pleural effusion with particular reference to its occurrence in nephrosis. J Can Assoc Radiol 10:24, 1959.
343a. Trackler RT, Brinker RA: Widening of the left paravertebral pleural line on supine chest roentgenograms in free pleural effusions. Am J Roentgenol 96:1027, 1966.
344. Petersen JA: Recognition of infrapulmonary pleural effusion. Radiology 74:34, 1960.
345. Barry WF Jr: Infrapulmonary pleural effusion. Radiology 66:740, 1956.
346. Kurlander GJ, Helmen CH: Subpulmonary pneumothorax. Am J Roentgenol 96:1019, 1966.
347. Friedman RL: Infrapulmonary pleural effusions. Am J Roentgenol 71:613, 1954.
348. Kafura PJ, Barnhard HJ: Ascites simulating subpulmonary pleural effusion. Radiology 101:525, 1971.
349. Teplick JG, Teplick SK, Goodman L, et al: The interface sign: A computed tomographic sign for distinguishing pleural and intraabdominal fluid. Radiology 144:359, 1982.
350. Feldman DJ: Localized interlobar pleural effusion in heart failure. JAMA 146:1408, 1951.
351. Weiss W, Boucot KR, Gefter WI: Localized interlobular effusion in congestive heart failure. Ann Intern Med 38:1177, 1953.
352. Pugatch RD, Faling LJ, Robbins AH, et al: Differentiation of pleural and pulmonary lesions using computed tomography. J Comput Assist Tomog 2:601, 1978.
353. Baber CE, Hedlund LW, Oddson TA, et al: Differentiating empyemas and peripheral pulmonary abscesses. The value of computed tomography. Radiology 135:755, 1980.
354. Stark DD, Federle MP, Goodman PC, et al: Differentiating lung abscess and emphysema: Radiography and computed tomography. Am J Roentgenol 141:163, 1983.
355. Shin MS, Ho K-J: Computed tomographic characteristics of pleural empyema. J Comput Tomogr 7:179, 1983.
356. Kerley P: In Shanks SC, Kerley P (eds): A Textbook of X-ray Diagnosis. 3rd ed, Vol II. Philadelphia, WB Saunders, 1962, p 403.
357. Higgins JA, Juergens JL, Bruwer AJ, et al: Loculated interlobar pleural effusion due to congestive heart failure. Arch Intern Med 96:180, 1955.
358. Fraser RG, Paré, JAPP: Diagnosis of Diseases of the Chest: An Integrated Study Based on the Abnormal Roentgenogram. Philadelphia, WB Saunders, 1970.
359. Jamison HW: An anatomic-roentgenographic study of the pleural domes and pulmonary apices: With special reference to apical subpleural scars. Radiology 36:302, 1941.
360. Renner RR, Markarian B, Pernice NJ, et al: The apical cap. Radiology 110:569, 1974.
361. McLoud TC, Isler RJ, Novelline RA, et al.: Review: The apical cap. Am J Roentgenol 137:299, 1981.
362. Berne AS, Heitzman ER: The roentgenologic signs of pedunculated pleural tumors. Am J Roentgenol 87:892, 1962.
363. Hutchinson WB, Friedenberg MJ: Intrathoracic mesothelioma. Radiology 80:937, 1963.
364. DeRienzo S: Radiologic Exploration of the Bronchus. Springfield, IL, Charles C Thomas, 1949.
365. MacEwan DW, Dunbar JS, Smith RD, et al: Pneumothorax in young infants—recognition and evaluation. J Can Assoc Radiol 22:264, 1971.
366. Gordon R: The deep sulcus sign. Radiology 136:25, 1980.

367. Rhea JT, vanSonnenberg E, McLoud, TC: Basilar Pneumothorax in the supine adult. Radiology 133:595, 1979.
368. Ziter FMH, Westcott JL: Supine subpulmonary pneumothorax. Am J Roentgenol 137:699, 1981.
369. Tocino IM: Pneumothorax in the supine patient: Radiographic anatomy. RadioGraphics 5:557, 1985.
370. Tocino IM, Miller MH, Fairfax WR: Distribution of pneumothorax in the supine and semirecumbent critically ill adult. Am J Roentgenol 144:901, 1985.
371. Christensen EE, Dietz GW: Subpulmonic pneumothorax in patients with chronic obstructive pulmonary disease. Radiology 121:33, 1976.
372. Schulman A, Dalrymple RB: Subpulmonary pneumothorax. Br J Radiol 51:494, 1978.
373. Axel L: A simple way to estimate the size of a pneumothorax. Invest Radiol 16:165, 1981.
374. Rhea JT, DeLuca SA, Greene RE: Determining the size of pneumothorax in the upright patient. Radiology 144:733, 1982.
375. Rohlfing BM: The shifting granuloma: An internal marker of atelectasis. Radiology 123:283, 1977.
376. Fraser RG, Hickey NM, Nicklason LT, et al: Dual-energy digital radiography in the detection of calcification in pulmonary nodules. Radiology 160:595, 1986.
377. West JB: Regional Differences in the Lung. New York Academic Press, 1977, p 239.
378. West JB: Regional Differences in the Lung. New York, Academic Press, 1977, pp 313–319.
379. Thomson KR, Eyssen GE, Fraser RG: Discrimination of normal and overinflated lungs and prediction of total lung capacity based on chest film measurements. Radiology 119:721, 1976.
380. Rabinov K, Stein M, Frank H: Tension hydrothorax—an unrecognized danger. Thorax 21:465, 1966.
381. Hanke R, Kretzschmar R: Round atelectasis. Semin Roentgenol 15:174, 1980.
382. Hanke VR, Kretzschmar R: Die Rundatelektasen. Fortschr Röntgenstr 138:151, 1983.
383. Khoury MB, Godwin JD, Halvorsen RA Jr, et al: CT of obstructive lobar collapse. Invest Radiol 20:708, 1985.
384. Naidich DP, Zerhouni EA, Siegelman SS: Lobar collapse. In Computed Tomography of the Thorax. New York, Raven Press, 1984, p 111.
385. LeRoux BT: Opacities of the middle and upper lobes in combination. Thorax 26:55, 1971.
386. Bergin CJ, Muller NL: CT of interstitial lung disease: A diagnostic approach. Am J Roentgenol 148:8, 1987.
387. Müller NL, Miller RR, Webb WR, et al: Fibrosing alveolitis: CT-pathologic correlation. Radiology 160:585, 1986.
388. Wandtke JC, Hyde RW, Fahey PJ, et al: Measurement of lung gas volume and regional density by computed tomography in dogs. Invest Radiol 21:108, 1986.
389. Stewart JG, MacMahon H, Vyborny CJ, et al: Dystrophic calcification in carcinoma of the lung: Demonstration by CT (case report). Am J Roentgenol 148:29, 1987.
390. Felson B: Thoracic calcifications. Dis Chest 56:330, 1969.
391. Sanders C, Frank M, Rutsky EA, et al: Metastatic calcification of the lungs in end-stage renal disease: Detection and quantitation by dual-energy digital chest radiography. Submitted to Invest Radiol, 1987.
392. Arnois D-C, Silverman FN, Turner ME: The radiographic evaluation of pulmonary vasculature in children with congenital cardiovascular disease. Radiology 72:689, 1959.
393. Connell DG, Crothers G, Cooperberg PL: The subpulmonic pleural effusion: Sonographic aspects. J Can Assoc Radiol 33:101, 1982.
394. Federle MP, Mark AS, Guillaumin ES: CT of subpulmonic pleural effusions and atelectasis: Criteria for differentiation from subphrenic fluid. Am J Roentgenol 146:685, 1986.

4

SUBJECT INDEX

Page numbers in *italics* indicate illustrations; page numbers followed by the letter t indicate a table.

NAME INDEX

Reference numbers are in **bold face** and are followed by the numbers of the pages on which they are cited.